Pathology of the Aging Human Nervous System

Pathology of the Aging Human Nervous System

SECOND EDITION

Edited by

SERGE DUCKETT, M.D. (Univ. Paris), Ph.D. (Univ. London),
Dr. ès Sciences (Univ. Paris)

Emeritus Professor of Neuropathology and Emeritus Associate Professor of Pathology
Jefferson Medical College of the Thomas Jefferson University
Philadelphia, Pennsylvania, USA

Invited Professor
Laboratoire de Neuropathologie R. Escourolle
Hôpital de la Salpêtrière, Université de Paris VI
Paris, France

J. C. DE LA TORRE, M.D. (Univ. Madrid), Ph.D. (Univ. Geneva)

Visiting Professor of Neuroscience
University of California San Diego
La Jolla, California, USA

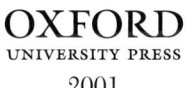

OXFORD
UNIVERSITY PRESS
2001

OXFORD
UNIVERSITY PRESS

Oxford   New York
Athens   Auckland   Bangkok   Bogotá   Buenos Aires   Calcutta
Cape Town   Chennai   Dar es Salaam   Delhi   Florence   Hong Kong   Istanbul
Karachi   Kuala Lumpur   Madrid   Melbourne   Mexico City   Mumbai
Nairobi   Paris   São Paulo   Shanghai   Singapore   Taipei   Tokyo   Toronto   Warsaw

and associated companies in
Berlin   Ibadan

Copyright © 2001 by Oxford University Press, Inc.

Published by Oxford University Press, Inc.
198 Madison Avenue, New York, New York 10016

Oxford is a registered trademark of Oxford University Press

All rights reserved. No part of this publication may be reproduced,
stored in a retrieval system, or transmitted, in any form or by any means,
electronic, mechanical, photocopying, recording, or otherwise,
without the prior permission of Oxford University Press.

Library of Congress Cataloging-in-Publication Data
Pathology of the aging human nervous system /
edited by Serge Duckett, J. C. de la Torre.—2nd ed.
p. ; cm.   Includes bibliographical references and index.
ISBN 0-19-513069-3 (cloth)
1. Geriatric neurology.   2. Nervous system—Diseases—Age factors.
I. Duckett, Serge.   II. De La Torre, J. C. (Jack C.), 1937–
[DNLM: 1. Nervous System Diseases—Aged.   2. Aging.   3. Nervous System—pathology—Aged.
WL 102 P197 2001]   RC346 .P34 2001   618.97'68—dc21   00-044082

The science of medicine is a rapidly changing field. As new research and clinical experience broaden our knowledge, changes in treatment and drug therapy do occur. The author and the publisher of this work have checked with sources believed to be reliable in their efforts to provide information that is accurate and complete, and in accordance with the standards accepted at the time of publication. However, in light of the possibility of human error or changes in the practice of medicine, neither the author, nor the publisher, nor any other party who has been involved in the preparation or publication of this work warrants that the information contained herein is in every respect accurate or complete. Readers are encouraged to confirm the information contained herein with other reliable sources, and are strongly advised to check the product information sheet provided by the pharmaceutical company for each drug they plan to administer.

1 3 5 7 9 8 6 4 2

Printed in the United States of America
on acid-free paper

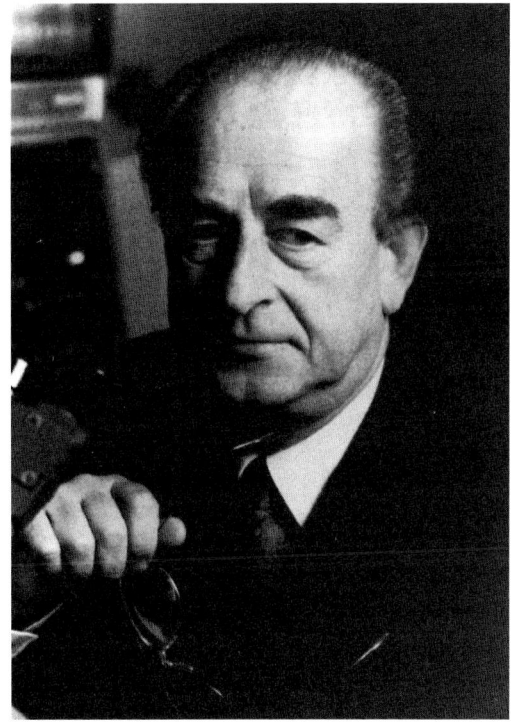
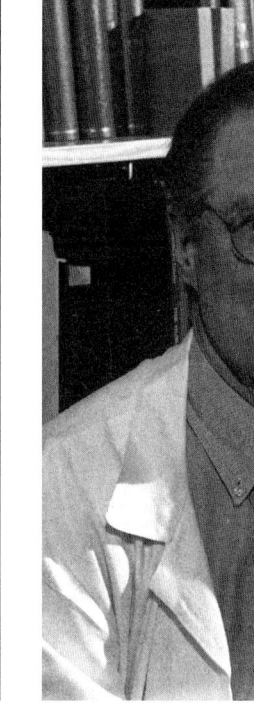

Henry M. Wisniewski   E. P. Richardson, Jr.

This book is dedicated to the masters of our trade, past and present, who contributed and are contributing to the topic of geriatric neuropathology: Alois Alzheimer, Franz Nissl, Walther Spielmeyer, William McMenemey, Sam Nevin, Richard G. Berry, Robert D. Terry, Serge Brion, and so many others. In fact, through presentations, discussions, and conversations with highly esteemed colleagues, all neuropathologists have contributed to our knowledge concerning this sometimes difficult topic. Two such colleagues left us last year: E. P. Richardson, Jr. and Henry Wisniewski. Another, Jean Lapresle, died a few days ago, December 9, 2000. We admired the quality of their work, and we liked them because they were gentlemanly, available, and kind.

Their accomplishments and biographies have been voiced eloquently in the medical press. (Terry RD. In Memoriam. Henry M. Wisniewski. (1931–1999). *J Neuropath Exp Neurol* 2000: 59 (1): 86–87) (DeGirolami U, Louis DV, Schoene WC, Vonsattel J-P, Hedley-Whyte T. In Memoriam. Edward Peirson Richardson, Jr. (1918–1998). *J Neuropath Exp Neurol* 1999: 58,506–507.)

Acknowledgments

We thank the members of our Senior Editorial Board for their availability, comments, and suggestions and for their contributions to our discipline. They are, in alphabetical order:

Raymond Adams
Ellsworth Alvord, Jr.
Richard G. Berry
Serge Brion
John B. Cavanagh
C. J. Gibbs, Jr.
Jean Lapresle
William Mair
Reinhart Friede
Robert D. Terry
Lord Walton of Detchant
Peter O. Yates
Wolfgang Zeman

We also thank Lauren M. Enck, Senior Editor, Clinical Medicine; Susan Hannan, Manager, Editing, Design & Production, Medicine; Laura T. Mitchell, Editorial Assistant; and Nancy Wolitzer, Senior Production Editor, Medicine of Oxford University Press, for their help, advice, and patience; and Shirley Sadak, for her spirited and continual availability, We also thank Professors J. J. Hauw and C. Duyckaert, Dr. D. Seilhan, Mrs. Claire Barnwell, Pierre and Caroline Bourgie, and Peter Eck for their support, criticism, and advice.

Foreword

LORD WALTON OF DETCHANT
Kt, TD, MA, MD, DSc, FRCP, FMedSci

Partly as a result of major advances in medicine in the 20th century, but also as a consequence of improving social circumstances in many, but not all, parts of the world, longevity in the human population is increasing steadily. Consequently, those diseases and afflictions that are particularly prevalent in the elderly are becoming more common and are presenting increasing problems to health care systems across the world. With greater and more precise understanding of the pathological, biochemical, and biological processes involved, the prospect of new forms of treatment to assuage the most dire effects of these diseases, and even in some cases to effect a cure, are becoming more practicable. In particular, developments of stem cell research and techniques of nuclear replacement, only recently approved in principle by the United Kingdom Parliament, carry outstanding prospects for the eventual amelioration of some of the worst effects of neurological disorders in the elderly.

The first edition of this book, edited by Serge Duckett and Jack de la Torre, was warmly welcomed by reviewers and by neurologists and neuropathologists around the world. I believe that this second edition, substantially modified and brought up to date, will be equally, if not even more, welcome. The concept and the structure of the book are admirable; the illustrations, as one would expect, are outstanding; and the coverage of the topics listed in the table of contents is comprehensive and complete. Normal aging, molecular biology, and functional imaging are considered at the outset, and subsequent chapters deal in depth with vascular diseases, basic mechanisms of neurodegeneration, the dementias, and with many of the progressive and as yet incurable degenerative disorders of the nervous system. The effects of malnutrition and alcoholism are reviewed, as are malignant diseases and neurometabolic disorders, while immunology, trauma, infection, and drug toxicity, as well as forensic neuropathology, are all handled by a distinguished team of expert authors. And, speaking as one who spent much of his professional lifetime in the investigation of neuromuscular disease, I was glad to note that disorders of peripheral nerves and of skeletal muscles are fully covered.

I am happy to recommend this outstanding volume to a wide audience of neurologists, geriatricians, and neuropathologists; indeed, physicians in all specialties may find much of interest to them within its pages. I am confident that this second edition of an outstanding and distinguished textbook is assured of success.

Preface

This volume is a new edition of one of the first books published on geriatric neuropathology. As in the first edition, the topics included reflect the multidisciplinary character of current neuropathology practice, including neuroimaging, immunology, genetics, microbiology, biochemistry, biophysics, epidemiology, and histology. In short, any process that is put to use in diagnosing human disease is discussed here. Neuroscientists in molecular biology, vascular dynamics, and pharmacology have also contributed to these chapters.

There are no "foreign" authors in this book—simply authors from various parts of the globe, and we wish there were more. We hope that with time, this book and other sources of medical information will reflect more widely the universality of medicine. There is a medical revolution afoot, which eventually will permit a physician anywhere in the world to diagnose and treat patients by consulting information provided through a computer. Moreover, software is being developed that will diffuse and translate medical or other information into any language. We have urged our contributors to write their chapters in simple, professional language because, as was evident with the first edition, our audience consists of a range of individuals who take care of neurologically impaired elderly individuals—from the professor or physician, to the visiting nurse who does rounds on a bicycle, to the layperson who takes care of a parent or a friend.

Concerning the discipline of neuropathology, there are fewer trainees in neuropathology fewer neuropathologists and neuropathology laboratories in the United States, Canada, France, United Kingdom, and Germany than ever before. This trend appears to be on the rise. Today, most practicing neuropathologists have general pathology responsibilities, with tumor pathology being their main neuropathological preoccupation. We were not able to determine the number of full-time neuropathologists in the countries noted above, but presumably there are few. There may be two reasons for this situation. The first concerns money: the high and rising costs of direct medical and surgical care and the lack of funds to support specialized diagnostic disciplines have reduced the overall number of specialists. Examples abound where the cost of one surgical case was higher than that of maintaining a minimally staffed neuropathology laboratory. The second reason is more positive: disciplines other than histopathology can now provide accurate diagnoses, sometimes with less pain for the patient and less expense. This trend will undoubtedly increase in the future. Does this presage a major restructuring of hospital laboratories in the pursuit of the least expensive way to render a correct diagnosis? Will a "new" neuropathology laboratory be born, directed by a multidisciplinarian neuropathologist who is a histopathologist, immunologist, geneticist, and radiologist wrapped into one?

Even with all this accumulation of new information we still have no dependable way to diagnose many mental disorders; this void of information must be filled because many of these cognitive conditions, including even loneliness, which in its most acute form may lead to passive suicide, as expressed in the bereavement and celibate syndromes, are the biggest killers of the elderly.

Paris, France S. D.
San Diego, California J. C. de la T.
September 2000

Contents

Contributors, xvii

1. The Normal Aging Human Brain, 1
   Serge Duckett

2. Molecular Biology of the Aging Nervous System, 16
   Mark P. Mattson

3. In Vivo Physiologic Imaging of Cerebral Ischemia, 42
   Jean-Claude Baron

4. Cerebrovascular Disease in the Elderly, 58
   Harry V. Vinters

5. Vascular Dementia, 101
   Jacqueline Mikol

6. Basic Mechanisms of Neurodegeneration in Dementia, 123
   Suzanne M. de la Monte and J. C. de la Torre

7. Dementia, 156
   Jean Paul G. Vonsattel and E. Tessa Hedley-Whyte
   The Neuroanatomical Basis of Dementia and Changes of Usual Aging

   Dementia with Lewy Bodies

   Paraneoplastic Limbic Encephalitis

   Creutzfeldt-Jakob Disease, Transmissible Spongiform Encephalopathies, and Prion Disease/ Jean Paul G. Vonsattel, Wendy Hobbs, and E. Tessa Hedley-Whyte

   Frontal and Frontotemporal Dementia

   Pick Disease/Jean Paul G. Vonsattel, G. Binetti, E. Tessa Hedley-Whyte, and John H. Growdon

8. Alzheimer's Disease, 207
   Jean-Jacques Hauw and Charles Duyckaerts

9. Parkinson's Disease, 264
   Tamas Revesz, Francoise Gray, and Francesco Scaravilli

10. The Scientific Basis of Parkinsonian Syndromes, 309
   Robert J. Schwartzman and Guillermo M. Alexander

11. Degenerative Diseases of the Cerebellum, 322
   Umberto De Girolami and Mel Feany

12. Immunocytochemistry and Molecular Genetics of Amyotrophic Lateral Sclerosis, 360
   Nicholas K. Gonatas

13. Huntington Disease with Emphasis on Late Onset and Aging, 369
   Jean Paul G. Vonsattel, E. Tessa Hedley-Whyte, and Marian DiFiglia

14. Effects of Malnutrition and Alcoholism on the Aging Nervous System, 392
   Clive Harper and Serge Duckett

15. Brain Tumors in the Elderly, 408
   Geoffrey J. Pilkington

16. Neurometabolic Disorders and the Aging Human Nervous System, 429
   Hans H. Goebel

17. Immunologic Diseases of the Aging Nervous System, 446
   Robert L. Knobler

18. Brain Trauma in the Elderly, 458
   J. C. de la Torre

19. Infectious Diseases, 474
   Leila Chimelli

20. Peripheral Neuropathies, 499
   Anne Vital and Claude Vital

21. The Aging Autonomic Nervous System, 527
   Robert E. Schmidt

22. Pathology of Skeletal Muscle in Aging, 546
   Cynthia Hawkins and Patrick Shannon

23. Drug Toxicity and the Aging Brain, 563
   Terumi A. Izukawa and Michael Gordon

24. Forensic Neuropathology, 572
   Jan E. Leestma

Appendix 1: Support Groups for the Neurologically Impaired Patients and Their Caretakers, 587

Appendix 2: The Diagnosis of the Creutzfeldt-Jakob Concept, 593

Index, 605

Contributors

GUILLERMO M. ALEXANDER, PH.D.
Professor of Neurology
Department of Neurology
Medical College of Pennsylvania Hahnemann
  University
Philadelphia, Pennsylvania

JEAN-CLAUDE BARON, M.D.
Director, INSERM Unit 320
Scientific Director, Cyceron PET Center
University of Caen School of Medicine
Caen, France

GIULIANO BINETTI, MD
Director, Neurobiology Laboratory
Alzheimer Research Unit
IRCCS S. Giovanni di Dio Fatebenefratelli
Brescia, Italy

LEILA CHIMELLI, M.D.
Professor of Pathology
Hospital Universitario C.F. Filho
Universidade Federal do Rio de Janeiro
School of Medicine
Rio de Janeiro, Brazil

SUZANNE M. DE LA MONTE, M.D., M.P.H.
Associate Professor of Medicine and Pathology
Department of Medicine and Pathology
Brown University School of Medicine
Providence, Rhode Island

J. C. DE LA TORRE, M.D., PH.D.
Visiting Professor of Pathology
Department of Pathology (Neuropathology)
UCSD-Pathology
Escondido, California

UMBERTO DE GIROLAMI, M.D.
Professor of Pathology
Director, Neuropathology Division
Brigham & Women's Hospital
Harvard Medical School
Boston, Massachusetts

MARIAN DiFIGLIA, PH.D.
Professor of Neurology
Department of Pathology (Neuropathology)
Massachusetts General Hospital
Harvard Medical School
Boston, Massachusetts

SERGE DUCKETT, M.D., PH.D.
Laboratoire de Neuropathologie R. Escourolle
Hôpital de la Salpêtrière
Paris, France

CHARLES DUYCKAERTS, M.D., PH.D.
Professor of Pathology
Laboratoire de Neuropathologie R. Escourolle
Hôpital de la Salpêtrière
Paris, France

MEL FEANY, M.D., PH.D.
Assistant Professor of Pathology
Department of Pathology
Division of Neuropathology
Brigham & Women's Hospital
Harvard Medical School
Boston, Massachusetts

HANS G. GOEBEL, M.D.
Professor of Neuropathology
Department of Neuropathology
Johannes Gutenberg University Medical Center
Mainz, Germany

NICHOLAS K. GONATAS, M.D.
Ralph and Sallie Weaver Professor of Research
  Medicine
Director, Division of Neuropathology
Department of Pathology & Laboratory Medicine
University of Pennsylvania Health System
Philadelphia, Pennsylvania

MICHAEL GORDON, M.D., F.R.C.P.C.
Head, Department of Geriatric and Internal
  Medicine
Baycrest Centre for Geriatric Care
Professor of Medicine, University of Toronto
North York, Ontario Canada

FRANCOISE GRAY, M.D. PhD.
Professor of Pathology
Department of Pathology (Neuropathology)
Faculte de Medicine de Paris Ouest
Garches, France

JOHN H. GROWDON, MD
Professor of Neurology
Department of Neurology
Massachusetts General Hospital
Harvard Medical School
Boston, Massachussetts

CLIVE HARPER, M.D.
Professor of Pathology (Neuropathology)
University of Sydney
Sydney, NSW, Australia

JEAN-JACQUES HAUW, M.D.
Professor and Director
Laboratoire de Neuropathologie R. Escourolle
Groupe Hospitalier Pitié-Salpêtrière
Paris, France

CYNTHIA HAWKINS, M.D.
Department of Pathobiology and Laboratory Medicine
University of Toronto
Division of Neuropathology, Toronto Western Hospital
Toronto, Canada

E. TESSA HEDLEY-WHYTE, M.D.
Professor of Pathology (Neuropathology)
C.S. Kubic Laboratory of Neuropathology
Massachusetts General Hospital
Harvard Medical School
Boston, Massachusetts

WENDY HOBBS, B.A.
Research Laboratory Supervisor
Molecular Neuropathology Laboratory
Massachusetts General Hospital East
Charlestown, Massachusetts

TERUMI A. IZUKAWA, M.D., F.R.C.P.C.
Deputy Head, Department of Geriatric and Internal Medicine
Baycrest Centre for Geriatric Care
North York
Ontario, Canada

ROBERT L. KNOBLER, M.D., PH.D.
Professor of Neurology (Neuroimmunology)
Department of Neurology
Jefferson Medical College
Philadelphia, Pennsylvania

JAN E. LEESTMA, M.D., M.M.
Associate Medical Director, Neuropathologist
Chicago Institute of Neurosurgery and Neuroresearch
Chicago, Illinois

MARK P. MATTSON, PH.D.
Chief of the Laboratory of Neurosciences
National Institute on Aging
Baltimore, Maryland

JACQUELINE MIKOL M.D.
Professor of Pathology
Department of Pathology (Neuropathology)
Hôpital Lariboisière
Paris, France

GEOFFREY J. PILKINGTON, BSc, PhD, CBiol, FIBiol, FRCPath
Professor of Experimental Neuro-oncology
The Maudsley Experimental Neuro-oncology Group
Institute of Psychiatry
London, United Kingdom

TAMAS REVESZ, PH.D
Senior Lecturer/Honorary Consultant
Department of Neuropathology
Institute of Neurology
National Hospital for Neurology & Neurosurgery
London, United Kingdom

FRANCESCO SCARAVILLI, M.D. PH.D
Professor and Director
Department of Neuropathology
National Hospital for Nervous Diseases
Queen Square
London, United Kingdom

ROBERT E. SCHMIDT, M.D., PH.D.
Professor of Pathology
Department of Pathology
Washington University School of Medicine
St. Louis, Missouri

ROBERT J. SCHWARTZMAN, M.D.
Professor and Chairman
Department of Neurology
Medical College of Pennsylvania Hahnemann University
Philadelphia, Pennsylvania

PATRICK SHANNON, M.D., F.R.C.P.C.
Staff Neuropathologist
Lecturer, University of Toronto
Department of Pathobiology and Laboratory Medicine
Toronto Western Hospital and University Health Network
Toronto, Canada

HARRY V. VINTERS, M.D.
Professor of Pathology/Neuropathology
Department of Pathology and Laboratory Medicine
Section of Neuropathology, Brain Research Institute & Neuropsychiatric Institute
UCLA Medical Center
Los Angeles, California

ANNE VITAL, M.D., PH.D.
Professor of Neuropathology
Neuropathology Laboratory
Université Victor Segalen
Bordeaux, France

CLAUDE VITAL, M.D.
Emeritus Professor of Pathology
Neuropathology Laboratory
Université Victor Segalen
Bordeaux, France

JEAN PAUL G. VONSATTEL, M.D.
Associate Professor of Pathology (Neuropathology)
C.S. Kubic Laboratory for Neuropathology
Massachusetts General Hospital
Harvard Medical School
Boston, Massachusetts

Pathology of the Aging Human Nervous System

1. The Normal Aging Human Brain

SERGE DUCKETT

The subject of this chapter—the normal aging brain—concerns the behavior, the health and its cost, population figures, and achievements of the 650 million humans over the age of 65 (65+) worldwide. The choice of 65 as the boundary between non-aging and aging is arbitrary and was made by Otto von Bismark, the founder of the Social Security system in 1881, and by Franklin Delano Roosevelt, who introduced it in the United States in 1935, for political and economic reasons. In those days politicians could wax eloquently during election time about their concern for the working human without worrying about post-election costs because only a very small minority of the population ever reached the age of 65. However, with the present 65+ population explosion and the increase in the cost of medical care, paid retirement has become a financial burden. Today the boundary between the non-old and the old is increasingly based on the expanding life expectancy. The real bar for old age has always been set by death, thus in 1900 one became old at 40, in 1950, at 55, and today at 74,[1] one day, presumably it will be 100.

Information that is valid today concerning the normal aging brain may not be so tomorrow; consequently, to keep abreast of recent advances in gerontology and geriatrics, *carpe diem*. Historically, the normal aging brain was considered an oxymoron because the concepts of normality and abnormality, namely cerebral degeneration, were linked together. Shakespeare's remark, "When the age is in, the wit is out," is an oft-cited truism not so randomly applied today.[2] The current medical view is that normal cerebral degeneration can be delayed in many cases through following simple, good health rules, which include getting proper nutrition and sufficient exercise, avoiding stress, and receiving medical attention and care. Thus when age sets in, the mind is not necessarily out. Still, the reality of aging remains, voiced by the sage of Broadway, Sophie Tucker, who said, "I have been young and I have been old and I would rather be young."

A few years ago the 65+ population was just emerging from a long period of characterization as a forgetful, amusing, but lamentable minority.[3] Now that perception has changed sharply as a result of the explosive growth in their (electoral) number; their increasing good health and its rising cost to taxpayers; the formation of organizations to protect their interests, such as the most powerful political lobby in the United States, the American Association of Retired People; the abolishment of forced retirement (Claude Pepper Act); and the fact that they form the wealthiest age-oriented population in the nation, even though 32% live below the poverty level. In short, they have gelt and clout.

RETIREMENT

The word *retirement* used to mean the permanent departure from a place of work, along with a secure, regular, check for the pursuit of "green, golf, and games" (the 3 G's) or "sun, sand, and sea" (the 3 S's) in warmer, friendlier, and quieter climates—the antechamber of the beyond. It also often signified the departure from active life and gradual mental and physical deterioration. The sentiment that financially secure retirement was the working man and woman's dream lasted from the introduction of Social Security until the 1980s, when retirees impatient with death's tardiness, usually in good health, bored with the 3 G's and the 3 S's and afternoon TV in sun-filtered rooms, and often financially squeezed because their unexpected longevity was proving too costly, went back to their former homes, family, and friends—"left the South and came back North."[3] That countermigration has increased steadily over the years as more retirees have gone back to work. At the same time, in the United States 40% of people 65+ and over have not retired and continue to contribute to Social Security. Others have used the security of retirement to make a change of life, to rest, or to realize an artistic and creative ambition—the Grandma Moses syndrome. Sadly enough, too many older humans' self-image has been hurt by negative external or media views, even though they know that their own experience and self-analysis contradict that impression.

The number of artists, painters, sculptors, designers, writers, woodworkers, cooks, etc. in the world who have begun their creative careers after retirement or after age 65+ is notable. Mrs. Anna Mary Robertson, known as "Grandma Moses," was a farmer's wife in upstate New York who brought up 10 children under difficult circumstances. She was 70, a widow alone, when someone gave her a box of paints. In a short time she started producing masterpieces of "naïve art" (*art naif*)—very colorful reminiscences, usually of pleasant events of her past in her native countryside, and she continued to do so until she died at the age of 101. Her early paintings were sold for $1 apiece; today they bring up to $1 million. There are elderly, genial naïve art painters, from all social classes, around the world, including a few who have achieved international recognition: Seraphine Louis, a cleaning lady; Auguste Bauchant, a gardener; Narcisse Belle, a butcher; Hector Hyppolite, a Voodoo priest; Ivan Laskovic, a postman; Dominique Lagru, a sheperd, Gertrude O'Brady, an expatriate heiress—and the list goes on.

NONAGENARIANS AND CENTENARIANS

Currently, the total U.S. population of those 90+ of age is 1,350,000, including 58,504 centenarians.[4] The population growth of the 85+ population rose 274% between 1960 and 1994, whereas it grew 45% in the general U.S. population. This group numbered 3 million in 1994, and will probably number 40 million in 2050.[4]

James Russell Wiggins, the editor of the local newspaper in Ellsworth, Maine, has been answering the phone in the editorial offices for the past 77 years, except when he was away serving as the chief U.S. delegate at the U.N. or editing the *Washington Post*. His response to the question of retiring is "Retire at 95? Ridiculous!" Mr. Wiggins is one of the 50,000 people aged 90+ employed in the United States today, this group represents about 3% of the total 90+ population.[5] According to studies of 1027 centenarians, 45.9% had normal brain function, 16.6% were very demented, and the rest were demented in varying lesser degrees. For people of age 110+ the death rate dropped back to that of people in their 80s.[6-11] In the New England Centenarian Study at Beth Israel–Deaconness Hospital and Harvard University Medical School, Silver and Perls noted that 80% of the centenarians were women, a disproportionate number of whom were women who had either never married or who had had children after the age of 40, and that the few men in the study were noticeably healthier than the women. They also found that extreme old age runs in families, and that the death rate leveled off in the nineties and decreased after age 100.[12,13]

REVOLUTION

Many of the 27 million able-bodied U.S. citizens age 65+ are partaking in the Gray Panther revolution, engaging in work, sports competition, and other physically demanding activities in addition to carrying on their usual responsibilities. They are also protesting, refusing and rejecting the clichéed characterizations of the aged as useless or demented. In general, this group of active elders feel that they possess those virtues gained by time and experience—namely education, diplomacy, dependability, and good judgment, qualities that should be exploited economically to their advantage and that of society. They reject the alternative that they be kept in publicly funded retirement and medical care programs at great cost to the nation—8% of the U.S. national budget. The most primitive tribes value the experience of their elders and use them. All civilizations, nations, and cultures have opted to nominate or elect older citizens for responsible tasks.

ACCOMPLISHMENTS AND CREATIVITY OF THOSE AGED 65+

The most dramatic demonstration of elderly mental prowess is the immense contribution to the arts by humans over the age of 65, which, when based on quality and permanence, competes very favorably with, and overwhelms, some would say, that of younger generations. The persistent creativity in the production of premier works of art, setting standards in their field, by older citizens is exemplified by the painting of the Last Judgement in the Sistine Chapel by Michaelangelo (1475–1564) when he was 59 to 66. He has been referred to as the "scourge of art" because of the immensity of his irreproducible talent. The death of this man while he was still in the full power of his genius marked the end of the greatest era of painting in human history—the Italian Renaissance. Old musicians, composers, and performers, whether of classical music or jazz, never die—they just fade away, be they Beethoven in his late 50s, Bach in his 60s, Duke Ellington and Ella Fitzgerald in his 70s, Horowitz in his 80s, or Benny Carter and Eubie Blake in their 90s.

In the physical world, the media sensation of 72-year-old Senator John Glenn's flight into space, parachute jumps by octagenarian veterans remembering the WWII Normandy landings, and sporting feats of elderly athletes have shown that physical accomplishments can be achieved by older citizens. However, accomplishments and creativity are preferentially sedentary in the older population. Creativity in older humans is proportional to the ability and ambition of the individual and can vary from gardening to the production of *Don Quixote*. Individuals aged 65+ have problems, tasks, issues, and motivations that are different from those of younger folk, thus their sense of creativity will be different. The ambition and will to perform and finish a creative act are motivated by stimuli that are usually different from and more generous than those of younger people. Older people may feel that they have less time left and develop an urge to accomplish a goal for which they will be remembered. Some individuals, such as Grandma Moses, have a burst of creativity that expresses or reaffirms past creative work or tendencies. Older citizens develop a sense of spiritual sufficiency often because they have to, and it is less dependant on external stimulation than for younger people. Such introspection can lead to meditation and reflection or contented solitude, and in gifted individuals it can result in creative masterpieces. The list of major accomplishments by women and men aged 65+ is long, and the following names illustrate this point.

Adams, John (1735–1826): Second president of the United States from the age of 62 to 66.

Adams, John Quincy (1767–1848): Sixth president of the United States from the age of 58 to 62, politically active until age 81.

Anthony, Susan B. (1820–1906): London International Council of Women delegate at age 79. National American Women Suffrage Association president until age 80.

Barton, Clara (1821–1912): Founder at age 80 of the National Association of First Aid and director until her death at 91.

Bellini, Giovanni (1430–1516): Painted the portrait of the doge Loredano at the age of 75.

Bernhardt, Sarah (1844–1923): Starred in *Daniel* in London at age 75, in Rostand's *La Gloire* at age 75, and in Verneuill's *Regine Armand* at 76, and made her final performance in *Daniel* at 78.

Boyd, William (1875–1979): Trained as a psychiatrist, Boyd established his reputation as a writer of pathology texts. He wrote his last edition of *The Introduction to the Study of Disease* at age 86, which went out of print in his 94th year. He was a lifelong lover of Scotch whiskey, a sentiment he expressed in his last words.

Buffon, G. L. (1707–1788): Writer of the 44 in-quarto texts on natural history concerning detailed descriptions and illustrations of all birds, fish, quadrupeds, and minerals known at the time. He finished and published these shortly before his death at 81.

Clemenceau, Georges. (1841–1929): Known as the "Tigre," he was the vigorous prime minister of France during WWI at age 76 to 79.

Cervantes, Saavedra, Miguel De (1547–1616): Completed *Don Quixote* in his 70s.

Churchill, Winston (1874–1865): Became wartime prime minister at 65 and again at 77; finished a six-volume of the war at age 70.

Corot, J. B. (1796–1875): Painted masterpieces such as *Head of an Italian Girl* and *The Blue Lady* at age 74.

Disraeli, Benjamin (1801–1888): Statesman, prime minister, and leader of his party in the United Kingdom until age 76.

Ellington, Edward Kennedy (Duke) (1899–1970): Composer of ballads, operas, and sacred works, orchestra leader and pianist. Fully active until his sudden death at 71.

Edison, Thomas A. (1847–1931): American inventor of the lightbulb and the phonograph who made conducted experiments and made improvments in his existing inventions until his last years.

Franklin, Benjamin (1706–1790): Represented the United States in France at age 76 to 79, was a member of the Constitutional Convention at 81, and was president of Pennsylvania from 79 to 82 years of age.

Galilei, Galileo (1564–1642): Physicist and astronomer engaged in the study of mechanics and projection, published his Dialogues at age 74.

Gladstone, W.E. (1809–1898): British statesman, orator, and author. Leader of the Conservative Party and was prime minister for the 4 fourth time from ages 83 to 85.

Goethe, Wolfgang von (1749–1832): Germany's greatest author. Completed his masterpiece *Faust* at age 82.

Hals, Franz (1584–1666): Painted *The Old Toper of Haarlem* and after 74 painted *The Young Man in the Flop Hat* and *Gardians of the Poorhouse*.

Hardy, Thomas (1840–1928): English poet and novelist, married at age 74, wrote a string of literary successes such as *Late Lyrics* at age 82, *Queen of Cornwall* at 83, *Human Shows* at 85, and *Christmas in the Elgin Room* at 87.

Holmes, O. W. (1809–1891): American poet, essayist, and physician. Published his *Medical Essays* and *Pages from an Old Volume of Life* at age 71, *Over the Teacups* at 75, and other works between the ages 75 and 80.

Hugo, Victor (1802–1885): French poet and novelist. Produced his greatest novels in his 70s. At 75 published the second series of *Légendes du Siécle* and *The Art of Being a Grandfather*. Continued to write until his death at 83.

Ingres, J.A.D. (1780–1867): Painted *La Source* when he was 76 and continued painting until his death.

Jefferson, Thomas (1743–1823): Third U.S. president at age 58, founded the University of Virginia at 76, devoted himself to his plans for the school until his death at 83.

Kuhn, Maggie (1905–1995): Founded the Gray Panthers, a social advocacy group for older adults, at the age of 65.

Mantegna, Andrea (1431–1506): Painted the *Madonna of Victory* at 65 and *Parnassus* at 70.

Madison, James (1751–1836): Fourth president of the U.S. at age 58, rector of the University of Virginia at 76, participated in the Virginia Constitutional Convention at 79, and wrote scholarly and influential articles until his death.

Michaelangelo Buanarroti (1475–1564): Considered the great painter of all time was also a sculptor and architect. Completed painting the Sistine Chapel in the Vatican between the ages of 72 and 89.

Newton, Sir Isaac (1642–1727): Mathematician and philosopher. Discoverer of the law of gravity. Worked productively until age 85.

Picasso, Pablo (1881–1974): Painting genius of the 20th century who created styles and masterpieces in a variety of media until the day before he died.

Rossini, G. A. (1792–1868): Produced a musical masterpiece *Petite Messe Solenelle* at age 76.

St. Saens, C. C. (1835–1921): Pianist, conductor, organist, and author; wrote an opera, an oratorio, and other compositions after age 76.

Shaw, G. B. (1856–1950): Dramatist and critic, wrote a series of successful plays and books after age 74, was an international radio commentator and critic until age 94.

Sophocles (495–406 BC): Dramatist and poet, produced *Philoctetus* and *Oedipus at Colonus* after age 74.

Tennyson, A. (1809–1892): Poet, who at 71 produced *Ballads and Poems*, at 75 became Lord, and published *Becke* at age 80 and *Demeter* and other notable works at 83.

Titian (Tiziano, V.) 1477–1576): Painter. After age 90 he painted a series of masterpieces, including *Transfiguration* and *Annunciation*; between ages 94 and 98 he painted *Battle of Lepanto* and he died at age 99 while working on the *Pieta*.

Tubman, Harriet (1820–1908): Freed more than 300 slaves through the Underground Railroad, and helped found a home for the poor in her 80s.

Verdi, G. (1813–1901): Musician. Composed *Othello* at 74, *Falstaff* at 80, and works on sacred subjects when he was 85.

Voltaire, J.F.A. (1694–1778): Author, free thinker, citizen of the world, who wrote profusely throughout his life, engaged in multiple occupations, including that of active farmer and manufacturer at age 80. Wrote and published *Irene* shortly before he died at age 84. As he lay dying, he suddenly woke up, saw a roaring fire in the fireplace and exclaimed, "Déjà!" ("already")—his last word.

MORPHOLOGY

The traditional methods of studying of the evolution of the normal aging human brain have been cross-sectional rather than longitudinal. The former is the comparative study of the macroscopy and microscopy of brains of various individuals; the latter is the repeated study of the brain of one individual over a period of time. Most studies have been done on the dead. The advent of modern imaging techniques has permitted the macroscopic study of the living brain.

Size of the Brain

In the nineteenth and early twentieth centuries there were numerous studies on the size, shape, regional prominence, and weight of the human brain and such information was drawn upon to deduce intelligence, character, and other virtues and deficiencies. Even recently there has been much media-scientific speculation about the possible significance of parietal lobe "hypertrophy" in Einstein's brain.

In 1972 Tomlinson wrote on the subject of morphologic brain changes in nondemented old humans.[14] He was dissatisfied with previous studies because he felt that the identification of normal and abnormal brains was unclear due to a lack of precise premortem information that reflected an erroneous clinical diagnosis. Together with Blessed and Roth, a joint study was devised consisting of a full physical and psychological examination and eventual postmortem examinations of the brains of 28 "nondemented" individuals, 16 women and 12 men, ages 65 to 92.[15] There was no histologic evidence in these brains to support a diagnosis of dementia. Neurofibrillary changes, senile plaques, and granulovacuolar changes were found in a small number of cases but never in significant amounts, and there was little evidence of cerebral softening. Cerebral atrophy was slight or absent in the majority and the brain weight and ventricular size did not differ greatly from those of younger subjects. The weight of the brain in male ranged from 1170 to 1430 g (with a mean of 1320 g; SD 77.9) and in females from 1080 to 1390 g (with a mean of 1213g; SD 91.8).[14] There was nothing in Tomlinson et al.'s review to suggest that the brain weight diminished markedly after the age of 65.

In another study the lateral ventricles were of normal size and appearance in 7 of 28 brains of elderly humans aged 65 to 92, and were slightly or moderately dilated in the rest.[14] The mean ventricular volume in 19 measured cases in that series was 26.6 ml and greater. These series do not support the notion that the ventricles of humans aged 65+ are larger than those of young adults. Davis and Wright[16] developed a technique that allows the examiner at autopsy to measure the ratio of the volume of the brain to that of the cranial vault. They examined 63 humans ages 7 to 82, and noted that the ratio was constant at about 0.92 until age 55, and then declined to 0.83 at age 90.

Radioimaging

Neuroradiology was revolutionized by computed tomographic (CT) reconstruction techniques, one of which is based on the use of X-rays (X-ray CT), the other being dependent on proton–molecule or proton–proton interactions—magnetic resonance imaging (MRI). X-ray CT and/or MRI permits the visualization of blood, blood vessels, fat, and water; and the identification of organs or structures in the living brain such as gray and white matter, pallidum, thalamus, and red nucleus and of pathological processes such as edema, demyelination, hemorrhages, dilatation of ventricles, and cerebral atrophy. These techniques, which permit the study of changes in living tissue at different stages of disease and during normal degeneration, have vastly expanded our understanding of the normal and pathologic nervous system, including early and often treatable diseases. After the introduction of CT scanning techniques and MRI, radiologists and neuroanatomists started studying of the normal and pathologic aging brain. These cross-sectional studies confirmed earlier studies and contributed more detailed information.

Recent longitudinal radioimaging studies[17,18] of the diminution of the size of the brain have confirmed previous observations and researchers have noted that the ventricular dilatation and cerebral atrophy begin during the fifth and sixth decades. The earliest signs of atrophy are in the cerebellar vermis. Widening of the cortical sulci, particularly in the frontal lobes and cisterns, appears at the start of the sixth decade and progresses slowly. Early on, the gray matter atrophies faster than white matter but by the early 60s this trend is reversed. This so-called normal process of cerebral atrophy is very slow and mostly clinically mute.[19,20]

Cells

There are no methods available at present that permit the histologic examination in situ of the brain without surgical intervention. Theoretically this type of study is possible by associating imaging methods and electron ion laser, or other types of probes or magnetic resonance done with elements other than hydrogen. The information concerning the morphology of the human brain, such as loss of cells and atrophy, has been based on cross-sectional studies and is therefore tentative. The finding of a loss of neurons in the human brain has been criticized because the brain in question was examined only once, usually after death, or because brain atrophy occurred without neuropathologic changes. These and other criticisms concerning the relationship between the morphology and function of a human brain and therefore the necessity of the examining both have been expressed in recent years, resulting in the amelioration of methods of brain study.[21,22]

Histologic examination of the normal aging brain has shown that there is a gradual minimal loss of neurons after age 50; although this loss may accelerate with advanced age, it is largely clinically mute. This neuronal loss is associated with a loss of dendrites, dendritic spines, and synapses in various parts of the cortex but not in the temporal lobe.[23–25] Recently, the discovery has been made that neurogenesis takes place in the injured temporal lobe.[26] It has been proposed that neural loss in the frontal cortex is the result rather than than the cause of the atrophy. Although there is an increasing loss of muscarinic cholinergic receptor bindings in the frontal cerebral cortex as humans age, there is no morphologic evidence of senile degeneration. In nondemented brains there have been only minimal nonspecific findings of cerebral degeneration.[24,25]

Terry and Hanson[23] compared the brain weight, cortical thickness, and cell count in the mid-frontal region and superior temporary gyrus of 18 patients with senile dementia of the Alzheimer type (SDAT) with those of 12 age-matched normal specimens between the ages of 70 and 89 years. The brain weight for the normal group was 930 to 1350 g (mean 1152 ± 45g) and that of the SDAT group was 918 to 1150 g (mean 1150 ± 20g), which indicates no significant statistical difference. There was no statistical difference in the size of cortical thickness, the packing density, or the number of cortical cells of both groups, as studied with a Quantimet image analyzer, except for the number of large neurons (>90 µm2) which was 40% fewer in SDAT brains. There were also more plaques in the SDAT brains. In Terry and Hansons[23] study of the morphologic parameters of brains of patients with Alzheimer's disease and those of brains of normal humans, they found that the neuronal loss per unit volume in the normal brain was much less than that previously reported and that the findings in patients with Alzheimer's disease at any age were clearly different from those for the normal controls.

Neurogenesis

The accepted view on aging of the brain is that the brain degenerates slowly and inevitably as we live beyond age 50 and toward 120. At first this degeneration occurs without noticeable clinical manifestations, but eventually it may lead to dementia. Today about 10%–12% of the 65+ population, or 3.5 million people are severely demented (e.g., with Alzheimer's disease), including ± 17% of the 58,504 centenarians.[7-11]. There has been little hope of changing that course of normal cerebral degeneration except to avert or minimize it by practicing a healthy lifestyle and receiving efficient medical care. However, recent studies have reported evidence that may alter the inevitability of cerebral degeneration and its clinical consequences.[27,28] A dent has been made in the classical dictum that adult human neurons do not replicate, through evidence showing that they reproduce in areas of the damaged adult human brain.[26] Additionally, the presence of apoptosis has been noted in the brains of humans afflicted with Azheimer's disease or the Creutzfelt-Jakob syndrome.[29] Tomei and Umansky have proposed that apoptosis is "the ultimate protective process for preservation of phenotypic fidelity in multicellular organisms," a process by which the organism detects damage and replaces defective cells.[30] These observations, presently the subject of debate,[31] permit the supposition that it is possible that both phenomena, neuronal reproduction and apoptosis, could be associated with repair of the pathologic brain and that cerebral degeneration is a normal apoptotic event that results in the replacement of old or sick neurons by new ones. Is there an age plateau, beyond which all organs will have the power to repair and renew themselves, yet to be reached? The present prolongation of life past 100 years is creating a sufficiently large population of old-old humans to investigate a possibly new and unknown "terra physiologica et biologica incognita," providing researchers with a brand new experimental laboratory in which to examine and exploit their and nature's adaptive talents.

It has been generally accepted that neurons do not replicate in the adult brain and that in early middle-life they naturally begin to disappear—at first slowly, then quickly after age 50, and when enough of them have disappeared, dementia results. In 1965 Altman and Das showed that neurogenesis did occur in the adult mouse brain,[32] and since then reports have appeared that support their discovery.[33-35] In 1998 came the news that neurogenesis does take place in the adult human brain, and even though it was observed in only one case, this finding was sufficient to open new vistas.[26]

CAUSES OF DEATH

According to the U.S. Bureau of Census, the causes of death in the U.S. elderly population changed considerably over the decades during the last century,[4] with the period 1950–1990 receiving the most extensive study.[36,37] Seven in 10 Americans who died in 1991 were elderly, i.e., 1.6 million out of 2.2 million, the main causes being heart disease, cancer, and stroke (Table 1–1). Since then death from heart disease has declined but that from cancer has increased.[36,38] Currently, The main causes of death in the elderly throughout the world are hunger and malnutrition (see Chapter 14).

POPULATION

There are roughly 6 billion humans on this earth today—double the number in 1959 and at least half the 10 billion in 2050—and if the birth rate remains at its 1990–1995 level, world population will be 15 billion in 2100 (Fig. 1–1 and Table 1–2).[40] Around the globe there are vast regional differences in wealth and life expectancy (a topic beyond the scope of this chapter): life expectancy for males is 40 years in Malawi, 58 in Russia, 68 in Europe, 74 in Western Europe, 73 in the United States, and 76 in Japan. These figures are higher for females.[41]

In the United States there are 35 million persons over the age of 65, 40% of whom are employed, and there will be 80 million in 50 years. The 65+ population will grow 2.8% annually between 2010 and 2030 when the baby boomers come on board.[4] The 65+ population has multiplied 11 times since 1900. The number of retired and nonretired persons will be equal by 2030, and there will be more humans age 65+ than those age 14 in 20 years' time. U.S. inhabitants who reach the age of 65 can expect to live 17 more years. By 2050, 20% of the U.S. population will be 65+ and if retirement advantages are extended to those aged 50–65+, that combined population will easily be the voting majority. Currently the 65+ population constitutes about 20% of the U.S. electorate (Table 1–3).[4]

Table 1-1. U.S. Deaths by Age and Leading Cause: 1994

Age and Leading Cause of Death	NUMBER OF DEATHS			DEATH RATE PER 100,000 POPULATION		
	Total	Male	Female	Total	Male	Female
All ages[a]	2,278,994	1,162,747	1,116,247	875.4	915.0	837.6
Leading Causes of Death						
Heart disease	732,409	361,276	371,133	281.3	284.3	2278.5
Malignant neoplasms (cancer)	534,310	280,465	253,845	205.2	220.7	190.5
Cerebrovascular disease (stroke)	153,306	60,225	93,081	58.9	47.4	69.8
Chronic obstructive pulmonary disease	101,628	53,729	47,899	39.0	42.3	35.9
Accidents	91,437	60,509	30,928	35.1	47.6	23.2
Pneumonia	81,473	37,339	44,134	31.3	29.4	33.1
Diabetes	56,692	24,758	31,934	21.8	19.5	24.0
HIV Infection	42,114	35,641	NA	16.2	28.0	NA
Suicide	31,142	25,174	NA	12.0	19.8	NA
Homicide and legal intervention	NA	19,707	NA	NA	15.5	NA
1 to 4 years old						
All causes	6,800	3,841	2,959	42.9	47.3	38.2
Leading Causes of Death						
Accidents	2,517	1,518	999	15.9	18.7	12.9
Congenital anomalies	714	354	360	4.5	4.4	4.6
Malignant neoplasms (cancer)	518	287	231	3.3	3.5	3.0
Homicide and legal intervention	473	265	208	3.0	3.3	2.7
Heart disease	285	146	139	1.8	1.8	1.8
Pneumonia and influenza	178	98	80	1.1	1.2	1.0
HIV Infection	199	98	101	1.3	1.2	1.3
5 to 14 years old						
All causes	8,464	5,182	3,282	22.5	26.9	17.9
Leading Causes of Death						
Accidents	3,508	2,305	1,203	9.3	12.0	6.6
Malignant neoplasms (cancer)	1,053	604	449	2.8	3.1	2.4
Congenital anomalies	434	232	202	1.2	1.2	1.1
Suicide	322	234	88	0.9	1.2	0.5
Homicide and legal intervention	572	357	215	1.5	1.9	1.2
Heart disease	327	174	153	0.9	0.9	0.8
Pneumonia and influenza	103	58	45	0.3	0.3	0.2
HIV Infections	182	96	86	0.5	0.5	0.5
15 to 24 years old						
All causes	35,241	26,758	8,483	98.0	145.8	48.2
Leading Causes of Death						
Accidents	13,898	10,417	3,481	38.7	56.8	19.8
Homicide and legal intervention	8,116	7,024	1,092	22.6	38.3	6.2
Suicide	4,956	4,302	654	13.8	23.4	3.7
Malignant neoplasms (cancer)	1,740	1,059	681	4.8	5.8	3.9
Cerebrovascular disease (stroke)	183	98	NA	0.5	0.5	NA
Chronic obstructive pulmonary disease	232	143	89	0.6	0.8	0.5

(*continued*)

Table 1-1.—Continued

Age and Leading Cause of Death	NUMBER OF DEATHS			DEATH RATE PER 100,000 POPULATION		
	Total	Male	Female	Total	Male	Female
Congenital anomalies	463	272	191	1.3	1.5	1.1
Heart disease	992	631	361	2.8	3.4	2.1
Pneumonia and influenza	221	115	106	0.6	0.6	0.6
HIV Infection	641	420	221	1.8	2.3	1.3
25 to 44 years old						
All causes	158,776	111,924	46,852	191.3	270.8	112.4
Leading Causes of Death						
Accidents	27,012	20,729	6,283	32.5	50.2	15.1
Malignant neoplasms (cancer)	21,899	10,091	11,808	26.4	24.4	28.3
Cerebrovascular disease (stroke)	3,519	1,845	1,674	4.2	4.5	4.0
HIV Infection	30,476	25,773	4,703	36.7	62.4	11.3
Heart disease	16,763	11,903	4,860	20.2	28.8	11.7
Pneumonia and influenza	2,155	1,341	814	2.6	3.2	2.0
Diabetes	2,467	1,480	987	3.0	3.6	2.4
Homicide and legal intervention	11,419	8,987	2,432	13.8	21.7	5.8
Suicide	12,729	10,265	2,464	15.3	24.8	5.9
45 to 64 years old						
All causes	375,016	231,647	143,369	736.9	942.6	544.8
Leading Causes of Death						
Malignant neoplasms (cancer)	132,839	71,165	61,674	261.0	289.6	234.4
Heart disease	102,956	72,623	30,333	202.3	295.5	115.3
Pneumonia and influenza	5,490	3,369	2,121	10.8	13.7	8.1
HIV Infection	9,822	8,659	1,163	19.3	35.2	4.4
Cerebrovascular (stroke)	14,932	8,179	6,753	29.3	33.3	25.7
Accidents	15,200	10,794	4,406	29.9	43.9	16.7
Chronic obstructive pulmonary disease	13,011	6,930	6,081	25.6	28.2	23.1
Chronic liver disease and cirrhosis	10,573	7,501	3,072	20.8	30.5	11.7
Diabetes	11,473	5,998	5,475	22.5	24.4	20.8
Suicide	7,108	5,427	1,681	14.0	22.1	6.4
65 years old and over						
All causes	1,662,573	765,270	897,303	5,014.1	5,679.2	4,558.8
Leading Causes of Death						
Heart disease	610,330	275,383	334,947	1,840.7	2,043.6	1,701.7
Malignant neoplasms (cancer)	376,186	197,220	178,966	1,134.5	1,463.6	909.2
Cerebrovascular (stroke)	134,340	49,910	84,430	405.2	370.4	429.0
Chronic obstructive pulmonary disease	87,048	45,945	41,103	262.5	341.0	208.8
Pneumonia and influenza	72,762	32,018	40,744	219.4	237.6	207.0
Diabetes	42,600	17,198	25,402	128.5	127.6	129.1
Accidents	28,314	14,152	14,162	85.4	105.0	72.0

HIV, human immunodeficiency virus; NA, not available.
[a] Includes those deaths with age not stated.
Source: U.S. National Center for Health Statistics, 1998;[51] annual and unpublished data.

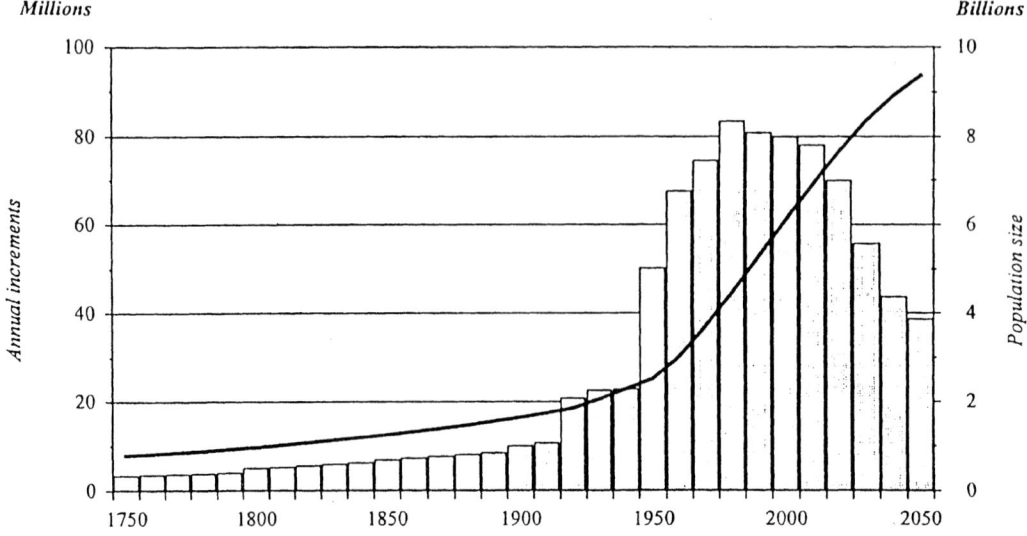

Figure 1–1. Long-term world population increments and population size, 1750–2050. From World Population Prospects, the 1996 Revision. New York: United Nations, 1998.[40]

Nine states have a population of people age 65+ of over one million: California, Florida, New York, Pennsylvania, Texas, Ohio, Illinois, New Jersey, and Michigan: these are also the most populated states. The states with the greatest proportions of elderly are Florida (19%) and Pennsylvania (16%).

The figures noted above are estimates projections, and statistics based on actual census counts. The projected figures are based on the present state of health care which does not take into account the potential effects on population growth of the eradication of diseases such as cancer, malnutrition, malaria, and TB,

Table 1–2. Past, Present, and Projected World Population in Millions

	1800	1900	1939	1997	2025
Asia	630	930	1244	3552	4914
Europe	155	293	380	582	575
Africa	100	150	191	743	1313
North America	12.4	94.6	163.4	393.7	512.8
South America	13.6	51.4	110.6	394	450.2
Total	911	1519.8	2089	5664.7	7567

Table 1–3. Population by Age and Gender in the United States, April 1, 1999

Age	Female	Male	Total
100+	48,163	10,341	58,504
90+	149,290	387,759	1,537,049
90	231,305	91,793	323,098
85+	2,918,250	1,225,354	4,143,704
80	691,539	446,349	1,137,888
70	1,022,103	830,184	1,852,287
65+	20,221,095	14,272,694	34,494,789
65	1,009,621	877,043	1,886,664

Source: U.S. Census Bureau. Population Estimates, Monthly Postcensal Residents and Armed Forces Overseas, 1999.[52]

pharmacologic and therapeutic discoveries, the potential benefits of gene therapy and the human history of killing one another.

HEALTH COSTS[42]

Senator Glenn's space flight in 1998 unleashed a great deal of media attention on the good mental and physical health of numerous folks aged 65+ and the public began to realize that the high cost of this group's retirement and health subsidies should be reviewed. Articles such as "The old aren't so old, and the young are plundered,"[43] and "Some solid research to demolish persistent myths of aging,"[44] appeared in the *New York Times*, and special television programs and town hall discussions across the country addressed the cost of health care and the number of workers available in 20 years to support each retiree. The financing of retirement and medical benefits has also attracted the attention of politicians. In 1999 President Clinton proposed a plan to exclude the wealthy from some Medicare benefits, lower some of its costs, and increase subsidies for prescription drug costs.[44-47] Today the average person aged 65 to 79 in the United States receives $12,000 in federal benefits (mainly Social Security and Medicare) and pays $4000 in taxes, whereas the average person aged 20 to 64 pays $8100 in taxes and receives $1500 in direct federal benefits (Table 1–4).

Currently there is no state-financed health care system covering the entire U.S. population as there is in all other Western countries. Medicare is limited to the population aged 65+. In 1999 there were 39 million Medicare beneficiaries and there will be 79 million more over the next three decades when the babyboomers qualify. There are also 15.5 million people who do not have drug coverage through their Medigap policies, retiree health plans or health maintenance organizations (Table 1–5). Because of a decrease in population growth due to the use of birth control programs, sex education, and humanitarian considerations, it is estimated that the number of people aged 60+ will be greater than that of those less than 60 years of age in the twenty-first century. Health planners and politicians are concerned about footing the health bill of the 65+ group or whatever age-group will be referred to as retired.

Until recently, the elderly were often viewed sympathetically and protectively as "on their way out." In 1997, Social Security, Medicare, and Medicaid cost 8% of the gross national income (GDP), and that share will rise to 13% by 2020, a 63% increase. The major portion of the costs of medical benefits in the past was for medical treatment. Since people

Table 1–4. Medicare Enrollees and Expenditures: 1980 to 1995

Item	1980	1985	1990	1991	1992	1993	1994	1995
Enrollees (millions)								
Total	28.5	31.1	34.2	34.9	35.6	36.3	36.9	37.5
Hospital insurance	28.1	30.6	33.7	34.4	35.2	35.9	36.5	37.1
Supplementary medical insurance	27.4	30.0	32.6	33.2	33.9	34.6	35.2	35.7
Expenditures (millions of dollars)								
Total	36,802	72,294	110,984	121,447	135,845	150,370	163,087	181,483
Hospital Insurance[a]	25,557	48,414	66,997	72,570	85,015	94,391	102,770	114,883
Inpatient hospital	24,116	44,940	59,451	62,777	71,147	76,402	80,788	87,503
Skilled nursing facility	395	548	2,575	2,652	4,119	5,780	7,056	9,142
Home health agency	540	1,913	3,666	5,327	7,579	10,049	12,136	14,895
Hospice	—	43	358	561	846	1,059	1,363	1,854
Supplementary medical insurance[a]	11,245	23,880	43,987	48,877	50,830	55,979	60,317	66,600
Physician	8,187	17,312	29,609	32,313	32,473	35,282	36,900	40,457
Outpatient hospital	1,897	4,319	8,482	9,783	10,894	11,539	14,034	15,405
Home health agency	234	38	74	65	79	112	154	182
Group practice prepayment	203	720	2,827	3,531	3,942	5,002	5,480	6,883
Independent laboratory	114	558	1,476	1,644	1,876	2,044	2,050	2,046

[a] Includes administrative expenses and, for hospital insurance, peer review activity, not shown separately.
Source: U.S. Health Care Financing Administration, Office of the Actuary; and U.S. National Center for Health Statistics, 1998.[51]

Table 1–5. Health Care Expenditures in Millions of Dollars by Type and State, 1993

State	Hospital Care	Physician Service	Purchases of Prescription Drugs[a]
U.S.	323,919	171,226	48,840
Northeast	19,056	9,250	2,710
Maine	1,376	601	213
New Hampshire	1,388	780	197
Vermont	562	265	108
Massachusetts	10,034	4,442	1,337
Rhode Island	1,314	575	206
Connecticut	4,380	2,587	650
Mid-Atlantic	57,854	25,238	7,219
New York	28,001	12,003	3,232
New Jersey	10,312	5,776	1,601
Pennsylvania	19,540	7,460	2,386
East–North Central	54,172	26,275	8,360
Ohio	14,305	7,118	2,095
Indiana	6,998	3,263	1,106
Illinois	15,621	6,970	2,206
Michigan	11,711	5,562	2,054
Wisconsin	5,537	3,362	899
West–North Central	22,252	10,987	3,195
Minnesota	4,796	3,617	739
Iowa	3,111	1,376	516
Missouri	7,652	2,958	975
North Dakota	903	445	103
South Dakota	920	342	104
Nebraska	2,003	825	293
Kansas	2,868	1,425	465
South Atlantic	56,711	30,041	9,412
Delaware	937	466	129
Maryland	5,926	3,704	1,140
District of Columbia	2,612	672	103
Virginia	7,031	3,769	1,343
West Virginia	2,346	988	412
North Carolina	7,801	3,717	1,392
South Carolina	4,221	1,685	665
Georgia	8,704	4,543	1,397
Florida	17,131	10,498	2,832
East–South Central	19,921	8,913	3,402
Kentucky	4,515	2,038	846
Tennessee	7,208	3,137	1,153

(*continued*)

Table 1–5.—Continued

State	Hospital Care	Physician Service	Purchases of Prescription Drugs[a]
Alabama	5,301	2,631	904
Mississippi	2,897	1,107	499
West–South Central	33,601	15,947	5,039
Arkansas	2,723	1,244	484
Louisiana	5,956	2,537	832
Oklahoma	3,329	1,610	569
Texas	21,592	10,526	3,153
Mountain	15,095	8,897	2,436
Montana	894	392	120
Idaho	900	486	182
Wyoming	417	160	64
Colorado	3,932	2,452	534
New Mexico	1,848	716	259
Arizona	3,999	2,799	728
Utah	1,743	864	302
Nevada	1,362	1,029	246
Pacific	45,259	35,677	7,067
Washington	5,305	3,720	853
Oregon	2,966	1,904	431
California	34,827	28,981	5,501
Alaska	701	301	85
Hawaii	1,460	771	197

[a] Covers spending for products purchased in retail outlets. The value of drugs and other products provided by hospitals, nursing homes, or other health professionals is included in estimates of spending for these providers' services.

Source: U.S. National Center for Health Statistics. *Health, United States, 1995;* U.S. National Center for Health Statistics, 1998.[51]

now live longer, more money is being spent yearly by Medicaid on prescription drugs than on doctor's services—$942 per person annually. Senator J. B. Breaux's committee that studied the future of Medicare came to a bipartisan conclusion that Medicare is antiquated because it does not cover the cost of prescription drugs. To tackle the issue of the increasing cost of Medicare and prescription drugs, President Clinton proposed a plan whereby the long-term cost of Medicare would be cut while the program to cover the cost of prescription drugs would be expanded, a proposition that claims to protect the Medicare program until 2027.[47]

In addition to the issue of providing adequate health care to the elderly is that of caring for those who suffer from senility. There are approximately 5.2 million demented elderly citizens in the United States, ±15% of the 35 million 65+ population, and the diagnosis of Alzheimer's disease is applicable to no more than 10% of that population. The cost of senility for the year 2000 is projected to be about $16.5 billion.

Wealth, social position, and education also play a role in the prolongation of life.[48,49] In 1967 a review of the mortality rates of 17,530 British male civil service employees over a period of 10 years revealed that the mortality rate varied highly with the service grade of the individual regardless of the cause of death.[50] All of these employees had had equal access to medical care under the British National Health System. Moreover, 25 years later a re-examination of the survivors showed that this social class gradient persisted among the elderly. These findings applied equally to smokers and nonsmokers.

I thank Mrs. Souad Aouad el Boustani, Service des Statistiques, UNESCO, Paris, France; M. Paula Bavasso, Paris; Mr. Alain Bissor, Bibliothèque de la Faculté de Médecine, Paris 6; Dr. Martine Deville-Velloz, Service de Documentation, Institut National d'Etudes Démographiques, Paris; Mde. V. Hugon-Leroux, Bibliothèque, Charcot, Hôpital de la Salpêtrière, Paris; M. Shirley Sadak, Jefferson Medical College, Philadelphia, PA; and M. Hava Tillipman of the U.S. Census Bureau, Bethesda, MD, for their advice and assistance in the preparation of this chapter.

REFERENCES

1. Goode E. New study finds middle age is prime of life. New York Times, 16 Feb, 1999; D 6.
2. Shakespeare W. Much Ado About Nothing, act III, scene 5, line 33.
3. Duckett S. The normal aging human brain. In: Duckett S, ed. The Pathology of the Aging Human Nervous System, 1 ed. Philadelphia, Lea and Febiger, 1991.
4. U.S. Census Bureau. Sixty-Five Plus in the United States. May 1995.
5. Retire at 95? Ridiculous, says Maine editor. International Herald Tribune, 14 May, 1999; 3.
6. Hilts PJ. Life at age 100 is surprisingly healthy. New York Times, 1 June, 1999; D 7.
7. Allard MA la Recherche du Secret des Centenaires. 100 Tableaux pour 100 Ans. Paris: Fondation Ipsen, 1991.
8. Mizutani T, Shimaza H. Neuropathological background of 27 centenarian brains. J Neurol Sci 1992; 108:168.
9. Fayuet G, Hauw JJ, Deleare Y, He Y, Duyckaerts C, et al. Neuropathologie de 20 centenaires. 1. Données cliniques. Rev Neurol (Paris) 1994; 150 (1) : 16.
10. Giannakopoulos P, Hof PR, Vallet PG, Giannakopoulos AS, Charnay Y, Bouras C. Quantitative analysis of neuropathologic changes in the cerebral cortex of centenarians. Prog Neuropsychopharmacol Biol Psychiatry 1995; 19 (4):577.
11. Ivan L. Neuropsychiatric examination of centenarians. In: Beregi E. Vol. 27 ed. Centenarians in Hungary. A Sociomedical and Demographic Study. Interdisciplinary Topics in Gerontology, vol. 27. Basel: Karger, 1990:53–64.
12. Silver M, Newell K, Hyman B, Growdon J, Hedley-Whyte ET, Perls T. Unraveling the mystery of cognitive changes in old age: correlation of neuropsychological evaluation with neuropathological findings in the extreme old. Int. Psychogeriatr 1998; 10(1):25.
13. Katzman R. The aging brain: limitations in our knowledge and future approaches. Arch Neurol 1997; 54(10): 1201.
14. Tomlinson BE. Morphological brain changes in nondemented old people. In: Van Progg HM, HF Kalverboer HF, eds. Aging of the CNS. Haarlem: De Erven F. Bohn, 1972:xx–xx.
15. Blessed G., Tomlinson BE, Roth M. The association between quantitative measures of dementia and of senile changes in the cerebral gray matter of elderly subjects. Br J Psychiatry 1968; 114:797.
16. Davis PJM, Wright EA. New method for measuring cranial cavity volume and its application to the assessment of cerebral atrophy at autopsy. Neuropathol Appl Neurobiol 1977; 3:341.
17. Schwartz M, et al. Computed tomographic analysis of brain morphometrics in 30 healthy men, aged 21 to 81 years. Ann Neurol 1985; 17 (2):146.
18. Nagata K. et al. A quantitative study of physiological cerebral atrophy with aging: a statistical analysis of the normal range. Neuroradiology 1987; 29:327.
19. Salonen O, Autti T, Raininko R, Ylikoski R, Erkinjuntti M, MRI of the brain in the neurologically healthy middle-aged and elderly individuals. Neuroradiology 1997; 39(8):537.
20. Wahlund LO, Almkvist O, Basun H, Julin P. MRI in successful aging, a 5-year follow-up study from the eight to the ninth decade of life. Magn Reson Imaging 1996; 14:601.
21. Fay, LA, de la Torre JC Effects of aging on the human nervous system. In: Principles and Practice of Geriatric Surgery. New York: Springer-Verlag, in press.
22. Martin GM. The biology of aging: what, why, and how? The new biology of aging. Presented at the SEP Symposium, University of Kansas, Kansas City, MO, September 26–29, 1999.
23. Terry RD, Hansen LA Some morphometric aspects of Alzheimer disease and of normal aging. In: Terry RD, ed. Aging and the Brain. New York: Raven Press, 1988:xx–xx.
24. Terry RD, DeTeresa R, Hansen LA. Neocortical cell counts in normal human adult aging. Ann Neurol 1987; 21(6):530.
25. Masliah E, Mallor M, Hansen L, DeTeresa R, Terry RD. Quantitative synaptic alterations in the human neocortex during normal aging. Neurology 1993; 43: 192–197.
26. Eriksson PS, Perflieva E, Bjork-Eriksson T, Alborn A-M, Nordborg C, Peterson DA, Gage FH. Neurogenesis in the adult human hippocampus. Nat Med 1998; 4(11):1313.
27. Rayl AJS Research turns another fact into myth. Scientist 1999; 13(4):16.
28. Editorial. Take comfort in human neurogenesis. Nat Med 1998; 4(11):1207.
29. Gray F, Adle-Biasette. H, Chretien F, Ereau T, Delisle MB, Vital C. Apoptose neuronale au cours des maladies à prions. Bull Acad Natl Med. 1999; 183(2): 305.
30. Tomei DL, Umansky SR. Aging and apoptosis control. Neurol Clin North Ame 1998; 16(3):735.
31. Perry G, Nunomura A. Apoptosis and Alzheimer's disease [letter to the editor] 1998; 282:1268.

32. Altman J, Das GD. Autoradiographic and histological evidence of postnatal hippocampal neurogenesis in rats. J Comp Neurol 1965; 124:319.
33. Kuhn HG, Dickinson-Anson H, Gage FH. Neurogenesis in the dentate nucleus of the adult rat: age-related decrease of neuromal progenitor proliferation. J Neurol Sci 1996; 16:2027.
34. Kaplan MS, Hinfd JW. Neurogenesis in the adult rat: electron microscopy analysis of light autoradiographs. Science 1977; 197:1092.
35. Kempermann G, Kuhn HG, Gage FH Genetic influence on neurogenesis in the dentate of adult mice. Proc Natl Acad Sci USA 1997; 94:10409.
36. (U.S. National Center for Health Statistics. Nat Vital Stat Rep 1998; 47(9):1.
37. Smith WE. Changing causes of death of elderly people in the United States. Gerontology 1998; 44:331
38. Lopez AD, Murray CCJL The global burden of disease. Nat Med 1998; 4(11):1241–1242.
39. National Center for Health Statistics: Vital Statistics of the United States, 1950, 1960, 1970, 1980, 1990. Washington DC: U.S. Public Health Service, 1953, 1963, 1974, 1985, 1994.
40. United Nations. World Population Prospects, 1996 revision. New York: United Nations Publications 1998.
41. United Nations. The Sex and Age Distribution of the World Populations, 1996 revision. New York: United Nations Publications, 1997.
42. Samuelson RI. The old aren't so old, and the young are plundered. New York Times, 6 Nov. 1998; ??.
43. Brody JE. Some solid research to demolish persistent myths of aging. New York Times, 20 April 1998; 12.
44. Pear R. Clinton planning to cut long-term cost of Medicare. New York Times, 27 June, 1999; 1.
45. Pear R. Clinton lays out plan to overhaul Medicare system. New York Times, 30 June 1999; 1.
46. Pear R. H.M.O.'s will raise Medicare premiums or trim benefits. New York Times, 2 July 1999; 1.
47. Hess D. Clinton pushes plan to cover prescriptions. Philadelphia Enquirer, 27 June 1999; 3.
48. Lachman ME, Weaver SL. Sociodemographic variations in the sense of control by domain. findings from the MacArthur studies of midlife. Psychol Aging 1998; 13(4):553.
49. Kubzansky LD, Berkman LF, Glass TA, Seeman TE. Is Educational attainment associated with shared determinants of health in the elderly? Findings from the MacArthur studies of successful aging. Psychosoc Med 1998; 60(5):578.
50. Smith GD, Shipley MJ, Rose G. Magnitude and causes of socioecenomic diferentials in mortality: further evidence from the Whitehall Study. J Epidemiol Commmun Health 1990; 44(4):265.
51. U.S. National Center for Health Statistics. Vital Statistics of the United States. Natl Vital Stat Rep 1998; 147(9).
52. U.S. Cencus Bureau. Population Estimates, Monthly Postcensal Residents and Armed Forces Overseas. 1999. April 1.

ADDITIONAL BACKGROUND LITERATURE

Akyama H, Meyer JS, Mortel KF, Terayama Y, Thornby JI, Kono S. Normal human aging: factors contributing to cerebral atrophy. J Neurol. Sci 1997; 152(1):39.
Cameron HA, Wooley CS, McEwen BS, Gould E. Differentiation of newly born neurons and glia in the dentate nucleus of the adult rat. Neuroscience 1993; 56:337.
Longévité et retraite. Popul Soci Bull INED Feb 1996; 310:10.
Gavazzi I. Collateral sprouting and responsiveness to nerve growth of aging neurons. Neurosci Lett 1995; 189(1):47.
Hachinski V. Decreased incidence and mortality of stroke. Stroke 1984; 15:376–378.
Kaye JA. Oldest-old healthy brain function: the genomic potential. Arch Neurol 1997; 54(10):1217.
Morsch R, Coleman SW. Neurons may live for decades with neurofibrillary tangles. J Neuropathol Exp Neurol 1999; 58(2):188.
Royal Commission on the Funding of Long Term Care. With respect to old age care—rights and responsibilities (Cmnd 4192–1). London: Stationary Office, 1999.
Toner R. Health care activists target women. New York Times, 14 Sept. 1999; 3.

2. Molecular Biology of the Aging Nervous System

MARK P. MATTSON

This chapter represents a synopsis of some of the salient changes at the molecular and cellular levels in the aging nervous system that likely contribute to the age-related alterations observed at the histological and functional levels. In light of the rapid increase in the application of molecular analyses to studies of aging and neurodegenerative disorders, it is impractical to attempt to cover in detail our current knowledge base in this area. There are common themes, however, that are emerging concerning age-related mechanisms of neuronal dysfunction and death—this chapter will focus on these aspects of the molecular basis of brain aging. Rapid progress in the identification of inherited genetic defects that cause age-related neurodegenerative disorders such as Alzheimer's and Huntington's diseases and in the elucidation of the pathogenic mechanisms of such mutations is providing a valuable framework for understanding mechanisms of nervous system aging in the absence of disease. The nervous system and other organ systems share many cellular and molecular aspects of aging, including increased oxidative damage to proteins, lipids, and DNA; protein aggregation; altered mitochondrial function and energy metabolism; and perturbed cellular ion homeostasis. However, because of the molecular complexity of the nervous system and the postmitotic nature of neurons, there are age-related changes unique to the nervous system. A variety of cellular signaling pathways (e.g., those involving neurotransmitters, cytokines, and neurotrophic factors) are altered during brain aging. An important consideration in studies of the aging nervous system concerns the interrelationships between the aging process and disease-specific alterations that lead to disorders such as Alzheimer's disease (AD), Parkinson's disease (PD), Huntington's disease (HD), amyotrophic lateral sclerosis (ALS), and stroke. An emerging theme from such studies is that oxidative stress, metabolic compromise, and perturbed cellular ion homeostasis interact in a feedforward manner to promote neuronal dysfunction and degeneration. The cell stress associated with aging may also engage adaptive signaling pathways involving (for example) neurotrophic factors and "stress" proteins that prevent neuronal degeneration and may promote synaptic remodeling. Such adaptive signaling mechanisms likely play important roles in individuals that age successfully (i.e., in the absence of neurological dysfunction).

STRUCTURAL CHANGES IN THE AGING NERVOUS SYSTEM

Structural changes in both neurons and glial cells occur during normal aging.[1–4] These changes include nerve cell death, dendritic retraction and expansion, synapse loss and remodeling, and glial cell reactivity. Many structural changes in the aging brain result from alterations in cytoskeletal proteins and the deposition of insoluble proteins such as amyloid in the extracellular space. The cytoskeleton of neurons and glial cells has been a particularly well-studied system with regard to aging of the nervous system and neurodegenerative disorders. The major cytoskeletal components include 6 nm–diameter actin microfilaments; 10–15 nm–diameter intermediate filaments consisting of one or more proteins that are different in different cell types (e.g., neurofilament proteins in neurons and glial fibrillary acidic protein in astrocytes); and 25 nm–diameter microtubules made of tubulin. In addition to the proteins that form cytoskeletal polymers, there are many different cytoskeleton-associated proteins that regulate the processes of filament assembly and depolymerization. For example, neurons express several microtubule-associated proteins (MAPs) that are differentially distributed within the complex architecture of the cells (e.g., tau is present in axons, whereas MAP-2 is present in dendrites but not in the axon).

During aging, and particularly in age-related neurodegenerative disorders, the neuronal cytoskeleton is altered.[5] Dramatic changes in levels of expression of the major cytoskeletal proteins do not occur during normal aging, although there is a clear increase in levels of glial fibrillary acidic protein, which may represent a reaction of astrocytes to subtle neurodegenerative changes.[6] There are changes in both the organization of the cytoskeletal proteins and in their post-translational modification that occur in the aging nervous system. For example, in many neurons cytoskeleton-associated proteins form insoluble filaments with a β-pleated sheet structure (Fig. 2–1). Increased levels of phosphorylation of the MAP tau occurs in some brain regions, particularly those regions, such as the entorhinal cortex and hippocampus, that are involved in learning and memory processes. Proteolysis of cytoskeletal proteins such as MAP-2

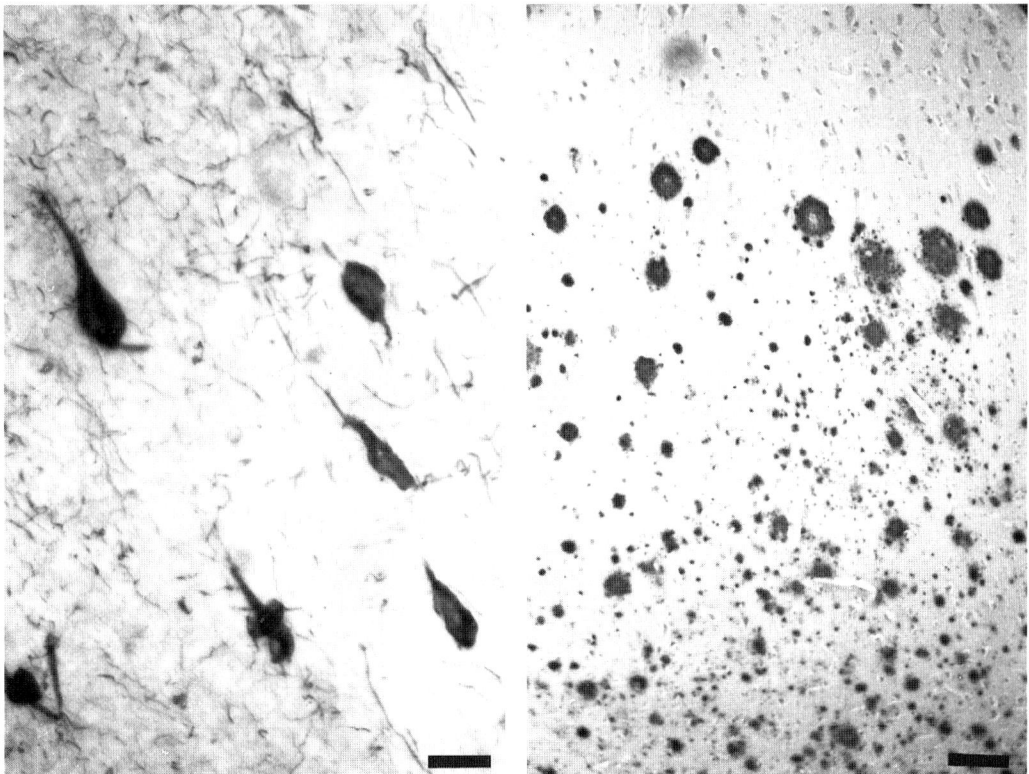

Figure 2–1. Histopathological alterations in Alzheimer's disease (AD). Sections of hippocampal tissue from a patient with AD immunostained with antibodies against either the microtubule-associated protein tau (*left*) or amyloid β-peptide (*right*). Note that the tau antibody binds strongly to degenerating "tangle-bearing" neuronal cell bodies and neurites, and that the amyloid β-peptide antibody stains neuritic plaques as well as smaller and more diffuse amyloid deposits. Scale bars: left, 20 μm; right, 100 μm.

and spectrin, mediated by calcium-activated proteases, is increased in some neuronal populations during aging. Cytoskeletal proteins are also subject to oxidative modification (e.g., glycation and covalent binding of lipid peroxidation products such as 4-hydroxynonenal) presumably because of the increased levels of oxidative stress that, as in other organ systems, are pervasive in the aging nervous system.[7]

Alterations in the neuronal cytoskeleton are particularly striking in age-related neurodegenerative disorders including AD, PD, and ALS. Neurofibrillary tangles, which are most prominent in AD,[8] are filamentous accumulations of tau that form in the cytoplasm of degenerating neurons (Fig. 2–1). Neurofibrillary tangle-bearing neurons exhibit decreased numbers of microtubules and altered compartmentalization of other cytosketal elements (e.g., MAP-2 accumulates in the cell body). Hyperphosphorylation of tau is a conspicuous feature of neurofibrillary tangles and may result from reduced dephosphorylation (due to altered phosphatase activity) or covalent modification by products of lipid peroxidation such as 4-hydroxynonenal.[7] In PD, neurons contain structures called *Lewy bodies*, which consist of abnormal accumulations of neurofilaments, MAPs (particularly MAP-1b), and actin-related proteins such as gelsolin.[9] Lower motor neurons in ALS patients exhibit massive accumulations of neurofilaments that congregate in inclusions in proximal regions of the axon.[10] Many of the disease-related cytoskeletal alterations are also observed at much lower frequencies during usual aging in the absence of disease, suggesting a contribution of the normal aging process to such changes. In this regard, it is interesting to note that evidence suggests that oxidative stress and perturbed cellular calcium homeostasis play major roles in altering the neuronal cytoskeleton in both usual aging and many different neurodegenerative disorders. Indeed, studies of experimental models of AD and ALS have shown that increased oxidative stress and perturbed calcium homeostasis can induce changes in the cytoskeleton similar to those seen in the human disorders.[7,11,12]

A unique aspect of the structure of the nervous system is the *synapse*, which is the site at which critical interneuronal signaling occurs. Synaptic signaling mediates fast neurotransmitter-mediated propagation of electrical activity in neuronal circuits as well as trophic interactions involving neurotrophic factors and cytokines. Alterations in synapses occur during aging and in neurodegenerative disorders. Analyses of synapses during the aging of rodents and humans suggest that there is a decrease in the number of synapses in some brain regions, but such decreases may be offset by increases in synaptic size.[13] Synaptic remodeling may occur during aging, and such breaking and making of synapses may represent responses to neuronal degeneration and dendritic regression or growth. Indeed, in several brain regions, synapse numbers are reduced while the size of individual synapses increase, presumably as the result of a compensatory mechanism. Synapse loss is a prominent feature of many different age-related neurodegenerative disorders including AD, PD, and HD.[2,14–16] It is believed that such synapse loss precedes neuron death, and that synaptic degeneration may result from age-and disease-related alterations (e.g., reduced energy availability and increased amyloid deposition) resulting in excitotoxic and oxidative damage.[17,18]

In addition to structural changes in neurons and glial cells with aging, the vessels that supply blood to the nervous system are subject to age-related atherosclerosis and arteriosclerosis.[19] The changes are essentially identical to those occurring in other organ systems and include basement membrane thickening, fibrosis, and accumulation of cholesterol-containing plaques. Such alterations render blood vessels susceptible to occlusion or rupture, which can manifest as stroke, a major cause of disability and death in the elderly population that often results in neurologic deficits and cognitive impairments. Reduced brain perfusion has been documented in aged individuals and may contribute to deficits in cognitive function. The cellular and molecular events that lead to vascular alterations in the nervous system during aging are likely to be similar to those that occur elsewhere in the body and include damage to endothelial cells by oxidized low-density lipoprotein (LDL) and a resultant inflammatory response. Indeed, the risk factors for cerebrovascular disease are essentially the same as those for atherosclerosis and include hypertension, hyperlipidemia, diabetes mellitus, apolipoprotein E genotype (the E-4 allele increases risk), and smoking. The blood–brain barrier is formed by tight junctions between vascular endothelial cells and requires interactions with astrocytes. Changes in the blood–brain barrier during aging include thinning of capillary walls and a decrease in number of mitochondria in endothelial cells. Compromise of the structural integrity of vascular endothelial cells may result in impaired transport functions such as the decreased glucose transport documented in aging and AD.[20]

MOLECULAR AND BIOCHEMICAL MARKERS OF AGING

An increasing number of genes expressed in the nervous system are being identified, and the expression of such genes in usual aging and in age-related neurodegenerative disorders is receiving greater scrutiny. However, even relatively crude analyses reveal generalized alterations in the major classes of macromolecules.[21] For example, the protein content of the brain decreases with aging and may play a major role in the age-related decrease in overall brain weight. In general, there is an increase in accumulation of insoluble aggregates of proteins in the brain during aging, with the cytoskeletal protein tau and amyloid β peptide (Aβ) being the two most closely linked to age-related neurodegeneration (see Protein Aggregation and Protease Activation, below). There is a progressive decrease in lipids (including cerebroside, choline phosphoglyceride, ethanolamine phosphoglyceride, and sphingomyelin) in the brain after the sixth decade of life. The increased accumulation of lipofuscin granules in cells of the nervous system is likely to be a structural correlate of damage to membrane lipids.[22] While little or no change in DNA content occurs in the brain during aging, there do appear to be region-specific changes in RNA levels such that RNA levels decrease in the nucleus basalis of Meynert and in several regions of cerebral cortex, but increase in the subicular region of the hippocampus.

Altered Gene Expression

Cells in the nervous system (particularly neurons) express upwards of 100 times the number of genes expressed in cells of other organ systems. It is therefore not surprising that some alterations in levels of gene expression have been documented in aging nervous systems. One example that appears to be quite consistent in studies of rodents and humans is an increase in levels of glial fibrillary acidic protein mRNA and protein,[6] which may reflect a response of astrocytes to age-related increases in oxidative stress and neuronal damage. Further evidence for astrocyte activation during aging comes from studies showing increased levels of the astrocyte-derived protein S-100β with aging in a sensescence-accelerated strain of mice.[23]

Altered transcriptional regulation in brain cells with increasing age is suggested by studies of transcription factor activities. Gel-shift analyses of NF-κB DNA binding activity in brain tissues from young and old rats showed an increase in constitutive levels of activated NF-κB in frontal cortex and cerebellum, but not in hippocampus.[24] Levels of the p50, p65, and p52 subunits of NF-κB proteins were unchanged, suggesting an enhanced activation rate of NF-κB which might result from age-related increases in levels of cellular oxidative and metabolic stress.[25,26] Gel-shift assays have shown that overall levels of activation of the transcription factor AP-1 are decreased in frontal cortex and hippocampus of aged rats and that there is a shift in the composition of AP-1, with Jun-Jun homodimers becoming predominant with increasing age.[27]

Additional data suggest that with increasing age their is a reduced ability of brain cells to cope with (oxidative and metabolic) stress. Overall levels of superoxide dismutase activity decreased with age in several different organs of rats, including the brain.[28] Levels of catalase activity in brain also decreased with age, wherease levels of glutathione peroxidase activity were unchanged. These age-related changes in antioxidant enzyme activities were paralleled by changes in levels of mRNAs encoding the enzymes. Such changes in antioxidant enzymes may contribute to age-related increases in levels of cellular oxidative stress. Levels of heat-shock protein 70 (HSP-70) mRNA increased in brain tissue from rats exposed to increasing temperatures and the magnitude of the HSP-70 response was reduced in old rats compared to that in young rats.[29] The latter findings suggest that aged animals may be less able to mount a stress response, which could, in theory, render neurons vulnerable to degeneration. Glucocorticoid administration results in increased levels of nerve growth factor (NGF) mRNA and protein in the cortex and hippocampus of young adult rats, but not in 24-month-old rats.[30] The latter studies also showed that glucocorticoid administration increases basic fibroblast growth factor (bFGF) mRNA levels to a similar extent in brain tissues from young and old rats. Levels of mRNAs encoding brain-derived neurotrophic factor (BDNF) and somatostatin were decreased in hippocampus, frontal cortex, motor cortex, and visual cortex of aged (>30 years old) monkeys compared to levels in young (2 years old) monkeys.[31]

Changes in levels of membrane transporters and receptors have also been documented in studies of aged humans and rodents. Chauhan and Siegel[32] reported that levels of mRNA encoding the α1 subunit of the Na^+/K^+-ATPase were increased by up to sevenfold in the dendritic fields of hippocampus of old rats compared to levels in young rats. In contrast, levels of the α3 subunit were decreased by about threefold in perikaryal layers of hippocampal pyramidal neurons. Mooradian and Shah[33] found that, whereas levels of mRNA encoding the glucose transporter GLUT-1 were similar in cerebral tissue from young and old rats, the in vitro translatability of GLUT-1 mRNA was reduced in tissue from old rats. Levels of the dopamine transporter mRNA were similar in substantia nigra tissue from young and middle-aged (18 to 57 year old) humans, but declined in a marked linear manner in subjects greater than 57 years old.[34] Such changes in dopamine transporter levels may contribute to age-related deficits in motor function. Additional alterations in specific neurotransmitter signaling pathways are suggested by studies of neurotransmitter receptor levels in young and aged animals. For example, levels of γ-aminobutyric acid (GABA) binding sites were decreased in cerebellum of aged (24-month-old) rats, and lifelong caloric restriction prevented the decrease.[35] Levels of mRNA encoding the α1-subunit of GABA-A receptors were unchanged in aged rats fed ad libitum, whereas levels of mRNA encoding the α2-subunit were decreased.

Finally, levels of expression of genes linked to a form of "programmed" cell death called *apoptosis* are increased in age-related neurodegenerative conditons. For example, levels of Par-4 (prostate apoptosis response-4; a leucine zipper and death domain-containing protein originally identified for its role in apoptosis of prostate cells[36]) mRNA and protein are increased in vulnerable regions (and to a lesser extent in nonvulnerable regions) of AD brain (Fig. 2–2). Approximately 40% of neurofibrillary tangle-bearing neurons are Par-4 immunoreactive, which suggests a direct relationship between increased Par-4 expression and neuronal degeneration in AD.[37] Recent immunohistochemical analyses of AD brain tis-

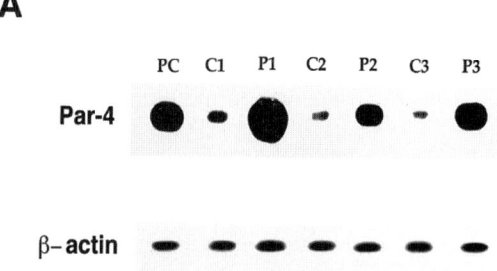

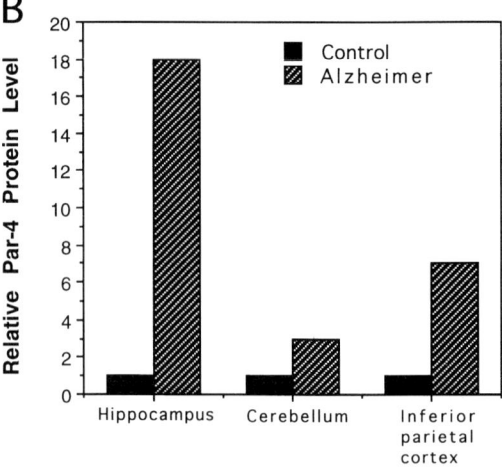

Figure 2–2. Expression of the apoptosis-related gene Par-4 is increased in brain tissue from patients with Alzheimer's disease (AD). *A.* Northern blot of Par-4 and β-actin mRNA levels in hippocampus from three control (C1–C3) and three AD (P1–P3) patients (PC, positive control). *B.* Par-4 protein levels (determined by densitometric analysis of Western blots) in different brain regions from control and AD patients. Values are the mean of determinations made in samples from 6 control and 6 AD patients. [Modified from Guo et al.[37]]

sue using antibodies against cell cycle–related proteins[38] are consistent with "abortive re-entry" of neurons into the cell cycle during aging and in AD.

Free Radical–Mediated Damage to Proteins, Lipids, and DNA

The definition of a *free radical* is any molecule with an unpaired electron in its outer orbital; in biological systems, oxygen-based molecules are the most important free radical species (Fig. 2–3). Mitochondria are the sites where most of the oxyradical production occurs in cells; superoxide anion radical ($O_2^{\cdot-}$) is generated during the electron transport process. Superoxide dismutases (MnSOD and Cu/ZnSOD) convert $O_2^{\cdot-}$ to hydrogen peroxide (H_2O_2), which is then converted to hydroxyl radical ($OH^{\cdot}$) via the Fenton reaction; this is catalyzed by Fe^{2+} and Cu^{+}. Another prominent oxyradical species is peroxynitrite ($ONOO^{-}$) which is formed when nitric oxide (NO) interacts with $O_2^{\cdot-}$. The enzyme nitric oxide synthase (NOS), which is activated by calcium/calmodulin, is responsible for generation of NO. Oxyradicals can cause direct damage to proteins and DNA, and several oxyradicals ($OH^{\cdot}$ and $ONOO^{-}$, in particular) can attack fatty acids in membranes, thereby initiating a highly destructive process called "lipid peroxidation." Studies of aging have provided compelling evidence that there is an increase in production and accumulation of oxyradicals in essentially all tissues in the body, including the nervous system.

Levels of protein oxidation, measured as protein carbonyls, are significantly elevated in

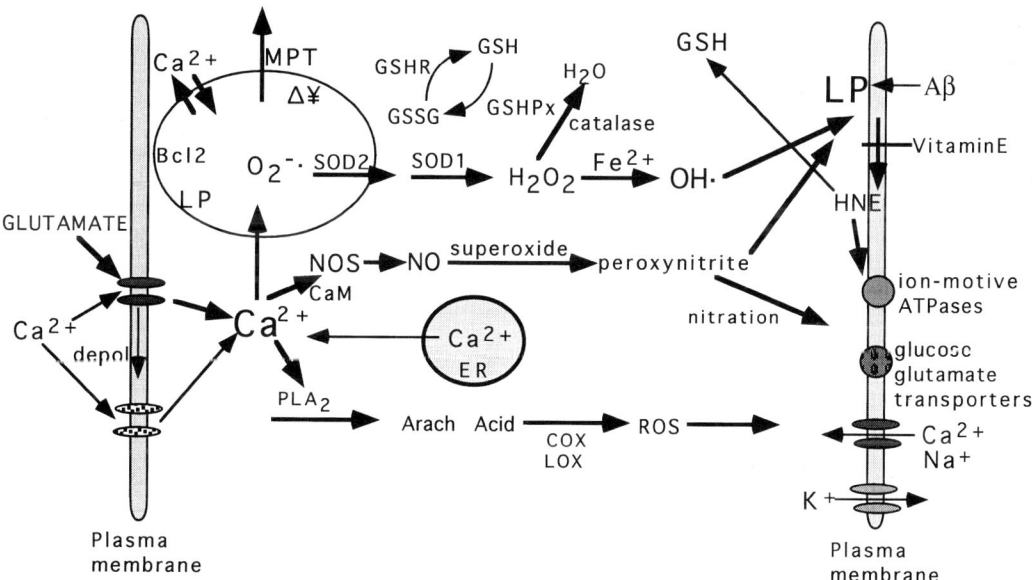

Figure 2–3. Sources of reactive oxygen species in neurons, and mechanisms for their removal, relevant to aging and neurodegenerative disorders. Superoxide anion radical $O_2^{\cdot-}$ is produced during the electron transport process in the mitochondria. Superoxide dismutase (SOD) converts $O_2^{\cdot-}$ to H_2O_2, which is converted to water by the enzymes catalase and glutathione peroxidase (GSHPx). Alternatively, highly reactive $OH^{\cdot}$ can be produced via Fenton chemistry in the presence of iron (Fe^{2+}). Amyloid β-peptide (Aβ) and Fe^{2+} induce membrane lipid peroxidation (LP), which results in generation of the toxic aldehyde 4-hydroxynonenal (HNE). HNE impairs the function of membrane ion-motive ATPases and glucose and glutamate transporters, which results in increased vulnerability of neurons to excitotoxicity. Elevation of $[Ca^{2+}]_i$ induced by glutamate or amyloid β-peptide, for example, promotes production of several different reactive oxygen species. Ca^{2+} binds calmodulin and thereby activates nitric oxide synthase (NOS) resulting in the generation of nitric oxide ($NO^{\cdot}$); NO interacts with $O2^{\cdot-}$ resulting in the formation of peroxynitrite, which can damage proteins. Ca^{2+} also promotes phospholipid hydrolysis via activity of phospholipase-A_2 (PLA_2). PLA_2 induces release of arachidonic acid, which is then attacked by lipoxygenases (LOX) and cyclooxygenases (COX) with resultant oxyradical formation. Elevated $[Ca^{2+}]_i$ also reduces mitochondrial transmembrane potential, which can lead to increased $O_2^{\cdot-}$ production. ER, endoplasmic reticulum.

the brains of aged rodents, and such age-associated protein oxidation can be prevented by administration of antioxidants.[39] Studies of membrane structure have provided evidence for oxidation-related alterations in membrane protein conformation in old rodents. Very little nuclear DNA damage occurs in the nervous system during usual aging, and its contribution to age-related dysfunction and neuronal degeneration may be minimal. In contrast, progressive and extensive oxidative damage to mitochondrial DNA occurs during aging, and may be exacerbated in neurodegenerative disorders. Mitochondria-derived oxyradicals are likely to play a central role in the cumulative oxidative damage to various cellular constituents that accrues with aging.[40] Age-related impairments in energy availability and metabolism may contribute to an acceleration of oxyradical production with aging (Table 2–1). The importance of mitochondrial oxyradical production in aging is underscored by recent studies of the mechanism through which caloric restriction extends lifespan in rodents and nonhuman primates (see Slowing Aging of the Nervous System by Dietary Restriction, below). Thus, one factor contributing to brain aging is simply the constant production of oxyradicals and resultant progressive damage to cellular components. In addition to the oxyradical damage that accrues with usual aging, there are specific initiators of oxidative stress that appear to play key roles in different age-related neurodegenerative disorders (see following sections on specific disorders). For example, in AD the increased generation and accumulation of Aβ may be a pivotal event that enhances oxidative stress in neurons,[41–43] and there is evidence that increased levels of Fe^{2+} and peroxynitrite in the substantia nigra play a role in the degeneration of dopaminergic neurons in victims of PD.[44,45] The damage to neurons in the brains of stroke victims is the result of a combination of factors including excessive calcium influx and the presence of blood components such as Fe^{2+} and thrombin. In HD the presence of trinucleotide repeats in the Huntingtin protein may induce oxidative stress in striatal neurons by a yet-to-be-determined mechanism.[46] The evidence that vulnerable neuronal populations in AD, PD, and HD are subjected to increased levels of oxidative stress is compelling.[47–49]

Levels of aldehydic products of membrane lipid peroxidation, such as malondialdehyde and 4-hydroxnonenal, are significantly elevated in the brain parenchyma and cerebrospinal fluid in AD.[50,51] Immunohistochemical analyses of brain tissue from AD and PD patients and of spinal cord tissue from ALS patients, using antibodies directed against 4-hydroxynonenal adducts, showed increased levels of this aldehyde in association with degenerating neurons. This increase suggests a role for lipid peroxidation in the neurodegenerative process.[52–54] Consistent with this role are data from experimental studies showing that 4-hydroxynonenal can induce neuronal apoptosis[55]; increase neuronal vulnerability to excitotoxicity[42]; impair glucose and glutamate transport[43,56]; and induce cross-linking of the protein tau and prevent its dephosphorylation.[7] Experimental studies in cell culture and animal models of AD and ALS have shown that lipid peroxidation can impair the function of the plasma membrane glucose and glutamate transporters; analyses of affected neural tissues in with patients AD and ALS indicate that glucose and glutamate transport are compromised.[41,54] A small percentage of cases of

Table 2–1. Factors that Promote or Suppress Oxidative Stress in the Aging Nervous System

Promote Oxidative Stress	Suppress Oxidative Stress
Mitochondrial ROS (superoxide)	Dietary restriction
Amyloidogenic peptides	Antioxidant vitamins and minerals
Iron accumulation	Neurotrophic factors
Metabolic compromise	Hormones (e.g., estrogen)
Glutamate receptor activation	Activity in neuronal circuits
Genetic aberrancies (disease-specific mutations and risk factors	
Hormones (e.g., glucocorticoids)	

ALS are caused by mutations in the antioxidant enzyme Cu/Zn-SOD; transgenic mice expressing ALS-linked Cu/Zn-SOD mutations develop lower motor neuron degeneration and a clinical phenotype similar to that of human ALS patients. Analyses of spinal cords of these mice have shown evidence for increased lipid peroxidation.[57] Chronic administration of vitamin E to these mice significantly delayed the onset of the clinical symptoms, suggesting a causal role for lipid peroxidation in the neurodegenerative process.[58]

Damage to nuclear DNA in striatum of HD patients,[59] the substantia nigra of PD patients,[60,61] and in hippocampus and vulnerable cortical regions of AD patients[62], has been documented. Specifically, levels of 8-hydroxyguanosine are increased. This DNA damage may be caused by several reactive oxygen molecules, with hydroxyl radical and peroxynitrite being the major culprits. The contribution of nuclear DNA damage to the neurodegenerative (cell death) process is not clear, but it could play a role in alterations in gene expression documented in the aging nervous system. Mitochondrial DNA damage is so extensive during normal aging because mitochondria are the site where the vast majority of free radicals are generated and because cells do not possess effective systems for repairing damaged mitochondrial DNA. Experiments in cultured cells and isolated mitochondria have shown that damage to mitochondrial DNA can lead to failure of mitochondrial electron transport and reduced ATP production. Moreover, the important calcium-sequestering function of mitochondria may be compromised as the result of age-related DNA damage, which may increase neuronal vulnerability to excitotoxicity and metabolic insults.

Protein Aggregation and Protease Activation

Aggregations of specific proteins inside neurons or in extracellular compartments have been documented in age-related chronic neurodegenerative disorders including AD, PD, HD, and ALS (Table 2–2). The *amyloid β peptide* (Aβ) is a 40–42 amino acid peptide that arises from a much larger membrane-spanning β-amyloid precursor protein (APP).[63] With normal aging, and to a much greater extent in AD, Aβ forms insoluble aggregates in the brain parenchyma and vasculature. Large (0.1–0.5 mm) aggregates are called "plaques" (Fig. 2–1). Two types of plaques can be discerned, a *diffuse form* consisting of nonfibrillar Aβ and not associated with neuronal degeneration, and a *compact fibrillar form* of plaque that is associated with degenerated neurons. Amyloid plaques accumulate to a greater extent in brain regions involved in learning and memory processes, such as the hippocampus and entorhinal cortex. Alterations in proteolytic processing of APP, which may result from age-related increases in cellular oxidative stress and impaired energy metabolism, may promote increased Aβ production and fibril formation.[63] The accumulation of Aβ in the brain in AD is roughly correlated with the amount of neuronal degeneration and with the severity of cognitive impairments. The cause(s) of the excessive Aβ accumulation in most cases of AD, which are "sporadic" (i.e., not resulting from specific inherited muta-

Table 2–2. Characteristics of Protein Aggregates in Age-Related Neurodegenerative Disorders

Disorder	Protein Involved	Characteristics of Aggregates
Alzheimer's disease	Amyloid β-peptide	Extracellular, β-sheet fibrils
	Tau	Intracellular, straight/twisted filaments
Parkinson's disease	α-synuclein	Intracellular/extracellular filaments
Huntington disease	Huntingtin	Cytoplasmic and nuclear, amorphous
Amyotrophic lateral sclerosis	Cu/Zn-SOD	Amorphous, cytoplasmic

tions), is unknown. However, in approximately 1% of AD cases, mutations in APP are responsible for the increased Aβ accumulation in the brain.

As with amyloid proteins in other age-related disorders (e.g., pancreatic amylin in diabetes mellitus), Aβ can damage cells. Cell culture studies have shown that Aβ can be neurotoxic and can increase neuronal vulnerability to metabolic, excitotoxic, and oxidative insults.[41,64] The adverse effects of Aβ on neurons are related to the propensity of Aβ to form fibrils; agents that prevent fibril formation, such as the dye Congo Red, block the toxic effects of Aβ. The sequence of events involved in Aβ-induced neuronal injury and death involves induction of membrane lipid peroxidation, which generates 4-hydroxynonenal.[65] 4-hydroxynonenal covalently modifies membrane proteins involved in maintenance of cellular ion homeostasis and energy metabolism, including the plasma membrane Na^+/K^+- and Ca^{2+}-ATPases, glucose transporters, and glutamate transporters. The oxidative stress induced in neurons by Aβ can eventually lead to excessive elevation of intracellular calcium levels, mitochondrial dysfunction, and a form of cell death called "apoptosis," in which the cell shrinks and its nucleus becomes condensed and its DNA fragments.[55] Oxidative stress in neurons, promoted by Aβ, can induce changes in the neuronal cytoskeleton similar to those seen in neurofibrillary tangles. Antioxidants such as vitamin E and glutathione can prevent apoptosis and neurofibrillary tangle-like changes in neurons exposed to Aβ42 (M.P. Mattson, unpublished data). Interestingly, certain neurotrophic factors (intercellular signaling proteins produced within the brain) can protect neurons against the damaging effects of Aβ by inducing the expression of genes that encode antioxidant enzymes.[66,67] In addition to its likely involvement in the neurodegenerative process, Aβ may also compromise neurotransmitter signaling pathways. For example, Aβ has been shown to impair coupling of muscarinic acetylcholine receptors to their downstream GTP-binding effector protein,[68] and it may also suppress acetylcholine production.[69] Such actions of Aβ could contribute to the well-established deficits in cholinergic signaling pathways in AD. Aβ may play a role in damage to the cerebral blood vessels and resulting deficits in nutrient transfer to the brain parenchyma. Extensive deposition of Aβ in cerebral vessels occurs in AD. Studies of cultured vascular endothelial cells have shown that Aβ can impair glucose transport and disrupt barrier functions in these cells.[20] Aβ induces oxidative stress in the endothelial cells, which can lead to their degeneration and death, and may also stimulate inflammatory processes in the brain.

In PD, a protein called "α-synuclein" forms fibrillar aggregates that are presumed to play a role in the neurodegenerative process,[70] although the underlying mechanisms are unexplored. In HD, the protein huntingtin forms intracellular aggregates that may accumulate in the nucleus.[71,72] Interestingly, in transgenic mice expressing ALS-linked Cu/Zn-SOD mutations the Cu/Zn-SOD protein may form aggregates.[73] It is of considerable interest that aberrant protein aggregation is a feature of many different age-related neurodegenerative disorders and that the location of the protein aggregates (e.g., extracellular, cytoplasmic or nuclear) can be quite different in the various disorders (Table 2–2).

Activation of several different proteases is increased in association with aging and age-related neurodegenerative disorders. For example, activity of calcium-dependent proteases called "calpains" is increased in several different tissues of aged humans (e.g., fibroblasts and red blood cells).[74,75] Calpain activity is also increased with aging in cortex and striatum of rats.[76] Nixon et al.[77] have provided evidence that the relative level of calpain I activation is increased in brains of patients with AD. It was also shown, using immunohistochemical methods, that levels of calpain II are increased in neurofibrillary tangle-bearing neurons in AD brain tissue. More recent studies have focused on the possible involvement of members of the caspase family of cysteine proteases in the pathogenesis of age-related neurodegenerative disorders. Studies of postmortem tissues from AD have provided evidence for increased caspase activation in vulnerable neuronal populations[78] (Fig. 2–4). Moreover, experimental data demonstrate that exposure of cultured neurons to disease-relevant insults and expression of AD-linked mutations in amyloid precursor protein and presenilins can promote caspase activation.[18,79]

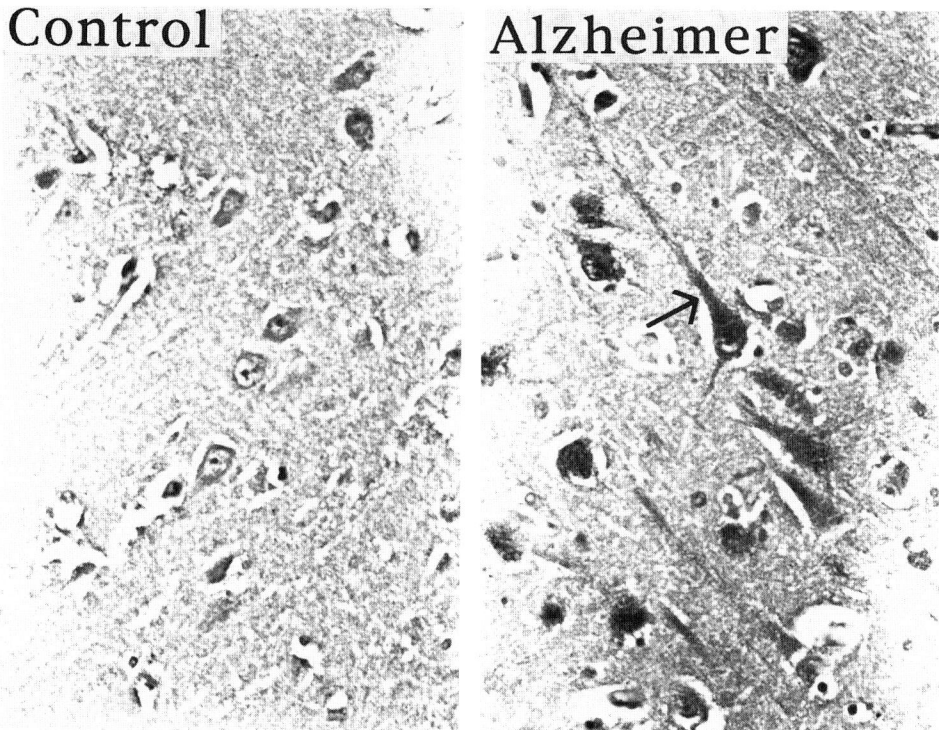

Figure 2–4. Sections of hippocampus from a neurologically normal control patient (*left*) and a patient with Alzheimer's disease (*right*) immunostained with an antibody that selectively recognizes activated caspase-3. Note increased levels of immunoreactivity in several neurons in the section from the Alzheimer's patient (e.g., arrow).

Alterations in Neurotransmitter Signaling Systems

A number of alterations in different neurotransmitter systems have been documented in studies of aging rodents and in analyses of brain tissues from humans with age-related neurodegenerative disorders.[80] While some of these alterations likely result from neuronal degeneration, others appear to occur in the absence of cell injury.

Acetylcholine is employed as a neurotransmitter in select populations of neurons in the brain and spinal cord. In the brain, basal forebrain neurons provide cholinergic input to widespread regions of neocortex and to the hippocampus; these cholinergic neurons are known to play key roles in learning and memory processes in humans and rodents. Many different studies have documented progressive deficits in multiple aspects of cholinergic signal transduction mechanisms with aging in some, but not all, brain regions (Fig. 2–5). Deficits in choline transport, acetylcholine synthesis, acetylcholine release, and coupling of muscarinic receptors to their GTP-binding effector proteins have been reported.[80] Cholinergic deficits are much more severe in AD patients and also differ qualitatively from the changes observed during normal aging. Particularly striking is a reduced ability of muscarinic agonists to activate GTP-binding proteins in cortical membranes prepared from postmortem brain tissue from AD patients (Fig. 2–5). Increased levels of membrane lipid peroxidation in neurons may contribute to impaired cholinergic signaling because exposure of cultured cortical neurons to $A\beta$, Fe^{2+}, and the lipid peroxidation product 4-hydroxynonenal results in impaired coupling of muscarinic receptors to the GTP-binding protein G_{q11}[81] (Fig. 2–5).

Very prominent reductions in both pre- and postsynaptic aspects of dopaminergic neuro-

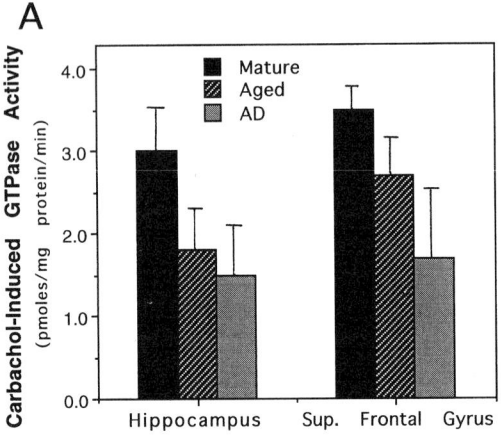

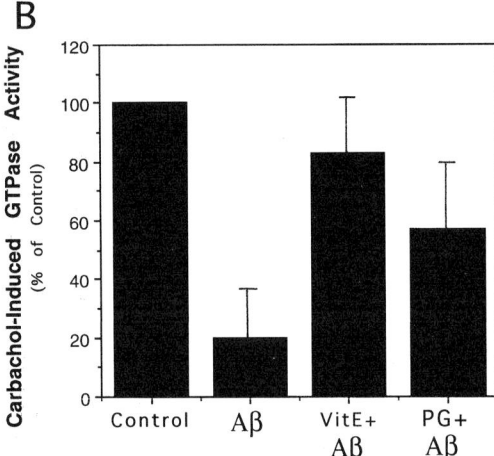

Figure 2–5. Evidence for impaired coupling of muscarinic receptors to GTP-binding protein in aging patients and those with Alzheimer's disease (AD). A. Levels of carbachol (muscarinic agonist)-induced GTPase activity in membranes from hippocampus and superior frontal gyrus of middle-aged, elderly normal (aged) and Alzheimer's (AD) patients. [Modified from Cutler et al.[161]] B. Levels of carbachol-induced GTPase activity in membranes from cultured rat cortical neurons that had been exposed to vehicle (Control), amyloid β-peptide (Aβ), vitamin E plus Aβ, or propyl gallate (PG) plus Aβ. [Modified from Kelly et al.[68]]

related impairment of coupling of dopamine receptors to their GTP-binding effector proteins. The contribution of oxidative stress to changes in dopaminergic signaling has not been established, although the prominent role of oxyradicals in the pathogenesis of PD makes a case for similar oxidative processes contributing to dopaminergic dysfunction during normal aging. These changes in dopaminergic signaling likely play a role in age-related deficits in motor control and may explain the fact that old humans and animals are suceptible to extrapyramidal effects of dopamine receptor antagonist drugs.

Norepinephrine and serotonin are the major monoamine neurotransmitters in the brain. Noradrenergic neurons are located primarily in the locus coeruleus and serotonergic neurons in the raphe nucleus; both types of neurons project to widespread regions of cerebral cortex. There are several subtypes of receptors for norepinephrine, each of which couples to GTP-binding proteins. There are also several subtypes of serotonin receptors, some of which couple to GTP-binding proteins and others of which are ligand-gated ion channels. There appear to be increased levels of norepinephrine with aging in some brain regions, while levels of α2 adrenergic receptors may decrease in cerebral cortex with advancing age in both rodents and humans.[80] Levels of serotonin decrease in the striatum, hippocampus, and cortex in the aging rat. Age-related decreases in levels of evoked serotonin release and of serotonin binding sites have been reported in both humans and rodents. Changes in serotonergic systems may play important roles in age-related changes in affect (e.g., increased depression).

The amino acid glutamate is the major excitatory neurotransmitter in the human brain. Glutamate stimulates ionotropic receptors that flux calcium and sodium; excessive activation of ionotropic glutamate receptors may play a role in the degeneration of neurons in several age-related disorders including stroke, AD, PD, and HD. Levels of ionotropic glutamate receptors have been reported to decrease with aging in humans and rodents.[82] However, these decreases may be the result of degeneration of the neurons expressing the receptors. The contribution of dysfunction of glutamatergic transmission, in the absence of neuronal death, to age- and disease-related

transmission occur during brain aging.[80] Decreases in dopamine levels and dopamine transporter levels in the striatum of humans and rats occur with advancing age. In both humans and rodents there is an age-related decrease in levels of D2 receptor binding sites in striatum. As with cholinergic signal transduction, there also appears to be an age-

deficits in brain function is unknown. The major inhibitory neurotransmitter in the human brain is γ-aminobutyric acid (GABA). Relatively little information is available concerning the impact of aging on GABAergic systems. However, in aged rodents levels of glutamate decarboxylase and GABA-A binding sites may be decreased. Interestingly, GABAergic interneurons are typically spared in various neurodegenerative disorders including AD.

Among the properties of neurons that set them apart from many other cell types is their excitability, which is regulated by a complex array of neurotransmitters and ion channels. Neurons express voltage-dependent sodium channels as well as multiple types of calcium and potassium channels that are differentially expressed among neuronal populations and are segregated in different cellular compartments (e.g., L-type calcium channels in the cell body, N-type calcium channels in the dendrites, and T-type calcium channels in presynaptic terminals). In addition, neurons possess membrane ion "pumps" that play critical roles in re-establishing ion gradients following neuronal stimulation. A variety of age-related alterations in electrophysiological parameters have been described in rodents and, in some cases, in humans.[83] The alterations range from increased thresholds for induction of action potentials in cranial nerves, to increased afterhyperpolarizations in hippocampal neurons, to impaired long-term potentiation of synaptic transmission in the hippocampus. Moreover, a generalized decrease in neuronal inhibition appears to occur during the aging process. Such alterations are correlated with diminutions in function of the corresponding neural circuits (e.g., hearing impairment in the case of the auditory nerve and cognitive impairment in the case of hippocampal circuits).

The calcium ion plays fundamental roles in regulating neuronal survival and plasticity in both the developing and adult nervous system. For example, calcium mediates the effects of neurotransmitters and neurotrophic factors on neurite outgrowth, synaptogenesis, and cell survival in many different regions of the developing nervous system. In the mature nervous system calcium influx into the presynaptic terminal is a stimulus for neurotransmitter release, while calcium influx into postsynaptic dendrites is a critical event in long-lasting synaptic changes associated with learning and memory processes. Studies of brains of aged rodents have provided evidence for alterations in neuronal systems that regulate calcium homeostasis. For example, age-related decreases in activity of the plasma membrane calcium ATPase and in levels of calcium-binding proteins have been documented. Aging also appears to be associated with increased calcium influx through voltage-dependent channels in hippocampal neurons in rats and with increased levels of calcium-dependent protease activity in neurons from humans with AD. Collectively, these changes would be expected to lead to increased levels of intracellular calcium in neurons. The factors that promote impaired calcium homeostasis in neurons in aging and age-related neurodegenerative disorders likely include increased levels of oxidative stress and metabolic compromise (see above). Indeed, experimental studies in animal and cell culture systems have shown that oxidative (e.g., exposure of neurons to Fe^{2+} or Aβ) and metabolic (e.g., glucose deprivation and exposure to mitochondrial toxins) insults disrupt neuronal calcium homeostasis.

Alterations in Neurotrophic Factor Signaling Systems

A variety of proteins that serve the functions of promoting neuronal survival and outgrowth and protecting the neurons against injury and death are produced by glia and neurons.[84] Examples include nerve growth factor (NGF), basic fibroblast growth factor (bFGF), brain-dervied neurotrophic factor (BDNF), insulin-like growth factor (IGF), and activity-dependent neurotrophic factor (ADNF). Neurotrophic factors are remarkable in that they have repeatedly been shown to protect neurons in cell culture and in vivo against a variety of insults relevant to the pathogenesis of age-related neurodegenerative conditions.[84,85] For example, bFGF can protect hippocampal and cortical neurons in cell culture against metabolic, oxidative, and excitotoxic insults and can greatly reduce brain damage in rodent models of stroke. One or more neurotrophic factors have also been shown to protect particular neuronal populations against neurodegenerative disorder-specific insults. Thus, BDNF protected dopaminergic neurons against 1-methyl-4-phenyl-1,2,3,6-tetrahydropyridine (MPTP) toxicity (PD model), while bFGF and sAPP protected hippocampal neurons against Aβ toxicity (AD model). There appear to be two general mechanisms through which neurotrophic factors prevent neuronal degeneration—namely by increasing cellular resistance to oxidative stress and by stabilizing cellular calcium homeostasis. These actions of neurotrophic factors appear to result from induction of the expression of antioxidant enzymes (e.g., superoxide dismutases and glutathione peroxidase) and calcium-regulating proteins (e.g., the calcium-binding protein calbindin).

While there is no clear evidence that aberrant neurotrophic factor signaling is a primary mechanism for age-related dysfunction and degeneration of neuronal circuits, it is very likely that neurotrophic factors can modulate such age-related processes. The ability of growth factors to prevent neuron degeneration in cell culture and animal models of age-related neurodegenerative conditions suggests that they play important roles in both successful brain aging and neurodegenerative disorders. Studies of neurotrophic factor expression in animals of different ages have documented age-related alterations. For example, levels of NGF mRNA and protein were reported to be reduced in the brain of aged rats.[86] Levels of NGF receptor protein may be decreased in the basal forebrain of both aged rats and aged humans.[87–88] Aged rats exhibit impaired performance on water maze tasks of visuospatial memory, and intraventricular administration of NGF to aged rats improves their cognitive function;[89] these findings suggest that decreased NGF levels may contribute to age-related cognitive dysfunction. Recent studies have shown that neurotrophic factors such as bFGF and ADNF can protect neurons against the death-promoting actions of AD-linked mutations in presenilin-1[90] (Fig. 2–6), which suggests that neurotrophic factors can interrupt neurodegenerative cascades involved in age-related neurodegenerative disorders.

The production of many different neurotrophic factors is increased by activity in neuronal circuits. Experimental findings suggest that such activity-dependent production of neurotrophic factors plays a major role in promoting neuronal survival and neurite outgrowth. For example, rats exposed to "en-

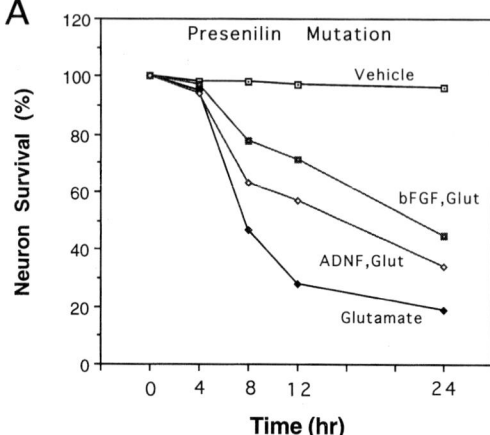

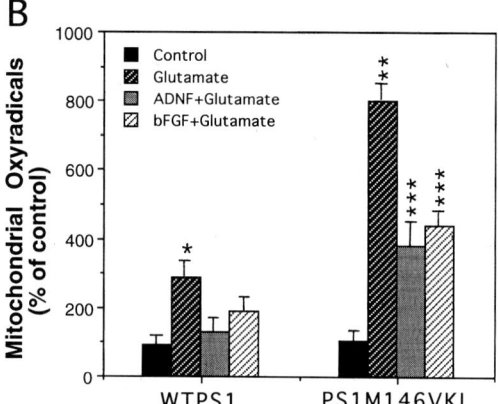

Figure 2–6. Neurotrophic factors protect neurons against genetic defects and environmental insults relevant to aging and the pathogenesis of Alzheimer's disease. A. Primary hippocampal cultures from PS-1 mutant knock-in mice were pretreated for 24 hr with vehicle, 100 ng/ml basic fibroblast growth factor (bFGF), or 0.1 pM activity-dependent neurotrophic factor (ADNF9). Cultures were then exposed for the indicated time periods to 100 μM glutamate, and neuron survival was quantified. B. Hippocampal cultures from wild-type mice (WTPS1) and PS-1 mutant knock-in mice (PS1M146VKI) were left untreated, or were pretreated for 24 hr with vehicle (control) 100 ng.ml bFGF or 0.1 pM ADNF9. Cultures were then exposed for 4 hr to 100 μM glutamate and levels of dihydrorhodamine 123 fluorescence (a measure of mitochondrial oxyradical levels) were quantified. [Modified from Guo et al.[90]]

riched" environments that include a variety of toys and climbing structures showed increased levels of NGF in hippocampus.[91] In addition, stimulation paradigms that induce long-term potentiation (LTP) of synaptic transmission in the hippocampus (believed to be a cellular correlate of learning and memory) also induced increases in NGF and BDNF mRNA levels,[92] and LTP was impaired in mice rendered genetically deficient in BDNF.[93] An additional neurotrophic factor that is upregulated in response to neuronal activity and may play roles in modulating learning and memory and preventing age-related neurodegeneration is the secreted form of APP.[94–96]

Rearing of rats in an intellectually enriched environment results in expansion of dendritic arbors and increased numbers of synapses in hippocampus and certain regions of cerebral cortex.[97,98] Moreover, epidemiological data suggest that humans with active minds have a reduced risk for developing AD as they age.[99] When taken together with data showing that neurotrophic factors can protect brain neurons against oxidative and metabolic insults relevant to brain aging and neurodegenerative disorders, these findings suggest a "use-it-or-lose-it" scenario of brain aging in which brain activity induces expression of neurotrophic factors, which in turn promote neuronal growth and plasticity (Fig. 2–7).

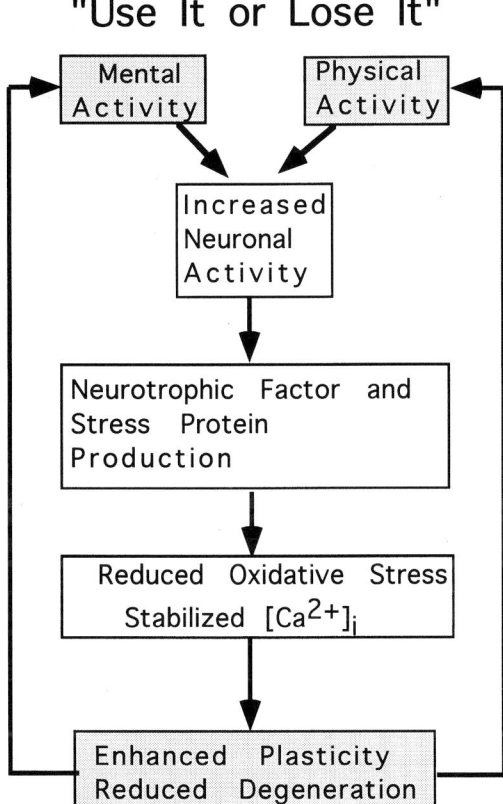

Figure 2–7. The "use-it-or-lose-it" hypothesis of successful brain aging and neurodegenerative disorders. Stimulation of activity in neuronal circuits by mental and physical activity increases the production of neurotrophic factors that enhance neuronal plasticity and function. Neurotrophic factors also protect neurons from age-related neurodegenerative cascades including excitotoxicity, energy deficits, and oxidative stress. In successful brain aging the enhanced mental and physical activity feeds back in a positive manner to stimulate the neurotrophic signaling pathways. Age-related neurodegenerative disorders may occur when levels of activation of neurotrophic signaling pathways are not able to override neurodegenerative cascades. [Modified from Mattson and Lindvall.[84]]

AGE-RELATED ALTERATIONS IN MITOCHONDRIAL FUNCTION AND ENERGY METABOLISM

Structural changes in synaptic mitochondria have been reported in studies of brain aging and include a decrease in numbers and increase in size and elongation.[40] During normal aging, levels of overall protein synthesis (including mitochondrial proteins) are unchanged. However, decreases in synthesis of specific mitochondrial proteins that are components of the the electron transport chain have been reported to occur in aged rodents. Evidence for mitochondrial dysfunction in usual aging and in neurodegenerative disorders is quite convincing[40] (Fig. 2–8). Mitochondrial dysfunction has been linked to several neurodegenerative disorders.[100] In PD there are clear mitochondrial enzyme dysfunctions including diminished activities of complex I and α-ketoglutarate dehydrogenase.[101] Exposure of cultured dopaminergic neurons to insults relevant to the pathogenesis of PD (e.g., MPTP and Fe^{2+}) causes mitochondrial dysfunction. In AD, cytochrome c oxidase and α-ketoglutarate dehydrogenase activity levels are markedly reduced in vulnerable brain regions.[102] Interestingly, mitochondrial deficits are also observed in non-neuronal cells, including platelets and fibroblasts, of AD patients. When mitochondria from platelets of AD patients are introduced into cultured neuroblastoma cells, levels of oxidative stress are

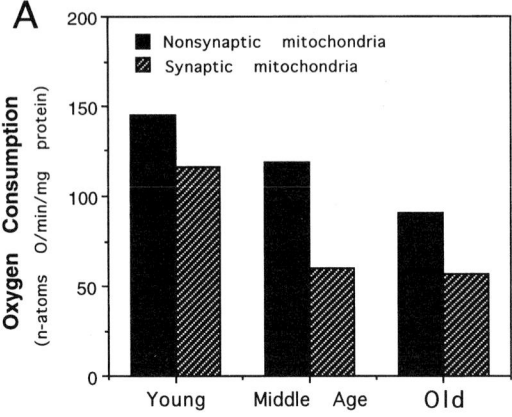

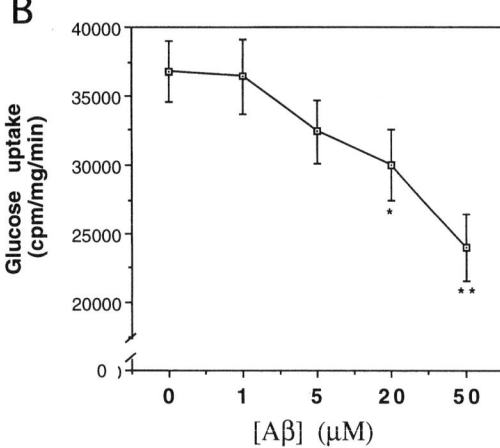

Figure 2–8. Evidence for perturbed neuronal energy metabolism in brain aging and in Alzheimer's disease. *A.* Levels of oxygen consumption, a measure of mitochondrial function, were measured in synaptic and nonsynaptic mitochondria from young (3 month), middle age (12 month) and old (24 month) rats. [Modified from Deshmukh et al.[162]] *B.* Levels of glucose uptake by cultured rat cortical neurons were measured following exposure to the indicated concentrations of amyloid β-peptide (Aβ). [Modified from Mark et al.[43]]

During the aging process changes that occur in the cerebral vasculature as well as in the neural cells themselves appear to result in reduced energy availability to neurons. These age-related changes may be accelerated in several different neurodegenerative disorders including AD and PD. While it is clear that cerebral metabolism decreases with aging, the underlying mechanisms are likely to be multifactorial. In addition to the vascular alterations described above, abnormalities in neuronal energy metabolism may accrue with aging and are exacerbated in age-related neurodegenerative conditions. These defects may result from age-associated oxidative damage to the DNA encoding these enzyme systems and/ or reduced activity of the proteins in these systems. However, in aging rodents levels of activity of complexes I, IV, and V appear to be unchanged during aging. Nevertheless, age-related neurodegenerative disorders such as AD and PD appear to involve widespread metabolic alterations, not only in the nervous system but also in many other organ systems. Indeed, metabolic abnormalities have been documented in circulating blood cells and in fibroblasts from AD and PD patients.[102] Studies of aging rodents have documented decreases in glucose and ketone body oxidation; oxygen consumption; local cerebral glucose utilization; and glycolytic compounds (e.g., fructose-1,6-diphosphate). Additional studies have shown that brain cells in older animals exhibit increased vulnerability to metabolic stresses. Incorporation of glucose into amino acids declines in the brains of aging mice, and older people are much more vulnerable to metabolic encephalopathy than are young people.

Another factor that may contribute to reduced neuronal energy metabolism is impairment of function of glucose transport proteins in neuronal and cerebrovascular cell membranes. Studies of postmortem brain tissues of AD patients have documented reduced levels of glucose transporters,[104] and experimental studies of cultured hippocampal neurons and synaptosomes have shown that insults relevant to the pathogenesis of AD (exposure to Aβ and oxyradical-generating agents) can impair glucose transport[43] (Fig. 2–8). Impairment of glucose transport and mitochondrial dysfunction would be expected to lead to ATP deple-

increased. This finding suggests an important conribution of mitochondrial alterations to the increased oxidative stress present in neurons in AD brain.[103] Moreover, exposure of cultured hippocampal neurons or cortical synaptosomes to insults relevant to the pathogenesis of AD (e.g., amyloid β-peptide (Aβ) and 4-hydroxynonenal (HNE)) causes mitochondrial dysfunction.[42–56]

tion and render neurons vulnerable to excitotoxicity.

IMMUNOLOGICAL AND HORMONAL ASPECTS OF THE AGING NERVOUS SYSTEM

Aberrant activation of immune cells is increasingly recognized as a contributing factor to age-related neurodegenerative disorders.[105-107] While the blood–brain barrier limits access of circulating lymphocytes to neurons in the brain, the brain is by no means spared from immune responses. The brain possesses resident immune effector cells called "microglia" that may respond to age- and disease-related neurodegenerative processes. Whereas alterations in peripheral immune functions with usual aging are well established, the involvement of the immune system in brain aging is not clear. A decline in peripheral immune function during aging may lead to an autoimmune-like phenomenon in the brain through which microglia are activated. Although inflammatory processes are limited in the brain during normal aging, there is abundant evidence that inflammatory processes are associated with and contribute to the neurodegenerative process in AD and other age-related neurodegenerative disorders. Activation of microglial cells in affected brain regions exhibits a characteristic pattern of increased local cytokine production (by glial cells) in association with the neuropathological changes, and activation of components of the complement cascade system occurs. In addition, epidemiologic and clinical data suggest that anti-inflammatory agents may suppress the development of AD. Collectively, the emerging data suggest a role for chronic inflammatory reactions in the pathogenesis of at least some neurodegenerative disorders.

Several age-related alterations in neuroendocrine systems during aging occur in both laboratory animals and humans. Age- and disease-related changes in levels of steroid hormones, particularly glucocorticoids and estrogens, have been well documented.[108,109] There is considerable evidence for age-related alterations in the diurnal regulation of circulating glucocorticoid levels and an increase in the mean level of glucocorticoids. Moreover, regulation of the hypothalamic–pituitary–adrenal axis is altered in AD patients such that plasma levels of glucocorticoids are increased. Animal studies have repeatedly shown that increased levels of glucocorticoids, including those induced by physiological or psychological stress, can increase the vulnerability of hippocampal neurons to injury and death induced by ischemic and excitotoxic insults. Collectively, these findings suggest that glucocorticoids may have a negative impact on the outcome of both acute (e.g., stroke) and chronic (e.g., AD) age-related neurological disorders. It has recently become quite clear that estrogen (17β-estradiol) has a beneficial effect on brain aging.[110] Moreover, elderly women who take estrogens perform better on cognitive tasks, and there is a markedly reduced risk of AD in postmenopausal women who take estrogen replacement therapy. Animal and cell culture studies have shown that 17β-estradiol can protect neurons from being damaged and killed by insults relevant to AD[111,112] (Fig. 2–9). The latter studies provide evidence that the neuroprotective mechanism of estrogen involves its inherent antioxidant proper-

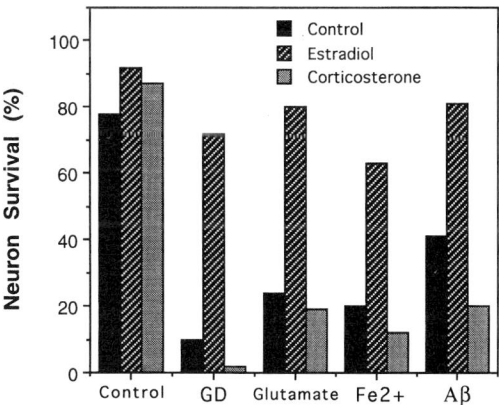

Figure 2–9. Estrogen protects cultured hippocampal neurons against metabolic, excitotoxic, and oxidative insults. Rat hippocampal cultures were pretreated for 2 hr with 0.2% dimethylsulfoxide (Control), 1 μM 17β-estradiol, or 1 μM corticosterone. Cultures were then exposed to vehicle (saline), glucose deprivation (GD), 50 μM glutamate, 5 μM FeSO$_4$ (Fe^{2+}) or 5 μM Aβ25–35. Neuronal survival was quantified at specified time points following each insult. Values are the mean of determinations made in at least four separate cultures. [Modified from Goodman et al.[111]]

ties that suppress neuronal membrane lipid peroxidation and preserve mitochondrial function.

NEURODEGENERATIVE DISORDER–SPECIFIC MOLECULAR ALTERATIONS

Individuals inherit two apolipoprotein E alleles, of which there are three isoforms (E2, E3, and E4). The E2 allele has been linked to increased lifespan and reduced incidence of AD[113]; this "longevity gene" may act, in part, by reducing atherosclerotic processes in the vasculature. Apolipoprotein E can also be considered a "predisposition" gene for which the E4 allele increases the risk for developing one or more age-related neurodegenerative disorders, including AD. Other genetic predisposition factors will undoubtedly be identified as work in this important area progresses.

Alzheimer's Disease

Three different genes have been identified in which mutations are causally linked to early-onset autosomal dominant familial AD.[114] The first gene for which mutations were causally linked to AD was that encoding APP.[63] The APP mutations result in amino acid changes adjacent to the N or C terminus of Aβ, or within the Aβ sequence. Analyses of cultured cells and transgenic mice expressing APP mutations suggest that the mutations result in altered proteolytic processing of APP such that cells produce more Aβ and less sAPPα (Fig. 2–10). As described above, increased levels of Aβ would be expected to induce oxidative stress and perturb calcium homeostasis in neurons. Decreased levels of sAPPα however, may promote neuronal degeneration because sAPPα activates neuroprotective signaling pathways.[94,95,115,116] sAPPα can protect cultured hippocampal neurons against glutamate toxicity, glucose deprivation, and oxidative insults that induce apoptosis, including exposure to Aβ[26,115,117] The neuroprotective actions of sAPPα are apparently mediated by a signaling pathway involving production of cyclic GMP. The sAPPα signaling pathway results in rapid activation of potassium channels that may play a role in preventing excitotoxicity.[94,95] In addition, the sAPPα signaling pathway activates NF-κB, which plays a role in preventing apoptosis.[25,26]

The presenilin-1 (PS-1) gene on chromosome 14 and the presenilin-2 (PS-2) gene on chromosome 1 can harbor mutations linked to many cases of early-onset inherited AD.[114] Expression of PS-1 or PS-2 mutations in cultured PC12 cells greatly increases their vulnerability to apoptosis induced by trophic factor withdrawal and Aβ.[118] The presenilin mutations somehow perturb calcium regulation in the endoplasmic reticulum (ER), which leads to enhanced calcium release when neurons are subjected to various apoptotic insults.[119,120]

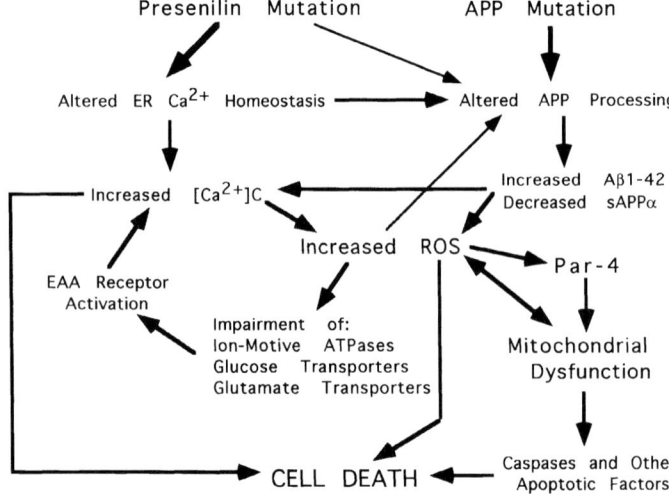

Figure 2–10. Proposed mechanisms by which presenilin and amyloid precursor protein mutations promote neuronal apoptosis and excitotoxicity. See text for discussion.

Calcium responses to agonists that induce calcium release from ryanodine- and IP_3-sensitive ER stores are enhanced in PC12 cells overexpressing mutant PS-1 compared to control cells overexpressing wild-type PS-1 or transfected with empty vector. Calcium responses to thapsigargin, an inhibitor of the ER Ca^{2+}-ATPase, are also enhanced in cells expressing PS-1 mutations. This response suggests that the mutations somehow result in an increased pool of ER calcium.[121] Inhibitors of calcium are released from ER (e.g., dantrolene), and blockers of voltage-dependent calcium channels (e.g., nifedipine) prevent Aβ-induced apoptosis in neurons expressing PS-1 mutations.[119,122] Recent studies of PS-1 mutant knock-in mice strengthen the case for an endangering action of PS-1 mutations that results from altered calcium homeostasis. Hippocampal neurons in PS-1 mutant knock-in mice exhibit increased vulnerability to apoptosis induced by Aβ,[79] and to excitotoxicity.[122] Hippocampal neurons expressing mutant PS-1 exhibit larger increases in levels of intracellular calcium and reactive oxygen species following exposure to glutamate.[79]

Other effects of PS-1 mutations that may be involved in their neurodegenerative action are being identified. For example, Kim et al.[123] found that presenilins can be cleaved by caspases, cysteine proteases that play a major role in apoptosis. Additional data suggest a role for interactions of PS-1 with β-catenin, a protein involved in cell adhesion and modulation of apoptosis in non-neuronal cells.[124] Mechanistic links between PS-1–β-catenin interactions, perturbed calcium homeostasis, and neuronal apoptosis remain to be determined.

Other Disorders

Although the mechanism(s) responsible for neuronal degeneration in PD remain unclear, data suggest important roles for increased levels of oxidative stress and mitochondrial dysfunction.[49,125] Studies of postmortem brain tissue from PD patients has revealed increased membrane lipid peroxidation, protein oxidation and protein nitration, and decreased mitochondrial complex I activity in the substantia nigra. Both environmental and genetic factors may sensitize dopaminergic neurons to age-related changes in the brain.[126,127] It was recently reported that mutations in the gene encoding α-synuclein are responsible for some cases of inherited PD.[128] Although such mutations are very rare, it has become evident that alterations in synuclein protein (i.e., aggregation and fibril formation) occur in most cases of PD. Aggregates of synuclein have been shown to induce apoptosis in cultured human neuroblastoma cells,[129] suggesting a cause–effect relationship between synuclein aggregation and neuronal degeneration in PD. Recent studies in animal models of PD have documented roles for classic apoptotic proteins, including Par-4 and caspases[130] in the pathogenesis of PD.

Several age-related inherited neurodegenerative conditions are caused by trinucleotide repeats in specific genes. The best known such disorder is HD, in which polyglutamine repeats in the huntingtin gene promote degeneration of neurons in the caudate/putamen and cerebral cortex. Other examples include spinal and bulbar muscular atrophy, fragile X syndrome, spinocerebellar ataxia type 1, and Machado-Joseph disease. Trinucleotide repeat mutations do not follow strict rules of Mendelian inheritance, as they are unstable and change size in successive generations. The mechanism(s) through which expansions of trinucleotide repeats causes neuronal degeneration have not been established, but recent findings suggest roles for protein aggregation and oxidative stress. For example, expression of mutant huntingtin protein in cultured cells and transgenic mice results in a neuropathology similar to that observed in striatal neurons in HD patients, including the formation of intranuclear inclusions of the huntingtin protein.[131,132]

A small percentage of cases of ALS are caused by mutations in the gene encoding the antioxidant enzyme Cu/Zn-SOD.[133] The mutations apparently alter the properties of the enzyme such that it becomes highly reactive with peroxides and thereby generates hydroxyl radical which can induce membrane lipid peroxidation and disrupt cellular calcium homeostasis.[134,135] The molecular genetics of stroke are very complex. Genetic risk factors for atherosclerosis and hypertension are also risk factors for stroke. An interesting genetic defect in the gene encoding notch-3 was recently identified as the cause of a syndrome called "CADASIL" (*c*erebral *a*utosomal *d*ominant *ar*-

teriopathy with *subcortical infarcts and leukoencephalopathy*), which results in recurrent strokes and early death.[136,137] The mutations result in substitution of other amino acids for cysteine residues in the notch-3. The mechanism responsible for the stroke-causing actions of the notch-3 mutations have not yet been determined, but they may result from effects of cerebrovascular cells.

SLOWING AGING OF THE NERVOUS SYSTEM BY DIETARY RESTRICTION

A well-documented method for increasing the lifespan of laboratory rodents is to reduce their dietary caloric intake.[138,139] Dietary restriction (DR) with maintenance of micronutrient intake reduces the development of age-related cancers and immune alterations and decreases levels of cellular oxidative stress in several organ systems.[140,141] Recent findings from studies of monkeys suggest similar benefits of DR in primates.[142,143] Although the mechanism by which DR increases resistance of cells to age-related pathology is not known, two possibilities are reduced mitochondrial oxyradical production[144] and induction of expression of cytoprotective stress proteins.[145–148] Whereas clear benefits of DR on several different organ systems have been demonstrated, its effects on the brain are largely unknown. Recent evidence suggests that, as in other organ systems, DR may slow age-related changes in the brain.[149] For example, age-related increases in levels of glial fibrillary acidic protein in the brain are suppressed in DR rats,[6] age-related loss of dendritic spines is retarded in DR rats,[150] aged DR rodents perform better on learning and memory tasks than ad-libitum fed (AL) age-matched rats,[151–153] and DR in adult rats may increase resistance of hippocampal and striatal neurons to excitotoxic and metabolic insults.[154] In addition, DR can reduce age-related alterations in dopaminergic signaling pathways.[155,156]

While the impact of DR on age-related neurodegenerative disorders is unknown, recent data from an epidemiological study suggest that PD patients have a history of higher daily calorie and fat intake than age-matched controls[157] (Fig. 2–11). Recent animal studies suggest that DR can increase resistance of neurons to degeneration associated with age-related disorders including AD, PD, and HD, and can improve outcome following stroke.[145,148,154] In one study, rats were either fed ad-libitum or were maintained on a DR diet (alternate-day feeding regimen) for 3–4 months.[154] The rats were then administered either kainic acid (a toxin that selectively damages hippocampal pyramidal neurons) or 3-nitropropionic acid (a toxin that selectively damages striatal neurons). In rats administered kainic acid the damage to hippocampal neurons was significantly reduced, and learning and memory deficits were ameliorated in DR rats (Fig. 2–11). In rats administered 3-nitropropionic acid the amount of damge to striatal neurons was decreased and motor deficits completely ameliorated in the rats maintained on the DR diet compared to control rats fed ad-libitum. In another study, mice maintained on a DR diet exhibited increased resistance to the damaging effects of MPTP, a toxin that selectively damages dopaminergic neurons in the substantia nigra.[145] The latter study also showed that "chemical DR," effected by administration of 2-deoxyglucose (2-DG; a nonmetabolizable analog of glucose), can protect dopaminergic neurons against MPTP-induced damage. Finally, a recent study using a rat model of focal ischemic brain injury showed that DR and 2-DG administration can reduce the extent of brain damage and improve behavioral outcome in this animal model of stroke[148] (Fig. 2–11). Collectively, these experimental findings strongly suggest that life-long reduction in food intake can provide a hedge against most (if not all) age-related neurodegenerative conditions.

Although the mechanism by which DR benefits the aging brain remains to be fully elucidated, accumulating data suggest that at least two mechanisms are likely operative. The first mechanism involves reduced production of (mitochondria-derived) free radicals. Thus, levels of cellular oxidative stress are decreased in many different tissues, including the brain, of rats and mice maintained on calorie-restricted diets.[141] The second mechanism involves induction of a mild stress response in neurons. Levels of the neuroprotective stress protein HSP-70 are increased in neurons in brains of rats subjected to DR, and levels of HSP-70 and GRP-78 (an endoplasmic reticulum stress protein) are also increased in several different brain regions of rats and in cultured neurons administered 2-DG.[146,148] Other studies have shown that increased levels of HSP-70 and GRP-78 can protect neurons against excitotoxic and metabolic insults relevant to brain aging and neurodegenerative disorders.[147,158] Although the specific mechanism by which HSP-70 and GRP-78 protect neurons is not yet established, high levels of expression of these proteins are correlated with enhanced cellular calcium homeostasis, improved mitochondrial function, and reduced levels of cellular oxidative stress. Finally, it was recently shown that DR increases levels of neurotrophic factors (particularly BONF) in several brain regions of rats and mice; the increase in BONF levels was associated with increased neurogenesis and increased resistance of neurons to excitotoxicity.[159,160]

CONCLUSIONS

A variety of structural changes occur in the brain during usual aging, and many such changes likely represent compensatory responses to adverse changes in cellular metabolism that occur during the aging process. There appear to be several shared processes that predispopse neurons to dysfunction and death in both usual aging and in age-related neurodegenerative disorders. At the cellular and molecular levels these changes include increased levels of oxidative stress; impaired mitochondrial function and energy metabolism; and dysregulation of neuronal calcium homeostasis. Disease-specific initiators of neuronal

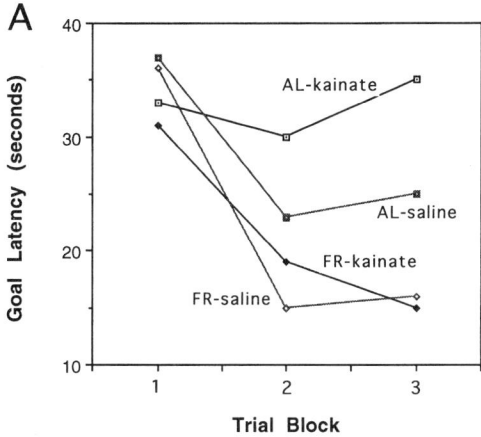

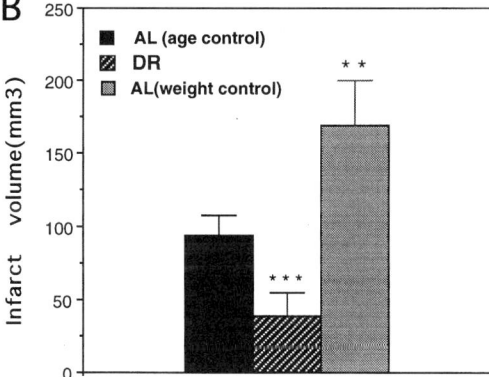

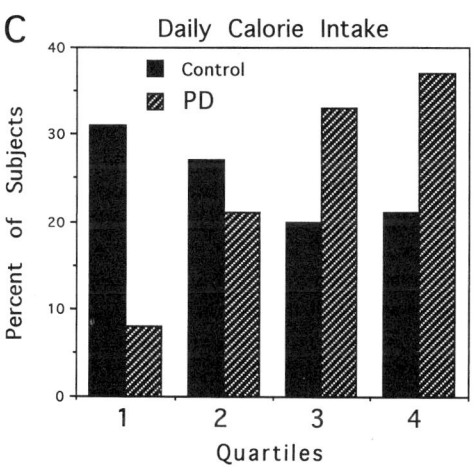

Figure 2–11. Evidence that food restriction (FR) increases resistance of neurons to age-related neurodegenerative disorders. *A.* Rats were maintained on either a FR diet or AL diets for 3 months. Rats were then administered kainate into the dorsal hippocampus bilaterally and were tested 24 hr later in the Morris water maze. Goal latency data showed that kainate causes severe impairment in the AL group, but not in the FR group. [Modified from Bruce-Keller et al.[154]] *B.* Rats maintained on dietary restriction (DR) exhibit reduced brain damage and improved behavioral outcome following focal ischemic brain injury. Brain infarct volumes are shown for DR rats ($n = 8$), age-matched AL-fed control rats ($n = 7$), and weight-matched AL-fed control rats ($n = 8$). Values are the mean and SD. ** $P < 0.01$, *** $P < 0.001$ compared to the AL age control value. [Modified from Yu et al.[148]] *C.* Average daily calorie intake in patients with Parkinson's disease (PD) and age-matched controls (data from a population-based case–control study). Quartile values for calorie intake were 1, <1022 kcal; 2, <1353 kcal; 3, <1652 kcal; 4, >1652 kcal. [Modified from Logroscino et al.[157]]

degeneration are being identified and include increased production of Aβ and reduced production of sAPPα in AD; trinucleotide repeat expansions in HD and related disorders; and dopamine- and Fe^{2+}-mediated free radical production in PD. As in many other organ systems, untoward changes in blood vessels may contribute greatly to age-related declines in cell function and tissue damage in the brain. A role for chronic inflammatory processes involving microglial activation are implicated in the pathogenesis of some neurodegenerative disorders. Intriguingly, neurotrophic signaling pathways that promote neuronal survival and adaptation are stimulated by brain activity, such that individuals with a high level of "intellectual" activity have a reduced risk for developing age-related neurodegenerative conditions such as AD. The collective research on brain aging strongly suggests that lifestyle principles that forestall age-related disorders in other organ systems (e.g., cardiovascular disease, cancers, and diabetes) will also promote successful brain aging. These principles include reduced calorie intake, increased exercise ("mental" and physical), and a diet enriched in antioxidants and sparse in fats.

REFERENCES

1. Katzman R, Terry RD. Normal aging of the nervous system. In: (Katzman R, Rowe JW, eds:) Principles of Geriatric Neurology. Philadelphia: FA Davis, 1992: 18–58.
2. Terry RD, Masliah E, Salmon DP, Butters N, DeTeresa R, Hill R, Hansen LA, Katzman R. Physical basis of cognitive alterations in Alzheimer's disease: synapse loss is the major correlate of cognitive impairment. Ann Neurol 1991; 30:572–580.
3. Hof PR, Giannakopoulos P, Bouras C. The neuropathological changes associated with normal brain aging. Histol Histopathol 1996; 11:1075–1088.
4. Dickson DW. Structural changes in the aged brain. In: Mattson MP, Geddes, eds. The Aging Brain. Greenwich, CT: JAI Press. Adv Cell Aging Gerontol 1997; 2:51–76.
5. Geddes JW, Matus AI. The neuronal cytoskeleton: changes associated with age, neurodegenerative disease and neuronal insult. In: Mattson MP, Geddes, JW, eds. The Aging Brain. Greenwich, CT: JAI Press. Adv Cell Aging Gerontol 1997; 2:23–50.
6. Morgan TE, Rozovsky I, Goldsmith SK, Stone DJ, Yoshida T, Finch CE. Increased transcription of the astrocyte gene GFAP during middle age is attenuated by food restriction: implications for the role of oxidative stress. Free Radic Biol Med 1997; 23:524–528.
7. Mattson MP, Fu W, Waeg G, Uchida K. 4-hydroxynonenal, a product of lipid peroxidation, inhibits dephosphorylation of the microtubule-associated protein tau. NeuroReport 1997; 8:2275–2281.
8. Braak H, Braak E. Neuropathological staging of Alzheimer-related changes. Acta Neuropathol 1991; 82:239–259.
9. Goedert M, Spillantini MG, Davies SW. Filamentous nerve cell inclusions in neurodegenerative diseases. Curr Opin Neurobiol 1998; 8:619–632.
10. Julien JP, Couillard-Despres S, Meier J. Transgenic mice in the study of ALS: the role of neurofilaments. Brain Pathol 1998; 8:759–769.
11. Mattson MP. Antigenic changes similar to those seen in neurofibrillary tangles are elicited by glutamate and calcium influx in cultured hippocampal neurons. Neuron 1990; 4:105–117.
12. Zhang B, Tu P, Abtahian F, Trojanowski JQ, Lee VM. Neurofilaments and orthograde transport are reduced in ventral root axons of transgenic mice that express human SOD1 with a G93A mutation. J Cell Biol 1997; 139:1307–1315.
13. Bertoni-Freddari C, Fattoretti P, Paoloni R, Caselli U, Galeazzi L, Meier-Ruge W. Synaptic structural dynamics and aging. Gerontology 1996; 42:170–180.
14. DeKosky ST, Scheff SW, Styren SD. Structural correlates of cognition in dementia: quantification and assessment of synapse change. Neurodegeneration 1996; 5:417–421.
15. Morgan DG May PC, Finch CE. Dopamine and serotonin systems in human and rodent brain: effects of age and neurodegenerative disease. J Am Geriatr Soc 1987; 35:334–345.
16. Zhan SS, Beyreuther K, Schmitt HP. Quantitative assessment of the synaptophysin immunoreactivity of the cortical neuropil in various neurodegenerative disorders with dementia. Dementia 1993; 4:66–74.
17. Mattson MP, Keller JN, Begley JG. Evidence for synaptic apoptosis. Exp Neurol 1998; 153:35–48.
18. Mattson MP, Partin J, Begley JG. Amyloid β-peptide induces apoptosis-related events in synapses and dendrites. Brain Res 1998; 807:167–176.
19. de la Torre JC. Cerebrovascular changes in the aging brain. In: Mattson MP, Geddes JW, eds. The Aging Brain. Greenwich, CT: JAI Press. Adv Cell Aging Gerontol 1997; 2:77–107.
20. Blanc EM, Toborek M, Mark RJ, Hennig B, Mattson MP. Amyloid β-peptide disrupts barrier and transport functions and induces apoptosis in vascular endothelial cells. J Neurochem 1997; 68:1870–1881.
21. Mrak RE, Griffin ST, Graham DI. Aging-associated changes in human brain. J Neuropathol Exp Neurol 1997; 56:1269–1275.
22. Sohal RS, Brunk UT. Lipofuscin as an indicator of oxidative stress and aging. Adv Exp Med Biol 1989; 266:17–26.
23. Griffin WS, Sheng JG, Mrak RE. Senescence-accelerated overexpression of S100β in brain of SAMP6 mice. Neurobiol Aging 1998; 19:71–76.
24. Korhonen P, Helenius M, Salminen A. Age-related changes in the regulation of transcription factor NF-κB in rat brain. Neurosci Lett (1997); 225:61–64.
25. Mattson MP, Goodman Y, Luo H, Fu W, Furukawa K. Activation of NF-κB protects hippocampal neurons against oxidative stress-induced apoptosis: evidence for induction of Mn-SOD and suppression of

peroxynitrite production and protein tyrosine nitration. J Neurosci Res 1997; 49:681–697.
26. Guo Q, Robinson N, Mattson MP. Secreted APPα counteracts the pro-apoptotic action of mutant presenilin-1 by activation of NF-κB and stabilization of calcium homeostasis J Biol Che 1998; 273:12341–12351.
27. Asanuma M, Kondo Y, Nishibayashi S, Iwata E, Nakanishi T, Ogawa N. Age-related changes in composition of transcription factor, AP-1 complex in the rat brain. Neurosci Lett 1995; 201:127–130.
28. Rao G, Xia E, Richardson A. Effect of age on the expression of antioxidant enzymes in male Fischer F344 rats. Mech Ageing Dev 1990; 53:49–60.
29. Blake MJ, Fargnoli J, Gershon D, Holbrook NJ. Concomitant decline in heat-induced hyperthermia and HSP70 mRNA expression in aged rats. Am J Physiol 1991; 260:R663–R667.
30. Colangelo AM, Follesa P, Mocchetti I. Differential induction of nerve growth factor and basic fibroblast growth factor mRNA in neonatal and aged rat brain. Mol Brain Res 1998; 53:218–225.
31. Hayashi M, Yamashita A, Shimizu K. Somatostatin and brain-derived neurotrophic factor mRNA expression in the primate brain: decreased levels of mRNAs during aging. Brain Res 1997; 749:283–289.
32. Chauhan NB, Siegel GJ. In situ analysis of Na^+/K^+-ATPase α1- and α3-isoform mRNAs in aging rat hippocampus. J Neurochem 1996; 66: 1742–1751.
33. Mooradian AD, and Shah GN. Age-related changes in glucose transporter-one mRNA structure and function. Proc Soc Exp Biol Med 1997; 216:380–385.
34. Bannon MJ, Poosch MS, Xia Y, Goebel DJ, Cassin B, Kapatos G. Dopamine transporter mRNA content in human substantia nigra decreases precipitously with age. Proc Natl Acad Sci USA 1992; 89:7095–7099.
35. Mhatre MC, Ticku MK. Caloric restriction retards the aging associated changes in γ-aminobutyric acidA receptor gene expression in rat cerebellum. Mol Brain Res 1998; 54:270–275.
36. Sells SF, Han SS, Muthukkumar S, Maddiwar N, Johnstone R, Boghaert E, Gillis D, Liu G, Nair P, Monnig S, Collini P, Mattson MP, Sukhatme VP, Zimmer SG, Wood DR, Jr, McRoberts JW, Shi Y, Rangnekar VM. Expression and function of the leucine zipper protein Par-4 in apoptosis. Mol Cell Biol 1997; 17:3823–3832.
37. Guo Q, Fu W, Xie J, Luo H, Sells SF, Geddes JW, Bondada V, Rangnekar V, Mattson MP. Par-4 is a mediator of neuronal degeneration associated with the pathogenesis of Alzheimer's disease. Nat Med 1998; 4:957–962.
38. Nagy Z, Esiri MM, Smith AD. The cell division cycle and the pathophysiology of Alzheimer's disease. Neuroscience 1998; 87:731–739.
39. Butterfield DA, Stadtman ER. Protein oxidation processes in aging brain. In: Mattson MP, Geddes JW, eds. The Aging Brain. Greenwich, CT: JAI Press. Adv Cell Aging Gerontol 1997; 2:161–191.
40. Benzi G, Moretti A. Contribution of mitochondrial alterations to brain aging. In: Mattson MP, Geddes JW, eds. The Aging Brain. Greenwich, CT: JAI Press. Adv Cell Aging Gerontol 1997; 2:129–160.
41. Mark RJ, Hensley K, Butterfield DA, Mattson MP. Amyloid β-peptide impairs ion-motive ATPase activities: evidence for a role in loss of neuronal Ca^{2+} homeostasis and cell death. J Neurosci 1995; 15:6239–6249.
42. Mark RJ, Lovell MA, Markesbery WR, Uchida K, Mattson MP. A role for 4-hydroxynonenal in disruption of ion homeostasis and neuronal death induced by amyloid β-peptide. J Neurochem 1997; 68:255–264.
43. Mark RJ, Pang Z, Geddes JW, Uchida K, Mattson MP. Amyloid β-peptide impairs glucose uptake in hippocampal and cortical neurons: involvement of membrane lipid peroxidation. J Neurosci 1997; 17: 1046–1054.
44. Good PF, Hsu A, Werner P, Perl DP, Olanow CW. Protein nitration in Parkinson's disease. J Neuropathol Exp Neurol 1998; 57:338–342.
45. Hirsch EC, Faucheux BA. Iron metabolism and Parkinson's disease. Mov Disord 1998; 13 (Suppl 1):39–45.
46. Alves-Rodrigues A, Gregori L, Figueiredo-Pereira ME. Ubiquitin, cellular inclusions and their role in neurodegeneration. Trends Neurosci 1998; 21:516–520.
47. Smith CD, Carney JM, Starke-Reed PE, Oliver CN, Stadtman ER, Floyd RA, Markesbery WR. Excess brain protein oxidation and enzyme dysfunction in normal aging and in Alzheimer disease. Proc Natl Acad Sci USA 1991; 88:10540–10543.
48. Smith MA, Taneda S, Richey PL, Miyata S, Yan S-D, Stern D, Sayre LM, Monnier VM, Perry G. Advanced maillard reaction end products are associated with Alzheimer disease pathology. Proc Natl Acad Sci USA 1994; 91:5710–5714.
49. Jenner P, Olanow CW. Understanding cell death in Parkinson's disease. Ann Neurol 1998; 44:S72–S84.
50. Lovell MA, Ehmann WD, Butler SM, Markesbery WR. Elevated thiobarbituric acid–reactive substances and antioxidant enzyme activity in the brain in Alzheimer's disease. Neurology 1995; 45:1594–1601.
51. Lovell MA, Ehmann WD, Mattson MP, Markesbery WR. Elevated 4-hydroxynonenal in ventricular fluid in Alzheimer's disease. Neurobiol Aging 1997; 18: 457–461
52. Yoritaka A, Hattori N, Uchida K, Tanaka M, Stadtman ER, Mizuno Y. Immunohistochemical detection of 4-hydroxynonenal protein adducts in Parkinson disease. Proc Natl Acad Sci USA 1996; 93:2696–2701.
53. Sayre LM, Zelasko DA, Harris PL, Perry G, Salomon RG, Smith MA. 4-Hydroxynonenal-derived advanced lipid peroxidation end products are increased in Alzheimer's disease. J Neurochem 1997; 68:2092–2097.
54. Pedersen WA, Keller JN, Fu W, Markesbery WR, Appel SH, Smith RG, Mattson MP. Protein modification by the lipid peroxidation product 4-hydroxynonenal in spinal cords of ALS patients. Ann Neurol 1998; 44: 819–824.
55. Kruman I, Bruce-Keller AJ, Bredesen D, Waeg G, and Mattson MP. Evidence that 4-hydroxynonenal mediates oxidative stress-induced neuronal apoptosis. J Neurosci 1997; 17:5089–5100.
56. Keller JN, Pang Z, Geddes JW, Begley JG, Germeyer A, Waeg G, Mattson MP. Impairment of glucose and glutamate transport and induction of mitochondrial oxidative stress and dysfunction in synaptosomes by amyloid β-peptide: role of the lipid peroxidation product 4-hydroxynonenal. J Neurochem 1997; 69:273–284.

57. Ferrante RJ, Shinobu LA, Schulz JB, Matthews RT, Thomas CE, Kowall NW, Gurney ME, Beal MF. Increased 3-nitrotyrosine and oxidative damage in mice with a human copper/zinc superoxide dismutase mutation. Ann Neurol 1997; 42:326–334.
58. Gurney ME, Cutting FB, Zhai P, Doble A, Taylor CP, Andrus PK, Hall ED. Benefit of vitamin E, riluzole, and gabapentin in a transgenic model of familial amyotrophic lateral sclerosis. Ann Neurol 1996; 39:147–157.
59. Browne SE, Bowling AC, MacGarvey U, Baik MJ, Berger SC, Muqit MM, Bird ED, Beal MF. Oxidative damage and metabolic dysfunction in Huntington's disease: selective vulnerability of the basal ganglia. Ann Neurol 1997; 41:646–653.
60. Alam ZI, Jenner A, Daniel SE, Lees AJ, Cairns N, Marsden CD, Jenner P, Halliwell B. Oxidative DNA damage in the parkinsonian brain: an apparent selective increase in 8-hydroxyguanine in substantia nigra. J Neurochem 1997; 69:1196–1203.
61. Alam ZI, Daniel SE, Lees AJ, Marsden DC, Jenner P, Halliwell B. A generalised increase in protein carbonyls in the brain in Parkinson's but not incidental Lewy body disease. J Neurochem 1997; 69:1326–1329.
62. Mococci P, MacGarvey MS, Beal MF. Oxidative damage to mitochondrial DNA is increased in Alzheimer's disease. Ann Neurol 1994; 36:747–751.
63. Mattson MP. Cellular actions of β-amyloid precursor protein, and its soluble and fibrillogenic peptide derivatives. Physiol Rev 1997; 77:1081–1132.
64. Mattson MP, Barger SW, Cheng B, Lieberburg I, Smith-Swintosky VL, Rydel RE. β-amyloid precursor protein metabolites and loss of neuronal calcium homeostasis in Alzheimer's disease. Trends Neurosci 1993; 16:409–415.
65. Mattson MP. Modification of ion homeostasis by lipid peroxidation: roles in neuronal degeneration and adaptive plasticity. Trends Neurosci 1998; 21:53–57.
66. Mattson MP, Lovell MA, Furukawa K, Markesbery WR. Neurotrophic factors attenuate glutamate-induced accumulation of peroxides, elevation of $[Ca^{2+}]_i$ and neurotoxicity, and increase antioxidant enzyme activities in hippocampal neurons. J Neurochem 1995; 65:1740–1751.
67. Mark RJ, Keller JN, Kruman I, Mattson MP. Basic FGF attenuates amyloid β-peptide-induced oxidative stress, mitochondrial dysfunction, and impairment of Na^+/K^+-ATPase activity in hippocampal neurons. Brain Res 1997; 756:205–214.
68. Kelly J, Furukawa K, Barger SW, Mark RJ, Rengen MR, Blanc EM, Roth GS, Mattson MP. Amyloid β-peptide disrupts carbachol-induced muscarinic cholinergic signal transduction in cortical neurons. Proc Natl Acad Sci USA 1996; 93:6753–6758.
69. Pedersen WA, Kloczewiak MA, Blusztajn JK. Amyloid beta-protein reduces acetylcholine synthesis in a cell line derived from cholinergic neurons of the basal forebrain. Proc Natl Acad Sci USA 1996; 93:8068–8071.
70. Conway KA, Harper JD, Lansbury PT. Accelerated in vitro fibril formation by a mutant alpha-synuclein linked to early-onset Parkinson disease. Nat Med 1998; 4:1318–1320.
71. Martindale D, Hackam A, Wieczorek A, Ellerby L, Wellington C, McCutcheon K, Singaraja R, Kazemi-Esfarjani P, Devon R, Kim SU, Bredesen DE, Tufaro F, Hayden MR. Length of huntingtin and its polyglutamine tract influences localization and frequency of intracellular aggregates. Nat Genet 1998; 18:150–154.
72. Perez MK, Paulson HL, Pendse SJ, Saionz SJ, Bonini NM, Pittman RN. Recruitment and the role of nuclear localization in polyglutamine-mediated aggregation. J Cell Biol 1998; 143:1457–1470.
73. Bruijn LI, Houseweart MK, Kato S, Anderson KL, Anderson SD, Ohama E, Reaume AG, Scott RW, Cleveland DW. Aggregation and motor neuron toxicity of an ALS-linked SOD1 mutant independent from wild-type SOD1. Science 1998; 281:1851–1854.
74. Peterson C, Goldman JE. Alterations in calcium content and biochemical processes in cultured skin fibroblasts from aged and Alzheimer donors. Proc Natl Acad Sci USA 1986; 83:2758–2762.
75. Schwarz-Ben Meir N, Glaser T, Kosower NS. Band 3 protein degradation by calpain is enhanced in erythrocytes of old people. Biochem J 1991; 275:47–52.
76. Kenessey A, Banay-Schwartz M, DeGuzman T, Lajtha A. Calpain II activity and calpastatin content in brain regions of 3- and 24-month-old rats. Neurochem Res 1990; 15:243–249.
77. Nixon RA, Saito KI, Grynspan F, Griffin WR, Katayama S, Honda T, Mohan PS, Shea TB, Beerman M. Calcium-activated neutral proteinase (calpain) system in aging and Alzheimer's disease. Ann NY Acad Sci 1994; 747:77–91.
78. Masliah E, Mallory M, Alford M, Tanaka S, Hansen LA. Caspase dependent DNA fragmentation might be associated with excitotoxicity in Alzheimer disease. J Neuropathol Exp Neurol 1998; 57:1041–1052.
79. Guo Q, Sebastian L, Sopher BL, Miller MW, Ware CB, Martin GM, Mattson MP. Increased vulnerability of hippocampal neurons from presenilin-1 mutant knock-in mice to amyloid β-peptide toxicity: central roles of superoxide production and caspase activation. J Neurochem 1999; 72:1019–1029.
80. Kelly JF, Roth GS. Changes in neurotransmitter signal transduction pathways in aging brain. In: Mattson MP, Geddes JW, eds. The Aging Brain. Greenwich, CT: JAI Press. Adv Cell Aging Gerontol 1997; 2:243–278.
81. Blanc EM, Kelly JF, Mark RJ, Mattson MP. 4-hydroxynonenal, an aldehydic product of lipid peroxidation, impairs signal transduction associated with muscarinic acetylcholine and metabotropic glutamate receptors: possible action on $G\alpha_{q/11}$. J Neurochem 1997; 69:570–580.
82. Magnusson KR. The aging of the NMDA receptor complex. Front Biosci 1998; 3:e70–e80.
83. Verkhratsky A, Shmigol A, Kirischuk S, Pronchuk N, Kostyuk P. Age-dependent changes in calcium currents and calcium homeostasis in mammalian neurons. Ann NY Acad Sci 1994; 747:365–381.
84. Mattson MP. Lindvall O. Neurotrophic factor and cytokine signaling in the aging brain. In: Mattson MP, Geddes JW, eds. The Aging Brain. Greenwich, CT: JAI Press. Adv Cell Aging Gerontol 1997; 2: 299–345.
85. Mattson MP, Furukawa K. Programmed cell life: antiapoptotic signaling and therapeutic strategies for neurodegenerative disorders. Restorative Neurol Neurosci 1996; 9:191–205.

86. Larkfors L, Ebendal T, Whittemore SR, Persson H, Hoffer B, Olson L. Decreased level of nerve growth factor (NGF) and its messenger RNA in the aged rat brain. Mol Brain Res 1987; 3:55–60.
87. Hefti F, Mash DC. Localization of nerve growth factor receptors in the normal human brain and in Alzheimer's disease. Neurobiol Aging 1989; 10:75–87.
88. Koh S, Chang P, Collier TJ, Loy R. Loss of NGF receptor immunoreactivity in basal forebrain neurons of aged rats: correlation with spatial memory impairment. Brain Res 1989; 498:397–404.
89. Fischer W, Gage FH, Bjorklund A. Degenerative changes in forebrain cholinergic nuclei correlate with cognitive impairments in aged rats. J Neurosci 1989; 1:33–45.
90. Guo Q, Sebastian L, Sopher BL, Miller MW, Glazner GW, Ware CB, Martin GM, Mattson MP. Neurotrophic factors interrupt excitotoxic neurodegenerative cascades promoted by a presenilin-1 mutation. Proc Natl Acad Sci USA 96:4125–4130.
91. Mohammed AH, Henriksson BG, Soderstrom S, Ebendal T, Olsson T, Seckl JR. Environmental influences on the central nervous system and their implications for the aging rat. Behav Brain Res 1993; 57:183–191.
92. Springer JE, Gwag BJ, Sessler FM. Neurotrophic factor mRNA expression in dentate gyrus is increased following in vivo stimulation of the angular bundle. Brain Res 1994; 23:135–143.
93. Korte M, Carroll P, Wolf E, Brem G, Thoenen H, Bonhoeffer T. Hippocampal long-term potentiation is impaired in mice lacking brain-derived neurotrophic factor. Proc Natl Acad Sci USA 1995; 92: 8856–8860.
94. Furukawa K, Barger SW, Blalock E, Mattson MP. Activation of K^+ channels and suppression of neuronal activity by secreted β-amyloid precursor protein. Nature 1996; 379:74–78.
95. Furukawa K, Sopher B, Rydel RE, Begley JG, Martin GM, Mattson MP. Increased activity-regulating and neuroprotective efficacy of α-secretase-derived secreted APP is conferred by a C-terminal heparin-binding domain. J Neurochem 1996; 67:1882–1896.
96. Ishida A, Furukawa K, Keller JN, Mattson MP. Secreted form of β-amyloid precursor protein shifts the frequency dependence for induction of LTD, and enhances LTP in hippocampal slices. NeuroReport 1997; 8:2133–2137.
97. Fiala BA, Joyce JN, Greenough WT. Environmental complexity modulates growth of granule cell dendrites in developing but not adult hippocampus of rats. Exp Neurol 1978; 59:372–383.
98. Greenough WT, Hwang HM, Gorman C. Evidence for active synapse formation or altered postsynaptic metabolism in visual cortex of rats reared in complex environments. Proc Natl Acad Sci USA 1985; 82: 4549–4552.
99. Evans DA, Hebert LE, Beckett LA, Scherr PA, Albert MS, Chown MJ, Pilgrim DM, Taylor JO. Education and other measures of socioeconomic status and risk of incident Alzheimer disease in a defined population of older persons. Arch Neurol 1997; 54: 1399–1405.
100. Bowling AC, Beal MF. Bioenergetic and oxidative stress in neurodegenerative diseases. Life Sci 1995; 56:1151–1171.
101. Schapira AH, Gu M, Taanman JW, Tabrizi SJ, Seaton T, Cleeter M, Cooper JM. Mitochondria in the etiology and pathogenesis of Parkinson's disease. Ann Neurol 1998; 44:S89–S98.
102. Gibson GE, Sheu KF, Blass JP. Abnormalities of mitochondrial enzymes in Alzheimer disease. J Neural Transm 1998; 105:855–870.
103. Swerdlow RH, Parks JK, Cassarino DS, Maguire DJ, Maguire RS, Bennett JP, Jr, Davis RE, Parker WD, Jr. Cybrids in Alzheimer's disease: a cellular model of the disease? Neurology 1997; 49:918–925.
104. Harr SD, Simonian NA, Hyman BT. Functional alterations in Alzheimer's disease: decreased glucose transporter 3 immunoreactivity in the perforant pathway terminal zone. J Neuropathol Exp Neurol 1995; 54:38–41.
105. McGeer PL, McGeer EG. The inflammatory response system of the brain: implications for therapy of Alzheimer and other neurodegenerative diseases. Brain Res Rev 1995; 21:195–218.
106. Kalaria RN, Harshbarger-Kelly M, Cohen DL, Premkumar DR. Molecular aspects of inflammatory and immune responses in Alzheimer's disease. Neurobiol Aging 1996; 17:687–693.
107. Zielasek J, Hartung HP. Molecular mechanisms of microglial activation. Adv Neuroimmunol 1996; 6: 191–222.
108. Meaney MJ, O'Donnell D, Rowe W, Tannenbaum B, Steverman A, Walker M, Nair NP, Lupien S. Individual differences in hypothalamic-pituitary-adrenal activity in later life and hippocampal aging. Exp Gerontol 1995; 30:229–251.
109. Simpkins JW, Green PS, Gridley KE, Singh M, de Fiebre NC, Rajakumar G. Role of estrogen replacement therapy in memory enhancement and the prevention of neuronal loss associated with Alzheimer's disease. Am J Med 1997; 103(3A):19S–25S.
110. McEwen BS, Gould E, Orchinik M, Weiland NG, Woolley CS. Oestrogens and the structural and functional plasticity of neurons: implications for memory, ageing and neurodegenerative processes. Ciba Found Symp 1995; 191:52–66.
111. Goodman Y, Bruce AJ, Cheng B, Mattson MP. Estrogens attenuate and corticosterone exacerbates excitotoxicity, oxidative injury and amyloid β-peptide toxicity in hippocampal neurons. J Neurochem 1996; 66:1836–1844.
112. Keller JN, Mattson MP. 17β-estradiol attenuates oxidative impairment of synaptic Na^+/K^+-ATPase activity, glucose transport and glutamate transport induced by amyloid β-peptide and iron. J Neurosci Res 1997; 50:522–530.
113. Saunders AM, Strittmatter WJ, Schmechel D, George-Hyslop PH, Pericak-Vance MA, Joo SH, Rosi BL, Gusella JF, Crapper-MacLachlan DR, Alberts MJ, Hulette C, Crain B, Goldgaber D, Roses AD. Association of apolipoprotein E allele epsilon 4 with late-onset familial and sporadic Alzheimer's disease. Neurology 1993; 43:1467–1472.
114. Hardy J. Amyloid, the presenilins and Alzheimer's disease. Trends Neurosci 1997; 20:154–159.
115. Mattson MP, Cheng B, Culwell A, Esch F, Lieberburg I, Rydel RE. Evidence for excitoprotective and intraneuronal calcium-regulating roles for secreted forms of β-amyloid precursor protein. Neuron 1993; 10: 243–254.

116. Lannfelt L, Basun H, Wahlund LO, Rowe BA, Wagner SL. Decreased α-secretase-cleaved amyloid precursor protein as a diagnostic marker for Alzheimer's disease. Nat Med 1995; 1:829–832.
117. Goodman Y, Mattson MP. Secreted forms of β-amyloid precursor protein protect hippocampal neurons against amyloid β-peptide-induced oxidative injury. Exp Neurol 1994; 128:1–12.
118. Mattson MP, Guo Q. Cell and molecular neurobiology of presenilins: a role for the endoplasmic reticulum in the pathogenesis of Alzheimer's disease? J Neurosci Res 1997; 50:505–513.
119. Guo Q, Furukawa K, Sopher BL, Pham DG, Robinson N, Martin GM, Mattson MP. Alzheimer's PS-1 mutation perturbs calcium homeostasis and sensitizes PC12 cells to death induced by amyloid β-peptide. NeuroReport 1996; 8:379–383.
120. Guo Q, Christakos S, Robinson N, Mattson MP. Calbindin blocks the pro-apoptotic actions of mutant presenilin-1: reduced oxidative stress and preserved mitochondrial function. Proc Natl Acad Sci USA 1998; 95: 3227–3232.
121. Guo Q, Sopher BL, Pham DG, Furukawa K, Robinson N, Martin GM, Mattson MP. Alzheimer's presenilin mutation sensitizes neural cells to apoptosis induced by trophic factor withdrawal and amyloid β-peptide: involvement of calcium and oxyradicals. J Neurosci 1997; 17:4212–4222.
122. Guo Q, Fu, W, Sopher BL, Miller MW, Ware CB, Martin GM, Mattson MP. Increased vulnerability of hippocampal neurons to excitotoxic necrosis in presenilin-1 mutant knockin mice. Nat Med 1999; 5: 101–107.
123. Kim T-W, Pettingell WH, Jung Y-K, Kovacs DM, Tanzi RE. Alternative cleavage of Alzheimer-associated presenilins during apoptosis by a caspase-3 family protease. Science 1997; 277:373–376.
124. Nishimura M, Yu G, Levesque G, Zhang DM, Ruel L, Chen F, Milman P, Holmes E, Liang Y, Kawarai T, Jo E, Supala A, Rogaeva E, Xu DM, Janus C, Levesque L, Bi Q, Duthie M, Rozmahel R, Mattila K, Lannfelt L, Westaway D, Mount HTJ, Woodgett J, Fraser PE, St. George-Hyslop P. Presenilin mutations associated with Alzheimer disease cause defective intracellular trafficking of β-catenin, component of the presenilin protein complex. Nat Med 1999; 5:164–169.
125. Dexter DT, Carter, CJ, Wells FR, Javoy-Agid F, Agid Y, Lees A, Jenner P, Marsden CD. Basal lipid peroxidation in substantia nigra is increased in Parkinson's disease. J Neurochem 1989; 52:381–389.
126. Bandmann O, Marsden CD, Wood NW. Genetic aspects of Parkinson's disease. Mov Disord 1998; 13: 203–211.
127. Langston JW. Epidemiology versus genetics in Parkinson's disease: progress in resolving an age-old debate. Ann Neurol 1998; 44:S45–S52.
128. Polymeropoulos MH, Lavedan C, Leroy E, Ide SE, Dehejia A, Dutra A, Pike B, Root H, Rubenstein J, Boyer R, Stenroos ES, Chandrasekharappa S, Athanassiadou A, Papapetropoulos T, Johnson WG, Lazzarini AM, Duvoisin RC, Di Iorio G, Golbe LI, Nussbaum RL. Mutation in the alpha-synuclein gene identified in families with Parkinson's disease. Science 1997; 276:2045–2047.
129. El-Agnaf OM, Jakes R, Curran MD, Middleton D, Ingenito R, Bianchi E, Pessi A, Neill D, Wallace A. Aggregates from mutant and wild-type alpha-synuclein proteins and NAC peptide induce apoptotic cell death in human neuroblastoma cells by formation of beta-sheet and amyloid-like filaments. FEBS Lett 1998; 440:71–75.
130. Duan W, Gash DM, Rangnekar V, Mattson MP. Participation of Par-4 in degeneration of dopaminergic neurons in models of Parkinson's disease. Ann Neurol 1999; 46:587–597.
131. Bates GP, Mangiarini L, Davies SW. Transgenic mice in the study of polyglutamine repeat expansion diseases. Brain Pathol 1998; 8:699–714.
132. Cooper JK, Schilling G, Peters MF, Herring WJ, Sharp AH, Kaminsky Z, Masone J, Khan FA, Delanoy M, Borchelt DR, Dawson VL, Dawson TM, Ross CA. Truncated N-terminal fragments of huntingtin with expanded glutamine repeats form nuclear and cytoplasmic aggregates in cell culture. Hum Mol Genet 1998; 7:783–790.
133. Cudkowicz ME, McKenna-Yasek D, Sapp PE, Chin W, Geller B, Hayden DL, Schoenfeld DA, Hosler BA, Horvitz HR, Brown RH, Jr. Epidemiology of mutations in superoxide dismutase in amyotrophic lateral sclerosis. Ann Neurol 1997; 41:210–221.
134. Wiedau-Pazos M, Goto JJ, Rabizadeh S, Gralla EB, Roe JA, Lee MK, Valentine JS, Bredesen DE. Altered reactivity of superoxide dismutase in familial amyotrophic lateral sclerosis. Science 1996; 271: 515–518.
135. Kruman I, Pedersen WA, Mattson MP. ALS-linked Cu/Zn-SOD mutation increases vulnerability of motor neurons to excitotoxicity by a mechanism involving increased oxidative stress and perturbed calcium homeostasis. Exp Neurol 1999; 160:28–39.
136. Joutel A, Corpechot C, Ducros A, Vahedi K, Chabriat H, Mouton P, Alamowitch S, Domenga V, Cecillion M, Marechal E, Maciazek J, Vayssiere C, Cruaud C, Cabanis EA, Ruchoux MM, Weissenbach J, Bach JF, Bousser MG, Tournier-Lasserve E. Notch3 mutations in CADASIL, a hereditary adult-onset condition causing stroke and dementia. Nature 1996; 383:707–710.
137. Joutel A, Vahedim K, Corpechot C, Troesch A, Hugues C, Vayssiere C, Cruaud C, Maciazek J, Weissenbach J, Bousser MG, Bach JF, Tournier-Lasserve E. Strong clustering and stereotyped nature of notch3 mutations in CADASIL patients. Lancet 1997; 350:1511–1515.
138. Weindruch RL, Walford S, Fligiel S, Guthrie D. The retardation of aging by dietary restriction: longevity, immunity and lifetime energy intake. J Nutr 1986; 116:641–654.
139. Jucker M, Ingram DK. Murine models of brain aging and age-related neurodegenerative diseases. Behav Brain Res 1997; 85:1–26.
140. Sohal RS, Ku HH, Agarwal S, Forster MJ, Lal H. Oxidative damage, mitochondrial oxidant generation and antioxidant defenses during aging and in response to food restriction in the mouse. Mech Ageing Dev 1994; 74:121–133.
141. Sohal RS, Weindruch R. Oxidative stress, caloric restriction, and aging. Science 1996; 273:59–63.
142. Lane MA, Baer DJ, Rumpler WV, Weindruch R, Ingram DK, Tilmont EM, Cutler RG, Roth GS. Cal-

orie restriction lowers body temperature in rhesus monkeys, consistent with a postulated anti-aging mechanism in rodents. Proc Natl Acad Sci USA 1996; 93:4159–4164.

143. Cefalu WT, Wagner JD, Wang ZQ, Bell-Farrow AD, Collins J, Haskell D, Bechtold R, Morgan T. A study of caloric restriction and cardiovascular aging in cynomolgus monkeys (*Macaca fascicularis*): a potential model for aging research. J Gerontol A Biol Sci Med Sci 1997; 52:B10–B19.

144. Dubey A, Forster MJ, Lal H, Sohal RS. Effect of age and caloric intake on protein oxidation in different brain regions and on behavioral functions of mouse. Arch Biochem Biophys 1996; 333:189–197.

145. Duan W, Mattson MP. Dietary restriction and 2-deoxyglucose administration improve behavioral outcome and reduce degeneration of dopaminergic neurons in models of Parkinson's disease. J Neurosci Res 1999; 57:195–206.

146. Lee J, Bruce-Keller AJ, Kruman I, Chan S, Mattson MP. 2-deoxy-D-glucose protects hippocampal neurons against excitotoxic and oxidative injury: involvement of stress proteins. J Neurosci Res 1999; 57:48–61.

147. Yu ZF, Luo H, Fu W, Mattson MP. The endoplasmic reticulum stress-responsive protein GRP78 protects neurons against excitotoxicity and apoptosis: suppression of oxidative stress and stabilization of calcium homeostasis. Exp Neurol 1999; 155:302–314.

148. Yu ZF, Mattson MP. Dietary restriction and 2-deoxyglucose administration reduce focal ischemic brain damage and improve behavioral outcome: evidence for a preconditioning mechanism. J Neurosci Res 1999; 57:830–839.

149. Finch CE, Morgan TE. Food restriction and brain aging. In: Mattson MP, Geddes JW, eds. The Aging Brain. Greenwich, CT: JAI Press. Adv Cell Aging Gerontol 1997; 2:279–297.

150. Moroi-Fetters SE, Mervis RF, London ED, Ingram DK. Dietary restriction suppresses age-related changes in dendritic spines. Neurobiol Aging 1989; 10:317–322.

151. Idrobo F, Nandy K, Mostofsky DI, Blatt L, Nandy L. Dietary restriction: effects on radial maze learning and lipofuscin pigment deposition in the hippocampus and frontal cortex. Arch Gerontol Geriatr 1987; 6:355–362.

152. Stewart J, Mitchell J, Kalant N. The effects of lifelong food restriction on spatial memory in young and aged Fischer 344 rats measured in the eight-arm radial and the Morris water mazes. Neurobiol Aging 1989; 10:669–675.

153. Pitsikas N, Algeri S. Deterioration of spatial and nonspatial reference and working memory in aged rats: protective effect of life-long calorie restriction. Neurobiol Aging 1992; 13:369–373.

154. Bruce-Keller AJ, Umberger G, McFall R, Mattson MP. Food restriction reduces brain damage and improves behavioral outcome following excitotoxic and metabolic insults. Ann Neurol 1999; 45:8–15.

155. Levin P, Janda JK, Joseph JA, Ingram DK, Roth GS. Dietary restriction retards the age-associated loss of rat striatal dopaminergic receptors. Science 1981; 214:561–562.

156. Diao LH, Bickford PC, Stevens JO, Cline EJ, Gerhardt GA. Caloric restriction enhances evoked DA overflow in striatum and nucleus accumbens of aged Fischer 344 rats. Brain Res 1997; 763:276–280.

157. Logroscino G, Marder K, Cote L, Tang MX, Shea S, Mayeux R. Dietary lipids and antioxidants in Parkinson's disease: a population-based, case–control study. Ann Neurol 1996; 39:89–94.

158. Lowenstein DH, Chan P, Miles M. The stress protein response in cultured neurons: characterization and evidence for a protective role in excitotoxicity. Neuron 1991; 7:1053–1060.

159. Lee J, Duan W, Long JM, Ingram DK, Mattson MP. Dietary restriction increases the number of newly generated neural cells, and induces BONF expression, in the dentate gyrus of rats. J Mol Neurosci 2000; 15:105–113.

160. Duan W, Lee J, Guoz, Mattson MP. Dietary restriction stimulates BONF production in the brain and thereby protects neurons against excitotoxic injury. J Mol Neurosci 2001; 16: in press.

161. Cutler R, Joseph JA, Yamagami K, Villalobos-Molina R, Roth GS. Area specific alterations in muscarinic stimulated low Km GTPase activity in aging and Alzheimer's disease: implications for altered signal transduction. Brain Res 1994; 664:54–60.

162. Deshmukh DR, Own OE, Patel MS. Effect of aging on the metabolism of pyruvate and 3-hydroxybutyrate in nonsynaptic and synaptic mitochondria from rat brain. J Neurochem 1980; 34:1219–1224.

3. In Vivo Physiologic Imaging of Cerebral Ischemia

JEAN-CLAUDE BARON

The advent of tomographic brain mapping techniques and especially of positron imaging of brain perfusion and metabolism in the late 1970s and early 1980s afforded new pathophysiologic insights into the understanding of acute cerebral ischemia, the hemodynamic and metabolic effects of carotid artery obstruction, and the neurobiological mechanisms underlying the clinical expression of stroke. Subsequent studies addressed the clinical correlates of such physiologic changes in terms of patient classification, clinical prognosis, and mechanisms of recovery. Recently, it has become possible to apply to large patient samples these concepts from positron emission tomography (PET) science, thanks to the availability of more accessible techniques such as single-photon emission computed tomography (SPECT) and stable xenon–computed tomography (Xe-CT), as well as magnetic resonance (MR)–based techniques such as proton and phosphorous spectroscopic imaging, and diffusion-weighted and perfusion imaging. The main findings will be briefly summarized in this chapter.

VARIABLES AND TECHNIQUES

Table 3–1 shows the main physiologic variables assessable by functional imaging in humans, together with their commonly used abbreviations. One hemodynamic variable not listed in Table 3–1 is the hemodynamic reserve, which expresses the vasodilatory capacity of the cerebrovascular bed, assessed with vasodilatation challenge such as inhalation of 5% CO_2 or intravenous (IV) injection of acetazolamide (Fig. 3–1)

Positron Emission Tomography

Using ^{15}O-labeled tracers such as H_2O, CO_2, CO, and O_2, and the glucose analogue ^{18}F-fluoro-2-deoxy-D-glucose (FDG), PET allows one to obtain quantitative tomographic maps of cerebral blood flow (CBF), cerebral blood volume (CBV), cerebral metabolic rate of oxygen ($CMRO_2$) and oxygen extraction fraction (OEF), and brain glucose utilization (CMRGlc), and as such is especially well suited for the investigation of ischemic stroke.[1] Access to CBF and CBV allows one to compute the CBV/CBF ratio, which represents the local circulatory mean transit time (t), and its corollary the CBF/CBV ratio, which reflects the local cerebral perfusion pressure (CPP).[2–4]

Single-Photon Emission Computed Tomography

This method of imaging is based on a tomographic principle akin to that of PET, but the use of single photons hampers the exact quantitation of physiological variables that are typical of PET and reduces the spatial resolution. Nevertheless, SPECT is a much simpler method than PET since the radiopharmaceuticals are commercially available, and the im-

Table 3–1. Physiologic Variables

Physiologic Variable	Abbreviation
Cerebral blood flow	CBF
Cerebral blood volume	CBV
Mean transit time	t
CBF/CBV ratio	CBF/CBV
Local tissue hematocrit	tHt
Cerebral metabolic rate of oxygen	$CMRO_2$
Cerebral metabolic rate of glucose	CMRGlc
Tissular pH	pHt
Oxygen extraction fraction	OEF
Glucose extraction fraction	GEF
Tissue partial O_2 tension	PtO_2

aging device is straightforward to use. Several SPECT perfusion tracers have been made available, especially ^{133}Xe, which requires the use of a dedicated tomograph but allows absolute CBF measurement, and ^{99m}Tc-hexamethyl-propyleneamine oxime (HMPAO), a nondiffusible perfusion-like radiotracer whose brain uptake is nonlinearly proportional to CBF in the normal brain, but may be dissociated from CBF in certain ischemic conditions and is difficult to quantify. Additional tracers include ^{99m}Tc-ECD, whose brain uptake appears sensitive to metabolic status as well as perfusion. In addition to perfusion, SPECT also enables the imaging of CBV, using red blood cell labeling.

Xenon–Computed Tomography

The cold Xe-CT method for measuring CBF relies on the enhancement of CT density through the use of nonradioactive xenon (inhaled at a near anesthetic dosage for several minutes) to calculate CBF on a pixel-by-pixel basis. This method has good spatial resolution but low sensitivity due to a poor signal-to-noise ratio, and is occasionally associated with cognitive side effects that have limited its use.

Specific Radiotracers

In addition to the above physiologic variables, PET also enables one to investigate specific binding sites or receptors by using, for instance, ^{11}C-flumazenil and ^{11}C-PK 11195, which serve as markers of neuronal death and glial proliferation, respectively. Corresponding SPECT tracers are now available for clinical use. Recently, ^{18}F-fluoromisonidazole has been developed as a tracer of hypoxic brain tissue and is being tested as a potential marker of the ischemic penumbra in acute stroke.[5]

NORMAL PHYSIOLOGY AND BASIC PATHOPHYSIOLOGY

Normal Brain

In physiological conditions, local values of CBF, CMRGlc, $CMRO_2$, and CBV match, according to linearly proportional relationships.[3,6] This reflects the metabolic regulation of the cerebral circulation, and explains why in physiological conditions the distribution of

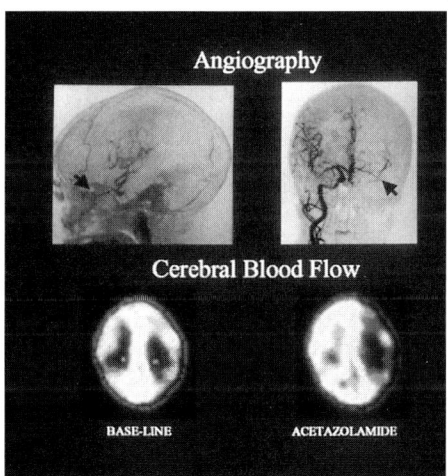

Figure 3–1. Impaired hemodynamic reserve. *Top:* Lateral view (*left*) of left carotid angiogram and anteroposterior view (*right*) of right carotid angiogram in a patient with repeated left internal carotid artery (ICA) territory transient ischemic attacks, showing left ICA occlusion with revascularization through the ipsilateral ophthalmic artery and the contralateral ICA. *Bottom:* Resting and post-acetazolamide PET scans of cerebral blood flow (CBF). Although the resting scan (*left*) showed little or no alteration in CBF in the affected hemisphere, the vasodilatation challenge with acetazolamide induced markedly asymmetric CBF (*right*). Clearly visible is a marked increase in CBF in the nonoccluded side, but a lack of increase in CBF on the occluded side along with a decrease in the posterior and anterior parts of the left carotid territory, respectively, suggests hemodynamic steal.

Table 3–2. Four Stages of Brain Hemodynamic and Metabolic Impairment as a Function of Severity in Cerebral Perfusion Pressure Drop

	Stage	CPP (%)	CBV	CBF	OEF	CMRO$_2$
1	Hemodynamic reserve (autoregulation)	60–100	moderate increase	no change	no change	no change
2	Perfusion reserve (oligemia)	40–60	marked increase	mild decrease	moderate increase	no change
3	Metabolic reserve (ischemic penumbra)	20–40	moderate increase	marked decrease	marked increase	mild-to-moderate decrease
4	Irreversible damage (ischemic necrosis)	< 20	decrease	very severe decrease	variable	marked decrease

CBF, cerebral blood flow; CBV, cerebral blood volume; CMRO$_2$, cerebral metabolic rate of oxygen; CPP, cerebral perfusion pressure; OEF, oxygen extraction fraction.

CBF is superimposable on that of CMRO$_2$ and CMRGlc.

Autoregulation and Hemodynamic Failure

Shown in Table 3–2 are the main hemodynamic and metabolic changes that occur in response to a fall in the CPP distal to an arterial obstruction; these stages are subdivided into four stages of increasing severity. The marked increase in CBV during the phase of *autoregulation* reflects the physiologic vasodilatation of resistance vessels, i.e., the hemodynamic reserve. As soon as the CPP falls below the lower threshold of autoregulation, the CBF starts to decline, but the CMRO$_2$ at first remains unaltered. This flow–metabolism uncoupling, which translates as a focal increase in the OEF up to the theoretical maximum of 1.00, has been termed "misery perfusion"[7] (Fig. 3–2). In the moderate stage of misery perfusion, the brain is able to maintain its CMRO$_2$ despite reduced CBF, although at the expense of tissue hypoxia (Fig. 3–2). During this phase, or *oligemia*, the perfusion reserve is called on. If the CPP drops further, neuronal function becomes impaired and the CMRO$_2$ falls despite maximally increased OEF, characterizing true ischemia, which comprises a reversible stage (the *ischemic penumbra*, see Fig. 3–3) and an irreversible one (*ischemic necrosis*, see Fig. 3–4).

Luxury Perfusion

Luxury perfusion is characterized by an oxygen supply in excess of demand,[8] and its hallmark is a focal reduction of the OEF.[9] It indicates full or partial re-establishment of perfusion within an ischemic or already irreversibly damaged tissue (Fig. 3–5). In luxury perfusion, the CBF may be increased (hyperperfusion), normal, or even decreased (relative luxury perfusion), although by definition in excess of prevailing CMRO$_2$, which itself may be normal, increased, or reduced.

LONG-STANDING ARTERIAL OBSTRUCTION: MAPPING HEMODYNAMIC FAILURE

The original observation of misery perfusion was in a patient with carotid artery occlusion and continuing reversible ischemic attacks, some triggered by orthostatism.[7] Since then, numerous imaging studies have documented that internal carotid artery disease may have hemodynamic consequences on the distal cerebral vascular bed.[2,10] The severity of such consequences is related both to the degree of obstruction (i.e., only > 50% stenosis or occlusion may have measurable effects) and to the compensation afforded by the circle of Willis (with the most marked effects seen when compensation is essentially or exclusively via the ipsilateral ophthalmic artery).

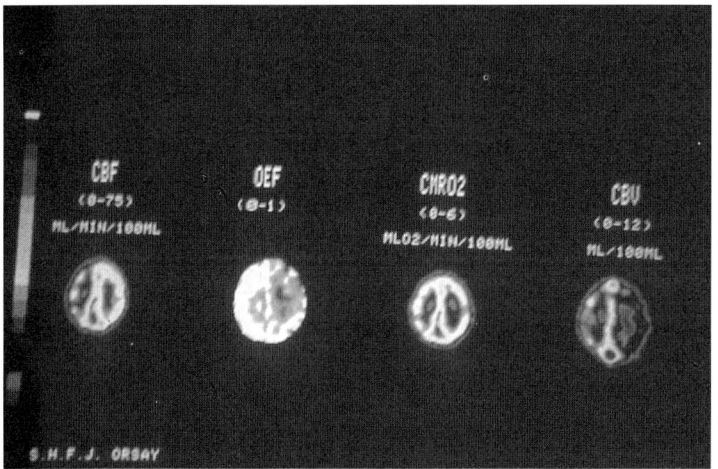

Figure 3–2. Misery perfusion: stage 2 of hemodynamic failure. Occlusion of the right internal carotid artery was diagnosed following an ipsilateral transient ischemic attack (TIA). Repeated TIAs followed despite closely supervised antiplatelet and then anticoagulant treatment. Some of the TIAs were triggered up on standing. Positron emission tomography (PET) performed several weeks later showed moderate hypoperfusion in the territory of the right carotid artery with a completely normal cerebral metabolic rate of oxygen ($CMRO_2$). As a result, the oxygen extraction function (OEF) was increased, causing "misery perfusion." These data suggest the inability of the collateral circulation to compensate fully for occlusion of the carotid artery, and that the pressure of the blood supply to the brain downstream of the circle of Willis is insufficient to maintain cerebral blood flow (CBF) (i.e., the local autoregulation mechanism has been overcome). This interpretation is supported by the observation of a marked increase in the cerebral blood volume on the side of the occlusion.

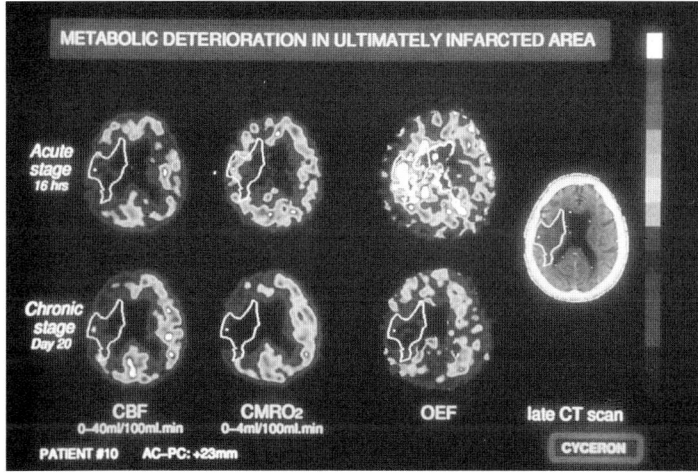

Figure 3–3. Acute misery perfusion (ischemic penumbra). Positron emission tomographic (PET) studies of cerebral blood flow (CBF), cerebral metabolic flow of oxygen ($CMRO_2$), and oxygen extraction function (OEF) performed 16 hr (*top row*) and 20 days (*bottom row*) after onset of middle cerebral artery (MCA) territory ischemic stroke in a 69-year-old patient, and co-registered late CT scan showing the contours of the hypodense lesion. In the acute stage, there is an area of misery-perfusion with markedly reduced CBF and increased OEF, but essentially unchanged $CMRO_2$, findings that are compatible with penumbra, i.e., pattern 2 of Marchal et al.[22] Part of this area also suffered metabolic deterioration at follow-up PET and infarction at late CT, indicating that this tissue was indeed at-risk. Note that parts of the ischemic tissue in the periphery escaped infarction despite similar physiology acutely. Note also the striking reversal of the OEF in the area destined to infarction, from very high acutely to very low subacutely.

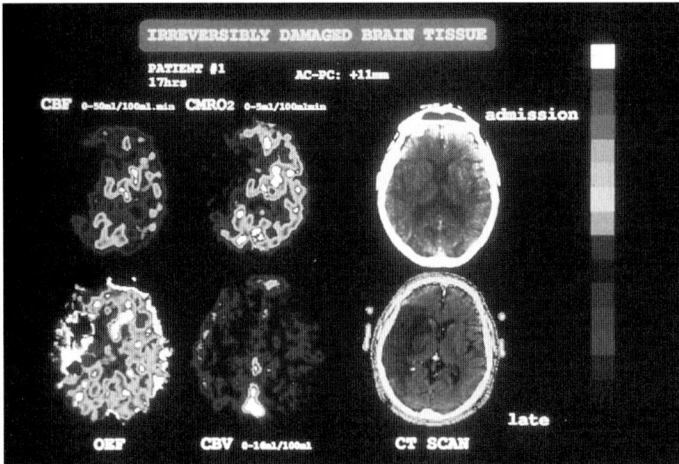

Figure 3–4. Early irreversible damage. Quantitative positron emission tomographic (PET) images of cerebral blood flow (CBF), cerebral metabolic rate of oxygen (CMRO$_2$), oxygen extraction fraction (OEF), and cerebral blood volume(CBV), obtained at the level of the basal ganglia in a 77-year-old patient, 17 hr after onset of right-sided middle cerebral artery (MCA) territory stroke. On the *right* are CT scans of this patient obtained at admission (*top*) and about 1 month later (*bottom*, co-registered three-dimensionally with PET). There was near-zero CBF and CMRO$_2$ in the whole affected (MCA) territory together with patchy OEF (black pixels represent unmeasurable OEF), representing presumably irreversible damage. The patient made a poor recovery and the initially severely hypometabolic area was infarcted at follow-up CT scan (*right*). This example illustrates pattern 1 of Marchal et al.[22]

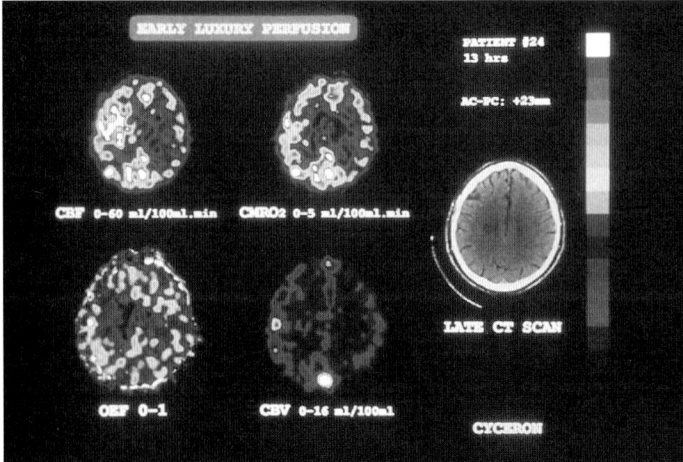

Figure 3–5. Early luxury-perfusion (spontaneous hyperfusion). Quantitative positron emission tomographic (PET) images of cerebral blood flow (CBF), cerebral metabolic rate of oxygen (CMRO$_2$), oxygen extraction fraction (OEF), and cerebral blood volume (CBV) obtained at the level of the corona radiata in a 61-year-old patient 15 hr after onset of left hemiparesis presumably due to right middle cerebral artery (MCA) embolism of cardiac origin. The pseudocolor scale in these images ranges from zero to a maximum pixel value of 60 ml/100 ml/min; and 16 ml/100 ml for CBF, CMRO$_2$, OEF, and CBV, respectively; the right side of the brain is on the reader's left side. The data demonstrate an area of increased perfusion with absolute hyperemia, documenting early reperfusion of previously ischemic tissue. The CMRO$_2$ is preserved or even slightly increased in the hyperperfused regions, which were morphologically intact at follow-up CT scan (obtained at day 62 post-stroke). This example illustrates pattern 3 of Marchal et al.[22]

Similar effects have been reported in patients with long-standing middle cerebral artery (MCA) stem stenosis or occlusion. The hemodynamic effects observed, which reflect the extent to which the CPP is reduced, range from simply autoregulated (Fig. 3–1) to true oligemia (Fig 3–2). Whatever their severity, these changes predominate in watershed (borderzone) territories. Furthermore, focal chronic misery perfusion has been documented to forerun the development of watershed infarction in some patients with tight carotid artery stenosis or occlusion.[11,12]

Although the clinical correlates of these hemodynamic changes can be straightforward, as in the rare instances of orthostatic transient ischemic attacks, they occasionally are difficult to ascertain. However, a relationship exists between the presence of high OEF and the occurrence of ipsilateral ischemic symptoms.[3] Several recent studies, including a prospective one,[14] indicate that, if cerebrovascular reactivity is severely impaired, there is a significantly increased risk of ipsilateral stroke despite the best medical treatment, which suggests that surgical revascularization may be warranted in such cases. Indeed, it has been amply documented that successful cerebral revascularization at least partially reverses the preoperatively observed hemodynamic compromise.[7,15-17] However, it has also been suggested that patients with the most compromised cerebrovascular physiology may also be those most at risk of perioperative complications such as low-pressure breakthrough of autoregulation (presumably as a result of long-term dysregulation of the cerebral circulation).[18] Thus, the results from functional imaging of each candidate for revascularization surgery need to be weighed carefully in relation to other clinical and instrumental data to assess the risk/benefit ratio of the surgical procedure under consideration.

ACUTE ISCHEMIC STROKE: MAPPING THE CORE, THE PENUMBRA, AND THE REPERFUSED TISSUE

By convention, the acute stage of stroke will be defined in the following discussion as the first 24 hr after onset of clinical symptoms, because available evidence suggests that this is the maximal time frame within which salvageable tissue may still be present.

Positron Emission Tomography Studies

Three findings in acute MCA territory stroke have been investigated in detail with respect to both their time course and their prognostic value for tissue and clinical outcome: the core of irreversibly damaged tissue, the penumbral tissue, and the hyperperfused tissue.

THE IRREVERSIBLY DAMAGED TISSUE

This tissue has been defined by means of PET as having a $CMRO_2$ below a threshold of about 1.4 ml/100 ml/min for gray matter regions,[6,19] or about 0.9 ml/100 ml/min for any voxel in brain tissue.[20] In a large proportion of patients, irreversible damage occurs very early in the striatocapsular area, in most instances in association with cortical misery perfusion.[21,22] Presumably because of the poor collaterals in the lenticulostriate territory, unlike in the cerebral cortex, this area constitutes the core of ischemia and rapidly suffers irreversible damage. However, in a subset of patients, the area of irreversible damage affects extensive parts of the cortical territory only hours into the stroke,[22] which suggests inadequate pial collaterals (Fig. 3–4). The profoundly hypometabolic areas express variable CBF and, in turn, variable OEF. In most instances, however, the CBF is also profoundly reduced, but partial reperfusion with variably reduced or even essentially normal CBF is occasionally encountered, especially in small deep infarcts.[23]

Marchal et al.[20] found that the volume of profoundly hypometabolic tissue as assessed by PET 5–18 hr post-onset of stroke was highly linearly correlated to final infarct volume, as measured by CT scan about 1 month later; the former, however, underestimated the latter by a factor of 2, because of subsequent metabolic deterioration of the surrounding penumbra (see below). Thus, mapping the profoundly hypometabolic tissue in the acute stage of stroke may provide an early assessment of already established damage and predict a *minimum* volume of final infarction.

PENUMBRAL TISSUE

One major finding from PET studies in both humans and in the baboon with MCA occlusion has been the demonstration, hours into the episode, of wide zones of cortex with still critically ischemic tissue[9,21,24] (Fig. 3–3). This tissue is characterized by reduced CBF (below the penumbral threshold of ~20 ml/100 g/min), massively increased OEF (usually above 0.80), and mildly to moderately reduced $CMRO_2$ (i.e., above the threshold for irreversibility described earlier). These alterations are consistent with at-risk but still recuperable (i.e., penumbral) tissue. Substantial cortical penumbra, reflecting efficient pial collaterals, has been reported in over 50% of patients studied within 9 hr of onset, in up to 25% of cases at 24 hr, and occasionally until 30 hr post-onset, suggesting a protracted window for therapeutic opportunity in a fraction of acute stroke cases. In one study, it was found that up to 52% of the ultimately infarcted tissue still exhibited physiological characteristics compatible with penumbra as late as 16 hr after onset of symptoms; this finding suggests that even delayed neuroprotection might have significantly altered the functional outcome in such cases.[23]

The transition of such "penumbral" areas to infarction has been documented within hours to days (Fig.3–3), and is signaled by a decline in $CMRO_2$ regardless of the local CBF, which may decline in parallel, remain stable, or even, at times, increase.[21,25,26] Within days, perfusion increases progressively in the necrotic tissue, representing neovascularization in the necrotic tissue, before decreasing again in the finally cavitated area.[9,27] This whole process is strikingly illustrated by the associated dramatic fall in the OEF, from initially very high to increasingly low values, signaling the exhaustion of the tissue's oxygen needs. Such a deleterious course of events does not always take place, however, and all or part of the penumbral tissue may eventually escape infarction,[25,28,29] consistent with the potential for reversibility that characterizes the penumbra. In this event, one hypothesis is that some favorable event (e.g., partial reperfusion) occurred after the PET study to save part or all of this tissue, a hypothesis recently confirmed in PET investigations of baboons.[24,30]

EARLY SPONTANEOUS HYPERPERFUSION

Early hyperperfusion, which suggests recanalization of the occluded artery, has been observed in up to one-third of cases studied between the fifth and the 18th hr after stroke onset[22,31] (Fig. 3–5). In most of the cases, hyperperfusion is not associated with reduced metabolism, but instead with a mildly increased $CMRO_2$, suggesting postischemic rebound of cellular energy-dependent processes.[26] However, the OEF is significantly reduced and the CBV significantly increased in these areas, indicating luxury perfusion with abnormal vasodilatation. In a sample of 10 such patients, no instance of MCA stem occlusion was recorded on transcranial Doppler examination, and the hyperperfused areas consistently exhibited intact morphology at chronic-stage CT.[26] Spontaneous recanalization of the occluded MCA artery may have occurred at some undefined time point before the PET study, resulting in efficient reperfusion of the previously ischemic and dysregulated, but still viable, tissue. Thus, contrary to the concept that sudden tissue reoxygenation might exacerbate ischemic damage, these findings in humans suggest that, consistent with some findings from animal studies, postischemic hyperperfusion is not detrimental (see ref. 32 for review). This is in turn consistent with the well-established notion that infarct size is reduced by early recanalization.

CLINICAL CORRELATES

Marchal et al.[22,31] conducted a prospective study in which the relationships between acute-stage PET findings and clinical outcome, were assessed. In their study of 30 patients with first-ever MCA territory stroke investigated with PET within 18 hr of symptom onset, each patient could be classified into one of three patterns of PET changes (Fig. 3–3 to 3–5), namely (1) pattern 1, characterized by a large subcorticocortical area of already extensive necrosis; (2) pattern 2, characterized by the presence of presumably penumbral tissue without associated irreversible damage, except possibly in the lenticulostriate area; and

(3) pattern 3, characterized by hyperperfusion without associated irreversible damage, except, again, possibly in a small area. There was a statistically highly significant relationship between PET patterns and subsequent neurological course. Thus, all patients classified as pattern 1 did poorly (early death from massive infarct, or poor outcome), while all patients classified as pattern 3 did well (complete or nearly complete recovery in all); patients classified as pattern 2 had a variable course, ranging from death to full recovery. These findings from functional imaging analysis are consistent with evidence from clinical studies that early recanalization is associated with rapid recovery, whereas persistence of MCA trunk occlusion is a risk factor for poor outcome and massive brain swelling. Consistent findings regarding hyperperfusion have been reported by Heiss et al.[33] who showed in a few cases both pre- and post-early IV thrombolysis that the occurrence of hyperperfusion was associated with good clinical and tissular outcome, unlike severe and persisting hypoperfusion.

ALLEVIATION OF PENUMBRA: ITS ROLE IN CLINICAL RECOVERY

Alleviation of penumbra has long been hypothesized as one major mechanism underlying early recovery from ischemic stroke. However, only recently was this mechanism directly documented in a quantitative way.[28] In Marchal et al.'s[31] sample, the degree of neurological recovery over the succeeding 2 months was positively correlated with the individual volume of acute-stage penumbral tissue that escaped infarction, as assessed by chronic stage CT. Somewhat unexpectedly, the best correlation was observed with 2-month recovery scores, which suggests that survival of the penumbra influences not only early but also late recovery. The hypothesis given to explain this finding was that survival of the penumbra not only allows for early return of function in the peri-infarct tissue but also provides an important opportunity for subsequent neural reorganization processes, in a synergistic rather than simply acumulative way. Thus, survival of the penumbra would appear to be an important early mechanism for subsequent functional recovery. Confirmatory results were reported recently by Heiss et al.[29] who found a significant positive relationship between the reduction in volume of critically hypoperfused tissue between pre-thrombolysis and post-thrombolysis PET, and the change in neurological scores between admission and 3 weeks.

Perfusion Studies with Single-Photon Emission Computed Tomography and Xenon–Computed Tomography

Because of the logistics involved, ^{133}Xe SPECT has been applied very little in studying acute stroke. Thus, essentially all studies have employed semiquantitative perfusion radiotracers, essentially ^{99m}Tc-HMPAO and, more recently, ^{99m}Tc-ECD. Overall, the findings have been consistent with the results described above from the PET studies, although with less accuracy due to poor spatial resolution, problems with reliability of the tracers as markers of perfusion, and lack of metabolic data. In close to 100% of patients with MCA territory stroke, acute-stage SPECT revealed a focally reduced tracer uptake, the extent of which was proportional to the severity of the neurological deficit assessed at the same time. Severe and extensive tracer hypofixation is almost invariably predictive of persistent MCA occlusion with subsequent large or malignant infarction,[34,35] while mild or moderate hypoperfusion carries a variable outcome but excludes death.[34,36] Profound hypoperfusion is also associated with increased risk of massive hemorrhagic transformation[37] or no reflow[38] following therapeutic thrombolysis. Conversely, normal uptake (with or without mild hyperfixation) is invariably associated with reversible neurological deficits.[34,39] Well-demarcated areas of massively increased tracer uptake appear to predict subsequent infarction,[40] but such hot spots may not necessarily represent true hyperperfusion but rather abnormal penetration of HMPAO in brain parenchyma due to an altered blood–brain barrier in an already severely damaged tissue.[41]

Either spontaneous or thrombolysis-induced early reperfusion of previously hypoperfused tissue is associated with better outcome,[38,42] and spectacular recovery is associated with complete, extensive reperfusion.[43] However, when the repeat SPECT is done >36–48 hr after onset, reperfusion may not always indicate good outcome because it may have occurred too late, in an already necrotic tissue.[44]

Studies with Xe-CT in acute MCA territory stroke are entirely consistent with the above findings from PET and SPECT. Thus, patients with normal or near-normal CBF had spontaneous resolution of their deficits, while those with considerably reduced CBF in the affected territories developed severe brain edema and herniation.[45,46]

Implications for Management and Therapy

All the above findings have major implications for management of the patient with acute stroke patient as well as for the design of pathophysiology-driven therapeutic trials in acute stroke. An especially important use of imaging studies is to provide an individual pathophysiologic diagnosis upon which decisions about therapy and medical management should ideally be based.[47]

REMOTE METABOLIC EFFECTS OF STROKE

Remote metabolic depression is characterized by coupled reductions in perfusion and metabolism in brain structures remote from, but connected with, the area damaged by the stroke. This effect is widely explained as depressed synaptic activity as a result of disconnection (either direct or transneural). Thus, through remote effects the disruption in distributed networks as a result of focal infarction can be tracked. Although these effects are often referred to collectively as "diaschisis,"[48] this term conceals a variety of cellular derangements, from reversible hypofunction to evolving Wallerian or transsynaptic degeneration, which all have the same PET expression. Importantly, some of these effects reflect purely functional, potentially recoverable synaptic derangement that may participate in both the acute clinical expression of stroke and the recovery from it.

Crossed Cerebellar Diaschisis

This phenomenon,[49] also known as "crossed cerebellar hypometabolism" (CCH), consists in a matched reduction in both perfusion and metabolism in the cerebellar hemisphere contralateral to supratentorial stroke (Fig. 3–6). It occurs in about 50% of patients with either cortical or subcortical stroke but is more frequent and severe with large hemispheric infarcts or with capsular stroke.[50] Evidence indicates CCH results from damage to the glutamatergic corticopontocerebellar system (CPCS), inducing transneuronal functional depression, although in rare instances it may result from retrograde cerebello-cortical effects.[51] Although CCH is correlated with both the presence and severity of hemiparesis,[50] this association is not systematic, and presumably merely reflects the anatomic intimacy of the pyramidal and corticopontine fibers. Observations of CCH after unilateral brain stem lesion at the level of the crus cerebri or basis pontis further support the CPCS mechanism.

In the vast majority of patients, CCH exhibits no tendency toward recovery,[27,50] and this chronicity suggests that CCH might evolve into transneuronal degeneration in the long run. However, the fact that CCH may develop within the first hours of stroke and subsequently disappear within a few days[52] indicates that it can also be a transient manifestation of deafferentation. This is further documented by the fact that CCH can transiently manifest in instances of reversible functional depression of the cerebral cortex, such as transient ischemic attacks, unilateral carotid infusion of barbiturates in epileptic patients,[53] or balloon occlusion of the internal carotid artery.[54] Finally, even in cases with chronic CCH from MCA stroke, crossed cerebellar atrophy is not demonstrated by MRI, even though ipsilateral atrophy of the cerebral peduncle is occasionally seen, which documents CPCS damage.[55]

Regarding the predictive value for neurological outcome, it has been shown that a lack of CCH in the acute stage of MCA territory stroke predicts good outcome, while its presence has little predictive value.[52] A relationship between CCH and ipsilateral ataxia would seem straightforward and has been reported anecdotally.[56] However, other studies indicate a lack of one-to-one association be-

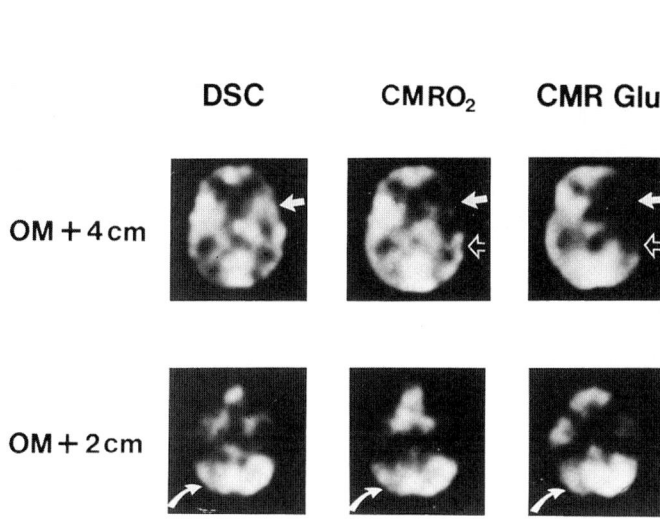

Figure 3-6. Crossed cerebellar diaschisis. Quantitative images of cerebral blood flow (CBF), cerebral metabolic rate of oxygen(CMRO$_2$), and cerebral metabolic rate of glucose (CMRGlc) obtained at two brain levels in a 37-year-old patient 6 days after massive right middle cerebral artery (MCA) infarction due to cardiac embolism. On these images, the right side of the brain is on the reader's right. The data show on level OM+ 4 cm a profoundly reduced CMRO$_2$ and CMRGlc in the infarcted area associated with a heterogeneous CBF showing combined areas of markedly reduced, moderately reduced, and increased flow (luxury perfusion, straight arrows). On level OM + 2 cm, a proportional reduction in flow, oxygen consumption, and glucose utilization in the entire left cerebellar hemisphere (crossed cerebellar diaschisis), demonstrating primary metabolic depression, is seen. This represents a remote transneuronal effect of right middle cerebral artery (MCA) infarction, which damages the crossed corticopontocerebellar pathway.

tween ataxia and CCH,[51] indicating that only ataxia due to CPCS damage will translate into CCH. Apart from ataxia, a significant relationship between CCH and ipsilateral flaccidity has been reported,[57] but again, this was not a one-to-one association.

Contralateral Cerebral Effects

Although contralateral cerebral effects have long been thought to underlie some "diffuse" symptoms of acute supratentorial stroke (such as agitation, confusion, and coma) and to exacerbate focal deficit, they have been difficult to document in either human or animal models because of many confounding factors—above all, the lack of adequate controls and the frequent use of CBF as the variable, despite this parameter's intrinsic variability. A recent study showed no relationship between changes in contralateral hemisphere CMRO$_2$ and early changes in neurological deficits.[58] Evidence is accumulating, however, that contralateral hemisphere hypometabolism develops in the subacute stage of MCA stroke, dissociated from the clinical recovery that takes place at this stage, and presumably this reflects the degeneration of severed transcallosal fibers.[58,59] Some data support the idea that in the chronic stage, slow recovery from contralateral hemisphere hypometabolism takes place and underlies late improvements in cognitive deficits.[59-61]

Subcortico Cortical Effects

SUBCORTICAL APHASIA

Earlier reports of mildly reduced cortical CMRGlc in small, deep infarcts[62,63] suggested that some aspects of language impairment of subcortical origin could be related to this remote effect. This was confirmed by findings showing significant hypometabolism of the whole left cortical mantle in patients with verbal impairment from left thalamic or thalamocapsular stroke[60] (Fig. 3-7). Metter et al.[64] documented that although the subcortical lesion itself did have a direct relation to some of the aphasia measures, left frontal and temporal hypometabolism played an indirect role in verbal fluency and comprehension tasks, respectively. Karbe et al.[65] also found a positive correlation between impairment in several aphasia items (oral and written comprehension, naming, and repetition) and left parietotemporal hypometabolism.

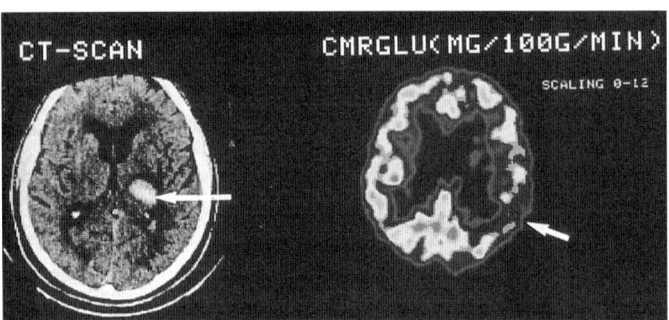

Figure 3–7. Thalamocortical diaschisis. In this chronically hypertensive patient who presented with sudden-onset right hemiparesis and speech difficulties, the CT scan (right-hand side) shows high density in the left thalamocapsular area (arrows) due to hemorrhage. The PET scan performed 2 weeks later to investigate cerebral glucose uptake shows hypometabolism in the left parietal and temporal cortex (arrows, in the axial plane at the level of the corona radiata). This phenomenon provides a mechanism for the speech difficulties of the patient, as it documents dysfunction of the thalamocortical system.

SUBCORTICAL NEGLECT

Marked ipsilateral cortical hypometabolism has been consistently reported after right-sided subcortical infarcts with left hemineglect.[60,66,67] Predominance of these effects over the frontal and parietal cortices, especially in the case of prominent motor hemineglect,[68] suggests involvement of the subcorticocortical network for directed attention, which involves parietofrontal interactions. Consistent with thin interpretation, motor neglect is characterized by sparing of the primary motor circuit (striatum, cerebellum, and motor strip) but hypometabolism of the "supramotor" circuit (i.e., premotor, prefrontal, cingulate, and parietal cortices).[69]

HEMIANOPIA

Damage to optic radiations induces a significant reduction in glucose utilization in the disconnected part of the ipsilateral primary visual cortex,[70] sometimes spreading to the visual association areas and even to the contralateral visual cortex.[71]

THALAMO-CORTICAL DIASCHISIS

As stated above, even small unilateral infarcts in the anterior, medial, or lateral thalamus almost invariably induce a metabolic depression of the entire ipsilateral cortical mantle, with lesser effects contralaterally.[60,72,73] Accentuation of this diffuse effect in the projection area corresponding to the apparent nuclear topography of the thalamic infarct suggests involvement of the thalamocortical excitatory projections from the intralaminar, anterior, ventral, and mediodorsal nuclei. A relation between cognitive impairment and cortical hypometabolism after thalamic stroke is supported by findings that, following ventrolateral thalamotomy, the decline in ipsilateral neocortical hypometabolism correlates significantly with the decline in cognitive performance.[60] Accordingly, posterolateral thalamic infarcts with pure sensorimotor stroke do not exhibit significant cortical hypometabolism.[74] As noted above, there are also significant relationships between the pattern of cortical hypometabolism and the aphasia profile or hemineglect after thalamic stroke.[60] Furthermore, preferential frontal cortex hypometabolism has been associated with frontal-like syndromes and global amnesia after right- or left-sided thalamic infarction.[72,73] In the bilateral paramedial thalamic infarction syndrome, which includes severe permanent amnesia and apathy, marked neocortical hypometabolism has been reported, which is consistent with the idea that thalamocortical deafferentation underlies "thalamic dementia."[75] Bogousslavsky et al[76] described isolated apathy in two patients with this syndrome, both of whom exhibited predominantly bifrontal hypoperfusion; this finding is consistent with the notion that the prefrontal–striatal–pallidal–thalamic loops play an important role in the control of behavior.

Ipsilateral Effects

Striatal and thalamic hypometabolism ipsilateral to corticosubcortical stroke is a frequent finding.[9,55,62] Thalamic hypometabolism develops a few days after the stroke and presumably represents active retrograde degeneration of the damaged thalamocortical neurons, while striatal hypometabolism probably reflects loss of glutamatergic input from the cortex. Left caudate and thalamic hypometabolism are significantly associated with Broca's (i.e., nonfluent) aphasia, but not with Wernicke's or conduction aphasia.[77] Thalamic hypometabolism has been associated with poor recovery of hand function after ischemic stroke.[78]

Ipsilateral cortical effects have been documented not only in case of subcortical stroke, as described above, but also after corticosubcortical infarcts, and the mechanism involved is disconnection via corticocortical pathways.[79,80]

Role of Cortical Hypometabolism in Behavioral Recovery from Stroke

Following subcortical stroke, both bilateral cortical metabolic depression and asymmetry tend to recover in an exponential fashion over the ensuing months, paralleling cognitive recovery.[60,81,82] Thus, following early transsynaptic depression, some mechanism of synaptic reorganization that underlies recovery from cognitive impairment slowly creeps in. Karbe et al.[83] found that patients with lesser defects in resting CMRGlc around Wernicke's and Broca's areas in the subacute stage of stroke had better outcome in terms of language comprehension and verbal fluency, respectively. An extensive longitudinal investigation of the relationship between cortical hypoperfusion and language performance in a large cohort of aphasic stroke patients (both cortical and subcortical) showed that initial language recovery within the first year post-onset[61] may be linked primarily to functional recovery in the dominant hemisphere, where an increase in CBF was observed at 9 months post-onset. The increased perfusion adjacent to the lesion may be crucial for early recovery from aphasia; this finding is consistent with that of Furlan et al.[28] regarding the fate of the penumbra as discussed above. Subsequent language recovery and long-term recovery in patients with aphasia may be related to slow and gradual compensatory functions in the contralateral hemisphere, specifically in the homotopic frontal and thalamic areas.[84] Taken together, the results from these investigations suggest that recovery of cortical metabolism, both ipsilateral and contralateral, at least in part subtends functional recovery after stroke and is one expression of neuronal reorganization after network damage.

White Matter Stroke and Subcortical Dementia

Studies of isolated white matter stroke, have shown an association between hypometabolism of the overlying cortex, which occurs as a result of disconnection, and cognitive impairment,[51] such as frontal lobe syndrome after capsular genu infarction[85] and neglect or aphasia after partial anterior choroidal artery stroke.[67] Similarly, leukoaraiosis, even when extensive, does not seem to greatly affect cortical metabolism unless cognitive impairment is present.[86-88] Accordingly, in Binswanger's dementia, neocortical metabolism is severely depressed, especially in the frontal lobe.[89] This finding also applies to bilateral paramedian thalamic infarction,[75] further highlighting the importance of strategic damage to subcorticocortical networks in the development of cognitive impairment of vascular origin.

RECEPTOR STUDIES IN VASCULAR DISORDERS

Neuronal Marker

^{11}C-flumazenil is an ideal potential in vivo marker of neuronal loss because it binds to the central benzodiazepine receptor, which is borne only by neurons, and is part of the GABA-A complex, which has widespread brain distribution. In both experimental and clinical stroke, loss of ^{11}C-flumazenil binding occurs hours after arterial occlusion in the ischemic core.[90,91] Several studies of the chronic stage have reported decreases in cortical binding of ^{11}C-flumazenil or its SPECT analog, ^{123}I-iomazenil, including in areas not showing frank infarction on structural imaging.[92] This finding has been taken as evidence for selective neuronal loss in the overlying cortex, which might in turn explain the neuropsychological deficits after subcortical infarction, e.g., language impairment; thus, benzodiazepine receptor imaging may enable the distinction of cortical dysfunction induced by diaschisis from that due to occult cortical damage. However, the finding of reduced flumazenil uptake in the cerebral cortex after striatocapsular infarction is not universal,[93] and histopathologic confirmation of neuronal loss has thus far been lacking. A recent experimental investigation using baboons suggested that reduced ^{11}C-flumazenil uptake in cortical zones overlying striato capsular infarction may not always correspond to cell loss,[94] and thus may reflect other functional processes, such as those resulting from deafferentation.

Glial Marker

[11]C-PK 11195 is a ligand of the peripheral benzodiazepine receptor, which is borne by microglia and macrophages and, as such, may be a good marker of glial proliferation after stroke. This hypothesis has been confirmed by studies in both humans and nonhuman primates, in which progressively increasing ^{11}C-PK11195 uptake occurred within the infarct that peaked at around 10–15 days.[90,95]

REFERENCES

1. Baron JC, Frackowiak RSJ, Herholz K, Jones T, Lammertsma AA, Mazoyer BM, Wienhardt K. Use of positron emission tomography in the investigation of cerebral hemodynamics and energy metabolism in cerebrovascular disease. J Cereb Blood Flow Metabol 1989; 9:723–742.
2. Gibbs JM, Wise RJS, Leenders KL, Jones T. Evaluation of cerebral perfusion reserve in patients with carotid-artery occlusion. Lancet 1984; 1:310–314.
3. Sette G, Baron JC, Mazoyer B, Levasseur M, Pappata S, Crouzel C. Local brain hemodynamics and oxygen metabolism in cerebro-vascular disease: positron emission tomography. Brain 1989; 112:931–951.
4. Schumann P, Touzani O, Young AR, Morello R, Baron JC, MacKenzie ET. Evaluation of the ratio of cerebral blood flow to cerebral blood volume as an index of local cerebral perfusion pressure. Brain 1998; 121:1369–1379.
5. Read SJ, Hirano T, Abbott DF, Sachinidis JI, Tochon-Danguy HJ, Chan JG, Egan GF, Scott AM, Bladin CF, McKay WJ, Donnan GA. Identifying hypoxic tissue after acute ischemic stroke using PET and 18F-fluoromisonidazole. Neurology, 1998; 51:1617–1621.
6. Baron JC, Rougemont D, Soussaline F, Bustany P, Crouzel C, Bousser MG, Comar D. Local inter relationship of cerebral oxygen consumption and glucose utilization in normal subjects and in ischemic stroke patients: a positron tomography study. Cereb Blood Flow Metab 1984; 4:140–149.
7. Baron JC, Bousser MG, Rey A, Guillard A, Comar D, Castaigne P. Reversal of focal "misery-perfusion syndrome" by extra-intracranial arterial bypass in hemodynamic cerebral ischemia: a case study with [15]O positron tomography. Stroke 1981; 12:454–459.
8. Lassen NA. The luxury perfusion syndrome and its possible relation to acute metabolic acidosis localised within the brain. Lancet 1966; 2:1113–1115.
9. Baron JC, Bousser MG, Comar D, Soussaline F, Castaigne P. Noninvasive tomographic study of cerebral blood flow and oxygen metabolism in vivo: potentials, limitations and clinical applications in cerebral ischemic disorders. Eur Neurol 1981; 20:273–284.
10. Powers WJ, Press GA, Grubb RL, Gado M, Raichle ME. The effect of hemodynamically significant carotid artery disesase on the hemodynamic status of the cerebral circulation. Ann Intern Med 1987; 106: 27–35.
11. Itoh M, Hatazawa J, Pozzilli C, Matsuzawa T, Abe Y, Fukuda H, Fujiwara T, Watanuki S, Ido T. Positron CT imaging of an impending stroke. *Neuroradiology* 1988; 30:276–279.
12. Yamauchi H, Fukuyama H, Fujimoto N, Nabatame H, Kimura J. Significance of low perfusion with increased oxygen extraction fraction in a case of internal carotid artery stenosis. Stroke 1992; 23:431–432.
13. Derdeyn CP, Yundt KD, Videen TO, Carpenter DA, Grubb RL, Powers WJ. Increased oxygen extraction fraction is associated with prior ischemic events in patients with carotid occlusion. Stroke 1998; 29:754–758.
14. Powers WJ, Derdeyn CP, Yundt KD, Carpenter DA, Videen TO, Fritsch SM, Spitznagel EL, Grubb RL. PET predicts subsequent stroke in patients with symptomatic carotid occlusion. Neurology 1998; 50: A195.
15. Gibbs JM, Wise RJS, Thomas DJ, Mansfield AU, Ross Russel RW. Cerebral haemodynamic changes after extracranial-intracranial bypass surgery. J Neurol Neurosurg Psychiatry 1987; 50:140–150.
16. Powers WJ, Martin WRW, Herscovitch P, Raichle ME, Grubb RL. Extracranial-intracranial bypass surgery: hemodynamic and metabolic effects. Neurology 1984; 34:1168–1174.
17. Samson Y, Baron JC, Bousser MG, Rey A, Derlon JM, David P, Comoy J. Effects of extra-intracranial arterial bypass on cerebral blood flow and oxygen metabolism in humans. Stroke 1985; 16:609–616.
18. Derlon JM, Bouvard G, Viader F, Petit MC, Dupuy B, Khoury S, Thenint JP, Houtteville JP. Impaired cerebral hemodynamics in internal carotid occlusion. Cerebrovasc Disord 2:72–81.
19. Powers WJ, Grubb RL Jr, Darriet D, Raichle ME. Cerebral blood flow and cerebral metabolic rate of oxygen requirements for cerebral function and viability in humans. J Cereb Blood Flow Metab 1985; 5: 600–608.
20. Marchal G, Benali K, Iglesias S, Viader F, Derlon JM, Baron JC. Voxel-based mapping of irreversible tissue damage by PET in the acute stage of ischemic stroke. Brain 1999, 123:2387–2400.
21. Wise RJS, Bernardi S, Frackowiak RSJ, Legg NJ,

Jones T. Serial observations on the pathophysiology of acute stroke. The transition from ischaemia to infarction as reflected in regional oxygen extraction. Brain 1983; 106:197–222.

22. Marchal G, Serrati C, Rioux P, Petit-Taboue MC, Viader F, De La Sayette V, Le Doze F, Lochon P, Derlon JM, Orgogozo JM, Baron JC. PET imaging of cerebral perfusion and oxygen consumption in acute ischaemic stroke: relation to outcome. Lancet 1993; 341: 925–927.

23. Marchal G, Beaudouin V, Rioux P, de la Sayette V, Le Doze F, Viader F, Derlon J-M, Baron J-C. Prolonged persistence of substantial volumes of potentially viable brain tissue after stroke: a correlative PET-CT study with voxel-based data analysis. *Stroke* 1996; 27:599–606.

24. Touzani O, Young AR, Derlon JM, Baron JC, MacKenzie ET. Progressive impairment of brain oxidative metabolism reversed by reperfusion following middle cerebral artery occlusion in anaesthetized baboons. *Brain Res* 1997; 767:17–25.

25. Heiss WD, Huber M, Fink GR, Herholz K, Pietryk U, Wagner R, Wienhard K. Progressive derangement of periinfarct viable tissue in ischemic stroke. J Cereb Blood Flow Metab 1992; 12:193–203.

26. Marchal G, Furlan M, Beaudouin V, Rioux P Hauttement JL, Serrati C, de la Sayette V, Le Doze F, Viader F, Derlon JM, Baron JC. Early spontaneous hyperperfusion after stroke: a marker of favorable tissue outcome. *Brain* 1996; 119:409–419.

27. Lenzi GL, Frackowiak RSJ, Jones T. Cerebral oxygen metabolism and blood flow in human cerebral ischemic infarction. J Cereb Blood Flow Metab 1982; 2: 231–235.

28. Furlan M, Marchal G, Viader F, Derlon J-M, Baron J-C. Spontaneous neurological recovery after stroke and the fate of the ischemic penumbra. Ann Neurol 1996; 40:216–226.

29. Heiss WD, Grond M, Thiel A, Von Stockhausen HM, Rudolf J, Ghaemi M, Löttgen J, Stenzel C, Pawlik G. Tissue at risk of infarction rescued by early reperfusion: a positron emission tomography study in systemic recombinant tissue plasminogen activator thrombolysis of acute stroke. *J Cereb Blood Flow Metab* 1998; 18:1298–1307.

30. Young AR, Sette G, Touzani O, Rioux P, Derlon JM, MacKenzie ET, Baron JC. Relationships between high oxygen extraction fraction in the acute stage and final infarction in reversible middle cerebral artery occlusion. An investigation in anaesthetized baboons with positron emission tomography. *J Cereb Blood Flow Metab* 1996; 16:1176–1188.

31. Marchal G, Rioux P, Serrati C, Furlan M, Derlon JM, Viader F, Baron JC. Value of acute-stage PET in predicting neurological outcome after ischemic stroke: further assessment. *Stroke* 1995; 26:524–525.

32. Marchal G, Young AR, Baron JC. Early postischaemic hyperperfusion: pathophysiological insights from positron emission tomography. J Cereb Blood Flow Metab 1999 lg: 467–482.

33. Heiss WD, Graf R, Löttgen J, Ohta K, Fujita T, Wagner R, Grond M, Wienhard K. Repeat positron emission tomographic studies in transient middle cerebral artery occlusion in cats: residual perfusion and efficacy of postischemic reperfusion J Cereb Blood Flow Metab 1997; 17:388–400.

34. Giubilei F, Lenzi GL, Di Piero V, Pozzilli C, Pantano P, Bastianello S, Argentino C, Fieschi C. Predictive value of brain perfusion single-photon emission computed tomography in acute ischemic stroke. Stroke 1990; 21:895–900.

35. Berrouschot J, Barthel H, von Kummer R, Knapp WH, Hesse S, Schneider D. 99m technetium-ethyl-cysteinate-dimer single-photon emission CT can predict fatal ischemic brain edema. Stroke 1998; 12: 2556–2562.

36. Limburg M, Van Royen EA, Hijdra A, De Bruïne JF, Verbeeten BWJ. Single-photon emission computed tomography and early death in acute ischemic stroke. Stroke 1990; 21:1150–1155.

37. Ueda T, Hatakeyama T, Kumon Y, Sakaki S, Uraoka T. Evaluation of risk of hemorrhagic transformation in local intra-arterial thrombolysis in acute ischemic stroke by initial SPECT. Stroke 1994; 25:298–303.

38. Herderschee D, Limburg M, van Royen EA, Hijdra K, Buller HR, Koster PA. Thrombolysis with recombinant tissue plasminogen activator in acute ischemic stroke: evaluation with rCBF-SPECT. *Acta Neurol Scand* 1991; 83:317–322.

39. Berrouschot J, Barthel H, Hesse S, Köster J, Knapp WH, Schneider D. Differentiation between transient ischemic attack and ischemic stroke within the first six hours after onset of symtoms by using 99mTc-ECD-SPECT. J Cereb Blood Flow Metab 1998; 18: 921–929.

40. Shimosegawa E, Hatazawa J, Inugami A, Fujita H, Ogawa T, Aizawa Y, Kanno I, Okudera T, Uemura K. Cerebral infarction within six hours of onset: prediction of completed infarction with technetium-99m-HMPAO SPECT. J Nucl Med 1994; 35:1097–1103.

41. Sperling B, Lassen NA. Hyperfixation of HMPAO in subacute ischemic stroke leading to spuriously high estimates of cerebral blood flow by SPECT. Stroke 1993; 24:193–194.

42. Barber PA, Davis SM, Infeld B, Baird AE, Donnan GA, Jolley D, Lichtenstein M. Spontaneous reperfusion after ischemic stroke is associated with improved outcome. Stroke 1998; 29:2522–2528.

43. Baird AE, Donnan GA, Austin MC, MacKay WJ. Early reperfusion in the "spectacular shrinking deficit" demonstrated by single-photon emission computed tomography. Neurology 1995; 45:1335–1339.

44. Jorgensen HS, Sperling B, Nakayama H, Raaschou HO, Olsen TS. Spontaneous reperfusion of cerebral infarcts in patients with acute stroke. Arch Neurol 1994; 51:865–873.

45. Firlik AD, Rubin G, Yonas H, Wechsler LR. Relation between cerebral blood flow and neurologic deficit resolution in acute ischemic stroke. Neurology 1998; 51:177–182.

46. Firlik AD, Yonas H, Kaufmann AM, Wechsler LR, Jungreis CA, Fukui MB, Williams RL. Relationship between cerebral blood flow and the development of swelling and life-threatening herniation in acute ischemic stroke. J Neurosurg 1998; 89:243–249.

47. Baron JC, von Kummer R, Del Zoppo GJ. Treatment of acute ischemic stroke: challenging the concept of a rigid and universal time window. *Stroke* 1995; 26: 2219–2221.

48. Feeney D, Baron JC. Diaschisis. Stroke 1986; 17:817–830.

49. Baron JC, Bousser MG, Comar D, Castaigne P.

Crossed cerebellar diaschisis in human supratentorial brain infarction. Trans Ame Neurol Assoc 1980; 105: 459–461.

50. Pantano P, Baron JC, Samson Y, Bousser MG, Derouesne C, Comar D. Crossed cerebellar diaschisis: further studies. Brain 1986; 109:677–694.

51. Pappata S, Mazoyer B, Tran-Dinh S, Cambon H, Levasseur M, Baron JC. Cortical and cerebellar hypometabolic effects of capsular, thalamo-capsular, and thalamic stroke: a positron tomography study. Stroke 1990; 21:519–524.

52. Serrati C, Marchal G, Rioux P, Viader F, Petit-Taboue MC, Lochon P, Luet D, Derlon JM, Baron JC. Contralateral cerebellar hypometabolism: a predictor for stroke outcome? J Neurol Neurosurg Psychiatry 1994; 57:174–179.

53. Kurthen M, Reichman K, Linke DB, Biersack HJ, Reuter BM, Durwen JF, Grunmann F. Crossed cerebellar diaschisis in intracarotid sodium amytal procedures: a SPECT study. Acta Neurol Scand 1990; 81: 416–422.

54. Brunberg JA, Frey KA, Horton JA, Deveikis JP, Ross DA, Koeppe RA [^{15}O]H$_2$O positron emission tomography determination of cerebral blood flow during balloon test occlusion of the internal carotid artery. AJNR Am J Neuroradiol 1994 15:725–732.

55. Pappata S, Tran Dinh S, Baron JC, Cambon H, Syrota A. Remote metabolic effects of cerebrovascular lesions: magnetic resonance and positron tomography imaging. Neuroradiology 1987; 29:1–6.

56. Tanaka M, Kondo S, Hirai S, Ishiguro K, Ishihara T, Morimatsu M. Crossed cerebellar diaschisis accompanied by hemiataxia: a PET study. J Neurol Neurosurg Psychiatry 1992; 55:121–125.

57. Pantano P, Formisano R, Ricci M, Di Piero V, Sabatini U, Barbanti P, Fiorelli M, Bozzao L, Lenzi GL. Prolonged muscular flaccidity after stroke. Morphological and functional brain alterations. Brain 1995; 118:1329–1338.

58. Iglésias S, Marchal G, Rioux P, Beaudouin V, Hauttement JL, De La Sayette V, Le Doze F, Derlon JM, Viader F, Baron JC. Do changes in oxygen metabolism in the unaffected cerebral hemisphere underlie early neurological recovery after stroke? A positron emission tomography study. Stroke 1996; 27:1192–1199.

59. Heiss WD, Kessler J, Karbe H, Fink GR, Pawlik G. Cerebral glucose metabolism as a predictor of recovery from aphasia in ischemic stroke. Arch Neurol 1993; 50:958–964.

60. Baron JC, D'Antona R, Pantano P, Serdaru M, Samson Y, Bousser MG. Effects of thalamic stroke on energy metabolism of the cerebral cortex. Brain 1986; 109:1243–1259.

61. Mimura M, Kato M, Kato M, Sano Y, Kojima T, Naeser M, Kashima H. Prospective and retrospective studies of recovery in aphasia. Changes in cerebral blood flow and language functions. Brain 1998; 121: 2083–2094.

62. Kuhl DE, Phelps ME, Kowell AP, Metter EJ, Selin C, Winter J. Effects of stroke on local cerebral metabolism and perfusion. Mapping by emission computed tomography of ^{18}FDG and ^{13}NH3. Ann Neurol 1980; 8:47–60.

63. Metter EJ, Wasterlain CG, Kuhl DE, Hanson WR, Phelps ME. FDG positron emission computed tomography in a study of aphasia. Ann Neurol 1981; 10: 173–183.

64. Metter EJ, Riege WH, Hanson WR, Jackson CA, Kempler D, Van Lancker D. Subcortical structures in aphasia. Arch Neurol 1988; 45:1229–34.

65. Karbe H, Szelies B, Herholz K, Heiss WD. Impairment of language is related to left parieto-temporal glucose metabolism in aphasic stroke patients. J Neurol 1990; 237:19–23.

66. Perani D, Vallar G, Cappa S, Messa C, Fazio F. Aphasia and neglect after subcortical stroke. A clinical/cerebral perfusion correlation study. Brain 1987; 110: 1211–1229.

67. Bogousslavsky J, Miklossy J, Regli F, Deruaz JP, Assal G, Delaloye G. Subcortical neglect: neuropsychological, SPECT, and neuropathological correlations with anterior choroidal artery territory infarction. Ann Neurol 1988; 23:448–452.

68. Fiorelli M, Blin J, Bakchine S, Laplane D, Baron JC. PET studies of cortical diaschisis in patients with motor hemi-neglect. J Neurol Sci 1991; 104:135–142.

69. Von Giesen HJ, Schlaug G, Steinmetz H, Benecke R, Freund HJ, Seitz RJ. Cerebral network underlying unilateral motor neglect: evidence from positron emission tomography. J Neurol Sci 1994; 125:29–38.

70. Bosley T, Rosenquist AC, Kushner M, Burke A, Stein A, Dann R, Cobbs W, Savino PJ, Schatz NJ, Alavi A, Reivich M. Ischemic lesions of the occipital cortex and optic radiations: positron emission tomography. Neurology 1985; 35:470–484.

71. Kiyosawa M, Bosley TM, Kushner M, Jamieson D, Alavi A, Reivich M. Middle cerebral artery strokes causing homonymous hemianopia: positron emission tomography. Ann Neurol 1990; 28:180–183.

72. Kuwert T, Hennerici M, Langen KL, Aulich A, Herzog H, Sitzer M, Feinendegen LE. Regional cerebral glucose consumption measured by positron emission tomography in patients with unilateral thalamic infarction. Cerebrovasc Diseases 1991; 1:327–336.

73. Szelies B, Herholz K, Pawlik G, Karbe H, Hebold I, Heiss WD. Widespread functional effects of discrete thalamic infarction. Arch Neurol 1991; 48:178–182.

74. Chabriat H, Levasseur M, Pappata S, Fiorelli M, Baron JC. Cortical metabolism in postero-lateral thalamic stroke: a PET study. Acta Neurol Scand 1992; 86:285–290.

75. Levasseur M, Baron JC, Sette G, Legault-Demare F, Pappata S, Mauguiere F, Benoit N, Tran-Dinh S, Degos JD, Laplane D, Mazoyer B. Brain energy metabolism in bilateral paramedian thalamic infarcts: a positron emission tomography study. Brain 1992; 115: 795–807.

76. Bogousslavsky J, Regli F, Delaloye G, Delaloye-Bischof A, Assal G, uske A. Loss of psychic self-activation with bithalamic infarction. Acta Neurol Scand 1991; 83:309–316.

77. Metter EJ, Kempler D, Jackson C, et al. Cerebral glucose metabolism in Wernicke's Broca's, and conduction aphasia. Arch Neurol 1989; 46:27–34.

78. Binkofski F, Seitz RJ, Arnold S, Classen J, Benecke R, Freund HJ. Thalamic metabolism and corticospinal tract integrity determine motor recovery in stroke. Ann Neurol 1996; 39:460–470.

79. Pantano P, Formisano R, Ricci M, Di Piero V, Sabatini U, Di Pofi B, Rossi R, Bozzao L, Lenzi

GL. Motor recovery after stroke. Morphological and functional brain alterations. Brain 1996; 119:1849–1857.
80. Iglesias S, Marchal G, Viader F, Baron JC. Delayed intrahemispheric remote hypometabolism: correlations with early recovery after stroke, Cerebrovascular Diseases, 2000, 10:391–402.
81. Baron JC, Levasseur M, Mazoyer B, Legault Demare F, Mauguiere F, Pappata S, Jedynak P, Derome P, Cambier J, Tran Dinh S, Cambon H. Thalamocortical diaschisis: PET study in humans. J Neurol Neurosurg Psychiatry 1992; 55:935–942.
82. Metter EJ, Jackson CA, Kempler D, Hanson WR. Temporoparietal cortex and the recovery of language comprehension in aphasia. Aphasiology 1992; 6:349–358.
83. Karbe H, Kessler J, Herholz K, Fink GR, Heiss WD. Long-term prognosis of poststroke aphasia studied with positron emission tomography. Arch Neurol 1995; 52:186–190.
84. Cappa SF, Perani D, Grassi F, Bressi S, Alberoni M, Franceschi M, Bettinardi V, Todde S, Fazio F. A PET follow-up study of recovery after stroke in acute aphasics. Brain Lang 1997; 56:55–67.
85. Tatemichi TK, Desmond DW, Prohovnik I, Cross DT, Gropen TI, Mohr JP, Stern Y. Confusion and memory loss from capsular genu infarction: a thalamocortical disconnection syndrome? Neurology 1992; 42:1966–1979.
86. Delpla PA, Zatorre R, Meyer E, Geraud G, Bes A, Etheir R, Hakim AM. Leucoaraïose et dysfonctionnement frontal précoce chez le sujet âgé non dément: approche neuropsychologique et par la caméra à positons. In: Bes A, Géraud G, eds. Cerveau et Hypertension Artérielle. Paris: J. Libbey, 1990:123–139.
87. Meguro K, Hatazawa J, Yamaguchi T, Itoh M, Matsuzauia T, Ono S, Miya zausa H, Hishihuma T, yanaik Sekitay. Cerebral circulation and oxygen metabolism associated with subclinical periventricular hyperintensity as shown by magnetic resonance imaging. Ann Neurol 1990; 28:378–383.
88. De Carli C, Murphy DG, Tranh M, Grady CL, Haxby JV, Gillette JA, Salerno JA, Gonzales-Aviles A, Horwitz B, Rapoport SI. The effect of white matter hyperintensity volume on brain structure, cognitive performance, and cerebral metabolism of glucose in 51 healthy adults. Neurology 1995; 45:2077–2084.
89. Yao H, Sadoshima S, Kuwabara Y, Ichiya Y, Fujishima M. Cerebral blood flow and oxygen metabolism in patients with vascular dementia of the Binswanger type. Stroke 1990; 21:1694–1699.
90. Sette G, Baron JC, Young AR, Myazawa H, Tillet I, Barré L, Travère JM, Derlon JM, MacKenzie ET. In vivo mapping of brain benzodiazepine receptor changes by positron emission tomography after focal ischemia in the anesthetized baboon. Stroke 1993; 24:2046–2058.
91. Heiss WD, Grond M, Thiel A, Ghaemi M, Sobesky J, Rudolf J, Bauer B, Wienhard K. Permanent cortical damage detected by flumazenil positron emission tomography in acute stroke. Stroke 1998; 29:454–461.
92. Nakagawara J, Sperling B, Lassen NA. Incomplete brain infarction of reperfused cortex may be quantitated with Iomazenil. Stroke 1997; 28:124–132.
93. Takahashi W, Ohnuki Y, Ohta T, Hamano H, Yamamoto M, Shinohara Y. Mechanism of reduction of cortical blood flow in striatocapsular infarction: studies using [123I]Iomazenil SPECT. NeuroImage 1997; 6:75–80.
94. Watanabe N, Young AR, Garcia JH, Liu K-F, Mézenge F, Derlon J-M, Lassen NA, Baron J-C. Focal cerebral ischaemia and chronic-stage reduced flumazenil uptake in anaesthetized baboons: a PET study with combined histological analysis. J Cereb Blood Flow Metab 1999; 19(Suppl. 1):S316.
95. Ramsay SC, Weiller C, Myers R, Cremer JE, Luthra SK, Lammertsma AA, Frackowiak RSJ. Monitoring by PET of macrophage accumulation in brain after ischaemic stroke. Lancet 1992; 239:1054–1055.

4. Cerebrovascular Disease in the Elderly

HARRY V. VINTERS

This chapter will deal with cerebrovascular diseases, especially those prone to cause significant morbidity and mortality in the geriatric population. Many forms of stroke and cerebrovascular disease pay little respect to arbitrary boundaries defined by age, whereas others (e.g., cerebral amyloid angiopathy [CAA]) are clearly more prevalent in the elderly than the young. Many principles important in understanding anoxic-ischemic brain injury can be applied to situations that affect the adult brain, regardless of age. The chapter is divided into a consideration of (*a*) cerebral infarcts and ischemic lesions, including anoxic-ischemic (hypoxic) encephalopathy, and (*b*) encephalic hemorrhage; vascular dementia is considered in Chapter 5. These divisions are admittedly somewhat artificial, since many of the disease processes discussed in this chapter may result, depending upon brain regions involved and the overall burden of cerebrovascular disease, in dementia. Throughout, I shall attempt to emphasize cerebrovascular problems that are especially likely to present in elderly individuals with an expanded discussion, whereas disease entities of less importance in the geriatric population (e.g., cerebral hemorrhage related to drug abuse, cerebrovascular complications of human immunodeficiency virus type 1 [HIV-1] infection, vein of Galen aneurysm, MELAS) will be de-emphasized. Any extensive review of human cerebrovascular disease and stroke owes a massive debt to the monograph of W. E. Stehbens,[1] which remains an authoritative classic in the field almost 30 years after its publication. More recent volumes and reviews on clinicopathologic aspects of cerebrovascular disease are also recommended to the interested reader;[2-7] as are sections devoted to stroke and cerebrovascular disease in standard textbooks of neuropathology.[8-10]

The magnitude of the stroke problem among the elderly is truly immense. In the United States there are approximately 0.5 million new strokes diagnosed annually, and some 3 million survivors of a previous stroke. As one recent review has stated, stroke is the third most frequent cause of death, the second most common cause of dementia found in a multidisciplinary memory clinic, and a major reason for severe (acquired) disability in developed nations; hence it has become a major public health issue.[11] Stroke has an incidence of 250–400 per 100,000 and a mortality of 25%–30%, and represents the third leading cause of death in industrialized countries.[12] The incidence of cerebrovascular disease increases substantially with age, being about 100/100,000 for individuals of age 45–54 years, but 1800/100,000 for those over 85 years of age.[8] Figures from the late 1960s comparing death rates (per 100,000 people) due to vascular disease of the central nervous system (CNS) showed a variation from 100 to 200. Among North American populations, brain infarcts are approximately 10 times as common as hemorrhages, whereas in the Orient spontaneous encephalic hemorrhage is almost as common as ischemic infarcts. In epidemiologic surveys, African-American men (ages 35–74 years) were 2.5 times and women 2.4 times as likely as whites to die of stroke.[13]

ANOXIA-ISCHEMIA (HYPOXIA) AND THE CENTRAL NERVOUS SYSTEM

A *cerebral infarct* can be defined as a region of necrosis showing irreversible injury to all cell types, usually within a specific vascular (arterial) territory of the brain. It often results from occlusion of a major artery or one of its branches, usually by a thrombus or embolus. By contrast, anoxic/hypoxic-ischemic encephalopathy (AIE) usually results from a sustained drop in cerebral perfusion pressure below the threshold for autoregulation (the situation of global brain ischemia) or perfusion of the brain by poorly oxygenated blood. Relative hyoxia may occur in the brain as a function of hypoxemic hypoxia (low oxygen content in the blood, e.g., CO poisoning, near drowning, respiratory arrest), stagnant hypoxia (an inadequate supply of oxygenated blood, e.g., cardiac arrest with prolonged asystole, intraoperative hypotensive episodes), or histotoxic hypoxia (inability of cerebral tissues to utilize oxygen, e.g., inhibition of mitochondrial enzymes involved in oxidative respiration as a result of cyanide and sulfide exposure with intoxication).

Within the brain, there is a hierarchy of susceptibility to anoxia of different cell type populations (e.g., neurons are more vulnerable than oligodendroglia, astrocytes, or microvascular endothelium) and different cells within a given set—especially neurons. Among neurons, the hierarchy of anatomic regions showing greatest to least vulnerability to anoxia (in adults) is hippocampus, neocortex, cerebellum, deep central gray matter, and brain stem. Within these structures, there is also variability of susceptibility to anoxia among different groups of neurons—e.g., the CA1 field of pyramidal cells in the hippocampus is vulnerable, the CA2 zone resistant, and within cerebellum the Purkinje cells show a remarkable susceptibility to anoxic injury not shared by the relatively resistant granule cells. Determinants of selective vulnerability are complex, but include (1) variable oxygen and energy requirements among different neurons, (2) glutamate receptor densities—glutamate acts as an excitotoxic neurotransmitter, and (3) activation of immediate early genes (e.g., heat shock protein) by ischemia-induced free radicals.[8,12] For an excellent review review of excitotoxicity, including the neuropathology and neurobiology of glutamate receptor subtypes, the reader is referred to reference 14.

An increase of extracellular calcium, acting as a second messenger, may initiate a series of cellular events (within both cytoplasm and nucleus) that influence the extent of tissue injury after either generalized or focal ischemia. These include activation of proteolytic enzymes that act to degrade both structural (cytoskeletal) and extracellular matrix (e.g., laminin) proteins. Lipid peroxidation and membrane damage may result from activation of phospholipase A_2 and cyclooxygenase, which in turn generates harmful free radicals. Nitric oxide (NO) made by nitric oxide synthase (NOS) may react with a superoxide anion to form peroxynitrite, a reactive species that promotes tissue damage.[12] In the case of focal cerebral ischemia, a cascade of events may result in a heavy burden of tissue damage, especially surrounding a region of complete necrosis. In and adjacent to this penumbra, there may be peri-infarct depolarizations, and subsequently (over hours or days) significant inflammation and even apoptosis, all of which may aggravate the neurologic deficit associated with even a comparatively small focal infarct. Indeed, many strategies for treating ischemic brain infarcts are aimed at minimizing tissue injury in the marginally perfused, but potentially salvageable, peri-infarct penumbra.[12] Blood insulin and glucose levels, for instance, may be important determinants of the extent of global and focal ischemia in various experimental and clinical settings.[15] Increasingly, there is interest in the inflammatory response to ischemic brain lesions, in particular because modifying this may be one rational approach to ameliorating the devastating sequelae of a stroke. Cytokines, leukocyte adhesion molecules, NO, and cyclooxygenase may all play major roles in this response.[16]

The diagnosis of acute AIE is made when neurons showing characteristic eosinophilic neuron change, with nuclear pyknosis, are seen either focally or distributed widely throughout the brain—especially in anoxia-sensitive structures (e.g., hippocampal pyramidal cell layer, Purkinje cells of the cerebellum). With time, these neurons disappear, leaving a glial scar. In particularly severe hypoxia or with profound hypotension (e.g., with prolonged cardiac arrest followed by resuscitation) regions of the brain may show laminar necrosis, characterized by patchy regions of necrosis of the deep cortical layers along one or more segments of the cortical ribbon (Fig. 4–1).[8] In severe cases, there may be essentially pancortical neuronal necrosis.

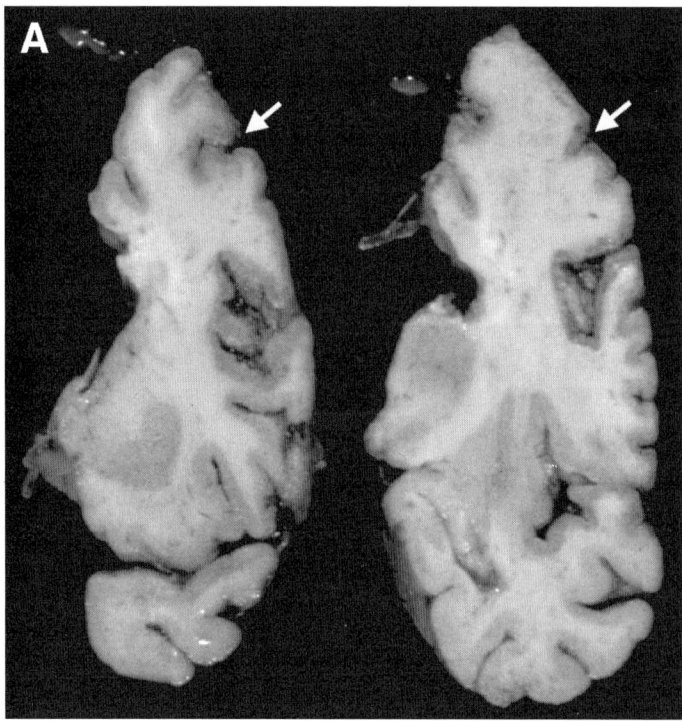

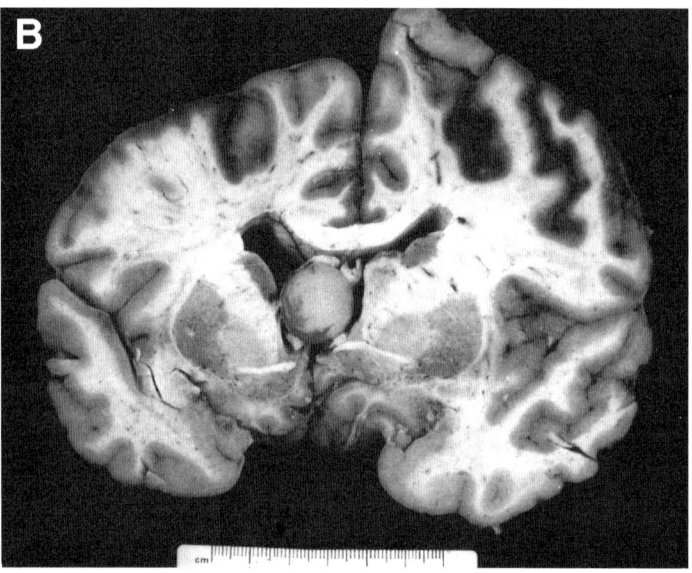

Figure 4–1. Cortical laminar necrosis (LN) and anoxic-ischemic encephalopathy. A: Coronal sections of brain at level of the temporal tip (*left*) and mammillary body (*right*). Note patchy, focally severe shrinkage and moth-eaten appearance of cortex (arrows), with sparing of other regions, e.g., temporal lobe. B: Anoxic-ischemic encephalopathy. Patient had experienced cardiorespiratory arrest while undergoing investigation for severe headaches, eventually found to be the result of a colloid cyst of the third ventricle (seen in this photograph). He died several hours later. Note multifocal regions of gray discoloration in the cortex, involving both cerebral hemispheres. The cortex–white matter junction is effaced in these regions. As in panel A, there is relative sparing of the temporal cortex.

PATHOPHYSIOLOGY OF ISCHEMIC BRAIN INFARCTS

Vascular Disease Causing Stroke

A somewhat simplistic classification of major types of cerebral vascular disease that may cause stroke and/or dementia is presented in Table 4–1. I accept the premise that subdividing vascular disease affecting the CNS into macro- and microvascular components may represent an oversimplification of the "real world" situation.[17] The two major forms of vasculopathy—especially atherosclerosis, arteriosclerosis and/or cerebral amyloid angiopathy (CAA)—often coexist in the elderly

Table 4–1. Major Categories of Arterial Disease That Affect the Human Nervous System

Arteriopathies Affecting (Primarily) Large Arteries
Atherosclerosis (simple/complicated)[a]
Fibromuscular dysplasia (FMD)
Moyamoya disease
Arterial dissection (cystic medial necrosis?)
HIV-associated vasculopathy
Vasculitis/angiitis/arteritis
    Giant cell (temporal) arteritis[a]
    Takayasu's arteritis

Arteriopathies Affecting Small Arteries
Arteriosclerosis/arteriolosclerosis/lipohyalinosis[a]
Cerebral amyloid (congophilic) angiopathy[a]
    Sporadic (associated with aging, AD/SDAT)[a]
    Familial CAA syndromes (HCHWA-D,[a] HCCAA or HCHWA-I, British CAA, transthyretin)
Vasculitis/angiitis/arteritis
    Primary (including granulomatous) angiitis of the CNS (often associated with CAA in the elderly)[a]
    Polyarteritis nodosa
    Wegener's granulomatosis
    Systemic lupus (SLE)
    Behçet disease
    Hypersensitivity vasculitis
    Lymphomatoid granulomatosis (LG)[b]
    Vasculitis secondary to systemic infection, connective tissue disease, malignancy, sarcoidosis
Associated with dementia
    Binswanger's subcortical (arteriosclerotic) leukoencephalopathy (BSLE)[a]
    CADASIL[a]
    Cerebral amyloid angiopathy (see above)[a]
Thrombotic thrombocytopenic purpura (TTP)
?MELAS (mitochondrial cytopathies with stroke-like episodes)
Cerebroretinal vasculopathy/HERNS (hereditary endotheliopathy, retinopathy, nephropathy, and stroke)

AD/SAT, Alzheimer's disease/senile dementia of the Alzheimer type; CAA, cerebral amyloid angiopathy; HCCAA, hereditary cystatin C amyloid angiopathy; HCHWA-D or -I, hereditary cerebral hemorrhage with amyloidosis, Dutch or Icelandic type.

[a] Entities of major clinical importance in the elderly. Neuropathologic entities that are an incidental finding at autopsy (e.g., siderocalcinosis of arteries in the basal ganglia) are not included in this table.

[b] Lymphomatoid granulomatosis is a controversial entity with features of both a vasculitis and a lymphoproliferative disorder.

and probably share major risk factors, an important one being mere aging. Co-morbidity from more than one form of angiopathy is common.

MACROANGIOPATHY

Atherosclerosis remains a leading factor contributing to the importance of cardiovascular and cerebrovascular disease as major causes of morbidity and mortality in most of the Western world, especially in the geriatric population. The pathogenesis (and, to some extent, etiology) of atherosclerosis is now understood in detail, thanks to advances in the evolution of animal models, and cell and molecular biological tools that can be utilized to study its initiating factors and progression, as summarized in several key reviews of recent years.[18–21] Early events that may precede the formation of atherosclerotic plaques have been suggested to include endothelial dysfunction (with abnormally increased permeability to lipoproteins and other plasma components), which is possibly mediated by NO and platelet-derived growth factor (PDGF), up-regulation of leukocyte adhesion molecules such as integrins and L-selectin and endothelial adhesion molecules, and migration of white blood cells (WBCs) into the arterial wall. Advanced lesions of complicated atherosclerosis develop after a fibrous cap forms over a fatty streak; this cap eventually overlies a necrotic core that includes a mixture of WBCs, lipids, and amorphous debris, and itself results from lipid accumulation, necrosis, and proteolytic activity.[18] Unstable plaques, often resulting in symptomatic plaque rupture, almost certainly result from thinning of the protective fibrous cap associated with the continued influx and activation of macrophages. Bleeding into this unstable plaque (with or without resultant rupture of atheroma into the arterial lumen) may occur from vasa vasorum or fragile microvessels within plaque itself. This may lead to mural or occlusive thrombus in an affected artery.

Atherosclerosis may involve major branches of the circle of Willis (Fig. 4–2). In Western populations atheromata tend to be most severe in the basal arteries, whereas in Japanese individuals, atherosclerosis is more severe in small peripheral arterial branches.[22] An arterial segment in or near the circle of Willis may undergo thrombosis with resultant brain infarct. Commonly, however, the brain is injured because of severely stenotic or occlusive atherosclerosis in the intracervical, extracranial carotid, and vertebral arterial systems.[23–26] The nature and extent of atheroma in neck arteries can be predicted with considerable success using ultrasonic and angiographic imaging techniques.[27–29] Carotid endarterectomy (CEA) is now routinely carried out as prophylaxis against stroke in patients with severe stenosis at the carotid bifurcation; not surprisingly, the surgical specimens that result from this procedure show typical features of complicated atheroma (Fig. 4–3).[30] Fragile, often ulcerated atheroma strategically located within cervical arteries may lead to artery-to-artery emboli of either platelet-fibrin or atheromatous material (Fig. 4–4), causing ischemic stroke.[31,32]

Patterns of ischemic brain infarcts resulting from thrombotic and embolic occlusions of the carotid arteries have been examined in a meticulous necropsy study of almost 1000 Norwegian patients.[33,34] Over 60% of the patients in this investigation were over 65 years old at the time of death. The close association between cardiovascular disease and severe carotid atherosclerosis was emphasized. Cerebral infarcts were found in 78% of patients with thromboembolic carotid occlusions; while the middle cerebral artery (MCA) territory of the cerebral hemisphere was most commonly infarcted in association with carotid occlusion, anterior and middle cerebral artery territories had also sometimes undergone necrosis.[26] In a companion investigation, the same workers analyzed the extent and clinicopathologic correlates of ischemic cerebrovascular disease within the brain—this was found in almost one-third of the 994 patients examined, with a mean age of 73.2 years for men and 75.6 years for women.[33,34]

Rarely, severe atheroma in the circle of Willis, especially the basilar artery, may cause ectasia or fusiform enlargement of the artery. This aneurysmal dilatation may result in symptoms because of extreme compression of nearby structures, e.g., the brain stem in the case of a basilar aneurysm.[35,36] Cross sections of these aneurysms show severe complicated atheroma, frequently with superimposed mural hemorrhage, rupture, and infiltration by chronic inflammatory cells. They may become occluded to produce devastating brain stem

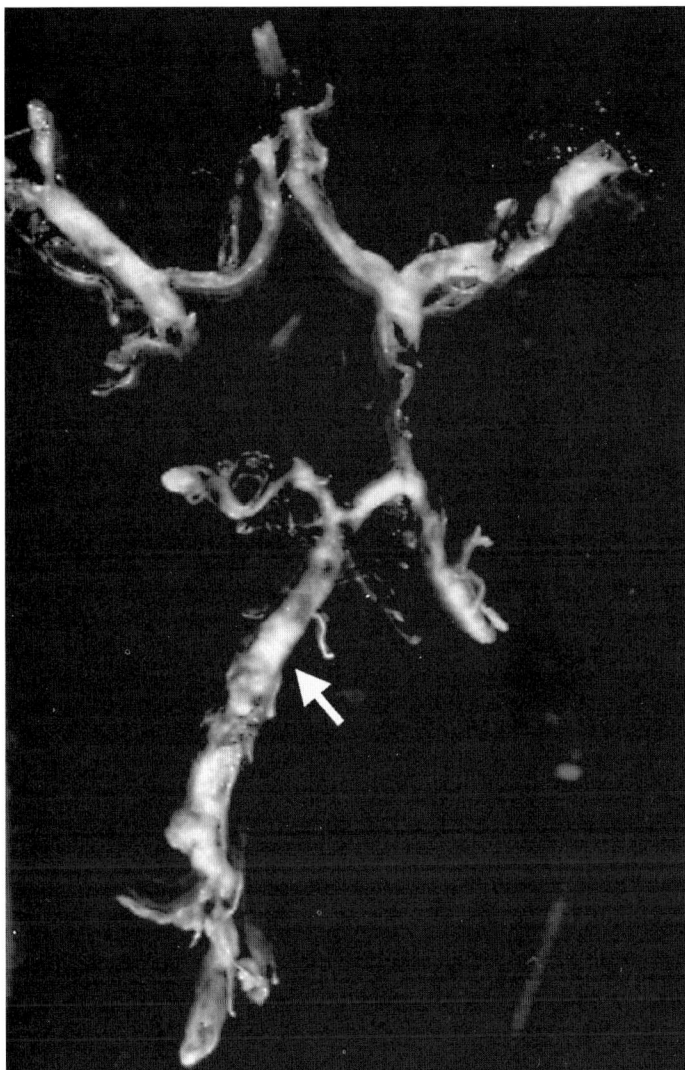

Figure 4–2. Atherosclerosis on the circle of Willis. Note patchy, focally accentuated atheroma on branches of the circle of Willis, e.g., mid-portion of the basilar artery (arrow) and the MCAs. The right posterior communicating artery was thin and fragmented during removal of the circle of Willis from the base of the brain.

and/or cerebellar infarcts. [see also Subarachnoid Hemmorrhage, below].

Other arteriopathies affecting large arteries (e.g., fibromuscular dysplasia [FMD], moyamoya disease, HIV-associated vasculopathy) are extremely rare causes of ischemic cerebrovascular disease in the elderly.[8,17,35] Instead, they are a major diagnostic consideration when ischemic stroke occurs in middle-aged and young adults or children.

MICROANGIOPATHY

By comparison with atherosclerosis, the molecular pathogenesis of arteriosclerosis/arteriolosclerosis (AS), one of the two most common forms of cerebral microangiopathy (the other being CAA, see discussion of intraparenchymal hemorrhage below, and Chapter 5), is poorly understood. There is scarcely uniform agreement on the the brain microvascular lesions best described by the term AS, thus its severity can be difficult to evaluate in a given case. However, the evolution of AS is strongly associated with a history of hypertension. Despite effective treatment in developed countries of severe hypertension, arteriosclerotic microvascular disease is still seen in autopsy brain specimens. A recent investigation has found that of 70 patients in whose

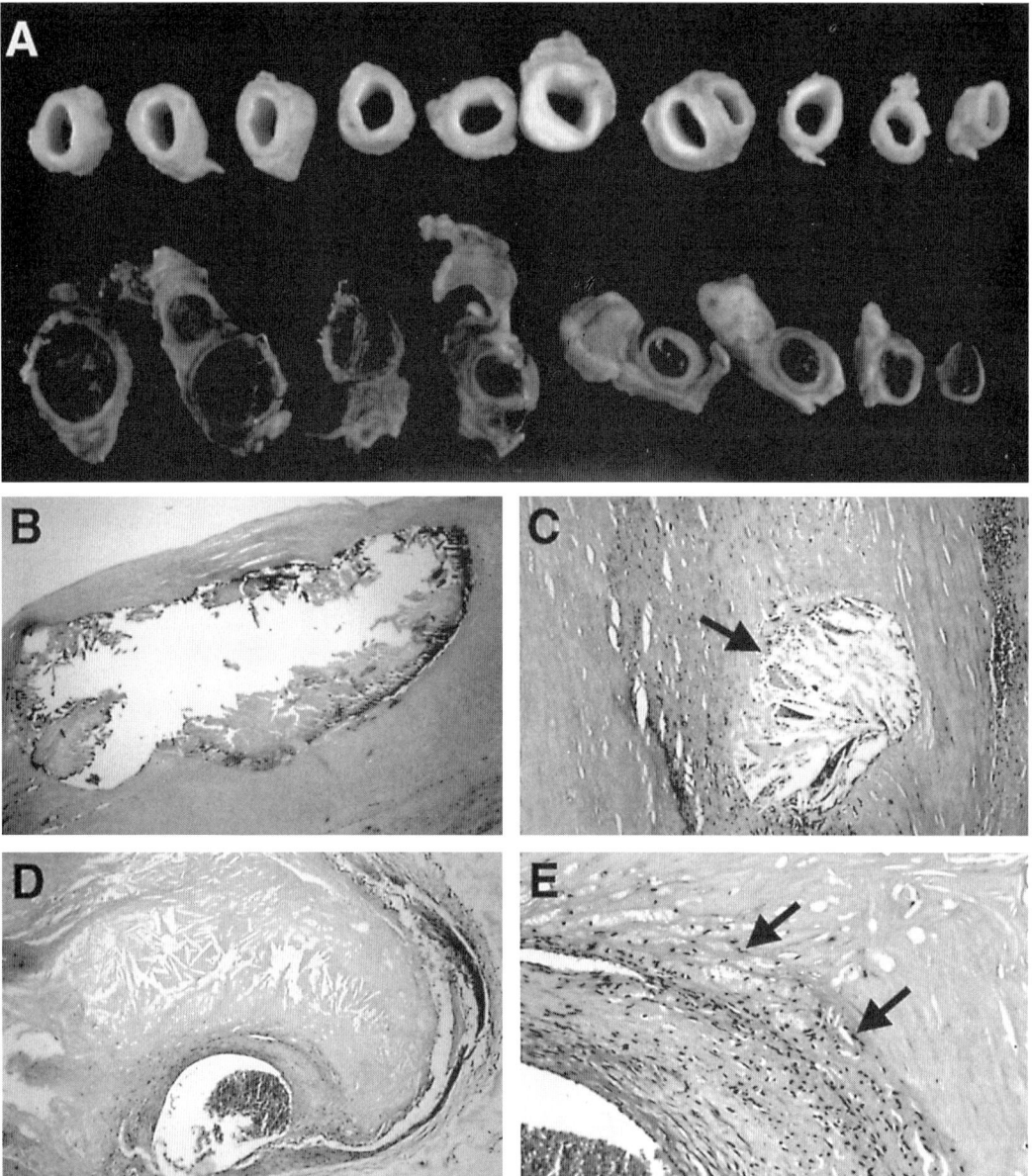

Figure 4–3. Atherosclerosis of the cervical carotid artery. *A:* Autopsy specimen from a 62-year-old male who had complete thrombosis of the left common carotid artery. Sections at top are of the ICA, showing moderate eccentric atheroma, including a semilunar area of intimal thickening, but relatively mild stenosis of the arterial lumen. Sections at bottom show thrombosed common and external carotid arteries. *B,C.* Histologic sections of carotid endarterectomy specimens from various patients. Panel B shows a prominently calcified portion of plaque, while panel C shows cholesterol clefts (arrow), also calcified, in a region of intimal fibromuscular hyperplasia. *D,E.* Severe atherosclerosis of intracranial arteries in a 78-year-old man with dementia. *D:* Low-power view of entire cross section of the artery, showing marked stenosis of the lumen and abundant cholesterol clefts within the atheroma. *E:* Magnified view; lumen is at lower left of the figure. Atheroma shows severe fibromuscular intimal hyperplasia and a large collection of foamy histiocytes (arrows) immediately deep to this. H&E, magnification: B,D, ×20; C, ×55, E, ×110.

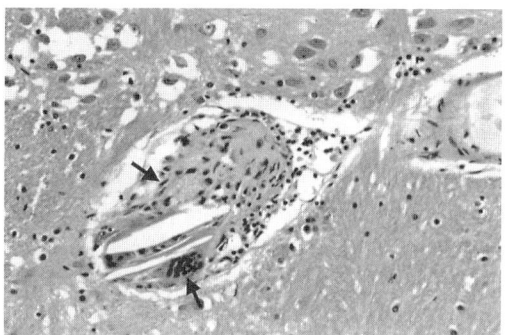

Figure 4–4. Atheroembolus. View of a brain section from patient who had experienced multiple stroke-like episodes over months prior to death. Small vessels occluded by atheromatous material (as in this section) were scattered throughout the brain. Note foamy histiocyte (arrow, top) and cholesterol cleft, surrounded by multinucleated giant cells (arrow, bottom), which are characteristic components of atheromatous plaque in situ. H&E, magnification: ×220.

brains significant cerebral small vessel disease was found at necropsy, almost one-third failed to meet stringent clinicopathologic criteria for hypertension. Cerebral microangiopathy was hypothesized to result, at least in part, from conditions that enhance small vessel permeability during life.[37] Microscopic features of AS, especially when severe, may include the following: hyaline thickening (sometimes with degeneration of the internal elastic lamina), intimal fibromuscular hyperplasia, variable degrees of lumenal narrowing, thinning of the media, concentric onion-skin type smooth muscle cell proliferation, and the presence of foamy macrophages in the arterial wall (Fig. 4–5).[1,17] Ultrastructural analysis of arterial medial injury in hypertensive patients who have experienced cerebral hemorrhage (before age 65) has shown atrophy and loss of smooth muscle cells (SMC) and accumulation of non-fatty debris and basement membrane materials.[38] Fibrinoid necrosis (Fig. 4–6) usually occurs only with malignant hypertension. Vascular lesions of AS thus show *some* similarities to those in advanced atherosclerosis. Obvious microatheroma may also be seen in medium-sized meningeal—and sometimes even intraparenchymal—arteries. Pathophysiologic mechanisms important in the genesis of cerebral AS have been the subject of relatively little systematic study. The term AS is sometimes used interchangeably with *lipohyalinosis* (LH), the latter deriving from an assumption of events likely to have been important in the pathogenesis of the microangiopathy—i.e., hyalinization and lipid deposition. Consequences of AS/LH, including lacunar infarcts and intracerebral hemorrhage, are discussed in the appropriate sections below.

Cerebral amyloid (Congophilic) angiopathy (CAA), a vascular lesion more commonly as-

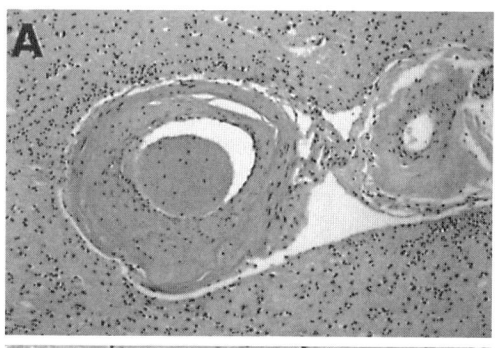
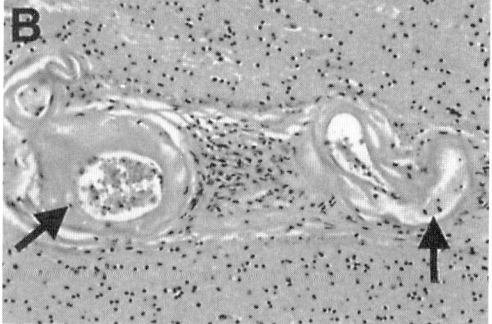
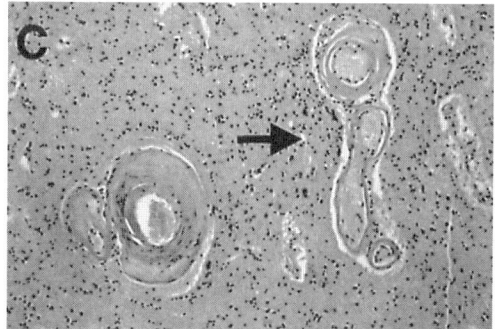

Figure 4–5. Severe arteriosclerotic change in an elderly patient with ischemic-vascular dementia. *A–C.* Extensive onion skin type and hyaline thickening of a severe degree. Cells noted within vessel wall (arrows, B) are probably histiocytes. In panel C, note old blood pigment immediately adjacent to a thickened arteriole (arrow), probably representing past leakage of blood from the lumen. H&E, magnification: A,C, ×55; B ×110.

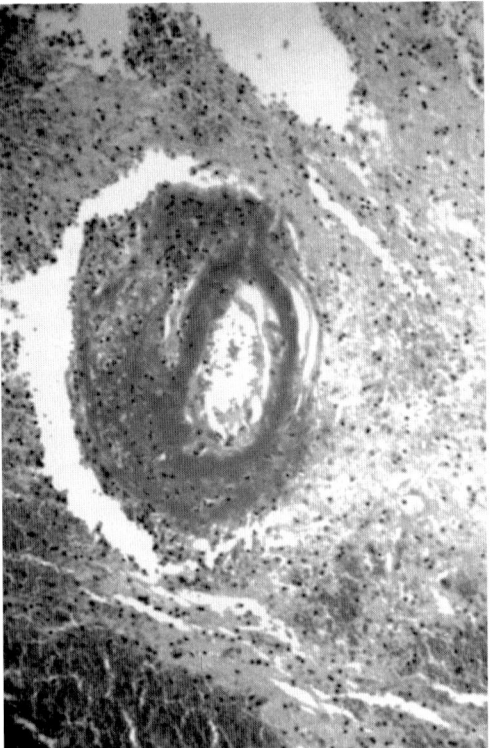

Figure 4–6. Fibrinoid necrosis of a brain parenchymal arteriole in a geriatric patient with combined CAA and arteriosclerotic cerebrovascular disease. Note replacement of cellular component of the vessel wall with eosinophilic, hyaline material; acute hemorrhage is noted in surrounding brain parenchyma. H&E, magnification: ×110.

sociated with brain hemorrhage than ischemia, both describes and defines a microvascular lesion that involves both parenchymal and leptomeningeal arterioles, whereby their medial and/or adventitial components are replaced by an eosinophilic hyaline fibrillar (at the ultrastructural level) material with distinctive biochemical properties.[39–41] Cerebral amyloid angiopathy is associated with both stroke and dementia. This microvascular lesion is included, with variable emphasis, as one of the key microscopic lesions that, when found in excess in the CNS, provide morphologic support for the clinical diagnosis of Alzheimer's disease/senile dementia of the Alzheimer type (AD/SDAT).[42] The most common form of CAA is that associated with deposition, within arterial walls, of amyloid β protein, a small, unique, approximately 4.2 kDa peptide cleaved from the amyloid precursor protein (APP), encoded by a gene on chromosome 21.[40,42] The disorder AD/SDAT is associated with excessive deposition of Aβ in both the brain parenchyma (as senile plaques [SPs]) and as CAA.

Relatively rare familial forms of CAA are also found in various geographic locations. In a circumscribed coastal region of the western Netherlands, a familial type of severe CAA (hereditary cerebral hemorrhage with amyloidosis, Dutch type/HCHWA-D) is attributed to a unique APP gene mutation (at codon 693). Massive Aβ deposition occurs within the media of cerebral arterioles, and fatal cerebral parenchymal hemorrhages frequently result.[43–46] An Icelandic form of CAA leading to hemorrhagic stroke, hereditary cerebral hemorrhage with amyloidosis, Icelandic type (HCHWA-I), results from mutation in the gene encoding cystatin C/γ-trace—hence this condition is also sometimes described as hereditary cystatin C amyloid angiopathy (HCCAA). It causes cerebral bleeds in young and middle-aged adults.[47,48] Brains from HCHWA-I patients show extensive deposition of γ-trace protein within arteriolar walls, associated with degeneration of the vessel walls.[48]

Setting aside the relatively rare examples of familial CAA, over 80% of brains originating from patients with autopsy-confirmed AD/SDAT show some degree of (Aβ) CAA, involving cerebral vessels in one or more cortical regions.[49] Brains with a moderate to severe degree of CAA show a significantly higher frequency of ischemic or hemorrhagic lesions than do those with negligible CAA. The CAA increases in extent and severity with advancing age. Moderate to severe CAA is found in as many as 12%–13% of brains from (unselected) patients over 85 years of age. Among consecutive autopsies on AD patients, however, moderate to severe CAA was noted in over 25%.[50,51] All regions of neocortex and overlying meninges may be affected by CAA, though there are minor variations in the distribution of affected arteries among lobes.[52,53] Whereas cerebellum and its meningeal covering are occasionally involved by CAA, the microvascular abnormality is virtually never found within deep central gray matter, subcortical white matter, or brain stem. The term CAA encompasses amyloid deposition within the walls of arterioles and capillaries, though the latter is sometimes described as dyshoric angiopathy, especially when, on histologic sections, amyloid appears to be "leaking" from the capillary wall into adjacent brain. Selected light microscopic and immunohistochemical features of CAA are highlighted in Fig. 4–7.

The severity of CAA within a region of brain or even a single affected arteriolar segment, can be graded, depending upon the degree of SMC replacement by amyloid within the media; grade 1 CAA defines deposition of amyloid protein among SMC in an otherwise intact arteriolar segment, whereas grade 3 CAA describes a situation whereby arteriolar media is entirely replaced by amyloid, and there is associated disruption of the vessel wall.[54] In general, the extent of amyloid deposition within vessel walls correlates with increasing risk of cerebral hemorrhage (see below).

A variety of CAA-associated microangiopathies (CAA-AM) have been described, including fibrosis, microaneurysm formation, chronic (including granulomatous) inflammation, "double-barreling," fibrinoid necrosis, and, very rarely, vessel wall calcification (Fig. 4–8).[41,55] Among patients with HCHWA-D, the severity of this secondary microvascular degeneration appears to correlate with the number of cerebrovascular lesions seen at autopsy.[45,46]

The pathogenesis of CAA is intriguing and incompletely understood. The SMCs appear to be able to synthesize APP mRNA and Aβ protein, assessed by in situ hybridization or immunohistochemistry in both human brain specimens and SMC cell cultures.[56–58] Various types of Aβ peptide, including ones that carry the amino acid substitution encoded by the

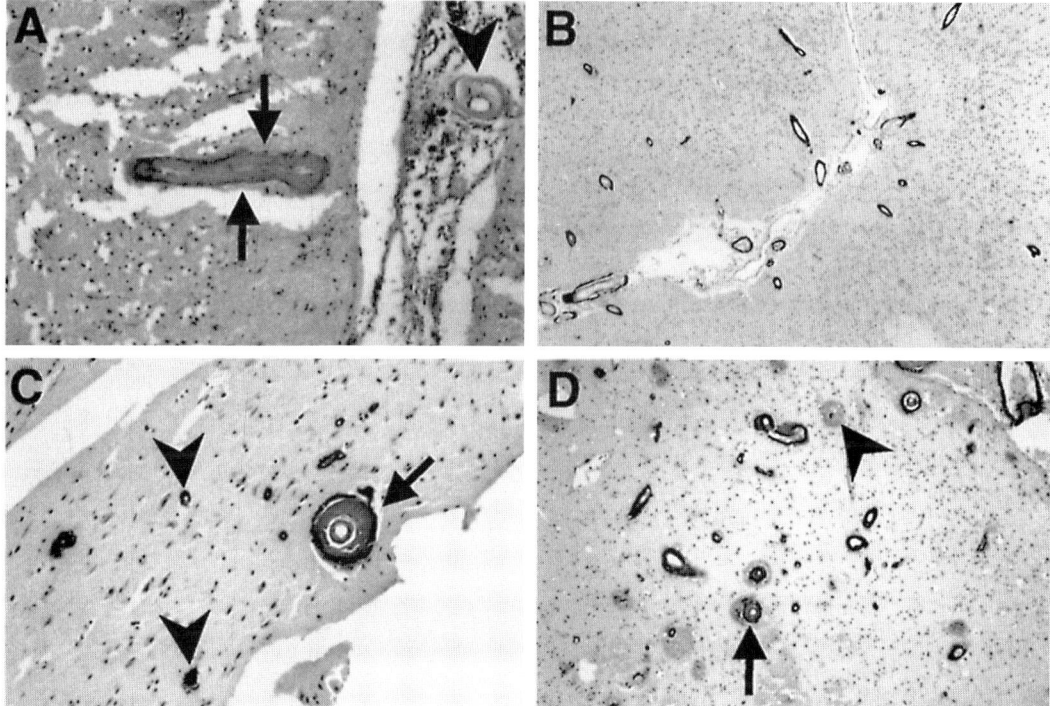

Figure 4–7. Cerebral amyloid angiopathy (CAA) *A:* Biopsy specimen from a patient with brain hemorrhage caused by CAA. Longitudinal section of an affected arteriole, stained with Congo red and viewed under nonpolarized light, shows thickening and is prominently stained (arrows). An affected leptomeningeal artery is less prominently stained (arrowhead). *B:* Brain section from a patient who experienced multiple bihemispheric parenchymal hematomas, immunostained with antibody to Aβ 1–40. Antibody labels only microvessels involved by CAA. *C:* Biopsy specimen from another patient stained with anti-Aβ 1–40. Several small capillaries are immunolabeled (arrowheads), as is a larger artery (arrow). Again, negligible plaque staining is present. By contrast, panel *D* (same case as illustrated in panel A), immunostained with anti-Aβ 1–42, shows scattered immunoreactive senile plaques (arrowhead) and a perivascular halo of Aβ immunoreactivity around several amyloid-laden arterioles (arrow). Magnification: A, D, ×55, B, ×20; C, ×110.

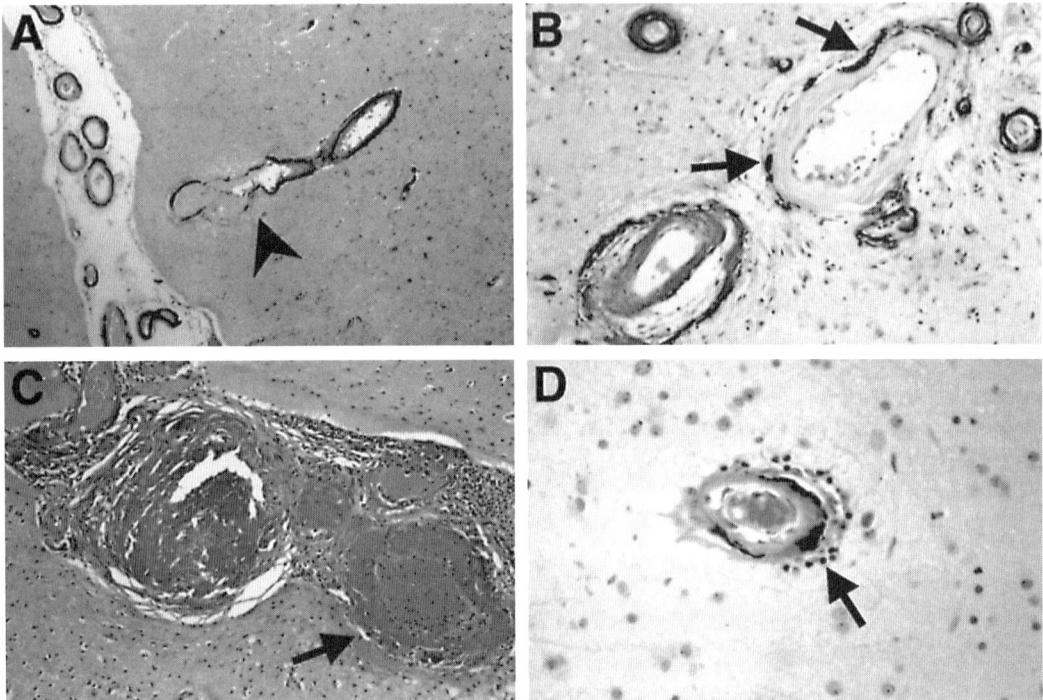

Figure 4–8. Cerebral amyloid angiopathy–associated microangiopathies (CAA-AM). All images are from sections of brain originating in patients with severe CAA, often associated with intraparenchymal hemorrhage. Panels A & B are micrographs from sections immunostained with primary antibodies to Aβ protein. *A:* Aneurysmal dilatation (arrowhead) in an arteriole, wall of which has been extensively replaced by Aβ protein. *B:* Severe thickening and fibrosis of an arteriole in which residual Aβ-immunoreactive material is seen (arrows). *C:* Extensive fibrinoid necrosis (arrow) of leptomeningeal arteries. *D:* Lymphocytes and foreign body giant cells (arrow) surround a microvessel involved by CAA. Magnification: A, ×20; B, ×110; C, ×55; D, ×120.

HCHWA-D codon 693 *APP* mutation, show pronounced cytotoxicity when added to SMC cultures.[59,60] Transgenic mouse models of Aβ overproduction in which CAA results are certain to clarify key pathogenetic questions.

VASCULITIS

As a cause of stroke in the elderly, vasculitis (angiitis) is much less common than either atherosclerosis or arteriosclerosis. However, because vasculitis is potentially treatable, recognizing its manifestations is crucial in patient management. The CNS may be affected by systemic vasculitides, or primary angiitis involving only the brain. Key reviews have summarized theories of pathogenesis of these comparatively rare conditions.[61–64] Whereas entities such as polyarteritis nodosa and Wegener granulomatosis commonly involve both the CNS and PNS, hypersensitivity vasculitis rarely (<10% of cases) results in neurologic dysfunction. From a pathologic perspective, vasculitic lesions are usually classified by (*a*) the size, type, and distribution of blood vessels affected, and (*b*) the nature of the inflammatory infiltrate that accompanies vessel wall injury or destruction (fibrinoid necrosis).

Large reviews of primary angiitis of the CNS (PACNS) report a preponderance of males among pathologically verified cases; the mean age at diagnosis (in both biopsy and autopsy studies) is usually in the fifth or sixth decade of life.[61–64] Patients with PACNS commonly experience a range of neurologic symptoms, varying from headaches or diffuse neurologic dysfunction to ischemic or hemorrhagic stroke (approximately 10%–15% each for the latter two). Histopathologic features of PACNS may vary from a dense lymphocytic infiltrate with or without fibrinoid necrosis to granulomatous inflammation with prominent multinucleated giant cells (Fig. 4–9). Over recent years it has been recognized that severe CAA in elderly patients may be associated with a relatively brisk granulomatous angiitis; thus in geriatric patients who show vasculitis on brain biopsy or in a fragment of brain evacuated together with clot material (from a patient with intraparenchymal hemorrhage), Congo red stains and/or Aβ immunohistochemistry are strongly indicated.[41,65]

Arguably the most common form of vasculitis encountered among the elderly is giant cell arteritis/angiitis (GCA). Its annual incidence has been estimated to be as high as 17–18 per 100,000 over the age of 50 years.[66] This form of angiitis is eminently responsive to steroid therapy. The multifocal nature of the angiitis is reflected in its various patterns of presentation, which may include headache, visual complaints, weight loss, and the syndrome of polymyalgia rheumatica.[67,68] Vessels commonly involved at autopsy include the aorta, coronary and cerebral arteries (including the central retinal artery), and arteries of the head and neck.[67–69] Devastating ischemic infarcts have been documented in patients with GCA who progress to develop occlusion of the MCA and anterior cerebral artery (ACA).[70] Frequently, patients undergo temporal artery biopsy to confirm the diagnosis. An affected vessel shows a transmural lymphohistiocytic infiltrate, among which multinucleated giant cells may be prominent (Fig. 4–9). "Skip" areas may occur in a biopsy, so special care must be taken in its detailed examination, often subserial sections through a tissue block must be used. Typical histopathologic features of GCA may persist in affected arteries even after successful corticosteroid therapy.[71]

The etiology of GCA is not well understood. An association between GCA and *Varicella zoster* infection of the arterial wall seems unlikely in view of detailed molecular and immunohistochemical studies that have failed to show either viral antigen or DNA within tissue specimens affected by the vasculitis.[72] Humoral immunity may be involved in the pathogenesis of GCA, given the finding of intra- and extracellular immunoglobulin and complement deposition within the inflamed arterial wall, though this may be relatively nonspecific. An autoimmune process has been suggested to be of importance, though it is unclear which antigen may be involved. The polyclonal lymphocytic infiltrate in GCA is mainly of T-cell types, with CD4 (T-helper) cells exceeding CD8 (T-suppressor) cells—i.e., cellular immunity also appears to be of significance in disease causation. Interleukin-1

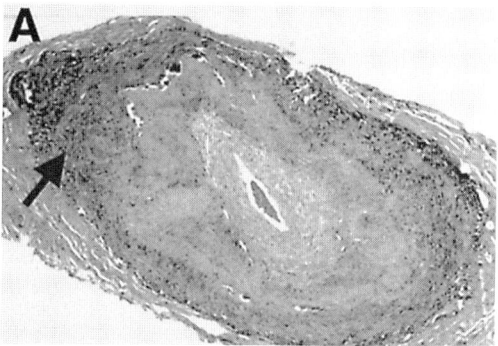
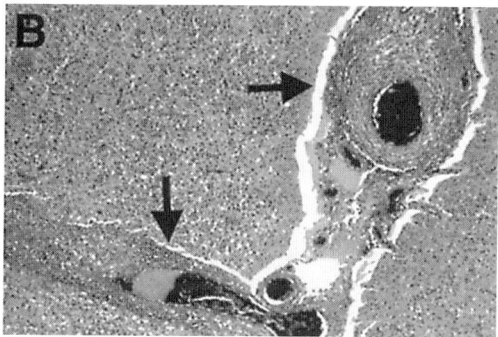
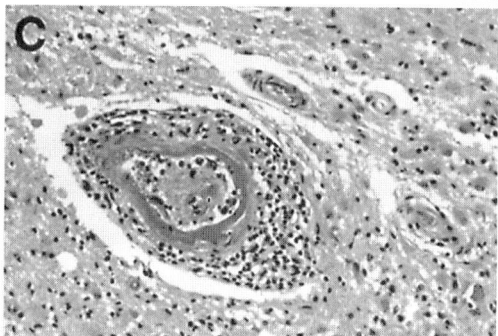

Figure 4–9. Angiitis/vasculitis. *A:* Temporal/giant cell arteritis (GCA). Note transmural inflammation through the wall of this temporal artery biopsy specimen. Scattered multinucleated giant cells (arrow) are present. *B:* Primary angiitis of the CNS (PACNS). Dense transmural mononuclear inflammatory cell infiltrates are in several meningeal vessels (arrows). Adjacent brain parenchyma (upper left) shows extensive encephalomalacia, and infiltration by mononuclear inflammatory cells. *C:* Same patient as shown in B. Note mixed inflammatory infiltrate around a vessel that shows fibrinoid necrosis. Surrounding brain parenchyma shows marked astrocytic gliosis. H&E, magnification: B, ×20 × C, ×110.

(IL-1) and IL-2 are present within GCA lesions, and serum IL-6 and thrombomodulin levels are elevated. The inflammatory infiltrate noted within affected arterial walls may represent a reaction to an as-yet unidentified microbial pathogen.[73,74]

Cerebral Embolism

Embolic infarcts may result whenever a mass of solid or undissolved material, usually (though not always) consisting of platelet-fibrin aggregates or thrombus, is carried in the bloodstream between two discontinuous sites and lodges in the distal site. In general, an embolic infarct may occur whenever any solid material forms within, or is introduced into, the arterial circulation, or forms in the venous circulation and has unrestricted passage to the arterial circulation, e.g., via a right-to-left cardiac shunt, such as a ventricular septal defect.[8] Most emboli that cause cerebral infarcts originate within either (a) atheromatous plaque (atheroemboli)[75] or (b) the heart. Other sources of emboli to the brain include fat (following bone fractures) and particulate material that enter the circulation during cardiothoracic surgical procedures, cerebral angiography, or interventional embolotherapy procedures.

Table 4–2 summarizes the most common sources of cardiogenic emboli that may cause cerebral infarct.[76-78] In most large series, embolic infarcts are less common than infarcts resulting from thrombi in the major cranial or cervical arteries; they probably account for 5%–25% of all ischemic brain infarcts. Unfortunately, patients at risk for thrombotic occlusion of a cervical or intracranial artery are also the same ones likely to develop a cardiac lesion, e.g., a hypokinetic myocardial wall segment with mural thrombus following a myocardial infarct, that may predispose to an embolic event. As many as 2.5% of patients with an acute myocardial infarct develop a new stroke within 2–4 weeks of the heart attack.[79] However, purely clinical criteria used to distinguish thrombotic from embolic stroke are inaccurate. Neurologic features suggestive of embolic (rather than thrombotic) brain infarct include abrupt onset of maximal neurologic deficit, headache and loss of consciousness at stroke onset, and clinical or imaging evidence for at least two distinct sites of embolization—either within the brain or the brain and an extra-CNS site. In one series, the mean age of patients encountered with a primary cardiac source of emboli was the mid-60s.[77] Nonrheumatic atrial fibrillation is clearly associated with an age-dependent stroke incidence that rises from 2.8% in the sixth decade of life to 7.1% in the ninth.[79]

Cardiogenic emboli usually migrate to the MCA bifurcation in the Sylvian fissure or to more distal MCA branches, less commonly to the vertebrobasilar system; in the latter tree, they often lodge at the basilar artery tip, frequently producing neurologic symptoms referrable to the calcarine (visual) cortex. In concluding whether an occluded artery has undergone embolic occlusion or in situ thrombosis, the pathologist must consider the degree of complicated atherosclerosis in the affected vessel. Thrombus superimposed on a large, focally calcified and ulcerated plaque—and attached to ulcerated intima—is more likely

Table 4–2. Potential Sources of Cardiogenic Emboli

Isolated Arrhythmias (40%–45%)
  Most commonly atrial fibrillation and sick sinus syndrome

Isolated Myocardial Abnormalities (25%–30%)
  Postmyocardial Infarct
    Global or focal left ventricular akinesia, with or without thrombus
    Ventricular aneurysm
  Patent foramen ovale
  Left atrial myxoma or thrombus

Isolated Valvular Abnormalities (20%–25%)
  Mitral valve prolapse or stenosis, prosthetic valve(s)
  Infectious and nonbacterial thrombotic (marantic) endocarditis
  Mitral annulus calcification
  Mitral valve prolapse/myxomatous degeneration

Arrhythmias and Myocardial Abnormalities (3%–5%)

Arrhythmias and Valvular Abnormalities (3%–5%)

Source: Adapted and modified from J. Bogousslavsky et al.[77]

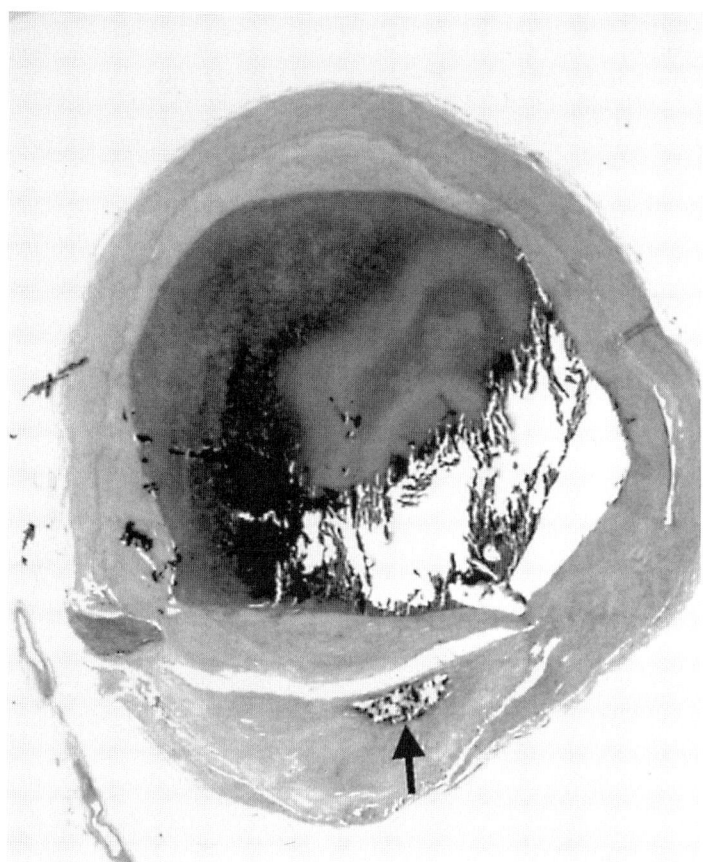

Figure 4–10. Embolus. An artery showing moderate atheroma (arrow indicates focally calcified region of intimal fibromuscular hyperplasia) in an artery that contains occlusive platelet-fibrin material. The relatively minimal atherosclerotic change in this artery and absence of intimal ulceration suggest that this is an embolus rather than in situ thrombosis. Magnification: ×20.

a thrombosis. A platelet-fibrin plug, clearly detached from the intima, in a relatively normal artery more likely represents an embolus (Fig. 4–10). Valvular abnormalities include the several types of lesions described below.

ENDOCARDITIS

Infective endocarditis (IE) may affect a native or prosthetic heart valve, usually the mitral, aortic, or both. Neurologic abnormalities may be the presenting feature of IE. Native valves most likely to develop IE are those which show either congenital or acquired abnormalities, e.g., from rheumatic valvular disease. Conversely, normal valves may become colonized by microorganisms as a consequence of intravenous drug use or hyperalimentation, immunosuppression, or nosocomial infection. An estimated 15%–25% of patients with IE develop embolic infarcts. While most brain infarcts associated with IE are comparatively small, those seen with *Staphylococcus aureus* infection may be massive. Other neurologic complications of IE include abscesses, mycotic (infectious) aneurysm, meningitis, encephalopathy, and intraparenchymal hemorrhage.

Nonbacterial thrombotic endocarditis (NBTE), also described as marantic endocarditis, an entity of uncertain etiology and pathogenesis, may complicate a wasting disease such as AIDS or widespread malignancy.[78–81] It is also seen with myriad non-neoplastic diseases that involve the heart, gastrointestinal tract, and lungs. The most common occurrence is in the seventh decade of life. Aortic and mitral valves are the ones most commonly affected; brain embolism is documented in approximately one-third of patients. Patients who come to necropsy following acute stroke in the presence of severe wasting or any condition that has placed them at risk for developing NBTE must be considered to have this entity unless proven otherwise by a thorough examination of the heart. Nonbacterial thrombotic endocarditis has been suggested to be of etiologic importance in 25%–30% of all ischemic strokes countered in cancer patients.[78]

Over recent decades, the prevalence of rheumatic heart disease has declined because of aggressive early treatment of group A streptococcal infection. The geriatric population is therefore one in which remnants of the disease are most likely to be encountered. It may cause scarring and deformation, sometimes with extensive calcification, of the mitral valve. Cerebral emboli in patients with rheumatic heart disease usually originate in the left atrium, often in association with atrial fibrillation. However, calcified debris or thrombus may embolize directly from the mitral valve.[78,82]

Mitral valve prolapse (MVP) is a controversial entity estimated to affect as many as 3–4% of males and over 5% of females.[78] Its importance as a cause of stroke, especially in young people, has been debated; it is a relatively insignificant cause of cardioembolic events in the elderly, if only because geriatric patients are far more likely to have numerous other serious vascular lesions that may produce ischemic brain infarcts. Calcification of the mitral annulus and calcific aortic stenosis may be found in as many as 25%–30% of those over 90 years of age. Mitral annular calcification is a surrogate marker for generalized complicated atherosclerosis and is also associated with other conditions that predispose to cardioembolic stroke, e.g., IE and arrhythmias.[78] Rarely, calcified embolic material that originates in such a calcified valve may migrate to the brain.

Prosthetic cardiac valves are either mechanical or constructed from biomaterials; emboli originating in both types are a major cause of brain infarct.[83] Mechanical valves are associated with a significantly higher risk of thromboembolism than are bioprostheses; hence patients with mechanical valves are usually maintained on long-term anticoagulation.[78,79] Obviously, when such patients develop an acute neurologic deficit, anticoagulant-related intraparenchymal cerebral hemorrhage is an important diagnostic consideration. Late prosthetic valve IE develops with roughly equal frequency on mechanical and bioprosthetic valves; however, major neurologic complications (with a higher mortality) are more common with mechanical valves, especially when replacing the native mitral valve.

NONCARDIOGENIC/ NONATHEROMATOUS EMBOLI

Fat emboli are usually associated with fractures of long bones or the pelvis (often after a motor vehicle accident), but may complicate soft tissue trauma or cardiothoracic surgical procedures. Patients over a broad age range may be affected.[8,84,85] Encephalopathic signs predominate, i.e., affected patients are usually restless, confused, stuporous, or comatose. Respiratory insufficiency often dominates the clinical picture, and some of the neurologic signs and symptoms are probably attributable to hyoxia. Cerebral findings at autopsy include widespread petechial hemorrhages confined to the white matter; fat emboli within small arteries may be demonstrable by fat stains carried out on frozen sections of involved brain regions.

Fragments of neoplasm may embolize to the brain in patients with widespread carcinomatosis or sarcomatosis. Parasites or parasitic ova may do likewise. Air embolism occurs with decompression sickness and with cardiac bypass surgery, the latter a scenario much more likely to be encountered among the elderly. Cardiac surgery may also result in unintentional embolization to the CNS of material or debris that is either released from a lesion or introduced during the procedure itself (Fig. 4–11). Emboli of intervertebral disc material have been reported in the spinal cord.[8] Finally, surgical and autopsy pathologists must keep in mind that intentional iatrogenic embolization is now an accepted way of treating many cerebral vascular malformations (especially arteriovenous malformations, see below) and even certain extra-axial brain tumors. These procedures have been in widespread use for at least 15–20 years; therefore materials injected into CNS lesions or ones that go 'astray' upon injection may be encountered years later in elderly individuals, because many of them are not effectively resorbed after placement within the brain. A large variety of embolotherapy materials are used, and many elicit a brisk granulomatous inflamma-

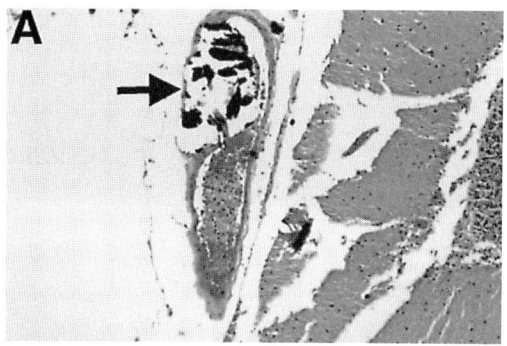

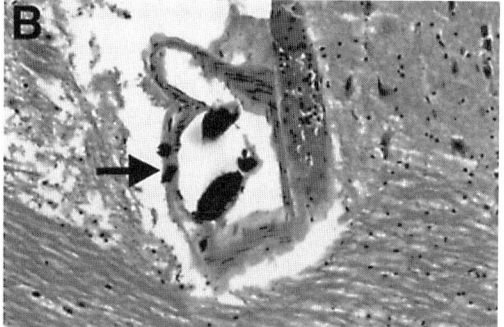

Figure 4–11. Sections of brain from a woman who had undergone coronary artery bypass graft surgery 8 days antemortem, during which severe calcification of the aortic and mitral valves was noted. An intra-aortic balloon pump was placed. At autopsy, calcified particulate material (arrows), frequently with overlying endothelium, was noted in the lumen of several meningeal and parenchymal arterioles, as illustrated in these two panels (A, cerebellum; B, pons). Only some of the particulate emboli were associated with parenchymal infarcts. H&E, magnification: A, ×55; B, ×110.

tory reaction that tends to persist for months or years (Fig. 4–12)[86–88]

Gross and Microscopic Features of Cerebral Infarcts

Cerebral infarcts can be subclassified as either hemorrhagic or nonhemorrhagic (bland or anemic), though in reality many have both components. Bland infarcts have historically been attributed to complete obstruction of blood flow to a given region of brain, whereas hemorrhagic infarcts have been thought to result from reperfusion of blood into an infarcted region of brain. Hemorrhagic infarcts more commonly result from emboli (see above) than in situ thrombosis.[6–10] Post-anoxic-ischemic tissue edema may lead to venous compression and elevated intravascular pressures, exacerbating the likelihood of hemorrhage into necrotic tissue.

Early changes of coagulative necrosis occur 8–48 hr after a region of brain is rendered ischemic.[8–10] The cortex–white matter junction becomes blurred or effaced, and affected cortex becomes dusky, secondary to hyperemia due to vascular dilatation. Cerebral edema reaches a maximum at 48–96 hr after an infarct has occurred—during this time the (clinical) risk of fatal brain herniation is maximal. Infarcted tissue becomes clearly delineated and a separation of necrotic from relatively normal brain may appear as a cracking artefact. Between 7 days and 3–4 weeks, liquefactive necrosis occurs. After approximately 3 weeks, cavitation of brain substance begins, and abundant macrophages may be seen within the necrotic tissue cavity by light microscopy. Eventually, the infarct is replaced by an irregular fluid-filled cyst traversed by fine blood vessels and gliotic trabeculae. Overlying meninges may become thickened and somewhat opaque. Usually, there is preservation of an intensely gliotic molecular layer of cortex overlying the infarct. If resolution of the infarct occurs, collapse and contraction of surrounding tissues may be prominent. The lining of a large cystic cavity resulting from an infarct (e.g., in the MCA territory) will often collapse as the brain is being removed from the calvarium at autopsy (Fig. 4–13).

Microscopic features of evolving infarct follow a characteristic sequence, though with substantial variation among patients (Fig. 4–14)[1,8–10] Between 6 and 24 hr after irreversible ischemia, neurons become shrunken and angulated and the cytoplasm takes on an intensely eosinophilic color (on H&E sections). Within white matter, axons become swollen and fragmented, myelin becomes pale, and eventually myelin sheaths disintegrate. Astrocytes and endothelial cells become swollen. Microvacuolation becomes visible, even by light microscopy. Polymorphonuclear leukocytes (PMNs) may migrate into the region of the infarct within 1–3 days after its occurrence, though in the author's experience this occurs much less consistently than after infarcts in other organs, e.g., the heart. Approximately 48 hr after the infarct, macrophages

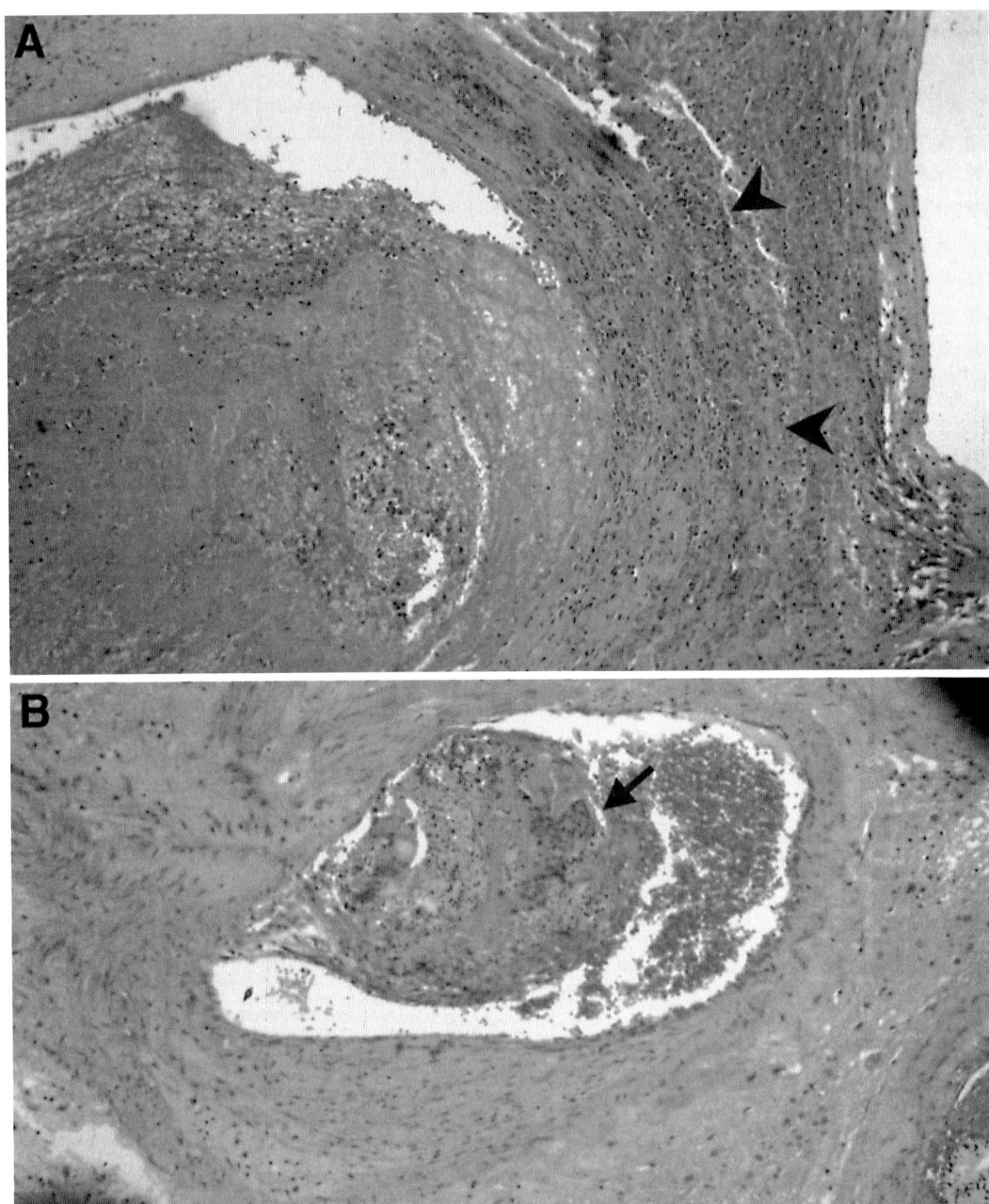

Figure 4–12. Intracranial arteriovenous malformations that have undergone preoperative (iatrogenic) embolization using a new agent. Note focal regions of angionecrosis (arrowheads, A). In another region from a different surgical specimen (B), a partially occlusive mural thrombus is seen; foreign body giant cells (arrow) surround embolotherapy material. H&E, magnification: A,B, ×110.

appear in increasing numbers at the edge of an infarct, phagocytose neuron, axon, and myelin breakdown products, and take on a foamy or granular appearance. Some macrophages are probably bone marrow–derived cells, whereas others may begin life as resident microglia within the brain.[89] Careful analysis of factors that initiate the microglial response

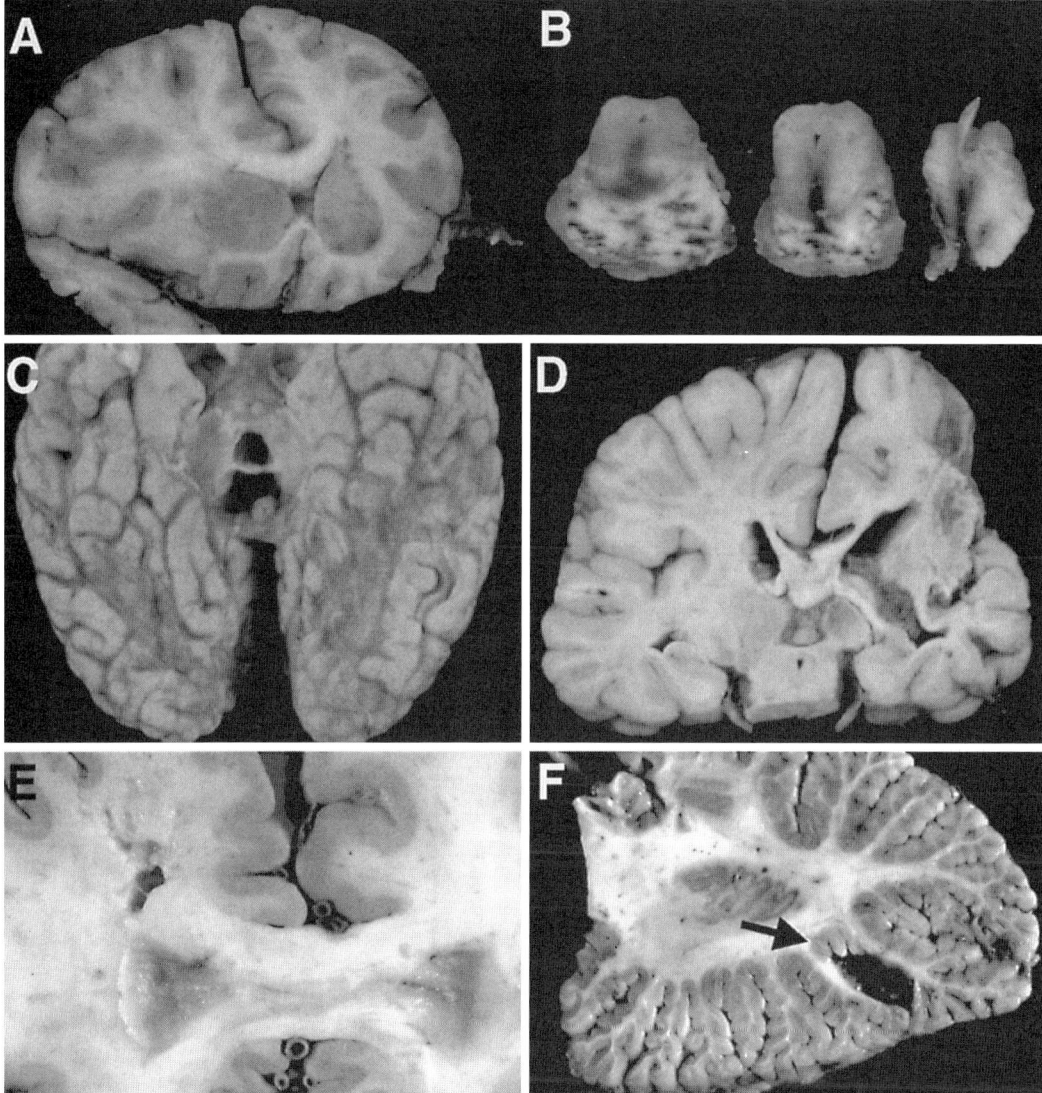

Figure 4–13. Appearance of a large cerebral infarct (at autopsy) varies with time interval between occurrence of the infarct and death of the patient. *A:* A relatively recent infarct (2–4 days prior to death) in the left cerebral hemisphere shows focal hemorrhagic transformation, multifocal blurring of the cortex–white matter junction, "cracking" artefact between infarcted and intact brain, and marked shift of midline structures from left to right, with pronounced subfalcine herniation. *B:* Fatal Duret brain stem hemorrhages that had resulted from this cerebral infarct, which had caused edema and herniations. *C:* Old cystic infarcts on undersurfaces of both temporal-occipital lobes, in the PCA territories of supply. *D:* Old cystic infarct in the right MCA territory (note sparing of mesial frontal cortex and white matter, which are supplied by the ACA). *E:* Old cystic infarct in left ACA territory, seen as multifocal cystic cavitation of white matter and the overlying cortex. *F:* Old cystic infarct in cerebellar cortex (arrow), probably resulting from vertebrobasilar thromboembolic disease.

after sublethal ischemic injury or neuronal damage has been undertaken in experimental settings.[90] Macrophages initially aggregate around capillaries. Macrophage density tends to be highest 2–3 weeks following an infarct; thereafter, they decrease in number, though in the author's experience many may be at the edges or center of an infarct that was clearly documented to have occurred years prior to a patient's death.

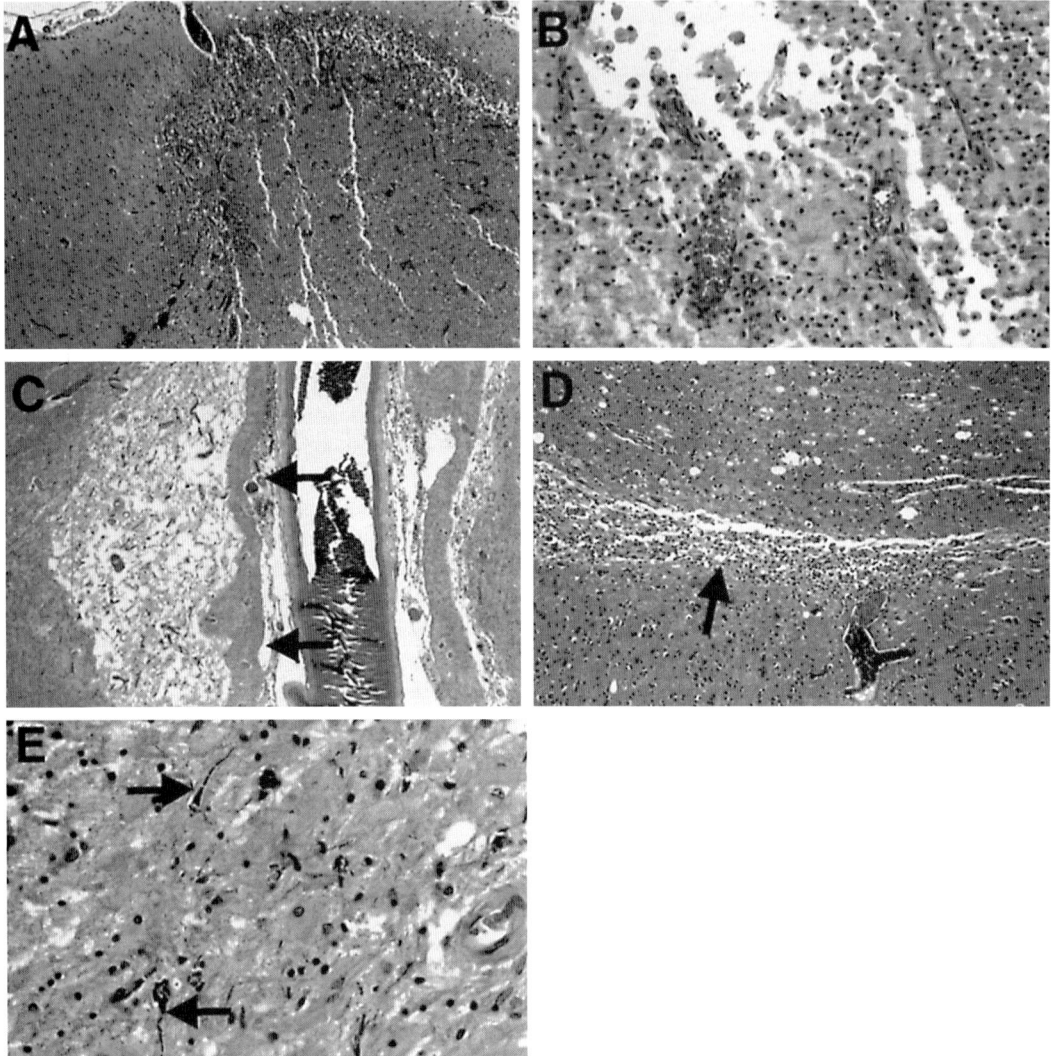

Figure 4-14. Cerebral infarcts, microscopic features. *A.* Relatively recent infarct (several days prior to death). Note clear line of demarcation between intact cortex (at left) and infarcted brain (at right). Junction between the two regions shows prominent microvascular endothelial proliferation. *B.* Detail from center of the area of encephalomalacia shows numerous macrophages. *C.* An old infarct shows typical preservation of the molecular layer (arrows) and underlying cystic cavity traversed by strands of glial and vascular tissue. *D.* An old (weeks to months) micro-infarct at cortex–white matter junction shows a slit-like cavity filled with macrophages (arrow) and surrounded by astrocytes. *E.* A frequent finding around old cystic infarcts is encrustation of dead neurons (arrows) and axons by calcium and iron (ferruginization). H&E, magnification: A, C, ×20; B, ×100; D, ×55; E, ×220.

Between two and four weeks after an infarct, endothelial proliferation with neovascularization occurs. Reactive astrocytes proliferate at the margins of an infarct and become hypertrophic, often taking on the appearance of gemistocytes. Eventually, 4–5 weeks after the infarct, capillaries become less prominent, necrotic debris and macrophages are less conspicuous or may disappear altogether, and a dense glial scar forms around the infarct cavity, whether it be large or small (e.g., a lacunar infarct).

WATERSHED OR BORDER ZONE INFARCTS

These occur along the boundaries between two arterial territories, generally major vessels such as the ACA and MCA; however, watershed infarcts may affect the brain stem, basal ganglia and cerebellum (Fig. 4–15).[91] When present in the cerebral hemispheres, border zone infarcts are often symmetrical bilaterally (in both location and extent) in the two cerebral hemispheres. Several hypotheses as to how or why they occur have been proposed, including profound hypotension and microemboli.[92,93] Watershed/border zone infarcts are most commonly associated with a sharp, often sustained, drop in systemic blood pressure—e.g., in an elderly individual with atherosclerosis undergoing major abdominal or cardiovascular surgery. Decrease in blood flow under such circumstances appears to be most severe in the arterial end fields. Emboli composed of cholesterol clefts or atheromatous debris from a more proximal plaque may occlude vessels within affected border zones.

LACUNAR INFARCTS

As mentioned above, arteriosclerosis (AS) or lipohyalinosis (LH) has been associated historically with two types of brain insult, viz., lacunar infarcts and intracerebral (*intraparenchymal*) hemorrhage. Lacunar infarcts are usually small (15 mm maximal dimension) regions of cystic cavitation most often seen within basal ganglia, thalamus, pons, internal capsule, and deep subcortical white matter (Fig. 4–16).[94–97] When found in abundance within the subcortical white matter, they are associated with the clinical syndrome of Binswanger's subcortical leukoencephalopathy (BSLE). Lacunar infarcts are to be distinguished from prominently enlarged perivascular spaces, which they may almost perfectly mimic on gross, and sometimes even microscopic, examination of the brain.[98] Lacunar infarcts have been associated with several distinctive stroke syndromes. Despite the historical association among lacunes, AS/LH, and high blood pressure, a documented history of hypertension is not found in as many as 35%–40% of individuals with these small, deep brain infarcts.[99] It has even been suggested that lacunes are the result of carotid atherosclerosis (e.g., through hemodynamic changes and/or atheroemboli) or even nonatheromatous emboli.[100] A large clinical study has found that, while lacunar syndromes are highly predictive of finding lacunes on appropriate neuroimaging studies, in approximately 25% of patients with lacunar syndromes (confirmed radiographically) the condition is associated with nonlacunar mechanisms of infarction.[101] Small areas of cystic cavitation resembling lacunar infarcts may result from nonhypertensive microvascular disease, e.g., in an octogenarian whose brain was examined because he was felt to have a mixed parenchymal/ischemic vascular dementia; sections of the brain showed multifocal areas resembling lacunes throughout the white matter, apparently the result of meningovascular syphilis rather than AS/LH (Fig. 4–17).

Occluded arteries of varying caliber may be found in close proximity to lacunar infarcts. When the abnormal artery has a diameter of 40–200 μm, it may show typical features of AS/LH, whereas a larger artery (up to 500 μm diameter) may contain microatheroma within its lumen and wall.[102,103] Defining clinicopathologic substrates of lacunes is especially diffi-

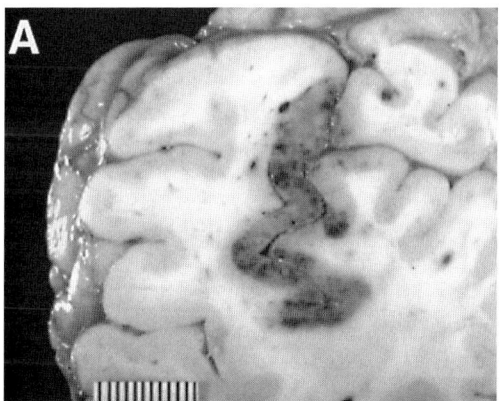
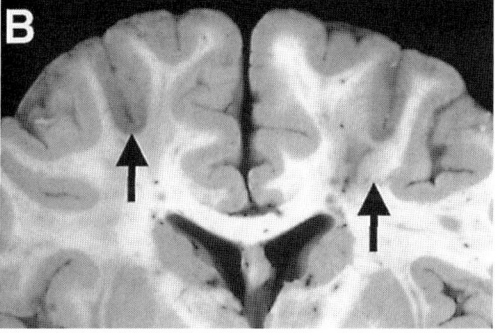

Figure 4–15. Watershed infarcts. *A.* Hemispheric infarct in the border zone between the left ACA and MCA territories. *B.* Symmetrical ACA/MCA border zone infarcts (arrows) in both cerebral hemispheres. Infarct on the right involves subcortical white matter as well as overlying cortex.

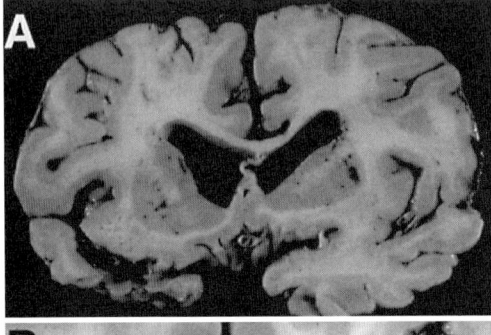

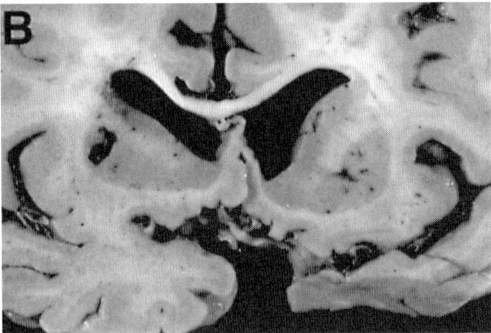

Figure 4–16. Lacunar infarcts (arrows) are commonly associated with a clinical history of hypertension. They typically involve the basal ganglia (as in this case; both panels represent coronal brain slices from the same patient), thalamus, and pons, and may extend into the internal capsule, resulting in focal neurologic signs.

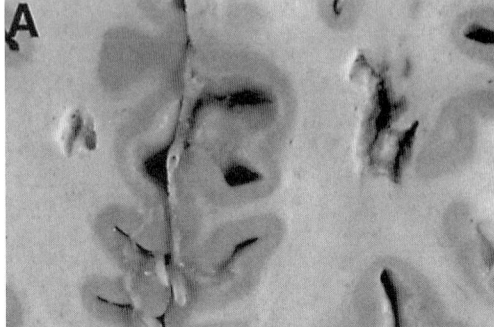

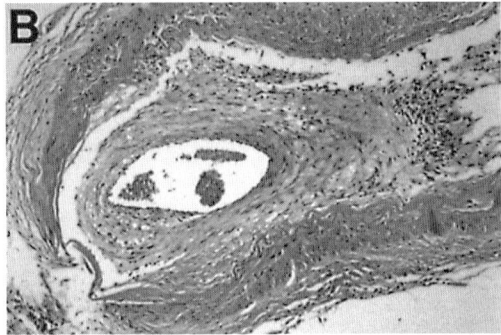

Figure 4–17. An elderly patient with a history of dementia and, at autopsy, typical features of meningovascular syphilis. *A.* Multiple cystic infarcts resembling lacunes are seen, especially within the subcortical white matter. *B.* Histologic sections showed typical features of Heubner's arteritis, involving meningeal arteries, as in this micrograph. H&E, magnification: B, ×55.

cult, given that the lesions are frequently asymptomatic.[104] Occurrence of AS/LH is also associated with intracerebral hemorrhage (see below). Miliary microaneurysms of Charcot-Bouchard (C-B) type have been discovered in hypertensive patients with parenchymal hemorrhage caused by hypertension.[105,106] More recent cytochemical and microradiagraphic study of cerebral microvessels in brains of hypertensive patients suggests that C-B aneurysms are rare and may sometimes simply represent arteriolar coils and twists that are interpreted as miliary microaneurysms.[107] It is the author's strong view that miliary (C-B type) microaneurysms (Fig. 4–18) are a nonspecific manifestation of microvascular or arteriolar degeneration, whether the result of AS/LH, CAA, or other less common entities such as CADASIL.

Infarcts in specific vascular territories, the result of atherosclerotic or embolic occlusion of major branches of the circle of Willis or more proximal segments of the carotid or vertebrobasilar systems, produce characteristic neurologic syndromes. A detailed discussion of these is beyond the scope of this chapter; the reader is referred to detailed descriptions of their clinicopathologic features.[1,4,108–113]

Venous (Including Sinus) Thrombosis

Thrombosis of dural venous sinuses occurs as an infrequent complication of various infectious and noninfectious processes, including polycythemia, sickle cell anemia (or trait), paroxysmal nocturnal hemoglobinuria, trauma, vasculitis, pregnancy, use of oral contraceptives, congenital heart disease, presence of lupus anticoagulants, dehydration, marasmus, and compression by mass lesions such as neoplasms or aneurysms; only a small proportion of which, e.g., septic thrombosis, are of importance in the geriatric population.[114–119] Recent reviews have emphasized that cerebral

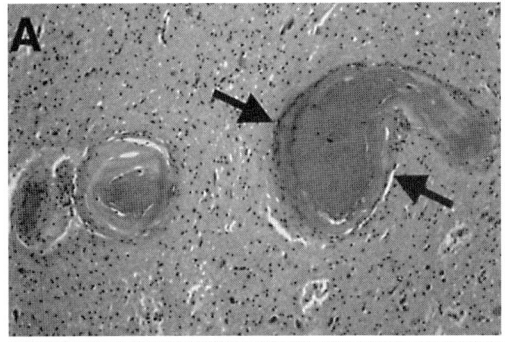
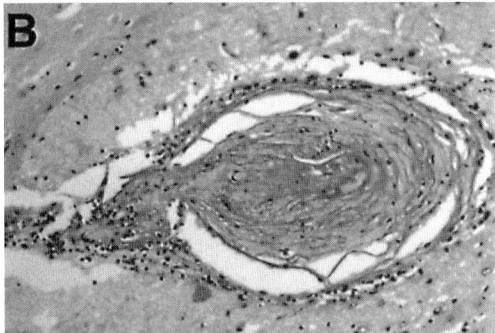
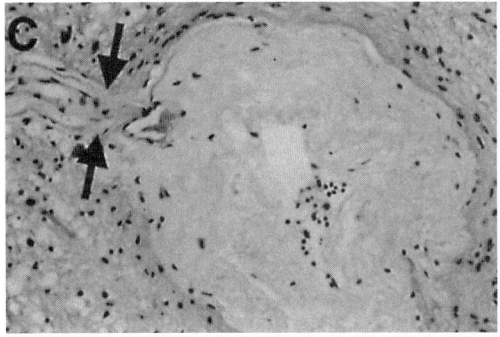

Figure 4–18. Charcot-Bouchard (C-B) microaneurysms, a characteristic complication of cerebral arteriolar degeneration, regardless of cause. *A.* Severe widespread cerebral arteriosclerosis. Aneurysmal dilatation (arrows) is noted in a markedly thickened arteriole. *B.* Cerebral amyloid angiopathy (CAA). Note balloon-like outpouching of an arteriole in a patient with widespread and severe CAA. *C.* C-B type microaneurysm in a patient with CADASIL. Neck of the aneurysm is indicated by arrows. H&E, magnification: A, ×55; B,C, ×110.

venous thrombosis (CVT) is far more common than previously thought, has a wide variety of clinical presentations and mode of onset, may have a favorable outcome, and is treatable using heparin or selective catheterization and urokinase.[120,121]

The cavernous sinuses, located at the skull base superior and lateral to the sphenoid sinuses, are the ones most commonly involved by septic thrombosis. The most common primary site of infection associated with cavernous sinus thrombosis is the medial face; common causal pathogens include gram-positive bacteria, especially *Staphylococcus aureus*.[114] Infection of the ethmoid and sphenoid air sinuses and dental infections are also conditions predisposing to septic cavernous sinus thrombosis.

Thrombosis in the cavernous sinus can extend to involve other dural sinuses, e.g., the petrosal, sigmoid, lateral, and inferior.[115] Spread of infection to the pituitary gland, with its resultant necrosis, has been described, as have associated findings such as meningitis, brain abscess, and cortical vein thrombosis with anemic or hemorrhagic brain infarction. Septic lateral sinus thrombosis is nearly always associated with spread of infection from the mastoid air cells after otitis media.[114,115] Pathogens usually associated with otitis media or mastoiditis include *Proteus* species, *Staph. aureus*, anaerobes or *Escherichia coli*. Septic superior sagittal sinus thrombosis occurs less commonly than thrombosis of the cavernous or lateral sinuses. The most common predisposing condition is bacterial meningitis, probably with associated spread of infection along diploic veins.

INTRACRANIAL HEMORRHAGE

Hemorrhage into the various intracranial compartments will be considered separately, beginning with the most superficial. This may be an arbitrary separation, since some etiologic mechanisms operative in (as one example) subarachnoid hemorrhage are also important in the pathogenesis of intraparenchymal hemorrhage. Also, bleeds into one compartment can easily extend into another—primary intraparenchymal bleeds may extend into the ventricular cavities, then into the subarachnoid space.

Extra-/Epidural Hemorrhage

Extra-/epidural hemorrhage (EDH) is more appropriately considered in relation to craniocerebral trauma, with which it is almost invariably linked; spontaneous EDH is an extraordinarily rare event.[8] In a large series of fatal head injuries from an Irish neurosurgical unit, neuropathologic findings included EDH in 18% of patients, acute intracerebral hematoma in 27%, subdural hematoma (SDH) in 45%, and skull fracture in 69% (patients not substratified by age).[122] Other studies suggest that over 90% of EDH patients are likely to have a skull fracture.[123] After a closed head injury, EDH presents as a rapidly evolving neurologic deficit, because the bleeding is usually from an arterial source (e.g., the middle meningeal artery) adjacent to a skull fracture. Less commonly, it results from tearing of a venous sinus. It may occur together with SDH. Extra-/epidural hemorrhage is found in 5%–15% of non-missile head injuries; the blood clot most commonly comes to occupy the temporal fossa in adults, the posterior fossa in children. Mortality from this condition is highest in the geriatric population. However, if treated early by drainage of the clotted blood, patients may make an uneventful recovery, provided substantial damage to the underlying brain tissue has not occurred.

Documentation of a fatal EDH must be carefully made at the time of necropsy; if this is *not* done during unroofing of the calvarium, another opportunity is unlikely to arise. It usually presents as a biconvex hematoma readily seen on removing the calvarium, before the dura is breached. As patients who have succumbed to EDH are often the subject of a forensic or medicolegal investigation, the size and site of any (causal) skull fracture and the volume of the hematoma should be assessed—bleeds of 75–100 ml are usually fatal. The pathologist should also document effects of the hematoma on the brain, e.g., distortion, herniations, and any associated contusions or lacerations of the brain substance.

Subdural Hemorrhage

This type of hemorrhage may be either acute or chronic, and is a major problem in the elderly. It has protean clinical manifestations, and frequently insidious evolution and presentation. Unlike EDH, SDH is not always associated with trauma—at least clinically perceived, documented or reported trauma. The clinical evolution of SDH may occur with a more indolent tempo, since bleeding is usually from a venous source, i.e., the bridging veins between the dura and the (leptomeningeal) brain surface. In a small number of patients, SDH may represent dissection of blood from the subarachnoid space, where it has originated from an arterial source such as a ruptured berry aneurysm or arteriovenous malformation (see below), into the subdural space.[1,8,9]

The pathogenesis of acute SDH is usually traumatic, resulting from the head being subjected to rapid acceleration or deceleration. Under these circumstances the brain, being a relatively inert structure, lags in movement in relation to that of the skull. This can cause traction on, and tearing of, the bridging veins between the brain surface and dura mater; the latter is tightly adherent to the inner table of the skull. Chronic SDH begins with rupture of the same bridging veins, but the acute hemorrhage is followed by cycles of organization and rebleeding due to the formation of richly vascular granulation tissue (or pseudomembrane) around the hematoma (Fig. 4–19).[8,9,124] Patients with impaired hemostasis (disease-

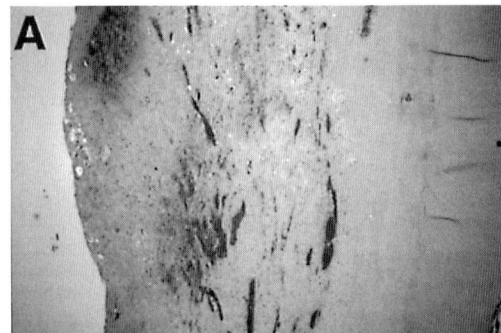
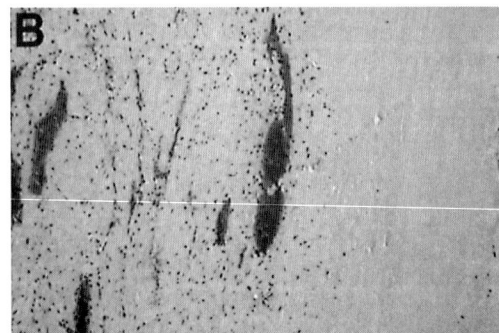

Figure 4–19. Subdural hematoma (SDH), organizing membrane. Both micrographs show dura (at right), and underlying this, richly vascularized granulation tissue, which can serve as nidus for repeated cycles of SDH. H&E, magnification: A, ×20; B, ×55.

associated or iatrogenic coagulopathy, platelet abnormalities) may develop spontaneous acute or chronic SDH, as may patients with dural tumors (metastases, meningiomas) or vascular malformations. In patients with hematologic malignancies or abnormal coagulation, smear subdural hematomas, of no clinical importance, are commonly found at autopsy.

Subdural hemorrhage, which may be bilateral, should be suspected in any patient who has experienced head trauma; the clinical diagnosis can be confirmed by appropriate neuroimaging studies. The unique problems involved with management of chronic SDH in the elderly are discussed in several publications.[125–127] Chronic SDH occurs most commonly in patients over the age of 50 years—in one study, the most common age-group affected (among both men and women) was 70–80 years old. The causal head injury may be trivial or not even recognized by the patient. Progression of clinical signs and symptoms may be stuttering or slow; in some patients, dementia may be the presenting feature of chronic SDH. Chronic SDH is especially common in people with cerebral atrophy due to aging or Alzheimer's disease, thus dementia secondary to the SDH may be difficult to differentiate from that due to underlying brain parenchymal disease. In patients who come to autopsy with SDH, the precise size and location of the clot and its impact on brain substance needs to be carefully evaluated; this can be done by weighing the subdural clot or estimating the volume of water it displaces.

Subarachnoid Hemorrhage

Hemorrhage into the subarachnoid space is a major cause of morbidity and mortality in people of all age-groups beyond childhood. Its somewhat less conspicuous profile in the elderly may simply reflect the fact that other types of intracranial cerebrovascular accident, usually related to atherosclerosis, hypertensive microvascular disease, or CAA (see above), are relatively more common in the geriatric age-group than in the young and middle-aged. Subarachnoid hemorrhage (SAH) may be secondary to intraparenchymal brain hemorrhage (IPH), i.e., when passage of blood occurs into the subarachnoid space, or it may represent the result of rupture of an aneurysm on the circle of Willis, one of its branches, or a distal arterial segment, a vascular malformation (hemangioma) within brain parenchyma or (rarely) on the circle of Willis, a neoplasm, or systemic causes.

BERRY/SACCULAR ANEURYSMS

An *aneurysm* may be defined as a localized and persistent pathologic dilatation of the heart or a blood vessel that results from the yielding of wall components.[1] Berry aneurysms, also referred to as saccular or congenital, usually occur at major bifurcation points on the circle of Willis (Fig. 4–20).) Over half occur on anterior portions of the circle of Willis, usually at the internal carotid (ICA)–posterior communicating artery or anterior choroidal artery junction, MCA bi -or trifurcation in the Sylvian fissure, and ACA—anterior communicating artery junction. Berry aneurysms may present with SAH at any age; in the Framingham Study, mean age at presentation with a SAH was essentially identical for men and women (62–63 years), whereas other studies suggest a mean age of aneurysmal rupture at around 55–60 years.[128,129] Most berry aneurysms present between the ages of 40 and 70 years, thus they appear as a more significant clinical problem in middle-aged than geriatric patients. Such aneurysms are approximately 1.5 to 2 times as common in women than men. From 10% to 30% of patients have multiple aneurysms.[130] Since a typical aneurysm expands gradually into the subarachnoid space, it rarely produces symptoms prior to rupture. However, cranial nerves may be compressed as they exit the brain stem, leading to isolated palsies. Giant aneurysms (usually larger than 2.5 cm in diameter) may present as space-occupying lesions within the brain, often with long-standing neurobehavioral abnormalities.[131] Warning signs of an impending SAH (usually a small hemorrhage or sentinel bleed) are described in as many as 20% of patients who progress to having a larger bleed.[130]

Though referred to as congenital, berry/saccular aneurysms are only rarely encountered in children or infants; however, this does not rule out the possibility that a fully developed aneurysm found in later life represents growth of a focus of mechanical weakening in a younger vessel. This theory has, however,

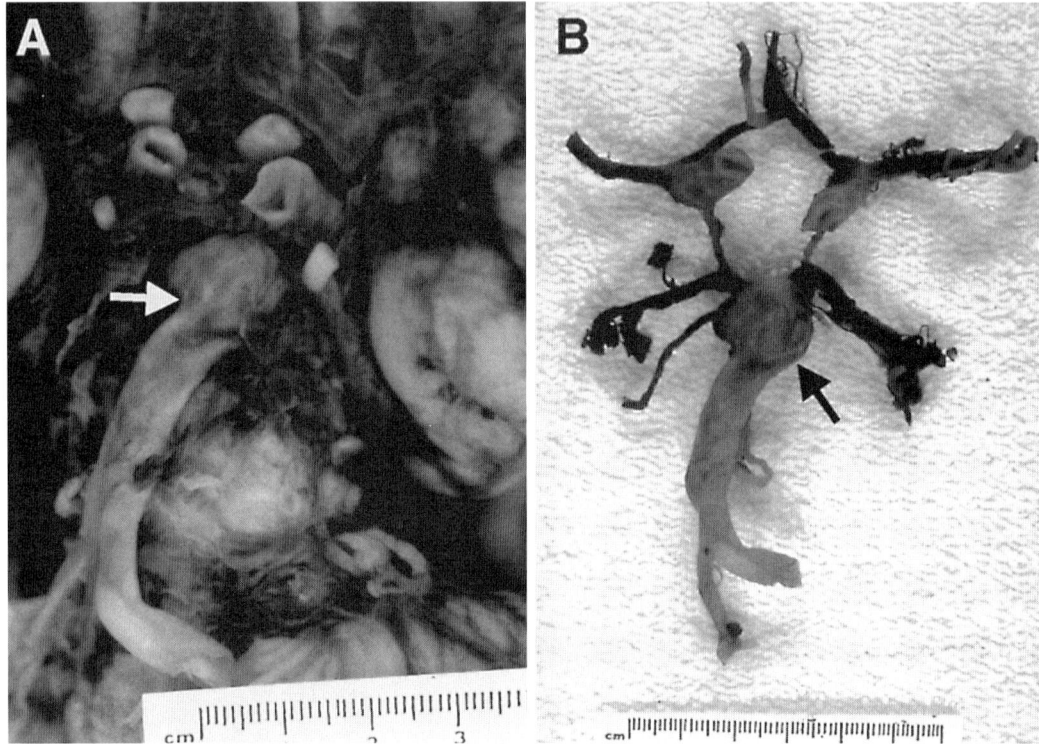

Figure 4–20. Berry (saccular) aneurysm of the basilar artery. Patient died of cerebral edema associated with massive subarachnoid hemorrhage. A. Aneurysm visible at base of the (fixed) brain (arrow); abundant subarachnoid hemorrhage is noted in adjacent basal cisterns. B. Circle of Willis dissected from the brain; note prominent aneurysm, which had undergone recent thrombosis, at the basilar artery tip (arrow).

been disputed.[1] Alternatively, berry aneurysms may develop as a result of degenerative changes within cerebral blood vessels, possibly secondary to loss of tensile strength due to weakening of connective tissues and/or elastica within their walls. Theories on the pathogenesis of berry aneurysms are abundant.[1,129,130] An increased incidence of intracerebral aneurysm is seen in many systemic diseases, including polycystic kidney disease, Marfan and Ehlers-Danlos syndromes, pseudoxanthoma elasticum, fibromuscular dysplasia, sickle cell disease, and coarctation of the aorta. African-Americans have approximately twice the risk of SAH seen in the Caucasian population.[130]

Rupture of a berry aneurysm usually produces life-threatening SAH (Fig. 4–21), though bleeding may occur directly into brain parenchyma, especially if the rupture site on the dome of the aneurysm is embedded within brain substance (Fig. 4–22). Intraventricular hemorrhage may also occur, though usually this is secondary to abundant blood within the subarachnoid space. Therefore, when an intraparenchymal hematoma is encountered in any patient, berry aneurysm should be considered in the etiologic differential diagnosis. The mortality from SAH secondary to a ruptured berry aneurysm is, unfortunately, high: it is estimated as 35%–50% in various studies.[132,133] Survivors of a SAH have major post-bleed morbidity, often associated with the development of hydrocephalus (secondary to scarring of the meninges) or rebleeding. Post-hemorrhage vasospasm, leading to multiple infarcts within the CNS, is a feared complication of a large SAH.[130,134] Successful clipping of an aneurysm by a skilled neurosurgeon with minimal postoperative complications may, however, be associated with an essentially normal life expectancy. These lesions are occasionally encountered in autopsies of elderly individuals

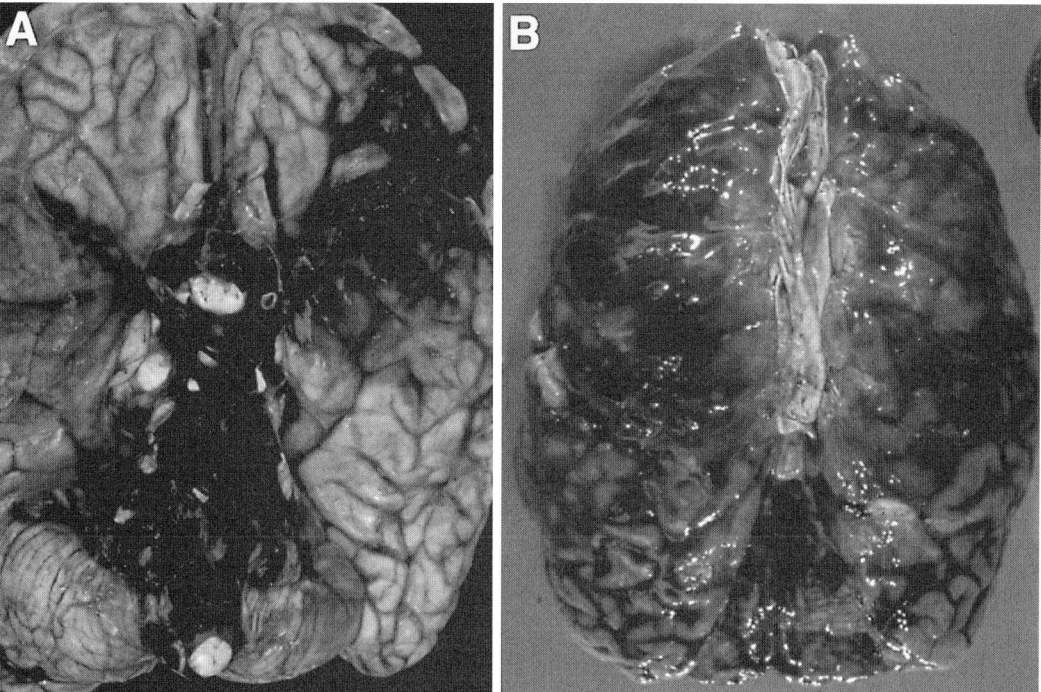

Figure 4–21. Massive fatal subarachnoid hemorrhage (SAH) in two different patients. A. Basal view of the brain, with clotted blood throughout basal cisterns and extending into the left Sylvian fissure. B. View of brain from the convexities; gyri and sulci are not visible because of massive acute SAH.

(Fig. 4–23),) even when no history of a SAH is available!

Berry aneurysms are encountered as an incidental finding at autopsy with an estimated frequency that varies tremendously—figures from 4% to 17% are quoted.[129,130] This variability probably reflects the size threshold accepted by a given pathologist for calling a lesion aneurysmal, or the care with which these tiny lesions are sought by the prosector. When seen in the elderly, incidental (unruptured) berry aneurysms often show significant superimposed atherosclerotic change (Fig. 4–24). There is controversy as to the factors (including, and especially, aneurysm size) that precipitate SAH. Aneurysms smaller than 10 mm in diameter have a low rate of rupture; location of an aneurysm also appears to be important in determining the likelihood of its bleeding, i.e., ICA–posterior communicating artery aneurysms and those within the vertebrobasilar system (especially located at the basilar artery tip) are more likely to hemorrhage than others.[135,136] Histologic sections of a berry aneurysm show loss of the elastica associated with thinning of the vascular media, especially around the rupture site (Fig. 4–25).

INFLAMMATORY (MYCOTIC) ANEURYSMS

These lesions, accounting for 3%–6% of all intracranial aneurysms, are almost always associated with subacute or acute bacterial endocarditis, less often with spread of infection from a contiguous site (e.g. meningitis, osteomyelitis) into the vessel wall.[8,129,137,138] Microorganisms causing the endocarditis may be varied and often are of low virulence; both bacteria and fungi can be responsible, the latter especially in immunocompromised patients and intravenous drug abusers. Inflammatory aneurysms (IAs), unlike berry aneurysms, usually occupy distal and peripheral branches of the arterial circulation. Rupture of an IA may result in SAH or IPH. An aneurysm, friable and weakened because of polymorphonuclear leukocytes in the vessel

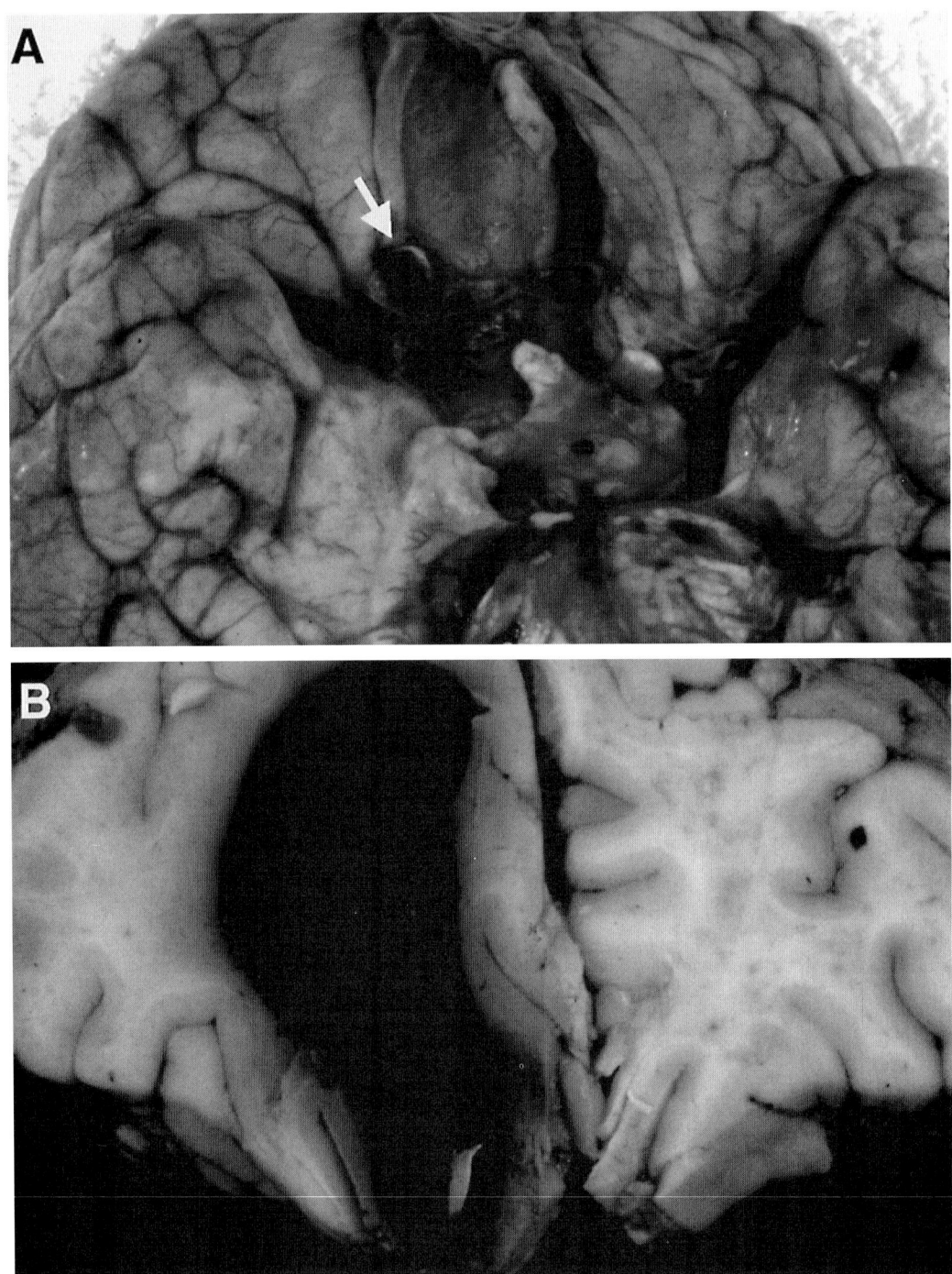

Figure 4–22. Right carotid–ophthalmic artery berry aneurysm in a 56-year-old woman. Balloon occlusion of the aneurysm was attempted. Basal view of (unfixed) brain in panel A shows the balloon (arrow), but surprisingly little subarachnoid hemorrhage. Coronal section of the fixed brain (B) shows large intraparenchymal hematoma in the right frontal lobe.

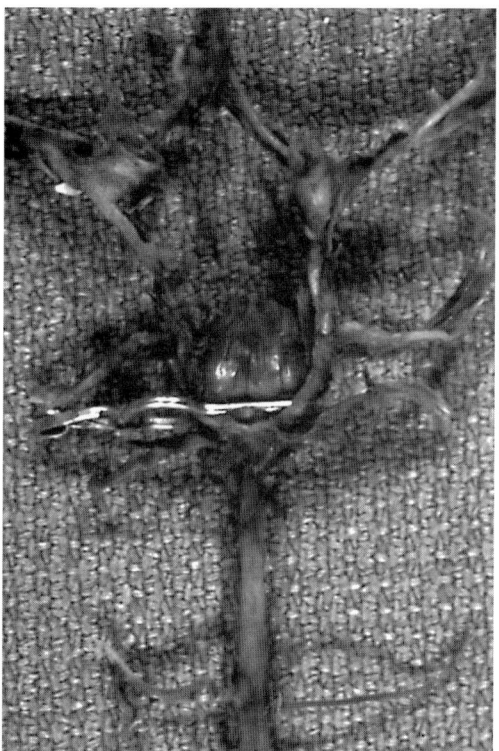

Figure 4–23. A large basilar tip aneurysm that had undergone clipping prior to patient's death.

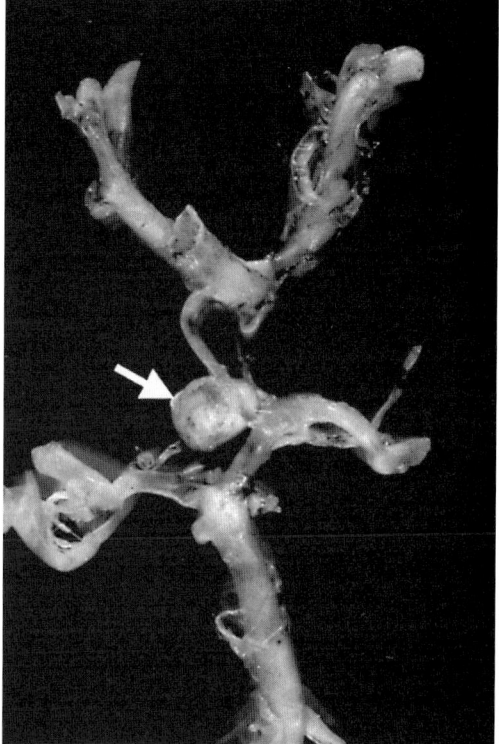

Figure 4–24. Berry aneurysm (arrow) identified in an elderly patient who underwent autopsy to establish the cause of dementia. The aneurysm showed extensive atheroma in its wall, but no evidence of previous rupture.

wall, is often resected in the course of removal of an intracerebral clot and must be sought in any such specimen that results from an at-risk patient. Stainable microorganisms may be seen among inflammatory cells on sections of an IA.

The pathogenesis of an IA due to endocarditis is hypothesized to result from a septic embolus that lodges within a branch of a cerebral artery, with subsequent extension of microorganisms from the embolus into the vessel wall. Septic emboli in individuals with infective endocarditis may lead to a pyogenic arteritis, not necessarily resulting in IAs, causing hemorrhagic transformation of an ischemic (bland) infarct or intracerebral hemorrhage.[139]

DISSECTING ANEURYSMS

These are almost always encountered in young and middle-aged patients (25–45 years old), only rarely in those over 65.[140–145] Dissection may occur in extracranial or intracranial branches of the carotid or vertebrobasilar system. Farrell et al.[140] have described autopsy findings in seven affected individuals with the syndrome of intracranial arterial dissection. When dissection had occurred in the anterior circulation, its site was between the internal elastic lamina and the media, with resultant intravascular thrombosis. When dissection had occurred in the posterior circulation, transmural dissection had often resulted in SAH. Variable degrees of acute inflammation were present at sites of dissection. Specific degenerative or inflammatory vasculopathies could not, however, be clearly identified. Clinically, arterial dissection is associated with trauma to the neck (often perceived as quite minimal), following exercise, after administration of heparin, or in the context of fibromuscular dysplasia, though none of these antecedent events or conditions may be present in a given patient. Intracerebral hemorrhage has been described in a 72-year-old man following transmural dissection of the ACA.[146]

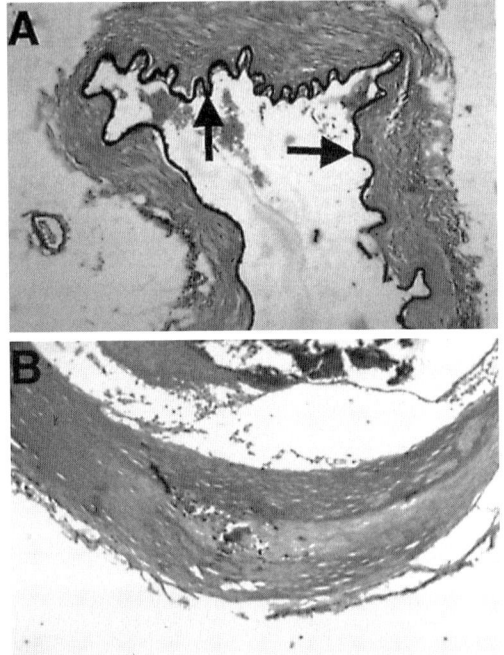

Figure 4–25. Histologic features of a berry/saccular aneurysm. Sections stained with elastica van Gieson. Portion of a normal intracranial artery (A) shows prominent internal elastic lamina (arrows). By contrast, a ruptured berry aneurysm from the same patient (B) shows complete absence of elastica in its wall and fibromuscular hyperplasia with focal calcification, i.e., atheromatous change. Magnification: A, ×55; B, ×20.

FUSIFORM ANEURYSMS

These lesions present (to the pathologist) as ectatic, often very tortuous or serpentine, basal arteries. They are unusual lesions, but of relatively greater clinical import in the geriatric population, largely because of their association with complicated atherosclerosis.[8,36] Conversely, in young patients they may be associated with deficiencies of the arterial muscularis and internal elastic lamina.[147] In one clinicopathologic review of the entity, seven autopsy cases presented over an age range of 56–65 years.[36] As their name implies, fusiform aneurysms result from enlargement and widening of an arterial segment along its length (Fig. 4–26). Most often, they are found on the basilar artery, though fusiform aneurysms may also occur on the anterior circulation.[147] In the older literature, they have been described as "arteriosclerotic aneurysms."[148,149] They may reach giant proportions (arbitrarily defined as larger than 2.5 cm) and often have laminated thrombi within their walls when examined in cross section; this probably results from severe complicated atheromatous change. Acute and chronic inflammatory change has been found within the walls of fusiform atherosclerotic aneurysms; this may be a primary cause of their becoming symptomatic, or it may be in response to severe atheromatous change or related thrombosis or rupture of the aneurysm.[36]

Fusiform aneurysms on the basilar artery can enlarge to the point where they cause significant brain stem displacement and compression, resulting in cranial nerve deficits. Because laminated thrombus is often present within their lumina, platelet-fibrin or atheromatous embolic material may travel distally in the circulation to produce transient ischemic attacks or infarcts in branches of the vertebrobasilar circulation. Such aneurysms may also rupture to produce SAH.

Intraparenchymal Hemorrhage

This may also be described as encephalic or brain hemorrhage, and defines primary bleeding into the brain substance rather than an adjacent compartment (see above) (Fig. 4–27). Obviously, IPH may extend into the ventricular cavities and the subarachnoid space. As a cause of stroke, IPHs are comparatively much less common (especially among the elderly) in Western populations than are infarcts resulting form atherothrombotic disease or even cerebral emboli.[8] The most common causes of IPH are, in roughly decreasing frequency, hypertension, CAA, anticoagulant administration, primary or secondary brain neoplasms, prescription or recreational drug use, arteriovenous malformations (AVMs) and aneurysms, and miscellaneous causes.[3] The discussion below will emphasize those conditions of greatest importance in the geriatric population. One study has suggested that spontaneous hematomas may readily occur within cerebral infarcts, and that primary IPH may thus be overdiagnosed.[150]

Given the increasing recognition and effective treatment of hypertension, a reasonable prediction would be that high blood pressure (HBP) should be in decline as a major cause of IPH; there is some evidence that this has

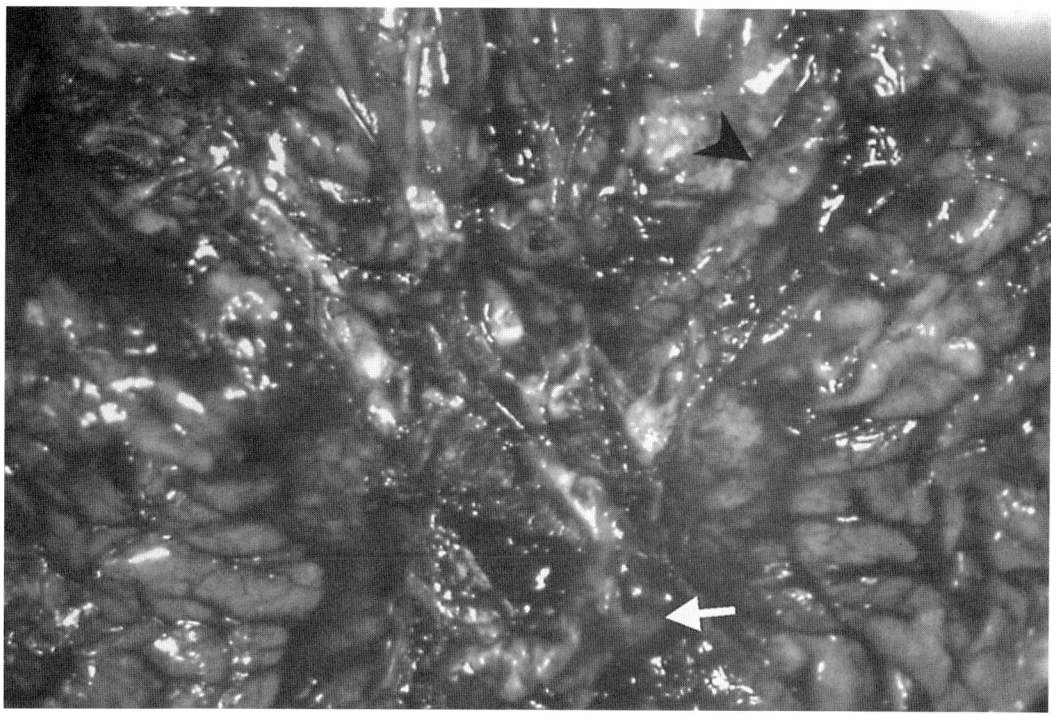

Figure 4–26. Basal view of (unfixed) brain from an elderly patient with severe atherosclerosis. Note marked atherosclerosis of all branches of the circle of Willis, but especially prominent within the basilar artery and left MCA. The basilar artery shows ectasia and tortuosity (lower arrow), whereas the left MCA shows fusiform enlargement (upper arrowhead). [Photograph courtesy of Prof. Michael A. Farrell, Dublin, Ireland].

been happening over recent decades.[3] Indeed, a population-based study from Japan has shown a diminution in the annual incidence of intracerebral hemorrhage between 1961 and 1983.[151] Among males over age 40 years, this figure decreased from 3.1/1000 (1961–1970) to 1.2/1000 (1974–1983). In autopsy series, the incidence of IPH varies markedly from center to center, as do apparent etiologies. This often reflects the unique clinical interests of a given center or the demographics of the population from which individuals are referred. In a setting where hematologic malignancies are treated aggressively in large numbers, for instance, IPH related to leukemia or thrombocytopenia would likely be disproportionately represented. Clinical and neuroimaging features of IPH are well described in recent and older reviews.[3–5,152]

HYPERTENSION

The assignment of the cause of primary IPH to HBP is usually done on the basis of (*a*) the presence within the brain of a patient who has experienced hemorrhage of microvascular changes (described above) as arteriosclerosis/lipohyalinosis (AS/LH), with or without Charcot-Bouchard (C-B) type microaneurysms, and/or (*b*) a clinical history of documented HBP, and/or (*c*) autopsy evidence for long-standing HBP, e.g., nephrosclerosis, or cardiomegaly with left ventricular hypertrophy. Typical locations for hypertensive IPH include the lateral or medial basal ganglia, thalamus, pons, and cerebellum, though hematomas may also be seen in the deep subcortical white matter (Fig. 4–28). The term "hypertensive hemorrhage" is sometimes applied to a given IPH with minimal support for the putative etiology.[153] The significance of increased heart weight (cardiomegaly) or left ventricular hypertrophy (LVH) found at autopsy is often not clear. Systemic hypertension is a common (perhaps the most common) cause of severe LVH, though other causes (e.g., aortic stenosis, ventricular septal defect, pericarditis, coronary artery disease) must al-

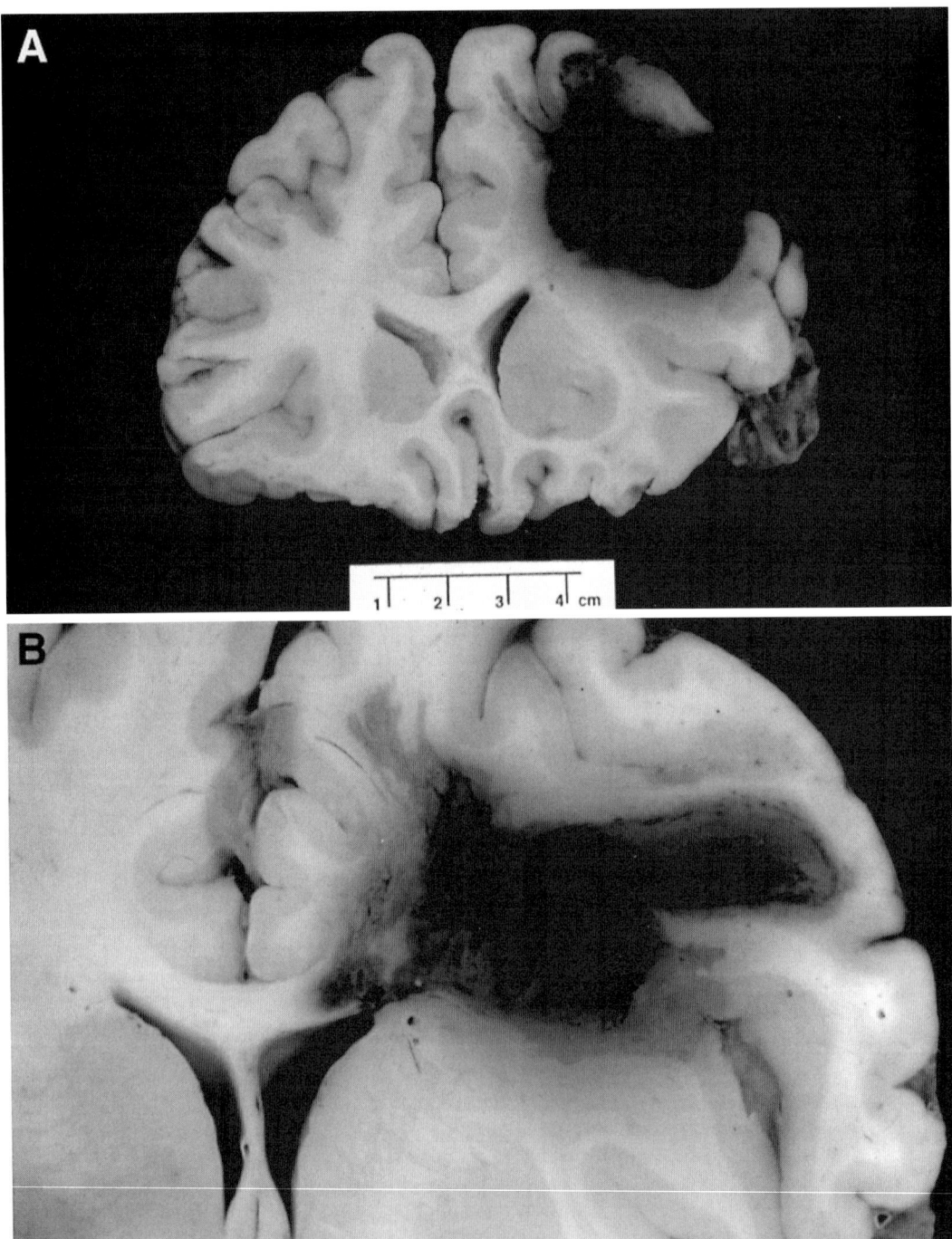

Figure 4–27. Intraparenchymal (IPH) (intracerebral) hemorrhage into the right frontal lobe, seen at two different levels. Precise etiology of the hemorrhage was not established, although histologic features of the brain parenchyma adjacent to the hematoma were suggestive of an occult vascular malformation. Patient was not hypertensive and did not have cerebral amyloid angiopathy. Note that the hemorrhage is in communication with both the subarachnoid space (A) and the right lateral ventricle (B).

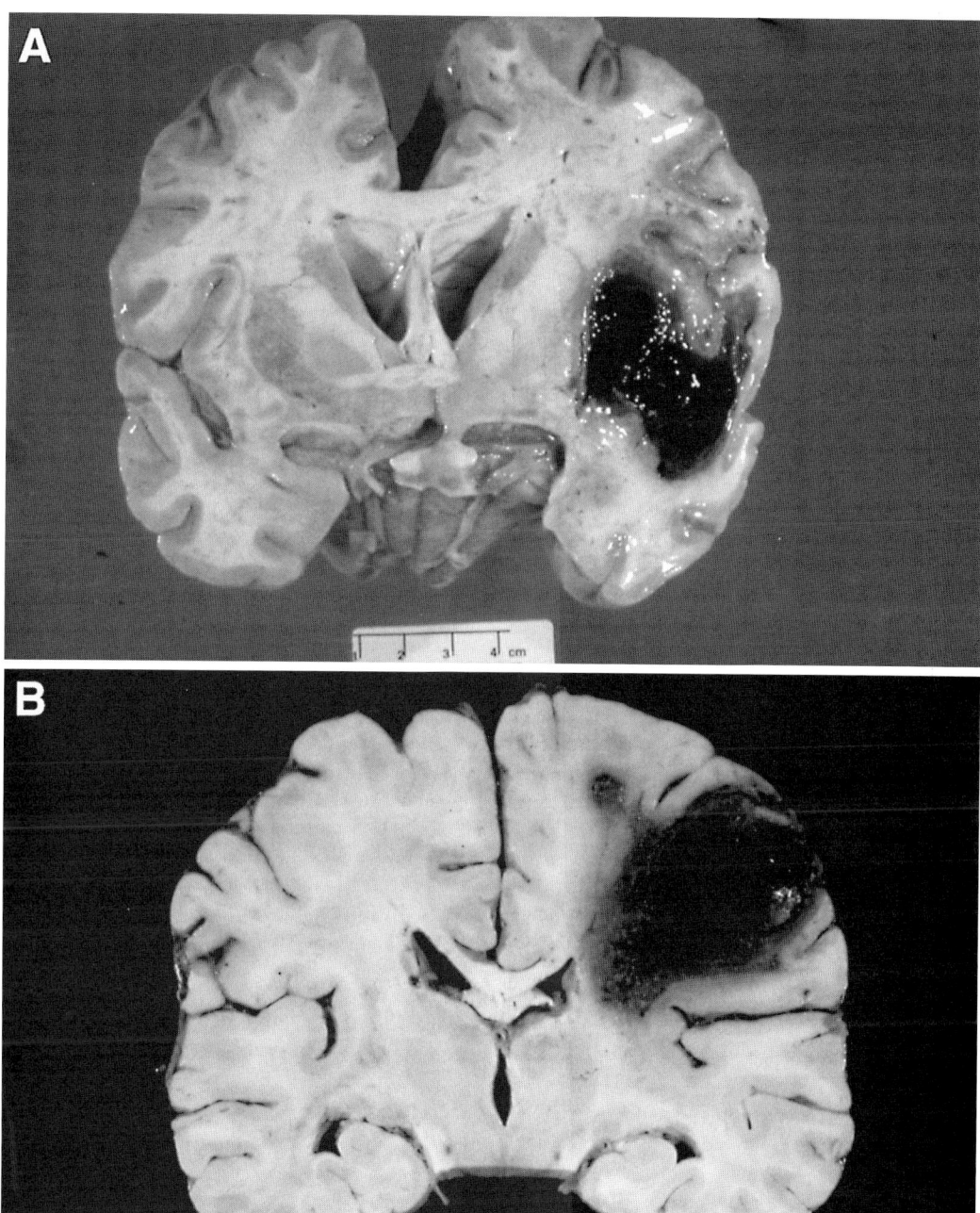

Figure 4–28. Hypertensive intraparenchymal hemorrhage *A.* Freshly cut brain shows subacute clotted blood in the right basal ganglia, extending into the right temporal lobe. Hemorrhage probably originated in the right putamen. *B.* Organizing right cerebral hypertensive hemorrhage in a 63-year-old patient.

ways be considered and ruled out by careful examination of the heart. Using a rigorous autopsy definition of apparent HBP, i.e., heart weight greater than the mean cardiac weight of necropsy controls +1.5 standard deviations, one investigator found that only 46% of patients with primary intracerebral hemorrhage had cardiac enlargement by this criterion.[154,155] Indeed, many patients with primary IPH had experienced relatively healthy lives without evidence of cardiovascular or cerebrovascular disease! Thus, HBP as a cause of IPH must be considered a diagnosis of exclusion.

Microscopic features of AS/LH associated with hypertensive IPH are discussed and illustrated above. Hypertensive IPH results from extravasation of blood from brain parenchymal arterioles that have become noncompliant and weakened by replacement of medial smooth muscle cells (SMC) by collagenous fibrous tissue, and because of fragmentation of the elastica. The C-B type microaneurysms may be found on affected arterioles, though they may be absent even when brain parenchyma around a putative hypertensive hemorrhage is sampled extensively.[156]

Typical appearances of hypertensive hematomas are shown in Figure 4-28. Appearance of a clot will vary, depending upon how long it has been in the brain between stroke onset and the patient's death. Hematomas that are months to years old will show (on gross inspection) a cystic cavity rimmed by yellowish–orange, scarred brain tissue representing the remnants of resorbed blood; the appearances may be quite similar to those of an old cystic infarct. Microscopic sections around the margins of a hematoma will show changes that also reflect the duration of the bleed: subacute hemorrhage (2–4 days) shows reactive microglia, while older bleeds contain hemosiderin-laden macrophages and abundant reactive astrocytes.

CEREBRAL AMYLOID ANGIOPATHY

The pathogenesis and microscopic features of this entity are discussed and illustrated above. It is worth re-emphasizing the patchy nature of CAA within brain cortex and leptomeninges, its segmental nature in a given arteriole, and its strong association with brain aging and AD/SDAT. The extent of amyloid deposition within vessel walls correlates with increasing risk of IPH. Cerebral amyloid angiopathy may have a variety of clinical and neuroradiographic manifestations, including no specific abnormality, but IPH is its most common stroke-related manifestation.[157–162] Other presentations of CAA include SAH without a component of IPH, leukoencephalopathy, angiitis, and recurrent transient neurologic symptoms (possibly due to microhemorrhages and/or microinfarcts within the CNS)—all of them rare.[40,41] An association between CAA and brain ischemic infarcts is less clearly established than that between CAA and IPH.

Cerebral amyloid angiopathy causes IPHs with highly distinctive clinicopathologic features (Fig. 4–29). Hematomas are typically found in patients within the eighth and ninth decades of life, many of whom have overt features of AD/SDAT. They occur within the cortex and subcortical white matter (lobar hemorrhages), and often dissect into the subarachnoid space, and less frequently, the ventricles. This anatomic predilection reflects the topography of CAA, a cortical and meningeal vasculopathy.[52] Heightened awareness of CAA as a likely etiology for cerebral (lobar) IPHs is also important for the surgical pathologist; CAA may be readily detected in fragments of brain parenchyma evacuated together with a hematoma.[163] Bleeds may occur, over months or years, into different lobes of the cerebral hemispheres. Cerebellum and brain stem (pons), common loci for hypertensive bleeds, are almost never a site for CAA-related hemorrhage.[41,55] As many as one-third of patients afflicted with CAA-related IPH may also have clinical evidence of HBP—mixed microangiopathies, with features of both AS/LH and CAA, may be found within brain of such individuals.[39,157]

There is a relatively clear difference between amyloid-laden vessels that are associated with hemorrhage and those that are not. Amyloid deposition in the arterial wall causes atrophy of the medial SMC layer in both leptomeningeal and parenchymal arteries, as the SMC are replaced by fibrillar amyloid.[164–166] These changes probably impair function of involved vessels by reducing their flexibility and compliance in response to fluctuations in arterial pressure. Fibrillar amyloid disrupts vascular architecture and weakens the affected arterial walls, causing cracks, focal fragmentation, and microaneurysm formation, with or

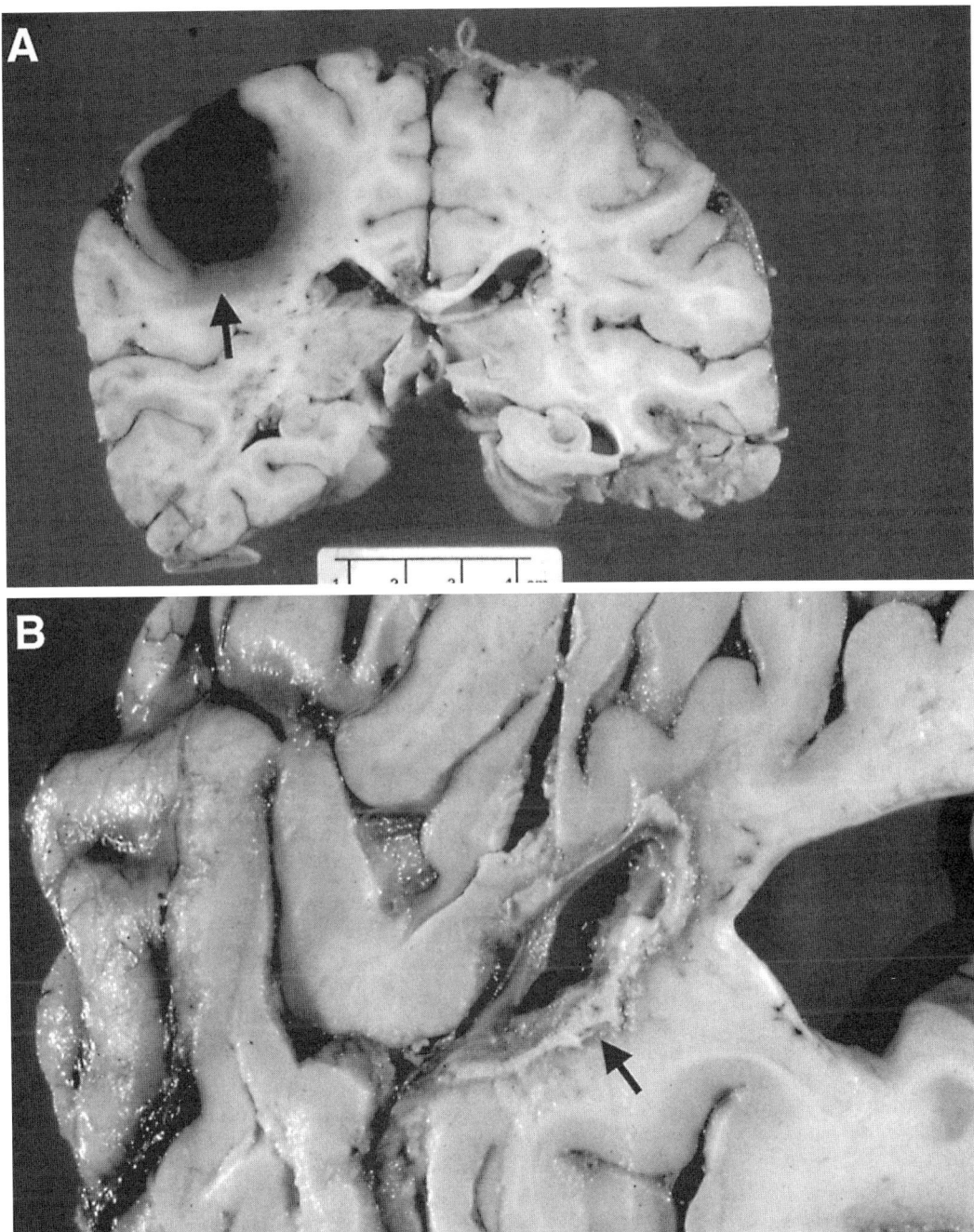

Figure 4–29. *A.* Subacute left frontal (lobar) hematoma (arrow) in the brain of a patient with severe cerebral amyloid angiopathy (CAA). Although CAA is a meningocortical microangiopathy, associated hemorrhages often extend into the subcortical white matter, as in this case. *B.* Old (lobar) hematoma (arrow) in a patient with long-standing Alzheimer's disease and severe CAA. The cavity resembles an old ischemic infarct, although overlying neocortex is spared.

without fibrinoid necrosis.[54,166] Amyloid deposits within CNS arteriolar walls appear to be comparatively well tolerated up to a threshold, e.g., CAA of grades 1 and 2 (see above). However, when grade 3 changes occur, the risk of IPH increases dramatically; in this situation, extrinsic, apparently trivial factors such as minor head trauma may trigger IPH.

VASCULAR MALFORMATIONS

These may involve the CNS parenchyma, overlying dura, or (rarely) both.[1,167-172] The most clinically important and "malignant" of these lesions, arteriovenous malformations (AVMs), rarely present beyond the age of 60 years, so they are a relatively minor problem in patients of advanced age. Arteriovenous malformations (also sometimes described, this author feels inappropriately, as arteriovenous aneurysms) may cause IPH and/or SAH; they are more frequently encountered as surgical specimens than at autopsy. They are usually found in the MCA territory, classically involving a wedge-shaped area of brain parenchyma and overlying leptomeninges, but may be seen anywhere in the CNS, including posterior fossa structures, and even on the circle of Willis. By definition, an AVM represents an abnormal direct communication between one or more arteries of the brain parenchyma and one or more draining veins, without an intervening capillary bed.[167] Its morphologic features, both grossly and microscopically, are characteristic (Fig. 4–30). An AVM consists of a collection of vascular channels of varying wall thickness and caliber or diameter, embedded within abnormal, gliotic, and occasionally malformed brain parenchyma.[8-10,167,170-172] The CNS parenchyma may or may not show morphologic evidence of old hemorrhage, but an absence of blood breakdown products (hemosiderin, hematoidin) in no way rules out the possibility that the AVM has bled prior to resection. Commonly, thrombosed and recanalized vascular channels are present within an AVM. Other intriguing abnormalities noted within AVMs are hyalinized, sometimes calcified (very rarely, ossified) arterial walls, and others that show foci of intimal fibromuscular hyperplasia. Infrequently, "foreign" particles, covered by endothelium and surrounded by foreign body type giant cells, are seen embedded within vessel walls; these are thought to represent material introduced into the circulation during cerebral angiography.[173]

Anteriovenous Malformations usually produce symptoms by bleeding (with reactive changes in surrounding brain parenchyma or leptomeninges), direct pressure on surround-

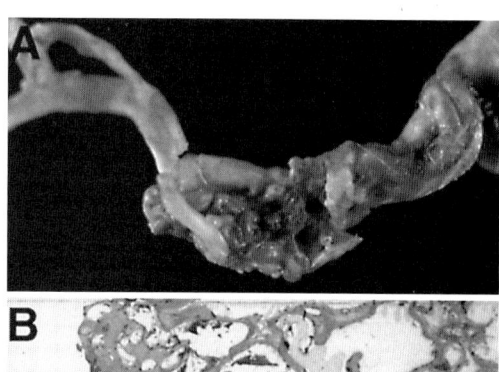

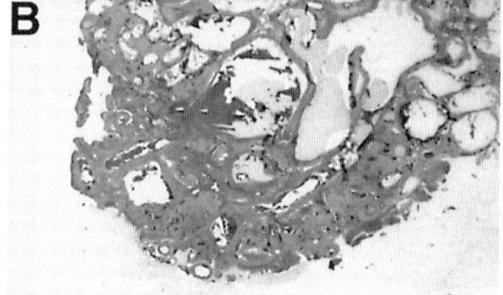

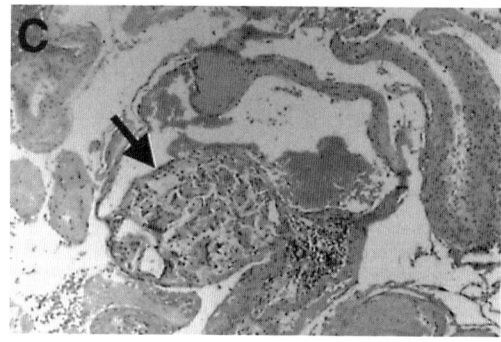

Figure 4–30. Arteriovenous malformation (AVM) of the brain. *A.* An AVM on the circle of Willis is seen as a tangle of vessels of varying caliber. *B.* Whole-mount specimen of a surgically resected, partly embolized AVM. Note again the marked variation in vessel lumen caliber and wall thickness—the vessels include arteries, veins, and arterialized veins showing fragmented, reduplicated, or absent internal elastic lamina. *C.* Microscopic detail of an AVM highlights the variation in component vessel wall thickness. Thin-walled channel at the center of the micrograph shows iatrogenic embolotherapy material (arrow), to which a foreign body giant cell reaction has developed; this material appears to have been incorporated into the vessel wall.

ing brain substance, or a "steal" of blood from normal anatomic structures because of a significant arteriovenous shunt through the AVM.[174] They are usually treated by excision or iatrogenic embolization therapy (performed with the intention of occluding and obliterating the AVM nidus), the latter resulting in a variety of tissue reactions to embolotherapy agents used (see Fig. 4–12).

Venous angiomas (VAs) consist of one or more dilated, often grossly apparent veins and their smaller tributaries, but without an obvious arterial component. A single tortuous vein (e.g., in the spinal subarachnoid space) may be described as a varix. Their component vessels are more dilated and have thicker walls than normal veins, and brain parenchyma between the vessels shows negligible reactive change or (old) hemorrhage.[8–10,167] They are usually found as an incidental lesion discovered at autopsy, as are capillary telangiectases, composed of multiple dilated capillaries without alterations of the surrounding brain substance. Both VAs and capillary telangiectases appear (at brain cutting) as small, fairly well-defined hemorrhagic lesions that initially suggest a localized region of bleeding.

Cavernous hemangiomas (CAs), though less common than AVMs, appear as closely packed blood vessels (of varying wall thickness) without intervening CNS parenchyma (Fig. 4–31).[8–10,167] They have a predilection for the pons, subcortical white matter, and the external capsule; in these regions, they may mimic primary CNS neoplasms and behave as space-occupying lesions, producing mass effect and irritation of surrounding brain that causes, for example, seizures. Though they do not usually

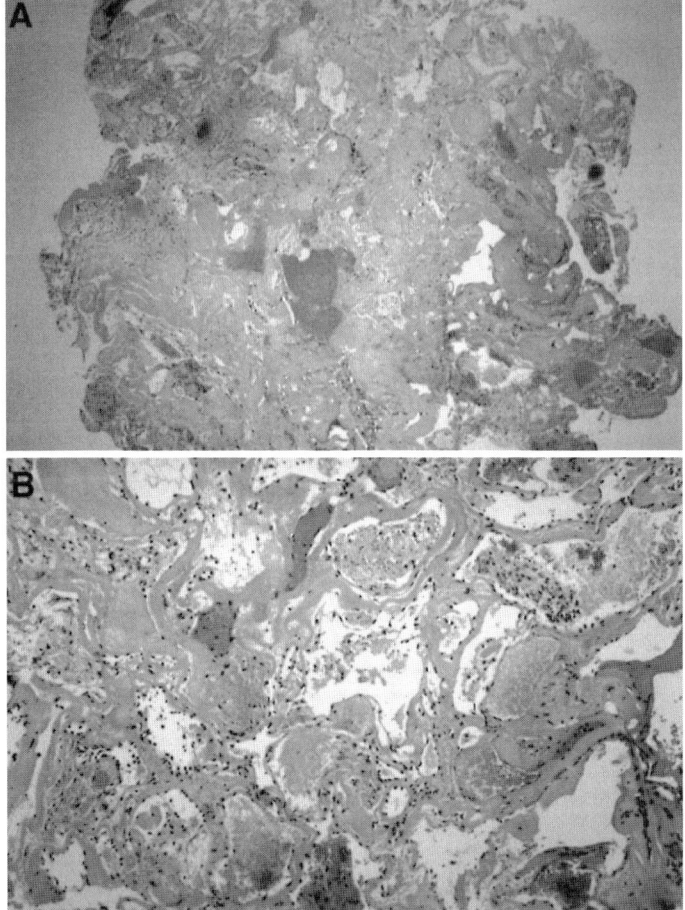

Figure 4–31. Cavernous hemangioma, shown at low (A) and intermediate (B) magnification. Note the prominently hyalinized vessels packed closely together. Surrounding brain parenchyma usually shows evidence of old hemorrhage. H&E, magnification: A, ×40; B, ×100.

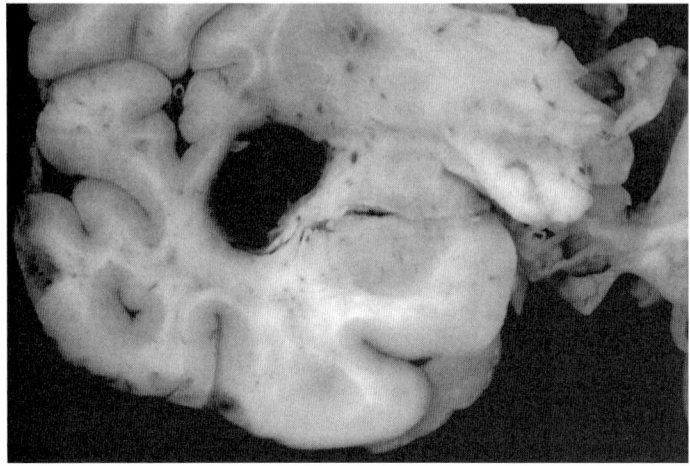

Figure 4–32. Intraparenchymal hemorrhage in left temporal lobe of a 55-year-old woman with heptatitis. Patient had no evidence for cerebral macrovascular or microvascular abnormalities.

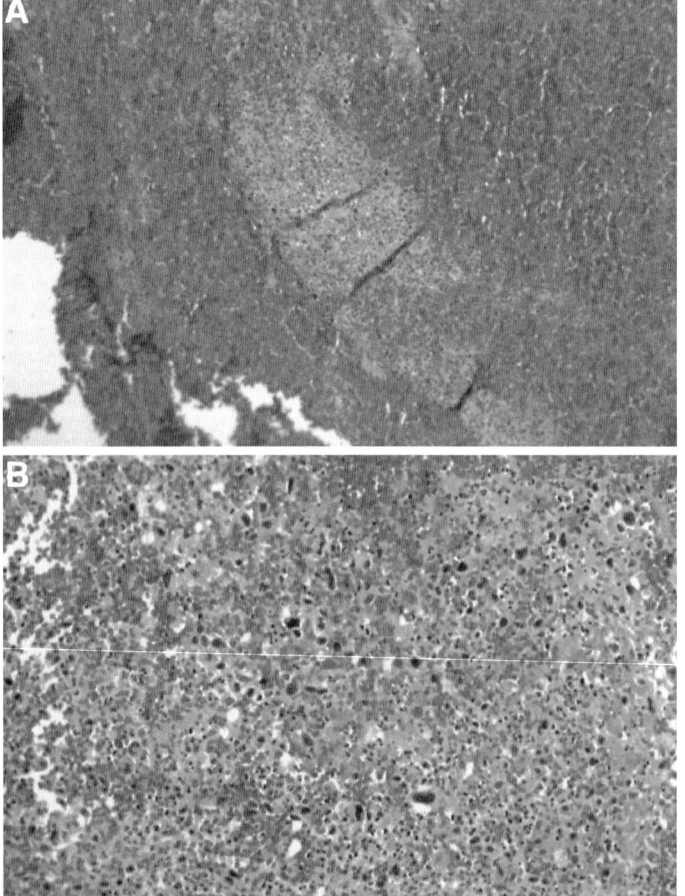

Figure 4–33. Acute cerebral hemorrhage into a metastatic tumor deposit. This surgical specimen was resected from a 77-year-old male with known lung carcinoma who developed an intraparenchymal hemorrhage. Abundant acute hemorrhage is noted (A). Highly atypical, somewhat cohesive, neoplastic cells are seen together with the blood (A,B). Hemorrhage into metastatic brain tumor deposits is well documented; occasionally, this is the presenting manifestation of the primary malignancy. H&E, magnification: A, ×100; B, ×205.

cause massive IPH, they are almost always surrounded by extensive deposits of hemosiderin on histologic sections, suggesting slow or recurrent leaks of blood from the component vessels. A familial syndrome of cavernous angiomas has recently been linked to a gene on chromosome 7q.[175,176] In the described kindreds, patients became symptomatic at an early age, usually the second or third decade of life.

SYSTEMIC AND MISCELLANEOUS FACTORS

An IPH may result from systemic factors and diseases such as thrombocytopenia, coagulopathy (either iatrogenic or secondary to hepatic failure), hemophilia, disseminated intravascular coagulation, leukemia, and abuse of recreational drugs such as cocaine.[4–10,177–179] Of these, anticoagulant-related bleeds and those associated with hematologic malignancies are relatively common in the geriatric population. In terms of topography and extent the bleeds may mimic, hematomas associated with HBP and CAA; they may also occur on a background of these common microangiopathies (Fig. 4–32).

Several structural lesions of the brain may also mimic primary IPH; the most common of these are primary or secondary neoplasms, and infections, in particular, those caused by microorganisms that have a propensity to invade vessel walls (e.g., Aspergillus). High-grade glial neoplasms (and low-grade oligodendrogliomas) probably bleed because of their content of thin-walled, fragile capillaries. Whereas infection-related bleeds usually occur on a background of sepsis and thus can be fairly readily differentiated, on clinical and neuroimaging grounds, from primary IPH, hemorrhage into a neoplasm may be its initial presentation, even in the case of metastases (Fig. 4–33).[180] The neoplasm may become apparent upon clot evacuation and careful scrutiny of its contents by a vigilant pathologist, or (if clot evacuation is not initially undertaken), after the hemorrhage is substantially resorbed and the tumor declares itself.

Work in the author's laboratory was supported by U.S. PHS grant P01 AG 12435 and P50 AG 16570. Carol Appleton prepared the figures, Annetta Pierro assisted with manuscript preparation, and Justine Garakian and Alexander Brooks cut and stained many of the sections from which micrographs were made.

REFERENCES

1. Stehbens WE. Pathology of the Cerebral Blood Vessels. St. Louis. C.V. Mosby, 1972.
2. Hachinski V, Norris JW. The Acute Stroke. Philadelphia. FA Davis, 1985.
3. Fisher M. Clinical Atlas of Cerebrovascular Disorders. London: Mosby-Year Book, 1994.
4. Barnett HJM, Mohr JP, Stein BM, Yatsu FM. (eds.) Stroke: Pathophysiology, Diagnosis, and Management. 3d ed. New York: Churchill Livingstone, 1998.
5. Batjer HH. (ed.) Cerebrovascular Disease. Philadelphia: Lippincott-Raven, 1997.
6. Caplan LR. Stroke: A Clinical Approach, 2nd ed. Boston: Butterworth-Heinemann, 1993.
7. Adams JH, Graham DI. Cerebrovascular disease. In: Anthony PP, Macsween RNM, eds. Recent Advances in Histopathology, Vol. 14. Edinburgh: Churchill Livingstone, 1989: 205–222.
8. Ellison D, Love S, Chimelli L, Harding B, Lowe J, Roberts GW, Vinters HV. Neuropathology: A Reference Text of CNS Pathology, Section 3. London: Mosby International, 1998.
9. Vinters HV, Farrell MA, Mischel PS, Anders KH. Diagnostic Neuropathology. New York: Marcel Dekker, 1998: 51–171.
10. Kalimo H, Kaste M, Haltia M. Vascular diseases. In: Graham DI, Lantos PL, eds. Greenfield's Neuropathology, Vol. 1, 6th ed. London: Arnold, 1997: 315–396.
11. Leys D, Lucas C, Henon H, Savoye C, Pasquier F, Pruvo J-P. Ischemic stroke in the elderly: is it necessary to look for a cause? In: Bruno A, Chollet F, Vellas BJ, Albarede JL, eds. Stroke in the Elderly. New York: Springer-Verlag, 1996: 23–40.
12. Dirnagl U, Iadecola C, Moskowitz MA. Pathobiology of ischaemic stroke: an integrated view. Trends Neurosci 1999; 22:391–397.
13. Gillum RF. Stroke in blacks. Stroke 1988; 19:1–9.
14. Whetsell WO Jr. Current concepts of excitotoxicity. J Neuropathol Exp Neurol 1996; 55:1–13.
15. Auer RN. Insulin, blood glucose levels, and ischemic brain damage. Neurology 1998; 51(Suppl. 3):S39–S43.
16. del Zoppo G, Ginis I, Hallenbeck JM, Iadecola C, Wang X, Feuerstein GZ. Inflammation and stroke: putative role for cytokines, adhesion molecules and iNOS in brain response to ischemia. Brain Pathol 2000; 10:95–112.
17. Vinters HV. Cerebral microvascular and macrovascular disease in the aging brain—similarities and differences. In: Verbeek MM, Vinters HV, de Waal RMW, eds. Cerebral Amyloid Augiopathy in Alzheimer's Disease and Related Disorders. Dordrecht: Kluwer, 2000: 59–78.
18. Ross R. Atherosclerosis—an inflammatory disease. N Engl J Med 1999; 340: 115–126.
19. Moore S. Cholesterol revisited: prime mover or a factor in the progression of atherosclerosis? Ann R. Coll Phys Surg Canada 1999; 32:198–204.
20. Ross R. The pathogenesis of atherosclerosis: a perspective for the 1990s. Nature 1993; 362:801–809.

21. Navab M, Berliner JA, Watson AD, Hama SY, Territo MC, Lusis AJ, Shih DM, Van Lenten BJ, Frank JS, Denver LL, Edwards PA, Fogelman AM. The yin and yang of oxidation in the development of the fatty streak. A review based on the 1994 George Lyman Duff Memorial Lecture. Arterioscler Thromb Vasc Biol 1996; 16:831–842.
22. Resch JA, Okabe N, Loewenson RB, Kimoto K, Katsuki S, Baker AB. Pattern of vessel involvement in cerebral atherosclerosis. A comparative study between a Japanese and Minnesota population. J Atheroscler Res 1969; 9:239–250.
23. Castaigne P, Lhermitte F, Gautier JC, Escourolle R, Derouesne C, Der Agopian P, Popa C. Arterial occlusions in the vertebro-basilar system. A study of 44 patients with post-mortem data. Brain 1973; 96:133–154.
24. Fisher CM, Gore I, Okabe N, White PD. Atherosclerosis of the carotid and vertebral arteries—extracranial and intracranial. J Neuropathol Exp Neurol 1965; 24:455–476.
25. Torvik A, Jörgensen L. Thrombotic and embolic occlusions of the carotid arteries in an autopsy material. Part 1. Prevalence, location and associated diseases. J Neurol Sci 1964; 1:24–39.
26. Torvik A, and Jörgensen L. (1966). Thrombotic and embolic occlusions of the carotid arteries in an autopsy series. Part 2. Cerebral lesions and clinical course. J Neurol Sci 1966; 3:410–432.
27. Droste DW, Karl M, Bohle RM, Kaps M. Comparison of ultrasonic and histopathological features of carotid artery stenosis. Neurol Res 1997; 19:380–384.
28. Post K, Eckstein H-H, Hoffmann E, Post S, Allenberg JR, Kauffmann GW. Degree of carotid artery stenosis. Comparison of selective and non-selective angiographic findings with surgical specimens. Eur J Radiol 1997; 25:9–13.
29. Manninen HI, Räsänen H, Vanninen RL, Berg M, Hippeläinen M, Saari T, Yang X, Karkolak, Kosina V-M. Human carotid arteries: correlation of intravascular US with angiographic and histopathologic findings. Radiology 1998; 206:65–74.
30. Morgenstern LB, Fox AJ, Sharpe BL, Eliasziw M, Barnett HJM, Grotta JC, for the North American Symptomatic Carotid Endarterectomy Trial (NASCET) Group. The risks and benefits of carotid endarterectomy in patients with near occlusion of the carotid artery. Neurology 1997; 48:911–915.
31. Masuda J, Ogata J, Yutani C, Miyashita T, Yamaguchi T. Artery-to-artery embolism from a thrombus formed in stenotic middle cerebral artery. Report of an autopsy case. Stroke 1987; 18:680–684.
32. Caplan LR, Amarenco P, Rosengart A, Lafranchise EF, Teal PA, Belkin M, DeWitt LD, Pessin MS. Embolism from vertebral artery origin occlusive disease. Neurology 1992; 42:1505–1512.
33. Jörgensen L, Torvik A. Ischaemic cerebrovascular diseases in an autopsy series. Part 1. Prevalence, location and predisposing factors in verified thrombo-embolic occlusions, and their significance in the pathogenesis of cerebral infarction. J Neurol Sci 1966; 3:490–509.
34. Jörgensen L, Torvik A. Ischaemic cerebrovascular diseases in an autopsy series. Part 2. Prevalence, location, pathogenesis, and clinical course of cerebral infarcts. J Neurol Sci 1969; 9:285–320.
35. Vinters HV. Pathology of cervical and intracranial atherosclerosis and fibromuscular dysplasia. In:Batjer, HH, eds. Cerebrovascular Disease. Philadelphia: Lippincott-Raven, 1997: 41–51.
36. Shokunbi MT, Vinters HV, Kaufmann JCE. Fusiform intracranial aneurysms. Clinicopathologic features. Surg Neurol 1988; 29:263–270.
37. Lammie AG, Brannan F, Slattery J, Warlow C. Non-hypertensive cerebral small vessel disease. An autopsy study. Stroke 1997; 28:2222–2229.
38. Takebayashi S, Kaneko M. Electron microscopic studies of ruptured arteries in hypertensive intracerebral hemorrhage. Stroke 1983; 14:28–36.
39. Vinters HV. Cerebral amyloid angiopathy—a critical review. Stroke 1987; 18: 311–324.
40. Vinters HV, Wang ZZ, Secor DL. Brain parenchymal and microvascular amyloid in Alzheimer's disease. Brain Pathol 1996; 6:179–195.
41. Vinters HV, and Vonsattel J-PG. Neuropathologic features and grading of Alzheimer-related and sporadic CAA. In: Verbeek MM, Vinters HV, de Waal RMW, eds. Cerebrovascular Amyloidosis in Alzheimer's Disease and Related Disorders. Dordrecht: Kluwer, 2000; 2000:137–155.
42. Vinters HV. Alzheimer's disease: a neuropathologic perspective. Curr Diagno Pathol 1998; 5:109–117.
43. Bornebroek M, Haan J, Maat-Schieman MLC, van Duinen SG, Roos RAC. Hereditary cerebral hemorrhage with amyloidosis—Dutch type (HCHWA-D): I. A review of clinical, radiologic and genetic aspects. Brain Pathol 1996; 6:111–114.
44. Maat-Schieman MLC, van Duinen SG, Bornebroek M, Haan J, Roos RAC. Hereditary cerebral hemorrhage with amyloidosis—Dutch type (HCHWA-D): II. A review of histopathological aspects. Brain Pathol 1996; 6:115–120.
45. Vinters HV, Natté R, Maat-Schieman MLC, van Duinen SG, Hegeman-Kleinn I, Welling-Graafland C, et al. Secondary microvascular degeneration in amyloid angiopathy of patients with hereditary cerebral hemorrhage with amyloidosis, Dutch type (HCHWA-D). Acta Neuropathol 1998; 95:235–244.
46. Natté R, Vinters HV, Maat-Schieman MLC, Bornebroek M, Haan J, Roos RAC, van Duinen SG. Microvasculopathy is associated with the number of cerebrovascular lesions in hereditary cerebral hemorrhage with amyloidosis, Dutch type. Stroke 1998; 29:1588–1594.
47. Ólafsson Í, Thorsteinsson L, Jensson Ó. The molecular pathology of hereditary cystatin C amyloid angiopathy causing brain hemorrhage. Brain Pathol 1996; 6:121–126.
48. Wang ZZ, Jensson O, Thorsteinsson L, Vinters HV. Microvascular degeneration in hereditary cystatin C amyloid angiopathy of the brain. APMIS 1997; 105: 41–47.
49. Ellis RJ, Olichney JM, Thal LJ, Mirra SS, Morris JC, Beekly D, Heyman A. Cerebral amyloid angiopathy in the brains of patients with Alzheimer's disease. The CERAD experience, part XV. Neurology 1996; 46: 1592–1596.
50. Greenberg SM. Cerebral amyloid angiopathy. Prospects for clinical diagnosis and treatment. Neurology 1998; 51:690–694.
51. Greenberg SM, Vonsattel J-PG. Diagnosis of cerebral amyloid angiopathy. Sensitivity and specificity of cortical biopsy. Stroke 1997; 28:1418–1422.

52. Vinters HV, Gilbert JJ. Cerebral amyloid angiopathy: incidence and complications in the aging brain. II. The distribution of amyloid vascular changes. Stroke 1983; 14:924–928.
53. Masuda J, Tanaka K, Ueda K, Omae T. Autopsy study of incidence and distribution of cerebral amyloid angiopathy in Hisayama, Japan. Stroke 1988; 19: 205–210.
54. Vonsattel JPG, Myers RH, Hedley-Whyte ET, Ropper AH, Bird ED, Richardson EP Jr. Cerebral amyloid angiopathy without and with cerebral hemorrhages: a comparative histological study. Ann Neurol 1991; 30:637–649.
55. Vinters HV. Cerebral amyloid angiopathy. In: Barnett HJM, Mohr JP, Stein BM, Yatsu FM, eds. Stroke: Pathophysiology, Diagnosis, and Management, 3rd, ed. New York: Churchill Livingstone, 1998:945–962.
56. Shoji M, Hirai S, Harigaya Y, Kawarabayashi T, Yamaguchi H. The amyloid beta-protein precursor is localized in smooth muscle cells of leptomeningeal vessels. Brain Res 1990; 530:113–116.
57. Natté R, de Boer WI, Maat-Schieman MLC, Baelde HJ, Vinters HV, Roos RAC, van Duinen SG. Amyloid beta precursor protein-mRNA is expressed throughout cerebral vessel walls. Brain Res 1999; 828:179–183.
58. Kawai M, Kalaria RN, Cras P, Siedlak SL, Velasco ML, Shelton ER, Chan HW, Greenberg BD, Perry G. Degeneration of vascular muscle cells in cerebral amyloid angiopathy of Alzheimer disease. Brain Res 1993; 623:142–146.
59. Davis J, van Nostrand WE. Enhanced pathologic properties of Dutch-type mutant amyloid beta-protein. Proc Natl Acad Sci USA 1996; 93:2996–3000.
60. Wang ZZ, Natté R, Berliner JA, van Duinen SG, Vinters HV. Toxicity of Dutch (E22Q) and Flemish (A21G) mutant amyloid beta proteins to human cerebral microvessel and aortic smooth muscle cells. Stroke 2000; 31:534–538.
61. Calabrese LH, Duna GF, Lie JT. Vasculitis in the central nervous system. Arthritis Rheum 1997; 40: 1189–1201.
62. Conn DL. Update on systemic necrotizing vasculitis. Mayo Clin Proc 1989; 64:535–543.
63. Moore PM, Cupps TR. Neurological complications of vasculitis. Ann Neurol 1983; 14:155–167.
64. Rhodes RH, Madelaire NC, Petrelli M, Cole M, Karaman BA. Primary angiitis and angiopathy of the central nervous system and their relationship to systemic giant cell arteritis. Arch Pathol Lab Med 1995; 119: 334–349.
65. Anders KH, Wang ZZ, Kornfeld M, Gray F, Soontornniyomkij V, Reed LA, Hart MN, Menchine M, Secor DL, Vinters HV. Giant cell arteritis in association with cerebral amyloid angiopathy: immunohistochemical and molecular studies. Hum Pathol 1997; 28:1237–1246.
66. Huston KA, Hunder GG, Lie JT, Kennedy RH, Elveback LR. Temporal arteritis. A 25-year epidemiologic, clinical, and pathologic study. Ann Intern Med 1978; 88:162–167.
67. Säve-Söderbergh J, Malmvall B-E, Andersson R, Bengtsson B-A. Giant cell arteritis as a cause of death. Report of nine cases. JAMA 1986; 255:493–496.
68. Gerber NJ. Giant cell arteritis and its variants. Eur Neurol 1984; 23:410–420.
69. Wilkinson IMS, Russell RWR. Arteries of the head and neck in giant cell arteritis. A pathological study to show the pattern of arterial involvement. Arch Neurol 1972; 27:378–391.
70. Imakita M, Yutani C, Ishibashi-Ueda H. Giant cell arteritis involving the cerebral artery. Arch Pathol Lab Med 1993; 117:729–733.
71. Evans JM, Batts KP, Hunder GG. Persistent giant cell arteritis despite corticosteroid treatment. Mayo Clin Proc 1994; 69:1060–1061.
72. Nordborg C, Nordborg E, Petursdottir V, LaGuardia J, Mahalingam R, Wellish M, Gilden DH. Search for varicella zoster virus in giant cell arteritis. Ann Neurol 1998; 44:413–414.
73. Ghanchi FD, Dutton GN. Current concepts in giant cell (temporal) arteritis. Surv Ophthalmol 1997; 42: 99–123.
74. Gordon LK, Levin LH. Visual loss in giant cell arteritis. JAMA 1998; 280: 385–386.
75. Kealy WF. Atheroembolism. J Clin Pathol 1978; 31: 984–989.
76. Hinchey JA, Furlan AJ, Barnett HJM. Cardiogenic brain embolism: incidence, varieties, and treatment. In: Barnett HJM, Mohr, JP, Stein BM, Yatsu FM, eds. Stroke: Pathophysiology, Diagnosis, and Management, 3rd ed. New York: Churchill Livingstone, 1998: 1089–1119.
77. Bogousslavsky J, Cachin C, Regli F, Despland P-A, Van Melle G, Kappenberger L (for the Lausanne Stroke Registry Group). Cardiac sources of embolism and cerebral infarction—clinical consequences and vascular concomitants: The Lausanne Stroke Registry. Neurology 1991; 41:855–859.
78. Vinters HV. Interactions between the heart and brain. In: Silver MD, ed. Cardiovascular Pathology, 2nd ed. New York: Churchill Livingstone, 1991: 1029–1071.
79. Cerebral Embolism Task Force. Cardiogenic brain embolism. The second report of the cerebral embolism task force. Arch Neurol 1989; 46:727–743.
80. Vinters HV, Anders KH. Neuropathology of AIDS. Boca Raton, FL: CRC Press, 1990.
81. Biller J, Challa VR, Toole JF, Howard VJ. Nonbacterial thrombotic endocarditis. A neurologic perspective of clinicopathologic correlations of 99 patients. Arch Neurol 1982; 39:95–98.
82. Furlan AJ. (ed.) The Heart and Stroke: Exploring Mutual Cerebrovascular and Cardiovascular Issues. London, Berlin: Springer-Verlag, 1987.
83. Usher BW. Cardiac valvular disease and stroke. Neurol Clin 1993; 11: 391–398.
84. Dines DE, Burgher LW, Okazaki H. The clinical and pathologic correlation of fat embolism syndrome. Mayo Clin Proc 1975; 50:407–411.
85. Kamenar E, Burger PC. Cerebral fat embolism: a neuropathological study of a microembolic state. Stroke 1980; 11:477–484.
86. Vinters HV, Lundie MJ, Kaufmann JCE. Long-term pathological follow-up of cerebral arteriovenous malformations treated by embolization with bucrylate. N Engl J Med 1986; 314:477–483.
87. Lanman TH, Martin NA, Vinters HV. The pathology of encephalic arteriovenous malformations treated by prior embolotherapy. Neuroradiology 1988; 30:1–10.
88. Schweitzer JS, Chang BS, Madsen P, Vinuela F, Martin NA, Marroquin CE, Vinters HV. The pathology of arteriovenous malformations of the brain treated by

embolotherapy. II. Results of embolization with multiple agents. Neuroradiology 1993; 35:468–474.
89. Thomas WE. Brain macrophages: evaluation of microglia and their functions. Brain Res Revi 1992; 17:61–74.
90. Kato H, Walz W. The initiation of the microglial response. Brain Pathol 2000; 10:137–143.
91. Torvik A. The pathogenesis of watershed infarcts in the brain. Stroke 1984; 15:221–223.
92. Adams JH, Brierley JB, Connor RCR, Treip CS. The effects of systemic hypotension upon the human brain. Clinical and neuropathological observations in 11 cases. Brain 1966; 89:235–268.
93. Brierley JB, Excell BJ. The effects of profound systemic hypotension upon the brain of *M. rhesus*: physiological and pathological observations. Brain 1966; 89:269–298.
94. Miller Fisher C. Lacunes: small, deep cerebral infarcts. Neurology 1965; 15: 774–784.
95. Miller Fisher C. Ataxic hemiparesis. A pathologic study. Arch Neurol 1978; 35:126–128.
96. Fisher CM. Pure sensory stroke involving face, arm, and leg. Neurology 1965; 15:76–80.
97. Miller Fisher C. Capsular infarcts. The underlying vascular lesions. Arch Neurol 1979; 36:65–73.
98. Challa VR, Bell MA, Moody DM. A combined hematoxylin-eosin, alkaline phosphatase and high-resolution microradiographic study of lacunes. Clin Neuropathol 1990; 9:196–204.
99. Miller VT. Lacunar stroke. A reassessment. Arch Neurol 1983; 40:129–134.
100. Waterston JA, Brown MM, Butler P, Swash M. Small deep cerebral infarcts associated with occlusive internal carotid artery disease. A hemodynamic phenomenon? Arch Neurol 1990; 47:953–957.
101. Gan R, Sacco RL, Kargman DE, Roberts JK, Boden-Albala B, Gu Q. Testing the validity of the lacunar hypothesis: the Northern Manhattan Stroke Study experience. Neurology 1997; 48:1204–1211.
102. Weisberg LA. Diagnostic classification of stroke, especially lacunes. Stroke 1988; 19:1071–1073.
103. Bamford JM, Warlow CP. Evolution and testing of the lacunar hypothesis. Stroke 1988; 19:1074–1082.
104. Tuszynski MH, Petito CK, Levy DE. Risk factors and clinical manifestations of pathologically verified lacunar infarctions. Stroke 1989; 20:990–999.
105. Cole FM, Yates P. Intracerebral microaneurysms and small cerebrovascular lesions. Brain 1967; 90:759–768.
106. Ross Russell RW. Observations on intracerebral aneurysms. Brain 1963; 86:425–442.
107. Challa VR, Moody DM, Bell MA. The Charcôt-Bouchard aneurysm controversy: impact of a new histologic technique. J Neuropathol Exp Neurol 1992; 51:264–271.
108. Devinsky O, Bear D, Volpe BT. Confusional states following posterior cerebral artery infarction. Arch Neurol 1988; 45:160–163.
109. Gacs G, Fox AJ, Barnett HJM, Vinuela F. Occurrence and mechanisms of occlusion of the anterior cerebral artery. Stroke 1983; 14:952–959.
110. Bogousslavsky J, Barnett HJM, Fox AJ, Hachinski VC, Taylor W, for the EC/IC Bypass Study Group. Atherosclerotic disease of the middle cerebral artery. Stroke 1986; 17:1112–1120.
111. Decroix JP, Graveleau Ph, Masson M, Cambier J Infarction in the territory of the anterior choroidal artery. A clinical and cumputerized tomographic study of 16 cases. Brain 1986; 109:1071–1085.
112. Helgason C, Caplan LR, Goodwin J, Hedges T, III. Anterior choroidal artery-territory infarction. Report of cases and review. Arch Neurol 1986; 43:681–686.
113. Kubik CS, Adams RD. Occlusion of the basilar artery—a clinical and pathological study. Brain 1946; 69:73–121.
114. DiNubile MJ. Septic thrombosis of the cavernous sinuses. Arch Neurol 1988; 45:567–572.
115. Southwick FS, Richardson EP Jr, Swartz MN. Septic thrombosis of the dural venous sinuses. Medicine 1986; 65:82–106.
116. Levine SR, Kieran S, Puzio K, Feit H, Patel SC, Welch KMA. Cerebral venous thrombosis with lupus anticoagulants. Report of two cases. Stroke 1987; 18:801–804.
117. Wechsler B, Vidailhet M, Piette JC, Bousser MG, Dell Isola B, Blétry O, Godeau P. Cerebral venous thrombosis in Behçet's disease: clinical study and long-term follow-up of 25 cases. Neurology 1992; 42:614–618.
118. Feldenzer JA, Bueche MJ, Venes JL, Gebarski SS. Superior sagittal sinus thrombosis with infarction in sickle cell trait. Stroke 1987; 18:656–660.
119. Bousser M-G, Barnett HJM. Cerebral venous thrombosis. In: Barnett HJM, Mohr JP, Stein BM, Yatsu FM, eds. Stroke: Pathophysiology, Diagnosis, and Management, 3rd ed. New York: Churchill Livingstone, 1998: 623–647.
120. Einhäupl KM, Villringer A, Meister W, Mehraein S, Garner C, Pellkofer M, et al. Heparin treatment in sinus venous thrombosis. Lancet 1991; 338:597–600.
121. Horowitz M, Purdy P, Unwin H, Carstens G, III, Greenlee R, Hise J, Kopitnik T, Batjer H, Rollins N, Samson D. Treatment of dural sinus thrombosis using selective catheterization and urokinase. Ann Neurol 1995; 38:58–67.
122. Bennett M, O'Brien DP, Phillips JP, Farrell MA. Clinicopathologic observations in 100 consecutive patients with fatal head injury admitted to a neurosurgical unit. Irish Med J 1995; 88:60–62.
123. Crooks DA. Pathogenesis and biomechanics of traumatic intracranial haemorrhages. Virchows Archiv A Pathol Anat 1991; 418:479–483.
124. Friede RL. Incidence and distribution of neomembranes of dura mater. J Neurol Neurosurg Psychiatry 1971; 34:439–446.
125. Drapkin AJ. Chronic subdural hematoma: pathophysiological basis for treatment. Br J Neurosurg 1991; 5:467–473.
126. Sprung Ch, Collmann H, Kazner E, Duisberg R. Chronic subdural hematoma in geriatric patients—factors affecting prognosis. Adv Neurosurg 1984; 12:204–211.
127. Heiss E. Results of treatment in chronic subdural hematomas. Adv Neurosurg 1984; 12:192–197.
128. Sacco RL, Wolf PA, Bharucha NE, Meeks SL, Kannel WB, Charette LJ McNamara PM, Palmer EP, D'Agostino R. Subarachnoid and intracerebral hemorrhage: natural history, prognosis, and precursive factors in the Framingham Study. Neurology 1984; 34:847–854.
129. Mohr JP, Kistler JP. Intracranial aneurysms. In: Bar-

nett HJM, Mohr JP, Stein BM, Yatsu FM, eds. Stroke: Pathophysiology, Diagnosis, and Management, 3rd ed. New York: Churchill Livingstone, 1998: 701–723.
130. Weaver JP, Fisher M. Subarachnoid hemorrhage: an update of pathogenesis, diagnosis and management. J Neurol Sci 1994; 125:119–131.
131. Bokemeyer C, Frank B, Brandis A, Weinrich W. Giant aneurysm causing frontal lobe syndrome. J Neurol 1990; 237:47–50.
132. Bonita R, Thomson S. Subarachnoid hemorrhage: epidemiology, diagnosis, management and outcome. Stroke 1985; 16:591–594.
133. Olafsson E, Hauser WA, Gudmundsson G. A population-based study of prognosis of ruptured cerebral aneurysm: mortality and recurrence of subarachnoid hemorrhage. Neurology 1997; 48:1191–1195.
134. Kassell NF, Sasaki T, Colohan ART, Nazar G. Cerebral vasospasm following aneurysmal subarachnoid hemorrhage. Stroke 1985; 16:562–572.
135. Caplan LR. Should intracranial aneurysms be treated before they rupture? N Engl J Med 1998; 339:1774–1775.
136. The International Study of Unruptured Intracranial Aneurysms Investigators. Unruptured intracranial aneurysms—risk of rupture and risks of surgical intervention. N Engl J Med 1998; 339:1725–1733.
137. Roach MR, Drake CG. Ruptured cerebral aneurysms caused by micro-organisms. N Engl J Med 1965; 273:240–244.
138. Salgado AV, Furlan AJ, Keys TF. Mycotic aneurysm, subarachnoid hemorrhage, and indications for cerebral angiography in infective endocarditis. Stroke 1987; 18:1057–1060.
139. Masuda J, Yutani C, Waki R, Ogata J, Kuriyama Y, and Yamaguchi T. Histopathological analysis of the mechanisms of intracranial hemorrhage complicating infective endocarditis. Stroke 1992 23:843–850.
140. Farrell MA, Gilbert JJ, Kaufmann JCE. Fatal intracranial arterial dissection: clinical pathological correlation. J Neurol Neurosurg Psychiatry 1985; 48:111–121.
141. Hart RG, Easton JD. Dissections. Stroke 1985; 16:925–927.
142. Pessin MS, Adelman LS, Barbas NR. Spontaneous intracranial carotid artery dissection. Stroke 1989; 20:1100–1103.
143. Hart RG. Vertebral artery dissection. Neurology 1988; 38:987–989.
144. Mokri B, Houser CW, Sandok BA, Piepgras DG. Spontaneous dissections of the vertebral arteries. Neurology 1988; 38:880–885.
145. Alexander CB, Burger PC, Goree JA. Dissecting aneurysms of the basilar artery in 2 patients. Stroke 1979; 10:294–299.
146. Guridi J, Gallego J, Monzon F, Aguilera F. Intracerebral hemorrhage caused by transmural dissection of the anterior cerebral artery. Stroke 1993; 24:1400–1402.
147. Little JR, St. Louis P, Weinstein M, Dohn DF. Giant fusiform aneurysm of the cerebral arteries. Stroke 1981; 12:183–188.
148. Courville CB. Arterioslcerotic aneurysms of the circle of Willis. Bull LA Neurol Soc 1962; 27:1–13.
149. Hayes WT, Bernhardt H, Young JM. Fusiform arteriosclerotic aneurysm of the basilar artery. Five cases including two ruptures. Vasc. Surgery 1967; 1:171–178.
150. Bogousslavsky J, Regli F, Uské A, Maeder P. Early spontaneous hematoma in cerebral infarct: is primary cerebral hemorrhage overdiagnosed? Neurology 1991; 41:837–840.
151. Ueda K, Hasuo Y, Kiyohara Y, Wada J, Kawano H, Kato I, Fujii I, Yanai T, Ornae T, Fujishima M. Intracerebral hemorrhage in a Japanese community, Hisayama: incidence, changing pattern during long-term follow-up, and related factors. Stroke 1988; 19:48–52.
152. Ransohoff J, Derby B, Kricheff I. Spontaneous intracerebral hemorrhage. Clin Neurosurg 1971; 18:247–266.
153. Brott T, Thalinger K, Hertzberg V. Hypertension as a risk factor for spontaneous intracerebral hemorrhage. Stroke 1986; 17:1078–1083.
154. Brewer DB, Fawcett FJ, Horsfield GI. A necropsy series of nontraumatic cerebral haemorrhages and softenings, with particular reference to heart weight. J Pathol Bacteriol 1968; 96:311–320.
155. Bahemuka M. Primary intracerebral hemorrhage and heart weight: a clinicopathologic case-control review of 218 patients. Stroke 1987; 18:531–536.
156. Fisher CM. Pathological observations in hypertensive cerebral hemorrhage. J Neuropathol Exp Neurol 1971; 30:536–550.
157. Okazaki H, Reagan TJ, Campbell RJ. Clinicopathologic studies of primary cerebral amyloid angiopathy. Mayo Clin Proc 1979; 54:22–31.
158. Gilles C, Brucher JM, Khoubesserian P, Vanderheagan JJ. Cerebral amyloid angiopathy as a cause of multiple intracerebral hemorrhages. Neurology 1984; 34:730–735.
159. Jellinger K. Cerebrovascular amyloidosis with cerebral hemorrhage. J Neurol 1977; 214:195–206.
160. Coria F, Rubio I. Cerebral amyloid angiopathies. Neuropathol Appl Neurobiol 1996; 22:216–227.
161. Vinters HV, Duckwiler GR. Intracranial hemorrhage in the normotensive elderly patient. Neuroimaging Clin North Am 1992; 2:153–169.
162. Gilbert JJ, Vinters HV. Cerebral amyloid angiopathy: incidence and complications in the aging brain. I. Cerebral hemorrhage. Stroke 1983; 14:915–923.
163. Yong WH, Robert ME, Secor DL, Kleikamp TJ, Vinters HV. Cerebral hemorrhage with biopsy-proved amyloid angiopathy. Arch Neurol 1992; 49:51–58.
164. Mandybur TI, Bates SRD. Fatal massive intracerebral hemorrhage complicating cerebral amyloid angiopathy. Arch Neurol 1978; 35:246–258.
165. Mandybur TI. Cerebral amyloid angiopathy: the vascular pathology and complications. J Neuropathol Exp Neurol 1986; 45:79–90.
166. Vinters HV, Secor DL, Read SL, Frazee JG, Tomiyasu U, Stanley TM, Ferreiro JA, Alkers M-A. The microvasculature in brain biopsy specimens from patients with Alzheimer's disease: an immunohistochemical and ultrastructural study. Ultrastruct Pathol 1994; 18:333–348.
167. Challa VR, Moody DM, Brown WR. Vascular malformations of the central nervous system. J Neuropathol Exp Neurol 1995; 54:609–621.
168. Mironov A. Classification of spontaneous dural ar-

teriovenous fistulas with regard to their pathogenesis. Acta Radiologica 1995; 36:582–592.
169. Mohr JP, Pile-Spellman J, Stein BM. Arteriovenous malformations and other vascular anomalies. In: Barnett HJM, Mohr JP, Stein BM, Yatsu FM, eds. Stroke: Pathophysiology, Diagnosis, and Management, 3rd ed. New York: Churchill Livingstone, 1998: 725–750.
170. Martin N, Vinters H. Pathology and grading of intracranial vascular malformations. In: Intracranial Vascular Malformations. Barrow DL, ed. Park Ridge, IL: American Association of Neurological Surgeons, 1990: 1–30.
171. McCormick WF, Hardman JM, Boulter TR. Vascular malformations ("angiomas") of the brain, with special reference to those occurring in the posterior fossa. J Neurosurg 1968; 28:241–251.
172. McCormick WF. The pathology of vascular ("arteriovenous") malformations. J Neurosurg 1966; 24:807–816.
173. Vinters HV, Kaufmann JCE, Drake CG. 'Foreign' particles in encephalic vascular malformations. Arch Neurol 1983; 40:221–225.
174. Costantino A, Vinters HV. A pathologic correlate of the 'steal' phenomenon in a patient with cerebral arteriovenous malformation. Stroke 1986; 17:103–106.
175. Gil-Nagel A, Dubovsky J, Wilcox KJ, Stewart JM, Anderson VE, Leppik IE, Orr HT Johnson EW, Weber JL, Rich SS. Familial cerebral cavernous angioma: A gene localized to a 15-cM interval on chromosome 7q. Ann Neurol 1996; 39:807–810.
176. Polymeropoulos MH, Hurko O, Hsu F, Rubenstein J, Basnet S, Lanek, Dietz H, Spetzler RF, Rigamont D. Linkage of the locus for cerebral cavernous hemangiomas to human chromosome 7q in four families of Mexican-American descent. Neurology 1997; 48:752–757.
177. McCormick WF, Rosenfield DB. Massive brain hemorrhage: a review of 144 cases and an examination of their causes. Stroke 1973; 4:946–954.
178. Levine SR, Welch KMA. Cocaine and stroke. Stroke 1987; 19:779–783.
179. Mody CK, Miller BL, McIntyre HB, Cobb SK, Goldberg MA. Neurologic complications of cocaine abuse. Neurology 1988; 38:1189–1193.
180. Mandybur TI. Intracranial hemorrhage caused by metastatic tumors. Neurology 1977; 27:650–655.

5. Vascular Dementia

JACQUELINE MIKOL

In 1894 Durand-Fardel[1] described cribriform damage in the brain of older adults that has since been known as "état criblé." Also at the end of the nineteenth century, a close relationship was established between vascular disease and dementia. Klippel[2] emphasized the role of atherosclerosis of the cerebral and extracerebral vessels in the development of dementia and Binswanger[3] described "encephalitis subcorticalis chronica progressiva," (1894) also later called "subcortical arteriosclerotic encephalopathy,"[4] or Binswanger disease. Subsequently, Marie (1901)[5] and Ferrand (1902)[6] described cerebral lacunae. Vascular dementia (VD) was considered to be related to diffuse lesions; it appeared as one of the main etiologies of mental disorders accompanying syphilis; Alzheimer's disease (AD) was considered a rare disorder.

The mechanism of vascular etiology was reanalyzed many years later by Tomlinson et al. (1971),[7] who showed that a volume of at least 100 ml of brain tissue had to be destroyed for dementia to occur. With the finding of multiple large and small cerebral infarcts Hachinski et al.[8] created the term "multi-infarct dementia" (MID), which was later substituted by the term "vascular dementia." Furthermore, the frequency of extracranial vascular disease due to thrombosis, embolism, or heart disease led investigators to give less importance to cerebral arteriosclerosis as a cause of VD.

The considerable progress of neuroimaging (see Chapter 3) has totally modified the study of VD. In 1987, Hachinski et al.[9] described the rarefaction of white matter under the term "leukoaraiosis," which since has been a great matter of debate. Recent data have shown that the roles of circulatory disturbances and abnormalities in small vessels deserve greater emphasis in the development of VD.

In this chapter, I shall address briefly the definition and epidemiology of vascular dementia and describe the different types of lesions and their mechanisms. Vascular dementia associated with AD will be described separately.

DEFINITION OF VASCULAR DEMENTIA

According to the supposed underlying mechanism, dementia, as related to vascular disturbances, was first described as "arteriosclerotic dementia";[10] this term was replaced by the terms "vascular dementia" and/or "multi-infarct dementia." More recently, the terms "dementia related to stroke,"[11] "post-stroke"[12] or "after-stroke dementia,"[13] "lacunar dementia"[14] or "hypoperfusion dementia"[15] have been suggested. "Vascular dementia," which is the term most currently used, will be used in this review. Many reports have tried to validate clinical criteria of VD, and all of them emphazise the disturbance of cognitive functions and the presence of focal deficits.[14,16,17] As with AD, for which satisfactory correlations between clinical and neuropathological data have been established and accepted, classifications of VD have been proposed. They include the revised *Diagnostic and Statistical Manual of Mental Disorders* (DSM) III[18] and DSM IV,[19] the 10th revision of the International Classification of Diseases (ICD 10; 1989), the Hachinski Ischemic Score, (HIS),[20] the National Institute of Neurological Association Disorders and Stroke–Association Internationale pour la Recherche et l'Enseignement en Neurosciences, (NINDS–AIREN); 1993,[15] the State of California Alzheimer's Disease Diagnostic and Treatment Centers, (ADDTC; 1992),[21] with probable, possible, and definite ischemic VD. This long list reflects the lack of consensus on diagnostic criteria for VD, which remain to be validated.[22] The risk factors are the same as those described in vascular pathology (see Chapter 4). Stroke and dementia are frequently associated in the same patient but it is often difficult to assess which is the supplementary factor(s) involved in the development of dementia. The risk of VD in relation to specific apolipoprotein E genotypes has also not been confirmed in neuropathological series.[23]

VASCULAR DEMENTIA

All authors agree that the incidence of VD increases with age and that half of these are observed in patients over 80 years of age.[24] The occurrence of VD is more common in Japan than in Western countries.[25] Men tend to have a higher incidence at a younger age than women.[26] However, it appears to be very difficult to give precise percentages. In an autopsy series of 87 patients from a dementia clinic, no VD was found.[27] In an another study including cases with progressive dementia from 10 university neuropathology laboratories, only six "pure" cases of VD were found.[28] These results were confirmed in a prospective series of 150 cases of dementia which included only 6 cases of VD (4%).[29] These results are lower than those given by clinical studies, in which rates of incidence were 20%,[24] and 6% to 25.5% 3 months after stroke, using different classifications.[30] There is a significant variability in the prevalence of the disorder.

NEUROIMAGING

Modern neuroimaging techniques have contributed extensively to our understanding of the lesions and pathophysiological mechanisms involved in VD. Pallor of the white matter, or leukoaraiosis, has been recognized as a frequent characteristic,[9] and rating scales for the location and severity of changes have been developed.[31,32] Cortical lesions have been distinguished from subcortical and periventricular hyperintensities, and MID has been set apart from lacunae alone or in association with leukoaraiosis, through the use of positron emission tomography (PET).[33] One group of patients with multiple large infarcts showed decreased regional cerebral blood flow and metabolic rate of oxygen, and another group had lacunae and leukoaraiosis in a state of "misery perfusion" in the deep structures as well as throughout the cerebral cortex, and a loss of the vascular reserve.

DIFFUSE FORMS OF VASCULAR DEMENTIA

Multiple Infarcts

Large cerebral infarcts that destroy cortical connections are sometimes observed in MID[10] (Figs. 5–1 and 5–2). They are often associated with focal or global cerebral atrophy, ventricular enlargement, and small lesions that can only be detected microscopically. A volume of 100 ml of cerebral softening, regardless of its distribution, is encountered in the demented patients; there is a positive correlation between reduced blood flow and degree of dementia.[7] The lesions are situated bilaterally in the cortex and white matter, the basal ganglia, and the brain stem, and they have rarely a laminar cortical distribution[34] (Fig. 5–3). Two groups of changes have been described.[34] In the oldest patients, the lesions were diffuse and predominantly in the periventricular white matter; clinically, the psychiatric features were similar to those observed in AD, although a history of strokes associated with cognitive function disturbances was also noticed. In the younger patients (presenile dementia) ischemic lesions were multiple but not usually present at the base of the brain; clinically they had been considered VD lesions.

Granular Atrophy of the Cerebral Cortex

Cortical granular atrophy is a rare form of MID that occurs in middle-aged or younger patients and has a recurrent clinical course of long duration characterized by intellectual im-

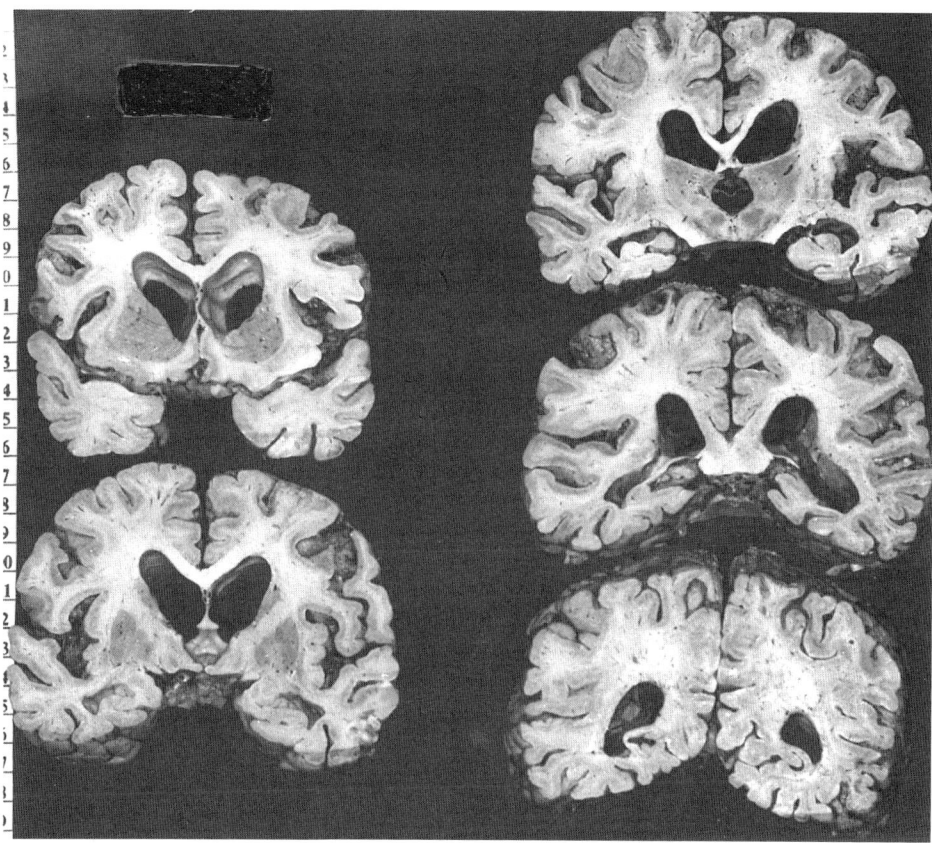

Figure 5–1. Multiple-infarct dementia. Coronal sections of the cerebral hemisphere show infarcts involving superficial gyri, basal ganglia, and thalamus. Note the enlarged ventricles. Myelin, Woelcke stain.

pairment and episodes of weakness or numbness of arms and legs; the face is spared.[35,36] Under macroscopic examination, some gyri appear shrunken and punctuated with many small depressions (Fig. 5–4A). The lesions are bilaterally symmetrical and located mainly along the border zone (watershed infarct) between the cortical areas of supply of the large cerebral arteries (Fig. 5–4B). The cortical gyri affected include the mid-frontal, the middle part of the ascending frontal and parietal, the posterior part of the superior parietal, the mid-temporal, and the middle and inferior occipital gyri; the cerebellar cortex is rarely involved (Fig. 5–4B).

Microscopically, the lesions correspond to small, triangular, transfixiant punctate areas of necrosis of the cortex that accompany occlusion of small, overlying leptomeningeal arteries[37–39] (Fig. 5–5). Lower motor neuron lesions and neurogenic muscle atrophy have also been observed.[40] Lacunae may also be present.

The original reports of cortical granular atrophy implicated thromboangeitis obliterans.[41] Subsequently, it was shown that stagnation or reduction in cerebral blood flow in relation to cardiac disturbances or atherosclerosis would also result in occlusion of the microvasculature.[42,43] Such lesions have been reported in three cases of generalized small vessel thrombosis (arteries and veins) in patients under 60 years of age. Ischemic lesions were found in the brain, and the main symptom was a progressive dementia.[44]

Watershed cerebral infarcts are brought on by either serious carotid artery disease or severe cardiopathy (valvular or ischemic heart disease) or both.[45]

Lacunae

Lacunae correspond to small infarcts that lie in the deeper part of the cerebrum and brain

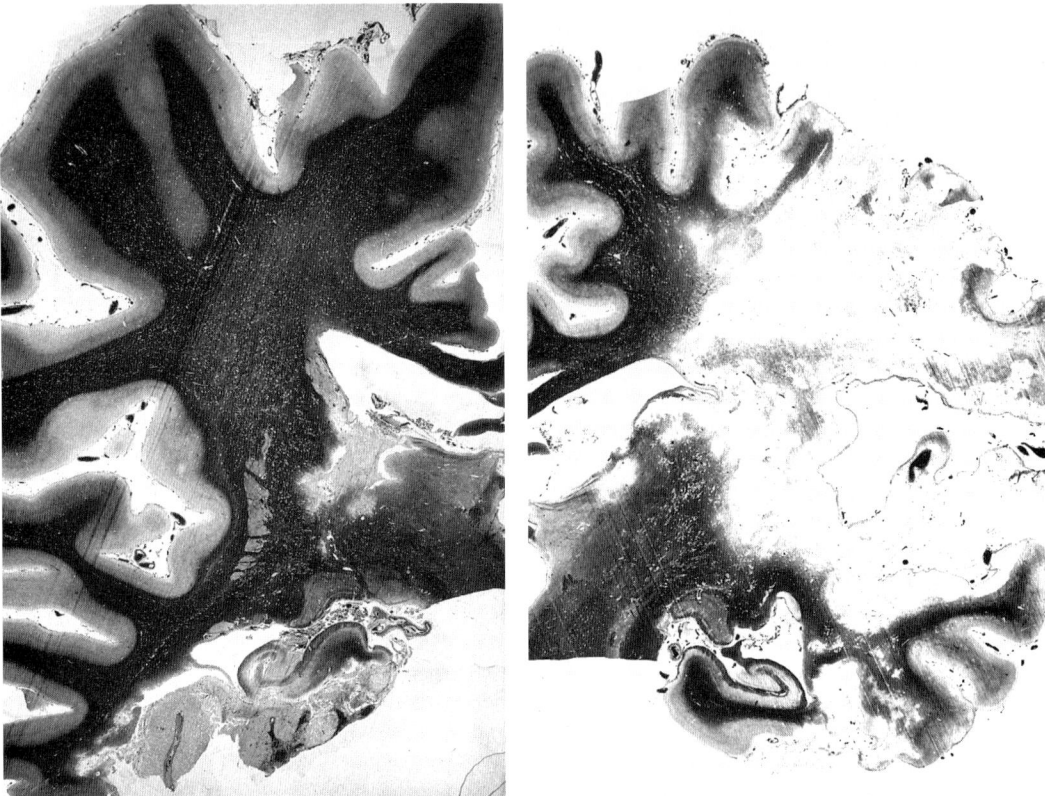

Figure 5–2. Multiple infarcts. Myelin preparation shows infarcts in both cerebral hemispheres of the same brain. Celloidin, Wolcke stain, ×1.75.

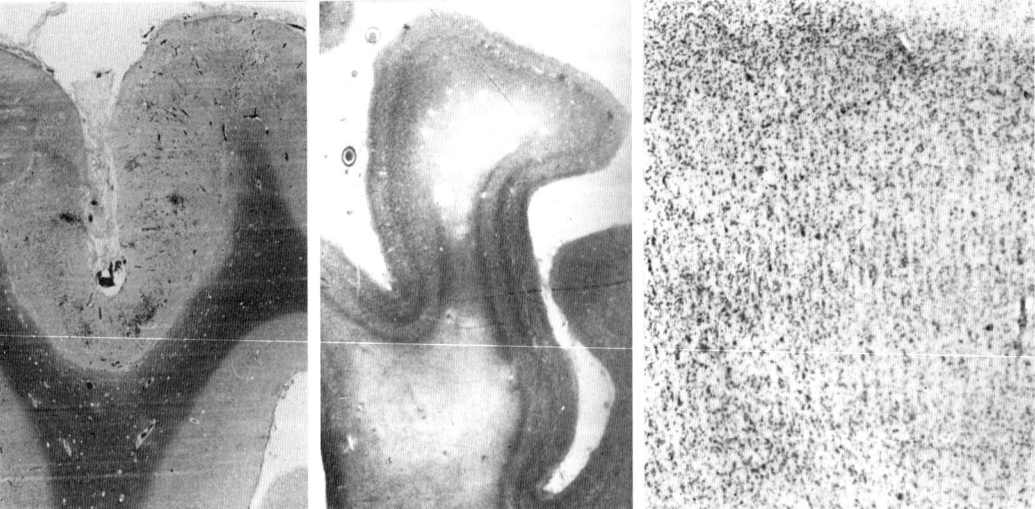

Figure 5–3. Multiple infarcts. *A.* Myelin preparation shows cortical hemorrhagic infarct. Celloidin, Wolcke stain, ×8.4. *B.* Infarcted white and gray matter; the spared IV lamina appears as a black line. Celloidin, hematein-phloxin-luxol fast blue (HPL), stain; ×5.6. *C.* Microscopic appearance of pale-staining area of cortical infarction. Celloidin, Nissl stain; ×82.5.

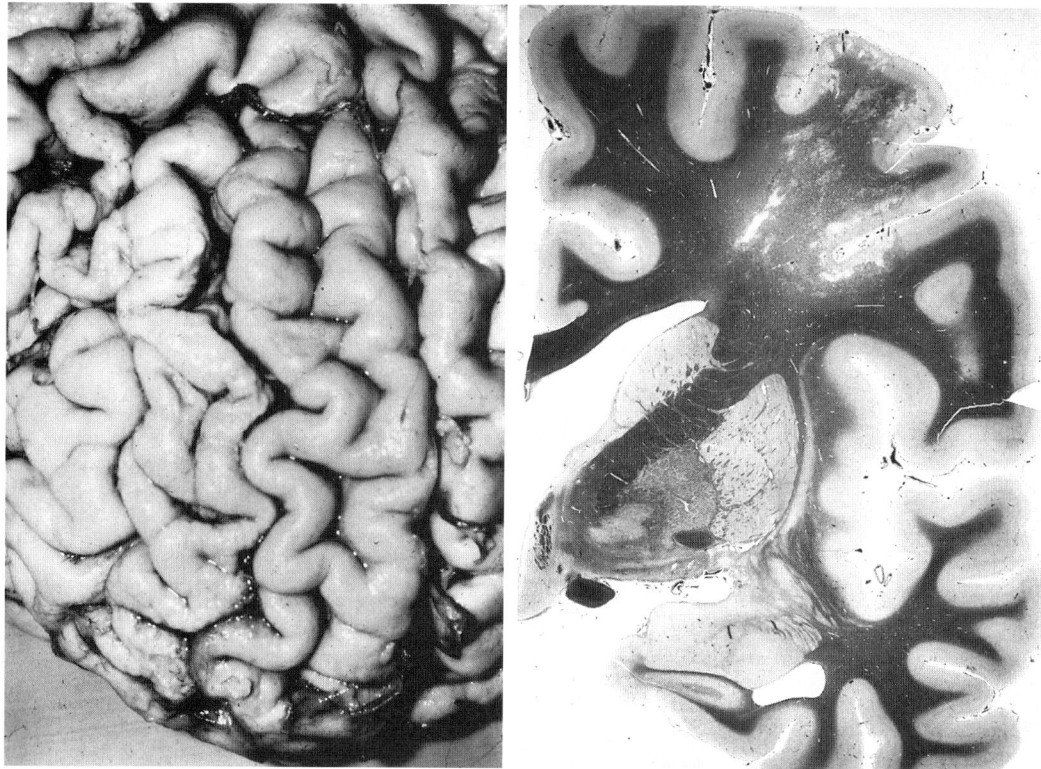

Figure 5–4. Granular atrophy of the cortex. A. Note the depressions of the surface after removal of the meninges. B. Myelin preparation shows numerous small infarcts in the boundary zone between the cortical territories of the anterior and middle cerebral arteries. Celloidin, Wolcke stain.

stem. The reports of Fisher[46,47] have perfectly demonstrated their characteristics: they range in size from large (1.5–2 cm) to very small (3–4 mm), and are often multiple (Fig. 5–6). The most common sites are the putamen, caudate nucleus, thalamus, and pons, and the white matter in the internal capsule. In large lacunae, the cause of the vascular occlusion is often atheromatous plaque located in a penetrating branch, 400–900 μm in diameter. In small lacunae, the occlusion may be due to an embolus, segmental arterial disorganization with or without enlargement by lipohyalinosis, or thrombosis of a fusiform microaneurysm.[47] A new classification of lacunae has been established.[48] The lacunae described by Fisher[46] are called type I lacunae, containing nonoccluded small vessels that pass through. Type II lacunae are the result of small hemorrhages; they are unique and situated in basal ganglia or cerebral white matter. Type III lacunae are dilatations of the perivascular spaces and are sieve-like (état criblé). Type IV lacunae are large and expansive, occupying much space.[49–51] This classification is not accepted by many authors. État criblé (type III) is frequently described separately.[52] This lesion is very small (1–2 mm) and consists of a dilation of Virchow-Robin perivascular space around a spiraled elongated arteriole; the space is filled with serum proteins that will be reabsorbed, inducing some degree of retraction and peripheral astrocytosis.[53] État criblé is preferentially present in white matter, basal ganglia, and the thalamus.

Dementia cannot always be correlated with the number and situation of the lacunae. However, in a series of 24 elderly patients with dementia who had cerebrovascular disease, severe cribriform change and microinfarction were the chief substrate of VD.[54] The lacunar etiology is more easily confirmed in localized lesions, for instance, in the thalamus.[29] In 90% of cases, lacunar infarcts are

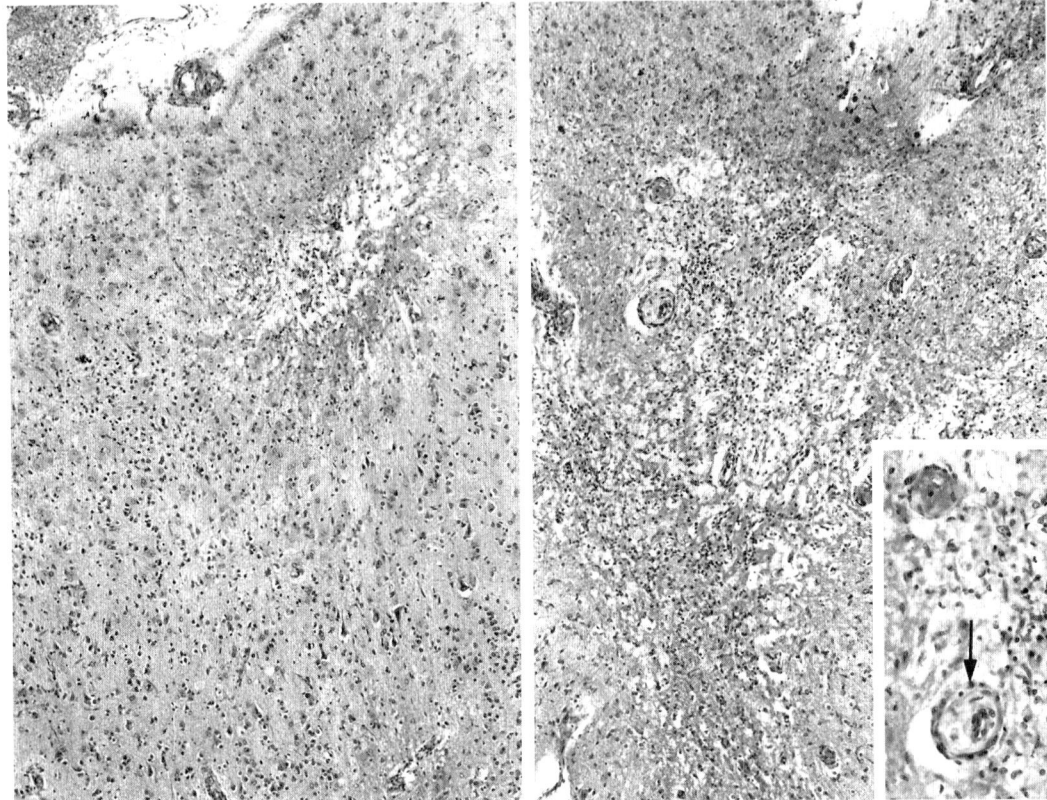

Figure 5–5. Granular atrophy of the cortex (corresponding to Fig. 5–4B). *A, B.* Small, triangular cortical infarcts under the surface. Note the endarteritis in the vessels observed in B. Celloidin, hematoxylin-eosin (H&E) stain; A,B, ×87.5; C, ×175.

associated with systemic arterial hypertension.[46]

Other vasculopathies such as Sneddon syndrome[55] or "thromboangiitis obliterans cerebrii" and sickle cell disease have been shown to be associated with dementia due to lacunar infarcts.

Binswanger Disease

Before the recent progress in neuroimaging results, subcortical arteriosclerosis encephalopathy was diagnosed only at necropsy. The main clinical symptoms are acute stroke, epileptic seizures, subacute accumulation of focal deficits, including pseudobulbar palsy, and pyramidal signs; alterations of mood, memory, and cognition proceed dementia.[56] Pre-existing hypertension and other factors known to predispose to vascular disease are also noted. A lengthy clinical course with clinical plateaus or intervals of improvement is usually observed.[4,57–59] Magnetic resonance (MR) images of the brain reveal diffuse patchy and homogeneous signals on both T1-weighted low-intensity and T2-weighted high-intensity changes in the subcortical and deep white matter bilaterally with or without a predominance.

At postmortem examination, externally the brain is normal. Atherosclerosis involves more or less the cervical extracranial vessels and the circle of Willis and its distal branches, with a variable reduction of the lumen in 93% of cases.[56] A 75% reduction in the lumina of carotid vessels and fresh thrombus of the vertebral arteries have been observed.[60] Upon gross examination, sections of the brain show bilateral large, patchy, soft regions of the white matter that appear whitish or yellow (Fig. 5–7). The lesions are situated primarily

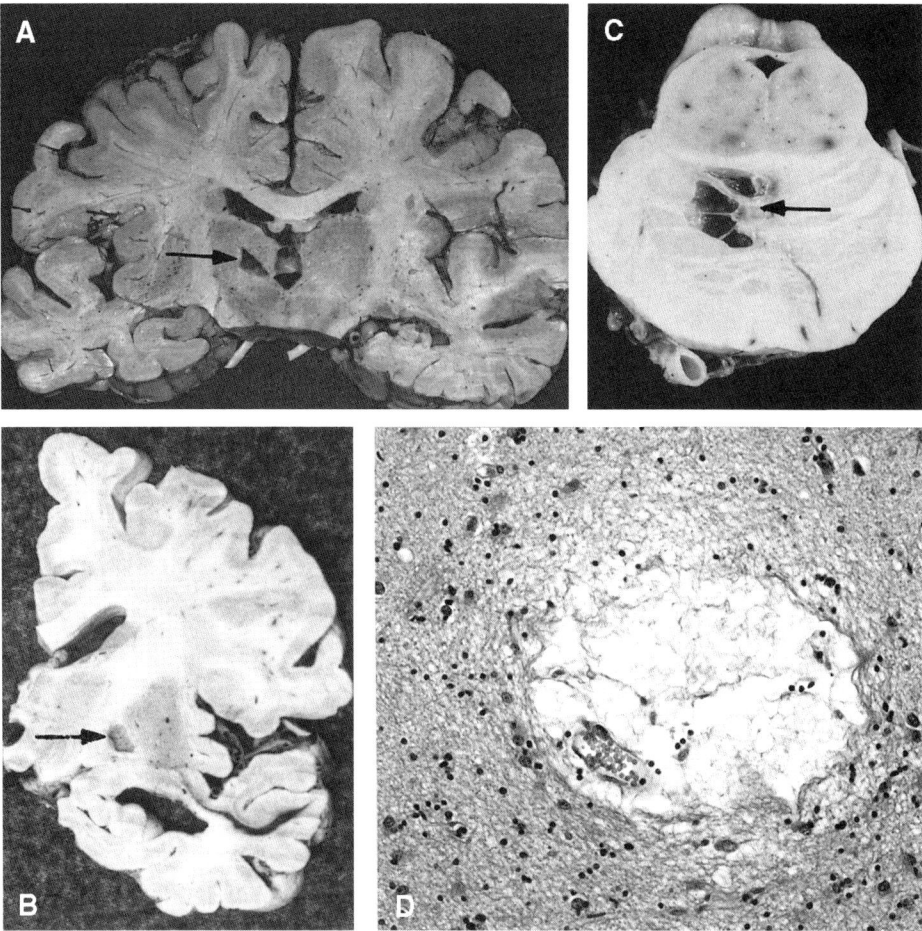

Figure 5–6. Lacunae. Coronal slices of the brain show large lacunae in the thalamus (A), the globus pallidus (B), and the pons (C). (D) Lacune (état criblé) in the putamen. Paraffin, H&E stain; ×175.

in the occipital or frontal lobe, particularly with unilateral predominance.[61] The ventricules are enlarged.

Histologic studies show various pathologic changes in the white matter: chronic progressive ischemia ranges from small areas of necrosis to large zones of myelin pallor with rarefied oligodendroglia and gliosis (Fig. 5–8); petechial hemorrhages may be present.[62] The arcuate U fibers are usually spared as well as the cortex (Fig. 5–8A, B). The terminal deep white matter arteries appear thickened and hyalinized with hypertrophy of the media,[63] and are often obliterated (Fig. 5–8C). They also contain fibrillary collagens.[64] Lacunae are especially frequent in the basal ganglia and thalamus (Fig. 5–9).

Binswanger disease (BD) is classically related to hypertension, but association has been reported with pseudoxanthoma elasticum,[65] and antiphospholipid antibody syndrome.[66] Possible but not proven associations include diabetes, polycythemia, syphilis, mucinous adenocarcinoma, thrombocytosis, severe hyperlipidemia, and hyperglobulinemia.[67]

Neuroimaging studies (lucencies on CT scan, lesions of high signal intensity on T2 MRI) have shown that a correlation of changes in white matter with only BD must be rejected. These changes have been observed in normal aging in up to 30% of asymptomatic individual.[33,68,69] Through CT scanning and MRI of fresh and fixed brains of elderly patients, including one who underwent MRI 11

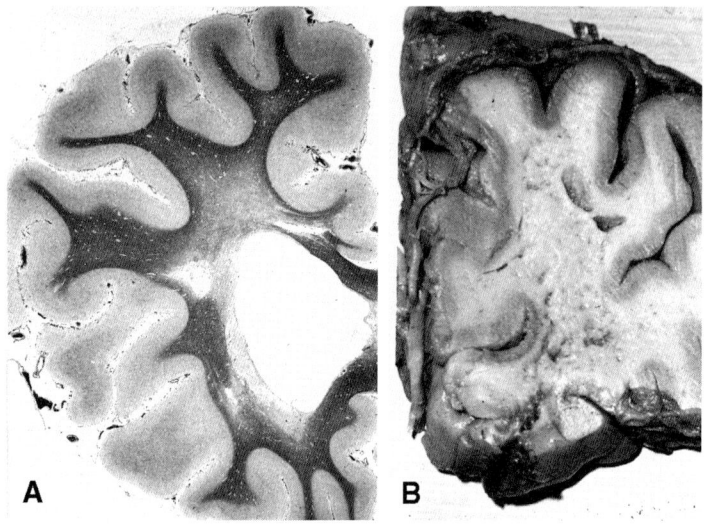

Figure 5–7. Binswanger's disease. *A.* Myelin preparation shows patchy demyelination of white matter in the frontal lobe. Celloidin, Wolcke stain. *B.* Cavitations and softenings of the white matter (occipital lobe).

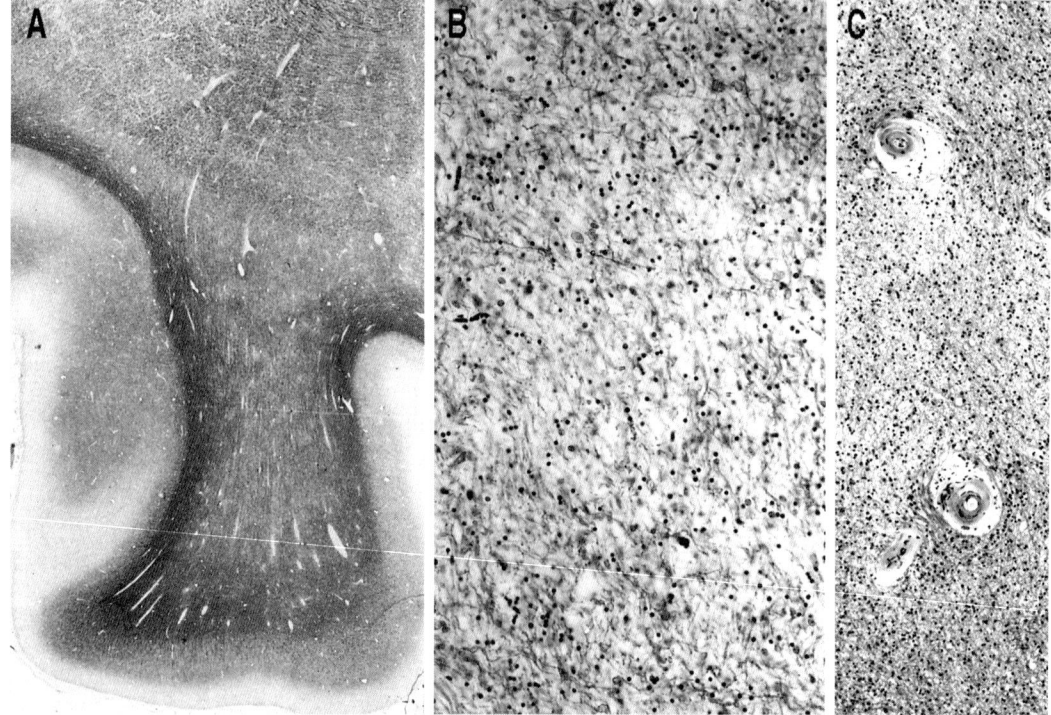

Figure 5–8. Binswanger's disease. *A.* Myelin preparation shows pallor of the white matter with sparing of the arcuate U fibers. Celloidin, Wolcke stain; ×4. *B.* Demyelination of the white matter. Celloidin, Wolcke stain; ×100. *C.* Arteriosclerotic vessels in the white matter. Celloidin, H&E stain; ×100.

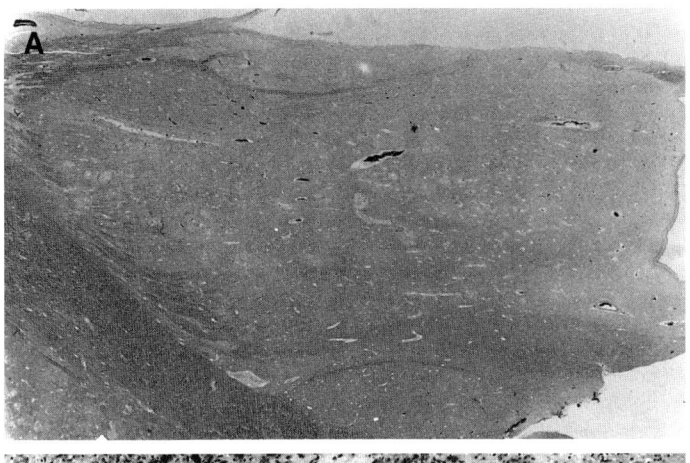
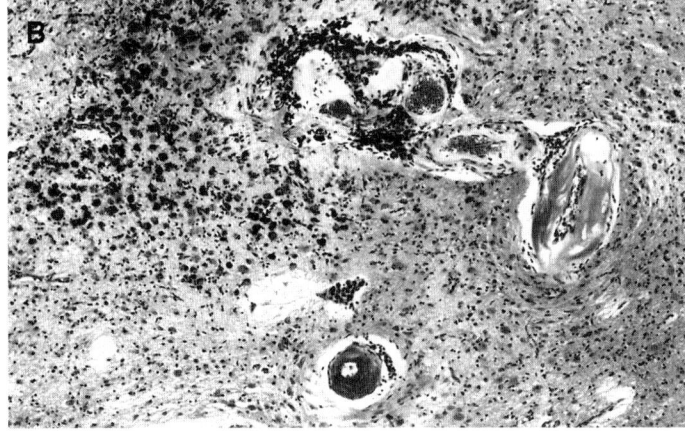

Figure 5–9. A. Note several small infarcts or hemorrhage in the thalamus. B. Higher-power view of a small hemorrhagic focus with hyaline thickening of the vessels. Celloidin, H&E stain; A, ×6.3; B, ×87.5.

days before death, subcortical MRI lesions were found to be associated with arteriosclerosis, dilated perivascular spaces, and vascular ectasia.[70] These changes have been observed in BD as well as in the lacunar state, systemic hypoperfusion, multiple strokes, and other leukoencephalopathies.[71] In descriptive terms, leukoaraisosis is a diminution of the density of the white matter; in physical terms, it represents an accumulation of extra- and intracellular water and of small protein molecules in the brain lattice.[72] Its morphological counterpart may consist of paraventricular loss of white matter, axon degeneration, secondary demyelination, multiple micro-infarcts, and perifocal gliosis,[73,74] but myelin and axon staining may be normal.[75] The data support "the uniform hypothesis that MRI provides a nonspecific index of brain parenchymal alterations caused by aging and chronic vascular disease."[76] Hachinski et al.[9] have shown that changes in white matter are indeed associated with intellectual impairment and somewhat, but not exclusively, with vascular disease, and that leukoaraiosis is a radiological term.

Various hypotheses regarding the distinguishing features and cause of BD have been considered. The disorder is a special vascular disease with tissue changes that are identical to those described in hypertensive arteriopathy, with a greater alteration of the vessels. Hypertensive encephalopathy is a factor in the development of edema, leading to fluid transsudation and demyelination; recently the role of poor perfusion of the white matter, caused by a drop in blood pressure, cardiac failure, or stenosis of large vessels in the presence of a wide zone of ischemia, has been emphasized in the occurrence of BD.[67] Repeated episodes of chronic or acute hypo- and hyperfusion and alteration in the blood–brain barrier, that is common to cerebral arteriopathic and amyloid angiopathies, have also been suggested.[77,78] Leukomalacia of periventricular and border zones is also considered to be the cause of BD, along with demyelination in the central semi-ovale which appears to be due to transient episodes of cardiac failure and chronic hypoxemia.[79,80] The use of current technics of clinical investigation have supported this hypothesis.[13] Subsequently, on the basis of critical analysis of over 100 publications (most appearing in the last decade), some authors concluded that BD did not exist.[81] Despite this controversy and although BD is a rare disease, it is a well-defined condition based on clinical, radiological, and neuropathological data. More than 100 cases were quoted in a review including 45 cases in Japan.[52,69]

Contributory factors have been reported for BD. The hypothesis of plasmatic viscosity, proposed in 1987,[82] was also highlighted by Caplan[67] among his criteria for the diagnosis of BD. A loss of synaptophysin immunoreactivity suggests a reduction in cortical synaptic population density,[83] but this result does not appear to be very specific, as it may be related to retrograde and/or anterograde degeneration. In 17 cases of BD, regressive changes in the astroglia and activation of microglia along with a decrease in oligodendroglia were found in the white matter in association with degradation of both myelin and axonal components.[84] These results indicate that there is some degree of inflammatory reaction and compromised axonal transport. No definitive conclusion has been accepted regarding the pathophysiology of BD, but the hypothesis of a defective regulation of blood flow and microcirculation associated with large-vessel disease and mechanical disturbances is an interesting one to consider.

Other Forms of Leukoencephalopathies

Other leukoencephalopathies may be difficult to differentiate from BD before histological examination. Following are descriptions of these disorders.

AMYLOID ANGIOPATHY

The role of cerebral amyloid angiopathy (CAA) in dementia has been discussed since the beginning of the century. Characterization of the disease is discussed in Chapter 4 (Figs. 5–10 and 5–11). Cerebral amyloid angiopathy is generally asymptomatic, but progression to an advanced stage can lead to vessel rupture and hemorrhage.[85] Leukoencephalopathy may be observed in diffuse hemorrhagic CAA.[86,87] Rapid progressive dementia is characterized by patchy demyelination, petechial cortical hemorrhages, and cortical infarcts with a variable degree of neuritic plaques.[88] When lesions are restricted to the white matter, only neuropathological examination can differentiate CAA leucoencephalopathy from BD.[89]

Familial forms of hereditary cerebral hemorrage with amyloidosis, dementia, and dominant autosomic transmission have also been individualized. Different proteins are involved, according to the family with disease. In CAA a mechanism of hypoperfusion of the distal white matter similar to that occurring in BD is involved.

CADASIL

Since the description of hereditary MID in Sweden,[90] this new disease has been observed all over the world. In 1993 Tounier Lasserve et al.[91] performed genetic linkage analysis of data from two unrelated French families with *c*erebral *a*utosomal *d*ominant *ar*teriopathy with *s*ubcortical *i*nfarcts and *l*eukoencephalopathy (CADASIL) and mapped the mutant gene to chromosome 1912. In 1996 the same group identified mutations in patients with CADASIL indicated that Notch 3 could be the defective protein.[92] The disease is characterized by recurrent episodes of focal brain dysfunction separated by remissions. It starts in mid-adulthood and leads in some patients to severe motor disability with pseudobulbar palsy and dementia.[93] Dementia of the subcortical type is the second most common clinical manifestation observed in one-third of symptomatic patients and it is present in 90% of patients before death.[94,95] No significant hypertension has been present in any of the patients. Results from MRI are always abnormal in symptomatic patients, showing leukoencephalopathy and small deep infarcts. Neuropathological studies have been reported in 23 cases. Gross examination shows ill-defined areas of malacia associated with lacunae in the basal ganglia. Hematoma was present in two cases, one in a patient subjected to anticoag-

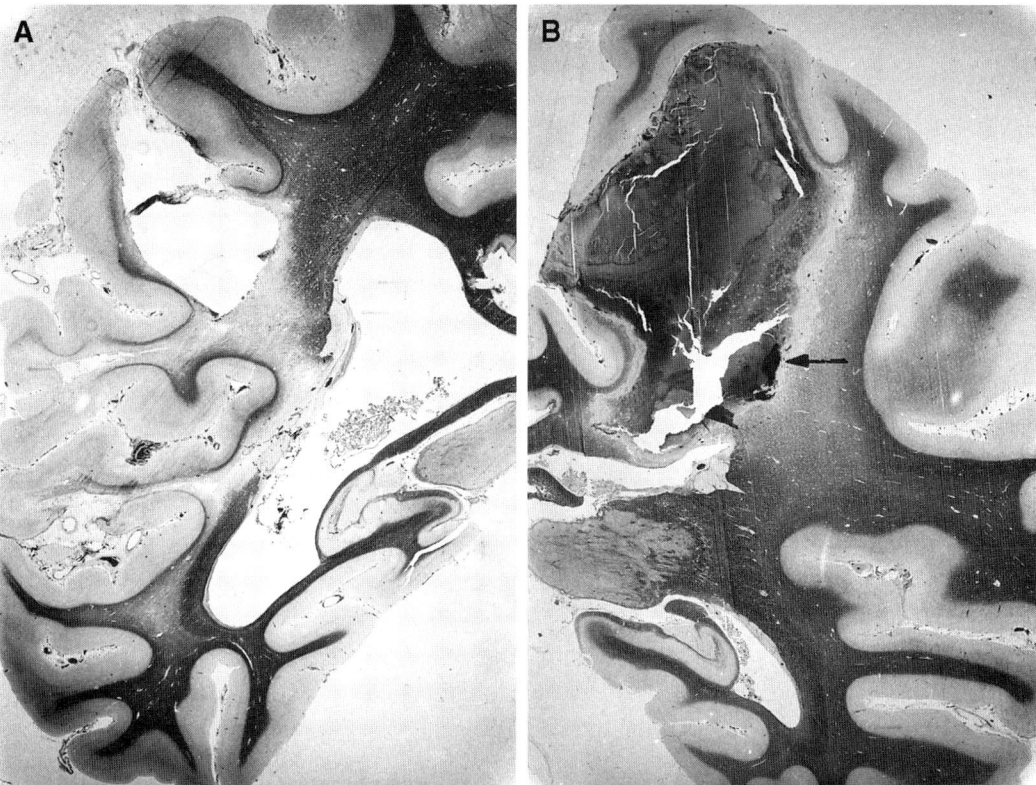

Figure 5–10. Amyloid angiopathy. Myelin preparations shows bilateral associated lesions in a demented patient: middle artery cerebral infarct (*A*) and frontoparietal hematoma (*B*). Celloidin, Woleke stain; ×1.7.

ulant therapy.[90,96] Histologically, the U fibers are preserved (Fig. 5–12A). Myelin and axonal loss increase from the subcortical to the periventricular zone, and is associated with small infarcts of the white matter, the basal ganglia, thalamus, brain stem, and, inconstantly, the cerebellum and spinal cord.[90,96]

The more specific lesion is a widespread vasculopathy of the small arteries penetrating the white matter and of some the leptomeningeal vessels. There is extensive noncongophilic (Fig 5–12B) material that thickens the media and reduplication of the internal elastic lamella. The myocytes are rarefied and appear as round, swollen cells.[97] No specific staining has been obtained except for faint immunopositivity for fragments of complement.[96,98,99] At the ultrastructural level this material is granular and osmiophilic without limiting membrane. Extracellularly it is close to the basal lamina of smooth muscle cells (Fig. 5–12C).

Although the precise nature of this deposit is unknown, it appears to be such a distinctive feature that diagnosis of CADASIL was confirmed in eight families on brain biopsies.[100–105] The observation of this granular material within the vessel walls of skin (Fig. 5–12D) muscle, and nerve[97,106] and, in some cases, of systemic viscera has greatly extended the recognition of this disease.[107,108] Very recent data have shown, using immunoelectron microscopy, the accumulation of the Notch 3 receptor ectodomain at the cytoplasmic membrane of vascular smooth muscle cells in close vicinity to the granular osmiophilic material.[108a]

Only one case was found to be associated with Alzheimer's disease.[109]

RARE DISEASES

Hereditary endotheliopathy with retinopathy, nephropathy, and stroke has been described in only one family.[110] Ultrastructural studies showed distinctive multilaminated vascular basement membranes in the brain and other tissues. Hereditary cerebral retinal was de-

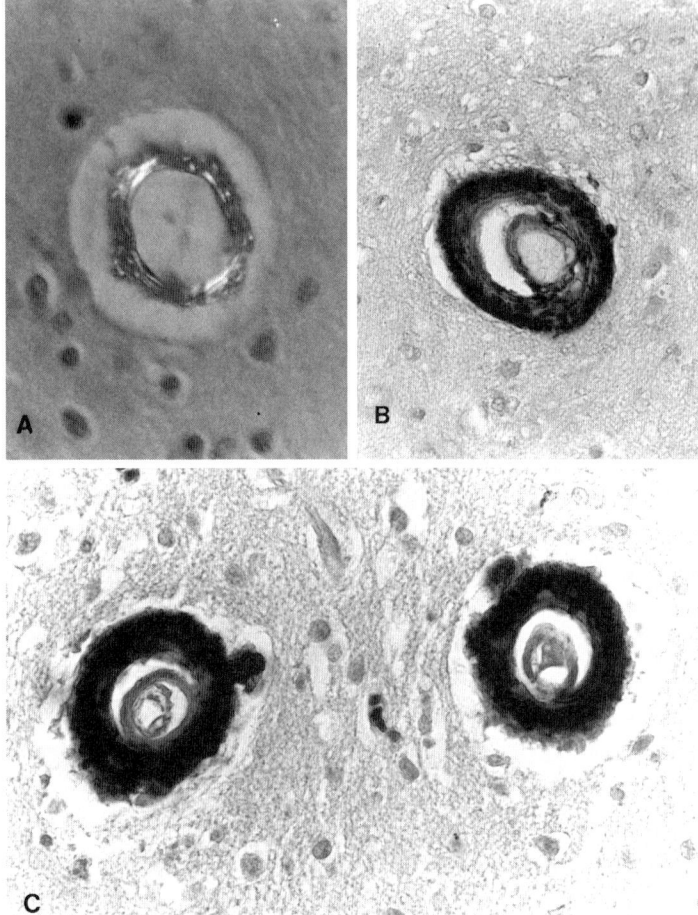

Figure 5–11. Amyloid angiopathy. A. Amyloid deposit observed with polarized light. B. Immunostaining with anti-apo E antibody (ABC complex-diaminobenzidin) showing the double barrow of the vessel wall. C. Immunostaining with anti-protein β A40 [gift of F. Chechler]. Paraffin; ×412.

scribed in two families.[111,112] Fibrinoid necrosis without inflammation was the basic vascular lesion. Subcortical vascular encephalopathy was also observed in a normal young Japanese adult with premature baldness and spondylitis deformans.[113] Arteriosclerosis was found in large and small vessels of the cortex and the white matter. Other Japanese cases have been reported[113a] characterized as CARASIL (cerebral autosomal recessive arteriosclerosis with subcortical infarcts and leukoencephalopathy).

Hemorrhagic Lesions

These lesions consist of large, multiple hematomas and/or small petechial foci. Most of them are associated with large and small infarcts. Lesions are related to hypertension and more frequently to CAA.

FOCAL FORMS OF VASCULAR DEMENTIA

Dementia is not always correlated with destruction of a large amount of tissue; it can be caused by focal lesions in relevant cerebral territories. The existence of asymmetrical or unilateral forms is not as well documented. These focal forms are rarely reported.

Bilateral Lesions

Most of lesions of localized forms are situated in the territory of the posterior cerebral artery. However, because the exact topography of the territory supplied by the intrinsic thalamic arteries has not been completely determined, the occipital, temporal, and thalamic dementias will be described separately.

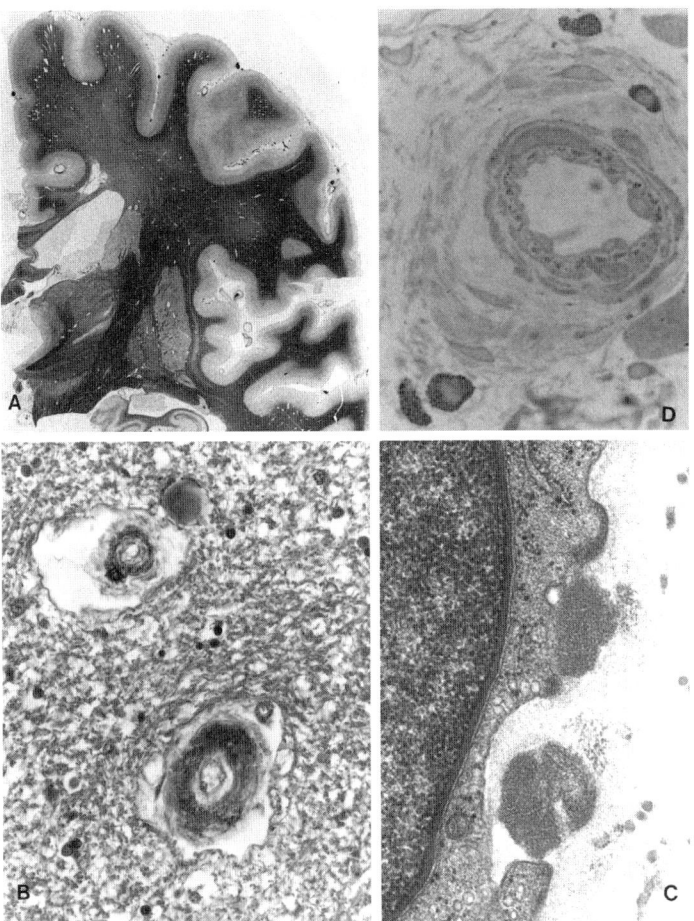

Figure 5–12. CADASIL. *A.* Pallor of the white matter of the frontal lobe associated with lacunae in the cingulate gyrus and thalamus. Celloidin, Wolcke stain; ×1.3. *B.* Granular deposits in the arterial walls of two small arteries. H&E stain; ×412. *C.* Electron micrograph of a skin biopsy: granular deposits are situated close to the smooth muscle cell membrane. Uranyl acetate–lead citrate stain; ×37200. *D.* Semithin section of skin biopsy shows the deposits at a light microscopic level. PAS stain; ×1030.

Occipital Lesions

Few observations of these lesions have been reported. The patient described by Dide and Botcazo[114] had Korsakoff syndrome with spatial disorientation, alexia, astereognosia, and hemianopsia. A bilateral infarct of the lingual lobe was present with extension into the left posterolateral thalamus; the anterior part of the limbic system was not described. The patient of Boudin et al.[115] had cortical blindness in addition to Korsakoff syndrome; anatomically bilateral inferomesial occipital infarcts were associated with lesions of the splenium of the corpus callosum and the posterior fornices.

Temporal Lesions

There are reports of demented patients with partial or complete lesions of the hippocampi, extending into neighboring temporal tissue with associate degenerations. However, even if these patients may have been considered demented,[116,117] in fact, most of them had only amnesia, except the patient described by Grunthal.[118] Amnesia has been the subject of many reports[34,119–122] and will not be discussed here.

Thalamic Lesions

There are several classical studies in which damage of the mediodorsal nucleus of the thalamus is regarded to be primarily responsible for amnesic or affective disorders, the role of the mammillothalamic bundle of Vicq-d' Azyr has also been discussed.[123] Clinical features of thalamic dementia have been identified on the basis of anatomical or neuroimaging correlations of published cases.[124,125] Behavioral disturbances are characterized by

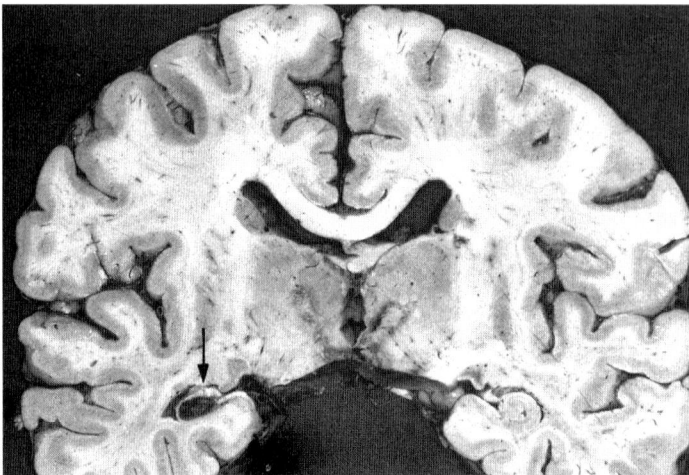

Figure 5–13. Focal form of vascular dementia. Coronal section of cerebral hemisphere shows bilateral paramedian infarcts in the thalami and hemorrhagic lesion of the Ammon's horn (arrow).

apathy, motor and verbal lack of spontaneity and responsiveness, affective indifference, and amnesia. Impaired attention is sometimes present. One patient presented with delusions without loss of memory and bilateral degenerative lesions of the mediodorsal nucleus.[126] Such findings accompany selective vascular or degenerative lesions of the thalamus involving the paramedian territories.[127] In most cases, paramedian infarcts affect the intralaminar and parafasicular nuclei, the inferior internal region of the mediodorsal nucleus, the inferior internal region of the central nucleus, and the superior internal pole of the red nucleus (Fig. 5–13). The frequency of focal thalamic lesions has been confirmed in recent series.[29,128]

Frontocingular Lesions

Dementia is frequently the clinical manifestation in primary cerebral degenerations or cerebral infections involving the frontocingulate gyrus, whereas its appears extremely rarely in vascular lesions affecting these gyri. The clinical manifestations are the result of infarcts in territories supplied by the anterior cerebral arteries. Clinically, in addition to paresis of lower limbs, there is some degree of mental disturbance, complex behavioral changes associated with the Korsakoff syndrome, mutism, akinesia,[29] loss of empathy or lack of attention. In Escourolle and Gray's[130] clinicopathological correlations of published cases, they emphasized the role of the complete disconnection between the frontal lobes and the components of the limbic system. The relevance of the circuitry of the frontal association cortex to dementia has also been analyzed.[100] Memory disturbances may be explained by damage to the fornices. The lesions are due to arteriosclerosis of the anterior cerebral artery, complications of aneurysms of the anterior communicating artery, surgery of tumors, or arteriovenous malformations situated in the anterior part of the skull in relation to vessels of the frontal lobe (see refs. 131 and 132 for review).

Asymmetrical Forms

Asymmetrical forms of lesions are rare, but analysis of the topography of these lesions has supported the notion that circuitry of the limbic system is involved. The first case of Dide and Pezet[133] included a left occipital infarct and a right thalamic lesion. The case of Victor et al.[117] was bitemporal and mostly confined to the left side with bilateral destruction of the hippocampomammillary connection. The case of Delay et al.[120] had a left temporo-occipital infarct, with secondary degeneration of the mammillary body and interruption of the right mammillothalamic bundle, i.e., a left pre-mammillary lesion and a right post-mammillary one. An asymmetry of lesions was also found in the case of Schenk,[134] who described destruction of the posterior right hippocampus and the left frontal lobe from the precentral area to the cingulate gyrus. Boudin et al.[135] reported a case of dementia with involvement of the left posterior pillar of the fornix and the right cingular gyrus.

Unilateral Forms

These forms of lesions are exceptional. The memory disturbances of the patient of Geschwind and Fusillo[136] disappeared after 2 months, even though he had a right hippocampal lesion. A minute controlateral lesion of the laterodorsal nucleus of the thalamus was noted in a number of cases. The role of this nucleus has been evaluated in the development of amnesia.[137,138] Dementia has also been reported as "strategic infarct dementia" after infarcts involving the inferior genu of the internal capsule; a thalamocortical disconnection has been suggested.[139] Unilateral lesions more often give rise to psychic disturbances than to real states of dementia. Such is the case, for instance, in the unilateral vascular lesions of the posterior part of the nondominant hemisphere, which produce, as a consequence, a pseudodementia of depressive type.[140]

PATHOGENESIS OF VASCULAR DEMENTIA

The various types of vascular lesions have already been discussed, so only a brief description of the pathogenesis of VD is given here. Vascular dementia may be the result of circulatory disturbances and/or abnormalities of the vessels walls.

Circulatory Disturbances

Cardiac diseases are the main etiology of systemic circulatory abnormalities. Although dementia can result from myxoma, infections, and marantic endocarditis, the hemodynamic type due to cardiac arrythmias and systemic hypotension is frequently noted. Unstable variations in arterial pressure and hypoperfusion induced by ischemia or hypoxia play an important role in the development of VD. These may be associated with hyperviscosity, abnormal hemostasis, and/or antiphospholipid antibodies syndrome[141] (Fig. 5–14). The role of blood-brain barrier abnormalities in VD is still a matter of debate. Most authors insist that the decrease in the cerebral vascular bed and modifications in the regulation process are involved.

The vascular diseases that cause dysfunction of the central nervous system CNS may simply be a manifestation of a systemic disease. Atherosclerosis is a disease process that most commonly affects the large arteries of the CNS. In recent theories on its pathogenesis, emphasis has been placed on the similitaries of the mechanisms and events involved to those of inflammation.[142] Various categories of risk factors have been postulated: age, genetic inheritance, gender, arterial hypertension, abnormalities of plasmal lipids, diabetes, and life style; hypertensive fibrinoid arteritis is less fre-

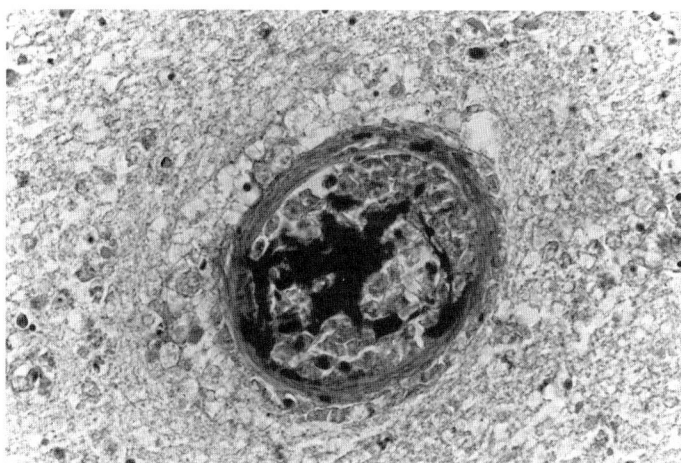

Figure 5–14. Disseminated intravascular coagulation (IVD) intravascular fibrin. Mallory staining, Paraffin; ×412.

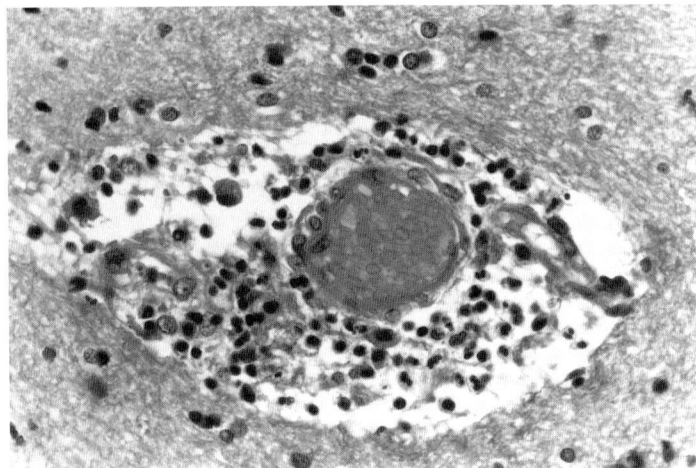

Figure 5–15. Primary cerebral angiitis. Inflammatory cells surround the vessel wall. (Biopsy) H&E stain paraffin; ×412.

quently a cause of VD because of the important progress in treatment of this disorder. Fisher[46] has attributed the diminution of lacunae, observed at postmortem examination, to the effective treatment of hypertension.

Abnormalities of Small Vessels

Abnormalities of small vessels consist of lipohyalinosis and fibrosis. Arterioles become spiraled and elongated and venules are frequently thickened and hyalinized. Amyloid angiopathy is discussed above. The relationship between dementia and angiitis has been established. Primary CNS vasculitis is also called noninfectious granulomatous angiitis;[46,143,144] this disorder is characterized by infiltration of small leptomeningeal and intraparenchymal arteries (200–500 úm in diameter) with lymphocytes, macrophages, and/or multinucleated giant cells, with a variable degree of fibrinoid necrosis. Parenchymal biopsy is sometimes necessary to confirm isolated cerebral angiitis before successfull treatment can occur (Fig 5–15).[145] Dementia is present in 40% of cases.[145] In patients with systemic necrotizing vasculitis, the most frequent concern is the group of polyarteritis nodosa.[144] Dementia related to giant cell arteritis is rare.[146,147] Dementia has also been seen in patients with rheumatoid arthritis, systemic lupus erythematosis (SLE)[148] alone, or in VD associated with antiphospholipid antibodies.

Dementia is rarely observed in fibromuscular dysplasia. It is present in moyamoya disease, which mostly affects young people. Several reports have demonstrated that there are common features between thromboangiitis obliterans cerebri, Sneddon sydrome, and corticomeningeal angiomatosis of Divry and Van Bogaert.[149] Dementia is found in 30% of Sneddon syndrome cases.[150] Although Sneddon syndrome is considered a thrombotic vasculopathy, the modifications of the small vessels of the brain appear inconstant.[151] One family with autosomal dominant inheritance has been reported.[152]

Neoplastic angioendotheliomatosis, a cause of subacute dementia, is now recognized as a true angiotropic lymphoma of B or T lineage.[153] Mitochondrial encephalomyopathy could be explained by a mitochondrial angiopathy of the pial arterioles and small arteries, as found in the (MELAS) (mitochondrial encephalopathy, lactic acidosis, and stroke-like episobles) syndrome.[54–156] Fabry disease may be also the source of dementia.[157,158] Dementia due to a thrombophlebitis of the superior sagittal sinus has also been observed.[159] Four cases were related to venous hypertensive encephalopathy caused by arteriovenous fistulas.[160–162]

VASCULAR DEMENTIA AND ALZHEIMER'S DISEASE

The frequency of "mixed" dementia was reported by Delay and Brion.[34] Recent studies have found concomitant cerebrovascular pathology in 36% of AD.[27,163] In some cases of dementia, stroke reveals asymptomatic AD.[12] Since white matter leukoaraiosis may be present in AD, many reports have tried to differentiate AD from BD through clinical and radiological criteria. These studies have shown that this type of diagnostic system cannot distinguish mixed AD/BD from BD.[164] Moreover loss of myelin with incomplete white matter infarction and reactive gliosis are "common histopathological findings in AD."[165] In these cases, only neuropathological examination alone can determine the nature of the dementia.

In these mixed lesions the mean volume of vascular lesions and density of neurofibrillary tangles and plaques in the superior temporal cortex were significantly lower than in VD and AD, respectively; these results might indicate additive effects.[166] The role of amyloid angiopathy has also been questioned in AD. In a retrospective study of 145 deceased patients, severe amyloid angiopathy was associated with an increased frequency of cerebral infarction in patients with AD; hypertension also had an important role.[167]

Three subgroups of VD are recognized: One is classical MID, including large and multiple foci of infarcts or hemorrhages that are mostly related to embolism or thrombosis of large vessels or cardiac events. The second subgroup includes lacunae, and état criblé alone or associated with leucoencephalopathy, i.e., lacunar dementia, that is associated with longer survival[168] and occurs more frequently than MID;[54] lesions of the thalamus are also associated with this type of VD. The third subgroup is mixed dementia associated with AD, which appears more frequently than dementia alone.

I thank V. Quinet and C. Martin, for typing the manuscript, and A. Chazalet for preparing figures.

REFERENCES

1. Durand-Fardel M. Traité Clinique et Pratique des Maladies des Vieillards. Paris: J. B. Baillière, 1984.
2. Klippel M. Caractères histologiques différentiels de la PG. Classification histologique des paralysies générales. Arch Med Exp 1891; 3:660–676.
3. Binswanger O. Die Abgrenzung der-allgemeinen progressiven paralysie. Berl Klin Wochenschr 1894; 31: 1103–1105; 1137–1139;1180–1186.
4. Olszewski J. Subcortical arteriosclerotic encephalopathy. World Neurol 1962; 3:359–375.
5. Marie P. Des foyers lacunaires de désintégration et de différents autres états cavitaires du cerveau. Rev Med 1901; 21:281–298.
6. Ferrand J. Essai sur l'hémiplégie des vieillards: les lacunes de désintégration cérébrale. Paris, 1902. Thesis Rousset.
7. Tomlinson BE, Blessed G, Roth M. Observations on the brains of demented old people. J Neurol Sci 1970; 11:205–242.
8. Hachinski VC, Lassen NA, Marshall J. Multi-infarct dementia. A cause of mental deterioration in the elderly. Lancet 1974; 14:207–210.
9. Hachinski VC, Potter P and Merskey H. Leukoaraiosis. Arch Neurol 1987; 44:21–23.
10. McMenemey WH. The dementias and progressive diseases of the basal ganglia. In: Greenfield JG, ed. Neuropathology, 3rd, ed London: E. Arnold, 1961: 475–521.
11. Tatemichi TK. How acute brain failure becomes chronic: a view of the mechanisms of dementia related to stroke. Neurology 1990; 40:1652–1659.
12. Pasquier F, Leys D. Why are stroke patients prone to develop dementia? J Neurol 1997; 244:135–142.
13. Moroney JT, Bagiella E, Desmond DW, Paik MC, Stern Y, Tatemichi TK. Risk factors for incident dementia after stroke. Role of hypoxic and ischemic disorders. Stroke 1996; 27:1283–1289.
14. De Reuck J, Santens P. The evolving concept of vascular dementia. In: Leys D, Pasquier F, Scheltens P, ed. Stroke and Alzheimer's Disease. The Hague: Holland Academic Graphics, 1998: 3–9.
15. Roman GC, Tatemichi TK, Erkinjuntti T, Cummings JL, Masdeu JC, Garcia JH, Amaducci L, Orgogozo JM, Brun A, Hofman A, Moody DM, O'Brien M, Yamaguchi T, Grafman J, Drayer BP, Bennett DA, Fischer M, Ogata J, Kokmen E, Bermejo J, Wolf PA, Gorelcik PB, Bick KL, Pajeau AK, Bell MA, Decarli C, Culebras A, Korczyn AD, Bogousslavsky J, Hartmann A, Scheinberg P. Vascular dementia: diagnostic criteria for research studies. Report of the NINDS-AIREN International Workshop Neurology 1993; 43: 250–260.
16. Erkinjuntti T. Vascular dementia: challenge of clinical diagnosis. Int Psychogeriatr 1997; 9 suppl 1:51–58.
17. Chabriat H, Bousser MG. Pure vascular dementia. In: Leys D, Pasquier F, Scheltens P, eds. Stroke and Alzheimer's Disease The Hague: Holland Academic Graphics, 1998: 28–43.
18. American Psychiatric Association Committee on Nomenclature and Statistics. Diagnostic and Statistical Manual of Mental Disorders (DSM-III-R). Washington, DC: American Psychiatric Association, 1987.
19. American Psychiatric Association Committee on Nomenclature and Statistics. Diagnostic and Statistical Manual of Mental Disorders (DSM-IV). Washington, DC: American Psychiatric Association, 1994.
20. Hachinski VC, Iliff L, Zihlka E, Du Boulay G, Mc Allister V, Marshall J, Russel R, Symon L. Cerebral blood flow in dementia. Arch Neurol 1975; 32:632–637.
21. Chui HC, Victoroff JI, Margolin D, Jagust W, Shankle R, Katzman R. Criteria for the diagnosis of ischemic vascular dementia proposed by the State of California

Alzheimer's Disease Diagnostic and Treatment Centers. Neurology 1992; 42:473–480.
22. Gold G, Giannokopoulos P, Montes-Paixao C, Jr, Herman Fr, Mulligan R, Michel JP, Bouras CC. Sensitivity and specificity of newly proposed clinical criteria for possible vascular dementia. Neurology 1997; 49:690–694.
23. Roses AD, and Saunders AM, ApoE, Alzheimer's disease, and recovery from brain stress. Ann N Y Acad Sci 1997; 26:200–212.
24. Parnetti L, Mari D, Mecocci P, Senin V. Pathogenetic mechanisms in vascular dementia. Int J Clin Lab Res 1994:24:15–22.
25. Jorm AF: Cross-national comparisons of the occurrence of Alzheimer's and vascular dementias. Eur Arch Psychiatry Clin Neurosci 1991; 240:218–222.
26. Jorm A, and Jolley D. The incidence of dementia: a meta-analysis. Neurology 1998:51:728–733.
27. Nolan KA, Lino M M, Seligmann AW, Blass JP. Absence of vascular dementia in an autopsy series from a dementia clinic. J Am Geriatr Soc. 1998; 46:597–604.
28. Hulette C, Nochlin D, McKeel D, Morris J, Mirra S, Sumi SM, Heyman A, Clinical-neuropathologic findings in multi-infarct dementia: a report of six autopsied cases. Neurology 1997; 48:668–672.
29. Jellinger KA. Clinical-neuropathologic findings in multi-infarct dementia: a report of six autopsied cases Neurology 1997; 49:1754–1755.
30. Pohjasvaara T, Erkinjuntti T, Vataja R, Kaste M. Dementia three months after stroke. Baseline frequency and effect of different definitions of dementia in the Helsinki Stroke Aging Memory Study (SAM) cohort. Stroke 1997; 28:785–792.
31. Scheltens P, Ravid R, Kamphorst W. Pathologic findings in a case of primary progressive aphasia. Neurology. 1994; 44:279–282.
32. Longstreth WT, Jr, Manolio TA, Arnold A, Burke GL, Bryan N, Jungreis CA, Enright PL, O'Leary D, Fried L. Clinical correlates of white matter findings on cranial magnetic resonance imaging of 3301 elderly people. The Cardiovascular Health Study Stroke. 1996; 27:1274–1282.
33. De Reuck J, Decco D, Marchau M, Santens P, Lemahieu I, Strijckmans K. Positron emission tomography in vascular dementia. J Neurol Sci. 1998; 154:55–61.
34. Delay J, Brion S. Les Démences Tardives. Paris: Masson, 1962.
35. Lindenberg R, Spatz H. Uber die Thromboendarteriitis Obliterans der Hirngefasse (cerebrale Form der V. Winiwarter Buergerschen Kranskheit). Virchows Arch Path Anat. 1939; 305:531–557.
36. Jellinger K. Neuropathological aspects of dementias resulting from abnormal blood and cerebral fluid dynamics. Acta Neurol Belg. 1976; 76:83–102.
37. Morel F, Meyra G. L'atrophie granulaire de l'écorce cérébrale. Contribution à l'étude de la forme systématisée de cette affection. Schweitz Arch Neurol Psychiatry 1944; 53:315–325.
38. Pentschew A. Die granulare Atrophie der Groshirnrinde. Arch Psychiat Nervenkr, 1933; 101:80–136.
39. Wildi E. Etat granulaire systématisé cardiopathique de l'écorce cérébrale (atrophie granulaire). Etude anatomo-clinique. Bull Acad Suisse Sci Med. 1959; 15 (suppl 1):18–83.
40. Kaplan JG, Katzman R, Horoupian DS, Fuld PA. Progressive dementia, visual deficits, amyotrophy, and micro-infarcts. Neurology (Minneapolis), 1985; 35:789–796.
41. Fischer CM. Cerebral thromboangiitis obliterans. Medicine (Baltimore) 1957; 35:169–209.
42. Romanul FCA, Abramowicz A. Changes in brain and pial vessels in arterial border zones. A study of 13 cases. Arch Neurol. 1961; 11:40–65.
43. Adams JH, Brierley JB, Connor RC, Treip CS. The effects of systemic hypotension upon the human brain. Clinical and neuropathological observations in 11 cases. Brain 1966: 89:235–238.
44. Torvik A, Endresen GKM, Abrahamsen AF, Godal HC. Progressive dementia caused by an unusual type of generalized small vessel thrombosis. Acta Neurol Scand. 1971; 47:137–150.
45. Evrard S, Woimant F, Le Coz P, Polivka M, Cousin C, Haguenau M. Watershed cerebral infarcts: retrospective study of 24 cases. Neurol Res 1992; 14:97–99.
46. Fisher CM. Lacunar strokes and infarcts: a review. Neurology (Minneapolis) 1982; 32:871–876.
47. Fisher CM. The arterial lesions underlying lacunes. Acta Neuro-pathol (Berl) 1969; 12:1–15.
48. Poirier J, Gray F, Gherardi R, Derouesne C: Cerebral lacunae. A new neuropathological classification. J Neuropath Exp Neurol 1985; 44:312.
49. Poirier J, Barbizet J, Gaston A, Merignac C. Démence thalamique. Lacunes expansives du territoire mésencéphalique paramédian. Hydrocéphalie par sténose de l'acqueduc de Sylvius Rev Neurol (Paris) 1983; 139:349–358.
50. Vital C, Julien J. Widespread dilatation of perivascular spaces: a leukoencephalopathy causing dementia Neurology, 1997; 48:1310–1313.
51. Benhaïem-Sigaux N, Gray F, Gherardi R, Roucayrol AM, Poirier J. Expanding cerebellar lacunes due to dilatation of the perivascular space associated with Binswanger's subcortical arteriosclerotic encephalopathy. Stroke 1987; 18:1087–1092.
52. Roman GC. From UBOs to Binswanger's disease. Impact of magnetic resonance imaging on vascular dementia research Stroke 1996; 27:1269–1273.
53. Braffman BH, Zimmerman RA, Trojanowski JQ, Konatas NK, Hickey WF, Schlaepfer WW. Brain MR: pathologic correlation with gross and histopathology. 1. Lacunar infarction and Virchow-Robin spaces. AJR Am J Roentgenol 1988; 151: 151–558.
54. Esiri M. Wilcock G, Morris J. Neuropathological assessment of the lesion of significance in vascular dementia. J Neurol Neurosurg Psychiatry 1997; 63:749–753.
55. Molaie M, Collins GH. Systemic non inflammatory vasculopathy with prominent CNS involvement. A case report. Angiology 1987; 38:686–695.
56. Babikian V, Ropper A. Binwanger's disease: a review. Stroke 1987; 18:2–12.
57. Caplan LR, Schoene WC. Clinical features of subcortical arteriosclerotic encephalopathy (Binswanger's disease). Neurology (Minneapolis) 1978; 28:1206–1215.
58. Garcin R, Lapresle J, Lyon G.: Encéphalopathie sous-corticale chronique de Binswanger. Etude anatomo-clinique de trois observations. Rev Neurol. 1960; 102:423–440.

59. Mikol J. Maladie de Binswanger et formes apparentées. Rev Neurol. 1968; 118:111–132.
60. Rosenberg GA, MK. Stovring, J, Bicknell JM. Subcortical arteriosclerotic encephalopathy (Binswanger): computerized tomography. Neurology (Minneapolis) 1979; 29: 1102–1106.
61. Ali Cherif A, Labrecque R, Pellissier JF, Ponset M, Boudouresques J. Encephalopathie sous-corticale de Binswanger. Rev Neurol. 1979; 135: 665–678.
62. Dupuis M, Brucher JM, Gonsette RE. Observation anatomo-clinique d'une encéphalopathie souscorticale artériosclereuse (maladie de Binswanger) avec hypodensité de la substance blanche au scanner cérébral. Acta Neurol Belg. 1984; 84: 131–140.
63. Okeda R. Correlative morphometric studies of cerebral arteries in Binswanger's encephalopathy and hypertensive encephalopathy. Acta Neuropath (Berl) 1973; 26:23–43.
64. Zhang WW, Olsson Y. The angiopathy of subcortical arteriosclerotic encephalopathy (Binswanger's disease): immunohistochemical studies using markers for components of extracellular matrix, smooth muscle actin and endothelial cells. Acta Neuropathol (Berl) 1997; 93:219–224.
65. Mayer SA, Tatemichi TK, Hair LS, Goldman JE, Camac A, Mohr JP. Hemineglect and seizures in Binswanger's disease: clinical-pathological report. J Neurol Neurosurg Psychiatry 1993; 56: 816–819.
66. Akiguchi I, Tomimoto H, Kinoshita M, Wakita H, Osaki A, Nishimura M, Kimura J. Effects of antithrombin on Binswanger's disease with antiphospholipid antibody syndrome. Neurology 1999; 52:398–401.
67. Caplan L.: Binswanger's disease-revisited. Neurology 1995; 45:626–633.
68. Davis PC, Mirra SS, Alazraki N. The brain in older persons with and without dementia: findings on MR PET, and SPECT images. AJR Am J Roentgenol 1994; 162:1267–1278.
69. Tomonaga M, Yamanouchi H, Toghi H, Kameyama M. Clinicopathological study of progressive vascular encephalopathy (Binswanger type) in the elderly. J Am Geriatr Soc 1982; 30:524–529.
70. Braffman BH, Zimmerman RA, Trojanowski JQ, Gonatas NK, Hickey WF, Schlaepper WW. Brain MR: pathologic correlation with gross and histophatology. 2 Hyperintense white-matter foci in the elderly. AJR Am J Roentgenol 1988; 151:559–566.
71. Erkinjuntti T. Types of multi-infarct dementia. Acta Neurol Scand 1987; 75:391–399.
72. Kowalski H, George AE, De Leon MJ, Mourino M, La Regina ME, Miler JD, Stylopoulos CA, Klinger A. Regional cerebral MRI T2 values. Effects of normal aging. Neurology (Minneapolis) 1988; 38 (suppl 1): 371.
73. Ferszt R, Bradac GB, Nassel F. Value of MRI in Diagnosing Alzheimer Versus Vascular Dementia. In: Cervos-Navarro J, Ferszt R, eds. Stroke and microcirculation. New York: Raven Press, 1987: 513–517.
74. Morgello S, Farrar JT, Heier LA. Periventricular hyperintense lesions on magnetic resonance scans. Neurology (Minneapolis) 1988; 38 (suppl 1): 139.
75. Grafton ST, Sumi SM, Stimac GK, Alvord EC Jr, Shaw CM, Nochlin D. Comparison of postmortem magnetic resonance imaging and neuropathologic findings in the cerebral white matter. Arch Neurol 1991; 48:293–298.
76. Awad IA, Spetzler RF, Hodak JA, Awad CA, Carey R. Incidental subcortical lesions identified on magnetic resonance imaging in the elderly. Correlation with age and cerebrovascular risk factors. Stroke 1986; 17:1084–1089.
77. Dubas F, Gray F, Roullet E, Escourolle R. Leucoencephalopathies artériopathiques. (17 cas anatomocliniques). Rev Neurol 1985; 141: 93–108.
78. Akiguchi I, Tomimoto H, Suenaga T, Wakita H, Budka H. Blood-brain barrier dysfunction in Binswanger's disease; an immunohistochemical study. Acta Neuropathol (Berl) 1998; 95:78–84.
79. De Reuck J, Vander Eecken HM. Periventricular leukomalacia in adults. Clinico-pathological study of four cases. Arch Neurol 1978; 35:517–521.
80. De Reuck J, Crevito L, De Coster W, Sieben G, Vander Eecken H. Pathogenesis of Binswanger chronic progressive subcortical encephalopathy. Neurology (Minneapolis) 1980; 30:920–928.
81. Pantoni L, Garcia JH. The significance of cerebral white matter abnormalities 100 years after Binswanger's report. A review. Stroke 1995; 26:1293–1301.
82. Schneider R, Ringelstein EB, Zeumer H, Kiesewetter H, Jung F. The role of plasma hyperviscosity in subcortical arteriosclerotic encephalopathy-Binswangers' disease. J Neurol 1987; 234:67–73.
83. Zhan SS, Beyreuther K, Schmitt HP. Synaptophysin immunoreactivity of the cortical neuropil in vascular dementia of Binswanger type compared with the dementia of Alzheimer type and nondemented controls. Dementia 1994; 5:79–87.
84. Akiguchi I, Tomimoto H, Suenaga T, Wakita H, Budka H. Alterations in glia and axons in the brains of Binswanger's disease patients. Stroke 1997; 28: 1423–1429.
85. Alonzo NC, Hyman BT, Rebeck GW, Greenberg SM. Progression of cerebral amyloid angiopathy: accumulation of amyloid-beta40 in affected vessels. J Neuropathol Exp Neurol 1998; 57:353–359.
86. Gray F, Dubas F, Roullet E, Escourolle R. Leukoencephalopathy in diffuse hemorrhagic cerebral amyloid angiopathy. Ann Neurol 1985; 18:54–59.
87. Yoshimura M, Yamanouchi H, Kuzuhara S, Mori H, Sugiura S, Mizutani T, Shimada H, Tomonaga M, Toyokura Y. Dementia in cerebral amyloid angiopathy: a clinicopathological study. J Neurol 1992; 239:441–450.
88. Greenberg SM, Vonsattel JP, Stakes, JW, Gruber M, Finklestein SP. The clinical spectrum of cerebral amyloid angiopathy: presentations without lobar hemorrhage. Neurology 1993; 43:2073–2079.
89. Bogucki A, Janczewska E, Koszewska I, Chmielowski M, Szymanska R. Evaluation of dementia in subcortical arteriosclerotic encephalopathy (Binswanger's disease). Eur Arch Psychiatry Clin Neurosci 1991; 241:91–97.
90. Sourander P, Walinder J. Hereditary multi-infarct dementia. Morphological and clinical studies of a new disease. Acta Neuropath (Berl) 1977; 39:247–254.
91. Tournier-Lasserve E, Joutel A, Melki J, Weissenbach J, Lathrop GM, Chabriat H, Mass JL, Cabanis EA, Baudrimont M, Maciazek J, Bach MA, Bousser MG. Cerebral autosomal dominant arteriopathy with subcortical infarcts and leukoencephalopathy maps to chromosome 19q12. Nat Genet 1993; 3:256–259.

92. Joutel A, Corpechot C, Ducros A, Vahedi K, Chabriat H, Mouton P, Alamowitch S, Domenga V, Cecillion M, Marechal E, Maciazek J, Vayssiere C, Cruaud C, Cabanis EA, Ruchoux MM, Weissenbach J, Bach JF, Bousser MG, Tournier-Lasserve E. Notch3 mutations in CADASIL, a hereditary adult-onset condition causing stroke and dementia. Nature 1996; 383:707–710.
93. Dichgans M, Mayer M, Uttner I, Bruning R, Muller-Höcker J, Rungger G, Ebke M, Klockgether T, Gasser T. The phenotypic spectrum of CADASIL: clinical findings in 102 cases. Ann Neurol 1998; 44:731–739.
94. Davous P. CADASIL: a review with proposed diagnostic criteria. Eur J Neurol 1998; 5:219–233.
95. Chabriat H, Vahedi K, Iba-Zizen MT, Joutel A, Nibbio A, Nagy T, Krebs MO. Clinical spectrum of CADASIL: a study of 7 families. Cerebral autosomal dominant arteriopathy with subcortical infarcts and leukoencephalopathy. Lancet 1995; 346:934–939.
96. Baudrimont M, Dubas F, Joutel A., Tournier-Lasserve E, Bousser MG. Autosomal dominant leukoencephalopathy and subcortical ischemic stroke. A clinicopathological study. Stroke 1993; 24:122–125.
97. Ruchoux MM, Guerouaou D, Vandenhaute B, Pruvo JP, Vermersch P, Leys D. Systemic vascular smooth muscle cell impairment in cerebral autosomal dominant arteriopathy with subcortical infarcts and leukoencephalopathy. Acta Neuropathol (Berl) 1995; 89:500–512.
98. Glusker P, Horoupian DS, Lane B. Familial arteriopathic leukoencephalopathy; imaging and neuropathologic findings. AJNR Am J Neuroradiol 1998; 19:469–475.
99. Nishio T, Arima K, Eto K, Ogawa M, Sunohara N. Cerebral autosomal dominant arteriopathy with subcortical infarcts and leukoencephalopathy-report of an autopsied Japanese case [in Japanese] Rinsho Shinkeigaku 1997; 37:910–916.
100. Goldman-Rakic PS. Circuitry of the frontal association cortex and its relevance to dementia. Arch. Gerontol Geriatr 1987; 6:299–309.
101. Adair JC, Hart BL, Kornfeld, M, Graham GD, Swanda RP, Ptacek LJ, Davis LE. Autosomal dominant cerebral arteriopathy: neuropsychiatric syndrome in a family. Neuropsychiatry Neuropsychol Behav Neurol 1998; 11:31–39.
102. Desmond DW, Moroney JT, Lynch T, Chan S, Chin SS, Shungu DC, Naini AB, Mohr JP. CADASIL in a North American family: clinical, pathologic, and radiologic findings. Neurology 1998; 51:844–849.
103. Estes ML, Chimowitz MI, Awad IA, Mc Mahon JT, Furlan AJ, Ratliff NB. Sclerosing vasculopathy of the central nervous system in nonelderly demented patients. Arch Neurol 1991; 48:631–636.
104. Lammie GA, Rakshi J, Rossor MN, Harding AE, Scaravilli F. Cerebral autosomal dominant arteriopathy with subcortical infarcts and leukoencephalopathy (CADASIL)—confirmation by cerebral biopsy in 2 cases. Clin Neuropathol 1995; 14:201–206.
105. Sabbadini G, Francia A, Calandriello L, Di Biasi C, Trasimeni G, Gualdi GF, Palladini G, Manfredi M, Frontali M. Cerebral autosomal dominant arteriopathy with subcortical infarcts and leucoencephalopathy (CADASIL). Clinical, neuroimaging, pathological and genetic study of a large Italian family. Brain 1995; 118:207–215.
106. Schroder JM, Sellhaus B, Jorg J. Identification of the characteristic vascular changes in a sural nerve biopsy of a case with cerebral autosomal dominant arteriopathy with subcortical infarcts and leukoencephalopathy (CADASIL). Acta Neuropathol (Berl) 1995; 89: 116–121.
107. Ruchoux MM, Maurage CA. Endothelial changes in muscle and skin biopsies in patients with CADASIL. Neuropathol Appl Neurobiol 1998; 24:60–65.
108. Ruchoux MM, Maurage CA. CADASIL: Cerebral autosomal-dominant arteriopathy with subcortical infarcts and leukoencephalopathy. J Neuropathol Exp Neurol 1997; 56:947–964.
108a. Joutel A, Andreux F, Gaulis S, Domenga V, Cecillon M, Battail N, Piga F, Chapon F, Godfrain C, Tournier-Lasserve E. The ectodomain of Notch3 receptor accumulates within the cerebrovasculature of CADASIL patients. J Clin Invest 2000; 105:597–605.
109. Gray F, Robert F, Labrecque R, Chretien F, Baudrimont M, Fallet-Bianco C, Mikol J, Vinters HV. Autosomal dominant arteriopathic leuko-encephalopathy and Alzheimer's disease. Neuropathol Appl Neurobiol 1994; 20:22–30.
110. Jen J, Cohen AH, Yue Q, Stout JT, Vinters HV, Nelson S, Baloh RW. Hereditary endotheliopathy with retinopathy, nephropathy, and stroke (HERNS). Neurology 1997; 49:1322–1330.
111. Grand MG, Kaine J, Fulling K, Atkinson J, Dowton SB, Farber M, Craver J, Rice K. Cerebroretinal vasculopathy. A new hereditary syndrome. Ophthalmology 1988; 95:649–659.
112. Gutmann DH, Fischbeck KH, Sergott RC. Hereditary retinal vasculopathy with cerebral white matter lesions. Am J Med Genet 1989; 34:217–220.
113. Yamamura T, Nishimura M, Shirabe T, Fugita M. Subcortical vascular encephalopathy in a normotensive, young adult with premature baldness and spondylitis deformans. A clinopathological study and review of the literature. J Neurol Sci 1987; 78:175–188.
113a. Fukutake T. Young-adult-onset hereditary subcortical vascular dementia: cerebral autosomal recessive arteriosclerosis with subcortical infarcts and leukoencephalopathy (CARASIL) [in Japanese]. Rinsho Shinkeigaku 1999; 39:50–52.
114. Dide H, Botcazo M. Amnésie continue, cécité verbale pure, perte du sens topographique, ramollissement double du lobe lingual. Rev Neurol 1902; 10: 676–680.
115. Boudin G, Barbizet J, Derouesné C, Amerongen P van. Cécité corticale et problème des "amnésies occipitales". Rev Neurol 1967; 116: 89–97.
116. Glees P, Griffith HG. Bilateral destruction of hippocampus (Cornu Ammonis) in a case of dementia. Monatschr Psychiatr Neurol 1952; 123:193–204.
117. Victor M, Angevine JB, Mancall EJ, Fischer CM. Memory loss with lesions of hippocampal formation. Report of a case with some remarks on the anatomical basis of memory. Arch Neurol 1965; 5:244–263.
118. Grunthal E. Ueber das Klinische Bild nach umschriebenem beiderseitigem Ausfall der Ammonshornrinde ein beitrag zur Kentniss der funktion des ammonshorns. Monatschr Psychiatr Neurol 1947; 113:1–16.

119. Brion S, Mikol J, Plas J. Neuropathologie des syndromes amnésiques chez l'homme. Rev Neurol 1985; 141:627–643.
120. Delay J, Brion S, Escourolle R, Marques JM. Démences artériopathiques Lésions du système hippocampomamillo-thalamique dans le déterminisme des troubles mnésiques. Rev Neurol 1961; 105: 22–33.
121. Horel JA. The neuro-anatomy of amnesia. A critique of the hippocampal memory hypothesis. Brain 1978; 101:403–445.
122. Squire LR. Memory and Brain. New York: Oxford University Press, 1987.
123. Delay J, Brion S. Le Syndrome de Korsakoff. Paris: Masson, 1969.
124. Cramon DY, Von Hebel N, Schuri U. A contribution to the anatomical basis of thalamic amnesia. Brain 1985; 108:993–1008.
125. Gloor P. The temporal lobe and limbic system. New York: Oxford University Press, 1997.
126. Bogaert LV, Martin L, Martin JJ. Sclérose latérale amyotrophique avec dégénérescence spino-cérébelleuse et délire épileptique. Contribution à l'étude des formes de passage des atrophies systématisées et des relations éventuelles entre l'état psychique et certaines atrophies thalamiques médianes. Acta Neurol Belg 1965; 65:845–872.
127. Castaigne P, Lhermitte F, Buge A, Escourolle R, Hauw JJ, Lyon-Caen O. Paramedian thalamic and midbrain infarcts clinical and neuropathological study. Ann Neurol 1981; 10: 127–148.
128. Bogousslavsky J, Regli F, Uske A. Thalamic infarcts: clinical syndromes, etiology, and prognosis Neurology 1988; 38:837–848.
129. Buge A., Escourolle R, Rancurel G, Poisson M. "Mutisme akinétique" et ramollissement bicingulaire. Trois observations anatomo-cliniques. Rev Neurol 1975; 131: 121–137.
130. Escourolle R, Gray F. Les accidents vasculaires du système limbique. In: Környey S, Tariska S, Gosztonyi G, eds. Proceedings of the VIIth International Congress of Neuropathology. Amsterdam: Excepta Medica, 1975: 195–202.
131. Brion S, Derome P, Guiot G, Teitgen J. Syndrome de Korsakoff par anévrysme de l'artère communicante antérieure; le probléme des syndromes de Korsakoff par hémorragie méningée. Rev Neurol 1968; 118: 293–299.
132. Brion S, Pragier G, Guerin R, Teitgen J. Syndrome de Korsakoff par ramollissement bilatéral du fornix. Le probléme des syndromes amnésiques par lésion vasculaire unilatérale. Rev Neurol 1969; 120:255–262.
133. Dide M, Pezet C. Syndrome occipital avec dyspraxie complète surajoutée. Bull Soc Clin Med Med 1913; 6:279–291.
134. Schenk V. Unilateral atrophy of the fornix. In: Biemond A, ed. Recent Findings in Neurological Sciences. The Hague: Elsevier 1959: 168–179.
135. Boudin G, Brion S, Pépin B, Barbizet J. Syndrome de Korsakoff d'étiologie artériopathique par lésion bilatérale asymétrique du systéme limbique. Rev Neurol 1968; 119:341–348.
136. Geschwind N, Fusillo M. Color naming defects association with alexia. Arch Neurol 1966; 15: 137–146.
137. Mikol J, Brion S, Derome P, De Pommery J, Gallissot MC. Connections of the latero-dorsal nucleus of the thalamus. II Experimental studies in Papio-Papio. Brain Res 1977; 138:1–16.
138. Mikol J, Menini M, Brion S, Guicharnaud L. Connexions du noyau latéro-dorsal du thalamus chez le singe. III Etude de ses efferences. Rev Neurol 1984; 140: 615–624.
139. Tatemichi TK, Desmond DW, Prohovnik I, Cross DROIT, Gropen TI, Mohr JP, Stern Y. Confusion and memory loss from capsular genu infarction: a thalamocortical disconnection syndrome? Neurology 1992; 42: 1966–1979.
140. Brion S, Chevalier JF, Guériot-Colasse C. Syndromes pseudo-démentiels par lésions de la partie postérieure de l'hémisphère mineur. In: Billé J, ed. L'actualité en Gérontologie. IVe Congrés de Neuro-Gériatrie et Géronto-Psychiatrie. Paris: Sandoz, 1980: 70–76.
141. Coull BM. Multiple cerebral infarctions and dementia associated with anticardiolipin antibodies. Stroke 1987; 18: 1107–1112.
142. Stary HC, Chandler AB, Dinsmore RE, Glagov S, Guyton JR, Insull W Jr, Rosenfeld ME, Shaffer SA, Schwartz CJ, Wagner WD, Wissler RW. A definition of advanced types of atherosclerotic lesions and a histological classification of atherosclerosis. A report from the Committee on Vascular Lesions of the Council on Arteriosclerosis, American Heart Association. Circulation 1995; 92: 1355–1374.
143. Lie JT. Primary (granulomatous) angiitis of the central nervous system: a clinicopathologic analysis of 15 new cases and a review of the literature. Human Pathol 1992; 23: 164–171.
144. Moore PM, Richardson B. Neurology of the vasculitides and connective tissue diseases. J Neurol Neurosurg Psychiatry 1998; 65: 10–22.
145. Chu CT, Gray L, Goldstein LB, Hulette CM. Diagnosis of intracranial vasculitis: a multi-disciplinary approach. J Neuropathol Exp Neurol 1998; 57: 30–38.
146. Caselli RJ, Hunder GG, Whisnant JP. Neurologic disease in biopsy proven giant cell (temporal) arteritis. Neurology (Minneapolis) 1988; 38: 352–359.
147. Inafuku T, Watanabe M, Takagi M, Hoshino H, Morinaga S, Koto A. Giant cell arteritis with bilateral obstruction of the internal carotid artery-report of an autopsy case [In Japanese]. Rinsho Shinkeigaku 1998; 38: 323–328.
148. Ellis SG, Verity MA. Central nervous system involvement in systemic lupus erythematosus. Semin Arthritis Rheum 1979; 8: 212–221.
149. Rebollo M, Val JF, Garijo F, Quintana F, Berciano J. Livedo reticularis and cerebrovascular lesions (Sneddon's syndrome). Clinical, radiological and pathological features in eight cases. Brain 1983; 106: 965–979.
150. Tourbah A, Piette JC, Iba-Zizen MT, Lyon-Caen O, Godeau P, Frances C. The natural course of cerebral lesions in Sneddon syndrome. Arch Neurol 1997; 54: 53–60.
151. Geschwind DH, FitzPatrick M, Mischel PS, Cummings JL. Sneddon's syndrome is a thrombotic vasculopathy: neuropathologic and neuroradiologic evidence. Neurology 1995; 45: 557–560.
152. Lossos A, Ben-Hur T, Ben-Nariah Z, Enk C, Gomori

153. M, Soffer D. Familial Sneddon's syndrome. J Neurol 1995; 242: 164–168.
154. Treves TA, Gadoth N, Blumen S, Korczyn AD. Intravascular malignant lymphomatosis: a cause of subacute dementia. Dementia 1995; 6: 286–293.
155. Lach B. Maternally inherited mitochondrial encephalomyopathy. A vasculopathy (abstract). Muscle Nerve 1986; 9: 13–33.
156. Ohama E, Ohara S, Ikuta F, Tanaka K, Nishizawa M, Miyatake T. Mitochondrial angiopathy in cerebral blood vessels of mitochondrial encephalomyopathy. Acta Neuropathol (Berl) 1987; 74: 226–233.
157. Zeviani M, Tiranti V, Piantadosi C. Mitochondrial disorders. Medicine (Baltimore) 1998; 77: 59–72.
158. Mendez MF, Stanley TM, Medel NM, Li Z, Tedesco DT. The vascular dementia of Fabry's disease. Dement Geriatr Cogn Disord 1997; 8: 252–257.
159. Mitsias P, Levine SR. Cerebrovascular complications of Fabry's disease. Ann Neurol 1996; 40:8–17.
160. Arne L, Guérin A, Julien J, Vital C. Sur un cas de leucoencéphalopathie subaiguë chez une malade ayant présenté une thrombophlébite des membres inférieurs. Rev Neurol 1965; 112:560–562.
161. Datta NN, Rehman SU, Kwok JC, Chan KY, Poon CY. Reversible dementia due to dural arteriovenous fistula: a simple surgical option. Neurosurg Rev 1998; 21: 174–176.
162. Hurst RW, Bagley LJ, Galetta, S, Glosser G, Lieberman AP, Trojanovski J, Sinson G, Stecker M, Zager E, Raps EC, Flamm ES. Dementia resulting from dural arteriovenous fistulas: the pathologic findings of venous hypertensive encephalopathy. AJNR Am J Neuroradiol 1998; 19: 1267–1273.
163. Jaillard A, Peres B, Hommel M. Neuropsychological features of dementia due to dural arteriovenous malformation. Cerebrovasc Dis 1999; 9: 91–97.
164. Premkumar DR, Cohen DL, Hedera P, Friedland RP, Kalaria RN. Apolipoprotein E-epsilon4 alleles in cerebral amyloid angiopathy and cerebrovascular pathology associated with Alzheimer's disease. Am J Pathol 1996; 148: 2083–2095.
165. Bennett DA, Wilson RS, Gilley DW, Fox JH. Clinical diagnosis of Binswanger's disease. J Neurol Neurosurg Psychiatry 1990; 53:961–965.
166. Brun A, Englund E. A white matter disorder in dementia of the Alzheimer type: a pathoanatomical study. Ann Neurol 1986; 19:253–262.
167. Zekry D, Duyckaerts C, Belmin J, Geoffre C, Vlaicu M, Sazdovithch V, Moulias R, Hauw JJ. Vascular, degenerative and mixed dementia. A clinicopathological study in 33 cases. Brain Pathol 1997; 7: 1213.
168. Olichney JM, Hansen LA, Hofstetter CR, Greendman M, Katzman R, Thal LJ. Cerebral infarction in Alzheimer's disease is associated with severe amyloid angiopathy and hypertension. Arch Neurol 1995; 52: 702–768.
169. Loeb C: Dementia due to lacunar infarctions: a misnomer or a clinical entity? Eur Neurol 1995; 35: 187–192.

6. Basic Mechanisms of Neurodegeneration in Dementia

SUZANNE M. DE LA MONTE AND J.C. DE LA TORRE

Dementia in Alzheimer's disease (AD) is ultimately mediated by cell loss, which studies have demonstrated occurs by several mechanisms including, apoptosis, impaired mitochondrial function, and possibly necrosis. Apoptosis is detectable in neurons, glial cells, cerebrovascular smooth muscle cells, and endothelial cells, indicating that either multiple cell types are adversely affected by neurodegeneration, or the loss of several cell types contributes to the overall disease process. A second major neuroanatomic correlate of dementia in AD is aberrant cortical neuritic sprouting with abundant proliferation of dystrophic neurites that are immunoreactive for phosphorylated neuronal cytoskeletal proteins, as well as other molecules such as growth-associated synaptic molecules and nitric oxide synthase-3. Whether the neuritic pathology represents a primary degenerative lesion, a secondary response to cell loss, or a combination of both, remains to be determined. There is growing evidence that AD, Pick's disease, Parkinson's disease, progressive supranuclear palsy, amyotrophic lateral sclerosis, and diffuse Lewy body disease share common features of neurodegeneration including the accumulation of intraneuronal filamentous inclusions, increased cell loss mediated in part by apoptosis, and increased neuritic sprouting. Within the last several years, extensive research aimed at determining the mechanisms of neuronal cell death has revealed important differences between aging and neurodegeneration of the CNS, with one of the critical distinctions being that brains with neurodegeneration exhibit heightened sensitivity to oxidative stress and free radical injury. Although genetic factors such as mutations in the presenilin or amyloid precursor protein genes, and the homozygous Apolipoprotein E_4 genotype predispose individuals to AD, sporadic (non-genetic) AD, which accounts for the vast majority of cases, is often associated with dysregulated expression genes that render the brain cells more susceptible to oxidative injury. For example, the aberrant gene expression of genes that encode superoxide dismutase I (SOD-1), nitric oxide synthase 3 (NOS-3), heme oxygenase-1, could lead to increased generation of free radicals and reduced CNS cellular resistance to oxidative stress, cytotoxic agents, and pro-apoptosis mechanisms. However, the progression of AD neurodegeneration has been linked to a variety of chronic disturbances in CNS function caused by impaired energy metabolism, cerebral hypoperfusion, amyloid-β toxicity, accumulation of non-amyloid-β precursor protein (α-synuclein), impaired calcium homeostasis, activation of pro-inflammatory cytokines, and impaired mitochondrial function due to mitochondrial DNA damage. Similar schemes are likely involved in other neurodegenerative diseases, including Parkinson's disease, amyotrophic lateral sclerosis, diffuse Lewy body disease, and Pick's disease. Therefore, a "multiple-hit" hypothesis could explain the development and progression of AD as well as other neurodegenerative diseases in the context of both aging and the aberrant expression of genes that promote oxidative stress within the CNS. The exciting conclusion drawn from this extensive review is that many of the factors likely to contribute to the progression of neurodegeneration are either preventable or treatable, suggesting that effective therapeutic measures could be developed to realistically reduce the incidence and prevalence of AD and other neurodegenerative diseases.

NEUROANATOMICAL SUBSTRATE FOR DEMENTIA AND IMPAIRED CENTRAL NERVOUS SYSTEM (CNS) FUNCTION WITH NEURODEGENERATION

Neuropathology of Alzheimer's Disease

Alzheimer's disease is associated with progressive cognitive impairment, memory loss, personality disorder, and behavioral disturbances. As the disease progresses, loss of function becomes more generalized and ultimately renders the subject vegetative and totally dependent upon external support. From the time of the initial case description by Alois Alzheimer, cerebral atrophy was a recognized feature of AD. Corresponding with the behavioral, personality, and cognitive dysfunction detected early in the course of disease, in vivo magnetic resonance imaging (MRI) studies combined with morphometric analysis studies have demonstrated initial atrophy of temporal lobe structures.[1-4] However, with progressive loss of function, the cerebral atrophy worsens and extends beyond corticolimbic structures and pathways. Postmortem cases with advanced or end-stage clinical dementia exhibit generalized cerebral atrophy with 25% to 40% reductions in cortical volume.[5-7] Similar reductions in tissue mass also occur in cerebral white matter[5,6] indicating that severe fiber loss is another important component of the disease.

The characteristic neuropathological abnormalities in AD include abundant neurofibrillary tangles, dystrophic neurites, senile plaques, and amyloid- deposition in the brain. The prominent localization of AD neurodegenerative lesions in corticolimbic structures accounts for some of the early clinical manifestations of disease.[8,9] Cognitive impairment in AD is correlated with neuronal loss, synaptic disconnection, and increased densities of filamentous lesions consisting of neurofibrillary tangles, dystrophic neurites, neuropil threads, and neuritic plaques. Filamentous neurodegenerative lesions are marked by accumulations of paired-helical and straight filaments[9] consisting of highly insoluble[10] 10-20 nm fibrils[11,12] that are largely composed of hyperphosphorylated tau, other cytoskeletal proteins, and ubiquitin.[13-17] Since paired helical and straight filaments can be generated in vitro from recombinant phospho-tau,[18] aberrant hyperphosphorylation of tau may have a critical role in the pathogenesis of cytoskeletal lesions associated with AD-type neurodegeneration.

Recent studies have focused on the potential role of mutations in the tau gene as a mechanism of neurodegeneration.[19,20] However, such "taupathies" are relatively rare compared with most cases of AD and other neurodegenerative diseases that exhibit sporadic occurrences. An alternative and highly attractive hypothesis is that perturbation of the regulatory mechanisms involved in tau phosphorylation, e.g., kinase and phosphatase activities, results in hyperphosphorylation, polymerization, and intraneuronal accumulation of tau. The constitutive activity levels of several kinases known to phosphorylate tau, including glycogen synthase kinase-3,[21,22] mitogen activated protein (MAP) kinase,[23,24] cyclin-dependent kinase-5[25-27] are currently under intense investigation in relation to AD and other neurodegenerative diseases.

Alzheimer-Type Neurodegeneration in Down Syndrome

Virtually all individuals with Down Syndrome (DS) who survive beyond 35 years of age exhibit neuropathological changes that closely resemble AD[28-31] and a small subset develops progressive dementia with clinical symptoms of AD.[32,33] Down syndrome is caused by overexpression of genes residing at the 21q22 segment, known as the Down locus. Several genes important for CNS function and linked to the development of AD-type neurodegeneration have been mapped to the Down locus, including those encoding the amyloid precursor protein (APP), protein S-100β, and Cu-Zn superoxide dismutase (SOD-1). Overexpression of the APP gene probably accounts for the early and abundant accumulation of amyloid-β in cells, senile plaques, and vessels in the brains of individuals with DS. Overexpression of S-100β occurs in hypertrophic astrocytes in DS brains. Since S-100β can induce neuritic growth, overexpression of the gene may contribute to the excessive proliferation of cortical neuropil neurites detectable beginning in the second decade of life. Finally, SOD-1 overexpression could cause excessive generation of free radicals and attendant production of hydrogen peroxide, thereby enhancing cellular susceptibility to oxidative stress. The nearly 50% higher levels of SOD-1 activity in DS than in control brains may be a critical factor governing accelerated aging and premature development of AD-type neurodegeneration.

Neuropathology of Non-Alzheimer's Disease Neurodegenerative Diseases

Like AD, other major neurodegenerative diseases, such as Pick's disease (PkD), Parkinson's disease (PD), progressive supranuclear palsy (PSP), amyotrophic lateral sclerosis (ALS), and diffuse Lewy body disease (DLBD), are characterized by neuronal loss and intraneuronal accumulations of insoluble fibrillar deposits derived from hyperphosphorylated tau, other cytoskeletal proteins, and ubiquitin.[8,34–36] However, these clinically distinct diseases are distinguished neuropathologically by the preferential cell loss and neurodegeneration involving particular structures within the CNS. In PkD, the targets of neurodegeneration include the frontal and temporal lobes, caudate nucleus, subthalamic nucleus, globus pallidus, thalamus, and substantia nigra. In DLBD, structures typically marred by neurodegeneration include monoaminergic and cholinergic neurons of the brain stem, basal forebrain, and diencephalon, the amygdala, globus pallidus, and corticolimbic structures and pathways. In PD, the neuropathology involves primarily the zona compacta of the substantia nigra, locus coeruleus, dorsal nucleus of the vagus, pedunuculopontine nucleus, thalamus, ventral tegmentum, basal ganglia, basal forebrain, and hypothalamus, but it can extend beyond these structures and overlap with AD or DLBD. In motor neuron disease due to ALS, neurodegeneration occurs mainly in the frontal cortex, hypoglossal nucleus, and ventral horn cells of the spinal cord, and the neuronal loss is accompanied by white matter gliosis and tract degeneration. However, neurodegeneration in ALS can also involve the striatum, thalamus, globus pallidus, subthalamic nucleus, or substantia nigra. The neuropathology of PSP mainly involves the basal ganglia, subthalamic nucleus, substantia nigra, red nucleus, brain stem tegmentum, superior colliculi, vestibular nuclei, and periaqueductal gray. Multiple systems atrophy (MSA) manifests heterogeneous pathology with prominent involvement of the globus pallidus, putamen, caudate nucleus, substantia nigra, pontine nuclei, inferior olives, dorsal nucleus of the vagus, and Purkinje cells in the cerebellum. Importantly, overlapping neurodegeneration with AD plus PD, ALS, or DLBD[8] contributes to the heterogeneous manifestations of disease.

CELL DEATH PATHWAYS IN NEURODEGENERATIVE DISEASES

Cell death occurs either by necrosis, apoptosis, or irreversible impairment of mitochondrial function. Apoptosis, or programmed cell death, involves a stereotyped cascade of altered gene expression and intracellular signaling that results in loss of cell volume, plasma membrane blebbing, and nuclear condensation, culminating in nucleosomal DNA fragmentation laddering.[300] Normal apoptosis is an important mechanism in to maintaining tissue architecture and controlling the number of cells in the body. However, apoptosis can become an important mediator of cell death under pathologic conditions and lead to the death of individual neurons[301] rather than clusters of neurons, which occurs with necrosis. By contrast, necrosis is mediated by massive influx of Ca^{2+} and Na^+ into cells, by loss of mitochondrial ATP, and by free radical formation in the cytosol. Impaired mitochondrial function can be mediated by extensive mitochondrial DNA damage caused by free radical injury. The biochemical events associated with necrosis cause lipid, protein and DNA peroxidation, that can quickly lead to cell swelling and plasma membrane rupture. One way to differentiate necrosis from apoptosis is to examine the uptake of fluorescent or vital dyes across cell membranes. For example, during the initial stages of necrosis, the plasma membrane integrity becomes compromised rendering the cells easily labeled with propidium iodide or trypan blue dyes, while cells in the initial stages of apoptosis do not take up these dyes. However, at later stages of apoptosis, the cell membranes do become leaky and more permeable to such dyes, making it difficult to differentiate them from necrosis. At later stages of cell damage, apoptotic identification can be made with agents such as Hoechst 33342, which stains live cells poorly but fluoresces brightly when taken up by the condensed chromatin found in the late stages of apoptotic cells. Other molecular probes for differentiating necrosis from apoptosis take advantage of the fact that DNA content becomes vulnerable during apoptosis. Special stains can be used to detect the reduced DNA content in cells, following leakage of low-molecular-weight DNA during apoptosis.

Atrophy of CNS structures in AD as well and other neurodegenerative diseases including DS, PkD, PD, DLBD, ALS, PSP, MSA, and Creutzfeldt-Jacob disease is to some degree mediated by apoptosis.[37–44] For example, brains with AD exhibit increased nicking and fragmentation of genomic DNA relative to aged control brains.[37–42] Of note is that apoptosis occurs in neurons as well as glial cells, suggesting that death of both cell types contributes to AD neurodegeneration. Similarly, apoptosis has been demonstrated to be an important mediator of both neuronal and glial cell death in other neurodegenerative disorders, but for each disease, apoptotic cell loss was most pronounced in the structures that were marred by neurodegeneration.[43]

The finding of increased genomic DNA fragmentation with neurodegeneration suggests that other factors and pre-existing conditions may precipitate or enhance cellular susceptibility to apoptosis. In this regard, increased apoptosis in neurodegenerative diseases is associated with up-regulation of pro-apoptotic genes such as *p53*, *CD95*, and *Bax*.[38,43,45–48] Cellular accumulation of pro-apoptotic gene products such as *Bax* and *p53*, or reduced levels of survival-promoting molecules such as Bcl-2[49–54] activate caspases. *Caspases* are a family of cysteine proteases that cleave cytoskeletal and other proteins required for maintenance of cell function. Caspase activation leads to nuclease release and fragmentation of genomic DNA. In AD, apoptosis may be mediated by intracellular signaling through caspases,[55] and in DS, caspase activation is detectable in glial cells years prior to the massive accumulation of AD-type neurodegenerative lesions.[56] Since apoptosis and apoptosis signaling pathways are currently under intense investigation, it is likely that the down-stream pathways that mediate apoptosis in AD may soon be thoroughly characterized. However, the larger and more critical problem is to delineate the upstream abnormalities responsible for activating apoptosis cascades and rendering CNS cells more susceptible to neurodegeneration.

POTENTIAL ROLE OF MITOCHONDRIAL DNA DAMAGE IN RELATION TO CELL LOSS

Although apoptosis is a demonstrated mechanism of cell loss in AD and other neurodegenerative diseases,[38,43,45,57–61] critics point out the lack of specificity of DNA fragmentation as a reliable marker of apoptosis[60] and the relative absence of apoptotic-specific protein to react with DNA-fragmented cells in AD hippocampal neurons.[62] Consequently, the DNA fragmentation found in AD brain neurons could reflect disturbances in the ante-mortem period which are not associated with apoptosis.[63] There is growing evidence that the increased apoptosis detected in postmortem AD brains actually reflects a marked increase in susceptibility to oxidative damage and free radical injury.[62,64–69] In this regard, it is noteworthy that in both familial and sporadic human neurodegenerative diseases, and in the transgenic mouse models of neurodegeneration, aging is the most significant factor correlated with the onset and progression of disease. Recent evidence suggests that aging and a number of prevalent age-associated diseases, including cancer, heart disease, and neurodegeneration, may be precipitated, propagated, or caused by impaired mitochondrial (Mt) function resulting from oxygen free-radical damage and accumulation of MtDNA mutations.[70–74] However, because of the broad impact that such conclusions could have on the strategies used to develop compounds for treating or preventing disease, detailed systematic studies using both human and experimental models are needed to formally prove this theory.

The major intracellular source of oxygen free radicals is the mitochondrial respiratory chain, since it continuously produces superoxide under normal physiological conditions. Metabolic disturbances in mitochondrial function result in electron escape from the electron transport chain, and attendant formation of hydroxyl radicals and hydrogen peroxide from superoxide. Increased oxidative stress causes further free radical damage to mitochondria and MtDNA. Mitochondrial DNA is not protected by histones or DNA-binding proteins. Mitochondrial DNA damage following exposure to high levels of reactive oxygen species and free radicals is mediated by intra-mitochondrial accumulation of 8-oxo-7,8-dihydro-2'-deoxyguanosine (8-OH-dG).[72,73] Incorporation of 8-OH-dG into MtDNA causes base mispairing, random point mutations, and deletions. Importantly, damaged mitochondria can replicate because the enzymes required for mitochondrial replication are encoded by genomic (Gn)DNA. Increased abundance of defective MtDNA that encodes respiratory enzymes may impair electron transport and enhance production of reactive oxygen species, leading to oxidative stress and further damage to mitochondria. The problem is compounded by increased peroxidation of lipids and oxidative modification of proteins by reactive oxygen species and hydrogen peroxide. The exponential age-related accumulations of intramitochondrial 8-OH-dG and mutated MtDNA suggest that the deterioration of organ function attributed to aging may be caused by somatically acquired MtDNA damage and impaired cellular energy production. Increased levels of reactive oxygen species and free radicals could lead to enhanced susceptibility apoptosis. In that context, apoptosis is mediated by opening of the mitochondrial permeability transition pores, cytochrome c release into the cytosol, and activation of caspases that mediate DNA fragmentation and cytoskeletal protein cleavage.

Impaired mitochondrial function and accumulation of MtDNA mutations could reduce cellular tolerance for free radical injury and thereby have a critical role in mediating cell loss in AD and other neurodegenerative diseases. To determine the potential relevance of MtDNA damage to neurodegeneration and cell loss in AD, we quantified the extent of nicking and fragmentation in MtDNA isolated[75] from postmortem AD (N = 20) and aged control (N = 12) temporal lobe samples using an end-labeling assay. The levels of [α-^{32}P]dCTP incorporated into the 3' ends of MtDNA using Klenow DNA polymerase were quantified with a scintillation counter. As shown in Figure 6–1A, the levels of end-labeled nicked or fragmented MtDNA were significantly higher in AD brains than in aged control brains. The increased MtDNA damage was associated with reduced mitochondrial protein content by Western blot analysis (Fig. 6–1B), and reduced mitochondrial protein immunoreactivity in cortical neurons by immunohistochemical staining (Fig. 6–1C, D). Aged control brains exhibited abundant coarse granular staining of neuronal perikarya and neuropil fibers (Fig. 6–1C), whereas brains with AD manifested strikingly reduced levels of mitochondrial immunoreactivity in cortical and hippocampal (CA1 and CA2) neurons and the adjacent neuropil fibers (Fig. 6–1D).

Mitochondrial DNA damage and impaired mitochondrial function can reduce the mitochondrial potential, which in turn could induce opening of a high conductance pore termed "mitochondrial permeability transition" (MPT). MPT causes mitochondrial depolarization and uncoupling of oxidative phosphorylation, reductions in ATP production, and finally cell death due to energy failure.[76,77] For example, oxidative stress can lead to ATP loss and cell necrosis, a likely mechanism of cell loss in AD. On the other hand, the administration of agents such as glutamine, that can raise cellular ATP levels, could be used to protect cells exposed to oxidative stress (78). Alternatively, cell death pathways in AD could be manipulated by targeting apoptosis-induced cell death with caspase inhibitors or the anti-apoptotic protein bcl-2 305. A number

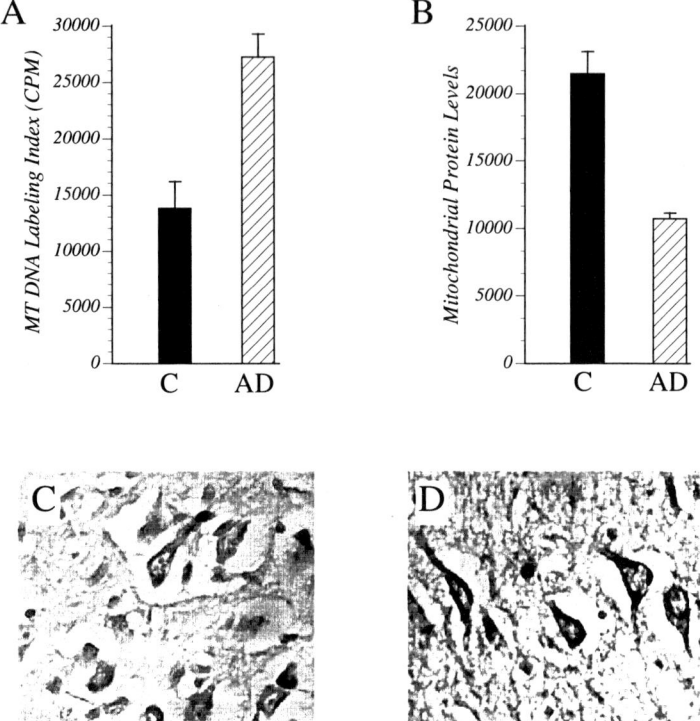

Figure 6–1. Increased mitochondrial DNA fragmentation (A) and reduced levels of mitochondrial protein immunoreactivity (B–D) in Alzheimer Disease (AD N = 20) relative to control (C; N = 12) temporal lobe tissue. A. Mitochondrial DNA was end-labeled with [α^{32}P]dCTP and Klenow DNA polymerase to detect nicking or fragmentation. [α^{32}P]dCTP incorporation was measured with a scintillation counter. The graphed levels reflect mean ± S.D. of cpm/100 ng of DNA. B. Reduced levels of mitochondrial protein in AD temporal lobe tissue measured by Western blot analysis and densitometry. Samples containing 60 μg of protein were subjected to Western blot analysis using monoclonal antibodies to human mitochondrial protein. A single ~65 kD molecule was detected in each sample. The levels of mitochondrial protein were assessed by densitometry, and the graph depicts the mean ± S.D. for AD and control (C) cases. C,D. Reduced levels of mitochondrial protein immunoreactivity in cortical neurons of AD brains (C) relative to control (D). Mitochondrial protein immunoreactivity was detected by immunohistochemical staining with the same antibodies used for Western blot analysis. Immunoreactivity was revealed using a biotinylated secondary antibody, avidin biotin horseradish peroxidase complexes, and TruBlue peroxidase substrate. The granular immunoreactivity represents the positive staining reaction.

of studies have already demonstrated that bcl-2 protein can be used effectively to apoptosis, since bcl-2 enhances the retention of cytochrome c within the mitochondria.[79,80] This pharmaco-molecular approach at targeting apoptosis-induced cell death may eventually prove to be useful since the levels of cytochrome c appear to be reduced in brains with AD.[81,82]

The observations summarized above suggest that MtDNA damage, mitochondrial depletion, and impaired mitochondrial function have important roles in AD neurodegeneration. The mechanism of MtDNA damage is not known, but contributing factors may include aberrant expression of genes that may promote oxidative stress by increasing the generation of reactive oxygen species and free radicals. Abnormalities in gene expression that result in chronic oxidative stress could lead to increased MtDNA damage and impaired mitochondrial function, and thereby have an important role in apoptotic cell loss or enhanced susceptibility to apoptosis in a number of different diseases.

MOLECULAR MECHANISMS OF APOPTOSIS WITH NEURODEGENERATION

There are several candidate genes and molecules that may either contribute to or cause heightened susceptibility to apoptosis in AD and other neurodegenerative diseases including, amyloid-β accumulation, mutated presenilins, and overactivity of SOD-1, NOS-3, or heme oxygenase-1 (HO-1). Although the potential roles of these molecules are discussed mainly in relation to AD, the comments here are likely to be relevant to other neurodegenerative diseases that exhibit intraneuronal accumulations of hyperphosphorylated cytoskeletal proteins and ubiquitin, increased apoptosis, activation of pro-apoptosis genes, and aberrant expression of the NOS 3 or HO-1 gene.

Amyloid-β

One of the characteristic neuropathological features of AD is the abundant accumulation of amyloid-β in the brain. In some autosomal dominant forms of AD, mutations of the amyloid precursor protein (APP) gene cause early and abundant amyloid-β deposition in the brain.[83,84] In the brains of transgenic mice, overexpression of mutant forms of the APP gene as detected in cases of familial AD, causes increased amyloid-β peptide deposition and neuronal cell death.[85–88] In addition, in transfected cells, overexpression of mutant APP increases cellular susceptibility to apoptosis,[89] and results in aberrant APP processing with accumulation of amyloid-β fibrils.[90,91]

A role for amyloid-β accumulation in relation to apoptosis in the brain is further suggested by the associated increased levels of Bax and p53 gene products in cell processes surrounding senile plaques.[38,45,92] Experimentally, amyloid-β has been shown to be neurotoxic,[64,93] to induce pro-apoptosis and inhibit cell survival gene expression,[94] and to activate oxidative stress-related genes.[95] However, amyloid-β- induced cellular degeneration can be rescued or prevented by treatment with antioxidant or free radical scavenger agents.[93] Together, these studies suggest that amyloid-β deposits in the brain may indirectly contribute to cell loss in AD due to activation of pro-apoptosis genes. Potential mechanisms by which amyloid-β peptides may promote apoptosis include (1) activation of pro-apoptosis genes or inhibition of apoptosis-suppressor genes.[94,96] (2) G-protein activation.[89] (3) increased production of superoxides and oxidative free radicals damage;[97–99] (4) synergistic effects with other neurotoxic or excitotoxic agents.[98] (5) disruption of intracellular ion homeostasis; and (6) interaction with mutated presenilin to perturb cellular calcium regulation and promote oxidative stress.[100,101]

Presenilins

Autosomal dominant, familial forms of AD are frequently associated with homozygous nonsense mutations (natural gene knockout) in the presenilin (PS-1, PS-2) genes.[102–104] The functions of presenilin genes are not known, but their widespread expression in normal brains,[105,106] and the increased apoptosis associated with expression of mutated forms of these molecules in transfected cells or brains of transgenic mice,[100,101,107–109] suggest a role for presenilins in cell survival or homeostasis. Presenilin-associated apoptosis has also been linked to increased susceptibility to the cytotoxic effects of amyloid-β peptide, oxidative stress, and trophic factor withdrawal.[100,101,108,109]

Superoxide dismutase I

Apoptosis in AD may be mediated by underlying abnormalities that render CNS cells more susceptible to oxidative stress-mediated apoptosis, since in AD, cell death frequently occurs at a distance from amyloid-β deposits.[37,38,110] The role of oxidative stress and free radical damage as major contributors to cell loss in AD and other neurodegenerative diseases,[111–119] has become a major focus of investigation. Importantly, both overexpression and mutation of the Cu-Zn-superoxide dismutase (SOD-1) gene have been linked to human neurodegenerative diseases, including DS +AD and ALS. Some familial forms of ALS are caused by mutation of the SOD-1 gene,[120,121] and transgenic mice that express mutant SOD-1 as occurs in familial ALS develop motor neuron disease.[122–124]

Superoxide dimutase I is a key enzyme in the metabolism of oxygen free radicals, and increased SOD-1 activity can generate free-radical stress through overproduction of hydrogen peroxide. Brains of individuals with DS exhibit substantially increased levels of SOD-1 activity. Transgenic mice that overexpress the SOD-1 gene in the brain exhibit neurodegeneration with impaired structure of synaptic terminals, proliferation of dystrophic neurites, and neurite retraction as occur in AD.[125,126] Under normal circumstances, increased SOD-1 activity with free radical production in the CNS activates adaptive responses such as increased gutathione peroxidase activity, but in DS, such adaptive responses are often inadequate.[127] In the absence of free radical scavenger agents, cells are rendered more vulnerable to oxidative stress. This phenomenon could account for the early onset of AD-type neurodegeneration, activation of pro-apoptosis genes, and apoptotic cell loss in brains of individuals with DS.[43] In sporadic AD, increased superoxide anion production and free radical generation are detectable in peripheral blood monocytes, although the mechanism does not involve mutation or over expression of the SOD-1 gene.[128]

Nitric Oxide Synthase-3

Nitric oxide synthase-3 (NOS-3)[129] and HO-1[130] represent two genes that are aberrantly expressed in AD, and whose gene products, when present in excess amounts can enhance cellular susceptibility to oxidative stress and freeradical injury. Recently, we demonstrated aberrant expression of NOS-3 in other neurodegenerative diseases including, PkD, PD, PSP, DLBD, ALS, MSA, and DS.[131] In each disease, including AD, aberrant NOS-3 expression and immunoreactivity are distributed mainly in structures that are marred by neurodegeneration and overlap with the distribution of apoptosis.[43,131] Normally, NOS activity generates NO through oxidation of a guanidino nitrogen of L-arginine.[132] However, over-expression of NOS gene(s), markedly increased enzyme activity, and cellular deficiencies in L-arginine, heme, or tetrahydrobiopterin promote the generation of H_2O_2, OH^- and superoxides.[133–136] In the various neurodegenerative diseases studied, high levels of NOS-3 gene expression and immunoreactivity were detected in degenerating and apoptotic neurons and glial cells.[38,43,129,131] suggesting a role for increased NOS activity with neurodegeneration.

Heme Oxygenase-1

Heme oxygenase-1 is an inducible microsomal enzyme that oxidatively cleaves heme, a pro-oxidant, to biliverdin, an antioxidant, and carbon monoxide, a potential neurotransmitter. Reduced HO-1 activity can result in accumulation of heme, whereas increased HO-1 activity can cause increased levels of CO, and possibly excitotoxic death of neurons.[137] Previous studies demonstrated increased levels of HO-1 mRNA and immunoreactivity in AD.[130,138] Since heme is a critical substrate for NO production, excessive oxidative cleavage of heme by HO-1 could encourage the generation of reactive oxygen species in cells with aberrantly high levels of NOS activity. Importantly, HO-1 and NOS expression can be co-localized in the same cells and induced by the same stimuli.[139–141] Therefore, the aberrantly increased expression of both NOS-3[129] and HO-1[130] in AD may contribute to the increased cellular susceptibility to oxidative stress and free radical injury.

NEURITIC PATHOLOGY AND SYNAPTIC DISCONNECTION IN AD

One of the most important correlates of dementia in AD is the extensive loss (approximately 30% or more) of neocortical synapses.[142–150] The loss of synapses exceeds that which occurs during normal aging, and is more extensive than the accompanying neuronal loss and accumulation of neurofibrillary tangles.[150] Synaptic pathology in AD has been characterized using silver impregnation techniques, immunohistochemical staining, confocal laser microscopy, and electron microscopy. Silver stains revealed a loss of dendritic spines in cortical layers II–IV, a loss of large pyramidal neurons, reduction in axonal collaterals, and increased numbers of intraneuronal neurofibrillary tangles, particularly in layers II and III.[151] Ultrastructural studies demonstrated the presence of abundant paired helical filaments, extensive synaptic alterations consisting of polymorphism of synaptic vesicles in the presynaptic terminals, dilation of synaptic clefts, and accumulation of osmiophilic material in postsynaptic terminals.[151] In addition, three broad categories of proliferated abnormal neuropil and plaque-associated neurites (presynaptic terminals) have been characterized (1) enlarged, vesicular; (2) dense, coarse; and (3) fine thread-like.[152,153] Quantitative immunohistochemical staining and three-dimensional reconstruction image analysis studies further documented (1) the severe loss (30–40%) of presynaptic terminals; (2) proliferation of dystrophic axon terminals; (3) increased densities of dendritic threads of variable thickness with disrupted cytoskeleton; (4) clustering of synapses around threads; and (5) apposition of presynaptic boutons to dendritic neuropil threads in AD neocortical structures.[152,154] The dystrophic axon terminals in the neuropil and near plaques exhibited immunoreactivity for synaptophysin and other synaptic proteins,[142,152,155] GAP-43,[153,156] and NOS-3,[129] whereas the dystrophic dendrites with disrupted cytoskeletons (neuropil threads) exhibited immunoreactivity for tau, neurofilament,[154,157,158] and p53.[38]

Dystrophic neurites primarily originate from presynaptic terminals,[152] and therefore represent degenerating axon terminals that project into the cortex and originate from neurons located in other structures.[159] Zilles et al. proposed that the stereotyped progression and clinical manifestations of AD may be attributed to propagation of synaptic loss and neurofibrillary tangle formation in distributions corresponding to stepwise disruption of major fiber connections between cortical areas, beginning first within the entorhinal–hippocampal connection, followed by the connection between the hippocampus and other limbic structures, and finally between association areas of neocortex.[160] One of the earliest abnormalities in AD is a loss of cholinergic input and choline acetyltransferase activity to the cerebral cortex due to loss of neurons in the nucleus basalis of Meynert.[161] As disease progresses, other neurotransmitter systems, including norepinephrine, dopamine, seratonin, and somatostatin, become affected.[162]

In addition to loss of synapses, AD neocortex and subcortical limbic structures are marred by the proliferation of dystrophic neurites representing both axons and dendrites. The increased size and synaptic contact length of residual axons also suggests concurrent sprouting and partially preserved plasticity.[143,148,154,162-164] Studies concerning the proliferation of neurites in relation to plaques demonstrated that presynaptic axonal neuritic sprouts (mainly cholinergic) exhibit acetylcholinesterase activity or synaptophysin immunoreactivity around diffuse plaques, but not mature plaques,[142,165] indicating that neuritic pathology may precede the development of mature amyloid-β plaques. Moreover, the detection of growth-associated synaptic proteins (GAP-43, synaptophysin, NOS-3, TGF-β1) in the neuropil and around plaques.[129,153,156,166-168] suggests that a subpopulation of the abnormal neurites may be sprouting (growing) rather than degenerating. This concept is supported by the findings in a recent study that showed some tau-positive neuropil and plaque-associated neurites in AD brains to be p53-positive (degenerating), and others, p53-negative (non-degenerating).[38]

Cotman and Anderson suggested that adaptive mechanisms involving regenerative sprouting may compensate for cell loss that occurs with aging, but with AD neurodegeneration, the system becomes overwhelmed.[169] For example, in normal aging, neuronal loss in the entorhinal cortex is not accompanied by synaptic loss, whereas in AD, there appears to be a progressive impairment in the ability to compensate for neuronal loss and re-establish synaptic connections.[170] Together, these observations suggest that in AD, neuritic sprouting is polymorphous and may represent primary neurodegeneration (dying back of axons), secondary neurodegeneration following cell loss and synaptic disconnection, or perhaps a regenerative or reparative response to injury as occurs in the normal brain. Importantly, if some of the neuritic sprouting in AD brains is indeed regenerative and therefore desirable, it would be important to distinguish the degenerating from the potentially healthy and viable cell populations.

NEURITIC PATHOLOGY IN NON–ALZHEIMER DISEASE NEURODEGENERATION

In AD, neuritic sprouting is a well-documented component of neurodegeneration and an important correlate of dementia.[153,158,171] In contrast, neuritic sprouting is not a generally recognized feature of most other dementing neurodegenerative diseases, although its presence has been demonstrated previously with antibodies to the growth-associated protein GAP-43[156] and by NADPH-diaphorase histochemistry.[172-175] NADPH-diaphorase corresponds to nitric oxide synthase (NOS),[176,177] and NOS-3 enzyme is localized in neuronal cell processes and growth cones during sprouting.[178] Further evidence of aberrant neuritic sprouting in non-AD neurodegenerative diseases was provided in a recent study that demonstrated clustered proliferation of both membranovesicular and granular/particulate NOS-3–immunoreactive sprouts in DLBD, PkD, PD, ALS, PSP, MSA, and DS+AD[131] as described previously in AD.[179] Experimentally, high levels of NO or increased NOS expression can either facilitate[180–185] or impair[186–190] neuritic sprouting, neuronal regeneration, neuronal viability, synaptic integrity, or synaptic plasticity, depending upon cell type. This suggests that aberrant NOS-3 immunoreactivity in neuritic processes may reflect either degenerative neuritic sprouting or a regenerative/reparative response to cell loss, synaptic disconnection, and trophic factor withdrawal in the context of neurodegeneration. Conceivably, both phenomena may co-exist with neurodegeneration since with increased NO production, some cell populations may respond to injury or cell loss by regenerating, whereas others may undergo degenerative sprouting and apoptosis.

GLIAL CELLS: INCREASED APOPTOSIS AND ABERRANT GENE EXPRESSION

In AD, AD+DS, and other neurodegenerative diseases, there is increasing evidence of white matter and glial cell pathology that may contribute to the overall disease processes. Alzheimer's disease, AD+DS, PD, DLBD, and Huntington's disease are all associated with cerebral white matter atrophy and fiber loss. In AD, the white matter atrophy is detectable early in the course of disease and precedes cortical atrophy.[6] In situ studies of apoptosis have demonstrated abundant labeling of both white matter and cortical glial cells in AD, PD, PkD, DLBD, PSP, MSA, and ALS.[43] Correspondingly, increased expression of pro-apoptosis genes such as *p53* and CD95/Fas receptor has been observed in glial cells in each of these diseases,[43] indicating that apoptosis cascades are activated in glia. In addition, in DS, increased levels of caspase 1 (interleukin-1β–converting enzyme) immunoreactivity are detectable in white matter glial cells years prior to the onset of AD-type neurodegeneration.[56]

Aberrant glial cell function appears to affect oligodendrocytes and protoplasmic (type 2) astrocytes. In AD as well as other neurodegenerative diseases, the abnormal protoplasmic astrocytes are marked by increased A_2B_5 immunoreactivity, and abnormal oligodendrocytes exhibit increased A_2B_5 and galactocerebroside immunoreactivity (Fig. 6–2). In addition, aberrant expression of GAP-43 and NOS-3 have been demonstrated in both oligodendrocytes and protoplasmic astrocytes in brains with AD, PkD, DLBD, PD, and DS+AD, primarily in regions with prominent neurodegeneration.[129,156] Increased NOS-3 expression in glial cells could result in high intracellular levels of NO and enhanced susceptibility to peroxynitrite-mediated apoptosis or cytotoxic cell death. Oligodendrocytes and protoplasmic astrocytes have important roles in supporting the structure and function of CNS axons and dendrites. Impaired function, degeneration, or apoptosis of these cell types could expose neuronal cell processes to an uncontrolled and potentially toxic extracellular fluid environment, and thereby represent an important and novel mechanism of axonal loss and synaptic disconnection in neurodegenerative diseases.

RATIONALE FOR EXPLORING OTHER GENE ABNORMALITIES IN ALZHEIMER'S DISEASE AND OTHER NEURODEGENERATIVE DISEASES

The aggregate findings suggest that the major abnormalities in cell biology and function associated with AD neurodegeneration include increased apoptosis, degeneration of presynaptic terminals, and aberrant neuritic sprouting, all of which contribute to progressive synaptic disconnection and dementia. The exciting aspect of these discoveries is that AD and other neurodegenerative diseases can now be approached in relation to early molecular abnormalities linked to impaired cellular function. For example, regardless of whether AD is familial or sporadic in occurrence, the major risk factor for developing clinically symptomatic disease is aging. Individuals with homozygous missence mutations in the presenilin genes live for six or eight decades before they develop AD. Even in trisomy 21 Down syndrome, in which virtually 100% of the individuals who survive beyond the fourth decade develop AD-type neurodegeneration, the aging process is accelerated and aging is still one of the most important variable involved. Thus, AD neurodegeneration probably repre-

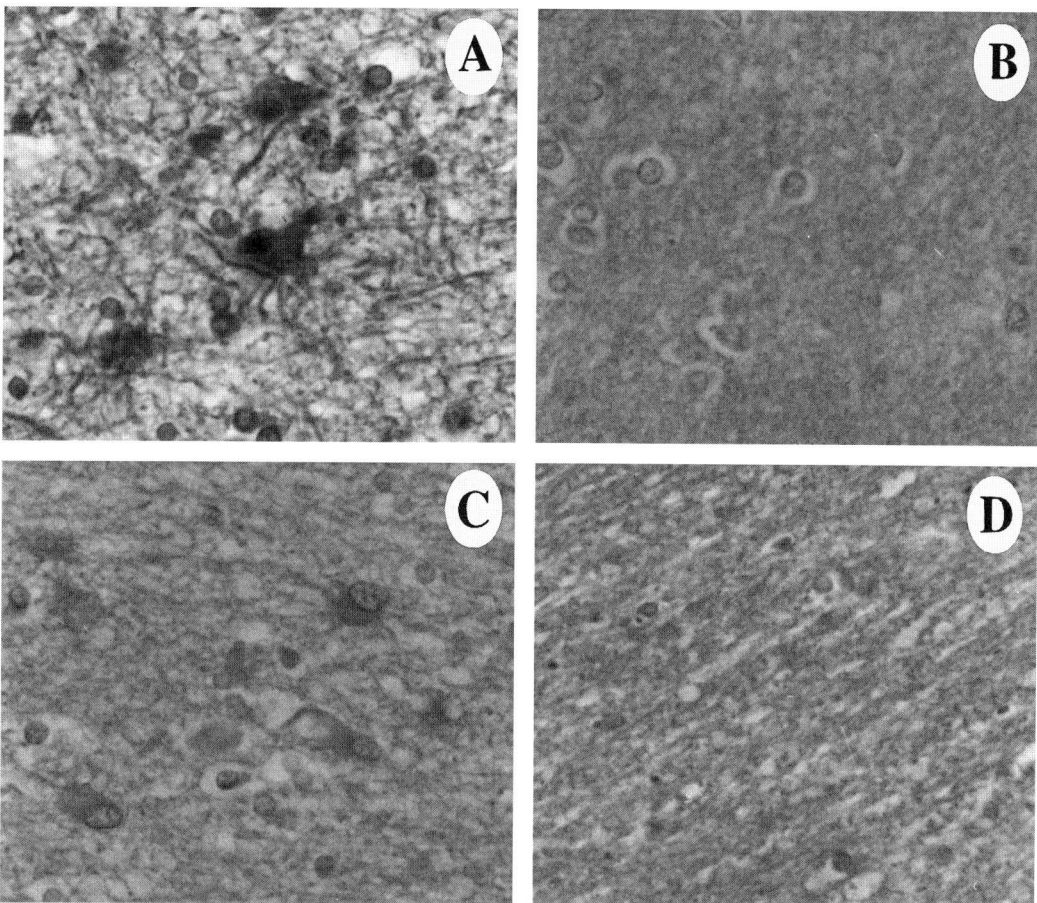

Figure 6–2. Glial cell abnormalities in Alzheimer's disease (AD) Paraffin sections from AD (A,C) and aged control (B,D) temporal lobe white matter were immunostained with monoclonal antibodies to galactocerebroside (A,B) or A_2B_5 (C,D) using the avidin-biotin horseradish complex method and diaminobenzidine co-precipitated with nickel chloride as the chromogen. Apart from the reactive gliosis associated with cell loss and proliferation of glial fibrillary acidic protein–immunoreactive hypertrophic astrocytes, both cerebral cortex and underlying white matter of regions with neurodegeneration exhibit increased galactocerebroside (A) and A_2B_5 (C) immunoreactivity in glial cells that represent oligodendrocytes or protoplasmic astrocytes. In contrast, control brains exhibit little or no cellular labeling with either antibody (B,D). Similarly increased levels of galactocerebroside and A_2B_5 immunoreactivity were observed in glial cells in brains with Pick's disease ($N = 6$), diffuse Lewy body disease ($N = 7$), amyotrophic lateral sclerosis ($N = 4$), and progressive supranuclear palsy ($N = 4$) (data not shown). However, for each disease, the abnormal glial cells were primarily distributed in structures that were marred by neurodegeneration.

sents a multistage process in which a number of factors contribute to pathologic events that culminate in increased cell death, neuritic sprouting, and synaptic disconnection. In this regard, AD neurodegeneration is likely to be precipitated by a cascade of events leading to altered gene expression and intracellular signaling which must be dissected to identify potential common pathways and mechanisms of therapeutic intervention. It is therefore important to identify prominent early abnormalities in gene expression that are likely to contribute to the stepwise process of AD neurodegeneration, particularly in relation to "sporadic" disease.

MOLECULAR ABNORMALITIES IN CEREBRAL BLOOD VESSELS IN AD

Recently, consideration has been paid to the potential contributions of cerebrovascular lesions such hemispheric infarcts, lacunes, hippocampal sclerosis, and leukoaraiosis to the clinical manifestations of dementia in AD.[191–201] For example, postmortem and neuroimaging studies suggest that AD may be complicated by vascular pathology in 20% to 40% of cases.[191,193,194,201] Moreover, there is evidence that vascular dementia is frequently accompanied by underlying, often clinically undetected, AD.[195,197–200] A survey of the of the Massachusetts General Hospital Alzheimer's Disease Research Center Brain Bank revealed the presence of cerebral micro-infarcts in approximately 30% of the AD cases. Like AD, cerebral infarction increases with age, and cerebrovascular lesions are most prevalent in individuals between 60 and 75 years of age. Neuronal loss and synaptic disconnection are responsible for the clinical deficits associated with both AD and cerebral infarction. Therefore, lesions caused by cerebrovascular disease could exacerbate the clinical course and contribute to the heterogeneity of AD. For examples, individuals with early, subclinical AD may develop cognitive impairment or dementia due to ischemic lesions and infarcts involving structures typically damaged by AD neurodegeneration.[198] If cerebral infarction does contribute to the progression of AD, early detection and treatment, as well as attention to risk factors such as systemic hypertension, history of stroke-like episodes, cerebral hypoperfusion as demonstrated by functional imaging studies, and apolipoprotein E (ApoE) genotype,[192,196,202–207] may help prevent, or delay the onset or mollify the course of clinically manifested AD in up to 30% of cases.

Vascular lesions correlated with dementia include microvascular brain injury with cribriform change,[8] subcortical white matter damage[8,208] and microinfarcts[8] with prominent involvement of the basal ganglia, thalamus, and deep white matter.[199] In a recent study, among patients with clinical AD-type dementia, a subset was identified as having relatively mild AD pathology plus abundant cerebrovascular lesions (AD+CVA) consisting of microvascular infarcts and ischemic lesions distributed in structures typically marred by AD neurodegeneration, in addition to deep cerebral white matter structures and subcortical nuclei.[209] Since dementia is ultimately caused by cell loss and synaptic disconnection, vascular-mediated as well as other types of injury could also impair cognitive function and exacerbate the clinical manifestations of AD if corticolimbic structures and pathways are involved.[160,193] In this regard, cerebral infarction or ischemia may acutely precipitate clinical dementia by exposing subclinical AD pathology.[198] Microvascular injury may further contribute to cognitive deterioration by causing disruption of the blood–brain barrier,[210,211] facilitating inadvertent development of autoantibodies to CNS cells,[212] and impairing cerebral blood flow, metabolic rate of oxygen, and oxygen extraction.[213,214]

With cerebral amyloid-β angiopathy, the frequencies of intracerebral hemorrhage and ischemic infarction are increased.[204] Experimental exposure of cerebrovascular smooth muscle cells to Aβ-1–42 peptide in vitro results in cellular degeneration,[215] and in vivo, leads to vascular disruption with damage to endothelial and smooth muscle cells and transvascular migration of leukocytes.[216,217] Experimental amyloid-β-induced vasculopathy can be prevented by treatment with free radical scavenger agents (216). Amyloid-β–induced vasculopathy may be mediated by apoptosis since increased levels of p53 immunoreactivity are detectable in smooth muscle and endothelial cells of cerebral vessels with prominent amyloid-β immunoreactivity (Fig. 6–3). Therefore, amyloid-β deposition may play a role in both neurite degeneration and vasculopathy in AD.

The Apo E-ε4 allele has been linked to a heightened risk of developing AD,[218–223] AD+CVA,[205,224–226] and cerebral amyloid angiopathy.[203,205,227] In contrast, the Apo E-ε2 allele is associated with a significantly lower risk for AD (202, 228, 229), and increased risk for vascular dementia.[202,230] Previous postmortem studies demonstrated a positive correlation between the Apo E-ε4 allele and amyloid-β deposition in cerebral vessels and senile plaques.[116,228,231] Experimentally, amyloid-β[85] and some forms of mutant amyloid precursor protein expressed in familial AD[232] have been demonstrated to be neurotoxic and to induce neuronal apoptosis. In addition, increased expression of the Bax pro-apoptosis gene has been found associated with amyloid-β deposits in senile plaques.[48] Moreover, in recent studies, microglial cell activation in relation to amyloid-β senile plaques and amyloid-β angi-

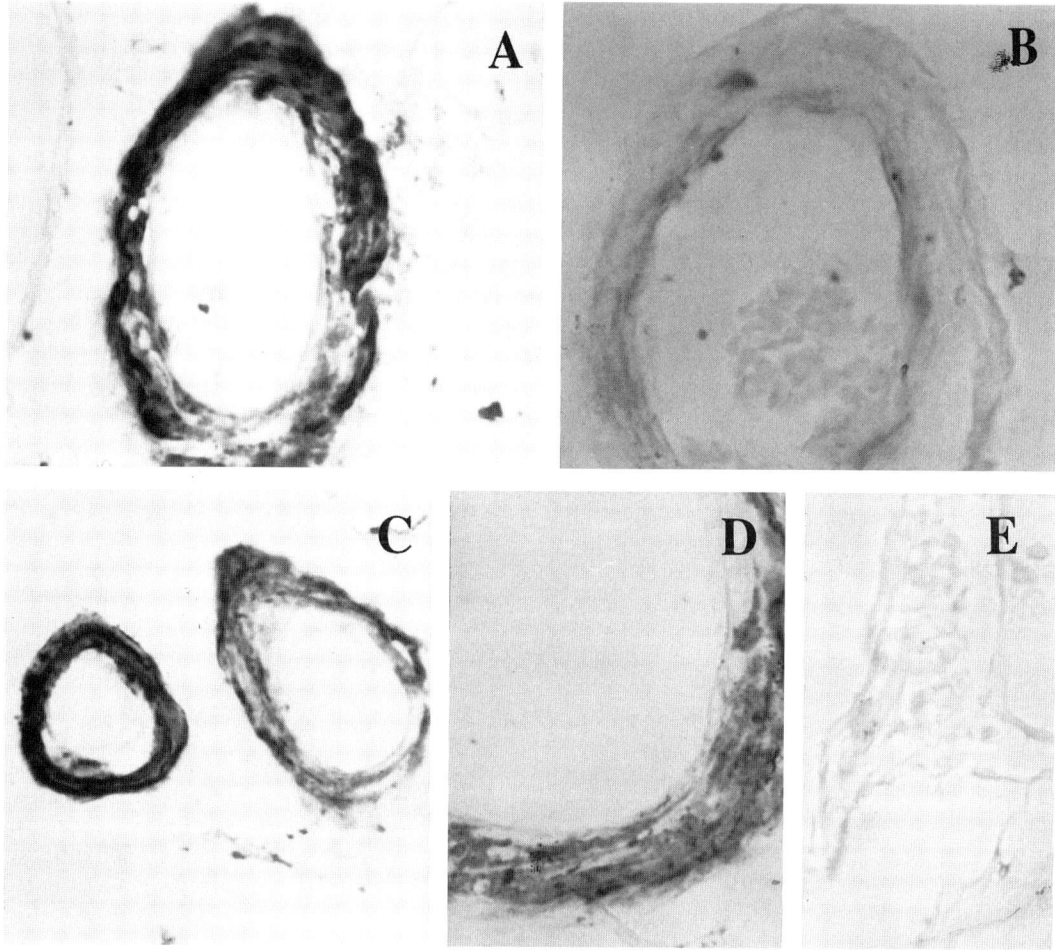

Figure 6–3. Co-localization of p53 pro-apoptosis gene product with Aβ in cerebrovascular smooth muscle cells in AD. Paraffin sections of AD (*A–D*) and control (*E*) temporal lobe were immunostained to detect Aβ using avidin-biotin horseradish peroxidase complex method and diaminobenzidine (brown) as the chromogen, and p53 using the avidin-biotin alkaline phosphatase complex method and BCIP/NBT (blue) as the chromogen. *A* Intense levels of Aβ immunoreactivity in smooth muscle cells of a superficial cortical vessel. *B,C* Co-localization of Aβ with p53 in medium-sized vessels. *D* Increased p53 and relatively low levels of Aβ in a cerebral vessel. *E* Control vessel with negative immunoreactivity for both Aβ-amyloid and p53.

opathy has been linked to the pathogenesis of AD neurodegeneration.[166,211,233]

ROLE OF CEREBRAL PERFUSION IN ALZHEIMER'S AND VASCULAR DEMENTIA

Vascular dementia (VD) is generally associated with multiple small and large infarcts involving mainly the white matter of the brain. White matter lesions (WML) are created in VD from an ischemic process secondary to a number of vascular risk factors that can be expressed with aging. Both VD and AD share many of the risk factors that can lead to WML. For example, VD and AD patients are at risk for WML in the presence of diabetes mellitus, atherosclerosis, hypotension/hypertension, atrial fibrillation, thrombogenic factors, hemorheologic abnormalities[63,234–236] and various conditions leading to heart disease (Table 6–1). Despite the conventional notion that AD is a primary neurodegenerative disorder that needs to be managed and treated as a separate

Table 6–1. Direct and Indirect Risk Factors for Alzheimer's Disease and Vascular Dementia that Are Known to Impair Optimal Cerebral Perfusion

Vascular Risk Factor	Dementia Affected
Ischemic stroke	Alzheimer's disease, vascular dementia
Diabetes mellitus	Alzheimer's disease, vascular dementia
Atrial fibrillation	Alzheimer's disease, vascular dementia
Atherosclerosis	Alzheimer's disease, vascular dementia
Thrombogenic factors	Alzheimer's disease, vascular dementia
Brain vessel wall pathology	Alzheimer's disease, vascular dementia
Hypertension/hypotension	Alzheimer's disease, vascular dementia
Amyloid angiopathy	Alzheimer's disease, vascular dementia
Blood–brain barrier dysfunction	Alzheimer's disease, vascular dementia
High serum fibrinogen levels	Alzheimer's disease, vascular dementia
Elevated serum viscosity	Alzheimer's disease, vascular dementia
Heart disease	Alzheimer's disease, vascular dementia
High homocysteine levels	Alzheimer's disease, vascular dementia
Oxidative stress	Alzheimer's disease, vascular dementia
Hyperlipidemia/high HDL-cholesterol	Alzheimer's disease, vascular dementia
Smoking/alcoholism	Alzheimer's disease, vascular dementia
Apolipoprotein E_4	Alzheimer's disease, vascular dementia

See text for details.

and distinct disease entity from VD, we will review recent evidence that points to a number of common risk factors shared by AD and VD that can result in the expression of either form of dementia. This evidence would have been dismissed a decade ago as unsubstantial and highly speculative since the argument that AD is caused by the formation of senile plaques/neurofibrillary tangles was and still is pervasive among many investigators.

The major risk factors associated with the development of cognitive failure in AD and VD are similar to those leading to the formation of WML. These vascular risk factors are summarized in Table 6–1. It can be seen from this table, that AD and VD share a substantial number of common vascular risk factors, a phenomenon that is highly suggestive but inconclusive as to the etiopathogenesis of AD.

It has been proposed that the pathogenesis of sporadic (nongenetic) AD and its heterogeneic disease pattern is due to two converging factors: (1) advanced age; and (2) presence of a vascular risk factor.[237] The first takes into account the generally-accepted findings that increased aging is inversely proportional to reduced cerebral blood flow; consequently, the more we age, the less blood flow reaches the brain. This physiologic process in and of itself should not create a problem for the aging individual unless an additional vascular-related burden, such as a condition that further reduces cerebral perfusion, is present during advanced aging (Table 6–1). At some point, when advanced age and a vascular risk factor converge, a critically attained threshold of cerebral hypoperfusion (CATCH hypothesis) is reached, which, over a chronic period of time, promotes cerebral capillary degeneration.[237] As a result, delivery of vital nutrients to the brain, including glucose and oxygen, is impaired.

Three events conspire to reduce substrate delivery required for the synthesis of ATP: (1) capillary structural distortion which moves less blood flow per μm^2 area (238), (2) compression and degeneration of endothelial cells at the capillary level which in turn reduce glucose delivery to neurons and glia via glucose transporter 1,[239,240] (3) "disturbed" (as opposed to "laminar") regional blood flow, which reduces substrate delivery across the blood-brain barrier.[192,241] The outcome of a constant and possibly progressive hemodynamic instability eventually compromises neuronal function, particularly in brain regions that are highly susceptible to ischemia, such as the CA1 hippocampal sector.[242] Being totally dependent on glucose and oxygen for energy, neurons and glia would be forced to reduce their mitochondrial oxidative phosphorylation and production of ATP, a condition that would likely create a biochemical cascade affecting all energy-dependent mechanisms within these cells. For example, since ATP is needed for the synthesis of acetylcholine and other neurotransmitters, impairment in neurotransmission results in subjects with AD.[239,240,242–244] The Na$^+$, K$^+$-ATPase pump, which requires 60% of all the ATP produced in the brain[243] cannot function optimally, while ion channels, including those regulating Ca^{2+} and glutamate flux, become disturbed, potentially creating a cytotoxic environment around the affected brain cells (Fig. 6–5). Chronically reduced cerebral blood flow can initiate cytokine release and induce inflammation of the brain tissue.[245] Continued ATP reductions will invariably lead to a series of pathological events, including impairment of slow and fast axonal transport, aberrant protein phosphorylation, protein synthesis changes, and loss of action potentials (Fig. 6–4). Synaptic loss and cell death likely follow the dysfunctional axonal transport system, an event that can result in the elaboration of abnormal proteins (for example, amyloid-β) as well as abnormal phosphorylation of tau and production of paired helical filaments (Fig. 6–4). The production of amyloid-β and paired helical filaments contributes to the deposition of senile plaques and neurofibrillary tangles in AD brains.

Below, we summarize the 10 major bodies of evidence that the above pathologic events are relevant to the pathogenesis of AD.

1. Upon review of a list of the major risk factors reported for AD (Table 6–1)—aging, cardiac disease, diabetes mellitus, stroke, head injury, hypertension and hypotension, transient ischemic attacks, atherosclerosis, high-serum cholesterol, menopause, atrial fibrillation and smoking. It is striking to observe that, despite their variable pathologic presentations, all these conditions share one common denominator: all are known to reduce or impair cerebral blood flow. Moreover, these risk factors in the presence of advanced aging may explain the clinical heterogeneity of Alzheimer's dementia.

2. Most medications reported thus far to delay the progress of AD, directly or indirectly, improve cerebral perfusion. Such medications include cholinomimetics, cholinergics, estrogen replacement therapy, NSAIDs, vitamin E, gingko biloba, and cholinesterase inhibitors.[246]

3. Single-photon-emisson computed tomographic (SPECT) measurements of cerebral blood flow in elderly subjects complaining of memory disturbances show that only those individuals with significant cerebral hypoperfusion in the hippocampal–amygdaloid region later developed AD after a 2-year longitudinal follow-up.[247] Other evidence has shown that cerebral blood flow decline correlates well with AD severity and may be present prior to abnormal metabolic or anatomic changes in the brains of these patients.[248–253]

4. Impaired cerebral blood flow in patients with AD is complicated by the presence of hemorheological abnormalities such as high-serum fibrinogen, reduced erythrocyte deformability, high plasma viscosity and decreased cerebrovascular reactivity. These hemorheologic abnormalities will further contribute to lowering blood flow to the brain.[254]

5. Brain hypoperfusion is associated with an increased oxygen extraction fraction and a preserved cerebral metabolic rate of oxygen as determined by positron emission tomographic (PET) studies of AD patients. This finding is suggestive of regional "misery perfusion" that may be possibly created by an abnormal or deficient microvasculature.[213,214,255]

6. Capillary degeneration in the brains of the majority of AD patients consist of basement membrane thickening, endothelial cell collapse, pericyte degeneration, vessel lumen distortions and collagen deposition throughout the basement membrane.[256–259] Such capillary changes can transform normal laminar blood flow into disturbed flow patterns that contribute to the impaired delivery of glucose and oxygen to neurons.[238] Many patients with AD in addition to the above capillary distortions also reveal amyloid angiopathy characterized by amyloid deposits within the microvasculature which ostensibly may add to impede optimal blood flow delivery to the brain.[260]

7. The AD susceptibility gene apo E$_4$ and the FAD gene PS-1 are associated with cerebral hypoperfusion, and in the case of PS-1, may herald AD symptoms.[247] Additional findings indicate that patients carrying the apo E$_4$ gene have the most severe regional cerebral hypoperfusion in the temporoparietal regions.[261]

8. Experimental evidence in rodents indicates that chronic brain hypoperfusion can lead to Alzheimer-like memory disturbances and these changes are associated with capillary distortions that mimic those in AD brains.[256] Moreover, other experimental data report that following chronic brain hypoperfusion in rodents, reduced levels of cytochrome oxidase in hippocampus (reflecting a neuronal energy deficiency and loss of Na^+, K^+-ATPase ionic pumping), MAP-2 loss in apical CA1 dendrites, and reduced glucose utilization are observed.[262–265]

9. Circulating soluble amyloid-β_{1-40} found in AD brain can cause cerebrovascular constriction and increased glial reactivity around cerebral blood vessels when injected intravenously in rodents.[266–268] Soluble amyloid-β deposits in AD brain may originate from the circulation, brain cells, or both, and its presence may precede the formation of toxic amyloid-β fibrils, suggesting that this peptide may be an immediate precursor of amyloid fibril deposition in Alzheimer's dementia. In addition, transgenic mice overexpressing mutant APP and deposition of amyloid-β showed a profound selective impairment of the neocortical microvasculature.[269] Alterations of cerebral blood flow in these rodent models are reminiscent of the cerebrovascular pathology observed in AD and could help explain how this abnormal physiologic process begins.

10. Successful treatment of VD may also benefit patients with AD and conversely, treatment aimed at AD may be useful in the treatment of VD.[270] The reason for this may lie in the considerable evidence indicating that AD and VD share many risk factors (see Table 6–1) and have a closely linked clinical presentation and cognitive profile. Since it is well accepted that VD is caused primarily by vascular insults to the brain, whereas AD is presumed to originate as a neurodegenerative disorder, the question arises as to whether an important overlap[271] or a common pathologic trigger is key in melding these two conditions so closely.[272] It is also fair to ask, in view of the evidence presented in this review, whether VD is a rogue variant of AD. Assuming that reducing risk factors for VD may also benefit AD, a common therapeutic target designed for either disorder may well prove beneficial for the other.

METABOLIC FACTORS IN DEMENTIA

Patients with AD suffer from a deficit in neuronal energy metabolism that has been well documented. To appreciate how this is thought to evolve and the functional consequences associated with progressive metabolic meltdown in such patients, a brief review of brain energy metabolism is warranted.

Glucose is the main and practically sole source of energy for the mammalian brain.[273] Glucose is known to regulate many brain functions, including memory and learning.[274] Plasma glucose is shuttled to the brain from the circulation where it diffuses into the brain parenchyma with the aid of glucose transporter 1, located in the endothelial cells of the capillary blood brain–barrier.[239] Once in the brain, glucose is further transported through glial and neuronal membranes by glucose transporter 3.[240] Under some pathologic conditions (e.g., hypoglycemia or anoxia), intracellular glucose levels can approach zero and brain glucose utilization becomes limited to glucose transport. Normally, glucose undergoes conversion to pyruvate in the brain cytosol via anaerobic glycolysis by enzymes that include hexokinase, phosphofructokinase and pyruvate kinase. The net gain in the anaerobic glycolytic energy production is 2 moles ATP for every mole of glucose. By contrast, glucose metabolism leading to conversion of pyruvate dehydrogenase complex and its oxidation to acetyl coenzyme A in mitochondria, results in oxidative phosphorylation and production of energy rich phosphates such as ATP, via aerobic glycolysis (also known as the citric acid cycle or Krebs cycle) (Fig. 6–4A). Consequently, 1 mole glucose yields 36 moles ATP from mitochondrial oxidative phophorylation, which constitutes 95% of all ATP generated in the brain.[273] Thus, oxidative phosphorylation yields about 18 times as much useful energy to brain cells as can be obtained from anaerobic glycolysis.[273] Since oxidative phoshorylation is dependent on the presence of glucose and oxygen to create ATP, any condition that reduces the delivery of oxygen (ischemia, hypoxia) or glucose (ischemia, hypoglycemia) can have extremely damaging effects on nerve cell function (6-4B). The reason for this lies in the energy-dependent processes that require ATP to maintain such cellular activities as Na^+, K^+-ATPase ion pumping, neuronal action potentials, slow/fast axonal transport, neurotransmitter synthesis release and uptake, Ca^{2+} transport, protein phosphorylation, transcription, translation, protein synthesis, and optimal synaptic function (Figure 6–4A).

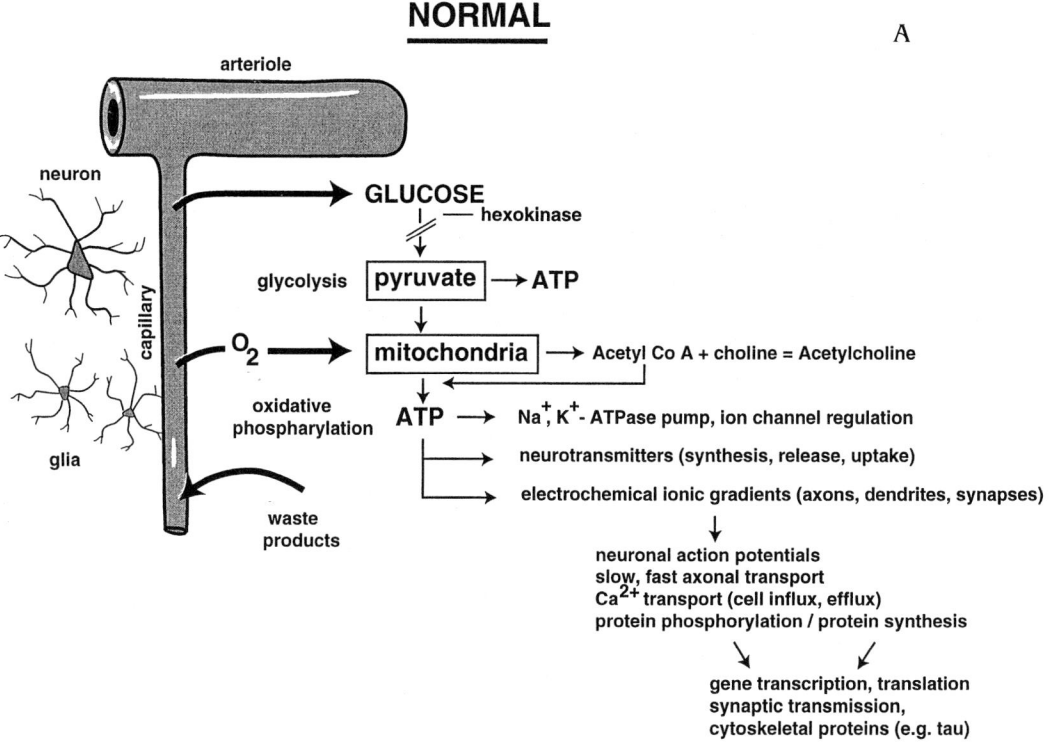
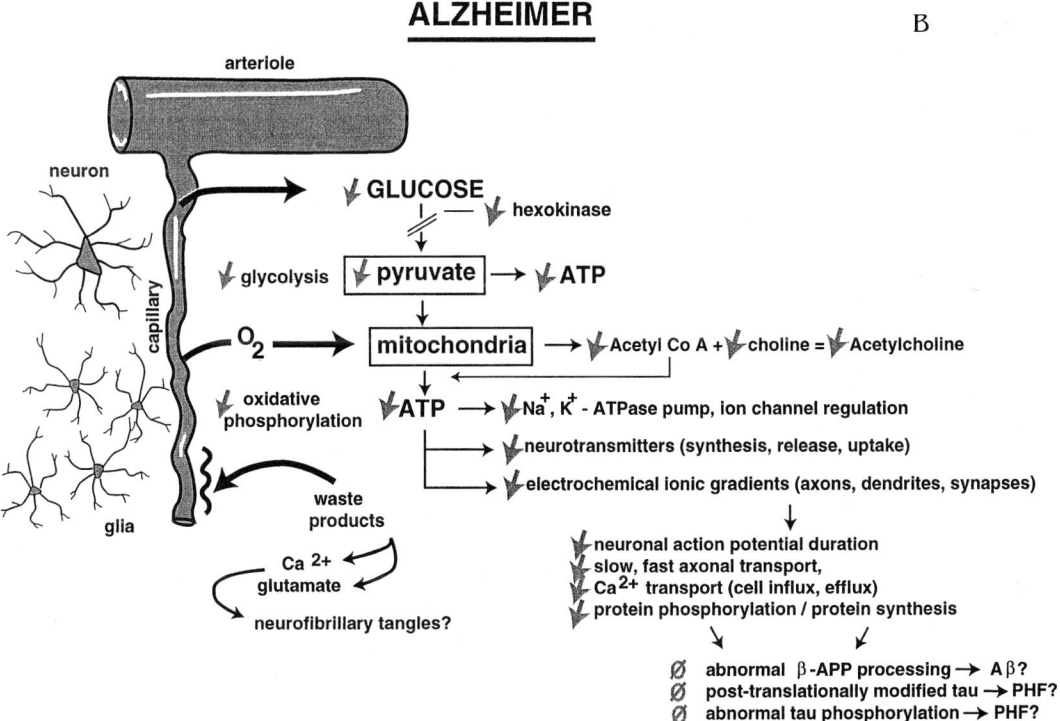

Figure 6–4. Cross section of a brain capillary during normal aging *(A)* and in Alzheimer's disease *(B)*. Structural capillary changes will cause the capillaries to distort and subsequently change the hemodynamic pattern of blood flow from laminar to "disturbed". The resulting hemodynamic change will impair optimal delivery of nutrients to brain cells. Consequences of impaired brain perfusion in Alzheimer's disease are schematically outlined above.

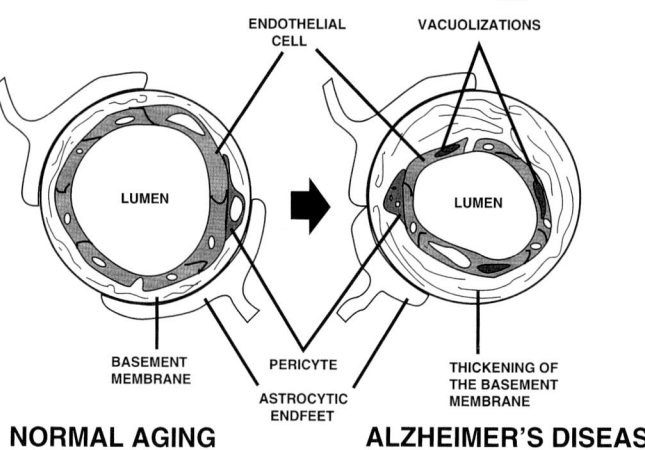

Figure 6–5. Typical cortical capillary degeneration found in Alzheimer brains at postmortem as sketched from electron micrographs. Thickened basement membrane is associated with compressed endothelial cell and pericyte degeneration. Distorted lumen provokes hemodynamic flow changes which impair energy substrate delivery to neurons.

All active cellular and molecular mechanisms in brain cells require a source of energy substrate to maintain optimal function, and this energy source is generally derived from ATP.

One of the means of evaluating oxidative phosphorylation in brain is to determine the activity of cytochrome oxidase, the terminal enzyme of the mitochondrial respiratory chain. The mitochondrial respiratory (O_2 consuming) chain is located on the inner membrane of the mitochondria which are the energy-producing organelles in neurons and glial cells. Levels of cytochrome oxidase in brain reflect endogenous neuronal activity[243] and are reported to be a useful marker of neuronal dysfunction and potential neurodegeneration.[244]

In AD, cytochrome oxidase and α-ketoglutarate dehydrogenase complex (α-KGDHC) are found reduced in the temporal cortex of postmortem material examined.[81] α-KGDHC is considered to be the rate-limiting enzyme of the citric acid cycle, so low levels of this enzyme suggest a cerebral metabolic abnormality and a deficient production of ATP. Since there is no such thing as a "mild" case of AD that does not rapidly progress, it must be assumed that the reduction of these two key energy-producing enzymes in AD is progressive and that neuronal activity and function in specific regions of the brain undergo neurodegeneration by way of a cell-death pathway that may involve necrosis, apoptosis, or both.

Down-regulation of oxidative phosphorylation in AD brain has been tied to regional reductions in glucose metabolism and to declining levels of cerebral blood flow.[250,275] Consequently, the level of depressed glucose metabolism and brain blood flow correlate well with dementia severity, particularly in the hippocampal region of the brain where cerebral perfusion appears most affected.[247,248,252] Glucose transporter 1 at the blood–brain barrier and glucose transporter 3 in brain tissue are also reduced in AD in regions where the neuropathological changes are most active.[239,240] The reduction of glucose transporter 1 in cerebral capillaries is relatively specific since other capillary enzymes are not affected. Neuronal depletion of glucose in AD occurs as a result of 4 main problems:

1. Decreased cerebral blood flow, thus glucose is delivered less to the brain[276]
2. Reduced glucose transporter 1 in microvessels[239,240]
3. Depressed hexokinase activity, the enzyme that catalyzes the reaction that phosphorylates glucose to glucose-6-phosphate during glycolysis[276]
4. Reduced glucose transporter 3 across brain cell membranes[240] impaired synthesis of acetyl coenzyme A and lowered levels of pyruvate dehydrogenase complex in the mitochondria;[81] both pro-

cesses are involved in the production of ATP via available intraneuronal glucose concentrations (Fig. 6–4B).

While the rate-limiting step for glucose utilization in the brain is assumed to be hexokinase, differential regulation of this enzyme and of the glucose transporters as well as phosphorylation of glucose could make all four mechanisms rate limiting.[240,277-279] Thus, substantial evidence indicates that at least in AD, and possibly other dementias, abnormal metabolic pathways characterized by a reduction in glucose turnover, is commonly present[250,275] which appears not to result from neurodegeneration but rather to contributes to it. This concept is a departure from the more dogmatic theory that amyloid-β deposition in the form of senile plaques is the cause of neurodegeneration in AD.

The "amyloid hypothesis" of AD has lost a substantial number of advocates in the past few years for the following reasons:

1. Amyloid-β deposition is not the earliest neuropathological event in AD[280]
2. Amyloid-β deposition does not correlate with disease severity or neuronal loss[146]
3. Many nondemented subjects have the same density of plaque formation at death as that in AD subjects[281,282]
4. Transgenic mice overexpressing mutant APP (Aβ) show cognitive deficits before amyloid-β deposition[283]
5. These same transgenicmice show no correlation between neuronal loss and amyloid-β depositon (see #1 above)[283,284]
6. These same transgenic mice also demonstrate no correlation between amyloid-β depositions and synaptic, metabolic, or cytoskeletal loss.[146,281,283]

It should be noted that the extent of neuronal and synaptic loss in AD appears to be a better correlate of disease severity than the relative density of senile plaques and neurofibrillary tangles which are considered to be the pathologic hallmarks of this dementia.[143,146] Consequently, a causal relationship between amyloid-β accumulation and AD has yet to be demonstrated. This conclusion leaves the door open to much speculation about the pathogenesis of AD and a host of other theories have been proposed to explain the void left by the amyloid hypothesis. A review of these proposals relative to the causality of AD is outlined below.

OTHER POSSIBLE FACTORS IN THE PATHOGENESIS OF DEMENTIA

Calcium Homeostasis

Calcium (Ca^{2+}) is an important intracellular messenger for many signal transduction pathways. Since several second messenger–generating systems can activate free, intracellular Ca^{2+}, many studies have focused on the cellular regulation of this crucial ion during aging and AD. Studies have shown that amyloid-β can disrupt Ca^{2+} homeostasis and increase neuronal vulnerability to excitotoxicity.[285] What makes Ca^{2+} an intriguing factor in the potential process of neurodegeneration is the modulating role it plays in the equilibrium controlling regeneration and degeneration. Thus, processes that disrupt the balance of cell growth and death may tip the balance towards cell death pathways when systems that regulate Ca^{2+} homeostasis break down.[257] The consequences of destabilizing Ca^{2+} homeostasis can lead to cell dysfunction, protein phosphorylation abnormalities (resulting in tau?), impairment of neurotransmission, membrane function damage, production of toxic glutamate levels, and countless other biochemical abnormalities affecting the neuroimmune and neuroendocrine systems.[285] Abnormalities of Ca^{2+} metabolism may also be associated with vascular dementia. However, the mechanisms resulting from this disturbance may be different from the intracellular homeostasis disbalance observed in AD.[257]

Non-Aβ Component of Alzheimer's Disease Amyloid / α-synuclein

The second major component of senile plaques in AD is a 35 amino acid peptide termed "non-amyloid-β component of AD amyloid" (NAC).[286] The cloned NAC precursor is a protein called "NACP" (or α-synuclein[287] which is found predominantly in presynaptic nerve terminals of the brain, where it can accumulate abnormally during the progress of AD.[288] Subsequent studies have shown the existence of two types of synuclein, α and β, and that NACP is homologous to α-synuclein.[289]

The role of α-synuclein is unclear, but its ratio with another presynaptic protein synaptophysin, doubles during the progress of AD.[289,290] NACP stimulates amyloid-β aggregation and binds amyloid-β.[290,291] A mutation in the α-synuclein gene has been shown to be associated with Lewy bodies in Parkinson's disease[292,293] and in the Lewy body variant of AD.[294] NACP is reported to accumulate abnormally in synaptic nerve terminals and senile plaques in AD brain[290], a finding that suggests a common link between these two neurodegenerative disorders. Accumulation of NACP appears to favor the center rather than the periphery of senile plaques[294,295] and may contribute to or cause amyloid-β aggregation in brain tissue from Alzheimer patients. The co-localization of NACP with synaptophysin found in Lewy bodies and the presence of Lewy bodies in PD and a variant of AD, suggest that these and other presynaptic proteins (such as chromogranin A, a major soluble protein in dense core secretory vesicles) may initiate or contribute to synaptic loss in these dementing disorders.[296]

Free Radicals

Evidence that oxidative stress and the formation of free radicals is an important mechanism in the evolution of AD has been accumulating at a fast rate over the past few years. Although it is debatable whether oxidative stress is the actual triggering event that leads to onset of cognitive and pathological changes in AD brains, it is nevertheless a crucial component in the evolution of this dementia. Oxidative stress has been shown to increase production of the AD pathologic marker amyloid-β, which in turn generates more oxidative stress.[297] These findings have been confirmed using transgenic mice that are made to produce amyloid-β and are then subjected to oxidative damage. Such transgenic mice show oxidative damage similar to that found in AD and this damage directly correlates with amyloid-β deposits in the brain.[297] Secondary factors, such as the formation of advanced glycation end products (AGEs), appear to integrate with oxidative stress and abnormal glucose metabolism to produce autotoxic superoxide radicals during AD.[298] The AGEs are reported to contribute to the formation of senile plaques and neurofibrillary tangles, the pathologic hallmarks found in Alzheimer's brains.[296,299] The cytotoxic effects of AGEs can be experimentally neutralized when energy metabolism is boosted with dose of α-ketoglutarate or pyruvate, two essential enzymes in the citric acid cycle.[300] The AGEs consequently elicit a wide range of cell-mediated responses that complicate the pathogenesis of dementia, including AD and vascular dementia.[301] The AGEs do this in several ways: (1) by direct production of free radicals[302] (2) by activation of signaling pathways,[303] and (3) by inducing activation of microglia.[304]

Lipid peroxidation is another activity associated with oxidative stress that has been implicated in AD. Increased lipid peroxidation has been detected in hippocampal, amygdaloid and parahippocampal regions of AD brains through the use of 4-hydroxynonenol, a marker of lipid peroxidation.[305] These brain regions are also known to undergo severe neuronal loss and tissue atrophy during AD, a finding suggestive of a link between neurodegeneration and lipid peroxidative products. Lipid peroxidation therefore, does not appear to be singularly characteristic of AD but can be found in other dementias such as PD, vascular dementia, and dementia with Lewy bodies.[306] The field of oxidative stress in dementia and neurodegeneration may offer viable leads in the search for solutions to these cognitive disorders; the reader is referred to a series of recently published reviews of the fundamental and clinical aspects of this rapidly expanding topic.[307–312]

Inflammation

Many key elements linking oxidative stress and inflammatory mechanisms appear to be present in AD. Such reactions as cell membrane attack, production of superoxide radicals, and excess glutamate production are reported to interact during neuronal expression of inflammation and oxidative damage.[313] These oxidative-inflammatory reactions are also present in other neurodegenerative disorders, such as Parkinson's dementia complex of Guam and amyotrophic lateral sclerosis.[314] The presumed process involving an inflammatory response in the development of AD is provided by reports of increased levels of cytokines and their receptors in AD brain tissue. For example, interleukin-1β (IL-1β), interleukin-6 (IL-6), type 8 interleukin-8 (IL-8) receptor, and the receptor for CSF-1 in brain or cerebrospinal fluid itself have been identified in Alzheimer postmortem brain tissue.[314] In this scheme, Aβ would stimulate the release of IL-6 and IL-8 by IL-1β-activated astrocytomas cells and by IL-8 monoctyes. Interleukin-1β is reported to regulate APP synthesis[315] and presumably could trigger enhanced APP production and Aβ deposition following various pathologic insults, including brain trauma.[316]

The major sites of IL-6 synthesis are neurons and glial cells, where this product can exert an opposite action. For example, IL-6 can trigger a process aimed at neuronal survival after injury, or it can result in a cell death pathway as described for AD.[317] In rodents, synapse and neuronal loss is observed following the constitutive expression of IL-6 induced by chronic infusion of lipopolysaccharide.[318] This model of neuroinflammatory reaction leads also to memory and learning loss.[319] Complement activation is known to lead to inflammation, cytolysis and opsomization (bacterial phagocytosis).[320] A potent activator of human complement in vitro is the senile plaque product Aβ1–42[321] which can alone induce the formation of C3a and C5a, powerful proinflammatory peptides.[322] C3 is present in diffuse plaques, this presence may be an early stage of mature senile plaque development and can activate microglial cells as part of the inflammatory reaction in brain tissue.[245,323] Microglia from postmortem AD brains have been shown to immunoreact positively with antibodies against IL-1β, IL-6, and tumor necrosis factor.[324] This evidence has stimulated a flurry of experiments in an attempt to demonstrate the role of inflammatory reactions in Alzheimer brains. The pragmatic intent of demonstrating a role for inflammation in AD as an "inflammatory brain response" lies in the possible benefit of using non-steroidal anti-inflammatory agents (NSAIDs) that may slow down the cognitive failure associated with this disorder and reduce the risk of developing AD. Several studies have indicated that, indeed, the use of NSAIDs can reduce risk and progression of this dementia.[314,324–327] However, several recent population-based studies were unable to confirm the benefits of NSAIDs in slowing the progression of or risk for AD.[328]

Genetics

Familial Alzheimer's disease (FAD) relates to the genetic component of this dementia and constitutes about 5% of all Alzheimer cases. Three genes have been identified so far that express mutant proteins that appear to result in clinical AD: (1) amyloid precursor protein (APP) on chromosome 21; (2) presenilin-1 (PS-1) on chromosome 14, and (3) presenilin-2 (PS-2) on chromosome 1.[329] Apolipoprotein E-4 (apo E-4) on chromosome 19 is considered a risk rather than a causal factor for the development of AD. Although the role of apo E-4 in the evolution of AD is far from clear, studies have shown that this protein plays a role in the modulation of Aβ production rate.[330]

Autosomal dominant AD can develop by mutations of APP, PS 1, and PS 2.[331] Mutant gene products are able to cause damage and death to vulnerable neuronal groups such as those localized in the CA1 hippocampal sector. The result of neuronal death in the hippocampal and entorhinal regions evolves into the initial clinical syndrome of AD, which is characterized by impairment of recent memory and visuospatial perception, and later in the disease process, disrupts judgement, language, abstraction, and problem solving. Most cases of FAD occur as early onset (< 65 years of age), but specific alleles of apo E-4 and α2-macroglobulins are associated with an increased risk for late-onset AD.[332–334] A common factor among FAD mutations is that they influence APP processing in a manner that increases the highly amyloidogenic production of amyloid-β1–43 peptides. These mutations have been successfully studied in transgenic mice that can generate wild-type PS 1, overexpress human APP, and produce accelerated amyloid-β deposits in their brain.[283,335] Thus, at least 3 known genes can influence amyloid-β deposition in FAD. Reduction of amyloid-β deposition is a viable therapeutic target and the use of transgenic mice has become a widely accepted experimental model for validating and screening potential treatments for AD.

CONCLUSIONS

Intensive study of the molecular and cellular basis of neurodegeneration in AD has led to the characterization of abnormalities in gene expression that mediate cell loss and synaptic disconnection in both sporadic and familial forms of the disease. Moreover, studies have provided tantalizing evidence that links molecular mechanisms of neurodegeneration among several diseases including, AD, diffuse Lewy body disease, Pick's disease, Parkinson's disease, and amyotrophic lateral sclerosis. Although the underlying mechanisms vary, cell loss in AD and other diseases is ultimately mediated by apoptosis, impaired mitochondrial function/mitochondrial DNA damage, necrosis, or cytotoxicity. Aging-associated cell loss is similarly mediated, but the degree of cell loss with neurodegeneration is significantly greater due to enhanced sensitivity to oxidative stress. In aggregate, there appears to be 3 dominant factors contributing to the enhanced sensitivity to oxidative stress in aged brains predisposed to neurodegeneration: (1) genetic factors such as presenilin or amyloid precursor protein gene mutations; (2) constitutively aberrant expression of genes with attendant increased generation of reactive oxygen species, e.g. nitric oxide synthase-3, superoxide dismutase I, and hemoxygenase-1; and (3) the occurrence of wide-ranging metabolic and cellular insults that compromise CNS function including, impaired energy metabolism, cerebral hypoperfusion, toxicity resulting from amyloid-β deposition, accumulation of non-amyloid-β precursor protein (α-synuclein), impaired calcium homeostasis, activation of pro-inflammatory cytokines, and impaired mitochondrial function due to mitochondrial DNA damage. The heterogeneous nature of AD from clinical, pathological, molecular, and physiological perspectives, is likely due to differential effects of the dominant influential factors which could act independently or synergistically to precipitate or propagate AD-type neurodegeneration. Therefore, we propose a "double-hit" hypothesis regarding the development and progression of AD. An important aspect of our hypothesis is that aging-associated impairment of mitochondrial function, induced by pathologic cerebral hypoperfusion and reduced energy substrate delivery to brain, could expose underlying defects that predispose the brain to AD-type neurodegeneration. This hypothesis is testable, and could be used to guide the development of effective measures to prevent and treat Alzheimer's disease and possibly other forms of neurodegeneration.

REFERENCES

1. Bartlett TQ, Vannier MW, McKeel DW, Jr., Gado M, Hildebolt CF, Walkup R. Interactive segmentation of cerebral gray matter, white matter, and CSF: photographic and MR images. Comput Med Imaging Graph 1994;18:449–460.
2. Erkinjuntti T, Lee DH, Gao F, Steenhuis R, Eliasziw M, Fry R, et al. Temporal lobe atrophy on magnetic resonance imaging in the diagnosis of early Alzheimer's disease. Arch Neurol 1993;50:305–310.
3. Koyama K, Hirasawa H, Karasawa A, Yoshimura M. [Use of MRI in the diagnosis of dementia of the Alzheimer type]. Nippon Ronen Igakkai Zasshi 1994;31:388–395.
4. Murphy DG, DeCarli CD, Daly E, Gillette JA, McIntosh AR, Haxby JV, et al. Volumetric magnetic resonance imaging in men with dementia of the Alzheimer type: correlations with disease severity. Biol Psychiatry 1993;34:612–621.
5. de la Monte SM, Hedley WE. Small cerebral hemispheres in adults with Down's syndrome: contributions of developmental arrest and lesions of Alzheimer's disease. J Neuropathol Exp Neurol 1990;49:509–520.
6. de la Monte SM. Quantitation of cerebral atrophy in preclinical and end-stage Alzheimer's disease. Ann Neurol 1989;25:450–459.
7. Hubbard BM, Anderson JM. A quantitative study of cerebral atrophy in old age and senile dementia. J Neurol Sci 1981;50:135–145.
8. Esiri M, Morris JE. The Neuropathology of Dementia. 1997.
9. Selkoe D. The molecular pathology of Alzheimer's disease. Neuron 1991;:487–498.
10. Selkoe D, Ihara Y, Salazar F. Alzheimer's disease: partial purification of paired helical filaments and demonstration of insolubility in SDS, urea, and guanidine. Science 1982;215:1243–1245.
11. Kidd M. Paired helical filaments in electron microscopy of Alzheimer's disease. Nature 1963;197:192–193.
12. Wisniewski H, Merz P, Iqbal K. Ultrastructure of paired helical filament of Alzheimer's neurofibrillary tangle. J Neuropathol Exp Neurol 1984;43:643–656.
13. Perry G, Rizzuto N, Autilio-Gambetti L, Gambetti P. Paired helical filaments from Alzheimer disease patients contain cytoskeletal components. Proc Natl Acad Sci USA 1985;82:3916–3920.

14. Grundke-Iqbal I, Iqbal K, Tung Y-C, Quinlan M, Wisniewski H, Binder L. Abnormal phosphorylation of the microtubule-associated protein (tau) in Alzheimer cytoskeletal pathology. Proc Natl Acad Sci USA 1986;83:4913–4917.
15. Kosik K, Joachim C, Selkoe D. Microtubule-associated protein, tau, is a major antigenic determinant of paired helical filaments in Alzheimer's disease. Proc Natl Acad Sci USA 1986;83:4044–4048.
16. Wood J, Mirra S, Pollock N, Binder L. Neurofibrillary tangles of Alzheimer disease share antigenic determinants with the axonal microtubule-associated protein tau (t). Proc Natl Acad Sci USA 1986;83:4040–4043.
17. Mori H, Kondo J, Ihara Y. Ubiquitin is a component of paired helical filaments in Alzheimer's disease. Science 1987;235:1641–1644.
18. Crowther RA, Olesen OF, Smith MJ, Jakes R, Goedert M. Assembly of Alzheimer-like filaments from full-length tau protein. FEBS Lett 1994;337:135–138.
19. Clark LN, Poorkaj P, Wszolek Z, Geschwind DH, Nasreddine ZS, Miller B, et al. Pathogenic implications of mutations in the tau gene in pallido-ponto-nigral degeneration and related neurodegenerative disorders linked to chromosome 17. Proc Natl Acad Sci U S A 1998;95:13103–13107.
20. Spillantini MG, Murrell JR, Goedert M, Farlow MR, Klug A, Ghetti B. Mutation in the tau gene in familial multiple system tauopathy with presenile dementia. Proc Natl Acad Sci U S A 1998;95(13):7737–77341.
21. Hanger DP, Hughes K, Woodgett JR, Brion JP, Anderton BH. Glycogen synthase kinase-3 induces Alzheimer's disease-like phosphorylation of tau: generation of paired helical filament epitopes and neuronal localisation of the kinase. Neurosci Lett 1992;147:58–62.
22. Lovestone S, Reynolds CH, Latimer D, Davis DR, Anderton BH, Gallo JM, et al. Alzheimer's disease-like phosphorylation of the microtubule-associated protein tau by glycogen synthase kinase-3 in transfected mammalian cells. Curr Biol 1994;4:1077–1086.
23. Drewes G, Lichtenberg-Kraag B, Doring F, Mandelkow EM, Biernat J, Goris J, et al. Mitogen activated protein (MAP) kinase transforms tau protein into an Alzheimer-like state. Embo J 1992;11:2131–2138.
24. Lu Q, Soria JP, Wood JG. p44mpk MAP kinase induces Alzheimer type alterations in tau function and in primary hippocampal neurons. J Neurosci Res 1993;35:439–444.
25. Brion JP, Couck AM. Cortical and brainstem-type Lewy bodies are immunoreactive for the cyclin-dependent kinase 5. Am J Pathol 1995;147:1465–1476.
26. Hosoi T, Uchiyama M, Okumura E, Saito T, Ishiguro K, Uchida T, et al. Evidence for cdk5 as a major activity phosphorylating tau protein in porcine brain extract. J Biochem (Tokyo) 1995;117:741–749.
27. Pei JJ, Grundke-Iqbal I, Iqbal K, Bogdanovic N, Winblad B, Cowburn RF. Accumulation of cyclin-dependent kinase 5 (cdk5) in neurons with early stages of Alzheimer's disease neurofibrillary degeneration. Brain Res 1998;797:267–277.
28. Mann DM. Alzheimer's disease and Down's syndrome. Histopathology 1988;13:125–137.
29. Mann DM. The pathological association between Down syndrome and Alzheimer disease. Mech Ageing Dev 1988;43:99–136.
30. Lai F, Williams RS. A prospective study of Alzheimer disease in Down syndrome. Arch Neurol 1989;46:849–853.
31. Schapiro MB. Dementia in Down's syndrome: cerebra glucose utilization, neuropsychological assessment, and neuropathology. Jeurology 1988;38:938–942.
32. Brugge KL. Cognitive impairment in adults with Down's syndrome: similarities to early cognitive changes in Alzheimer's disease. Neurology 1994;44:232–238.
33. Devenny DA. Normal ageing in adults with Down's syndrome: a longitudinal study. J Intellect Disabil Res 1996;40(Pt 3):208–221.
34. Halliday G, Davies L, McRitchie D, Cartwright H, Pamphlett R. Ubiquitin-positive achromatic neurons in corticobasal degeneration. Acta Neuropathol (Berl) 1995;90:68–75.
35. Lennox G, Lowe J, Morrell K, Landon M, Mayer R. Ubiquitin is a component of neurofibrillary tangles in a variety of neurodegenerative disease. Neurosci Lett 1988;94:211–217.
36. Love S, Saitoh T, Quijada S, Cole G, Terry R. Alz-50, ubiquitin and tau immunoreactivity of neurofibrillary tangles, Pick bodies and Lewy bodies. J Neuropathol Exp Neurol 1988;47:393–405.
37. Lassmann H, Bancher C, Breitschopf H, Wegiel J, Bobinski M, Jellinger K, et al. Cell death in Alzheimer's disease evaluated by DNA fragmentation in situ. Acta Neuropathol (Berl) 1995;89:35–41.
38. de la Monte SM, Sohn YK, Wands JR. Correlates of p53- and Fas (CD95)-mediated apoptosis in Alzheimer's disease. J Neurol Sci 1997;152:73–83.
39. Dragunow M, Faull RL, Lawlor P, Beilharz EJ, Singleton K, Walker EB, et al. In situ evidence for DNA fragmentation in Huntington's disease striatum and Alzheimer's disease temporal lobes. Neuroreport 1995;6:1053–1057.
40. Anderson AJ, Su JH, Cotman CW. DNA damage and apoptosis in Alzheimer's disease: colocalization with c-Jun immunoreactivity, relationship to brain area, and effect of postmortem delay. J Neurosci 1996;16:1710–1719.
41. Smale G, Nichols NR, Brady DR, Finch CE, Horton WJ. Evidence for apoptotic cell death in Alzheimer's disease. Exp Neurol 1995;133:225–230.
42. Su JH, Anderson AJ, Cummings BJ, Cotman CW. Immunohistochemical evidence for apoptosis in Alzheimer's disease. Neuroreport 1994;5:2529–2533.
43. de la Monte SM, Sohn YK, Ganju N, Wands JR. p53- and CD95-associated apoptosis in neurodegenerative diseases. Lab Invest 1998;158:1001–1009.
44. Jesionek-Kupnicka D, Buczynski J, Kordek R, Sobow T, Kloszewska I, Papierz W, et al. Programmed cell death (apoptosis) in Alzheimer's disease and Creutzfeldt-Jakob disease. Folia Neuropathol 1997;35:233–235.
45. Su JH, Deng G, Cotman CW. Bax protein expression is increased in Alzheimer's brain: correlations with DNA damage, Bcl-2 expression, and brain pathology. J Neuropathol Exp Neurol 1997;56:86–93.
46. Nagy ZS, Esiri MM. Apoptosis-related protein ex-

pression in the hippocampus in Alzheimer's disease. Neurobiol Aging 1997;18:565–571.
47. Nishimura T, Akiyama H, Yonehara S, Kondo H, Ikeda K, Kato M, et al. Fas antigen expression in brains of patients with Alzheimer-type dementia. Brain Res 1995;695:137–145.
48. MacGibbon GA, Lawlor PA, Sirimanne ES, Walton MR, Connor B, Young D, et al. Bax expression in mammalian neurons undergoing apoptosis, and in Alzheimer's disease hippocampus. Brain Res 1997;750: 223–234.
49. Allen RT, Cluck MW, Agrawal DK. Mechanisms controlling cellular suicide: role of Bcl-2 and caspases. Cell Mol Life Sci 1998;54:427–445.
50. Chen YC, Lin-Shiau SY, Lin JK. Involvement of reactive oxygen species and caspase 3 activation in arsenite-induced apoptosis [In Process Citation]. J Cell Physiol 1998;177:324–333.
51. Eskes R, Antonsson B, Osen-Sand A, Montessuit S, Richter C, Sadoul R, et al. Bax-induced cytochrome C release from mitochondria is independent of the permeability transition pore but highly dependent on Mg2+ ions [In Process Citation]. J Cell Biol 1998; 143:217–224.
52. Kitamura Y, Shimohama S, Kamoshima W, Ota T, Matsuoka Y, Nomura Y, et al. Alteration of proteins regulating apoptosis, Bcl-2, Bcl-x, Bax, Bak, Bad, ICH-1 and CPP32, in Alzheimer's disease. Brain Res 1998;780:260–269.
53. Rosse T, Olivier R, Monney L, Rager M, Conus S, Fellay I, et al. Bcl-2 prolongs cell survival after Bax-induced release of cytochrome c [see comments]. Nature 1998;391:496–499.
54. Widmann C, Gibson S, Johnson GL. Caspase-dependent cleavage of signaling proteins during apoptosis. A turn-off mechanism for anti-apoptotic signals. J Biol Chem 1998;273:7141–7147.
55. Desjardins P, Ledoux S. Expression of ced-3 and ced-9 homologs in Alzheimer's disease cerebral cortex. Neurosci Lett 1998;244:69–72.
56. Griffin WS. Brain interleukin 1 and S-100 immunoreactivity are elevated in Down syndrome and Alzheimer disease. Proc Natl Acad Sci USA 1989;86: 7611–7615.
57. Erro E, Tunon T. [Preliminary results of the study of neuronal death and the expression of bcl-2 protein in Alzheimer's disease]. Rev Med Univ Navarra 1997;41: 28–33.
58. Su JH, Satou T, Anderson AJ, Cotman CW. Up-regulation of Bcl-2 is associated with neuronal DNA damage in Alzheimer's disease. Neuroreport 1996;7: 437–440.
59. Mullaart E, Boerrigter ME, Ravid R, Swaab DF, Vijg J. Increased levels of DNA breaks in cerebral cortex of Alzheimer's disease patients. Neurobiol Aging 1990;11:169–173.
60. Perry G, Nunomura A, Lucassen P, Lassmann H, Smith MA. Apoptosis and Alzheimer's disease [letter; comment]. Science 1998;282:1268–1269.
61. Troncoso JC, Sukhov RR, Kawas CH, Koliatsos VE. In situ labeling of dying cortical neurons in normal aging and in Alzheimer's disease: correlations with senile plaques and disease progression. J Neuropathol Exp Neurol 1996;55:1134–1142.
62. Stadelmann C, Bruck W, Bancher C, Jellinger K, Lassmann H. Alzheimer disease: DNA fragmentation indicates increased neuronal vulnerability, but not apoptosis. J Neuropathol Exp Neurol 1998;57:456–464.
63. Ott A, Stolk RP, Hofman A, van Harskamp F, Grobbee DE, Breteler MM. Association of diabetes mellitus and dementia: the Rotterdam Study. Diabetologia 1996;39:1392–1397.
64. Sayre LM, Zagorski MG, Surewicz WK, Krafft GA, Perry G. Mechanisms of neurotoxicity associated with amyloid beta deposition and the role of free radicals in the pathogenesis of Alzheimer's disease: a critical appraisal. Chem Res Toxicol 1997;10:518–526.
65. Sayre LM, Zelasko DA, Harris PL, Perry G, Salomon RG, Smith MA. 4-Hydroxynonenal-derived advanced lipid peroxidation end products are increased in Alzheimer's disease. J Neurochem 1997;68:2092–2097.
66. Smith MA, Harris PL, Sayre LM, Perry G. Iron accumulation in Alzheimer disease is a source of redox-generated free radicals. Proc Natl Acad Sci U S A 1997;94(18):9866–8.
67. Smith MA, Perry G. Free radical damage, iron, and Alzheimer's disease. J Neurol Sci 1995;134 Suppl:92–94.
68. Smith MA, Perry G, Richey PL, Sayre LM, Anderson VE, Beal MF, et al. Oxidative damage in Alzheimer's [letter]. Nature 1996;382:120–121.
69. Yan SD, Yan SF, Chen X, Fu J, Chen M, Kuppusamy P, et al. Non-enzymatically glycated tau in Alzheimer's disease induces neuronal oxidant stress resulting in cytokine gene expression and release of amyloid beta-peptide. Nat Med 1995;1:693–699.
70. Ozawa T. Mitochondrial DNA mutations associated with aging and degenerative diseases. Exp Gerontol 1995;30:269–290.
71. Ozawa T. Genetic and functional changes in mitochondria associated with aging. Physiol Rev 1997;77: 425–464.
72. Richter C. Reactive oxygen and DNA damage in mitochondria. Mutat Res 1992;275:249–255.
73. Richter C. Oxidative damage to mitochondrial DNA and its relationship to ageing. Int J Biochem Cell Biol 1995;27:647–653.
74. Schapira AHV. Mitochondrial dysfunction in neurodegenerative disorders and aging. In: Schapira AHV, DiMauro S, editors. Mitochondrial Disorders in Neurology. London: Butterworth-Heinemann Ltd; 1994. p. 227–224.
75. Higuchi Y, Linn S. Purification of all forms of HeLa cell mitochondrial DNA and assessment of damage to it caused by hydrogen peroxide treatment of mitochondria or cells. J Biol Chem 1995;270:7950–7956.
76. Lemasters JJ. V. Necrapoptosis and the mitochondrial permeability transition: shared pathways to necrosis and apoptosis. Am J Physiol 1999;276(1 Pt 1):G1–G6.
77. Lieberthal W, Koh JS, Levine JS. Necrosis and apoptosis in acute renal failure. Semin Nephrol 1998;18: 505–518.
78. Lelli JL, Jr., Becks LL, Dabrowska MI, Hinshaw DB. ATP converts necrosis to apoptosis in oxidant-injured endothelial cells. Free Radic Biol Med 1998;25:694–702.
79. Kluck RM, Bossy-Wetzel E, Green DR, Newmeyer DD. The release of cytochrome c from mitochondria: a primary site for Bcl-2 regulation of apoptosis [see comments]. Science 1997;275(5303):1132–1136.
80. Yang J, Liu X, Bhalla K, Kim CN, Ibrado AM, Cai J,

et al. Prevention of apoptosis by Bcl-2: release of cytochrome c from mitochondria blocked [see comments]. Science 1997;275(5303):1129–1132.
81. Kish SJ. Brain energy metabolizing enzymes in Alzheimer's disease: alpha- ketoglutarate dehydrogenase complex and cytochrome oxidase. Ann N Y Acad Sci 1997;826:218–228.
82. Parker WD, Jr., Filley CM, Parks JK. Cytochrome oxidase deficiency in Alzheimer's disease. Neurology 1990;40(8):1302–1303.
83. Price DL, Sisodia SS, Gandy SE. Amyloid beta amyloidosis in Alzheimer's disease. Curr Opin Neurol 1995;8:268–274.
84. Querfurth HW, Wijsman EM, St G, Hyslop PH, Selkoe DJ. Beta APP mRNA transcription is increased in cultured fibroblasts from the familial Alzheimer's disease-1 family. Brain Res Mol Brain Res 1995;28:319–337.
85. LaFerla FM, Hall CK, Ngo L, Jay G. Extracellular deposition of beta-amyloid upon p53-dependent neuronal cell death in transgenic mice. J Clin Invest 1996;98(7):1626–1632.
86. Oster GM, McPhie DL, Greenan J, Neve RL. Age-dependent neuronal and synaptic degeneration in mice transgenic for the C terminus of the amyloid precursor protein. J Neurosci 1996;16(21):6732–6741.
87. Hsiao KK, Borchelt DR, Olson K, Johannsdottir R, Kitt C, Yunis W, et al. Age-related CNS disorder and early death in transgenic FVB/N mice overexpressing Alzheimer amyloid precursor proteins. Neuron 1995;15:1203–1218.
88. Sandhu FA, Salim M, Zain SB. Expression of the human beta-amyloid protein of Alzheimer's disease specifically in the brains of transgenic mice. J Biol Chem 1991;266:21331–21334.
89. Giambarella U, Yamatsuji T, Okamoto T, Matsui T, Ikezu T, Murayama Y, et al. G protein betagamma complex-mediated apoptosis by familial Alzheimer's disease mutant of APP. Embo J 1997;16:4897–4907.
90. Essalmani R, Macq AF, Mercken L, Octave JN. Missense mutations associated with familial Alzheimer's disease in Sweden lead to the production of the amyloid peptide without internalization of its precursor. Biochem Biophys Res Commun 1996;218:89–96.
91. Maruyama K, Terakado K, Usami M, Yoshikawa K. Formation of amyloid-like fibrils in COS cells overexpressing part of the Alzheimer amyloid protein precursor. Nature 1990;347(6293):566–569.
92. Tortosa A, Lopez E, Ferrer I. Bcl-2 and Bax protein expression in Alzheimer's disease. Acta Neuropathol (Berl) 1998;95:407–412.
93. Prehn JH, Bindokas VP, Jordan J, Galindo MF, Ghadge GD, Roos RP, et al. Protective effect of transforming growth factor-beta 1 on beta-amyloid neurotoxicity in rat hippocampal neurons. Mol Pharmacol 1996;49:319–328.
94. Paradis E, Douillard H, Koutroumanis M, Goodyer C, LeBlanc A. Amyloid beta peptide of Alzheimer's disease downregulates Bcl-2 and upregulates bax expression in human neurons. J Neurosci 1996;16(23):7533–7539.
95. Pappolla MA, Chyan YJ, Omar RA, Hsiao K, Perry G, Smith MA, et al. Evidence of oxidative stress and in vivo neurotoxicity of beta-amyloid in a transgenic mouse model of Alzheimer's disease: a chronic oxidative paradigm for testing antioxidant therapies in vivo. Am J Pathol 1998;152:871–877.
96. Forloni G, Bugiani O, Tagliavini F, Salmona M. Apoptosis-mediated neurotoxicity induced by beta-amyloid and PrP fragments. Mol Chem Neuropathol 1996;28:163–171.
97. Behl C, Sagara Y. Mechanism of amyloid beta protein induced neuronal cell death: current concepts and future perspectives. J Neural Transm Suppl 1997;49:125–134.
98. Gray CW, Patel AJ. Neurodegeneration mediated by glutamate and beta-amyloid peptide: a comparison and possible interaction. Brain Res 1995;691:169–179.
99. Sopher BL, Fukuchi K, Kavanagh TJ, Furlong CE, Martin GM. Neurodegenerative mechanisms in Alzheimer disease. A role for oxidative damage in amyloid beta protein precursor-mediated cell death. Mol Chem Neuropathol 1996;29:153–168.
100. Guo Q, Furukawa K, Sopher BL, Pham DG, Xie J, Robinson N, et al. Alzheimer's PS-1 mutation perturbs calcium homeostasis and sensitizes PC12 cells to death induced by amyloid beta-peptide. Neuroreport 1996;8:379–383.
101. Guo Q, Sopher BL, Furukawa K, Pham DG, Robinson N, Martin GM, et al. Alzheimer's presenilin mutation sensitizes neural cells to apoptosis induced by trophic factor withdrawal and amyloid beta-peptide: involvement of calcium and oxyradicals. J Neurosci 1997;17:4212–4222.
102. Levy LE, Poorkaj P, Wang K, Fu YH, Oshima J, Mulligan J, et al. Genomic structure and expression of STM2, the chromosome 1 familial Alzheimer disease gene. Genomics 1996;34:198–204.
103. Levy-Lahad E, Wasco W, Poorkaj P, Romano DM, Oshima J, Pettingell WH, et al. Candidate gene for the chromosome 1 familial Alzheimer's disease locus [see comments]. Science 1995;269(5226):973–977.
104. Sherrington R, Rogaev EI, Liang Y, Rogaeva EA, Levesque G, Ikeda M, et al. Cloning of a gene bearing missense mutations in early-onset familial Alzheimer's disease. Nature 1995;375:754–759.
105. Cribbs DH, Chen LS, Bende SM, LaFerla FM. Widespread neuronal expression of the presenilin-1 early-onset Alzheimer's disease gene in the murine brain. Am J Pathol 1996;148:1797–806.
106. Suzuki T, Nishiyama K, Murayama S, Yamamoto A, Sato S, Kanazawa I, et al. Regional and cellular presenilin 1 gene expression in human and rat tissues. Biochem Biophys Res Commun 1996;219:708–713.
107. Janicki S, Monteiro MJ. Increased apoptosis arising from increased expression of the Alzheimer's disease-associated presenilin-2 mutation (N141I). J Cell Biol 1997;139:485–495.
108. Mattson MP, Guo Q, Furukawa K, Pedersen WA. Presenilins, the endoplasmic reticulum, and neuronal apoptosis in Alzheimer's disease. J Neurochem 1998;70:1–14.
109. Wolozin B, Iwasaki K, Vito P, Ganjei JK, Lacana E, Sunderland T, et al. Participation of presenilin 2 in apoptosis: enhanced basal activity conferred by an Alzheimer mutation. Science 1996;274(5293):1710–1713.
110. Bancher C, Lassmann H, Breitschopf H, Jellinger KA. Mechanisms of cell death in Alzheimer's disease. J Neural Transm Suppl 1997;50:141–152.

111. Simonian NA, Coyle JT. Oxidative stress in neurodegenerative diseases. Annu Rev Pharmacol Toxicol 1996;36:83–106.
112. Markesbery WR. Oxidative stress hypothesis in Alzheimer's disease. Free Radic Biol Med 1997;23:134–147.
113. Olanow CW, Arendash GW. Metals and free radicals in neurodegeneration. Curr Opin Neurol 1994;7:548–558.
114. Mukherjee SK, Adams JJ. The effects of aging and neurodegeneration on apoptosis-associated DNA fragmentation and the benefits of nicotinamide. Mol Chem Neuropathol 1997;32:59–74.
115. Jenner P. Oxidative stress in Parkinson's disease and other neurodegenerative disorders. Pathol Biol (Paris) 1996;44:57–64.
116. Chandrasekaran K, Giordano T, Brady DR, Stoll J, Martin LJ, Rapoport SI. Impairment in mitochondrial cytochrome oxidase gene expression in Alzheimer disease. Brain Res Mol Brain Res 1994;24:336–340.
117. Le-Prince G, Delaere P, Fages C, Lefrancois T, Touret M, Salanon M, et al. Glutamine synthetase (GS) expression is reduced in senile dementia of the Alzheimer type. Neurochem Res 1995;20:859–862.
118. Gotz ME, Kunig G, Riederer P, Youdim MB. Oxidative stress: free radical production in neural degeneration. Pharmacol Ther 1994;63:37–122.
119. Beal MF. Mitochondria, free radicals, and neurodegeneration. Curr Opin Neurobiol 1996;6:661–666.
120. Ince PG, Tomkins J, Slade JY, Thatcher NM, Shaw PJ. Amyotrophic lateral sclerosis associated with genetic abnormalities in the gene encoding Cu/Zn superoxide dismutase: molecular pathology of five new cases, and comparison with previous reports and 73 sporadic cases of ALS. J Neuropathol Exp Neurol 1998;57:895–904.
121. Chou SM. Neuropathology of amyotrophic lateral sclerosis: new perspectives on an old disease. J Formos med Assoc 1997;96:488–498.
122. Morrison BM, Janssen WG, Gordon JW, Morrison JH. Time course of neuropathology in the spinal cord of G86R superoxide dismutase transgenic mice. J Comp Neurol 1998;391:64–77.
123. Dal Canto MC, Gurney ME. Development of central nervous system pathology in a murine transgenic model of human amyotrophic lateral sclerosis. Am J Pathol 1994;145:1271–1279.
124. Dal Canto MC, Gurney ME. Neuropathological changes in two lines of mice carrying a transgene for mutant human Cu, Zn SOD, and in mice overexpressing wild type human SOD: a model of familial amyotrophic lateral sclerosis (FALS). Brain Res 1995;676:25–40.
125. Groner Y, Elroy-Stein O, Avraham KB, Yarom R, Schickler M, Knobler H, et al. Down syndrome clinical symptoms are manifested in transfected cells and transgenic mice overexpressing the human Cu/Zn-superoxide dismutase gene. J Physiol 1990;84:53–77.
126. Groner Y, Elroy-Stein O, Avraham KB, Schickler M, Knobler H, Minc-Golomb D, et al. Cell damage by excess CuZnSOD and Down's syndrome. Biomed Pharmacother 1994;48:231–240.
127. Antila E, Westermarck T. On the etiopathogenesis and therapy of Down syndrome. Int J Dev Biol 1989;33:183–188.
128. Margaglione M, Garofano R, Cirillo F, Ruocco A, Grandone E, Vecchione G, et al. Cu/Zn superoxide dismutase in patients with non-familial Alzheimer's disease. Aging (Milano) 1995;7:49–54.
129. de la Monte SM, Bloch KD. Aberrant expression of the constitutive endothelial nitric oxide synthase gene in Alzheimer disease. Mol Chem Neuropathol 1997;30:139–159.
130. Premkumar DR, Smith MA, Richey PL, Petersen RB, Castellani R, Kutty RK, et al. Induction of heme oxygenase-1 mRNA and protein in neocortex and cerebral vessels in Alzheimer's disease. J Neurochem 1995;65:1399–1402.
131. Sohn YK, Ganju N, Bloch KD, de la Monte SM. Neuritic sprouting with aberrant expression of the nitric oxide synthase 3 gene in neurodegenerative diseases. J Neurol Sci 1999:(In Press).
132. Schmidt H, Walter U. NO at work. Cell 1994;78:919–925.
133. Leist M, Fava E, Montecucco C, Nicotera P. Peroxynitrite and nitric oxide donors induce neuronal apoptosis by eliciting autocrine excitotoxicity. Eur J Neurosci 1997;9:1488–1498.
134. Pou S, Pou W, Bredt D, Snyder S, Rosen G. Generation of superoxide by purified brain nitric oxide synthase. J Biol Chem 1992;267:24173–24176.
135. Stamler J. Nitration and related target interactions of nitric oxide (Review). Cell 1994;78:931–936.
136. Xia Y, Dawson V, Dawson T, Snyder S, Zweier J. Nitric oxide synthase generates superoxide and nitric oxide in arginine-depleted cells leading to peroxynitrite-mediated cellular injury. Proc Natl Acad Sci USA 1996;93:6770–6774.
137. Maines MD. Heme oxygenase: function, multiplicity, regulatory mechanisms, and clinical applications. FASEB J 1988;2:2557–2568.
138. Schipper HM, Cisse S, Stopa EG. Expression of heme oxygenase-1 in the senescent and Alzheimer-diseased brain. Ann Neurol 1995;37:758–768.
139. Durante W, Christodoulides N, Cheng K, Peyton KJ, Sunahara RK, Schafer AI. cAMP induces heme oxygenase-1 gene expression and carbon monoxide production in vascular smooth muscle. Am J Physiol 1997;273(1 Pt 2):H317–H323.
140. Kurata S, Matsumoto M, Yamashita U. Concomitant transcriptional activation of nitric oxide synthase and heme oxygenase genes during nitric oxide-mediated macrophage cytostasis. J Biochem (Tokyo) 1996;120:49–52.
141. Seki T, Naruse M, Naruse K, Yoshimoto T, Tanabe A, Imaki T, et al. Interrelation between nitric oxide synthase and heme oxygenase in rat endothelial cells. Eur J Pharmacol 1997;331:87–91.
142. Masliah E, Terry RD, DeTeresa RM, Hansen LA. Immunohistochemical quantification of the synapse-related protein synaptophysin in Alzheimer disease. Neurosci Lett 1989;103:234–239.
143. DeKosky ST, Scheff SW. Synapse loss in frontal cortex biopsies in Alzheimer's disease: correlation with cognitive severity. Ann Neurol 1990;27:457–464.
144. DeKosky ST, Scheff SW, Styren SD. Structural correlates of cognition in dementia: quantification and assessment of synapse change. Neurodegeneration 1996;5:417–421.

145. Scheff SW, Price DA. Synapse loss in the temporal lobe in Alzheimer's disease. Ann Neurol 1993;33:190–199.
146. Terry RD, Masliah E, Salmon DP, Butters N, DeTeresa R, Hill R, et al. Physical basis of cognitive alterations in Alzheimer's disease: synapse loss is the major correlate of cognitive impairment. Ann Neurol 1991;30:572–580.
147. Scheff SW, Sparks L, Price DA. Quantitative assessment of synaptic density in the entorhinal cortex in Alzheimer's disease [see comments]. Ann Neurol 1993;34:356–361.
148. Scheff SW, Sparks DL, Price DA. Quantitative assessment of synaptic density in the outer molecular layer of the hippocampal dentate gyrus in Alzheimer's disease. Dementia 1996;7:226–232.
149. Samuel W, Terry RD, DeTeresa R, Butters N, Masliah E. Clinical correlates of cortical and nucleus basalis pathology in Alzheimer dementia. Arch Neurol 1994;51:772–778.
150. Davies CA, Mann DM, Sumpter PQ, Yates PO. A quantitative morphometric analysis of the neuronal and synaptic content of the frontal and temporal cortex in patients with Alzheimer's disease. J Neurol Sci 1987;78:151–164.
151. Baloyannis SJ, Manolidis SL, Manolidis LS. The acoustic cortex in Alzheimer's disease. Acta Otolaryngol Suppl (Stockh) 1992;494:1–13.
152. Masliah E, Hansen L, Albright T, Mallory M, Terry RD. Immunoelectron microscopic study of synaptic pathology in Alzheimer's disease. Acta Neuropathol (Berl) 1991;81:428–433.
153. Masliah E, Mallory M, Hansen L, Alford M, Albright T, DeTeresa R, et al. Patterns of aberrant sprouting in Alzheimer's disease. Neuron 1991;6:729–739.
154. Masliah E, Ellisman M, Carragher B, Mallory M, Young S, Hansen L, et al. Three-dimensional analysis of the relationship between synaptic pathology and neuropil threads in Alzheimer disease. J Neuropathol Exp Neurol 1992;51:404–414.
155. Lassmann H, Weiler R, Fischer P, Bancher C, Jellinger K, Floor E, et al. Synaptic pathology in Alzheimer's disease: immunological data for markers of synaptic and large dense-core vesicles. Neuroscience 1992;46:1–8.
156. de la Monte SM, Ng SC, Hsu DW. Aberrant GAP-43 gene expression in Alzheimer's disease. Am J Pathol 1995;147:934–946.
157. de la Monte SM, Spratt RA, Chong J, Ghanbari HA, Wands JR. Immunohistochemical and histopathologic correlates of Alzheimer's disease-associated Alz-50 immunoreactivity quantified in homogenates of cerebral tissue. Am J Pathol 1992;141:1459–1469.
158. de la Monte SM, Wands JR. Diagnostic utility of quantitating neurofilament-immunoreactive Alzheimer's disease lesions. J Histochem Cytochem 1994;42:1625–1634.
159. Lassmann H, Fischer P, Jellinger K. Synaptic pathology of Alzheimer's disease. Ann N Y Acad Sci 1993;695:59–64.
160. Zilles K, Qu M, Schleicher A, Schroeter M, Kraemer M, Witte OW. Plasticity and neurotransmitter receptor changes in Alzheimer's disease and experimental cortical infarcts. Arzneimittelforschung 1995;45(3A):361–366.
161. Whitehouse PJ, Price DL, Struble RG, Clark AW, Coyle JT, Delon MR. Alzheimer's disease and senile dementia: loss of neurons in the basal forebrain. Science 1982;215(4537):1237–1239.
162. Dewan MJ, Gupta S. Current concepts in the treatment of Alzheimer's disease. Clin Ther 1992;14:2–10.
163. Adams IM. Structural plasticity of synapses in Alzheimer's disease. Mol Neurobiol 1991;5:411–419.
164. Bertoni FC, Fattoretti P, Casoli T, Meier RW, Ulrich J. Morphological adaptive response of the synaptic junctional zones in the human dentate gyrus during aging and Alzheimer's disease. Brain Res 1990;517:69–75.
165. Struble RG, Cork LC, Whitehouse PJ, Price DL. Cholinergic innervation in neuritic plaques. Science 1982;216(4544):413–415.
166. Peress NS, Perillo E. Differential expression of TGF-beta 1, 2 and 3 isotypes in Alzheimer's disease: a comparative immunohistochemical study with cerebral infarction, aged human and mouse control brains. J Neuropathol Exp Neurol 1995;54:802–811.
167. Masliah E, Mallory M, Hansen L, DeTeresa R, Alford M, Terry R. Synaptic and neuritic alterations during the progression of Alzheimer's disease. Neurosci Lett 1994;174:67–72.
168. Masliah E, Mallory M, DeTeresa R, Alford M, Hansen L. Differing patterns of aberrant neuronal sprouting in Alzheimer's disease with and without Lewy bodies. Brain Res 1993;617:258–266.
169. Cotman CW, Anderson KJ. Synaptic plasticity and functional stabilization in the hippocampal formation: possible role in Alzheimer's disease. Adv Neurol 1988;47:313–335.
170. Lippa CF, Hamos JE, Pulaski SD, DeGennaro LJ, Drachman DA. Alzheimer's disease and aging: effects on perforant pathway perikarya and synapses. Neurobiol Aging 1992;13:405–411.
171. McKee AC, Kosik KS, Kowall NW. Neuritic pathology and dementia in Alzheimer's disease. Ann Neurol 1991;30:156–165.
172. Good P, Werner P, Hsu A, OIlanow C, Perl D. Evidence of neuronal oxidative damage in Alzheimer's disease. Am J Pathol 1996;149:21–28.
173. Kuljis R, Schelper R. Alterations in nitrogen monoxide-synthesizing cortical neurons in amyotrophic lateral sclerosis with dementia. J Neuropathol Exp Neurol 1996;55:25–35.
174. Hunot S, Boissiere F, Faucheux B, Brugg B, Mouatt-Prigent A, Agid Y, et al. Nitric oxide synthase and neuronal vulnerability in Parkinson's disease. Neuroscience 1996;72:355–363.
175. Benzing W, Mufson E. Increased number of NADPH-d-positive neurons within the substantia innominata in Alzheimer's disease. Brain Res 1995;670:351–355.
176. Dawson T, Bredt D, Fotuhi M, Hwang P, Snyder S. Nitric oxide synthase and neuronal NADPH diaphorase are identical in brain and peripheral tissues. Proc Natl Acad Sci USA 1991;88:7797–7801.
177. Wolf G, Wurdig S, Shunzel G. Nitric oxide synthase in rat brain is predominantly located at neuronal endoplasmic reticulum: an electron microscopic demonstration of NADPH-diaphorase activity. Neurosci Lett 1992;147:63–66.
178. Moroz L, Winlow W, Turner R, Bulloch A, Luko-

wiak K, Syed N. Nitric oxide synthase-immunoreactive cells in the CNS and periphery of Lymnaea. Neuroreport 1994;5:1277–1280.
179. Son H, Hawkins R, Kiebler M, Huang P, Fishman M, Kandel E. Long-term potentiation is reduced in mice that are doubly mutant in endothelial and neuronal nitric oxide synthase. Cell 1996;87:1015–1023.
180. Bredt D, Snyder S. Transient nitric oxide synthase neurons in embryonic cerebral cortical plate, sensory ganglia, and olfactory epithelium. Neuron 1994;13:301–313.
181. Nowicky A, Bindman L. The nitric oxide synthase inhibitor, N-monomethyl-L-arginine blocks induction of a long-term potentiation-like phenomenon in rat medial frontal cortical neurons in vitro. J Neurophysiol 1993;70:1255–1259.
182. Peunova N, Enikolopov G. Nitric oxide triggers a switch to growth arrest during differentiation of neuronal cells. Nature 1995;375:68–73.
183. Ward S, Shuttleworth C, Kenyon J. Dorsal root ganglion neurons of embryonic chicks contain nitric oxide synthase and respond to nitric oxide. Brain Res 1994;648:249–258.
184. Yezierski R, Liu S, Ruenes G, Busto R, Dietrich W. Neuronal damage following intraspinal injection of a nitric oxide synthase inhibitor in the rat. J Cereb Blood Flow Metab 1996;16:996–1004.
185. Farinelli S, Park D, Greene L. Nitric oxide delays the death of trophic factor-deprived PC12 cells and sympathetic neurons by a cGMP-mediated mechanism. J Neurosci 1996;16:2325–2334.
186. Mesenge C, Verrecchia C, Allix M, Boulu R, Plotkine M. Reduction of the neurological deficit in mice with traumatic brain injury by nitric oxide synthase inhibitors. J Neurotrauma 1996;13:11–16.
187. Klatt P, Schmidt K, Uray G, Mayer B. Multiple catalytic functions of brain nitric oxide synthase. Biochemical characterization, cofactor requirement, and the role of Nw-hydroxy-L-arginine as an intermediate. J Biol Chem 1993;268:14781–14787.
188. Nishikawa T, Kirsch J, Koehler R, Bredt D, Snyder S, Traystmann R. Effect of nitric oxide synthase inhibition on cerebral blood flow and injury volume during focal ischemia in cats. Stroke 1993;24:1717–1724.
189. Ferriero D, Holtzman D, Black S, Sheldon R. Neonatal mice lacking neuronal nitric oxide synthase are less vulnerable to hypoxic-ischemic injury. Neurobiol Dis 1996;3:64–71.
190. Dawson V, Kizushi V, Huang P, Snyder S, Dawson T. Resistance to neurotoxicity in cortical cultures from neuronal nitric oxide synthase-deficient mice. J Neurosci 1996;16:2479–2487.
191. Crystal HA, Dickson DW, Sliwinski MJ, Lipton RB, Grober E, Marks NH, et al. Pathological markers associated with normal aging and dementia in the elderly. Ann Neurol 1993;34:566–573.
192. de la Torre J. Impaired brain microcirculation may trigger Alzheimer's disease. Neurosci Biobehav Rev 1994;18:397–401.
193. Dickson DW, Davies P, Bevona C, Van HK, Factor SM, Grober E, et al. Hippocampal sclerosis: a common pathological feature of dementia in very old (> or = 80 years of age) humans. Acta Neuropathol (Berl) 1994;88:212–221.
194. Frisoni GB, Beltramello A, Binetti G, Bianchetti A, Weiss C, Scuratti A, et al. Computed tomography in the detection of the vascular component in dementia. Gerontology 1995;41:121–128.
195. Ince PG, McArthur FK, Bjertness E, Torvik A, Candy JM, Edwardson JA. Neuropathological diagnoses in elderly patients in Oslo: Alzheimer's disease, Lewy body disease, vascular lesions. Dementia 1995;6:162–168.
196. Kawamura J, Meyer JS, Terayama Y, Weathers S. Leuko-araiosis and cerebral hypoperfusion compared in elderly normals and Alzheimer's dementia. J Am Geriatr Soc 1992;40:375–380.
197. Nagy Z, Esiri MM, Jobst KA, Morris JH, King EM, McDonald B, et al. The effects of additional pathology on the cognitive deficit in Alzheimer disease. J Neuropathol Exp Neurol 1997;56:165–70.
198. Pasquier F, Leys D. Why are stroke patients prone to develop dementia? J Neurol 1997;244:135–42.
199. Snowdon DA, Greiner LH, Mortimer JA, Riley KP, Greiner PA, Markesbery WR. Brain infarction and the clinical expression of Alzheimer disease. The Nun Study [see comments]. JAMA 1997;277:813–817.
200. Victoroff J, Mack WJ, Lyness SA, Chui HC. Multicenter clinicopathological correlation in dementia. Am J Psychiatry 1995;152:1476–1484.
201. Zahner B, Lang CJ, Engelhardt A, Thierauf P, Neundorfer B. A case of Alzheimer's disease with extensive focal white matter changes. Dementia 1995;6:294–300.
202. Betard C, Robitaille Y, Gee M, Tiberghien D, Larrivee D, Roy P, et al. Apo E allele frequencies in Alzheimer's disease, Lewy body dementia, Alzheimer's disease with cerebrovascular disease and vascular dementia. Neuroreport 1994;5:1893–1896.
203. Kalaria RN, Cohen DL, Premkumar DR. Apolipoprotein E alleles and brain vascular pathology in Alzheimer's disease. Ann N Y Acad Sci 1996;777:266–270.
204. Olichney JM, Hansen LA, Hofstetter CR, Grundman M, Katzman R, Thal LJ. Cerebral infarction in Alzheimer's disease is associated with severe amyloid angiopathy and hypertension. Arch Neurol 1995;52:702–708.
205. Premkumar DR, Cohen DL, Hedera P, Friedland RP, Kalaria RN. Apolipoprotein E-epsilon4 alleles in cerebral amyloid angiopathy and cerebrovascular pathology associated with Alzheimer's disease. Am J Pathol 1996;148:2083–2095.
206. Sevush S, Durara R, Rivero J, Pascal S, Barker WW. Clinicopathologic study of probable Alzheimer disease: assessment of criteria for excluding cerebrovascular disease. Alzheimer Dis Assoc Disord 1995;9:208–212.
207. Yoshitake T, Kiyohara Y, Kato I, Ohmura T, Iwamoto H, Nakayama K, et al. Incidence and risk factors of vascular dementia and Alzheimer's disease in a defined elderly Japanese population: the Hisayama Study. Neurology 1995;45:1161–1168.
208. Pantoni L, Garcia JH. Cognitive impairment and cellular/vascular changes in the cerebral white matter. Ann N Y Acad Sci 1997;826:92–102.
209. Etiene D, Kraft J, Ganju N, Gomez-Isla T, Gemelli B, Hyman BT, et al. Cerebrovascular pathology contributes to the heterogeneity of Alzheimer's disease. J Alz Dis 1998;1:1–16.

210. Tomimoto H, Akiguchi I, Suenaga T, Nishimura M, Wakita H, Nakamura S, et al. Alterations of the blood-brain barrier and glial cells in white-matter lesions in cerebrovascular and Alzheimer's disease patients [see comments]. Stroke 1996;27:2069–2074.
211. Tomimoto H, Akiguchi I, Wakita H, Suenaga T, Nakamura S, Kimura J. Regressive changes of astroglia in white matter lesions in cerebrovascular disease and Alzheimer's disease patients. Acta Neuropathol (Berl) 1997;94(2):146–52.
212. Lopez OL, Rabin BS, Huff FJ, Rezek D, Reinmuth OM. Serum autoantibodies in patients with Alzheimer's disease and vascular dementia and in nondemented control subjects. Stroke 1992;23:1078–1083.
213. Nagata K, Buchan RJ, Yokoyama E, Kondoh Y, Sato M, Terashi H, et al. Misery perfusion with preserved vascular reactivity in Alzheimer's disease. Ann N Y Acad Sci 1997;826:272–281.
214. Tohgi H, Yonezawa H, Takahashi S, Sato N, Kato E, Kudo M, et al. Cerebral blood flow and oxygen metabolism in senile dementia of Alzheimer's type and vascular dementia with deep white matter changes. Neuroradiology 1998;40:131–137.
215. Van Nostrand WE, Davis SJ, Saporito IS. Amyloid beta-protein induces the cerebrovascular cellular pathology of Alzheimer's disease and related disorders. Ann N Y Acad Sci 1996;777:297–302.
216. Thomas T, Thomas G, McLendon C, Sutton T, Mullan M. beta-Amyloid-mediated vasoactivity and vascular endothelial damage [see comments]. Nature 1996;380:168–171.
217. Thomas T, Sutton ET, Bryant MW, Rhodin JA. In vivo vascular damage, leukocyte activation and inflammatory response induced by beta-amyloid. J Submicrosc Cytol Pathol 1997;29:293–304.
218. Corder EH, Saunders A, Strittmatter WJ, al. e. Gene dosage of apolipoprotein E type 4 allele and the risk for Alzheimer's in late onset families. Science 1993; 261:921–923.
219. Farlow M, Murrell J, Ghetti B, Unverzagt F, Zeldenrust S, Benson M. Confirmation of the epsilon 4 allele of the apolipoprotein E gene as a risk factor for late-onset Alzheimer's disease [see comments]. Neurology 1994;44:342–344.
220. Marx J. Gene dose of apolipoprotein E type 4 allele and the risk of Alzheimer's disease in late onset families [see comments]. Science 1993;261:921–923.
221. Mayeux R, Stern Y, Ottman R, al. e. The apolipoprotein e4 allele in patients with Alzheimer's disease. Ann Neurol 1993;34:752–754.
222. Noguchi S, Murakami N, Yamada N. Apolipoprotein E genotype and Alzheimer's disease. Lancet 1993; 342:342–347.
223. Strittmatter WJ, Saunders A, Schmechel D, al. e. Apolipoprotein E: high affinity binding to b/A4 amyloid and increased frequency of type 4 allele in familial Alzheimer's disease. Proc Natl Acad Sci USA 1993;90:1977–1981.
224. Palumbo B, Parnetti L, Nocentini G, Cardinali L, Brancorsini S, Riccardi C, et al. Apolipoprotein-E genotype in normal aging, age-associated memory impairment, Alzheimer's disease and vascular dementia patients. Neurosci Lett 1997;231:59–61.
225. Treves TA, Bornstein NM, Chapman J, Klimovitzki S, Verchovsky R, Asherov A, et al. APOE-epsilon 4 in patients with Alzheimer disease and vascular dementia. Alzheimer Dis Assoc Disord 1996;10:189–91.
226. Wieringa GE, Burlinson S, Rafferty JA, Gowland E, Burns A. Apolipoprotein E genotypes and serum lipid levels in Alzheimer's disease and multi-infarct dementia. Int J Geriatr Psychiatry 1997;12:359–362.
227. Zubenko GS, Stiffler S, Stabler S, Kopp U, Hughes HB, Cohen BM, et al. Association of the apolipoprotein E epsilon 4 allele with clinical subtypes of autopsy-confirmed Alzheimer's disease. Am J Med Genet 1994;54:199–205.
228. Perry RT, Go RC, Harrell LE, Acton RT. Apolipoprotein E in the genetics and epidemiology of Alzheimer's disease. Am J Med Genet 1995;60:456–460.
229. Haan J, Van BC, van DC, Voorhoeve E, van HF, van SJ, et al. The apolipoprotein E epsilon 4 allele does not influence the clinical expression of the amyloid precursor protein gene codon 693 or 692 mutations. Ann Neurol 1994;36:434–437.
230. Bergem AL, Lannfelt L. Apolipoprotein E type epsilon4 allele, heritability and age at onset in twins with Alzheimer disease and vascular dementia. Clin Genet 1997;52:408–413.
231. Evans KC, Berger EP, Cho CG, Weisgraber KH, Lansbury PJ. Quantitative analysis of senile plaques in Alzheimer disease: observation of log-normal size distribution and molecular epidemiology of differences associated with apolipoprotein E genotype and trisomy 21 (Down syndrome). Proc Natl Acad Sci U S A 1995;92:3586–3590.
232. Yamatsuji T, Okamoto T, Shizu T, Murayama Y, Tanaka N, Nishimoto I. Expression of V642 APP mutant causes cellular apoptosis as Alzheimer train-linked phenotype. EMBO 1996;15:498–509.
233. Zarow C, Barron E, Chui HC, Perlmutter LS. Vascular basement membrane pathology and Alzheimer's disease. Ann N Y Acad Sci 1997;826:147–60.
234. Hofman A, Ott A, Breteler MM, Bots ML, Slooter AJ, van Harskamp F, et al. Atherosclerosis, apolipoprotein E, and prevalence of dementia and Alzheimer's disease in the Rotterdam Study [see comments]. Lancet 1997;349:151–154.
235. Schneider R, Ringelstein EB, Zeumer H, Kiesewetter H, Jung F. The role of plasma hyperviscosity in subcortical arteriosclerotic encephalopathy (Binswanger's disease). J Neurol 1987;234:67–73.
236. Skoog I, Palmertz B, Andreasson LA. The prevalence of white-matter lesions on computed tomography of the brain in demented and nondemented 85-year-olds. J Geriatr Psychiatry Neurol 1994;7: 169–75.
237. de la Torre JC. Critical threshold cerebral hypoperfusion causes Alzheimer's disease? Acta Neuropathol (Berl) 1999;98:1–8.
238. de la Torre JC, Mussivand T. Can disturbed brain microcirculation cause Alzheimer's disease? Neurol Res 1993;15:146–53.
239. Kalaria RN, Harik SI. Reduced glucose transporter at the blood-brain barrier and in cerebral cortex in Alzheimer disease. J Neurochem 1989;53:1083–1088.
240. Simpson IA, Chundu KR, Davies-Hill T, Honer WG, Davies P. Decreased concentrations of GLUT1 and GLUT3 glucose transporters in the brains of patients with Alzheimer's disease [see comments]. Ann Neurol 1994;35:546–551.

241. de la Torre JC. Cerebromicrovascular pathology in Alzheimer's disease compared to normal aging. Gerontology 1997;43:26–43.
242. Bobinski M, de Leon MJ, Tarnawski M, Wegiel J, Reisberg B, Miller DC, et al. Neuronal and volume loss in CA1 of the hippocampal formation uniquely predicts duration and severity of Alzheimer disease. Brain Res 1998;805:267–269.
243. Wong-Riley MT. Cytochrome oxidase: an endogenous metabolic marker for neuronal activity. Trends Neurosci 1989;12:94–101.
244. Abdollahian NP, Cada A, Gonzalez-Lima F, de la Torre JC. Cytochrome oxidase: a predictive marker of neurodegeneration. In: Gonzalez-lima F, editor. Cytochrome Oxidase in Neuronal Metabolism and Alzheimer's Disease. New York: Plenum Press; 1998. p. 233–261.
245. Eikelenboom P, Zhan SS, van Gool WA, Allsop D. Inflammatory mechanisms in Alzheimer's disease. Trends Pharmacol Sci 1994;15:447–450.
246. de la Torre JC. Hemodynamic consequences of deformed microvessels in the brain in Alzheimer's disease. Ann N Y Acad Sci 1997;826:75–91.
247. Johnson KA, Jones K, Holman BL, Becker JA, Spiers PA, Satlin A, et al. Preclinical prediction of Alzheimer's disease using SPECT. Neurology 1998;50:1563–1571.
248. Jagust WJ, Eberling JL, Reed BR, Mathis CA, Budinger TF. Clinical studies of cerebral blood flow in Alzheimer's disease. Ann N Y Acad Sci 1997;826:254–262.
249. Celsis P, Agniel A, Cardebat D, Demonet JF, Ousset PJ, Puel M. Age related cognitive decline: a clinical entity? A longitudinal study of cerebral blood flow and memory performance. J Neurol Neurosurg Psychiatry 1997;62(6):601–608.
250. Meier-Ruge W, Bertoni-Freddari C. The significance of glucose turnover in the brain in the pathogenetic mechanisms of Alzheimer's disease. Rev Neurosci 1996;7:1–19.
251. Prohovnik I, Mayeux R, Sackeim HA, Smith G, Stern Y, Alderson PO. Cerebral perfusion as a diagnostic marker of early Alzheimer's disease. Neurology 1988;38:931–937.
252. Waldemar G, Hogh P, Paulson OB. Functional brain imaging with single-photon emission computed tomography in the diagnosis of Alzheimer's disease. Int Psychogeriatr 1997;9(Suppl 1):223–7; discussion 247–252.
253. Montaldi D, Brooks DN, McColl JH, Wyper D, Patterson J, Barron E, et al. Measurements of regional cerebral blood flow and cognitive performance in Alzheimer's disease. J Neurol Neurosurg Psychiatry 1990;53:33–38.
254. Ajmani RS, Metter EJ, Jaykumar R, Ingram DK, Spangler EL, Abugo O, et al. Hemodynamic changes during aging associated with cerebral blood flow and impaired cognitive function. Neurobiol Aging 2000;21:257–269.
255. Yamaji S, Ishii K, Sasaki M, Imamura T, Kitagaki H, Sakamoto S, et al. Changes in cerebral blood flow and oxygen metabolism related to magnetic resonance imaging white matter hyperintensities in Alzheimer's disease. J Nucl Med 1997;38:1471–1474.
256. De Jong GI, Farkas E, Stienstra CM, Plass JR, Keijser JN, de la Torre JC, et al. Cerebral hypoperfusion yields capillary damage in the hippocampal CA1 area that correlates with spatial memory impairment. Neuroscience 1999;91:203–10.
257. Eckert A, Forstl H, Zerfass R, Oster M, Hennerici M, Muller WE. Changes of intracellular calcium regulation in Alzheimer's disease and vascular dementia. J Neural Transm Suppl 1998;54:201–210.
258. Mancardi GL, Perdelli F, Rivano C, Leonardi A, Bugiani O. Thickening of the basement membrane of cortical capillaries in Alzheimer's disease. Acta Neuropathol 1980;49:79–83.
259. Kalaria RN, Hedera P. Differential degeneration of the cerebral microvasculature in Alzheimer's disease. Neuroreport 1995;6:477–480.
260. Joachim CL, Morris JH, Selkoe DJ. Clinically diagnosed Alzheimer's disease: autopsy results in 150 cases [see comments]. Ann Neurol 1988;24:50–56.
261. Lehtovirta M, Kuikka J, Helisalmi S, Hartikainen P, Mannermaa A, Ryynanen M, et al. Longitudinal SPECT study in Alzheimer's disease: relation to apolipoprotein E polymorphism. J Neurol Neurosurg Psychiatry 1998;64(6):742–746.
262. Tsuchiya M, Sako K, Yura S, Yonemasu Y. Local cerebral glucose utilisation following acute and chronic bilateral carotid artery ligation in Wistar rats: relation to changes in local cerebral blood flow. Exp Brain Res 1993;95:1–7.
263. Ni JW, Matsumoto K, Li HB, Murakami Y, Watanabe H. Neuronal damage and decrease of central acetylcholine level following permanent occlusion of bilateral common carotid arteries in rat. Brain Res 1995;673:290–296.
264. de la Torre JC, Cada A, Nelson N, Davis G, Sutherland RJ, Gonzalez-Lima F. Reduced cytochrome oxidase and memory dysfunction after chronic brain ischemia in aged rats. Neurosci Lett 1997;223:165–168.
265. de la Torre JC, Fortin T. A chronic physiological rat model of dementia. Behav Brain Res 1994;63:35–40.
266. Suo Z, Humphrey J, Kundtz A, Sethi F, Placzek A, Crawford F, et al. Soluble Alzheimers beta-amyloid constricts the cerebral vasculature in vivo. Neurosci Lett 1998;257:77–80.
267. Su GC, Arendash GW, Kalaria RN, Bjugstad KB, Mullan M. Intravascular infusions of soluble beta-amyloid compromise the blood-brain barrier, activate CNS glial cells and induce peripheral hemorrhage. Brain Res 1999;818:105–117.
268. Crawford F, Suo Z, Fang C, Sawar A, Su G, Arendash G, et al. The vasoactivity of A beta peptides. Ann N Y Acad Sci 1997;826:35–46.
269. Iadecola C, Zhang F, Niwa K, Eckman C, Turner SK, Fischer E, et al. SOD1 rescues cerebral endothelial dysfunction in mice overexpressing amyloid precursor protein. Nat Neurosci 1999;2:157–161.
270. Mielke R, Moller HJ, Erkinjuntti T, Rosenkranz B, Rother M, Kittner B. Propentofylline in the treatment of vascular dementia and Alzheimer-type dementia: overview of phase I and phase II clinical trials. Alzheimer Dis Assoc Disord 1998;12(Suppl 2):S29–S35.
271. Wallin A. The overlap between Alzheimer's disease and vascular dementia: the role of white matter changes. Dement Geriatr Cogn Disord 1998;9 Suppl 1:30–35.
272. Englund E. Neuropathology of white matter changes

273. Erecinska M, Silver IA. ATP and brain function. J Cereb Blood Flow Metab 1989;9:2–19.
274. Winocur G, Gagnon S. Glucose treatment attenuates spatial learning and memory deficits of aged rats on tests of hippocampal function. Neurobiol Aging 1998;19:233–241.
275. Meier-Ruge WA, Bertoni-Freddari C. Pathogenesis of decreased glucose turnover and oxidative phosphorylation in ischemic and trauma-induced dementia of the Alzheimer type. Ann N Y Acad Sci 1997; 826:229–241.
276. Hoyer S. Oxidative metabolism deficiencies in brains of patients with Alzheimer's disease. Acta Neurol Scand Suppl 1996;165:18–24.
277. Whitesell RR, Ward M, McCall AL, Granner DK, May JM. Coupled glucose transport and metabolism in cultured neuronal cells: determination of the rate-limiting step. J Cereb Blood Flow Metab 1995; 15: 814–826.
278. Liguri G, Taddei N, Nassi P, Latorraca S, Nediani C, Sorbi S. Changes in Na+,K(+)-ATPase, Ca2(+)-ATPase and some soluble enzymes related to energy metabolism in brains of patients with Alzheimer's disease. Neurosci Lett 1990;112:338–342.
279. Pardridge WM. Glucose transport and phosphorylation: which is rate limiting for brain glucose utilization? [editorial; comment] [see comments]. Ann Neurol 1994;35(5):511–2.
280. Braak H, Braak E. Diagnostic criteria for neuropathologic assessment of Alzheimer's disease. Neurobiol Aging 1997;18(4 Suppl):S85–S88.
281. Arriagada PV, Marzloff K, Hyman BT. Distribution of Alzheimer-type pathologic changes in nondemented elderly individuals matches the pattern in Alzheimer's disease [see comments]. Neurology 1992;42:1681–1688.
282. Robakis NK. In: Terry RD, Katzman R, Bick KL, editors. Alzheimer's Disease. New York: raven Press; 1994. p. 317–326.
283. Hsiao K, Chapman P, Nilsen S, Eckman C, Harigaya Y, Younkin S, et al. Correlative memory deficits, Abeta elevation, and amyloid plaques in transgenic mice [see comments]. Science 1996;274:99–102.
284. Irizarry MC, Soriano F, McNamara M, Page KJ, Schenk D, Games D, et al. Abeta deposition is associated with neuropil changes, but not with overt neuronal loss in the human amyloid precursor protein V717F (PDAPP) transgenic mouse. J Neurosci 1997;17:7053–7059.
285. Mattson MP, Cheng B, Davis D, Bryant K, Lieberburg I, Rydel RE. beta-Amyloid peptides destabilize calcium homeostasis and render human cortical neurons vulnerable to excitotoxicity. J Neurosci 1992;12: 376–389.
286. Ueda K, Fukushima H, Masliah E, Xia Y, Iwai A, Yoshimoto M, et al. Molecular cloning of cDNA encoding an unrecognized component of amyloid in Alzheimer disease. Proc Natl Acad Sci U S A 1993; 90:11282–11286.
287. Jakes R, Spillantini MG, Goedert M. Identification of two distinct synucleins from human brain. FEBS Lett 1994;345:27–32.
288. Jensen PH, Hojrup P, Hager H, Nielsen MS, Jacobsen L, Olesen OF, et al. Binding of Abeta to alpha- and beta-synucleins: identification of segments in alpha-synuclein/NAC precursor that bind Abeta and NAC. Biochem J 1997;323(Pt 2):539–46.
289. Iwai A, Masliah E, Yoshimoto M, Ge N, Flanagan L, de Silva HA, et al. The precursor protein of non-A beta component of Alzheimer's disease amyloid is a presynaptic protein of the central nervous system. Neuron 1995;14:467–475.
290. Masliah E, Iwai A, Mallory M, Ueda K, Saitoh T. Altered presynaptic protein NACP is associated with plaque formation and neurodegeneration in Alzheimer's disease. Am J Pathol 1996;148:201–210.
291. Yoshimoto M, Iwai A, Kang D, Otero DA, Xia Y, Saitoh T. NACP, the precursor protein of the non-amyloid beta/A4 protein (A beta) component of Alzheimer disease amyloid, binds A beta and stimulates A beta aggregation. Proc Natl Acad Sci U S A 1995; 92:9141–9145.
292. Polymeropoulos MH, Lavedan C, Leroy E, Ide SE, Dehejia A, Dutra A, et al. Mutation in the alpha-synuclein gene identified in families with Parkinson's disease [see comments]. Science 1997;276:2045–2047.
293. Spillantini MG, Schmidt ML, Lee VM, Trojanowski JQ, Jakes R, Goedert M. Alpha-synuclein in Lewy bodies [letter]. Nature 1997;388:839–840.
294. Takeda A, Mallory M, Sundsmo M, Honer W, Hansen L, Masliah E. Abnormal accumulation of NACP/alpha-synuclein in neurodegenerative disorders. Am J Pathol 1998;152:367–372.
295. Iwai A, Masliah E, Sundsmo MP, DeTeresa R, Mallory M, Salmon DP, et al. The synaptic protein NACP is abnormally expressed during the progression of Alzheimer's disease. Brain Res 1996;720: 230–234.
296. Nishimura M, Tomimoto H, Suenaga T, Nakamura S, Namba Y, Ikeda K, et al. Synaptophysin and chromogranin A immunoreactivities of Lewy bodies in Parkinson's disease brains. Brain Res 1994;634: 339–344.
297. Smith MA, Hirai K, Hsiao K, Pappolla MA, Harris PL, Siedlak SL, et al. Amyloid-beta deposition in Alzheimer transgenic mice is associated with oxidative stress. J Neurochem 1998;70:2212–2215.
298. Munch G, Schinzel R, Loske C, Wong A, Durany N, Li JJ, et al. Alzheimer's disease—synergistic effects of glucose deficit, oxidative stress and advanced glycation endproducts. J Neural Transm 1998;105: 439–461.
299. Vitek MP, Bhattacharya K, Glendening JM, Stopa E, Vlassara H, Bucala R, et al. Advanced glycation end products contribute to amyloidosis in Alzheimer disease. Proc Natl Acad Sci U S A 1994;91:4766–4770.
300. Loske C, Neumann A, Cunningham AM, Nichol K, Schinzel R, Riederer P, et al. Cytotoxicity of advanced glycation endproducts is mediated by oxidative stress. J Neural Transm 1998;105:1005–1015.
301. Bierhaus A, Hofmann MA, Ziegler R, Nawroth PP. AGEs and their interaction with AGE-receptors in vascular disease and diabetes mellitus. I. The AGE concept. Cardiovasc Res 1998;37:586–600.
302. Mullarkey CJ, Edelstein D, Brownlee M. Free radical generation by early glycation products: a mechanism for accelerated atherogenesis in diabetes. Biochem Biophys Res Commun 1990;173:932–939.

303. Vlassara H, Li YM, Imani F, Wojciechowicz D, Yang Z, Liu FT, et al. Identification of galectin-3 as a high-affinity binding protein for advanced glycation end products (AGE): a new member of the AGE-receptor complex. Mol Med 1995;1:634–646.
304. McMillian M, Kong LY, Sawin SM, Wilson B, Das K, Hudson P, et al. Selective killing of cholinergic neurons by microglial activation in basal forebrain mixed neuronal/glial cultures. Biochem Biophys Res Commun 1995;215:572–577.
305. Markesbery WR, Lovell MA. Four-hydroxynonenal, a product of lipid peroxidation, is increased in the brain in Alzheimer's disease. Neurobiol Aging 1998;19:33–36.
306. Owen AD, Schapira AH, Jenner P, Marsden CD. Indices of oxidative stress in Parkinson's disease, Alzheimer's disease and dementia with Lewy bodies. J Neural Transm Suppl 1997;51:167–173.
307. Hoyer S, Lannert H. Inhibition of the neuronal insulin receptor causes Alzheimer-like disturbances in oxidative/energy brain metabolism and in behavior in adult rats. Ann N Y Acad Sci 1999;893:301–303.
308. Jenkins BG, Chen YI, Kuestermann E, Makris NM, Nguyen TV, Kraft E, et al. An integrated strategy for evaluation of metabolic and oxidative defects in neurodegenerative illness using magnetic resonance techniques. Ann N Y Acad Sci 1999;893:214–242.
309. Grunewald T, Beal MF. Bioenergetics in Huntington's disease. Ann N Y Acad Sci 1999;893:203–213.
310. Mattson MP, Pedersen WA, Duan W, Culmsee C, Camandola S. Cellular and molecular mechanisms underlying perturbed energy metabolism and neuronal degeneration in Alzheimer's and Parkinson's diseases. Ann N Y Acad Sci 1999;893:154–175.
311. Rapoport SI. Functional brain imaging in the resting state and during activation in Alzheimer's disease. Implications for disease mechanisms involving oxidative phosphorylation. Ann N Y Acad Sci 1999;893:138–153.
312. Sheu KF, Blass JP. The alpha-ketoglutarate dehydrogenase complex. Ann N Y Acad Sci 1999;893:61–78.
313. McGeer PL, McGeer EG. Mechanisms of cell death in Alzheimer disease—immunopathology. J Neural Transm Suppl 1998;54:159–166.
314. McGeer EG, McGeer PL. The importance of inflammatory mechanisms in Alzheimer disease. Exp Gerontol 1998;33:371–378.
315. Vandenabeele P, Fiers W. Is amyloidogenesis during Alzheimer's disease due to an IL-1-/IL-6- mediated 'acute phase response' in the brain? [see comments]. Immunol Today 1991;12:217–219.
316. Royston MC, Rothwell NJ, Roberts GW. Alzheimer's disease: pathology to potential treatments? Trends Pharmacol Sci 1992;13:131–133.
317. Gadient RA, Otten UH. Interleukin-6 (IL-6)—a molecule with both beneficial and destructive potentials. Prog Neurobiol 1997;52:379–390.
318. Campbell IL, Abraham CR, Masliah E, Kemper P, Inglis JD, Oldstone MB, et al. Neurologic disease induced in transgenic mice by cerebral overexpression of interleukin 6. Proc Natl Acad Sci U S A 1993;90:10061–10075.
319. Heyser CJ, Masliah E, Samimi A, Campbell IL, Gold LH. Progressive decline in avoidance learning paralleled by inflammatory neurodegeneration in transgenic mice expressing interleukin 6 in the brain. Proc Natl Acad Sci U S A 1997;94:1500–1505.
320. McPhaden AR, Waley K. the complement system and inflammation. In: Immunology and Medicine Series. Dordrecht: Kluwer Academic Publishers; 1992.
321. Webster S, Bradt B, Rogers J, Cooper N. Aggregation state-dependent activation of the classical complement pathway by the amyloid beta peptide. J Neurochem 1997;69:388–398.
322. Bradt BM, Kolb WP, Cooper NR. Complement-dependent proinflammatory properties of the Alzheimer's disease beta-peptide. J Exp Med 1998;188:431–438.
323. Eikelenboom P, Rozemuller JM, van Muiswinkel FL. Inflammation and Alzheimer's disease: relationships between pathogenic mechanisms and clinical expression. Exp Neurol 1998;154:89–98.
324. Dickson DW, Lee SC, Mattiace LA, Yen SH, Brosnan C. Microglia and cytokines in neurological disease, with special reference to AIDS and Alzheimer's disease. Glia 1993;7:75–83.
325. Breitner JC, Gau BA, Welsh KA, Plassman BL, McDonald WM, Helms MJ, et al. Inverse association of anti-inflammatory treatments and Alzheimer's disease: initial results of a co-twin control study. Neurology 1994;44:227–232.
326. Rogers J, Kirby LC, Hempelman SR, Berry DL, McGeer PL, Kaszniak AW, et al. Clinical trial of indomethacin in Alzheimer's disease. Neurology 1993;43:1609–1611.
327. Stewart WF, Kawas C, Corrada M, Metter EJ. Risk of Alzheimer's disease and duration of NSAID use [see comments]. Neurology 1997;48:626–632.
328. in 't Veld BA, Launer LJ, Hoes AW, Ott A, Hofman A, Breteler MM, et al. NSAIDs and incident Alzheimer's disease. The Rotterdam Study [see comments]. Neurobiol Aging 1998;19:607–611.
329. Mann DM, Iwatsubo T, Pickering-Brown SM, Owen F, Saido TC, Perry RH. Preferential deposition of amyloid beta protein (Abeta) in the form Abeta40 in Alzheimer's disease is associated with a gene dosage effect of the apolipoprotein E E4 allele. Neurosci Lett 1997;221:81–84.
330. Jordan J, Galindo MF, Miller RJ, Reardon CA, Getz GS, LaDu MJ. Isoform-specific effect of apolipoprotein E on cell survival and beta- amyloid-induced toxicity in rat hippocampal pyramidal neuronal cultures. J Neurosci 1998;18:195–204.
331. Thinakaran G, Regard JB, Bouton CM, Harris CL, Price DL, Borchelt DR, et al. Stable association of presenilin derivatives and absence of presenilin interactions with APP. Neurobiol Dis 1998;4:438–453.
332. Strauss S, Bauer J, Ganter U, Jonas U, Berger M, Volk B. Detection of interleukin-6 and alpha 2-macroglobulin immunoreactivity in cortex and hippocampus of Alzheimer's disease patients. Lab Invest 1992;66:223–230.
333. Blacker D, Wilcox MA, Laird NM, Rodes L, Horvath SM, Go RC, et al. Alpha-2 macroglobulin is genetically associated with Alzheimer disease [see comments]. Nat Genet 1998; 19:357–360.

334. Roses AD. Apolipoprotein E alleles as risk factors in Alzheimer's disease. Annu Rev Med 1996;47:387–400.
335. Games D, Adams D, Alessandrini R, Barbour R, Berthelette P, Blackwell C, et al. Alzheimer-type neuropathology in transgenic mice overexpressing V717F beta-amyloid precursor protein [see comments]. Nature 1995;373:523–527.

7. Dementia

JEAN PAUL G. VONSATTEL AND E. TESSA HEDLEY-WHYTE

The growing awareness of the early signs of mental decline has increased the incidence of the diagnosis of dementia. Likewise, the increasing life expectancy with the growing number of elderly individuals raises the prevalence of dementing illnesses since dementia occurs primarily late in life.[1] The prevalence of Alzheimer's disease (AD), the most common cause of dementia, is age dependent and is estimated to be between 3 and 11 per 100 persons older than 65 years.[2,3] Thus, dementia is a growing problem facing modern society and care providers.

Dementia is characterized by acquired, cognitive impairments with intact arousal causing disruption of independent life. Memory, language, and judgment fail. Dementia occurs in association with more than 55 medical, psychiatric, or neurologic conditions.[1,4] The most important cause of dementia is primary degeneration of the brain, including AD; Pick disease, frontotemporal dementia; dementia with Lewy bodies, including Alzheimer's disease Lewy body variant; and dementia associated with amyotrophic lateral sclerosis, prion diseases, and hippocampal sclerosis.[5,6] Furthermore, dementias may be caused by infections, trauma; and genetic, metabolic, or neoplastic disease, e.g., limbic encephalitis.[7–11] Treatable causes of dementias include thyroid disease,[2] syphilis, fungal and viral infections, vitamin deficiencies (B-12), tumor, subdural hematoma[2,12] hydrocephalus including normal pressure hydrocephalus,[13,14] neurosarcoidosis,[15,16] and vasculitis.[17] Depression may mimic dementia. In depression, it is often the patient who defines the mental deficits, whereas in AD it is usually the family who is aware of the problem.[1] Dementia may occur as a sequel to encephalitis, hypoxia, carbon monoxide intoxication, or trauma.[8]

In the first part of this chapter we briefly define the principal, pathological hallmarks occurring in selected dementing illnesses and we address their overlaps with changes that appear during usual aging. First, we consider the topography of the relative, selective vulnerability in dementing illnesses. Second, we define the major, microscopical characteristics observed in usual aging and dementing illnesses.

In the succeeding segments of this chapter we focus on the non-Alzheimer's and non-vascular dementias resulting from primary degeneration of the central nervous system with emphasis on their neuropathological features. The dementing diseases selected are: dementia with Lewy bodies, paraneoplastic limbic encephalitis, Creutzfedlt-Jakob disease (CJD), and Pick disease (PcD). The discussion also corvers frontotemporal dementia (FTD), diffuse Lewy body disease (DLBD), and Alzheimer's disease Lewy body variant (ADLBV); Creutzfeldt-Jakob disease (CJD): fatal familial insomnia (FFI), bovine spongiform encephalopathy (BSE), or "mad cow disease," and Gerstmann-Sträussler-Scheinker disease or syndrome (GSSS); and hippocampal sclerosis. We include dementia secondary to paraneoplastic limbic encephalitis because it can mimic any of the neurodegenerative dementing illnesses listed above and should be included in the differential diagnosis at least early in the course of the ailment.

The Neuroanatomical Basis of Dementia and Changes of Usual Aging

The pathological substratum of primary degeneration of the brain usually occurs without acute or chronic inflammatory infiltrates, although scattered microgliocytes are often present.[19-21] It may include volume loss, neuronal shrinkage, neuronal loss, myelin loss, reactive astrocytosis, formation of neurofibrillary tangles of Alzheimer's, neuropil threads, and neuronal and glial inclusions.[22] By the time the patient dies, the changes are usually widespread but tend to predominate in one area from which they appear to have spread.[23,24] The primary degeneration may in turn trigger remote secondary changes. For example, severe atrophy of the hippocampal formation is often associated with myelin and fiber loss involving the fornix and the mammillothalamic tract, and neuronal loss involving the anterior nucleus of the thalamus. Likewise, severe atrophy of the frontal lobe may cause shrinkage of the medial third of the cerebral peduncle. The symptoms may reflect the relative, selective topography of the degenerative process. Yet, dementia may result from degeneration of many structures either individually or in combination, which include the cerebral cortex, cerebral white matter, hippocampal formation, entorhinal region, amygdala, nucleus basalis of Meynert, striatum, thalamus, mesencephalon with substantia nigra, and cerebellum.[25] In addition, there are instances in which the selective distribution of the pathological changes can clearly explain the dementia, as in limbic encephalitis.[9]

CEREBRAL CORTEX

Cerebral, cortical degeneration is a major cause of dementia and is somewhat selective.

The *cerebral cortex* is composed of the *allocortex* and the phylogenetically more recent, *neocortex*. This phylogenetic subdivision includes the following regions, which are useful in assessing the topographic characteristics associated with the dementia:

ALLOCORTEX
- *Archicortex* Hippocampal formation (presubiculum, subiculum prosubiculum, cornu ammonis, dentate fascia)
- *Paleocortex* Pyriform cortex (entorhinal area)

NEOCORTEX
- *Homotypical* Cortex with six distinctive layers (e.g., parietal lobe)
- *Heterotypical* Agranular (BA4 = motor cortex) Granular (BA17 = visual cortex)

The allocortical regions are particularly prone to degeneration in usual aging and, more extensively, in dementing illnesses.[26-32] Indeed, the large pyramidal neurons, especially those of the Sommer sector of the *hippocampal formation,* are susceptible to neurofibrillary tangle formation, granulovacuolar degeneration, and Hirano body formation in usual aging.[32-34] The stellate neurons of layer 2 of the entorhinal cortex are highly susceptible to neurofibrillary tangle formation.[29] These changes are conspicuous in AD and ADLBV. The large and small pyramidal neurons and the granule neurons of the fascia dentata are susceptible to Pick body formation in PcD.[35-37]

Within the neocortex, in many dementing diseases the homotypical cortex is usually more involved than the heterotypical cortex.[38] (Figs. 7–1 and 7–2). Neocortical neurons can be categorized as pyramidal and nonpyramidal. The pyramidal neurons have extensive intracortical and extracortical connections; and it is these neurons that are most affected in dementing, degenerative diseases.[33]

CEREBRAL WHITE MATTER

The white matter or centrum semi-ovale occupies much of each cerebral hemisphere. Age-related volume loss of the brain involves the white mater more than the gray matter[39] Dementing illnesses with destructive or a demyelinating process include progressive multifocal leukoencephalopathy,[40-42] the encepha-

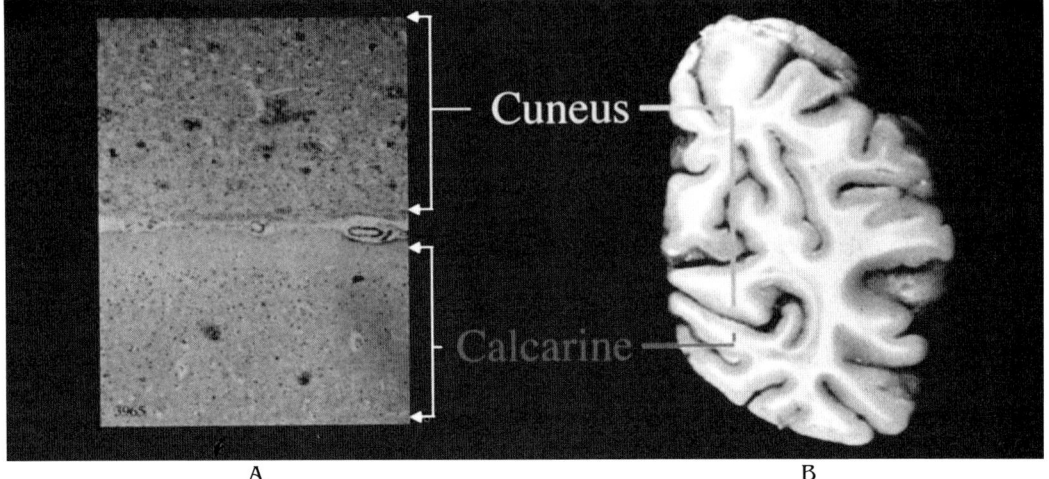

Figure 7–1. *A.* Relative, selective vulnerability of homotypical versus heterotypical cortex. The density of silver-stained neuritic plaques is higher in the homotypical, cuneal neocortex (upper half) than in the heterotypical, calcarine neocortex (lower half). Bielschowsky stain; original magnification before reduction, ×3. *B.* Coronal section of the cerebral hemisphere showing the site selected for the microphotograph depicted in A.

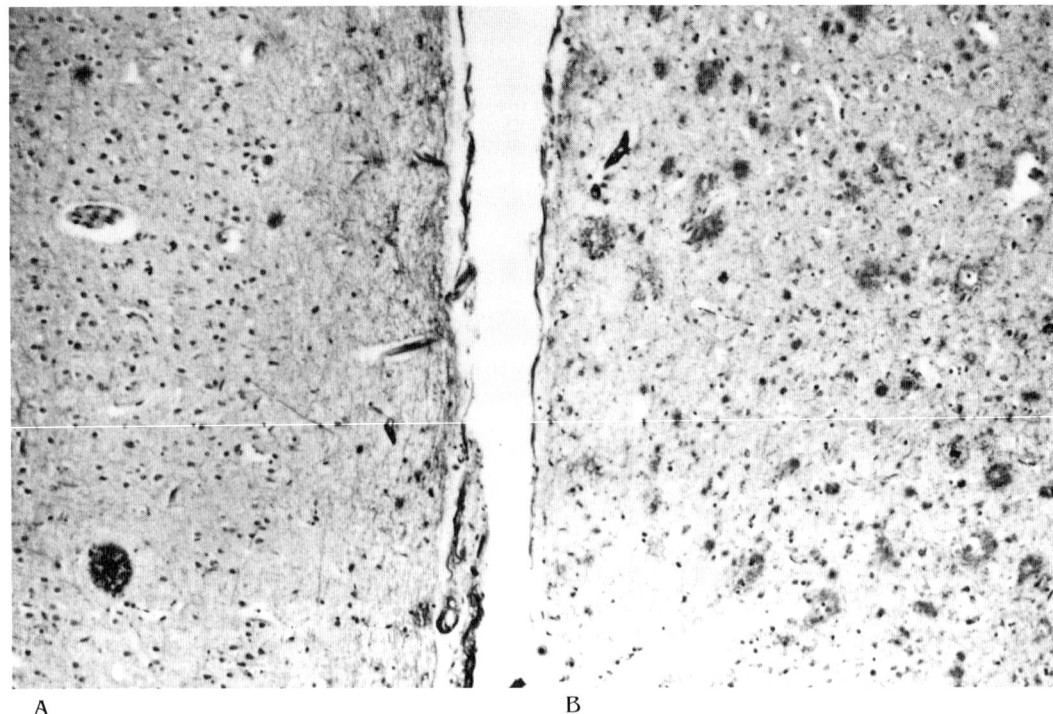

Figure 7–2. Microphotograph (same as in Fig. 7–1) showing the calcarine cortex (*A*) and cuneal cortex (*B*). Note the high density of neuritic plaques in the cuneal, homotypical cortex in contrast to that in the calcarine, heterotypical cortex. Modified Bielschowsky stain; original magnification, ×3.

lopathy of the acquired immune deficiency syndrome (AIDS),[43] and multiple sclerosis.[44] White matter loss with dementia may be caused by vasculopathies. For example, nearly 30% of individuals with *cerebral autosomal dominant arteriopathy with subcortical infarcts and leukoencephalopathy* (CADASIL) developed dementia.[45] Hypertensive vascular changes may result in loss of subcortical white matter and cause dementia as in Binswanger disease.[46–49] Some demented patients with severe cerebral amyloid angiopathy (CAA) have white matter loss without other changes that could account for the dementia.[50–52] Callosal dementia, recently described by Ghika-Schmidt et al., may occur following focal myelinolysis involving the corpus callosum and adjacent white matter.[53]

SUBCORTICAL NUCLEI AND DEMENTING ILLNESSES

The *amygdala* often shows severe pathological changes in dementing diseases, e.g., AD (neuronal loss, neurofibrillary tangles, neuritic plaques and gliosis), DLBD (neuronal loss, neurons with Lewy body, spongiform changes), herpes simplex encephalitis (neuronal loss, gliosis, hemosiderin), or limbic encephalitis (neuronal loss, vacuolated neurons, lymphocytic infiltrates). The *nucleus basalis of Meynert* is the site of degeneration in AD, LBD including ADLBV and DLBD, Parkinson disease, and progressive supranuclear palsy.

The large neurons of the *neostriatum* (caudate nucleus, nucleus accumbens and putamen) undergo neurofibrillary degeneration in AD.[54–56] Likewise, neostriatal tangles occur in progressive supranuclear palsy.[57–60] Furthermore, the *striatum* bears the brunt of the cerebral atrophy in Huntington's disease, which is characterized by dementia and movement disorder.[61]

The dorsomedian and the anterior nuclei of the *thalamus* are especially prone to neuronal loss with or without the formation of neuritic plaques or neurofibrillary tangles or both in several neurodegenerative diseases.[62,63] The centrum medianum is gliotic in the late stage of Huntington disease. The rostral third or half of the thalamus may be atrophic (usually medial > lateral) in PcD.[35,64,65] These thalamic changes are almost always encountered in the context of dementia. In addition, unilateral thalamic infarct or hemorrhage may cause dementia.[66,67]

BRAIN STEM AND DEMENTING ILLNESSES

The *brain stem* often shows degenerative changes in dementing illnesses. Neuronal loss involves the

- *substantia nigra pars compacta* in LBD including DLBD and ADLBV, PcD (in up to 70% of cases), Parkinson disease, and progressive supranuclear palsy;
- *nucleus coeruleus* in AD, DLB, and Parkinson disease;
- *dorsal and median raphe nuclei* in AD, LBD, Parkinson disease, and progressive supranuclear palsy.

Widespread *cerebellar* damage may occur in Creutzfeldt-Jakob disease, GSSS, and olivopontocerebellar atrophy.

In summary, the areas that are especially prone to degeneration in dementing illnesses are the amygdala, entorhinal and pyriform cortices, hippocampal formation, mammillary bodies, anterior and dorsomedian nuclei of thalamus, neocortex (homotypical > heterotypical) and neostriatum (Fig. 7–3), nucleus coeruleus, and raphe nuclei.

PATHOLOGICAL HALLMARKS OF DEMENTING DISEASES AND USUAL AGING

Cerebral Atrophy

Cerebral atrophy is expressed by narrowing of the gyri and widening of the sulci, resulting in up to 20% to 30% weight loss. Cerebral atrophy may occur in cognitively normal subjects as an expression of usual aging.[32] Atrophy may be lacking or may be subtle early in the course of any neurodegenerative process. Atrophy is often conspicuous in advanced dementia, but it may be absent despite the presence of extensive, microscopic degenerative changes.[25,68] Severe dementia with little or no

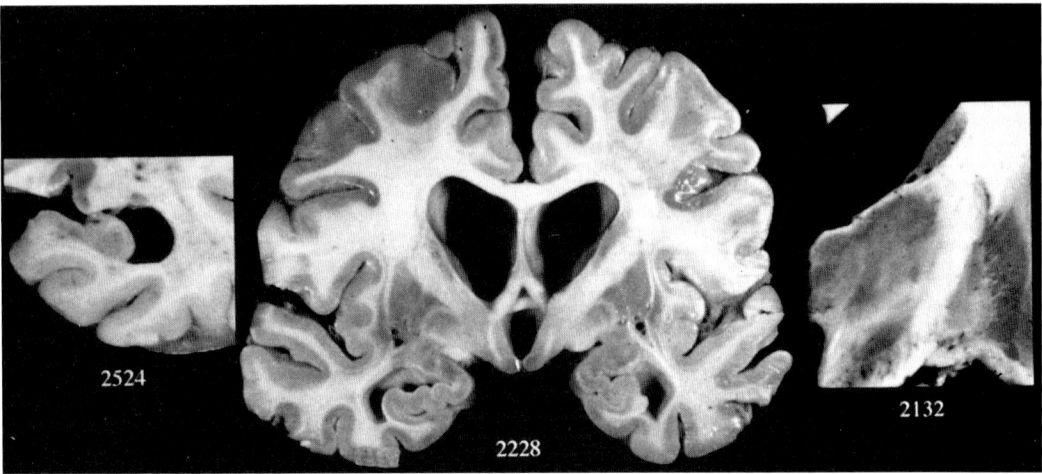

Figure 7–3. Sites that are especially prone to degeneration in dementing illnesses are hippocampal formation (*left*); mammillary body, amygdaloid nucleus, uncus, entorhinal cortex, and isocortex (*center*); and dorsomedian and anterior nuclei of thalamus (*right*).

atrophy usually occurs in DLBD or in occasional patients with AD, especially those who are older then 80 at death.[69–71] Tomlinson et al. recorded four brains weighing > 1300 g among 16 brains from patients with AD; one of which weighed 1510 g, and concluded that brain weights are of no significance for the pathological diagnosis of dementia in old age.[71] Other examples of severe dementia that may not have atrophic brains on neuroimaging or postmortem gross examination are dementia lacking distinctive histology,[72–74] Creutzfeldt Jakob disease or prion diseases,[75] and AIDS encephalopathy.[76,77] The atrophy tends to be diffuse with or without regional accentuation in AD or ADLBV.[78–80] The atrophy may be disproportionately severe in one or more cerebral lobes; and on one side more than the other.[81] Typical examples of dementia with circumscribed atrophy are Pick disease with or without amyotrophic lateral sclerosis and hippocampal sclerosis.[5,6] Examples of regional atrophy without or with mild to moderate dementia are corticobasal degeneration,[35,64,81–83] and multiple system atrophy.[84,85]

Dementia may occur in conditions with prominent atrophy of deep gray nuclei: atrophy of the striatum as in Huntington disease,[86–88] atrophy of the substantia nigra pars compacta as in end-stage Parkinson's disease,[89] or atrophy of both the pars compacta and pars reticulata of the substantia nigra in progressive supranuclear palsy.[90]

Ventricular Enlargement

The volume of each lateral ventricle is about 7.0–10.0 cc in individuals without neurological or psychiatric diseases, and can reach up to 50 cc in demented people; the severity and topography of the ventricular widening tend to match that of the parenchymal atrophy.

Neuritic Plaques

Neuritic plaques (or senile plaques, amyloid argyrophilic plaques) are abundant in AD and to a lesser extent in many intellectually normal older subjects.[32,91–93] Neuritic plaques develop in the cerebral cortex, amygdala, hippocampal formation, and striatum, especially in the nucleus accumbens. They may also occur in the thalamus particularly within the dorsomedian and anterior nuclei and in the cerebellar cortex.[94]

Practically, three stages of morphologically distinct plaques can be identified: (*1*) the classical, or neuritic, plaques, (*2*) the immature plaques, and (*3*) the diffuse, or preamyloid, plaques. The *classical*, or *neuritic*, *plaques* are

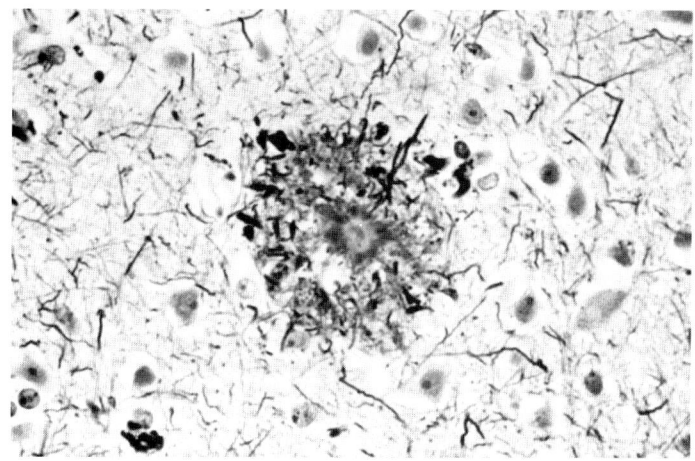

Figure 7–4. Neuritic plaque with a centrally located amyloid core, surrounded by a halo of argyrophilic, dystrophic neurites, which is in contrast to kuru plaque (see Creutzfeldt-Jakob Disease, Spongiform Encephalopathies). Modified Bielschowsky stain; original magnification, ×500.

composed of a centrally located Congo red–positive amyloid core (Fig. 7–4). This core is surrounded by a halo of distorted neurites containing argyrophilic, paired helical filaments (dystrophic neurites). Rod-shaped microglial cells and macrophages can be seen within the plaques, while reactive astrocytes tend to be at the periphery of the plaques, or in the parenchyma surrounding the plaques. *Immature plaques* are oval or spherical amyloid-containing areas with sharp borders, neuropil changes such as discrete amyloid fibers, and swollen, argyrophilic neurites, but without compact amyloid core. The *diffuse*, or *pre-amyloid, plaques* are polymorphous, usually round, oval, or cuneiform, weakly argyrophilic areas without apparent structural changes of the neuropil. Thus, diffuse plaques lack the argyrophilic, dystrophic neurites characteristically present in classical plaques. Immature plaques and diffuse plaques contain amyloid, which is not in the β-pleated sheet conformation; therefore, in contrast to neuritic plaques, immature and diffuse plaques do not stain with Congo red. However, they do react with antibodies to β-A4 amyloid.

Neurofibrillary Changes

Neurofibrillary changes are due to the cytoplasmic or intracellular accumulation of paired helical filaments whose formation is mainly secondary to the hyperphosphorylation of tau.[95,96] Tau is a microtubule-associated protein that promotes tubulin assembly in vitro and stabilizes microtubules in vivo.[97] Neurofibrillary changes consist of tortuous, argyrophilic, tau-positive fibrils found in the neuropil (neuropil threads), in the halo of neuritic plaques (dystrophic neurites), in the cytoplasm of pyramidal (flame-shaped neurofibrillary tangles) or oval neurons (globose tangles) and in the cytoplasm of oligodendrocytes or astrocytes (glial cytoplasmic tangles). Tau-labeled glial cytoplasmic inclusions have been observed in certain forms of familial frontotemporal dementia associated with parkinsonism due to a mutation involving the tau gene on chromosome 17.[98–102]

Granulovacuolar Degeneration

Granulovacuolar degeneration consists of the presence of one or more cytoplasmic granules, 1–2 μm across, surrounded by an optically empty rim, or vacuole, measuring 3–5 μm in diameter (Fig. 7–5). They most frequently involve the hippocampal pyramidal neurons of the Sommer sector (CA1) and subiculum. They may also be seen in cortical and subcortical neurons. They can occur in elderly individuals with normal cognition, although to a lesser extent than in patients with Alzheimer's disease. Tomlinson et al. reported severe involvement of the pyramidal cells of Sommer sector in every demented patient and that "some degree" of this change was found in 70% of the control brains.[71]

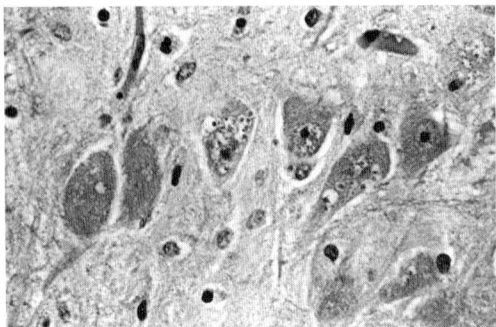

Figure 7–5. Pyramidal cells of the Sommer sector (CA1) with granulovacuolar degeneration. Luxol fast blue counterstained with hematoxylin and eosin; original magnification, ×500.

Hirano Bodies

Hirano bodies are ovoid, or rod-shaped, eosinophilic, amorphous structures 10–30 μm in length, that are found among, usually adjacent to, or in the cytoplasm of hippocampal pyramidal neurons, especially in CA-1[34] (Fig. 7–6). They can be found from youth to old age in both normal and demented subjects. Their number increases with age, and they are more frequent in people with dementia than in intellectually normal subjects. They may derive from an age-related alteration of the microfilamentous system.

Lewy Bodies

In contrast to general belief, it is G. Marinesco and not F. Lewy who provided the first description of cytoplasmic inclusions now called "Lewy bodies." The description of these cytoplasmic inclusions is included in Marinesco's report on the nuclear inclusions occurring in the pigmented neurons of the substantia nigra now referred to as "Marinesco bodies."[103,104] About 10 years after Marinesco's publication, F. Lewy described the occurrence of cytoplasmic inclusions in the substantia innominata while reporting on his findings in the lenticular nucleus of individuals with parkinsonism.[105,106] Trétiakoff, who perhaps was not aware that Marinesco described not only the nuclear but also the cytoplasmic inclusions occurring in the pars compacta of the substantia nigra, rediscovered the nigral, cytoplasmic inclusions and coined the term "Lewy body."[107]

The precise role of Lewy bodies in the neuronal dysfunction in Parkinson's disease and in other dementing, degenerative diseases associated with the accumulation of many Lewy bodies is unclear.[108,109] They may also occur in neuroaxonal dystrophy and Hallervorden Spatz disease.[108,110–112] and in many patients with Down syndrome.[113] Occasional Lewy bodies can be encountered in normal elderly subjects.[69,114]

Lewy bodies are neuronal, cytoplasmic, eosinophilic inclusions that are weakly argyrophilic. They are labeled with antibodies directed against ubiquitin or α-synuclein but not with antibodies directed against tau.[108,115–118]

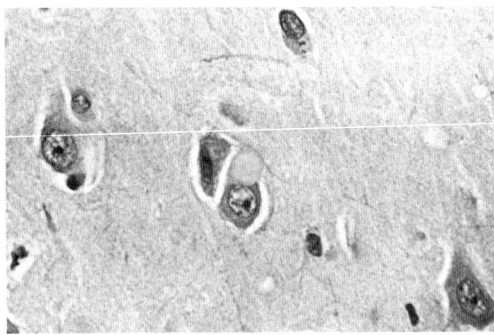

Figure 7–6. Pyramidal cell (center) of the Sommer sector (CA1), which contains a Hirano body consisting of an eosinophilic, homogeneous structure. Note cytoplasmic, granulovacuolar degeneration involving the neuron that is near the upper border of the picture. Luxol fast blue counterstained with hematoxylin and eosin; original magnification, ×500.

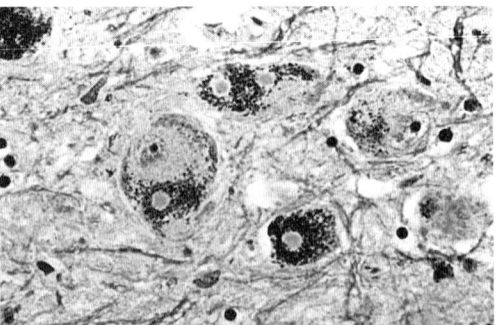

Figure 7–7. Three pigmented neurons with one or more brain stem–type Lewy bodies. Luxol fast blue counterstained with hematoxylin and eosin; original magnification, ×500.

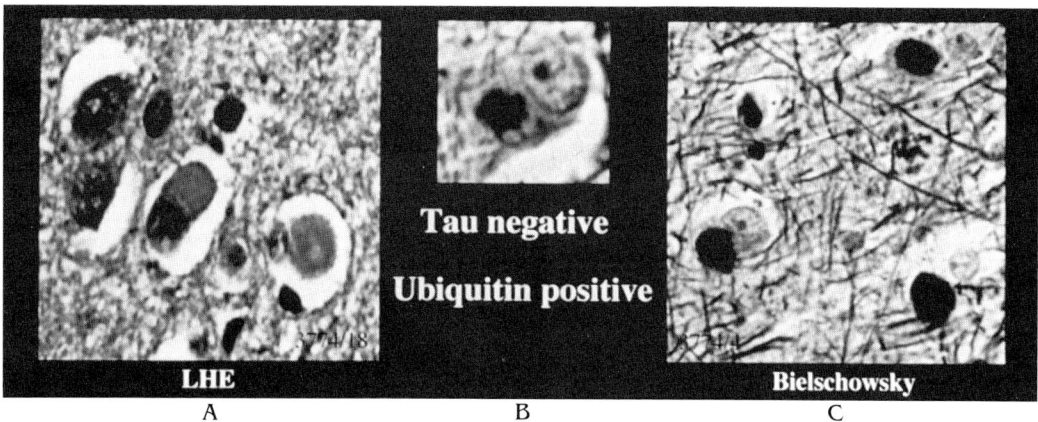

Figure 7–8. Cortical Lewy bodies. *A.* Two atrophic, cortical neurons, each containing a single Lewy body. Luxol fast blue counterstained with hematoxylin and eosin (LHE). *B.* A cortical neuron labeled with antibody directed against ubiquitin. In contrast to Pick bodies, Lewy bodies are not labeled with antibodies directed against tau. *C.* Cortical neurons with argyrophilic Lewy bodies. Modified Bielschowsky stain. The argyrophilia of Lewy bodies may vary, and at times they may be indistinguishable from Pick bodies (see Fig. 7–10). Original magnification, ×313.

Their morphology varies, so two types of Lewy body can be distinguished: the brain stem, or classical, type (Fig. 7–7) and the cortical type (Fig. 7–8).

The *brain stem–type* Lewy bodies are round and 8–30 μm in diameter and consist of a hyalin core with or without concentric, lamellar bands and with a peripheral, pale halo.[103] Brain stem–type Lewy bodies are most commonly found in the pigmented neurons of the brain stem, including the pars compacta of the substantia nigra and nucleus coeruleus (Fig 7–7), in the Edinger-Westphal nucleus, dorsal motor nucleus of the vagus, thalamus, hypothalamus, substantia innominata, olfactory bulb, and autonomic ganglions.[108] At times, a few neurons, especially pigmented ones, contain more than one Lewy body.

The *cortical-type* Lewy bodies are less distinct and are smaller than brain stem–type Lewy bodies. They are pale and eosinophilic with ill-defined borders and without a hyalin core or concentric lamellae (Fig. 7–8). Neocortical neurons prone to contain cortical-type Lewy bodies are those located in layers V and VI. Affected cortical neurons contain only one Lewy body. The sites of predilections for cortical-type Lewy bodies are the cingulate gyrus, insula, entorhinal cortex, parahippocampal gyrus, occipitotemporalis gyrus, and amygdala.

Marinesco Bodies

Marinesco bodies are homogeneous, eosinophilic, round, intranuclear structures 2.0–10.0 μm in diameter that are found in the pars compacta of the substantia nigra and, to a lesser extent, in the nucleus coeruleus[103,119] (Fig. 7–9). They are labeled with antibodies directed against ubiquitin.[120] Their occurrence increases with age.[119]

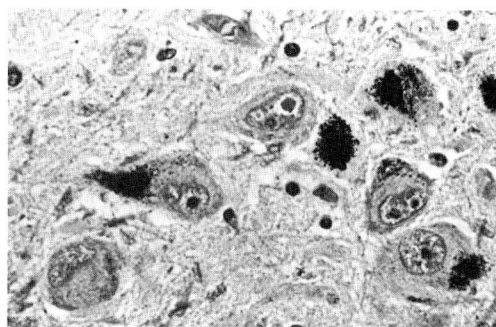

Figure 7–9. Pigmented neurons of the pars compacta of the substantia nigra. Two neurons have a nucleus with a single, eosinophilic, round inclusion or Marinesco body that is near the nucleolus. The Marinesco body of the neuron located in the upper center of the picture is smudgy and surrounded by a clear zone compared to the sharply demarcated nucleolus. Luxol fast blue counterstained with hematoxylin and eosin; original magnification, ×500.

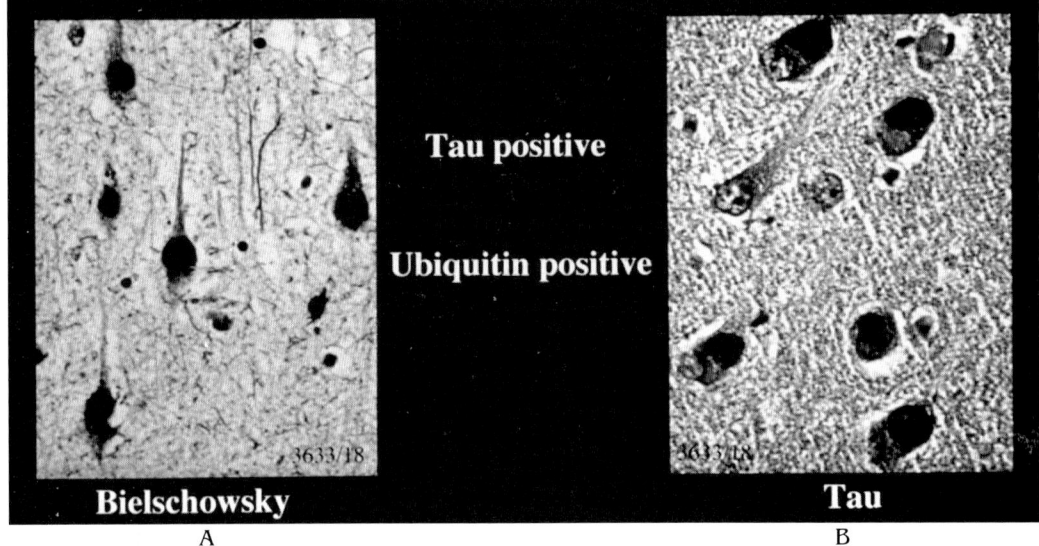

Figure 7–10. A. Argyrophilic, cytoplasmic inclusions or Pick bodies involving pyramidal neurons of the hippocampal formation. Modified Bielschowsky stain. B. Cortical neurons containing Pick bodies labeled with antibodies directed against tau. In contrast to Pick bodies, Lewy bodies are not labeled with anti-tau antibodies (see Fig. 7–8). Original magnification, ×313.

Pick Bodies

Pick bodies are round or oval, well-outlined, argyrophilic, tau-positive, ubiquitin-positive, synuclein-negative, intracytoplasmic bodies measuring 10–15 μm across[91,121,122] (Fig. 7–10). They are found in cortical pyramidal neurons and in the hippocampal formation and in the amygdala. They can also occur in the striatum and brain stem. Pick bodies are found in about 30% to 50% (or more depending on sampling and methods of evaluation) of brains with circumscribed atrophy from demented patients. Pick body–like inclusions can be encountered in the dentate fascia in Alzheimer's disease. Additional data on PcB are to be found in the section on Pick disease (page 197).

Ballooned Neurons (Pick Cells)

Ballooned neurons (BN), also referred to as Pick cells, are swollen neurons with convex contours, homogeneous glassy, pale, eosinophilic cytoplasm, and eccentric nuclei.[123,124] The cytoplasm is diffusely argyrophilic with variable intensity. At times, cytoplasmic vacuoles with or without a centrally located granule are present (Fig. 7–11). Ballooned neurons are found in 60% of brains with circumscribed atrophy and they also occur in corticobasal degeneration, progressive supranuclear palsy, AD, and Creutzfeldt-Jakob disease. Additional details on ballooned neurons are provided in the section on Pick disease (pag 200).

Status Spongiosus versus Spongiform Changes

Status spongiosus consists of irregular cavitation of the neuropil in the presence of a dense glial meshwork (Fig. 7–12). It is nonspecific and characteristically is the manifestation of end-stage gliosis.[125] *Spongiform changes* consist of the presence of small, round, or ovoid vacuoles within the neuropil (Fig. 7–13), which are hallmarks of the spongiform encephalopathies, and are characteristically accompanied by a discrete reactive astrocytosis.[125,126]

To some extent, spongiform changes (with, or without little reactive astrocytosis) are also observed in LBD,[127] ADLBV,[78,128,129] and in some cases of AD.[130] At times, the spongiform changes occurring in DLBD, ADLBV, or even in AD are indistinguishable from those observed in spongiform encephalopathies.[131]

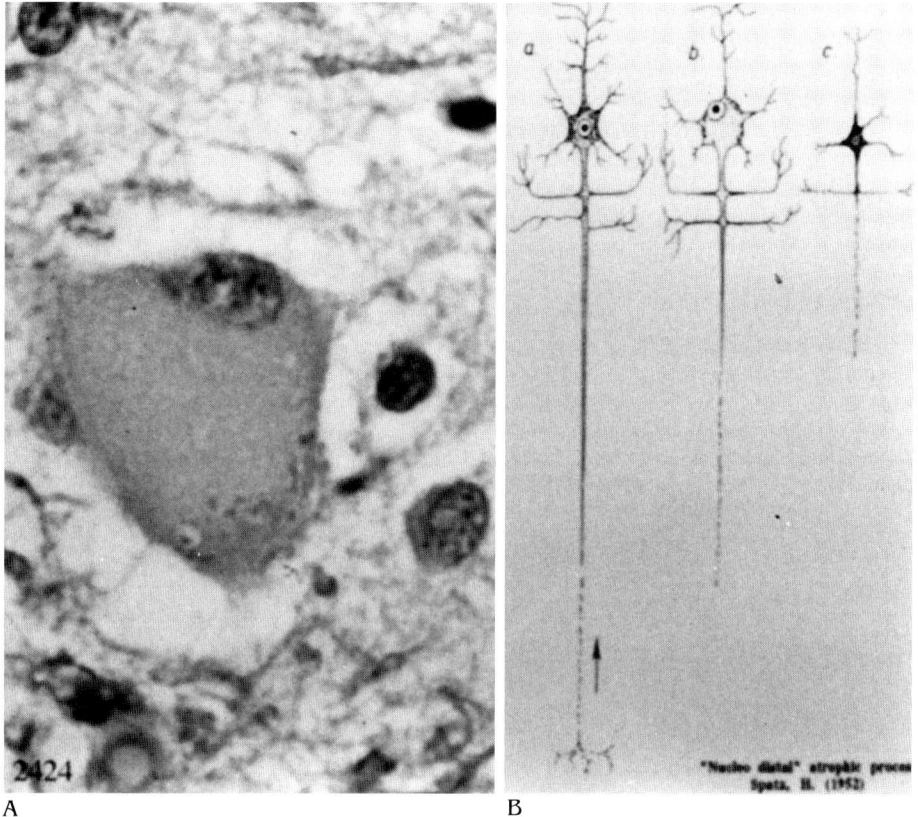

Figure 7–11. *A*. Ballooned neuron or Pick cell with granulovacuolar degeneration. Luxol fast blue counterstained with hematoxylin and eosin; original magnification, ×500. *B*. Spatz's hypothesis regarding the formation of ballooned neurons. According to this hypothesis, the degenerative process occurs first at the distal end of the axon and gradually moves toward the cell body, which undergoes dilatation (swollen phase) followed by shrinkage, and then neuronophagia (nucleodistal atrophy).

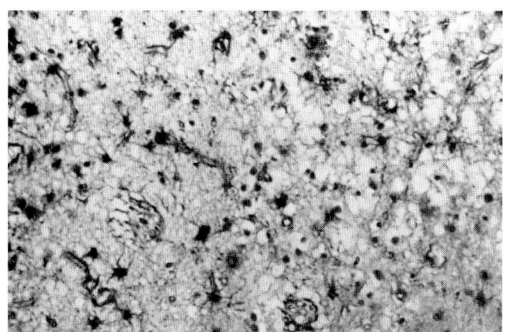

Figure 7–12. Status spongiosus involving the second–third cortical layers of the prefrontal cortex. There is severe neuronal loss and astrocytosis. GFAP counterstained with hematoxylin; original magnification, ×200.

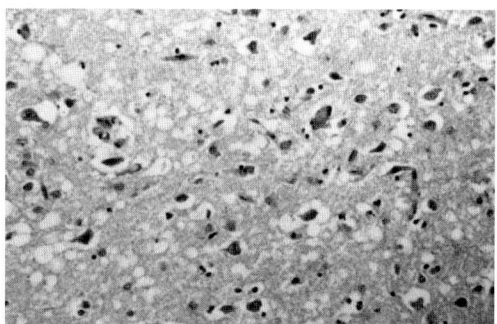

Figure 7–13. Spongiform changes with neuronal loss and gliosis involving the cortex. Luxol fast blue counterstained with hematoxylin and eosin; original magnification, ×200.

Accurate diagnostic categorization of the cause of the dementia is essential for the patients, patients' families, choice of therapies, and research. Careful integration of clinical and pathological findings, including topography of the brunt of the degeneration and identification of microscopical hallmarks are often crucial for optimal, diagnostic precision.

We thank Larry Cherkas for his assistance and advice. We are truly grateful to T. Wheelock for his help. We express our appreciation to the numerous pathologists who referred case material to the Harvard Brain Tissue Resource Center, and the Alzheimer Disease Research Center; this work would not have been possible without their assistance. We are especially grateful to the families of the patients for providing brain tissue for research. This work was supported in part by NIH grants NINCDS 31862 (Harvard Brain Tissue Resource Center, J.P.V.); NS 16367 (Huntington's Disease Center Without Walls, J.P.V.); and NIA 2P50-AGO 5134 (J.P.V., E.T.H.-W.).

REFERENCES

1. Geldmacher DS, Whitehouse PJ. Evaluation of dementia. N Engl J Med 1996; 335:330–336.
2. Corey-Bloom J, Thal LJ, Galasko D, Folstein M, Drachman D, Raskind M, Lanska DJ. Diagnosis and evaluation of dementia. Neurology 1995; 45:211–218.
3. Van Broeckhoven CL. Molecular genetics of Alzheimer disease: identification of genes and gene mutations. Eur Neurol 1995; 35:8–19.
4. Growdon JH, Rossor MN. The dementias. In Blue Books of Practical Neurology. Boston: Butterworth/Heinemann, 1999:XXV–XVII.
5. Corey-Bloom J, Sabbagh MN, Bondi MW, Hansen L, Alford MF, Masliah E, Thal LJ. Hippocampal sclerosis contributes to dementia in the elderly. Neurology 1997; 48:154–160.
6. Dickson DW, Davies P, Bevona C, Van Hoeven KH, Factor SM, Grober E, Aronson MK, Crystal HA. Hippocampal sclerosis: A common pathological feature of dementia in very old (≥ 80 years of age) humans. Acta Neuropathol 1994; 88:212–221.
7. Corsellis JAN, Goldberg GJ, Norton AR. "Limbic encephalitis" and its association with carcinoma. Brain 1968; 91:481–496.
8. Bakheit AMO, Kennedy PGE, Behan PO. Paraneoplastic limbic encephalitis: Clinico-pathological correlations. J Neurol Neurosurg Psychiatry 1990; 53:1084–1088.
9. Richardson EP Jr, Hedley-Whyte ET. Case Records of the Massachusetts General Hospital. Case 30–1985. N Engl J Med 1985; 313:249–257.
10. Koroshetz WJ, McKee AC. Case Records of the Massachusetts General Hospital. Case 39–1988. N Engl J Med 1988; 319:849–860.
11. Dubas F, Gray F, Escourolle R, Castaigne P. Poliencéphalomyélites subaiguës avec cancer. Six cas anatomo-cliniques et revue de la littérature. Rev Neurol 1982; 138:725–742.
12. Mizutani T, Shimada H. Neuropathological background of twenty-seven centenarian brains. J Neurol Sci 1992; 108:168–177.
13. Adams RD, Fisher CM, Hakim S, Ojemann RG, Sweet WH. Symptomatic occult hydrocephalus with "normal" cerebrospinal-fluid pressure. A treatable syndrome. N Engl J Med 1965; 273:117–126.
14. Vanneste JAL. Three decades of normal pressure hydrocephalus: are we wiser now? J Neurol Neurosurg Psychiatry 1994; 57:1021–1027.
15. Winkler GF, Vonsattel JP. Case Records of the Massachusetts General Hospital. Case 6–1990. Rapidly developing confusion, impaired memory, and unsteady gait in an elderly man. N Engl J Med 1990; 322:388–397.
16. Delaney P. Neurologic manifestations in sarcoidosis. Ann Intern Med 1977; 87:336–345.
17. Chu CT, Gray L, Goldstein LB, Hulette CM. Diagnosis of intracranial vasculitis: a multi-disciplinary approach. J Neuropathol Exp Neurol 1998; 57:30–38.
18. van Duijn CM. Epidemiology of the dementias: recent developments and new approaches. J Neurol Neurosurg Psychiatry 1996; 60:478–488.
19. McGeer PL, Itagaki S, Tago H, McGeer EG. Reactive microglia in patients with senile dementia of the Alzheimer type are positive for the histocompatibility glycoprotein HLA-DR. Neurosci Lett 1987; 79:195–200.
20. Paulus W, Bancher C, Jellinger K. Microglial reaction in Pick's diseae. Neurosci Lett 1993; 161:89–92.
21. Kreutzberg W. Microglia: a sensor for pathological events in the CNS. Trends Neurosci 1996; 19:312–318.
22. Spielmeyer W. Histopathologie des Nervensystems. Berlin: Julius Springer, 1922.
23. von Braunmühl A. Über eine eigenartige hereditärfamiliäre Erkrankung des Zentralnervensystems. Arch Psychiatrie Z Neurol 1954; 191:419–449.
24. Spatz H. Die "systematischen Atrophien". Eine wohlgekenzeichnete Gruppe der Erbkrankheiten des Nervensystems. Arch Psychiatrie 1938; 108:1–18.
25. Grabowski TJ, Damasio AR. Definition, clinical features and neuroanatomical basis of dementia. In: Esiri MM, Morris JH, eds. The Neuropathology of Dementia. Cambridge: Cambridge University Press, 1997:1–20.
26. Selkoe DJ. Aging, amyloid, and Alzheimer disease. N Engl J Med 1989; 320:1484–1487.
27. Katzman R. The aging brain. Limitations in our knowledge and future approaches. Arch Neurol 1997; 54:1201–1205.
28. Giannakopoulos P, Hof PR, Kövari E, Vallet PG, Herrmann FR, Bouras C. Distinct patterns of neuronal loss and Alzheimer's disease lesion distribution in elderly individuals older than 90 years. J Neuropathol Exp Neurol 1996; 55:1210–1220.
29. Gómez-Isla T, Price JL, McKeel DW, Jr, Morris JC, Growdon JH, Hyman BT. Profound loss of layer II entorhinal cortex neurons occurs in very mild Alzheimer's disease. J Neurosci 1996; 16:4491–4500.
30. Morris JC, Storandt M, McKeel DW, Jr., Rubin EH, Price JL, Grant EA, Berg L. Cerebral amyloid deposition and diffuse plaques in "normal" aging: Evi-

dence for presymptomatic and very mild Alzheimer's disease. Neurology 1996; 46:707–719.
31. Kaye JA. Oldest-old healthy brain function. The genomic potential. Arch Neurol 1997; 54:1217–1221.
32. Davis DG, Schmitt FA, Wekstein DR, Markesbery WR. Alzheimer neuropathologic alterations in aged congnitively normal subjects. J Neuropathol Exp Neurol 1999; 58:376–388.
33. Morrison BM, Hof PR, Morrison JH. Determinants of neuronal vulnerability in neurodegenerative diseases. Ann Neurol 1998; 44(Suppl 1):S32–S44.
34. Hirano A. Hirano bodies and related neuronal inclusions. Neuropathol Appl Neurobiol 1994; 20:3–11.
35. Binetti G, Growdon JH, Vonsattel J-PG. Pick's disease. In: Growdon JH, Rossor MN, eds. Blue Books of Practical Neurology. The Dementias (19). Boston: Butterworth-Heinemann, 1998:7–44.
36. Delacourte A, Sergeant N, Wattez A, Gauvreau D, Robitaille Y. Vulnerable neuronal subsets in Alzheimer's and Pick's disease are distinguished by their τ isoform distribution and phosphorylation. Ann Neurol 1998; 43:193–204.
37. Armstrong RA, Cairns NJ, Lantos PL. Quantification of pathological lesions in the frontal and temporal lobe of ten patients diagnosed with Pick's disease. Acta Neuropathol 1999; 97:456–462.
38. Suvà D, Favre I, Kraftsik R, Esteban M, Lobrinus A, Miklossy J. Primary motor cortex involvement in Alzheimer disease. J Neuropathol Exp Neurol 1999; 58: 1125–1134.
39. Filley CM. The behavioral neurology of cerebral white matter. Neurology 1998; 50:1535–1540.
40. Aström K-E, Mancall EL, Richardson EP, Jr. Progressive multifocal leuko-encephalopathy. A hitherto unrecognized complication of chronic lymphatic leukaemia and Hodgkin's disease. Brain 1958; 81:93–111.
41. Richardson EP Jr. Progressive multifocal leukoencephalopathy. N Engl J Med 1961; 265:815–823.
42. Perentes E, Vonsattel JP. La leucoencephalopathie multifocale progressive. Rev Med Suisse Romande 1979; 99:829–839.
43. Glass JD, Wesselingh SL, Selnes OA, McArthur JC. Clinical-neuropathologic correlation in HIV-associated dementia. Neurology 1993; 43:2230–2237.
44. Fontaine B, Seilhean D, Tourbah A, Daumas-Duport C, Duyckaerts C, Benoit N, Devaux B, Hauw JJ, Rancurel G, Lyon-Caen O. Dementia in two histologically confirmed cases of multiple sclerosis: one case with isolated dementia and one case associated with psychiatric symptoms. J Neurol Neurosurg Psychiatry 1994; 57:353–359.
45. Dichgans M, Mayer M, Uttner I, Brüning R, Müller-Höcker J, Rungger G, Ebke M, Klockgether T, Gasser T. The phenotypic spectrum of CADASIL: clinical findings in 102 cases. Ann Neurol 1998; 44:731–739.
46. Fisher CM. Binswanger's enephalopathy: a review. J Neurol 1989; 236:65–79.
47. Caplan LR, Schoene WC. Clinical features of subcortical arteriosclerotic encephalopathy (Binswanger disease). Neurology 1978; 28:1206–1215.
48. Olszewski J. Subcortical arteriosclerotic encephalopathy. Review of the literature on the so-called Binswanger's disease and presentation of two cases. World Neurol 1962; 3:359–375.
49. Hansen LA, Crain B. Making the diagnosis of mixed and non-Alzheimer's disease. Arch Pathol Lab Med 1995; 119:1023–1031.
50. DeWitt LD, Louis DN. Case Records of the Massachusetts General Hospital. Case 27–1991. A 75-year-old man with dementia, myoclonic jerks, and tonic-clonic seizures. N Engl J Med 1991; 325:42–54.
51. Dubas F, Gray F, Roullet E, Escourolle R. Leucoencéphalopathies artériopathiques (17 cas anatomocliniques). Rev Neurol 1985; 141:93–108.
52. Loes DJ, Biller J, Yuh WTC, Hart MN, Godersky JC, Adams HP, Jr., Keefauver SP, Tranel D. Leukoencephalopathy in cerebral amyloid angiopathy: MR imaging in four cases. AJNR 1990; 11:485–488.
53. Ghika-Schmid F, Ghika J, Assal G, Bogousslavsky J. Démence callosale. Troubles du comportement lors de myélinolyse centro- et extra-pontique. Rev Neurol 1999; 155:367–373.
54. Herz E, Fünfgeld E. Zur Klinik und Pathologie der Alzheimerschen Krankheit. Arch Psychiatrie 1928; 84: 633–664.
55. Schottky J. Über präsenile Verblödung. Z Ges Neurol Psychiatrie (Berl) 1932; 140:333–397.
56. Selden N, Mesulam M-M, Geula C. Human striatum: the distribution of neurofibrillary tangles in Alzheimer's disease. Brain Res 1994; 658:327–331.
57. Probst A, Luginbühl M, Langui D, Ulrich J, Landwehrmeyer B. Pathology of the striatum in progressive supranuclear palsy: abnormal tau proteins in astrocytes and cholinergic interneurons. Neurodegeneration 1993; 2:183–193.
58. Lantos PL. The neuropathology of progressive supranuclear palsy. J Neural Transm [Suppl] 1994; 42: 137–152.
59. Cervós-Navarro J, Schumacher K. Neurofibrillary pathology in progressive surpanuclear palsy (PSP). J Neural Transm 1994; [Suppl] 42:153–164.
60. Steele JC, Richardson JC, Olszewski J. Progressive supranuclear palsy. Arch Neurol 1964; 10:333–359.
61. Vonsattel J-PG, DiFiglia M. Huntington disease. J Neuropathol Exp Neurol 1998; 57:369–384.
62. Deymeer F, Smith TW, DeGirolami U, Drachman DA. Thalamic dementia and motor neuron disease. Neurology 1989; 39:58–61.
63. Katz DA, Naseem A, Horoupian DS, Rothner AD, Davies P. Familial multisystem atrophy with possible thalamic dementia. Neurology 1984; 34:1213–1217.
64. Vonsattel J-PG, Binetti G, Kelley LM. Pick disease. In: Wasco W, Tanzi RE, eds. Molecular Mechanisms of Dementia. Totowa, NJ: Humana Press, 1997:253–269.
65. von Bagh K. Klinische und pathologisch-anatomische Studien an 30 Fällen systematischer umschriebener Atrophie der Grosshirnrinde (Pickscher Krankheit). Ann Acad Sci Fennicae Ser A V Med Anthropol 1946; 10:1–132.
66. Wallesch CW, Kornhuber HH, Kunz T, Brunner RJ. Neuropsychological deficits associated with small unilateral thalamic lesions. Brain 1983; 106:141–152.
67. Guard O, Bellis F, Mabille JP, Dumas R, Boisson D, Devic M. Démence thalamique après lésion hémorragique unilatérale du pulvinar droit. Rev Neurol 1986; 142:759–765.
68. Beal MF, Vonsattel J-P. Case Records of the Massachusetts General Hospital. Case 7–1998. A 74-year-old man with dementia, Parkinsonism, and an insular lesion. N Engl J Med 1998; 338:603–610.

69. Okazaki H, Lipkin LE, Aronson SM. Diffuse intracytoplasmic ganglionic inclusions (Lewy type) associated with progressive dementia and quadriparesis in flexion. J Neuropathol Exp Neurol 1961; 20:237–244.
70. Sima AAF, Clark AW, Sternberger NA, Sternberger LA. Lewy body dementia without Alzheimer changes. Can J Neurol Sci 1986; 13:490–497.
71. Tomlinson BE, Blessed G, Roth M. Observations on the brains of demented old people. J Neurol Sci 1970; 11:205–242.
72. Knopman DS, Mastri AR, Frey WH, Sung JH, Rustan T. Dementia lacking distinctive histologic features: a common non-Alzheimer degenerative dementia. Neurology 1990; 40:251–256.
73. Giannakopoulos P, Hof PR, Bouras C. Dementia lacking distinctive histopathology: Clinicopathological evaluation of 32 cases. Acta Neuropathol 1995; 89:346–355.
74. Michel B, Didic M, Gambarelli D, Viallet F, Gastaut JL. Deux cas de démence frontale avec lésions histologiques non spécifiques: discussion clinico-pathologique et nosologique. Rev Neurol 1996; 152:669–677.
75. Kropp S, Schulz-Schaeffer WJ, Finkenstaedt M, Riedemann C, Windl O, Steinhoff BJ, Zerr I, Kretzschmar HA, Poser S. The Heidenhain variant of Creutzfeldt-Jakob disease. Arch Neurol 1999; 56:55–61.
76. Seilhean D, Michaud J, Duyckaerts C, Hauw J-J. Physiopathologie de l'infection du système nerveux par le VIH-1 et de la démence du SIDA. Rev Neurol 1998; 154:830–842.
77. Bell JE. The neuropathology of adult HIV infection. Rev Neurol 1998; 154:816–829.
78. Lippa CF, Smith TW, Swearer JM. Alzheimer's disease and Lewy body disease: a comparative clinicopathological study. Ann Neurol 1994; 35:81–88.
79. Förstl H, Burns A, Luthert P, Cairns N, Levy R. The Lewy-body variant of Alzheimer's disease. Clinical and pathological findings. Br J Psychiatry 1993; 162:385–392.
80. Hely MA, Reid WGJ, Halliday GM, McRitchie DA, Leicester J, Joffe R, Brooks W, Broe GA, Morris JGL. Diffuse Lewy body disease: clinical features in nine cases without coexistent Alzheimer's disease. J Neurol Neurosurg Psychiatry 1996; 60:531–538.
81. Boeve BF, Maraganore DM, Parisi JE, et al. Pathologic heterogeneity in clinically diagnosed corticobasal degeneration. Neurology 1999; 53:795–800.
82. Rebeiz JJ, Kolodny EH, Richardson EP, Jr. Corticodentatonigral degeneration with neuronal achromasia. Arch Neurol 1968; 18:20–33.
83. Gibb RG, Luthert PJ, Marsden CD. Corticobasal degeneration. Brain 1989; 112:1171–1192.
84. Lantos PL, Papp MI. Cellular pathology of multiple system atrophy: a review. J Neurol Neurosurg Psychiatry 1994; 57:129–133.
85. Feldman RG, McKee AC. Case Records of the Massachusetts General Hospital. Case 46–1993. A 75-year-old man with right-sided rigidity, dysarthria, and abnormal gait. N Engl J Med 1993; 329:1560–1567.
86. Hayden MR. Huntington's Chorea. Berlin Heidelberg New York: Springer-Verlag, 1981.
87. Folstein SE. Epidemiology. In: Folstein SE, ed. Huntington's Disease. A Disorder of Families. Baltimore: The Johns Hopkins University Press, 1989:88–105.
88. Harper PS, Houlihan GD, Jones AL, et al. Psychiatric aspects of Huntington's disease. In: Harper PS, ed. Huntington's Disease. Major Problems in Neurology, 31, 2nd ed. Philadelphia : W.B. Saunders Company, 1996:73–121.
89. Rinne JO, Rummukainen J, Paljärvi L, Rinne UK. Dementia in Parkinson's disease is related to neuronal loss in the medial substantia nigra. Ann Neurol 1989; 26:47–50.
90. Gearing M, Olson DA, Watts RL, Mirra SS. Progressive supranuclear palsy: neuropathologic and clinical heterogeneity. Neurology 1994; 44:1015–1024.
91. Alzheimer A. Über eigenartige Krankheitsfälle des späteren Alters. Z Ges Neurol Psychiatrie (Berl) 1911; 4:356–385.
92. Alzheimer A. Über eine eigenartige Erkrankung der Hirnrinde. Allg Z Psychiatr Psychol Gerichtl Med 1907; 64:146–148.
93. Simchowicz T. Sur la signification des plaques séniles et sur la formule sénile de l'écorce cérébrale. Rev Neurol 1924; 1:221–227.
94. Dickson DW. The pathogenesis of senile plaques. J Neuropathol Exp Neurol 1997; 56:321–339.
95. Portier M-M. Progrès neurologique. Le cytosquelette neuronal: aspects structuraux, fonctionnels et dynamiques. Rev Neurol 1992; 148:1–19.
96. Tolnay M, Probst A. Review: tau protein pathology in Alzheimer's disease and related disorders. Neuropathol Appl Neurobiol 1999; 25:171–187.
97. Iwatsubo T, Hasegawa M, Ihara Y. Neuronal and glial tau-positive inclusions in diverse neurologic diseases share common phosphorylation characteristics. Acta Neuropathol 1994; 88:129–136.
98. Feany MB, Dickson DW. Widespread cytoskeletal pathology characterizes corticobasal degeneration. Am J Pathol 1995; 146:1388–1396.
99. Chin SS-M., Goldman JE. Glial inclusions in CNS degenerative diseases. J Neuropathol Exp Neurol 1996; 55:499–508.
100. Mirra SS, Murrell JR, Gearing M, Spillantini MG, Goedert M, Crowther RA, Levey AI, Jones R, Green J, Shoffner JM, Wainer BH, Schmidt ML, Trojanowski JQ, Ghetti B. Tau pathology in a family with dementia and a P301L mutation in tau. J Neuropathol Exp Neurol 1999; 58:335–345.
101. Spillantini MG, Goedert M, Crowther RA, Murrell JR, Farlow MR, Ghetti B. Familial multiple system tauopathy with presenile dementia: a disease with abundant neuronal and glial tau filaments. Proc Natl Acad Sci USA 1997; 94:4113–4118.
102. Goedert M, Crowther RA, Spillantini MG. Tau mutations cause frontotemporal dementias. Neuron 1998; 21:955–958.
103. Marinesco G. Sur la présence des corpuscules acidophiles paranucléolaires dans les cellules du locus niger et du locus coeruleus. CR Acad Sci 1902; 135:1000–1002.
104. Janota I. Widespread intranuclear neuronal corpuscles (Marinesco bodies) associated with a familial spinal degeneration with cranial and peripheral nerve involvement. Neuropathol Appl Neurobiol 1979; 5:311–317.

105. Lewy FH. Paralysis Agitans. I. Pathologische Anatomie. In: Lewandowsky M, ed. Handbuch der Neurologie (Dritter Band, Spezielle Neurologie II). Berlin: Julius Springer, 1912:920–933.
106. Lewy FH. Zur pathologischen Anatomie der Paralysis agitans. Dtsch Z Nervenheilkd 1913; 50:50–55.
107. Trétiakoff C. Contribution à l'étude de l'anatomie pathologique du locus niger de Soemmering avec quelques déductions relatives à la pathogénie des troubles du tonus musculaire et de la maladie de Parkinson. Paris: Jouve & Cie, Éditeurs, 1919.
108. Forno LS. Neuropathology of Parkinson's disease. J Neuropathol Exp Neurol 1996; 55:259–272.
109. McKeith IG, Galasko D, Kosaka K, Perry EK, Dickson DW, Hansen LA, Salmon DP, Lowe J, Mirra SS, Byrne EJ, Lennox G, Quinn NP, Edwardson JA, Ince PG, Bergeron C, Burns A, Miller BL, Lovestone S, Collerton D, Jansen ENH, Ballard C, de Vos RAI, Wilcock GK, Jellinger KA, Perry RH. Consensus guidelines for the clinical and pathologic diagnosis of dementia with Lewy bodies (DLB): Report of the consortium on DLB international workshop. Neurology 1996; 47:1113–1124.
110. Gibb WRG, Lees AJ. The relevance of the Lewy body to the pathogenesis of idiopathic Parkinson's disease. J Neurol Neurosurg Psychiatry 1988; 51:745–752.
111. Forno LS. Concentric hyalin intraneuronal inclusions of Lewy type in the brains of elderly persons (50 incidental cases): relationship to parkinsonism. J Am Geriatr Soc 1969; 17:557–575.
112. Newell KL, Boyer P, Gomez-Tortosa E, Hobbs W, Hedley-Whyte ET, Vonsattel JP, Hyman BT. α-Synuclein immunoreactivity is present in axonal swellings in neuroaxonal dystrophy and acute traumatic brain injury. J Neuropathol Exp Neurol 1999; 58:263–268.
113. Lippa CF, Schmidt ML, Lee VM-Y, Trojanowski JQ. Antibodies to α-synuclein detect Lewy bodies in many Down's syndrome brains with Alzheimer's disease. Ann Neurol 1999; 45:353–357.
114. Lipkin LE. Cytoplasmic inclusions in ganglion cells associated with parkinsonian states. A neurocellular change studied in 53 cases and 206 controls. Am J Pathol 1959; 35:1117–1133.
115. Pollanen MS, Dickson DW, Bergeron C. Pathology and biology of the Lewy body. J Neuropathol Exp Neurol 1993; 52:183–191.
116. Spillantini MG, Schmidt ML, Lee VM-Y, Trojanowski JQ, Jakes R, Goedert M. α-Synuclein in Lewy bodies. Nature 1997; 388:839–840.
117. Irizarry MC, Growdon W, Gomez-Isla T, Newell K, George JM, Clayton DF, Hyman BT. Nigral and cortical Lewy bodies and dystrophic nigral neurites in Parkinson's disease and cortical Lewy body disease contain α-synuclein immunoreactivity. J Neuropathol Exp Neurol 1998; 57:334–337.
118. Baba M, Nakajo S, Tu P-H, Tomita T, Nakaya K, Lee VM-Y, Trojanowski JQ, Iwatsubo T. Aggregation of α-synuclein in Lewy bodies of sporadic Parkison's disease and dementia with Lewy bodies. Am J Pathol 1998; 152:879–884.
119. Yuen P, Baxter DW. The morphology of Marinesco bodies (paranucleolar corpuscles) in the melanin-pigmented nuclei of the brain-stem. J Neurol Neurosurg Psychiatry 1963; 26:178–183.
120. Ii K, Ito H, Tanaka K, Hirano A. Immunocytochemical co-localization of the proteasome in ubiquitinated structures in neurodegenerative diseases and the elderly. J Neuropathol Exp Neurol 1997; 56:125–131.
121. Brion S, Plas J, Jeanneau A. La maladie de Pick. Point de vue anatomo-clinique. Rev Neurol 1991; 147:693–704.
122. Feany MB, Mattiace LA, Dickson DW. Neuropathologic overlap of progressive supranuclear palsy, Pick's disease and corticobasal degeneration. J Neuropathol Exp Neurol 1996; 55:53–67.
123. Williams HW. The peculiar cells of Pick's disease. Their pathogenesis and distribution in disease. Arch Neurol Psychiatry 1935; 34:508–519.
124. Dickson DW, Yen S-H, Suzuki KI, Davies P, Garcia JH, Hirano A. Ballooned neurons in select neurodegenerative diseases contain phosphorylated neurofilament epitopes. Acta Neuropathol 1986; 71:216–223.
125. Masters CL, Richardson EP Jr. Subacute spongiform encephalopathy (Creutzfeldt-Jakob disease). The nature and progression of spongiform change. Brain 1978; 101:333–344.
126. Collinge J, Palmer MS, Sidle KCL, Mahal SP, Campbell T, Brown J, Hardy J, Brun AE, Gustafson L, Bakker E, Roos R, Groen JJ. Familial Pick's disease and dementia in frontal lobe degeneration of non Alzheimer type are not variants of prion disease. J Neurol Neurosurg Psychiatry 1994; 57:762.
127. Ince PG, Perry EK, Morris CM. Dementia with Lewy bodies. A distinct non-Alzheimer dementia syndrome? Brain Pathology 1998; 8:299–324.
128. Hansen L, Salmon D, Galasko D, et al. The Lewy body variant of Alzheimer's disease: a clinical and pathologic entity. Neurology 1990; 40:1–8.
129. Kazee AM, Han LY. Cortical Lewy bodies in Alzheimer's disease. Arch Pathol Lab Med 1995; 119:448–453.
130. Smith TW, Anwer U, DeGirolami U, Drachman DA. Vacuolar change in Alzheimer's disease. Arch Neurol 1987; 44:1225–1228.
131. Budka H, Aguzzi A, Brown P, Brucher J-M, Bugiani O, Gullotta F, Haltia M, Hauw J-J, Ironside J-W, Jellinger K, Kretzschmar HA, Lantos PL, Masullo C, Schlote W, Tateishi J, Weller RO. Neuropathological diagnostic criteria for Creutzfeldt-Jakob disease (CJD) and other human spongiform encephalopathies (Prion diseases). Brain Pathol 1995; 5:459–466.

Dementia with Lewy Bodies

Synonyms for dementia with Lewy bodies (DLB) include dementia associated with Lewy bodies, diffuse Lewy body disease, cortical Lewy body disease, Lewy body dementia, and senile dementia of Lewy body type.

Alzheimer's disease Lewy body variant (ADLBV) is the condition usually referred to when the pathological hallmarks of dementia with Lewy bodies coexist with that of Alzheimer's disease (AD).

Early comprehensive reports on DLB are that by Okazaki et al., published in 1961,[1] and that by Woodward, published in 1962.[1,2] Subsequent studies led to coherent, clinical, and pathological descriptions of DLB; however, the pathological basis for the dementia and the etiology are still unknown. A definitive diagnosis requires microscopical examination; the presence of cortical and subcortical Lewy bodies are the hallmark of DLB.[3-7]

Lewy body dementia accounts for 15% to 30% of all dementias.[7,8] In our series of 613 brains from demented patients, 81% had changes of pure AD. The series included 74 brains (12%) with changes of AD and cortical and subcortical Lewy bodies (ADLBV) (Table 7–1). In addition, there were 40 (6.5 %) that met the criteria for diffuse Lewy body disease (Table 7–2). Thus, 114 (18.6%) among 613 brains from demented patients contained cortical and subcortical Lewy bodies with or without coexistent Alzheimer's changes of an extent to meet the criteria for AD. Among brains categorized as DLBD, 82 % were from men (Table 7–2), and among brains categorized as ADLBV, 54% were from men (Table 7–1). This is in accordance with a series of 39 patients with DLBD, in which 24 (62%) were men[9]. Thus, LBD is more frequent in men than in women, especially when Alzheimer's changes are minimal or lacking.

SYMPTOMS

The core features of DLB that distinguish it from AD include (1) fluctuating cognitive loss with episodic delirium, (2) psychiatric symptoms including depression and visual hallucinations, and (3) extrapyramidal signs that are either spontaneous or a side effect of neuroleptics. According to recent guidelines, the clinical diagnosis of DLB requires the presence of at least one of these three features.[6] Secondary features that support the diagnosis include falls, syncope, transient loss of consciousness, and sensitivity to neurolpetics. Early in the course of the disease, episodes of cognitive decline alternate with episodes during which cognition is either normal or nearly normal. Short-term memory decline is more prominent than long-term memory loss. The features of parkinsonism are usually mild and include rigidity, bradykinesia, a mask-like facies, stooped posture, and a slow, shuffling gait. Parkinsonism may occur before dementia or vice-versa.[10] Psychiatric symptoms may result from involvement of the amygdala, limbic, and temporal cortex; extrapyramidal signs from the degeneration of pars compacta of the substantia nigra; and dysphagia from the changes involving the dorsal nucleus of vagus.[11]

GENETICS

Lewy bodies are hallmarks of Parkinson's disease and LBD.[12,13] Studies of an Italian family

Table 7–1. Alzheimer's Disease Lewy Body Variant

	N	Mean	Range	SD
Age				
All	74	78.9 years	62–98 years	6.8 years
Men	40	76.7 years	62–88 years	6.4 years
Women	34	81.3 years	69–98 years	6.4 years
Brain weight	74	1201 g	920–1580 g	135 g

Table 7–2. Lewy Body Dementia (Diffuse Lewy Body Disease)

	N	Mean	Range	SD
Age				
All	40	75 years	60–87 years	6.5 years
Men	33	74.2 years	60–84 years	6.2 years
Women	7	78 years	67–87 years	7.6 years
Brain weight	40	1249 g	1020–1550 g	126 g

with Parkinson's disease led to the mapping of a Parkinson disease susceptibility gene to the 4q21–23 genomic region, which encodes a presynaptic nerve terminal protein, α-synuclein.[14,15] α-synuclein is a major component of Lewy bodies and dystrophic neurites associated with Parkinson's disease and DLB.[17,16–19] To our knowledge, the α-synuclein mutations have not been found in cases of LBD, including a family with autosomal inheritance.[20]

NEUROPATHOLOGICAL DIAGNOSTIC CLASSIFICATION

Controversy exists as to whether Parkinson's disease and DLB, including ADLBV (see below), represent two entities or whether they belong to the spectrum of a single disorder.[21–23] We use the following categories for brains with Lewy bodies: Parkinson's disease, ADLBV, and diffuse Lewy body disease or DLB. These three categories include brains that have in common the presence of Lewy bodies with neuronal loss involving the substantia innominata, hypothalamus, amygdala, midbrain raphé, pars compacta of the substantia nigra, nucleus coeruleus, and dorsal nucleus of the vagus.

In Parkinson's disease brains, atrophy is absent or mild and cortical Lewy bodies are either rare,[13,24–27] not found, or absent.[22] In ADLBV, the changes of AD coexists with that of diffuse Lewy body disease. Kosaka coined the term "DLB common form" when the changes of LBD coexists with the presence of many plaques or tangles or both.[3] Thus, brains from demented patients with concomitant Alzheimer's changes that meet the neuropathological criteria for the diagnosis of AD and changes characteristic of DLB are best categorized as ADLBV.[28,29] Unfortunately, the categorization DLBD vs. ADLBV varies greatly depending on the neuropathological, diagnostic criteria used for AD.[29] Earlier categorizations for these brains included the dual denomination of AD with Parkinson's disease.

Alzheimer's disease Lewy body variant may represent mixed AD–Parkinson's disease. The frequent presence of occasional Lewy bodies in the neocortex of individuals with idiopathic Parkinson disease supports this hypothesis. Perhaps the coexistence of AD favors the formation of neocortical Lewy bodies in individuals developing Parkinson's disease.[4,22]

NEUROPATHOLOGY OF DEMENTIA WITH LEWY BODIES

Gross Examination

The brains of patients with diffuse Lewy body disease usually lack atrophy (Fig. 7–14). If present, the cerebral atrophy is mild, despite severe dementia.[11] (Table 7–2). The pars compacta of the substantia nigra and the nucleus coeruleus are pale (Fig. 7–14).

Microscopical Examination

Brain stem– and cortical-type Lewy bodies are considered essential for a pathologic diagnosis of DLB.[30] Brain stem–type Lewy bodies occur mainly in the pigmented neurons of the brain stem, especially those of the pars compacta of the substantia nigra, nucleus coeruleus and dorsal nucleus of vagus. It is our

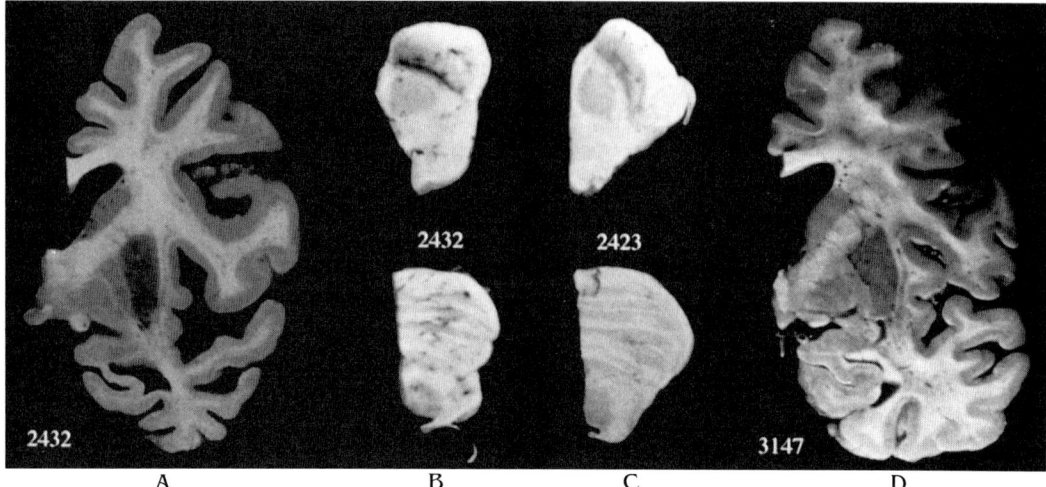

Figure 7–14. Comparative features between Alzheimer's disease (A,B) and diffuse Lewy body disease (C,D). A. Coronal section of the right cerebral hemisphere passing through the amygdaloid nucleus of a 89-year-old woman with Alzheimer's disease. The brunt of the atrophy involves the temporal lobe, especially the amygdaloid nucleus and rostral hippocampal formation. B. Transverse section of the mesencephalon (*top*) and upper portion of the metencephalon (*bottom*). The pars compacta of the substantia nigra is well pigmented; in contrast, the nucleus coeruleus cannot be distinguished, which is typical of Alzheimer's disease. However, since the amount of pigment is age related, its detection does not always reflect the actual neuronal density, especially in patients older than 80 years. C. Same structures and sites as in B, as they appear at postmortem examination of patients with Alzheimer's disease Lewy body variant or with diffuse Lewy body disease. Both the pars compacta of the substantia nigra and nucleus coeruleus are pale. D. Coronal section of the right cerebral hemisphere passing through the amygdaloid nucleus of a 63-year-old man with diffuse Lewy body disease. The atrophy is mild compared to the more prominent atrophy in Alzheimer's disease (A).

experience that in LBD, as in idiopathic Parkinson disease, there are more neurons with Lewy bodies in the nucleus coeruleus than in the pars compacta of the substantia nigra as judged by conventional methods of examination.[31] Other areas with neurons containing Lewy bodies are the hypothalamus, substantia innominata, amygdaloid nucleus, and entorhinal cortex; and parahippocampal and occipitotemporal gyri. Cortical-type Lewy bodies (Fig. 7–15) occur mostly in neurons of the cingulate gyrus, parahippocampal gyrus

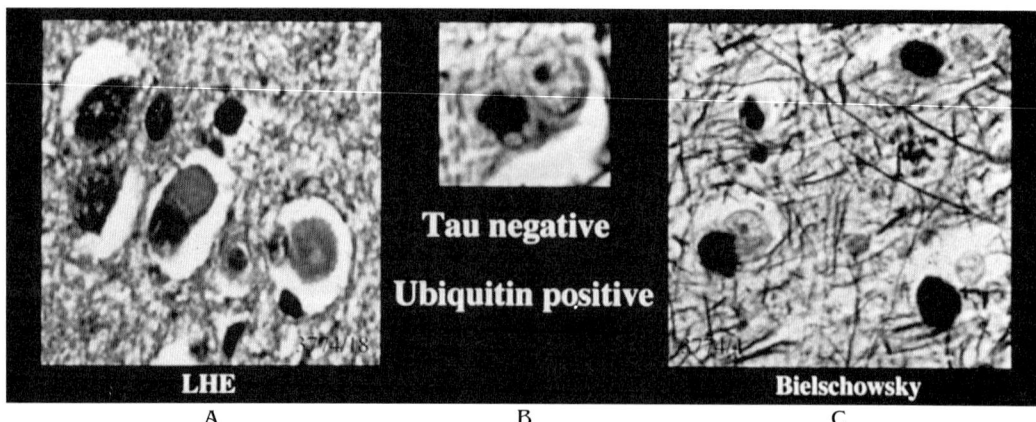

Figure 7–15. Cortical Lewy bodies. A. Two atrophic, cortical neurons, each containing a single Lewy body. Luxol fast blue, counterstained with hematoxylin and eosin (LHE). B. A cortical neuron labeled with antibody against ubiquitin. C. Cortical neurons with argyrophilic Lewy bodies. Modified Bielschowsky stain); original magnification, ×313.

(Fig. 7–16), insula, and temporal, parietal, and frontal cortices.[4,24] They are rare or absent in the occipital lobe especially in the visual cortex. They are occasionally present in the subiculum; however, they are not found in the hippocampal dentate gyrus.[4] Lewy bodies occur preferentially in small and medium sized pyramidal neurons of the fifth and sixth cortical layers, and rarely in the third layer.[4] The neocortex may have up to three to five neurons with cortical-type Lewy bodies per 100× microscopic field. Lewy bodies are argyrophilic and resemble Pick bodies especially in sections prepared with modified Bielschowsky stain, and both are labeled with anti-ubiquitin antibodies. However, in contrast to Pick bodies, Lewy bodies are not labeled with antibodies directed against tau (Fig. 7–15). Woodward listed the following changes involving cortical neurons with Lewy bodies: swelling, hyalinization, cytoplasmic eosinophilia, vacuoles, nuclear lobulation, and nuclear swelling.[2] The density of cortical neurons is usually within normal limits or slightly decreased.

In contrast to the neocortex, neuronal loss may be marked in the paleocortex or entorhinal area, parahippocampal and occipitotemporalis gyri; and amygdaloid nucleus. The three sites where neuronal loss and reactive gliosis are usually conspicuous are the pars compacta of the substantia nigra, the nucleus coeruleus, and the dorsal nucleus of vagus.

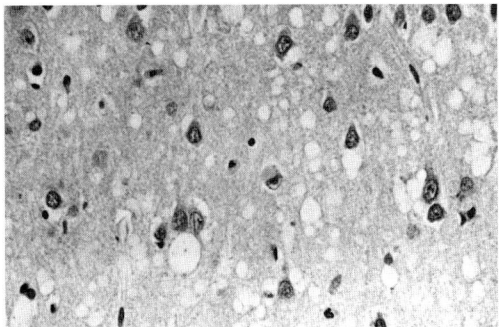

Figure 7–16. Spongiform changes in diffuse Lewy body disease. Third cortical layer of the parahippocampal gyrus. The neuropil has scattered optically empty vacuoles. Note the absence of reactive gliosis. Neuronal density is slightly decreased. Centrally located is a neuron with a cytoplasmic, glassy round inclusion (Lewy body) molding the nucleus, the chromatin of which is condensed against the nuclear membrane. Luxol fast blue, counterstained with hematoxylin and eosin; original magnification, ×200.

The severity of neuronal loss in the substantia innominata varies from mild to severe.[4,24]

Alzheimer's changes (neuritic plaques or tangles or both) are either absent or mild. It is this constellation that Osaka referred to as "DLB pure form."[3]

Additional findings include Lewy-related neurites (LRN). Lewy-related neurites consist of aggregates of proteins that are invisible in sections stained with hematoxylin and eosin or most silver impregnation, but are labeled with antibodies directed against ubiquitin and α-synuclein. Lewy-related neurites also occur in the amygdaloid nucleus, substantia innominata, dorsal nucleus of vagus, and other brain stem nuclei. Of interest is the selective damage of the CA2–CA3 sectors of the hippocampal formation in contrast to AD.[32,33] This may or may not be visible using conventional silver impregnation, e.g. Bielschowsky methods, depending on the quality of the techniques.[32,34] Similar changes involving CA1–CA3 sectors of hippocampal formation may occur in idiopathic Parkinson's disease and progressive supranuclear palsy, thus they are not specific for LBD.[22,33]

Spongiform changes (Fig. 7–16) usually without reactive gliosis (in contrast to Creutzfeldt-Jakob disease) are often prominent, especially in the entorhinal cortex, parahippocampal and occipitotemporalis gyri, neocortex ventral to the nucleus accumbens, insula, and in amygdaloid nucleus.[35] Rarely, spongiform changes are transcortical and associated with mild gliosis, which mimics Creutzfeldt-Jakob disease.[35]

Cortical Lewy bodies have been found in most brains that were referred to as "plaque-only" AD, as mentioned before.[36,37]

In our series of 74 demented subjects with Lewy bodies, the patients with LBD (Table 7–2) tended to be younger than patients with ADLBV (Table 7–1). The preponderance of men in the group with LBD is much more striking than in the group with ADLBV. Finally, brain atrophy is less pronounced in the group with DLB than in the group with ADLBV.

REFERENCES

1. Okazaki H, Lipkin LE, Aronson SM. Diffuse intractytoplasmic ganglionic inclusions (Lewy type) associated with progressive dementia and quadriparesis

1. in flexion. J Neuropathol Exp Neurol 1961; 20:237–244.
2. Woodward J. Concentric hyaline inclusion body formation in mental disease analysis of twenty-seven cases. J Neuropathol Exp Neurol 1962; 21:442–449.
3. Kosaka K. Diffuse Lewy body disease in Japan. J Neurol 1990; 237:197–204.
4. Gibb RG, Esiri MM, Lees AJ. Clinical and pathological features of diffuse cortical Lewy body disease (Lewy body dementia). Brain 1987; 110:1131–1153.
5. Hely MA, Reid WGJ, Halliday GM, et al. Diffuse Lewy body disease: clinical features in nine cases without coexistent Alzheimer's disease. J Neurol Neurosurg Psychiatry 1996; 60:531–538.
6. McKeith IG, Galasko D, Kosaka K, Perry EK, Dickson DW, Hansen LA, Salmon DP, Lowe J, Mirra SS, Byrne EJ, Lennox G, Quinn NP, Edwardson JA, Ince PG, Bergeron C, Burns A, Miller BL, Lovestone S, Collerton D, Jansen ENH, Ballard C, de Vos RAI. Wilcock GK, Jellinger KA, Perry RH. Consensus guidelines for the clinical and pathologic diagnosis of dementia with Lewy bodies (DLB): report of the consortium on DLB international workshop. Neurology 1996; 47:1113–1124.
7. Kosaka K. Diffuse Lewy body disease. Rinsho Shinkeigaku Clini Neurol 1995; 35:1455–1456.
8. Perry RH, Irving D, Blessed G, Perry EK, Fairbairn AF. Clinically and neuropathologically distinct form of dementia in the elderly. Lancet 1989; 1:166.
9. Ala TA, Yang K-H, Frey WH, II. Hallucinations and signs of parkinsonism help distinguish patients with dementia and cortical Lewy bodies from patients with Alzheimer's disease at presentation: a clinicopathological study. J Neurol Neurosurg Psychiatry 1997; 62:16–21.
10. Byrne EJ, Lennox G, Lowe J, Godwin-Austen RB. Diffuse Lewy body disease: clinical features in 15 cases. J Neurol Neurosurg Psychiatry 1989; 52:709–717.
11. Beal MF, Vonsattel J-P. Case Records of the Massachusetts General Hospital. Case 7-1998. A 74-year-old man with dementia, Parkinsonism, and an insular lesion. N Engl J Med 1998; 338:603–610.
12. Gray F. Neuropathologie des syndromes parkinsoniens. Rev Neurol 1988; 144:229–248.
13. Forno LS. Neuropathology of Parkinson's disease. J Neuropathol Exp Neurol 1996; 55:259–272.
14. Polymeropoulos MH, Lavedan C, Leroy E, Ide SE, Dehejia A, Dutra A, Pike B, Root H, Rubenstein J, Boyer R, Stenroos ES, Chandrasekharappa S, Athanassiadou A, Papapetropoulos T, Johnson WG, Lazzarini AM, Duvoisin RC, Di Iorio G, Golbe LI, Nussbaum RL. Mutation in the α-synuclein gene identified in families with Parkinson's disease. Science 1997; 276:2045–2047.
15. Polymeropoulos MH. Autosomal dominant Parkinson's disease and α-synuclein. Ann Neurol 1998; 44(Suppl 1):S63–S64.
16. Irizarry MC, Growdon W, Gomez-Isla T, et al. Nigral and cortical Lewy bodies and dystrophic nigral neurites in Parkinson's disease and cortical Lewy body disease contain α-synuclein immunoreactivity. J Neuropathol Exp Neurol 1998; 57:334–337.
17. Spillantini MG, Schmidt ML, Lee VMY, Trojanowski JQ, Jakes R, Goedert M. α-Synuclein in Lewy bodies. Nature 1997; 388:839–840.
18. Trojanowski JQ, Lee VMY. Aggregation of neurofilament and α-synuclein proteins in Lewy bodies. Arch Neurol 1998; 55:151–152.
19. Baba M, Nakajo S, Tu P-H, Tomita T, Nakaya K, Lee VM-Y, Trojanowski JQ, Iwatsubo T. Aggregation of α-synuclein in Lewy bodies of sporadic Parkinson's disease and dementia with Lewy bodies. Am J Pathol 1998; 152:879–884.
20. Denson MA, Wszolek ZK, Pfeiffer RF, Wszolek EK, Paschall TM, McComb RD. Familial parkinsonism, dementia, and Lewy body disease: study of family G. Ann Neurol 1997; 42:638–643.
21. Litvan I, MacIntyre A, Goetz CG, Wenning GK, Jellinger K, Verny M, Bartko JJ, Jankovic J, McKee A, Brandel JP, Chaudhuri KR, Lai EC, D'Olhaberriague L, Pearce RKB, Agid Y. Accuracy of the clinical diagnoses of Lewy body disease, Parkinson disease, and dementia with Lewy bodies. Arch Neurol 1998; 55:969–978.
22. Brown DF, Dababo MA, Bigio EH, Risser RC, Eagan KP, Hladik CL, White CL. Neuropathologic evidence that the Lewy body variant of Alzheimer disease represents coexistence of Alzheimer disease and idiopathic Parkinson disease. J Neuropathol Exp Neurol 1998; 57:39–46.
23. Ince PG, Perry EK, Morris CM. Dementia with Lewy bodies. A distinct non-Alzheimer dementia syndrome? Brain Pathol 1998; 8:299–324.
24. Gibb WRG, Luthert PJ, Janota I, Lantos PL. Cortical Lewy body dementia: clinical features and classification. J Neurol Neurosurg Psychiatry 1989; 52:185–191.
25. Hughes AJ, Daniel SE, Kilford L, Lees AJ. Accuracy of clinical diagnosis of idiopathic Parkinson's disease: a clinico-pathological study of 100 cases. J Neurol Neurosurg Psychiatry 1992; 55:181–184.
26. Hughes AJ, Daniel SE, Blankson S, Lees AJ. A clinicopathologic study of 100 cases of Parkinson's disease. Arch Neurol 1993; 50:140–148.
27. Gibb WRG, Lees AJ. The relevance of the Lewy body to the pathogenesis of idiopathic Parkinson's disease. J Neurol Neurosurg Psychiatry 1988; 51:745–752.
28. Samuel W, Galasko D, Masliah E, Hansen LA. Neocortical Lewy body counts correlate with dementia in the Lewy body variant of Alzheimer's disease. J Neuropathol Exp Neurol 1996; 55:44–52.
29. Hansen LA, Samuel W. Criteria for Alzheimer's disease and the nosology of dementia with Lewy bodies. Neurology 1997; 48:126–132.
30. Ellis RJ, Olichney JM, Thal LJ, Mirra SS, Morris JC, Beekly D, Heyman A. Cerebral amyloid angiopathy in the brains of patients with Alzheimer's disease: The CERAD experience, part XV. Neurology 1996; 46:1592–1596.
31. den Hartog Jager WA, Bethlem J. The distribution of Lewy bodies in the central and autonomic nervous systems in idiopathic paralysis agitans. J Neurol Neurosurg Psychiatry 1960; 23:283–290.
32. Dickson DW, Ruan D, Crystal H, Mark MH, Davies P, Kress Y, Yen S-H. Hippocampal degeneration differentiates diffuse Lewy body disease (DLBD) from Alzheimer's disease: light and electron microscopic

immunocytochemistry of CA2-3 neurites specific to DLBD. Neurology 1991; 41:1402–1409.
33. Kim H, Gearing M, Mirra S. Ubiquitin-positive CA2/3 neurites in hippocampus coexist with cortical Lewy bodies. Neurology 1995; 45:1768–1770.
34. Lippa CF, Smith TW, Swearer JM. Alzheimer's disease and Lewy body disease: a comparative clinicopathological study. Ann Neurol 1994; 35:81–88.
35. Burkhardt CR, Filley CM, Kleinschmidt-deMasters BK, de la Monte S, Norenberg MD, Schneck SA. Diffuse Lewy body disease and progressive dementia. Neurology 1988; 38:1520–1528.
36. Hansen LA, Masliah E, Galasko D, Terry RD. Plaque-only Alzheimer disease is usually the Lewy body variant, and vice versa. J Neuropathol Exp Neurol 1993; 52:648–654.
37. Terry RD, Hansen LA, DeTeresa R, Davies P, Tobias H, Katzman R. Senile dementia of the Alzheimer type without neocortical neurofibrillary tangles. J Neuropathol Exp Neurol 1987; 46:262–268.

Paraneoplastic Limbic Encephalitis

Dementia associated with carcinoma may be secondary to a destructive, inflammatory process of the brain affecting the limbic system, a condition referred to as "paraneoplastic limbic encephalitis."[1,2]

Paraneoplastic limbic encephalitis can be misdiagnosed as Alzheimer disease, especially in the elderly.[1,3] Paraneoplastic syndromes affecting the nervous system are due to an immune reaction against antigens shared by the tumor and the nervous system.[4,5] For example, paraneoplastic limbic encephalitis is often associated with antineuronal antibodies such as anti-Hu.[6] Pulmonary, mammary, intestinal, renal, and gynecological carcinomas may also be coupled with paraneoplastic limbic encephalitis.[3,7–9] Furthermore, limbic encephalitis may occur without detectable primary tumor or infectious agents, although a cryptic neoplasm cannot be ruled out unequivocally.[10] In such instances, etiologies of limbic encephalitis to investigate are herpes simplex or lyssa virus (rabies), which have a neurotropism for the mesiotemporal regions. However, the course of the viral limbic encephalitis is faster than that of the paraneoplastic limbic encephalitis.

NEUROPATHOLOGY

Gross Examination

The brain of a patient with paraneoplastic limbic encephalitis may appear normal or may display atrophy of the medial, temporal lobe, with or without dirty-gray, usually linear, discoloration of the hippocampal formation and uncus[3] (Fig. 7–17). The amygdaloid nucleus

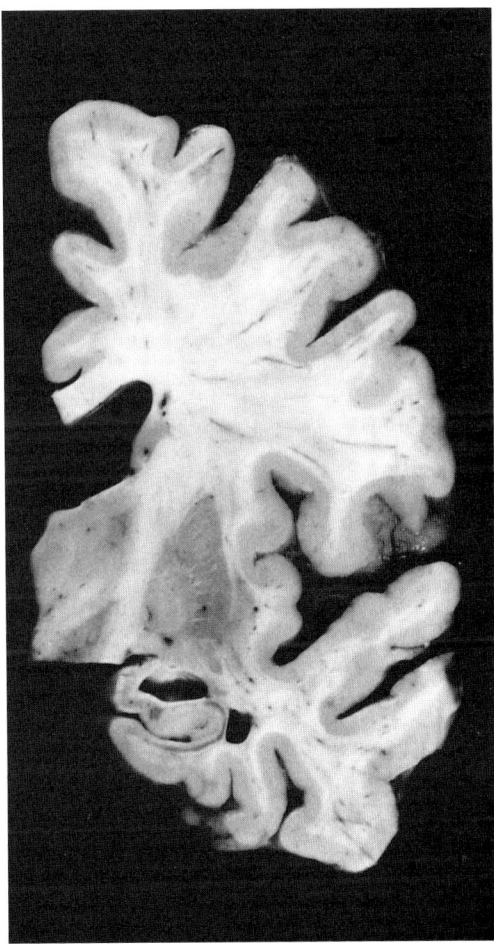

Figure 7–17. Paraneoplastic limbic encephalitis in an 81-year-old woman with clinical diagnosis of Alzheimer disease made 8 months before her death. A small cell carcinoma of the lung was found at autopsy. Shown here is the coronal section of the right cerebral hemisphere passing through the subthalamic nucleus. Note the linear discoloration of the hippocampal formation involving especially the Sommer sector (CA1) and subiculum.

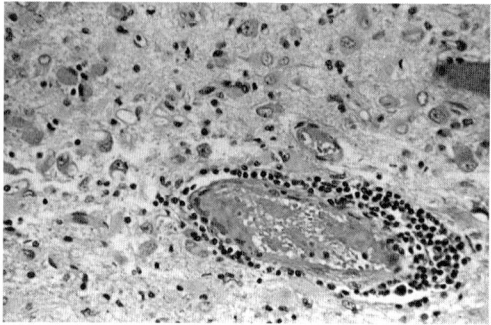

Figure 7-18. Parahippocampal cortex with perivenular lymphocytic infiltrates including rare plasmocytes, scattered lymphocytes within the neuropil, and reactive gliosis. Note the presence of optically empty vacuoles in neurons. Luxol fast blue counterstained with hematoxylin and eosin; original magnification, ×100.

may appear darker than normally expected. The demarcation between gray and white matter of the affected areas may be sharp or blurred.

Microscopical examination

Perivascular, primarily perivenular, chronic inflammatory infiltrates, mainly lymphocytes with plasmocytes, are more prominent in the gray than in the white matter. Rare lymphocytes may be dispersed within the parenchyma. Scattered, microglial nodules, neuronophagia, neurons with optically empty cytoplasmic vacuoles, and astrocytosis are also prominent (Fig. 7-18). Especially vulnerable are the hippocampal formation, medial temporal lobe including amygdala, mammillary body, cingulate gyrus, and inferior olivary nucleus.[9] The brain stem, notably the metencephalon and myelencephalon, may be extensively involved.[3]

Paraneoplastic limbic encephalitis mimics Alzheimer disease. Thus, the diagnosis of paraneoplastic limbic encephalitis should be included in the differential diagnoses of dementias, especially at the onset of the mental decline. The diagnosis of paraneoplastic limbic encephalitis may be difficult, even daring, when the underlying cancer is still unknown.[11] The presence of antineuronal antibodies in the cerebrospinal fluid or serum or both may unveil a carcinoma while still asymptomatic.[12] For example, anti-Hu antibodies in the cerebrospinal fluid or in serum, which binds to a nuclear protein of neurons and tumor cells, suggest a small cell carcinoma of the lung.

REFERENCES

1. Corsellis JAN, Goldberg GJ, Norton AR. "Limbic encephalitis" and its association with carcinoma. Brain 1968; 91:481-496.
2. Richardson EP Jr, Hedley-Whyte ET. Case Records of the Massachusetts General Hospital. Case 30-1985. N Engl J Med 1985; 313:249-257.
3. Koroshetz WJ, McKee AC. Case Records of the Massachusetts General Hospital. Case 39-1988. N Engl J Med 1988; 319:849-860.
4. Delattre JY, Davila L, Vega F, Poisson M. Autoimmunité et syndromes neurologiques paranéoplasiques. Rev Neurol 1991; 147:549-556.
5. Scaravilli F, An SF, Groves M, Thom M. The neuropathology of paraneoplastic syndromes. Brain Pathol 1999; 9:251-260.
6. Alamowitch S, Graus F, Uchuya M, Reñé R, Bescansa E, Delattre JY. Limbic encephalitis and small cell lung cancer. Clinical and immunological features. Brain 1997; 120:923-928.
7. Rosenblum MK. Paraneoplasia and autoimmunologic injury of the nervous system: the anti-Hu syndrome. Brain Pathol 1993; 3:199-212.
8. Tsukamoto T, Mochizuki R, Mochizuki H, Noguchi M, Kayama H, Hiwatashi M, Yamamoto T. Paraneoplastic cerebellar degeneration and limbic encephalitis in a patient with adenocarcinoma of the colon. J Neurol Neurosurg Psychiatry 1993; 56:713-716.
9. Dubas F, Gray F, Escourolle R, Castaigne P. Poliencéphalomyélites subaiguës avec cancer. Six cas anatomo-cliniques et revue de la littérature. Rev Neurol 1982; 138:725-742.
10. Dubas F, Gray F, Henin D, Foncin JF, Escourolle R, Castaigne P. Polioencéphalomyélites subaiguës sans cancer. Quatre cas anatomo-cliniques et revue de la littérature. Rev Neurol 1982; 138:743-753.
11. Dalmau JO, Posner JB. Paraneoplasic syndromes. Arch Neurol 1999; 56:405-408.
12. Giometto B, Taraloto B, Graus F. Autoimmunity in paraneoplastic neurological syndromes. Brain Pathol 1999; 9:261-273.

Creutzfeldt-Jakob Disease, Transmissible Spongiform Encephalopathies, and Prion Disease

JEAN PAUL G. VONSATTEL, WENDY HOBBS, AND E. TESSA HEDLEY-WHYTE

In memory of Dr. Edward Peirson Richardson, Jr.

Synonyms for Creutzfeldt-Jakob disease (CJD) include spongiform encephalopathies, transmissible spongiform encephalopathies (TSE), slow virus diseases, and prion diseases. Transmissible spongiform encephalopathies are sporadic or genetic, fatal, neurodegenerative disorders that occur in humans and animals and are caused by infectious agents.[1,2] They include three major groups: (1) acquired (kuru, iatrogenic CJD, and new-variant CJD); (2) sporadic Creutzfeldt-Jakob disease (S-CJD); and (3) inherited, which encompasses the familial form of CJD (F-CJD), the Gerstmann-Sträussler-Scheinker syndrome (GSSS), and fatal familial insomnia (FFI).

Spongiform change is an important pathological hallmark of TSE.[3,4] However, it may or may not occur in FFI.[5–8] Other pathological features common to the TSE are gliosis, neuronal loss with or without amyloid deposition, and lack of chronic or acute inflammatory infiltrates. The distribution of the changes is primarily in the gray matter and it differs according to the group, however, with considerable overlap.[3,9–11] The extent of the changes is variable from brain to brain.

Commonly, the condition referred to as "Creutzfeldt-Jakob disease" (CJD) is a rare form of rapidly worsening dementia with extrapyramidal syndrome, myoclonus, and, in the brain, spongiform change, astrocytosis, and neuronal loss with amyloid plaques in 10% of cases.[3,12] The iatrogenic form of CJD resulted from the use of contaminated electrodes, following cadaveric grafts of dura mater, cornea, or eardrums, cadaveric pituitary-derived human growth hormone therapy, and maybe after blood transfusion.[13–18] The autosomal dominant GSSS is characterized by extrapyramidal and often cerebellar signs, dementia, and amyloid deposits in the cerebellar and cerebral cortices.[10,19–21] Fatal familial insomnia is a dominantly inherited form of thalamic dementia associated with insomnia, dysautonomia, and movement disorders with the brunt of the pathology involving the thalamus.[5,22–24] The definitive diagnosis of TSE relies on neuropathology.[6]

PRION PROTEIN AND GENETICS

The causative agent of TSE is probably a host, highly conserved, 35 kDa glycoprotein referred to as "prion protein" (PrP) that became pathogenic perhaps due to an expansion of its β-pleated configuration.[25] The normal prion protein, PrP^C, is ubiquitous, soluble, and digestible by proteinase K. It is a constitutive protein of cell membranes and highly expressed in neurons. The PrP gene, *PRNP*, maps to the short arm of chromosome 20. The polymorphism of codon 129 of *PRNP* gene influences both the risk of developing the disease and its phenotype (see below).[26,27] The alteration of the prion particle is rare and may occur independently of any nucleic acids. It may result from post-translational changes of the PrP^C structure. The conversion renders the protein pathogenic—denoted as PrP^{Sc}, PrP^{CJD}, or PrP^{res}—infectious, partially resistant to protease, insoluble, and resistant to prolonged heating to 100°C (212°F). Moreover, data[25] suggest that prions multiply by conversion of PrP^C into PrP^{CJD}.[25] The available antibodies do not distinguish between PrP^C and PrP^{CJD}. However, in contrast to PrP^{CJD}, PrP^C can be easily digested with protease. Thus, subjecting histologic sections to proteinase K prior to immunohistochemistry reveals whether the tissue contains the pathogenic form of PrP. Current consensus is that detection of PrP^{CJD} in brain tissue sections using immunoperoxidase methods is the most reliable diagnostic marker for TSE.[28] The acquired, sporadic, and inherited TSE are apparently caused by alteration of PrP^C, although the proof that PrP^C converts into infectious PrP^{CJD} is still lacking. Thus, one cannot absolutely exclude that causative mechanisms or agents other than PrP^{CJD} may trigger TSE.

The routes of transmission of TSE are only partially elucidated. The spread of bovine spongiform encephalopathy (BSE) in the United Kingdom, France, Germany, Ireland, and Switzerland may have been linked to feeding cattle with meat and bone meal contaminated with sheep scrapie. Iatrogenic transmission through contaminated surgical electrodes and through grafts of dura, cornea, or growth hormone obtained from CJD cadavers has been well documented.[13-18]

The incubation period is 1–5 years in sheep,[29] 2.5–8 years in cattle,[2] over 10 and up to 20 years in humans,[16,17,30] and 2 to 12 months in experimental rodents.[2,4]

The inherited group includes forms that have been linked to point mutations or base-pair repeats within the *PRNP* reading frame.[31,32] The translation product of the *PRNP* gene is polymorphic with methionine (Met) or valine (Val) at codon 129 and glutamic acid or lysine (Lys) at codon 178. In the United Kingdom, 38% of the normal population are homozygous Met/Met, 12% are Val/Val, while 51% are heterozygous (Met/Val) at the codon 129 locus of the *PRNP* gene.[33] As alluded to before, the polymorphism at codon 129 affects both the risk and the phenotype of F-CJD and S-CJD.[26] An association exists between the iatrogenic form of CJD and homozygosity at codon 129. For example, the Met/Met genotype at codon 129 is the most frequent in S-CJD and is also found in the new variant of CJD including BSE.[34] The Met/Met genotype at codon 129 favors cortical involvement and little or no amyloid deposition. The Val-Val genotype favors involvement of the deep gray nuclei and the formation of amyloid deposits. The Met/Val genotype (Fig. 7–19) favors the formation of kuru plaques.[33,34]

Many families with CJD or FFI are linked to a mutation at codon 178 of the *PRNP* gene. When this mutation at locus 178 is coupled with valine at locus 129, it causes CJD. However, when the mutation at codon 178 is coupled with methionine at position 129, it causes FFI.[26] Further mutations at codons 102, 117, 198, 200, and 217 have been found in associ-

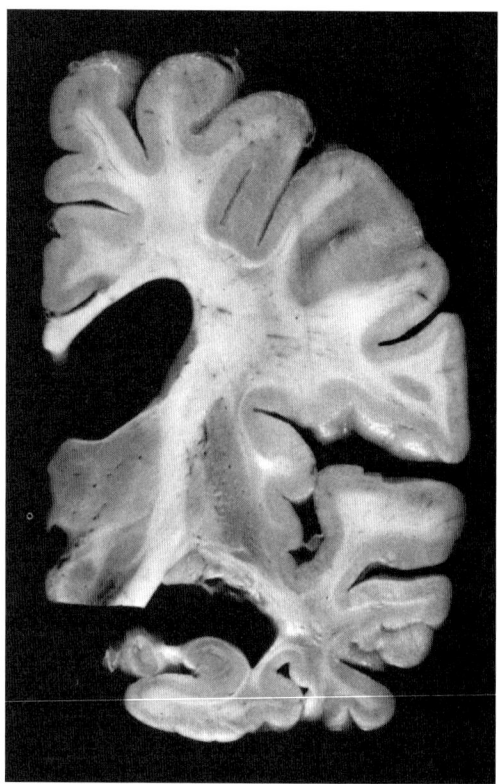

Figure 7–19. Coronal section passing through the subthalamic nucleus of the right cerebral hemisphere of a 53-year-old woman with sporadic Creutzfeldt-Jakob disease, heterozygosity Met/Val at codon 129 of prion protein gene (*PRNP*), and with PrP^{res} type 2 (*MV2*).[27,55] Symptom onset occurred at age 47 years. Symptoms included depression, hypoactivity, weight gain, impaired short memory, urinary incontinence and unstable gait.[41] The striatum (caudate nucleus, putamen and globus pallidus) and white matter including corpus callosum are atrophic, mimicking Huntington disease. Cortical thickness is apparently normal.

ation with prion disease in large pedigrees including GSSS.[1,32,35–38]

CLINICAL COURSE

Creutzfeldt-Jakob disease is rare and may present as a sporadic (S-CJD), genetic (F-CJD), or infectious illness. Sporadic CJD accounts for 85% percent of cases and F-CJD, which is autosomal dominant, accounts for the rest.[2,39] The prevalence and incidence of CJD has varied in part because of the increasing awareness of the illness. The prevalence, incidence, and mortality rate are 0.5 to 1.0 per million per year in the United States, Western Europe, Israel, and Australia.[32,39,40] Women and men are equally prone to develop the disease. In a series of 94 patients (83 with sporadic and 11 with F-CJD) there were 51 men and 43 women.[39] The mean age at onset is symmetrically distributed around the mean of 60 years.[11] Symptoms include visuospatial disorders, rapidly worsening dementia, myoclonus, motor dysfunction, and paroxysmal bursts of high-voltage slow waves on electroencephalography (EEG). Patients with F-CJD exhibiting chorea may be misdiagnosed with Huntington disease.[31] The mean total duration of illness of the series of 94 patients mentioned above was 7.3 months (SD 7.5 months, range 1.5 to 55.0 months). The mean age at death was 57 years (SD 10.2 years, range 27 to 78 years).[39] Six patients were aged 80 or more. The mean age at death of the 11 patients with F-CJD was 51 years (SD 11.7 years, range 35 to 69 years), and that of the 83 patients with S-CJD was 58 years (SD 9.7, range 27 to 78 years).[39] Billette et al. reported that the mean age at death of patients with S-CJD was 61.5 years, that of 31 patients with iatrogenic CJD was 30.5 years, and that of 18 patients with CJD putatively due to cadaveric growth hormone therapy was 23.5 years.[14] As a rule, 80% of the patients die within 12 months of onset of symptoms and the rest have a long course up to 5 years or more.[11,41]

New variant CJD differs from classic CJD in that the patients are younger (mean age 27 years), and psychiatric symptoms including depression or sensory disturbances or both predominate at onset, followed by dementia and ataxia or choreoathetosis.[42,43] The characteristic EEG changes are lacking and the course of the disease has an average of 14 months.

Kuru, which means 'trembling' in the Fore language, is confined to Papua New Guinea. Kuru is characterized by tremor, cerebellar ataxia, movement disorders, dysarthria, and mutism, and death often occurs within 1 year from onset of symptoms.[2] Both the incidence and prevalence of kuru are steadily decreasing since the practice of cannibalism ended in the 1960s.

Slowly worsening cerebellar ataxia followed by dementia characterize the Gerstmann-Sträussler-Scheinker syndrome (GSSS).[16,19,44] Usually ataxia is the predominating symptom and dementia may or may not be severe or may occur only late in the course of the illness.[45] The mean age at onset of symptoms of 15 individuals with definite GSSS was 44.3 years (SD 8.3 years, range 31 to 62years). The mean of the duration of the disease in 14 patients was 6.6 years (SD 5.1 years, range 2 to 17 years). The age at death of 18 patients was 52.8 years (SD 7.5 years, range 31 to 62 years).[44]

Fatal familial insomnia (FFI), first described in 1986, is an atypical prion disease in which insomnia, dysautonomia, motor abnormalities, and weight loss are the salient signs usually followed by mental decline.[5,8,22,46] Age at onset of symptoms is 20 to 60 years, duration of the disease varies between 7 to 36 months.[5,8,47] Some familial progressive subcortical gliosis and some familial thalamic dementias may belong to the TSE category. Petersen et al. reported a family with progressive subcortical gliosis linked to chromosome 17 and characterized by the presence of protease-resistant PrP that lack a mutation in the coding region of the *PRPN* gene, suggesting that other genes influence the propriety of PrP.[48] Thus, inherited prion disease should be excluded by *PRNP* gene evaluation and protease digestion of tissue samples in any patient with atypical dementia and ataxia.

NEUROPATHOLOGY

The brain in TSE may or may not show atrophy. The cut surfaces of the cerebral hemispheres and brain stem are apparently normal or show variable degrees of atrophy (Fig. 7–

19) pallor of the substantia nigra, blurred demarcation between gray and white matter, and rarely, discoloration of the centrum semi ovale. The vermis is often atrophic. The intensity and distribution of pathological changes vary from case to case. Richardson and Masters focused on the clinicopathological correlation, which is a practical approach for both clinicians and neuropathologists.[11] In the Heidenhain variants of CJD, visual symptoms and occipital involvement predominate. In the striatal variants, chorea or choreoathetosis and striatal involvement prevail and mimic Huntington disease both clinically and pathologically (Fig. 7–19). In the thalamic variants, which include FFI, the brunt of the lesions involves the thalamus and hypothalamus. The cerebellar variants resemble kuru and are typified by severe involvement of the cerebellum. The variants with oculomotor dysfunction mimic progressive supranuclear palsy. In the panencephalopathic variants, both gray and white matter are undergoing degeneration.

As mentioned before, the three features detected under the microscope, that are characteristic of TSE are spongiform change, neuronal loss, and fibrillary astrocytosis involving gray matter and, to a much lesser extent, white matter with or without amyloid deposits.[3] The region of the brain where the changes prevail determines the variant as defined by the clinicopathological correlation listed above. Thus, in planning a brain biopsy or in opting for a restrictive postmortem examination to reduce the risk of contamination, one should be aware of the topographic variations of the parenchymal degeneration occurring in TSE.

Spongiform change (Fig. 7–20) consists of the presence of countless small, round, or ovoid, 1.0 to 25.0 μm in diameter, optically empty vacuoles within the neuropil and the cytoplasm of neurons, at times molding the nucleus.[1,3,41] Spongiform change in TSE may occur before the onset of symptoms.[9,18] Experimentally, spongiform change was first observed 13 weeks after inoculation and consisted of two types of membrane-bound vacuoles in neuronal elements.[4] One type of vacuole, developing within myelinated axons (myelinated vacuoles), contained secondary vacuoles and vesicles with or without membrane fragments. The other type of vacuole was found within neuronal processes lacking myelin (unmyelinated vacuole).[4] Figure 7–21

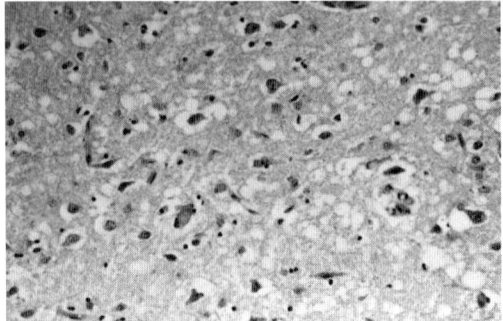

Figure 7–20. Micorphotograph of temporal cortex (same patient as in Fig. 7–19) showing spongiform change, decreased neuronal density, and reactive gliosis. Luxol fast blue counterstained with hematoxylin and eosin; original magnification, ×200.

depicts the ultrastructure of both myelinated and unmyelinated vacuoles in a brain biopsy sample from a patient with S-CJD. The striatum may be the site where spongiform change occurs first.[18] According to Hauw, the only constant location for spongiform change in CJD is the head of the caudate nucleus.[6] Spongiform change involves sequentially the deeper before the superficial cortical layers; however, transcortical involvement occurs in patients with protracted illness.[3] Furthermore, with time, severe neuronal loss occurs and small vacuoles may merge to form large, optically empty, coarse spaces of up to 50 or more μm across, separated by astrocytic pro-

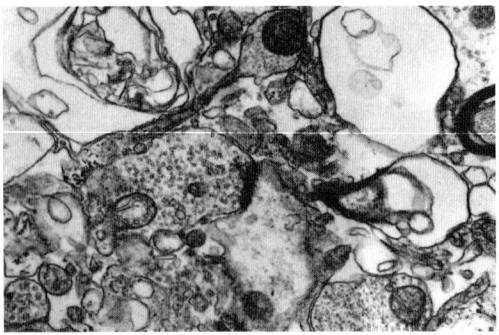

Figure 7–21. Ultrastructural features of cerebral cortical biopsy of a 78-year-old woman with sporadic Creutzfeld-Jakob disease. A large, C-shaped unmyelinated vacuole contains two secondary vacuoles (upper left). Myelinated axons show large vacuoles in axoplasm (upper right). Note the presence of small myelinated and unmyelinated vacuoles. [Courtesy of Dr. Howard Chang, M.D., Massachusetts General Hospital, Boston].

cesses, thus developing status spongiosus.[3] Both single and coalescent vacuoles of variable sizes encircle a focus of compact amyloid—a complex referred to as "florid' plaque"—in the new variant of CJD.

Fibrillary astrocytosis appears after the formation of vacuoles within neurons and within the neuropil.[9] The degree of gliosis is proportional to neuronal loss.[3] Spongiform change and fibrillary astrocytosis are usually more prominent in the dorsal medial nucleus of the thalamus than in the other thalamic nuclei. At postmortem examination, the cerebellum of patients with CJD frequently shows spongiform change confined to the molecular layer.[3] The dentate gyrus is spared while the subiculum shows spongiform change in patients with a chronic course of illness. Spongiform change may be lacking or subtle, especially in FFI, in which neuronal loss and gliosis involve mainly the anterior and dorsomedian nuclei of the thalamus with possible extension within other adjacent nuclei including the pulvinar.[5–7,22–24,46,47]

Optically empty spaces around neurons, oligodendrocytes, and vessels both in gray and white matter are artifacts produced by improper paraffin embedding and are not to be confused with spongiform change.[49]

Amyloid occurs in 10% of CJD brains, especially those from patients with a chronic course. Amyloid is found in all brains from patients with GSSS. Amyloid deposits in TSE produce two distinctive type of plaques: the kuru plaque (Fig. 7–22) and the multicentric plaque (Fig. 7–23) or Gerstmann-Sträussler-Scheinker (GSS) plaque. Amyloid plaques in CJD are similar to amyloid plaques in kuru, thus they are often referred to as "kuru plaques." Kuru and GSS plaques can be found in both gray and white matter. Kuru plaques have an eosinophilic, periodic acid-Schiff (PAS)–positive, round core 50 to 100 μm in diameter with radiating spikes at their periphery (Fig. 7–22). Multicentric amyloid plaques or GSS plaques are the neuropathological hallmark of GSSS. They consist of a spherical aggregate of irregular, moderately argyrophilic masses of amyloid (Fig. 7–23), with or without a larger mass centrally located.[19,21] Although GSS plaques are characteristically found in brains from patients with GSSS, they may be encountered in brains from patients with CJD (Fig. 7–23). In contrast to neuritic plaques,

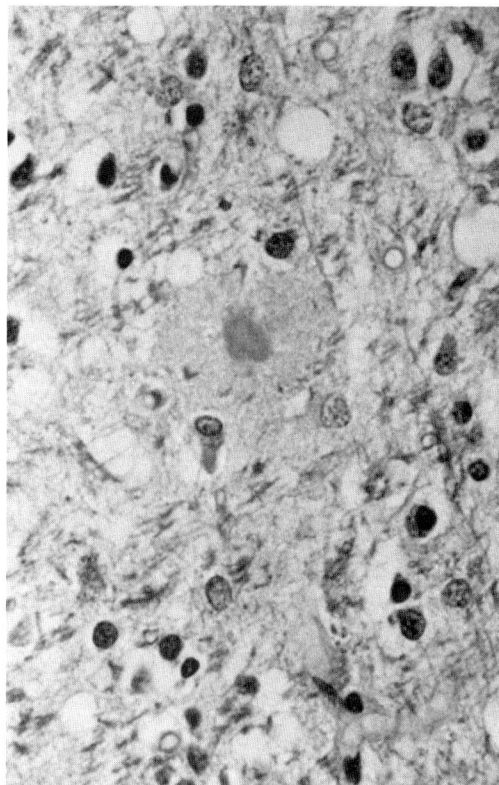

Figure 7–22. Microphotograph of the calcarine cortex (same patient as in Fig. 7–19) showing a kuru plaque (center) neuronal loss, reactive astrocytes, and scattered vacuoles. Luxol fast blue counterstained with hematoxylin and eosin; original magnification, ×500.

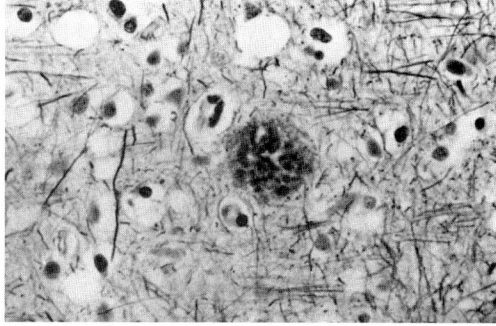

Figure 7–23. Microphotograph of the calcarine cortex (same patient as in Fig. 7–19) showing a multicentric amyloid plaque. Note the absence of dystrophic neurites. Modified Bielschowsky stain; original magnification, ×500.

kuru and GSS plaques are devoid of dystrophic neurites, or if present, abnormal neurites are scant.[50] The amyloid core consists of compact PrP[CJD] arranged in a β-pleated configuration, hence the kuru core is congophilic although weak compared to the β-amyloid core of neuritic plaques. Under polarized light, the amyloid core of kuru plaque has a Maltese cross appearance.[10,31] Kuru and GSS plaques are alike ultrastructurally. They are composed of irregularly arranged fibrils of 10 nm in diameter.[45] The amyloid of kuru and GSS plaques is immunoreactive with PrP antibodies but not with β-amyloid antibodies. However, kuru and GSS-plaques may coexist with β-amyloid–containing plaques.[31,51] Recently, plaques containing both PrP and β-amyloid were identified in five brains from affected members of a family with hereditary Alzheimer's disease.[52]

Although CJD primarily affects gray matter, the white matter may show severe involvement in rare instances.[53,54] The white matter degeneration, which coexists with gray matter involvement, includes myelin loss, fibrillary astrocytosis, scattered macrophages, and spongiform change.[53,54]

Recently, Parchi et al. provided a detailed analysis of molecular and clinicopathological features in a series of 300 subjects with CJD.[27,55] Accordingly, the polymorphic codon 129 of the PRNP (Met/Met, Val/Val, or Met/Val), and two types of PrP[CJD] (type 1 and type 2) strongly influence the variability encountered in CJD.[26] The Met/Met at codon 129 with type 1 PrP[CJD] (M1M1) and Met/Val with type 1 PrP[CJD] (MV1) account for 70% of their series of S-CJD and include the cases classified as typical CJD of the myoclonic type and the Heidenhain variant. The Met/Val at codon 129 with type 2 PrP[CJD] (MV2) (Fig. 7–19) is characterized by longer mean duration of symptoms and the presence of kuru plaques (Fig. 7–22). This molecular–clinicopathological correlation has the potential to unveil key steps of the pathogenesis of the transmissible spongiform encephalopathies.

We thank Larry Cherkas for his assistance and advice. We express our appreciation to the pathologists who referred case material to the Harvard Brain Tissue Resource Center, and the Alzheimer Disease Research Center; this work would not have been possible without their assistance. We are grateful to the families of the patients for providing brain tissue for research. This work was supported in part by NIH grants NINCDS 31862 (Harvard Brain Tissue Resource Center, J.P.V.); NS 16367 (Huntington's Disease Center Without Walls, J.P.V., W.H.); and NIA 2P50-AG0 5134 (J.P.V., E.T.H.-W.).

REFERENCES

1. Prusiner SB. Genetic and infectious prion diseases. Arch Neurol 1993; 50:1129–1153.
2. Gajdusek DC. Subacute spongiform encephalopathies: transmissible cerebral amyloidosis caused by unconventional viruses. In: Fields BN, Knipe DM, eds. Virology, 2nd ed. New York: Raven Press, 1990: 2289–2324.
3. Masters CL, Richardson EP, Jr. Subacute spongiform encephalopathy (Creutzfeldt-Jakob disease). The nature and progression of spongiform change. Brain 1978; 101:333–344.
4. Liberski PP, Yanagihara R, Asher DM, Gibbs CJ, Jr, Gajdusek DC. Reevaluation of the ultrastructural pathology of experimental Creutzfeldt-Jakob disease. Serial studies of the Fujisaki strain of Creutzfeldt-Jakob disease virus in mice. Brain 1990; 113:121–137.
5. Seilhean D, Duyckaerts C, Hauw J-J. Insomnie fatale familiale et maladies à prions. Rev Neurol 1995; 151: 225–230.
6. Budka H, Aguzzi A, Brown P, Brucher J-M, Bugiani O, Gullotta F, Haltia M, Hauw J-J, Ironside J-W, Jellinger K, Kretzschmar HA, Lantos PL, Masullo C, Schlote W, Tateishi J, Weller RO. Neuropathological diagnostic criteria for Creutzfeldt-Jakob disease (CJD) and other human spongiform encephalopathies (Prion diseases). Brain Pathol 1995; 5:459–466.
7. Silburn P, Cervenáková L, Varghese P, Tannenberg A, Brown P, Boyle R. Fatal familial insomnia: a seventh family. Neurology 1996; 47:1326–1328.
8. Almer G, Hainfellner JA, Brücke T, Jellinger K, Kleinert R, Bayer G, Windl O, Kretzschmar HA, Hill A, Sidle K, Collinge J, Budka H. Fatal familial insomnia: a new Austrian family. Brain 1999; 122:5–16.
9. Masters CL, Kakulas BA, Alpers MP, Gajdusek DC, Gibbs CJ. Preclinical lesions and their progression in the experimental spongiform encephalopathies (kuru and Creutzfeldt-Jakob disease) in primates. J Neuropathol Exp Neurol 1976; 35:593–605.
10. Masters CL, Gajdusek DC, Gibbs CJ Jr. Creutzfeldt-Jakob disease virus isolations from the Gerstmann-Sträussler syndrome with an analysis of the various forms of amyloid plaque deposition in the virus-induced spongiform encephalopathies. Brain 1981; 104:559–588.
11. Richardson EP, Jr, Masters CL. The nosology of Creutzfeldt-Jakob disease and conditions related to the accumulation of PrP[CJD] in the nervous system. Brain Pathol 1995; 5:33–41.
12. Johnson RT. Prion disease. N Engl J Med 1992; 326: 486–487.
13. Marzewski DJ, Towfighi J, Harrington MG, Merril CR, Brown P. Creutzfeldt-Jakob disease following pituitary-derived human growth hormone therapy: a new American case. Neurology 1988; 38:1131–1133.
14. Billette De Villemeur T, Gourmelen M, Beauvais P,

14. Rodriguez D, Vaudour G, Deslys J-P, Dormont D, Richard P, Richardet J-M. Maladie de Creutzfeldt-Jakob chez quatre enfants traités par hormone de croissance. Rev Neurol 1992; 148:328–334.
15. Patry D, Curry B, Easton D, Mastrianni JA, Hogan DB. Creutzfeldt-Jakob disease (CJD) after blood product transfusion from a donor with CJD. Neurology 1998; 50:1872–1873.
16. Brown P. Human growth hormone therapy and Creutzfeldt-Jakob disease: a drama in three acts. Pediatrics 1988; 81:85–92.
17. Croxson M, Brown P, Synek B, et al. A new case of Creutzfeldt-Jakob disease associated with human growth hormone therapy in New Zealand. Neurology 1988; 38:1128–1130.
18. New MI, Brown P, Temeck JW, Owens AB, Hedley-Whyte ET, Richardson EP. Preclinical Creutzfeldt-Jakob disease discovered at autopsy in a human growth hormone recipient. Neurology 1988; 38:1133–1134.
19. Gerstmann J, Sträussler E, Scheinker I. Über eine eigenartige hereditär-familiäre Erkrankung des Zentralnervensystems. Zugleich ein Beitrag zur Frage des vorzeitigen lokalen Alterns. Z Ges Neurol Psychiatrie (Berl) 1936; 154:736–762.
20. von Braunmühl A. Über eine eigenartige hereditär-familiäre Erkrankung des Zentralnervensystems. Arch Psychiatrie Z Neurol 1954; 191:419–449.
21. Seitelberger F. Eigenartige familiär-hereditäre Krankheit des Zentralnervensystems in einer niederösterreichischen Sippe. (Zugleich ein Beitrag zur vergleichenden Neuropathologie des Kuru). Wien Klin Wochenschr 1962; 74:687–691.
22. Lugaresi E, Montagna P, Baruzzi A, Cortelli, P, Tinuper P, Zucconi M, Gambetti PL, Medori R. Insomnie familiale à évolution maligne: une nouvelle maladie thalamique. Rev Neurol 1986; 142:791–792.
23. Julien J, Vital C, Deleplanque B, Lagueny A, Ferrer X. Atrophie thalamique subaiguë familiale. Troubles mnésiques et insomnie totale. Rev Neurol 1990; 146:173–178.
24. Medori R, Tritschler H-J, LeBlanc A, Villare F, Manetto V, Chen HY, Xue R, Leal S, Montagna P, Cortelli P, Tinuper P, Avoni P, Mochi M, Baruzzi A, Hauw JJ, Ott J, Lugaresi E, Autilio-Gambetti L, Gambetti P. Fatal familial insomnia, a prion disease with a mutation at codon 178 of the prion protein gene. N Engl J Med 1992; 326:444–449.
25. Cohen FE, Pan K-M, Huang Z, Baldwin M, Fletterick RJ, Prusiner SB. Structural clues to prion replication. Science 1994; 264:530–531.
26. Monari L, Chen SG, Brown P, Parchi P, Petersen RB, Mikol J, Gray F, Cortelli P, Montagna P, Ghetti B, Goldfarb LG, Gajdusek DC, Lugaresi E, Gambetti P, Autilio-Gambetti L. Fatal familial insomnia and familial Creutzfeldt-Jakob disease: different prion proteins determined by a DNA polymorphism. Proc Natl Acad Sci USA 1994; 91:2839–2841.
27. Parchi P, Giese A, Capellari S, Brown P, Schulz-Schaeffer W, Windl O, Zerr I, Budka H, Kopp N, Piccardo P, Poser S, Rojiani A, Streichemberger N, Julien J, Vital C, Ghetti B, Gambetti P, Kretzschmar H. Classification of sporadic Creutzfeldt-Jakob disease based on molecular and phenotypic analysis of 300 subjects. Ann Neurol 1999; 46:224–233.
28. Kretzschmar HA, Ironside JW, DeArmond SJ, Tateishi J. Diagnostic criteria for sporadic Creutzfeldt-Jakob disease. Arch Neurol 1996; 53:913–920.
29. Cuillé J, Chelle P-L. La maladie dite tremblante du mouton est-elle inoculable? Comptes Rendus Acad Sci 1936; 203:1552–1554.
30. Prusiner SB, Gajdusek DC, Alpers MP. Kuru with incubation periods exceeding two decades. Ann Neurol 1982; 12:1–9.
31. Collinge J, Brown J, Hardy J, Mullan M, Rossor MN, Baker H, Crow TJ, Lofthouse R, Poulter M, Ridley R, Owen F, Bennett C, Dunn G, Harding AE, Quinn N, Doshi B, Roberts, GW, Honavar M, Janota I, Lantos PL. Inherited prion disease with 144 base pair gene insertion. Brain 1992; 115:687–710.
32. Brown P. The phenotypic expression of different mutations in transmissible human spongiform encephalopathy. Rev Neurol 1992; 148:317–327.
33. MacDonald ST, Sutherland K, Ironside JW. Prion protein genotype and pathological phenotype studies in sporadic Creutzfeldt-Jakob disease. Neuropathol Appl Neurobiol 1996; 22:285–292.
34. Tranchant C, Geranton L, Guiraud-Chaumeil C, Mohr M, Warter JM. Basis of phenotypic variability in sporadic Creutzfeldt-Jakob disease. Neurology 1999; 52:1244–1249.
35. Tranchant C, Doh-Ura K, Steinmetz G, Chevalier Y, Kitamoto T, Tateishi J, Warter JM. Mutation du codon 117 du gène du prion dans une maladie de Gerstmann-Sträussler-Scheinker. Rev Neurol 1991; 147:274–278.
36. Goldgaber D, Goldfarb LG, Brown P, Asher DM, Brown WT, Lin S, Teener JW, Feinstone SM, Rubenstein R, Kascsak RJ, Boellaard JW, Gajdusek DC. Mutations in familial Creutzfeldt-Jakob disease and Gerstmann-Sträussler-Scheinker's syndrome. Exp Neurol 1989; 106:204–206.
37. Mallucci GR, Campbell TA, Dickinson A, Beck J, Holt M, Plant G, de Pauw KW, Hakin RN, Clarke CE, Howell S, Davies-Jones GAB, Lawden M, Smith CML, Ince P, Ironside JW, Bridges LR, Dean A, Weeks I, Collinge J. Inherited prion disease with an alanine to valine mutation at codon 117 in the prion protein gene. Brain 1999; 122:1823–1837.
38. Bertoni JM, Brown P, Goldfarb LG, Rubenstein R, Gajdusek DC. Familial Creutzfeldt-Jakob disease (Codon 200 mutation) with supranuclear palsy. JAMA 1996; 268:2413–2415.
39. Masters CL, Harris JO, Gajdusek DC, Gibbs CJ, Bernoulli C, Asher DM. Creutzfeldt-Jakob disease: patterns of worldwide occurrence and the significance of familial and sporadic clustering. Ann Neurol 1979; 5:177–188.
40. Cathala F, Brown P, Raharison S, Chatelain J, Lacanuet P, Castaigne P, Gibbs CJ, Jr., Gajdusek DC. Maladie de Creutzfeldt-Jakob en France. Contribution à une recherche épidémiologique. Rev Neurol 1982; 138:39–51.
41. Growdon JH, Vonsattel JP. Case Records of the Massachusetts General Hospital. Case 17–1993. A 53-year-old woman who died after several years of a dementing illness with intermittent generalized seizures and abnormal movements of the extremities and head. N Engl J Med 1993; 328:1259–1266.
42. Brown P. The risk of bovine spongiform encephalopathy ('mad cow disease') to human health. JAMA 1997; 278:1008–1011.

43. Will RG, Ironside JW, Zeidler M, Cousens SN, Estibeiro K, Alperovitch A, Poser S, Pocchiari M, Hofman A, Smith PG. A new variant of Creutzfeldt-Jakob disease in the UK. Lancet 1996; 347:921–925.
44. Hainfellner JA, Brantner-Inthaler S, Cervenáková L, Brown P, Kitamoto T, Tateishi J, Diringer H, Liberski PP, Regele H, Feucht M, Mayr N, Wessely P, Summer K, Seitelberger F, Budka H. The original Gerstmann-Sträussler-Scheinker family of Austria: divergent clinicopathological phenotypes but constant PrP genotype. Brain Pathol 1995; 5:201–211.
45. Hudson AJ, Farrell MA, Kalnins R, Kaufmann JCE. Gerstmann-Sträussler-Scheinker disease with coincidental familial onset. Ann Neurol 1983; 14:670–678.
46. Nagayama M, Shinohara Y, Furukawa H, Kitamoto T. Fatal familial insomnia with a mutation at codon 178 of the prion protein gene: first report from Japan. Neurology 1996; 47:1313–1316.
47. Rossi G, Macchi G, Porro M, Giaccone G, Bugiani M, Scarpini E, Scarlato G, Molini GE, Sasanelli F, Bugiani O, Tagliavini F. Fatal familial insomnia. Genetic, neuropathologic, and biochemical study of a patient from a new Italian kindred. Neurology 1998; 50:688–692.
48. Petersen RB, Tabaton M, Chen SG, Monari L, Richardson SL, Lynches T, Manetto V, Lanska DJ, Markesbery WR, Currier RD, Autilio-Gambetti L, Wilhelmsen KC, Gambetti P. Familial progressive subcortical gliosis: presence of prions and linkage to chromosome 17. Neurology 1995; 45:1062–1067.
49. Smith TW, Anwer U, DeGirolami U, Drachman DA. Vacuolar change in Alzheimer's disease. Arch Neurol 1987; 44:1225–1228.
50. Genthon R, Gray F, Salama J, Duyckaerts C, Belin C, Brucher JM, Baron H, Delaporte P. Maladie de Gerstmann-Sträussler-Scheinker. Étude pathologique et généalogique. Rev Neurol 1992; 148:335–342.
51. Hainfellner JA, Wanschitz J, Jellinger K, Liberski PP, Gullotta F, Budka H. Coexistence of Alzheimer-type neuropathology in Creutzfeldt-Jakob disease. Acta Neuropathol 1998; 96:116–122.
52. Leuba G, Saini K, Savioz A, Charnay Y. Early-onset familial Alzheimer disease with coexisting β-amyloid and prion pathology. JAMA 2000; 283:1689–1691.
53. Krüger H, Meesmann C, Rohrbach E, Müller J, Mertens HG. Panencephalopathic type of Creutzfeldt-Jakob disease with primary extensive involvement of white matter. Eur Neurol 1990; 30:115–119.
54. Park TS, Kleinman GM, Richardson EP. Creutzfeldt-Jakob disease with extensive degeneration of white matter. Acta Neuropathol 1980; 52:239–242.
55. Parchi P, Castellani R, Capellari S, Ghetti B, Young K, Chen SG, Farlow M, Dickson DW, Sima AAF, Trojanowski JQ, Petersen RB, Gambetti P. Molecular basis of phenotypic variability in sporadic Creutzfeldt-Jakob disease. Neurology 1996; 39:767–778.

Frontal and Frontotemporal Dementia

The frontotemporal dementias (FTD) are an ill-defined group of non-Alzheimer, neurodegenerative, dementing diseases with frontal lobe symptoms of variable severity.[1,2] Forty to fifty percent of the patients have affected members in their families.[3] Onset of symptoms usually occurs between age 50 and 65 years. Duration of the disease from onset of symptoms until death varies between 6 to 12 years. Symptoms include apathy, disinhibition, euphoria, hyperorality, bulimia, and aphasia. As in Pick disease (which clinically cannot be distinguished reliably from FTD[2]), the following three syndromes summarize the clinical findings often observed in FTD: (1) moriatic syndrome (or moria: foolishness or dullness of comprehension, frivolity, joviality, inability to take anything seriously), (2) PES syndrome (palilalia, echolalia, stereotypia), (3) or PEMA syndrome (palilalia, echolalia, mutism, and amimia).[4,5] An increasingly recognized subtype is FTD associated with amyotrophic lateral sclerosis (FTD-ALS). The onset of dementia is insidious and occurs often before the age of 65 years, and usually precedes the associated, gradual neurogenic muscular atrophy.[6] Patients with FTD-ALS typically develop dementia of frontal lobe type with or without symptoms of motor neuron disease, although their brains contain neuronal, ubiquitin-labeled inclusions identical to those observed in the non-motor areas in classical motor neuron disease.[7–9] In a review article, Hudson[10] reported that 18 patients with ALS and with dementia had lower motor neuron degeneration at postmortem examination.

GENETIC ASPECTS OF FRONTAL LOBE DEMENTIAS

Recently, Spillantini et al. described an autosomal, dominant, dementing illness referred to as "familial multiple system tauopathy with presenile dementia," and "frontotemporal dementia and parkinsonism linked to chromosome 17" (FTDP-17), which belong to the group of FTD until otherwise proven.[11,12] This condition is linked to chromosome 17q21–22 and shows widespread neuronal and glial tau protein deposits. The authors identified 41 affected subjects spread over seven generations in a pedigree of 383 individuals. The mean age at onset of symptoms was 49 years with a range of 10 years. Symptoms include imbalance, memory loss, bradykinesia, axial and limb rigidity, superior gaze palsy, and dysphagia. There is diffuse brain atrophy with frontotemporal predominance. Neuronal loss and fibrillary lesions involve the cerebral cortex, hippocampal formation, substantia nigra, hypothalamus, periaqueductal gray, third and fourth cranial nerve nuclei, and reticular nuclei. In addition, there is myelin and axonal loss in the propriospinal tract, ventral and lateral spinothalamic tracts, and lateral vestibulopsinal tract with mild neuronal loss and neurofibrillary changes involving the anterior and posterior spinal gray matter.[11,12] Currently many families with dementia linked to chromosome 17 have been identified.[13] In chromosome 17–linked dementia, atrophy involves chiefly the frontal and temporal regions, striatum (caudate nucleus > putamen), amygdala, and substantia nigra compacta and reticulata with relative preservation of the nucleus coeruleus.[14–16]

Additional individuals with familial dementia linked to chromosome 17 have been reported. The conditions have clinical and pathological features that currently cannot be distinguished reliably from the FTD group. Examples of these conditions are the disinhibition dementia parkinsonism amyotrophy complex (DDPAC);[15] the rapidly progressive autosomal dominant parkinsonism and dementia with pallido pontonigral degeneration (PPND) and marked pyramidal tract dysfunction;[17,18] and the hereditary dysphasic disinhibition dementia (HDDD).[19,20]

Bird et al.[21] reported three separate families that shared identical mutation of the tau gene, the affected members of which had severe behavioral abnormalities with frontal lobe atrophy. Onset of symptoms and neuropathological findings between members of these families were different despite their identical mutation, which suggests that modifying genes or environment may play a role. For example, ballooned neurons were present in one brain but were not found in another brain from affected members. Furthermore, one brain had argyrophilic perinuclear rings that were not found in another brain, both from affected subjects; and one brain showed tangles, the distribution of which mimicked that found in progressive supranuclear palsy.[21] Argyrophilic perinuclear rings involving neurons in the frontal and temporal cortices were identified with Pick bodies in the granular layer of the dentate gyrus of individuals from six families with frontal lobe dementia and parkinsonism linked to chromosome 17q21–22 (FTDP-17) with a mutation in the tau gene.[22] Widespread neuronal and glial inclusions, neuropil threads, and astrocytic plaques as seen in corticobasal degeneration were reported in two individuals with FTD and parkinsonism linked to chromosome 17.[23] These examples emphasize the heterogeneity of symptoms and pathological findings in individuals with a mutation in the tau gene. The clinical and pathological spectra of dementias linked to chromosome 17 could be narrowed and thus gain in specificity through improvement of the identification and interpretation of symptoms, pathological features, and topography.

NEUROPATHOLOGY

Gross Examination

The external surface of the brain is either normal or shows mild to moderate atrophy.[24] The atrophy may be confined to the frontal lobe or may involve both the frontal and temporal lobes and sometimes includes the parietal lobes (Fig. 7–24). The transition between the atrophic and apparently normal areas is ill defined. The cut surfaces of the coronal sections of the brain may appear normal or may show slight to moderate cortical and white matter atrophy, especially of the anterior third of both the frontal and temporal lobes (Fig. 7–25). The neostriatum (caudate nucleus, putamen and nucleus accumbens) and thalamus may be mildly to moderately smaller than normal (Fig. 7–26). The substantia nigra is pale (Fig 7–26) in about 50% of the brains in contrast to the nucleus coeruleus, which tends to be relatively preserved.

A comprehensive description of the neuropathological findings in FLD-17 is provided by Sima et al. who studied six brains with this disorder.[25] Briefly, the brain weight of their series ranged from 970 to 1350g. The atrophy involved mainly the anterior ventral regions of

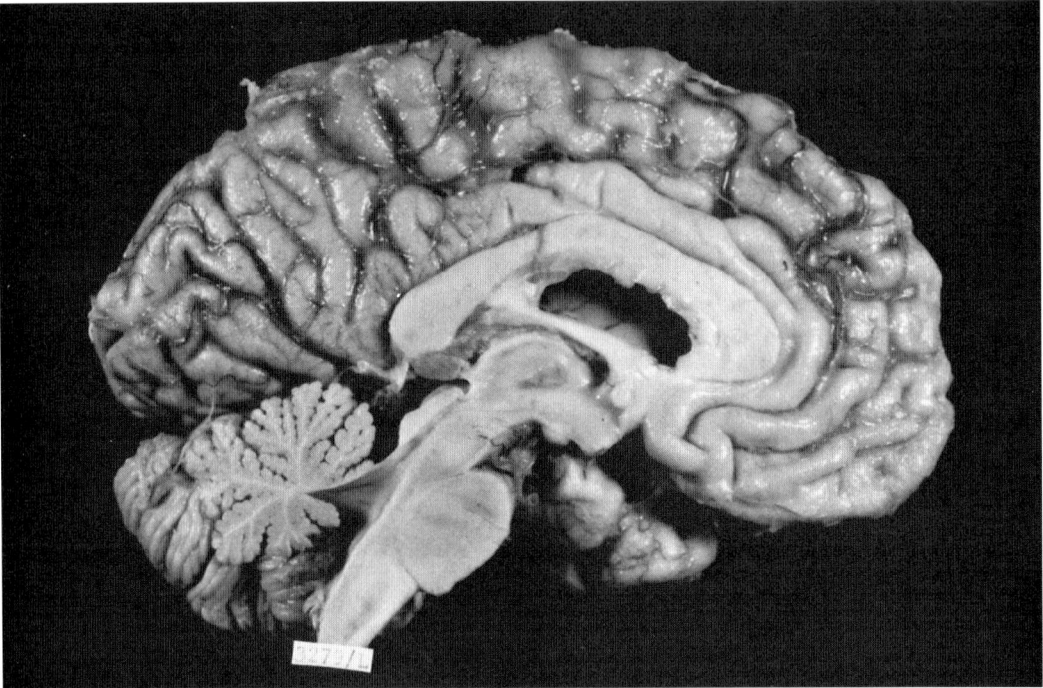

Figure 7–24. Medial aspect of the left half brain of a 74-year-old demented woman with a family history of non-Alzheimer's, frontal type dementia. Atrophy was moderate and diffuse. Main microscopical findings included scattered vacuoles with shrunken pyramidal neurons in the upper frontal cortical layers (see Fig. 7–27), marked neuronal loss involving the internal segment of globus pallidus, substantia nigra pars reticulata, and compacta (see Fig. 7–26), locus coeruleus, subthalamic nucleus, red nucleus, and pons. The hippocampal formation and amygdaloid nucleus were unremarkable. Neither neuritic plaques nor tangles were found.

the temporal lobe and the prefrontal and anterior cingulate gyrus with normal appearance of the posterior frontal, parietal, and occipital areas. The hippocampal formation was normal. The ventral anterior neostriatum was atrophic with mild brown discoloration. The substantia nigra was pale.

Microscopical Examination

The main findings are status spongiosus involving the upper cortical layers (I–III), notably of the frontal, temporal, and parietal lobes, with mild gliosis at the corticosubcortical junction (cortical layer VI and U fibers), and scattered, atrophic, pyramidal neurons (Fig. 7–27) within these regions.[24] The rostral portion of the neostriatum shows mild or moderate neuronal loss with scattered reactive astrocytes usually involving the head of the caudate nucleus more than the adjacent putamen. Gliosis may involve both segments of the globus pallidus, dorsally more than ventrally, or may be confined to the external segment. When the substantia nigra is involved, both the compacta and reticulata show neuronal loss and gliosis, with the brunt of the changes being within the compacta. The frontopontine fibers of the cerebral peduncle may show myelin loss with rare macrophages. Mild gliosis may be seen within the subthalamic nucleus, red nucleus, and the pons. Neuritic plaques and neurofibrillary tangles of Alzheimer's are rare or absent (Fig. 7–27). Thus, the atrophy in FTD is mild to moderate and usually confined to the anterior two-thirds of the telencephalon with ill-defined transition between the atrophic and relatively preserved area.

On microscopical examination, the main findings provided by Sima et al. on FLD-17

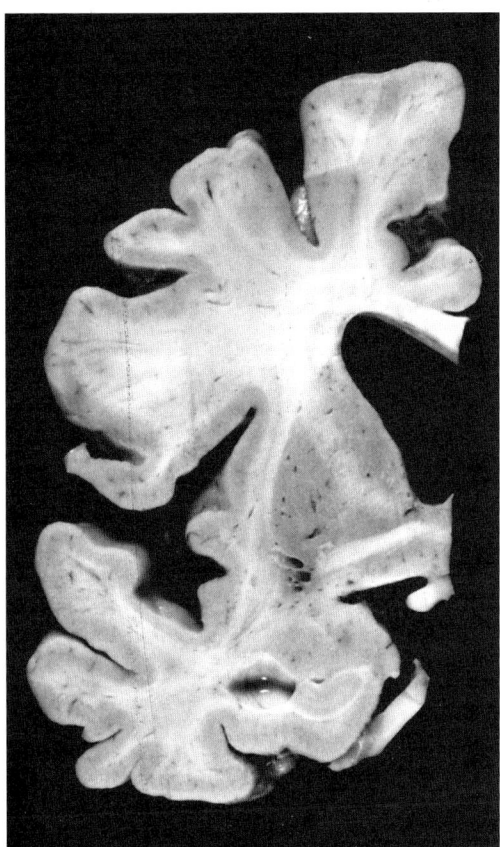

Figure 7–25. Coronal section of the left cerebral hemisphere passing through the anterior white commissure of the same patient as in Figure 7–24. The sulci and lateral ventricle are wider than normal. The amygdala and neostriatum are mildly atrophic. The globus pallidus is slightly discolored. The anterior white commissure has normal thickness.

Argyrophilic neurons were present in the third cranial nerve nucleus, dorsal raphe nucleus, ventral hypothalamus, subthalamic nucleus, periaqueductal gray, pars compacta of the substantia nigra, red nucleus, and globus pallidus. Oligodendrocytes with argyrophilic cytoplasm, which labeled with ubiquitin and tau, were found in the white matter, external capsule, ansa lenticularis, corpus callosum, and brain stem.[25]

included scattered, ballooned neurons and mild, neuronal loss involving the CA1 to CA3 areas, subiculum, and prosubiculum of the otherwise normal hippocampal formation. Neuronal loss and gliosis were noticed in the following structures in a descending order of severity: amygdaloid nucleus, substantia nigra, ventral portion of globus pallidus, periaqueductal gray, ventral putamen, ventral hypothalamus, and caudate nucleus. The nucleus coeruleus showed mild neuronal loss. The red nucleus, thalamus, and substantia innominata were minimally involved, if at all. Neocortical and hippocampal neurofibrillary tangles of Alzheimer and neuritic plaques were very rare.

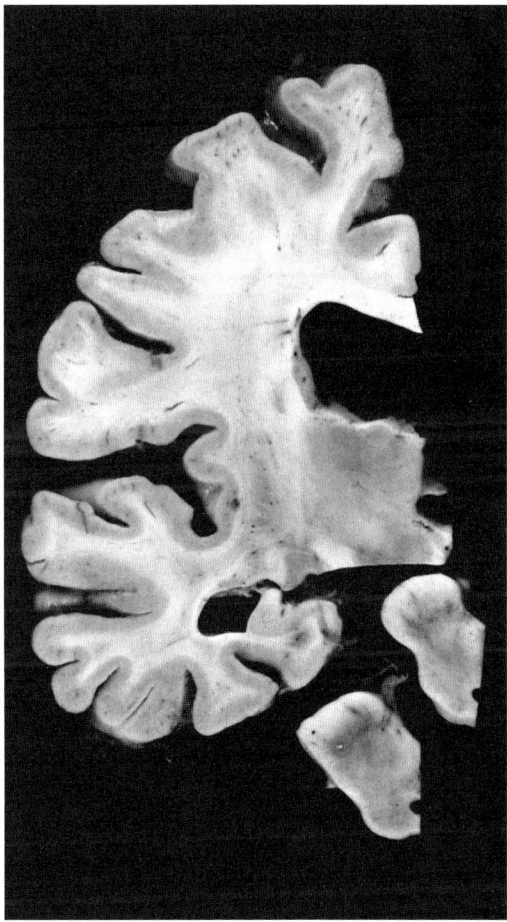

Figure 7–26. Coronal section of the left cerebral hemisphere passing through the lateral geniculate body, and two transverse sections through the left hemimesencephalon of the same patient as in Figure 7–24. The hippocampal formation is moderately atrophic. The sulci and ventricular system are wider than normal. The thalamus is within normal limits. The pars compacta of the substantia nigra is moderately pale.

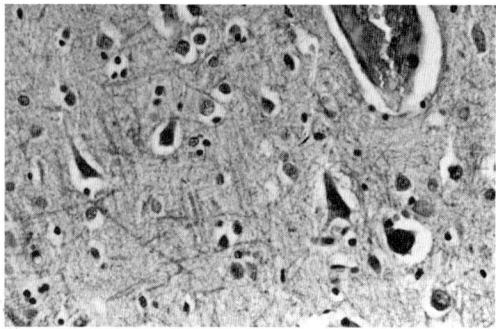

Figure 7-27. Microphotograph of third layer of prefrontal cortex (same patient as in Figure 7-24) showing scattered, shrunken neurons. Note the absence of neurofibrillary tangles of Alzheimer's and of neuritic plaques. Modified Bielschowsky stain; original magnification, ×312.

Frontal Lobe Dementia versus Pick Disease

In 1994 the Lund and Manchester Groups distinguished the FLD from Pick disease using the following two clinical and neuropathological criteria:

[In FLD there is] slight symmetrical convolutional atrophy in frontal and anterior temporal lobes, neither circumscribed nor of a knife blade type; atrophy can be severe in a few cases . . . "Two types of histological changes underly the atrophy and both share an identical anatomical distribution in the frontal and temporal lobes. The commonest pathology is that of nerve cell loss and microvacuolation, together with a mild or moderately severe astrocytic gliosis in the outer cortical layers, and is designated frontal lobe degeneration. This is to distinguish it from the typical Pick-type histology characterized by intense astrocytic gliosis in the presence of intraneuronal inclusion bodies and inflated neurons in all cortical layers. Cases of frontotemporal dementia with a similar level of astrocytosis but without inclusions or inflated neurons should be best included in this Pick-type category pending a more definitive histological identification."[26]

This excerpt highlights the overlap between FLD and Pick disease. A key point is that the atrophy in FTD is mild to moderate and is usually confined to the anterior two-thirds of the telencephalon with ill-defined transition between the atrophic and the relatively preserved area. This is in contrast to Pick disease, which is characterized by the presence of diffuse, moderate atrophy of the cerebrum with superimposed, circumscribed, severe atrophy of the frontal, frontotemporal, or frontotemporoparietal regions. Furthermore, in Pick disease, the transition between the severely atrophic and the relatively preserved areas is abrupt. The lack of universal consensus on the diagnostic criteria for FTD and for Pick disease causes confusion, as discussed in more detail in the section on Pick disease.

Some investigators emphasize the clinical findings whereas others emphasize the pathological findings in their attempts to define FTD. The clinical inference of FTD suggests that the cerebral atrophy is confined to the frontal or frontotemporal regions. However, on postmortem examination, the cerebral atrophy is rarely restricted to the frontal or frontotemporal regions. Hence, the functional map of the brain only partially supports the correlation between symptoms and damaged regions as implied by the designation FTD. Arnold Pick's focus was mainly twofold: (1) to determine whether cerebral, circumscribed atrophy was secondary to vascular insufficiency or to primary degeneration; and (2) to check whether there was a correlation between the loss of functions and the circumscribed atrophy.[27-30] The modern literature on FLD stresses the clinical and molecular biology findings, which are now the prevailing factors in the choice of the terminology used for these dementias. These different approaches spawned a plethora of labels to refer to non-Alzheimer's dementias with frontal lobe symptoms, mild to moderate frontotemporal atrophy, and without Pick bodies. Examples of terms referring to this type of dementias are listed in the section on Pick disease.

Pick disease is characterized by mild or moderate, diffuse atrophy of the brain with superimposed, severe, circumscribed frontal, or frontotemporal or frontotemporal-parietal atrophy. Thus, atrophy of the frontal or frontotemporal region occurs in both FTD and PcD, a distinctive feature being the extent of the severity of the atrophy in PcD brains. The atrophy is severe and circumscribed in PcD whereas it is mild to moderate in FTD. Unfortunately, the confusion resulting from the lack of consensus on the diagnostic criteria for FTD and PcD persists despite the availability of a detailed inventory of clinicopathological findings, including results from precise microscopical evaluations. Since the determination of the presence or absence of Pick bodies or ballooned neurons or both requires either biopsy specimens or postmortem examination of the brain, a definite, clinical diagnosis of PcD is quasi-impossible intra vitam. Requiring the presence of Pick bodies for diagnosing PcD would undercut the clinical diagnosis of PcD during life (see section on Pick disease).

NEUROPATHOLOGICAL CATEGORIZATION: A PRACTICAL APPROACH

Our methods for categorizing brains from patients with non-Alzheimer dementia and frontal lobe symptoms are as follows: brains with moderate, diffuse atrophy and with superimposed, severe, frontal, or frontotemporal, or frontoparietal-temporal, circumscribed atrophy with or without Pick bodies or ballooned neurons are categorized as Pick disease. These brains are subcategorized as Pick disease type A if both Pick bodies and ballooned neurons are present. Pick disease type B is assigned if ballooned neurons are present without Pick bodies. In the absence of both Pick bodies and ballooned neurons they are categorized as Pick disease C.

By exclusion, brains from patients with non-Alzheimer's dementia, which show moderate atrophy involving the frontal, or frontotemporal, or frontotemporoal parietal regions with neither Pick bodies, ballooned neurons, nor Lewy bodies are categorized as FTD. Brains without visible atrophy or with mild frontal or frontotemporal or parietal atrophy are assigned the diagnosis of dementia lacking distinctive histology (DLDH).[1] The minimum criteria for the neuropathological diagnosis of DLDH are (1) frontal and temporal or parietal neocortical cell loss and astrocytosis; (2) subcortical cell loss and astrocytosis involving at least the substantia nigra; and (3) absent or rare neuritic plaque and neurofibrillary tangles of Alzheimer's, and neither Pick bodies nor Lewy bodies.[1,25] When appropriate, the specimens are subcategorized on the basis of salient, detectable features.

REFERENCES

1. Knopman DS, Mastri AR, Frey WH, Sung JH, Rustan T. Dementia lacking distinctive histologic features: a common non-Alzheimer degenerative dementia. Neurology 1990; 40:251–256.
2. Mann DMA. Dementia of frontal type and dementias with subcortical gliosis. Brain Pathol 1998; 8:325–338.
3. Stevens M, van Duijn CM, Kamphorst W, de Knijff P, Heutink P, van Gool WA, Scheltens P, Ravid R, Oostra BA, Niermeijer MF, van Swieten JC. Familial aggregation in frontotemporal dementia. Neurology 1998; 50:1541–1545.
4. Tissot R, Constantinidis J, Richard J. La Maladie de Pick. Paris: Masson, 1975.
5. Miller BL, Ikonte C, Ponton M, Levy M, Boone K, Darby A, Berman N, Mena I, Cummings JL. A study of the Lund-Manchester research criteria for frontotemporal dementia: clinical and single-photon emission CT correlations. Neurology 1997; 48:937–942.
6. Mitsuyama Y. Presenile dementia with motor neuron disease. Dementia 1993; 4:137–142.
7. Vercelletto M, Bertout C, Geffriaud J, Labat JJ, Magne C, Fève JR. Démence de type frontal et sclérose latérale amyotrophique. Trois cas avec étude en tomographie d'émission monophotonique (HmPAO Tc^{99m}). Rev Neurol 1995; 151:640–647.
8. Okamoto K, Hirai S, Yamazaki T, Sun X, Nakazato Y. New ubiquitin-positive intraneuronal inclusions in the extra-motor cortices in patients with amyotrophic lateral sclerosis. Neurosci Letters 1991; 129:233–236.
9. Jackson M, Lennox G, Lowe J. Motor neurone disease-inclusion dementia. Neurodegeneration 1996; 5:339–350.
10. Hudson AJ. Amyotrophic lateral sclerosis and its association with dementia, parkinsonism and other neurological disorders: a review. Brain 1981; 104:217–247.
11. Spillantini MG, Goedert M, Crowther RA, Murrell JR, Farlow MR, Ghetti B. Familial multiple system tauopathy with presenile dementia: a disease with abundant neuronal and glial tau filaments. Proc Natl Acad Sci USA 1997; 94:4113–4118.
12. Spillantini MG, Bird TD, Ghetti B. Frontotemporal dementia and parkinsonism linked to chromosome 17: a new group of tauopathies. Brain Pathol 1998; 8:387–402.
13. Poorkaj P, Bird TD, Wijsman E, Nemeans E, Garruto RM, Anderson L, Andreadis A, Wiederholt WC, Raskind M, Schellenberg GD. Tau is a candidate gene for chromosome 17 frontotemporal dementia. Ann Neurol 1998; 43:815–825.
14. Foster LN, Wilhelmsen K, Sima AAF, Jones MZ, D'Amato CJ, Gilman S, Conference Participants. Frontotemporal dementia and parkinsonism linked to chromosme 17: a consensus conference. Ann Neurol 1997; 41:706–715.
15. Lynch T, Sano M, Marder KS, Bell KL, Foster NL, Defendini RF, Sima AAF, Keohane C, Nygaard TG, Fahn S, Mayeux R, Rowland LP, Wilhelmsen KC. Clinical characteristics of a family with chromosome 17-linked disinhibition–dementia–parkinsonism–amyotrophy complex. Neurology 1994; 44:1878–1884.

16. Reed LA, Schmidt ML, Wszolek ZK, Balin BJ, Soontornniyomkij V, Lee VM-Y, Tojanowski JQ, Schelper RL. The neuropathology of a chromosome 17–linked autosomal dominant parkinsonism and dementia ("pallido-ponto-nigral degeneration"). J Neuropathol Exp Neurol 1998; 57:588–601.
17. Wijker M, Wszoleck ZK, Wolters ECH, Rooimans MA, Pals G, Pfeiffer RF, Lynch T, Rodnitzky RL, Wilhelmsen KC, Arwert F. Localization of the gene for rapidly progressive autosomal dominant parkinsonism and dementia with pallido-ponto-nigral degeneration to chromosome 17q21. Hum Mol Genet 1996; 5:151–154.
18. Baker M, Kwok JBJ, Kucera S, Crook R, Farrer M, Houlden H, Isaacs A, Lincoln S, Onstead L, Hardy J, Wittenberg L, Dodd P, Webb S, Hayward N, Tannenberg T, Andreadis A, Hallupp M, Schofield P, Dark F, Hutton M. Localization of frontotemporal dementia with parkinsonism in an Australian kindred to chromosome 17q21–22. Ann Neurol 1997; 42:794–798.
19. Morris JC, Cole M, Banker BQ, Wright D. Hereditary dysphasic dementia and the Pick–Alzheimer spectrum. Ann Neurol 1984; 16:455–466.
20. Lendon CL, Lynch T, Norton J, McKeel DW, Busfield F, Craddock N, Chakraverty S, Gopalakrishnan G, Shears SD, Grimmett W, Wilhelmsen KC, Hansen L, Morris JC, Goate AM. Hereditary dysphasic disinhibition dementia. A frontotemporal dementia linked to 17q21–22. Neurology 1998; 50:1546–1555.
21. Bird TD, Nochlin D, Poorkaj P, Cherrier M, Kaye J, Payami H, Peskind E, Lampe TH, Nemens E, Boyer PJ, Schellenberg GD. A clinical pathological comparison of three families with frontotemporal dementia and identical mutations in the tau gene (P301L). Brain 1999; 122:741–756.
22. van Swieten JC, Stevens M, Rosso SM, Rizzu P, Joosse M, de Koning I, Kamphorst W, Ravid R, Spillantini MG, Niermeijer MF, Heutink P. Phenotypic variation in hereditary frontotemporal dementia with tau mutations. Ann Neurol 1999; 46:617–626.
23. Mirra SS, Murrell JR, Gearing M, Spillantini MG, Goedert M, Crowther RA, Levey AI, Jones R, Green J, Shoffner JM, Wainer BH, Schmidt ML, Trojanowski JQ, Ghetti B. Tau pathology in a family with dementia and a P301L mutation in tau. J Neuropathol Exp Neurol 1999; 58:335–345.
24. Gustafson L, Brun A, Passant U. Frontal lobe degeneration of non-Alzheimer type. In: Rossor MN, ed. Baillière's Clinical Neurology. International Practice and Research. Unusual dementias. London: Baillière Tindall / W.B. Saunders, 1992:559–582.
25. Sima AAF, Defendini R, Keohane C, D'Amato C, Foster NL, Parchi P, Gambetti P, Lynch T, Wilhelmsen KC. The neuropathology of chromosome 17-linked dementia. Ann Neurol 1996; 39:734–743.
26. The Lund and Manchester Groups. Clinical and neuropathological criteria for frontotemporal dementia. J Neurol Neurosurg Psychiatry 1994; 57:416–418.
27. Pick A. Ueber die Beziehungen der senilen Hirnatrophie zur Aphasie. Prag Med Wochenschr 1892; 16:165–167.
28. Pick A. Senile Hirnatrophie als Grundlage von Herderscheinungen. Wien Klin Wochenschr 1901; 14:403–404.
29. Pick A. Zur Symptomatologie des linksseitigen Schläfenlappenatrophie. Monatsschr Psychiatr Neurol 1904; 16:378–388.
30. Pick A. Über einen weiteren Symptomenkomplex im Rahmen der Dementia senilis, bedingt durch umschriebene stärkere Hirnatrophie (gemischte Aparxie). Monatsschr Psychiatr Neurol 1906; 19:97–108.

Pick Disease

JEAN PAUL G. VONSATTEL, G. BINETTI, E. TESSA HEDLEY-WHYTE, AND JOHN H. GROWDON

We recently published a review on Pick disease (PcD) from which this report is derived.[1] Between 1892 and 1906, Arnold Pick (Fig. 7–28A) reported on four women and two men with dementia in an attempt to understand the relationship between topography and function of the brain.[2-5] Pick's original idea was to evaluate patients whose brains showed a mild, diffuse atrophy with superimposed, circumscribed areas of intense atrophy in certain lobes or convolutions (Fig. 7–28B). At first, Pick was inclined to attribute the atrophy to vascular disturbances. However, he gradually was convinced that "circumscribed

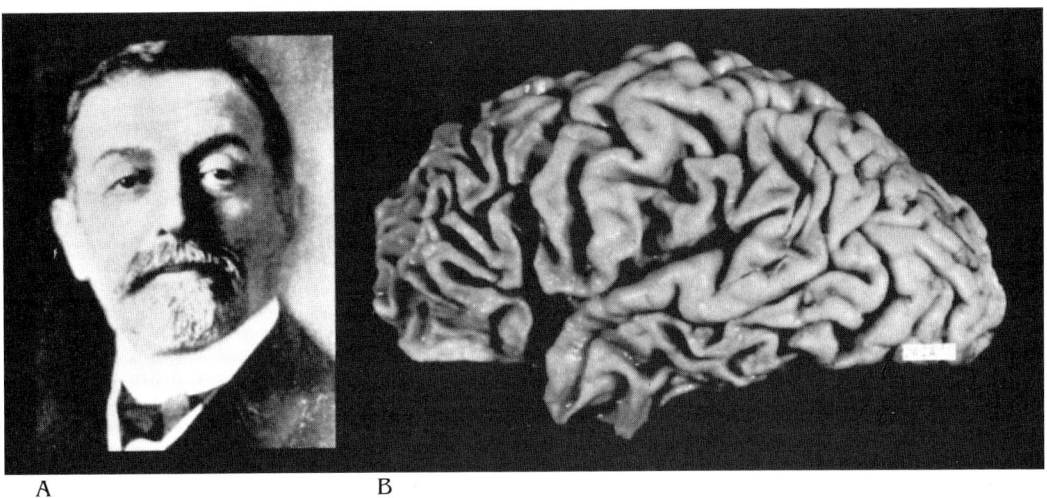

Figure 7–28. A. Arnold Pick (1851–1924). B. Lateral aspect of the left, cerebral hemisphere of a 71-year-old woman with Pick disease (type A). The hemisphere shows diffuse, moderate atrophy with superimposed, severe atrophy involving the frontal, inferior parietal, and temporal lobes. Note the relative preservation of the caudal two-thirds of the superior temporal gyrus (see Fig. 7–30 for medial aspect and coronal sections of the same specimen).

atrophy" resulted from primary degeneration rather than from vascular disorders.[2,3] Eventually, Pick claimed that in some instances, "senile brain atrophy" was circumscribed, challenging the belief that senile, cerebral atrophy was a diffuse process.[3,5] To support his claim, Pick presented clinical data and the gross findings of the evaluation performed by Chiari on the brains of August H., who died at the age of 71 years,[2] and of Josef Vlasak, who died at the age of 60 years.[5] Onset of symptoms in August H. occurred 2 years before death and included mental weakness, aggressiveness, apathy, and speech difficulties. His brain weighed 1150 g (right hemisphere 500 g; left hemisphere 470 g) and showed diffuse atrophy, which was graded as marked except for the temporal lobe where it was severe, and more conspicuous on the left side than on the right; no microscopical findings were provided.[2]. Josef Vlasak's clinical data included family burden of mental illness involving at least a sister, "amnesic" aphasia with preserved ability to recite the months serially, memory loss, stereotypy, and apraxia. His brain (1105 g [right hemisphere 485 g; left hemisphere 460 g]) showed severe atrophy involving the frontal lobes and left inferior parietal lobule, mild atrophy involving the right inferior parietal lobule and the bilateral temporal and occipital lobes, and no atrophy of the precentral gyri or superior parietal lobules. No microscopical evaluation was performed.[5,6]

In 1918, Richter documented severe, circumscribed, asymmetric (left > right), frontal atrophy in a demented, 49-year-old woman, corroborating Pick's observations.[7] These publications emphasized that cerebral degeneration can be circumscribed and asymmetric, that specific symptoms can be correlated with regional, cerebral atrophy, and that the condition might be hereditary. These findings, despite limited neuropathological data, still constitute the solid basis of PcD as noted by Lüers and Spatz in 1957,[8] and Tissot et al. in 1975.[9]

The first description of both Pick bodies and ballooned neurons and their association with circumscribed atrophy were provided by Alzheimer.[10] He was puzzled that neuritic plaques were absent in the brain of Therese Mühlich, who had dementia.[11] Furthermore, Alzheimer noticed that there was relative preservation of the superior temporal gyrus as compared to the severely atrophic middle and inferior temporal gyri.[10] In contrast to a recent claim, Therese Mühlich was not evaluated clinically by Arnold Pick.[12] Thus, it is not known whether Pick bodies or ballooned neurons were present in the brains of the patients described by Arnold Pick.

Altman confirmed Alzheimer's observation with his report on two brains with circumscribed atrophy, Pick bodies, and ballooned neurons.[13] Altman noticed that the superficial, neocortical layers were more prone to degeneration than the deep ones. He described the relative preservation of the hippocampus, which contrasted with the severe atrophy of the subiculum and nearby temporal gyri, atrophy of the medial thalamus and of the frontopontine fibers, and the abrupt transition between severely atrophic and relatively preserved regions of the cerebral hemispheres. Altman established that the circumscribed atrophy could include the temporal lobes in addition to the frontal lobes. Richter illustrated ballooned neurons in his report on frontal, circumscribed atrophy; however, he did not mention the presence or absence of neuronal inclusions or Pick bodies.[7]

Gans referred to the frontal atrophy as "Pick atrophy," which was to become a source of confusion.[14] While Arnold Pick saw a match between the circumscribed atrophy and the cerebral areas that are ontogenetically the latest to myelinate, Gans hypothesized that the regions to atrophy were those phylogenetically recent. Gans referred to the Edinger's school, which pointed out the vulnerability of the phylogenetically newer parts of the brain in neurodegeneration, while Onari and Spatz reported that the atrophy often encroaches or includes phylogenetically old parts as well, and they coined the term "Pick disease."[11]

Stertz tried to characterize the symptoms that result from chiefly frontal or chiefly temporal atrophy.[15] Stertz's report is interesting because the patients he described played a crucial role in the characterization of PcD: the brains of patients Bradt (no Pick body, no ballooned neuron), Mühlich, and Ruge (both with Pick bodies and ballooned neurons) were all studied by Onari and Spatz.[11] Furthermore, the brain of patient Mühlich was evaluated by Alzheimer, which led him to the first description of both Pick bodies and ballooned neurons.[10] Thus, between 1922 and 1929, PcD gained acceptance as an entity typified by gradual dementia that could be distinguished from presenile or senile dementia by its symptomatology, the presence of circumscribed atrophy, and the absence or scarcity of plaques or tangles or both. This entity was referred to either as "Pick atrophy,"[14,15] "Pick lobar sclerosis,"[16] or "Pick diseas."[11,16-20]

Striatal and nigral atrophy in PcD was emphasized by von Braunmühl, who reported the findings made in three patients with an akinetic-hypertonic syndrome.[21] Von Braunmühl's hypothesis was that the atrophy of the striatum and of the substantia nigra was a primary process and not secondary to the cortical degeneration, a claim supported later by Grünthal.[21,22] Von Bagh's PcD study included 30 brains with circumscribed atrophy (7 mainly frontal, 9 mainly temporal; 14 mainly frontotemporal) without any mention of Pick bodies. In 8 of those 30 brains he found severe atrophy of the anterior striatum (caudate nucleus > putamen) and in 7, severe atrophy of the thalamus (rostral > caudal, and medial > lateral).[17,18]

In 1922, Gans claimed that "Pick atrophy" was probably a heredodegenerative disease.[14] Familial occurrences of PcD gained acceptance following the reports by von Braunmühl and Leonhard, Grünthal, and Schmitz and Meyer.[22-24] Von Braunmühl and Leonhard described the findings of two sisters (29 and 31 years old at onset of symptoms, and 32 and 35 years old, respectively, at death) whose brains displayed circumscribed atrophy, Pick bodies, and ballooned neurons and whose mother might have had PcD.[23] The circumscribed atrophy of the sister with the shorter course of the disease encompassed the frontal lobe, while that of the sister with the longer course of the disease included the frontal, temporal, and parietal lobes (especially on the left side). Severe atrophy of the striatum was noticed in both brains along with atrophy and pallor of the substantia nigra.[23] Grünthal further emphasized the familial occurrence of PcD by describing two demented brothers (45 and 42 years old at onset of symptoms and 50 and 45 years old at death) whose brains showed circumscribed atrophy including the orbital region, insula, temporal pole, hippocampal formation (with relative preservation of the Sommer sector), caudate nucleus, medial thalamus, and substantia nigra, but there were neither Pick bodies nor ballooned neurons.[22] Schmitz and Meyer described a woman (52 years old at onset of symptoms and 56 at the time of death) with gradual dementia and aphasia. Although her brain showed severe circumscribed frontal atrophy including striatum, and ballooned neurons, there were neither Pick bodies nor tangles nor neuritic plaques. The father and two sisters of the patient had the same symptoms and clinical course; however, they were not evaluated pathologically.[24]

Schneider provided a comprehensive summary of the neuropathological features of PcD in 1927 and 1929.[19,20] Schneider presented four new patients: patient Greppmager (neither Pick body nor ballooned neuron), patient Jatzel (with ballooned neurons, but without Pick body), patient Moser (without reference to Pick body or ballooned neuron), and patient Naumann (with ballooned neuron, but without Pick body). Furthermore, Schneider reviewed already reported patients, including Ruge (with Pick bodies and with ballooned neurons) and Mielich (or Mühlich), initially described by Alzheimer.[10] Patients Ruge and Mühlich had circumscribed atrophy, Pick bodies, and ballooned neurons, and both had been studied by Onari and Spatz,[11] with clinical data provided by Stertz.[15] Schneider summarized patterns of cerebral atrophy in PcD: rostral > caudal; gyrus fusiformis or parahippocampal gyrus > middle temporal gyrus > inferior temporal gyrus, or instances where the brunt of the atrophy was in the poles of the superior and middle frontal gyri, with relative preservation of the motor strip. Furthermore, Schneider performed quantitative studies in the brains of patients Jatzel, Ruge, and Mielich (or Mühlich) and concluded that the less marked the atrophy, the higher the number of ballooned neurons. Ballooned neurons were located mainly in the superficial cortical layers early in the course of the disease, while later they were also found in the deep cortical layers. Schneider noticed that Pick bodies were present in four (there is an apparent discrepancy between this statement and the neuropathological descriptions) of the six brains containing ballooned neurons. He remarked that Pick bodies might be difficult to find and that their distribution matched that of the ballooned neurons.[19]

Grünthal suggested that the circumscribed atrophy had one (or rarely more) starting locus, which he referred to as the "primary shrinkage center," from which the degenerative process gradually extends and that this site could vary from brain to brain.[22] Von Bagh claimed that often this center involves the medial, caudal portion of the orbital–gyrus rectus region and, less frequently, the frontal pole.[18] The joint occurrence of PcD and amyotrophic lateral sclerosis was first observed by von Braunmühl in 1932.[25]

Most of these reports, from Pick to von Bagh, illustrate the efforts of investigators to establish detailed clinicopathological correlation to understand the occurrence and course of the cerebral circumscribed atrophies, or PcD.

CLINICAL ASPECTS

A broad analysis of clinical aspects of PcD with emphasis on the features that distinguish it from Alzheimer's disease (AD) is provided by Binetti et al.[1,26] Currently, the reliability of the diagnosis of PcD depends on both the clinical course and the pathological findings. Most clinical data about PcD patients with detailed postmortem evaluations are derived from individuals having discrete frontotemporal atrophy, either with or without parietal involvement, Pick bodies, or mild concomitant Alzheimer pathology. Therefore, this brief clinical review reflects data obtained from series of patients categorized as having PcD according to the criteria described by Tissot et al.,[9] or according to criteria closely resembling them, since Pick bodies or ballooned neurons are not sensitive indicators of the whole range of reported PcD.[8,27,28]

Pick disease is rare, and is often confused with AD; clarification is then brought by postmortem evaluation.[26,29] Reliable estimates of the incidence or prevalence of PcD cannot be determined because of the lack of universally accepted diagnostic criteria, awareness of the entity, possible clinical overlaps with AD and frontal lobe dementia, and uncertainties regarding the placement of PcD under the broad term "frontotemporal lobar degeneration."[1,30] Based on clinical evaluations, PcD has been reported to be three to five times less frequent than AD.[31,32] In individuals aged 65 or older, the prevalence of PcD is estimated to be 5 to 6 per 1000 persons,[33] whereas the prevalence of AD is estimated to be between 3 and 11 per 100 persons in this same age-group.[34,35] In some studies, women are more often involved than men at a ratio of up to 2:1.[8,9,28,33] In other studies, men are more often involved than women.[18,26]

Onset of symptoms usually occurs during the fifth or sixth decades of life;[8,9] however, patients as young as 27[23,36–38] or older than 80 years at onset of symptoms have been reported.[9,39] Patients with early onset of symptoms have a shorter clinical course, increased familial incidence, and more severe pathology (involvement of the deep gray nuclei) than patients with late onset.[8,40] The symptoms observed in PcD are predominantly determined by the circumscribed frontotemporal or frontotemporoparietal atrophy.

The earliest symptoms are variable, and include language impairment and changes in the personality or character of the patients rather than their formal intelligence.[8,26] Binetti et al. reported memory loss as being a major symptom occurring early in the course of the disease.[26] Behavioral disturbances, personality changes (socially inappropriate activity including disinhibition), hyperorality, excessive manual exploration, euphoria, jocularity, irritability, emotional blunting, apathy, depression, echolalia, and mutism are reported as early symptoms.[41] In contrast to AD, perception and orientation (visuospatial skills) are relatively preserved; e.g., the bulimic PcD patient looks for food in an organized fashion.[26,27,41–43]

Pyramidal signs may occur when the circumscribed atrophy includes the precentral gyrus.[44] Extrapyramidal signs (truncal rigidity, cogwheel rigidity, stooped posture, festinating gait, tremor, choreoathetosis) are less frequently observed than would be expected since striatopallidonigral degeneration is observed in 62% to 78% of the PcD brains (see below).[18,40,45] Three syndromes are often observed in PcD: moriatic syndrome (or moria), PES syndrome (palilalia, echolalia, stereotypia), and PEMA syndrome (palilalia, echolalia, mutism, amimia).[9,27,46]

Heston et al. estimated that the mean survival time for men was 6.3 years and for women, 8.4 years.[47] Survival from onset of symptoms to death ranges from 1 to 15 years.[9,27,44] The mean age of death in our neuropathological series was 73.6 ($\pm$10.9) years.[1]

The youngest patient of the von Bagh's series ($n = 30$) was 33 years old and the oldest, 77 years old at death.[17]

THE GENETICS OF PICK DISEASE

Sporadic PcD is more frequent than familial.[8,9,22–24,28,36,44,48–50] The two families described by Löwenberg et al.[36] and by Malamud and Waggoner[48] showed a dominant pattern of inheritance. Autopsies revealed severe atrophy involving the frontal, parietal, and temporal lobes with relative preservation of the superior temporal gyrus. Pick bodies and ballooned neurons were present.

In 1982, Groen and Endtz analyzed the data published on families with more than one PcD patient per generation and with at least one member with the disease confirmed neuropathologically.[44] They identified 26 families, including the Dutch Schenk family. In these families, autosomal dominant transmission was the most likely mode of inheritance.[49] The Dutch Schenk family had 25 members with PcD across six generations. Of these 25 members, the diagnosis of PcD was confirmed pathologically in 14. The Schenk family continues to be evaluated and now includes 34 affected relatives across seven generations.[51] This family may help our understanding of the molecular genetics of PcD because it is one of three Dutch families (family II in the report by Heutink et al.[51]) linked to chromosome 17 and reported as "hereditary frontotemporal dementia" (HFTD).

Chromosome 17 has also been associated with other neurodegenerative dementing disorders, including dysphasic disinhibition dementia,[52] disinhibition–dementia–parkinsonism–amyotrophy complex (DDPAC),[53,54] progressive subcortical gliosis (PSG),[55] pallidopontonigral degeneration (PPND),[56] chromosome 17–linked dementia,[57,58] and familial multiple system tauopathy with presenile dementia.[59]

There are no known causes of sporadic PcD. Possession of the apolipoprotein E-ε4 allele is a risk factor for AD; however, in PcD, the incidence of the E-ε4 allele is either slightly increased,[60] or identical to that of the control population.[61]

NEUROPATHOLOGY

Brain Weight and Lateral Ventricular Volume

The average Pick brain weight reported is 900–1000 g for women and 1000–1220 g for men.[9,28] In our postmortem series of 35 patients (20 women and 15 men; 23 with Pick bodies), the average brain weight and volume of one lateral ventricle are as follows: women, 955 g ± 174 g; 26 ± 13 cc (normal 7–10 cc); men, 1085 g ± 172 g; 29 cc ± 15 cc.[1]

Gross Examination

The brain in Pick disease is characterized by circumscribed, severe atrophy, which is superimposed upon a mild to moderate diffuse atrophy.[18] (Figs. 7–28 and 7–29). In the part involved by the circumscribed atrophy, the gyri may resemble a knife edge, or "Nussrelief."[62]

The circumscribed atrophy is usually bilateral, asymmetric or symmetric, panlaminar (see below) frontal, frontotemporal, or frontoparietotemporal, and may or may not include parietal involvement (Table 7–3). Up to 60% of the PcD brains show more atrophy on one side than the other, most frequently on the left.[18,28] Exceptionally, the atrophy also involves the occipital lobe[41] or is mainly confined to the parietal lobe on one side.[63,64] Unilateral, parietal, circumscribed atrophy (with Pick bodies) has been observed.[63] When multiple lobes are involved (at times referred to as mixed atrophy), the atrophy can be equally severe among lobes or can predominate in any one of them. The involvement can encompass the whole lobe or part of it (Fig. 7–28). It might be more severe medially than laterally, or vice-versa. The transition between the atrophic and relatively preserved areas is abrupt (Fig. 7–29), or when gradual, is usually confined over a narrow band. Often, the caudal third of the superior temporal gyrus is relatively preserved (Figs. 7–28 and 7–30). Spatz claimed that the circumscribed atrophy is an

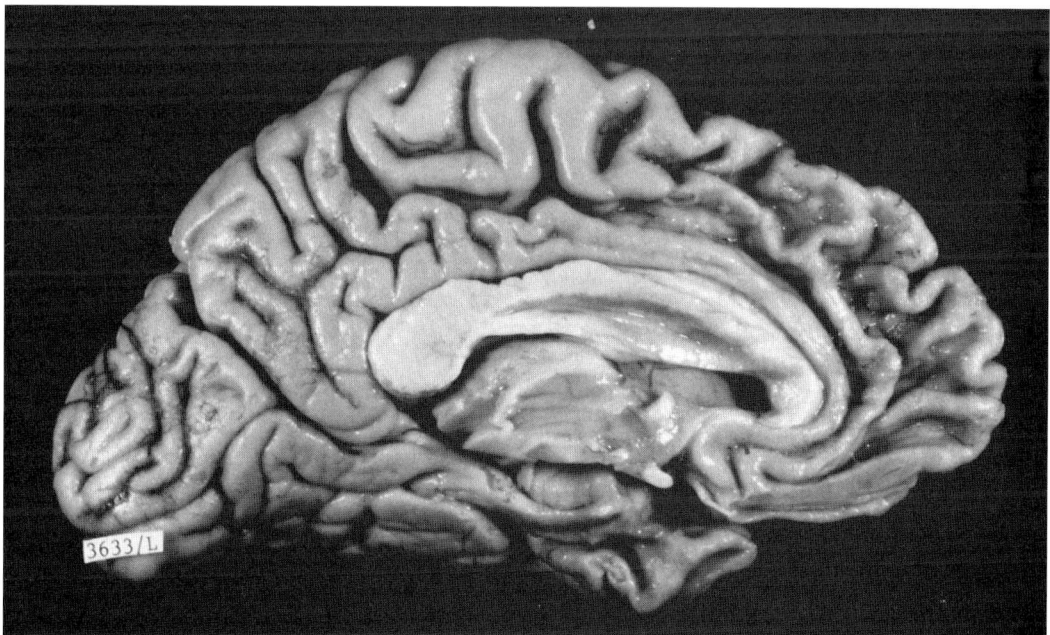

Figure 7–29. Medial aspect of the left, cerebral hemisphere of an 82-year-old man with Pick disease (type A). The brunt of the atrophy includes the frontal lobe and anterior two-thirds of the temporal lobe. Note the abrupt transition between the atrophic and preserved, rostral edge of the paracentral lobule. Both the rostrum and body of the corpus callosum are severely shrunken while the splenium is apparently normal. The gyrus rectus shows knife-edge atrophy ("Nussrelief").

Table 7–3. Gross Examination of Pick Disease Brain

Characteristics

Mild to Moderate, Diffuse Atrophy with

Superimposed, circumscribed atrophy involving frontal, frontotemporal, or frontoparietotemporal lobes

Panlaminar atrophy of all structures included in the circumscribed, atrophic portion of the brain, e.g., neocortex, center semi-ovale and deep gray nuclei

Relative preservation of caudal third of superior temporal gyrus, precentral gyrus (BA4), occipital lobe

Transition between severely atrophic and relatively preserved areas is often abrupt.

---

essential diagnostic feature of PcD,[62] a claim that has gained acceptance.[12]

Panlaminar atrophy refers to the shrinkage of all the structures included in the portion of the brain bearing the brunt of the atrophy (Table 7–3). For example, if the lobar atrophy extends from the frontal pole to the precentral gyrus, including the temporal lobe, usually the pathological changes will be conspicuous in the cortex, white matter, rostral striatum and thalamus with mesencephalic extension, amygdala, and hippocampal formation (Fig. 7–30). When involved, the thalamus is more atrophic rostrally than caudally and the dorsomedian and anterior nuclei usually are more prone to degeneration than the other nuclei.[13,21,65] The same observations were made by Löwenberg et al. in a 25-year-old patient (with both Pick bodies and ballooned neurons); however, in addition, they found that the pulvinar was involved.[36]

In contrast to Huntington disease, the atrophy of the rostral portion of the neostriatum can be extreme while the caudal portion is relatively preserved (see Chapter 13).[66] Furthermore, the head of the caudate nucleus and the nucleus accumbens are more atrophic than the nearby putamen, which shows more pathological changes along the internal capsule than along the external capsule.

The frequency of involvement of deep gray nuclei as recorded in 32 brains (10 with Pick bodies) from patients diagnosed with PcD are summarized in Table 7–4.[9,33,67] Striatopallidonigral degeneration was found in 78% percent of the 41 brains (11 with Pick bodies) evaluated by Kosaka et al.[45] Usually, in PcD the nucleus coeruleus is relatively preserved even when there is severe pallor of the pars com-

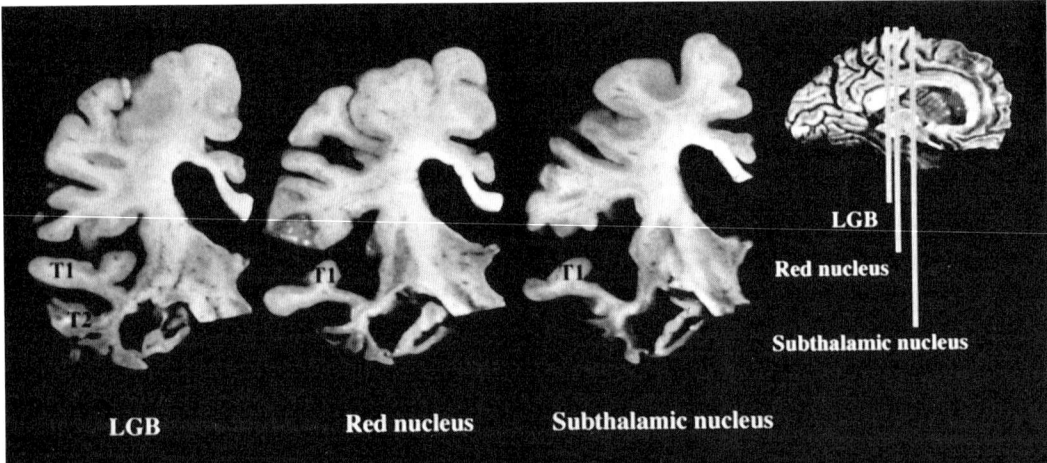

Figure 7–30. Medial aspect (upper right) of the same cerebral hemisphere as that shown in Figure 7–28. The vertical lines indicate the sites where the cuts were performed to obtain the three coronal sections of the hemisphere with indication of the anatomical landmark chosen for each section. The brunt of the atrophy includes the cingulate gyrus, striatum, thalamus, and temporal lobes with relative preservation of the superior temporal gyrus (T1). Although the coronal sections shown include the relatively preserved part of the frontal lobe, there is evidence of panlaminar atrophy (see text).

Table 7–4. Frequency and Distribution of Atrophy in Deep Gray Nuclei in Pick Disease

Sites	%	Distribution of Atrophy
Thalamus	62	Rostral > caudal Medial > lateral
Caudate nucleus and putamen	69	Rostral > caudal Head of caudate nucleus > putamen
Globus pallidus	56	Both segments; rostral > caudal
Amygdala	66	Diffuse, in contrast to Alzheimer's disease
Substantia nigra	59	Pars compacta and reticulata; rostral > caudal (relative preservation of nucleus coeruleus)

pacta of the substantia nigra. Hulette and Crain reported four patients with "Pick syndrome," but without movement disorder, whose brains showed severe, circumscribed, frontotemporal atrophy and marked atrophy of the caudate nucleus (neither Pick body nor ballooned neuron was found).[68] In addition to the nigral damage, atrophy of the crus cerebri and inferior olivary nucleus may occur.[8,9,13]

Microscopical Examination

Neuronal loss, cortical status spongiosus (Fig. 7–31), myelin and axonal loss, and astrogliosis are obvious in the atrophic areas. Scattered neurons with Pick bodies (Fig. 7–32) or ballooned neurons (Fig. 7–11) may or may not be present.[11] Furthermore, neurofibrillary tangles of Alzheimer's and neuritic plaques are rare or absent.[11]

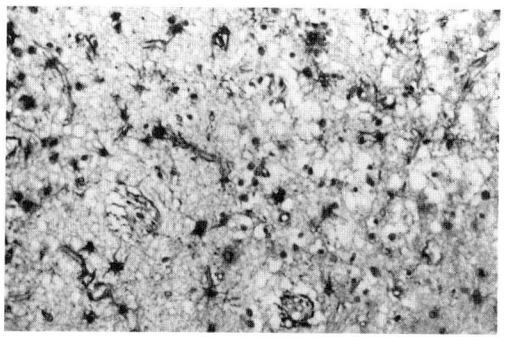

Figure 7–31. Status spongiosus involving the second–third cortical layers of the prefrontal cortex. There is severe neuronal loss and astrocytosis. GFAP counterstained with hematoxylin; original magnification, ×200.

The three outer cortical layers are more prone to degeneration than the inner layers. Proliferation of microglial cells was found to be conspicuous in both atrophic cortex and white matter using the microgliocyte marker KiM1lP.[69,70] Scattered astrocytes and oligodendrocytes with tau-positive inclusions were observed.[71–73] In contrast to AD, the amygdala in PcD tends to be diffusely damaged without apparent nuclear selectivity.[41] The density of neurons, fibers, or myelin may be apparently normal in nonatrophic areas. The substantia innominata is usually preserved.[74] Neuronal density of the substantia innominata was apparently normal in 18 of our 35 postmortem series with PcD; the rest showed mild ($n = 11$) or marked ($n = 6$) decrease of the neuronal density.

Cortical or corticosubcortical argyrophilic grains are often present in neurodegenerative diseases, including PcD.[75,76] They consist of small, spindle-shaped argyrophilic grains loosely scattered in the neuropil. They may be interconnected by coiled bodies of silver-stained filaments and are accompanied by elongated argyrophilic glial cytoplasmic inclusions located especially in the subcortical white matter and subiculum.[76] Argyrophilic grains and coiled bodies contain dense accumulations of straight filaments with a diameter of about 9.0 nm.[75]

PICK BODIES

Pick bodies (Fig. 7–32) were first described by Alois Alzheimer following the evaluation of the brain of Therese Mühlich who was one of his demented patients.[10,11,15,19] Thus, in con-

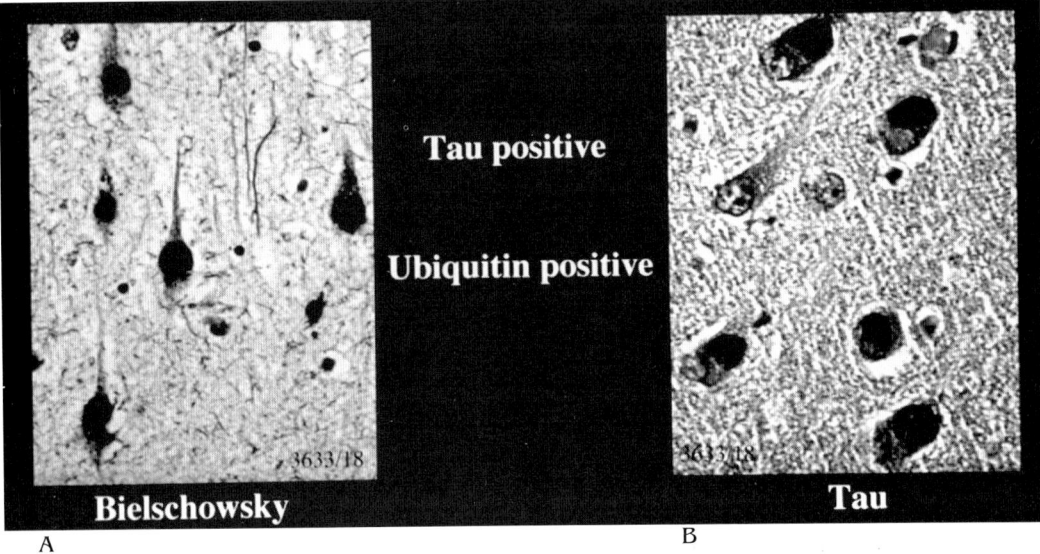

Figure 7–32. *A.* Argyrophilic, cytoplasmic inclusions or Pick bodies involving pyramidal neurons of the hippocampal formation. Modified Bielschowsky stain. *B.* Cortical neurons containing Pick bodies labeled with antibodies directed against tau. In contrast to Pick bodies, Lewy bodies are not labeled with anti-tau antibodies; original magnification, ×313.

trast to a recent claim, Therese Mühlich was not a patient of Arnold Pick.[12] The neuropathological evaluations of Arnold Pick's patients were essentially macroscopical, therefore, it is not known whether their brains harbored Pick bodies or ballooned neurons or both.[11] Part of the confusion about PcD diagnostic criteria is due to the false belief that Pick bodies were originally identified in brains of patients described by Arnold Pick.

Alzheimer's description of Pick bodies is as follows:

Sections prepared with Bielschowsky method show small pyramidal cells containing an argyrophilic, sometimes structureless ball near the nucleus, whose size varies from half to twice that of the nucleus. The inclusion is either above or below the nucleus, which is displaced accordingly downward or upward. Fibrillary changes are absent in the rest of the cell, the protoplasm and the axonal process are partially visible.

This description is accompanied by a figure illustrating five neuronal inclusions; four inclusions are round or slightly oval but differ by their size, while one inclusion is clearly oval, larger than the others, and contains optically empty vacuoles or pale foci.[10] In addition to being argyrophilic, Pick bodies are weakly eosinophilic. Alzheimer's description of the Pick body is that of the classic inclusion corresponding with the appearance of the majority of the inclusions seen at the postmortem examination. However, a minority of Pick bodies, or Pick body–like inclusions, are smaller or larger than the usual ones with apparent uneven features as depicted by Alzheimer in his original drawing of Pick bodies.[10] The smaller Pick body–like inclusions tend to be present in the early stage of the disease or in the areas with little degenerative changes. They may be as small as the nucleolus and tend to abut the cytoplasmic aspect of the slightly argyrophilic nuclear membrane or argyrophilic perinuclear ring (APR) (Fig. 7–33). At times, the cytoplasm of the neurons containing these small Pick body–like inclusions is weakly discolored a dirty gray with the modified Bielschowsky stain. The larger Pick body–like inclusions tend to occupy most of the neuronal cytoplasm; they may be lobulated and express variable argyrophilia or immunoreactivity (Fig. 7–32, right). Argyrophilic Pick bodies that appear as basophilic spheroids containing an eosinophilic core in hematoxylin and eosin–stained sections are referred to as "compound Pick bodies."[77] Ultrastructurally, the inclusions lack membranes and are com-

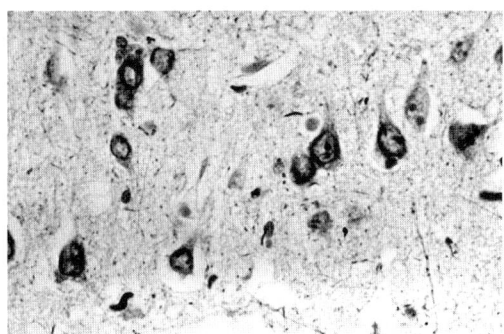

Figure 7–33. Hippocampal, dentate gyrus with neurons containing small, argyrophilic, intracytoplasmic, round inclusions (? small Pick bodies), perinuclear argyrophilic rings, or both. Modified Bielschowsky stain; original magnification, ×313.

posed of straight filaments 15–18 nm in diameter without sidearm or fuzzy material attached to them.[40,78,79]

The sites of predilection for Pick bodies are the hippocampal formation (stratum granulosum of the dentate gyrus, Sommer sector [CA1], subiculum, and indusium griseum), entorhinal cortex, amygdala, septal nuclei, and in the second, third, and sixth cortical layers of the frontal, cingulate, and temporal neocortices.[9,80–82] Armstrong et al. found the highest density of Pick bodies in the stratum granulosum of the dentate gyrus and, to a lesser extent, in the CA1 region.[83] Rare Pick bodies may be identified in otherwise normal cortical areas, suggesting that their presence may precede the apparent neuronal loss or that their visualization at postmortem examination may partially depend on the course of the disease as suggested by Schneider.[1,19,20] Pick bodies that are apparently free in the neuropil are occasionally present in the cortical areas displaying extreme atrophy.[9] Pick bodies may be prominent in the anterior neostriatum (caudate nucleus, putamen and nucleus accumbens) and hypothalamus,[9,40] but are rarely found in the globus pallidus (JPV, personal observation). They were observed in the nucleus coeruleus.[84]

Pick bodies are stained with antibodies to ubiquitin, chromogranin A,[85,86] phosphorylated neurofilament epitopes, tau (Fig. 7–32), or to A2B5, which recognizes neuronal surface ganglioside, indicating that membrane proteins may be incorporated into the inclusions.[71,73,87] They also react with the N-terminal and the intermediate segments of amyloid precursor protein (APP).[88] However, Pick body immunocytochemical inconsistencies have been reported, such as lack of affinity with antibodies directed against ubiquitin.[89,90] Pick bodies are not labeled with antibodies directed against α-synuclein.[91]

In the classification of Tissot et al., Pick bodies are found in 31% of brains with lobar atrophy[9] at about the same frequency as reported earlier.[8] We systematically evaluated 35 brains with circumscribed lobar atrophy; 22 of them had definite Pick bodies (many in 12, rare in 10) detected with modified Bielschowsky silver impregnation. However, using antibodies for tau and ubiquitin, scattered cortical or limbic Pick bodies, although rare, were detected in 5 of the 13 brains in which no Pick bodies could be found with the modified Bielschowsky method during the initial evaluation.[1] These "Bielschowsky false-negative" brains were those with the most severe pathology. Pick bodies might fail to stain when silver impregnation is not optimal, and this "false negativity" may result from the lack of standardization of the silver staining techniques.[9,72] Furthermore, Pick bodies stain poorly with silver and with antibodies to neurofilaments or microtubules, in addition to straight filaments, when they contain granular material possibly derived from ribosomes.[40] Perhaps Pick bodies are hard to find when the pathology is extreme, in the way neurofibrillary tangles can be difficult to detect in brains of patients with very severe AD.[92] The presence of Pick bodies (and ballooned neurons) may be a transient event and no longer apparent in the late stages of the disease,[19,23,28,93] although many Pick bodies may be observed even in severely involved areas in some brains, illustrating the heterogeneity of this degenerative disorder.[23,82]

Alternative splicing of RNA transcripts generates six tau isoforms that can be identified in Western immunoblots of normal brains. They contain either three (3R) of four microtubule-binding domains (4R). Immunoblot evaluation of brain samples containing Pick bodies shows only phosphorylated 3R-tau isoforms. They aggregate into phosphorylated 55 and 64 kDa tau protein doublets. This differs from the triplet tau profile (55, 64, and 69) of the paired helical filaments in AD, where all six tau isoforms are phosphorylated with equal amounts of 3R and 4R tau.[94,95] Buée-Scherrer et al. confirmed this particular tau profile in brains with Pick bodies but without neurofibrillary tangles of Alzheimer's; however, they also demonstrated that the tau profile of brains containing both Pick bodies and neurofibrillary tangles of Alzheimer's was similar to that of AD (tau 55, 64, and 69).[96] In some instances, cortical Lewy bodies are strongly argyrophilic and therefore may be difficult to differentiate from Pick bodies by usual staining methods; hence, discrimination between cortical Lewy bodies and Pick bodies may require ultrastructural evaluation.[79]

BALLOONED NEURONS (PICK CELLS)

Ballooned neurons or Pick cells are swollen neurons with convex contours, homogeneous, glassy, pale, eosinophilic cytoplasm, and eccentric nuclei (Fig. 7.11). The cytoplasm is diffusely argyrophilic with variable intensity. At times, cytoplasmic vacuoles with or without a centrally located granule are present.[19,27,28,97,98] Ultrastructurally, ballooned neurons have variable features. Some are filled with straight filaments similar to those found in Pick bodies, while others contain normal elements with admixed straight filaments of variable density.[28,40,78] Ballooned neurons can be distinguished from swollen chromatolytic neurons, suggesting a different pathogenesis. Irregular dilatation of proximal neuronal processes and cytoplasmic vacuoles characterize ballooned neurons, but not chromatolytic neurons.[98] Spatz hypothesized that the process of ballooned neuron formation in PcD is identical to that of the retrograde reaction of the cell body following axonal injury[62] During chromatolysis, there is transient neuronal swelling in reaction to the axonal degeneration, which is thought to start at the periphery; this process is then followed by shrinkage and eventually disappearance of the neuron[8,62] (Fig. 7.11).

In the classification of Tissot et al., ballooned neurons are found in 62 % of brains with lobar atrophy.[9,33] They are scattered especially in the intermediary zones between the severely affected and the relatively preserved areas of the neocortex and entorhinal cortex.[19] They are frequently observed in the anterior cingulate gyrus, insular cortex, and claustrum. At times, they are found in the anterior neostriatum.[9] Ballooned neurons apparently do not occur in the dentate gyrus.[83] They share most of the immunocytochemical characteristics of the filaments in Pick bodies.[28,86,98] Many ballooned neurons in PcD are positive with antibodies to β-crystallin; they may or may not stain with antibodies to ubiquitin,[72,99] or Alz-50.[100]

STATUS SPONGIOSUS

In the atrophic areas, the parenchyma is severely gliotic with coarse, irregular vacuoles that give a loose texture to the tissue under the microscope; these changes are referred to as status spongiosus (Fig. 7–31). The outer layers of the atrophic cortex are especially involved. As mentioned before, *status spongiosus* is defined as follows: "nonspecific, and characteristically is the manifestation of end-stage gliosis; it consists of irregular cavitation of the neuropil in the presence of a dense glial meshwork."[101]

Neuropathological Diagnostic Criteria of Pick Disease

As yet, there is no consensus on the neuropathological diagnostic criteria for PcD. The first published, comprehensive criteria for the neuropathological diagnosis of PcD we found are those proposed by Onari and Spatz in 1922.[11] They suggested that the anatomical diagnosis of PcD be made when these hallmarks are present: (*1*) circumscribed atrophy, (*2*) severe loss of all constituents of the neuronal parenchyma involving especially the upper cortical layers, (*3*) absence of neurofibrillary tangles of Alzheimer's and neuritic plaques in both atrophic and relatively preserved cortices, and (*4*) possible occurrence of Pick bodies with predominant temporal or frontal atrophy; however, they may be lacking and their absence would not change the overall picture.

Currently, for some investigators, the presence of lobar atrophy, gliosis, and neuronal loss with mild or no Alzheimer's pathology, and with or without Pick bodies, is the prerequisite for diagnosing PcD.[6,8,9,26–28,33,39,45,60,62,67,90,99,100,102–107] Others require that Pick bodies and ballooned neurons be present in addition to the circumscribed atrophy and neuronal loss and that neurofibrillary tangles of Alzheimer's and neuritic plaques be absent or rare.[12,40,47,72,81–83, 86,94,108–111] For these investigators, the brains from demented patients with lobar atrophy, but without Pick bodies, are categorized in groups with designations such as " 'atypical' PcD,"[112] "fronto-temporal degeneration,"[105] "frontal lobe dementia,"[46,113] "frontal lobe dementia of non-Alzheimer's type,"[46,114] "frontal lobe degeneration,"[99] "dementia of frontal lobe type,"[113–115] "primary progressive aphasia,"[116–118] or "dementia lacking distinctive histopathology."[112,119–121] Of interest is that Pick bodies were found in at least one brain of a patient from the Schenk family with hereditary, frontotemporal dementia linked to chromosome 17.[49,51,107]

Munoz-Garcia et al. proposed subcategorizing PcD brains into two groups (classic and generalized) on the basis of the involvement of the subcortical structures including the distribution and histochemical, immunochemical, and ultrastructural characteristics of the Pick bodies.[40] According to this scheme, the "classic" group includes those brains with predominantly cortical atrophy and with Pick bodies that stain with antibodies to neurofilament proteins and tubulin. The "generalized" group includes those brains with subcortical and cortical atrophy and with weakly argyrophilic RNA-containing Pick bodies, which stain poorly with antibodies to neurofilaments or microtubules.

It is controversial whether Pick bodies must be present for diagnosing PcD, or conversely, whether the lack of Pick bodies rules out the diagnosis of PcD. From a practical neuropathological point of view, the requirement of the presence of Pick bodies for the diagnosis of PcD is seductive, yet perhaps too rigid. Such a requirement would undercut the clinical diagnosis during life.[37,68] It would disqualify Pick's original six patients, who were reported between 1892 and 1906, in which clinicopathological correlation was based only on the gross examination of the brains without reference to neuronal inclusions.[2–5] Indeed, these inclusions were not identified until 1911; furthermore, the original description of Pick bodies did not result from the evaluation of the brains of patients evaluated by A. Pick.[10]

In the face of this confusing terminology, we prefer the classification scheme proposed

Table 7–5. Diagnostic and Neuropathological Classification of Pick Disease

Pathological Features	Type A	Type B	Type C
Lobar, circumscribed atrophy	+	+	+
Ballooned neurons (Pick cells)	+	+	
Pick bodies	+		

Modified from Tissot R, Constantinidis J, Richard J. La maladie de Pick. Paris: Masson, 1975.[9]

by Tissot et al.[9,33] This classification embraces three subgroups (Table 7–5) of non-Alzheimer's dementia brains with lobar, or circumscribed atrophy: (1) group A includes those brains with Pick bodies and ballooned neurons, (2) group B includes those brains with ballooned neurons and no Pick bodies, and (3) group C includes those brains with neither Pick bodies nor ballooned neurons.[9,33,67] In the International Classification of Diseases (ICD-10) there is no reference to Pick bodies in the definition of PcD, and the neuropathological picture is described as a selective atrophy of the frontal and temporal lobes without the occurrence of neuritic plaques and neurofibrillary tangles in excess of what is seen in normal aging. As pointed out earlier, there are brains from patients that are clinically and pathologically indistinguishable from those categorized as "typical" PcD (PcD type A) except for the absence of Pick bodies. These should be referred to as PcD type B, or PcD type C, according to Tissot et al.[9]

More recent diagnostic concepts on PcD are discussed by Baldwin and Förstl[108] and by Jellinger.[86] According to these concepts, PcD should not be diagnosed on the basis of frontotemporal degeneration alone. The presence of ballooned neurons is not specific to PcD as ballooned neurons are seen in many other neurodegenerative conditions,[8,97] including corticobasal degeneration, AD, primary progressive aphasia, chromosome 17–linked dementia, Creutzfeldt-Jakob disease, and progressive supranuclear palsy.[51,57,58,73,93,98,116,122–129] However, special emphasis is given to the presence of Pick bodies for diagnosing "typical" PcD since Pick bodies are almost never identified in conditions other than those combining dementia and circumscribed cerebral atrophy. Pick body–like inclusions may, however, be encountered in AD or other neurodegenerative diseases.[130–132] Furthermore, Sparks et al. reported Pick bodies and ballooned neurons in the grossly normal brain of a non-demented patient, suggesting that neuropathological features of PcD may precede the occurrence of symptoms.[133]

The neuropathological features that are usually accepted as being characteristic of PcD may be summarized as follows: circumscribed, asymmetric or symmetric, frontal, frontotemporal, or frontotemporoparietal atrophy (lobar atrophy often including the hippocampal formation, amygdala, and deep gray nuclei, especially in the anterior portion of the striatum, with relative preservation of the caudal third of the superior temporal gyrus), status spongiosus, reactive gliosis, and neuronal loss in the atrophic areas with or without the presence of Pick bodies or ballooned neurons, and with rare or without the presence of neurofibrillary tangles of Alzheimer's or neuritic plaques.

We owe a special debt of gratitude to Wendy Hobbs, who did so much to help us in the preparation of this review. We thank Larry Cherkas for his assistance and advice. We express our appreciation to the numerous pathologists who referred case material to the Harvard Brain Tissue Resource Center, and the Alzheimer Disease Research Center; this work would not have been possible without their assistance. We are especially grateful to the families of the patients for providing brain tissue for research. This work was supported in part by NIH grants NINCDS 31862 (Harvard Brain Tissue Resource Center, J.P.V.); NS 16367 (Huntington's Disease Center Without Walls, J.P.V.); and NIA 2P50-AG0 5134 (J.P.V., G.B., E.T.H.W., J.H.G.)

REFERENCES

1. Binetti G, Growdon JH, Vonsattel J-PG. Pick's disease. In: Growdon JH, Rossor MN, eds. Blue Books of Practical Neurology. The Dementias (19). Boston: Butterworth-Heinemann, 1998:7–44.
2. Pick A. Ueber die Beziehungen der senilen Hirnatrophie zur Aphasie. Prag Med Wochenschr 1892; 16:165–167.
3. Pick A. Senile Hirnatrophie als Grundlage von Herderscheinungen. Wien Klin Wochenschr 1901; 14:403–404.
4. Pick A. Zur Symptomatologie des linksseitigen Schläfenlappenatrophie. Monatsschr Psychiatr Neurol 1904; 16:378–388.
5. Pick A. Über einen weiteren Symptomenkomplex im Rahmen der Dementia senilis, bedingt durch umschriebene stärkere Hirnatrophie (gemischte Aparxie). Monatsschr Psychiatr Neurol 1906; 19:97–108.
6. Vonsattel J-PG, Binetti G, Kelley LM. Pick disease. In: Wasco W, Tanzi RE, eds. Molecular Mechanisms of Dementia. Totowa, NJ: Humana Press, 1997:253–269.
7. Richter H. Eine besondere Art von Stirnhirnschwund mit Verblödung. Z Ges Neurol Psychiatrie (Berl) 1918; 38:127–160.
8. Lüers T, Spatz H. Picksche Krankheit (Progressive umschriebene Grosshirnatrophie). In: Lubarsch O, Henke F, Rössle R, Scholz W, eds. Handbuch der speziellen pathologischen Anatomie und Histologie (XIII/1 Bandteil A). Heidelberg: Springer-Verlag, 1957:614–715.
9. Tissot R, Constantinidis J, Richard J. La maladie de Pick. Paris: Masson, 1975:1–122.
10. Alzheimer A. Über eigenartige Krankheitsfälle des späteren Alters. Z Ges Neurol Psychiatrie (Berl) 1911; 4:356–385.
11. Onari K, Spatz H. Anatomische Beiträge zur Lehre von der Pickschen umschriebenen Grosshirnrinden-Atrophie ("Picksche Krankheit"). Z Ges Neurol Psychiatrie (Berl) 1926; 101:470–511.
12. Dickson DW. Pick's disease: a modern approach. Brain Pathol 1998; 8:339–354.
13. Altman E. Über die umschriebene Gehirnatrophie des späteren Alters. Z Ges Neurol Psychiatrie (Berl) 1923; 83:610–643.
14. Gans A. Betrachtungen über Art und Ausbreitung des krankhaften Prozesses in einem Fall von Pickscher Atrophie des Stirnhirns. Z Ges Neurol Psychiatrie (Berl) 1922; 80:10–28.
15. Stertz G. Über die Picksche Atrophie. Ges Neurol Psychiatrie (Berl) 1926; 101:729–747.
16. Korbsch H. Picksche und Huntingtonsche Krankheit bei Geschwistern. Arch Psychiatrie 1933; 100:326–349.
17. von Bagh K. Über anatomische Befunde bei 30 Fällen von systematischer Atrophie der Grosshirnrinde (Pickscher Krankheit) mit besonderer Berücksichtigung der Stammganglien und der langen absteigenden Leitungsbahnen. Eine vorläufige Mitteilung. Arch Psychiatrie 1941; 114:68–70.
18. von Bagh K. Klinische und pathologisch-anatomische Studien an 30 Fällen systematischer umschriebener Atrophie der Grosshirnrinde (Pickscher Krankheit). Ann Acad Sci Fennicae Ser A V Med Anthropolo 1946; 10:1–132.
19. Schneider C. Über Picksche Krankheit. Monatsschr Psychiatr Neurol 1927; 65:230–275.
20. Schneider C. Weitere Beiträge zur Lehre von der Pickschen Krankheit. Z Ges Neurol Psychiatrie (Berl) 1929; 120:340–384.
21. von Braunmühl A. Über Stammganglienveränderungen bei Pickscher Krankheit. Z Ges Neurol Psychiatrie (Berl) 1930; 124:214–221.
22. Grünthal E. Über ein Brüderpaar mit Pickscher Krankheit. Eine vergleichende Untersuchung, zugleich ein Beitrag zur Kenntnis der Verursachung und des Verlaufs der Erkrankung. Z Ges Neurol Psychiatrie (Berl) 1930; 129:350–375.
23. von Braunmühl A, Leonhard K. Über ein Schwes-

ternpaar mit Pickscher Krankheit. Zeitschr Ges Neurol Psychiatrie (Berl) 1934; 150:209–241.
24. Schmitz HA, Meyer A. Über die Pickscher Krankheit, mit besonderer Berücksichtigung der Erblichkeit. Arch Psychiatrie 1933; 99:747–761.
25. von Braunmühl A. Picksche Krankheit und amyotrophische Lateralsklerose. Allg Z Psychiatr Psychol Gerichtl Med 1932; 96:364–366.
26. Binetti G, Locascio JJ, Corkin S, Vonsattel JP, Growdon JH. Differences between Pick disease and Alzheimer disease in clinical appearance and rate of cognitive decline. Arch Neurol 2000; 57:225–232.
27. Brion S, Plas J, Jeanneau A. La maladie de Pick. Point de vue anatomo-clinique. Rev Neurol 1991; 147:693–704.
28. Brown J. Pick's disease. In: Rossor MN, ed. Baillière's Clinical Neurology. International Practice and Research. Unusual Dementias. London: Baillière Tindall/W.B. Saunders, 1992:535–557.
29. Galton CJ, Patterson K, Xuereb JH, Hodges JR. Atypical and typical presentations of Alzheimer's disease: a clinical, neuropsychological, neuroimaging and pathological study of 13 cases. Brain 2000; 123:484–498.
30. van Duijn CM. Epidemiology of the dementias: recent developments and new approaches. J Neurol Neurosurg Psychiatry 1996; 60:478–488.
31. Terry RD. Dementia. A brief and selective review. Arch Neurol 1976; 33:1–4.
32. Heston LL. The clinical genetics of Pick's disease. Acta Psychiatr Scand 1978; 57:202–206.
33. Tissot R, Constantinidis J, Richard J. Pick's disease. In: Frederiks JAM, ed. Handbook of Clinical Neurology, Vol. 2 (46): Neurobehavioural Disorders. Amsterdam: Elsevier Science Publishers, 1985:233–246.
34. Corey-Bloom J, Thal LJ, Galasko D, Folstein M, Drachman D, Raskind M, Lanska DJ. Diagnosis and evaluation of dementia. Neurology 1995; 45:211–218.
35. Van Broeckhoven CL. Molecular genetics of Alzheimer disease: identification of genes and gene mutations. Eur Neurol 1995; 35:8–19.
36. Löwenberg K, Boyd DA, Salon DD. Occurrence of Pick's disease in early adult years. Arch Neurol Psychiatry 1939; 41:1004–1020.
37. Rana Mowadat HR, Kerr EE, St Clair D. Sporadic Pick's disease in a 28-year-old woman. Br J Psychiatry 1993; 162:259–262.
38. Stewart JT, Ware MR, Bauer RM, Hoffman MK, Lefler LA. A case of early-onset Pick's disease. J Clin Psychiatry 1992; 53:380.
39. Binns JK, Robertson EE. Pick's disease in old age. J Mental Sci 1962; 108:804–810.
40. Munoz-Garcia D, Ludwin SK. Classic and generalized variants of Pick's disease: a clinicopathological, ultrastructural, and immunocytochemical comparative study. Ann Neurol 1984; 16:467–480.
41. Cummings JL, Duchen LW. Klüver-Bucy syndrome in Pick disease: clinical and pathologic correlations. Neurology 1981; 31:1415–1422.
42. Holland AL, McBurney DH, Moossy J, Reinmuth OM. The dissolution of language in Pick's disease with neurofibrillary tangles: a case study. Brain Lang 1985; 24:36–58.
43. Hodges JR, Gurd JM. Remote memory and lexical retrieval in a case of frontal Pick's disease. Arch Neurol 1994; 51:821–827.
44. Groen JJ, Endtz LJ. Hereditary Pick's disease second re-examination of a large family and discussion of other hereditary cases, with particular reference to electroencephalography and computerized tomography. Brain 1982; 105:443–459.
45. Kosaka K, Ikeda K, Kobayashi K, Mehraein P. Striatopallidonigral degeneration in Pick's disease: a clinicopathological study of 41 cases. J Neurol 1991; 238:151–160.
46. Gustafson L, Brun A, Passant U. Frontal lobe degeneration of non-Alzheimer type. In: Rossor MN, ed. Baillière's Clinical Neurology. International Practice and Research. Unusual Dementias. London: Baillière Tindall/W.B. Saunders, 1992:559–582.
47. Heston LL, White JA, Mastri AR. Pick's disease. Clinical genetics and natural history. Arch Gen Psychiatry 1987; 44:409–411.
48. Malamud N, Waggoner RW. Genealogic and clinicopathologic study of Pick's disease. Arch Neurol Psychiatry 1943; 50:288–303.
49. Schenk VWD. Re-examination of a family with Pick's disease. Ann Hum Gen 1959; 23:325–333.
50. Collinge J, Palmer MS, Sidle KCL, Mahal SP, Campbell T, Brown J, Hardy J, Brun AE, Gustafson L, Bakker E, Roos R, Groen JJ. Familial Pick's disease and dementia in frontal lobe degeneration of non-Alzheimer type are not variants of prion disease. J Neurol Neurosurg Psychiatry 1994; 57:762.
51. Heutink P, Stevens M, Rizzu P, Bakker E, Kros JM, Tibben A, Niermeijer MF, van Duijn CM, Oostra BA, van Swieten JC. Hereditary frontotemporal dementia is linked to chromosome 17q21-q22: a genetic and clinicopathological study of three Dutch families. Ann Neurol 1997; 41:150–159.
52. Lendon CL, Lynch T, Norton J, McKeel DW, Busfield F, Craddock N, Chakraverty S, Gopalakrishnan G, Shears SD, Grimmett W, Wilhelmsen KC, Hansen L, Morris JC, Goate AM. Hereditary dysphasic disinhibition dementia. A frontotemporal dementia linked to 17q21–22. Neurology 1998; 50:1546–1555.
53. Lynch T, Sano M, Marder KS, Bell KL, Foster NL, Defendini RF, Sima AAF, Keohane C, Nygaard TG, Fahn S, Mayeux R, Rowland LP, Wilhelmsen KC. Clinical characteristics of a family with chromosome 17-linked disinhibition–dementia–parkinsonism–amyotrophy complex. Neurology 1994; 44:1878–1884.
54. Baker M, Kwok JBJ, Kucera S, Crook R, Farrer M, Houlden H, Isaacs A, Lincoln S, Onstead L, Hardy J, Wittenberg L, Dodd P, Webb S, Hayward N, Tannenberg T, Andreadis A, Hallupp M, Schofield P, Dark F, Hutton M. Localization of frontotemporal dementia with parkinsonism in an Australian kindred to chromosome 17q21–22. Ann Neurol 1997; 42:794–798.
55. Petersen RB, Tabaton M, Chen SG, Monari L, Richardson SL, Lynches T, Manetto V, Lanska DJ, Markesbery WR, Currier RD, Autilio-Gambetti L, Wilhelmsen KC, Gambetti P. Familial progressive subcortical gliosis: presence of prions and linkage to chromosome 17. Neurology 1995; 45:1062–1067.
56. Wijker M, Wszoleck ZK, Wolters ECH, Rooimans MA, Pals G, Pfeiffer RF, Lynch T, Rodnitzky RL, Wilhelmsen KC, Arwert F. Localization of the gene for rapidly progressive autosomal dominant parkinsonism and dementia with pallido-ponto-nigral degen-

eration to chromosome 17q21. Hum Mol Genet 1996; 5:151–154.
57. Sima AAF, Defendini R, Keohane C, D'Amato C, Foster NL, Parchi P, Gambetti P, Lynch T, Wilhelmsen KC. The neuropathology of chromosome 17-linked dementia. Ann Neurol 1996; 39:734–743.
58. Bird TD, Nochlin D, Poorkaj P, Cherrier M, Kaye J, Payami H, Peskind E, Lampe TH, Nemens E, Boyer PJ, Schellenberg GD. A clinical pathological comparison of three families with frontotemporal dementia and identical mutations in the tau gene (P301L). Brain 1999; 122:741–756.
59. Spillantini MG, Goedert M, Crowther RA, Murrell JR, Farlow MR, Ghetti B. Familial multiple system tauopathy with presenile dementia: a disease with abundant neuronal and glial tau filaments. Proc Natl Acad Sci USA 1997; 94:4113–4118.
60. Schneider JA, Gearing M, Robbins RS, de l'Aune W, Mirra SS. Apolipoprotein E genotype in diverse neurodegenerative disorders. Ann Neurol 1995; 38:131–135.
61. Gomez-Isla T, West HL, Rebeck GW, Harr SD, Growdon JH, Locascio JJ, Perls TT, Lipsitz LA, Hyman BT. Clinical and pathological correlates of apolipoprotein Eε4 in Alzheimer's disease. Ann Neurol 1996; 39:62–70.
62. Spatz H. La maladie de Pick, les atrophies systématisées progressives et la sénescence cérébrale prématurée localisée. In: The Proceedings of the First International Congress of Neuropathology, Vol. 2. Torino: Rosenberg and Sellier, 1952:375–406.
63. Cambier J, Masson M, Dairou R, Henin D. Étude anatomo-clinique d'une forme pariétale de la maladie de Pick. Rev Neurol 1981; 137:33–38.
64. Lang AE, Bergeron C, Pollanen MS, Ashby P. Parietal Pick's disease mimicking cortico-basal ganglionic degeneration. Neurology 1994; 44:1436–1440.
65. Lüers Th. Über fronto-thalamische Syndrome bei der Pickschen Krankheit. Dtsch Z Nervenheilkd 1950; 164:179–198.
66. Vonsattel J-P, Myers RH, Stevens TJ, Ferrante RJ, Bird ED, Richardson EP, Jr. Neuropathological classification of Huntington's disease. J Neuropathol Exp Neurol 1985; 44:559–577.
67. Constantinidis J. Pick dementia: anatomical correlations and pathophysiological considerations. Interdiscipl Top Gerontol 1985; 19:72–97.
68. Hulette CM, Crain BJ. Lobar atrophy without Pick bodies. Clin Neuropathol 1992; 11:151–156.
69. Paulus W, Bancher C, Jellinger K. Microglial reaction in Pick's disease. Neurosci Lett 1993; 161:89–92.
70. Hollister RD, Xia M, McNamara MJ, Hyman BT. Neuronal expression of class II major histocompatibility complex (HLA-DR) in 2 cases of Pick disease. Arch Neurol 1997; 54:243–248.
71. Iwatsubo T, Hasegawa M, Ihara Y. Neuronal and glial tau-positive inclusions in diverse neurologic diseases share common phosphorylation characteristics. Acta Neuropathol 1994; 88:129–136.
72. Dickson DW, Feany MB, Yen S-H, Mattiace LA, Davies P. Cytoskeletal pathology in non-Alzheimer degenerative dementia: new lesions in diffuse Lewy body disease, Pick's disease, and corticobasal degeneration. J Neural Transm 1996; (Suppl) 47:31–46.
73. Feany MB, Mattiace LA, Dickson DW. Neuropathologic overlap of progressive supranuclear palsy, Pick's disease and corticobasal degeneration. J Neuropathol Exp Neurol 1996; 55:53–67.
74. Tagliavini F, Pilleri G. Basal nucleus of Meynert. A neuropathological study in Alzheimer's disease, simple senile dementia, Pick's disease and Huntington's chorea. J Neurol Sci 1983; 62:243–260.
75. Braak H, Braak E. Cortical and subcortical argyrophilic grains characterize a disease associated with adult onset dementia. Neuropathol Appl Neurobiol 1989; 15:13–26.
76. Martinez-Lage P, Munoz DG. Prevalence and disease associations of argyrophilic grains of Braak. J Neuropathol Exp Neurol 1997; 56:157–164.
77. Sam M, Gutmann L, Schochet SS, Doshi H. Pick's disease: a case clinically resembling amyotrophic lateral sclerosis. Neurology 1991; 41:1831–1833.
78. Wisniewski HM, Coblentz JM, Terry RD. Pick's disease. A clinical and ultrastructural study. Arch Neurol 1972; 26:97–108.
79. Tiller-Borcich JK, Forno LS. Parkinson's disease and dementia with neuronal inclusions in the cerebral cortex: Lewy bodies or Pick bodies. J Neuropathol Exp Neurol 1988; 47:526–535.
80. Ball MJ. Topography of Pick inclusion bodies in hippocampi of demented patients. A quantitative study. J Neuropathol Exp Neurol 1979; 38:614–620.
81. Hof PR, Bouras C, Perl DP, Morrison JH. Quantitative neuropathologic analysis of Pick's disease cases: cortical distribution of Pick bodies and coexistence with Alzheimer disease. Acta Neuropathol 1994; 87:115–124.
82. Jellinger KA. Quantitative neuropathologic analysis of Pick's disease cases. Acta Neuropathol 1994; 87:223–224.
83. Armstrong RA, Cairns NJ, Lantos PL. Quantification of pathological lesions in the frontal and temporal lobe of ten patients diagnosed with Pick's disease. Acta Neuropathol 1999; 97:456–462.
84. Fukui T, Sugita K, Kawamura M, Shiota J, Nakano I. Primary progressive apraxia in Pick's disease: a clinicopathologic study. Neurology 1996; 47:467–473.
85. Dickson DW, Wertkin A, Kress Y, Ksiezak-Reding H, Yen S-H. Ubiquitin immunoreactive structures in normal human brains. Distribution and developmental aspects. Lab Invest 1990; 63:87–99.
86. Jellinger KA. Neuropathological criteria for Pick's disease and frontotemporal lobe dementia. In: Cruz-Sánchez FF, Ravid R, Cuzner ML, eds. Neuropathological Diagnostic Criteria for Brain Banking. Amsterdam: IOS Press, 1995:35–54.
87. Yasuhara O, Matsuo A, Tooyama I, Kimura H, McGeer EG, McGeer PL. Pick's disease immunohistochemistry: new alterations and Alzheimer's disease comparisons. Acta Neuropathol 1995; 89:322–330.
88. Yasuhara O, Aimi Y, McGeer EG, McGeer PL. Accumulation of amyloid precursor protein in brain lesions of patients with Pick disease. Neurosci Lett 1994; 171:63–66.
89. Wechsler AF, Verity MA, Rosenschein S, Fried I, Scheibel AB. Pick's disease. A clinical, computed tomographic, and histologic study with Golgi impregnation observations. Arch Neurol 1982; 39:287–290.
90. Yokoo H, Oyama T, Hirato J, Sasaki A, Nakazato Y. A case of Pick's disease with unusual neuronal inclusions. Acta Neuropathol 1994; 88:267–272.

91. Mezey E, Deheijia A, Harta G, Papp MI, Polymeropoulos MH, Brownstein MJ. Alpha synuclein in neurodegenerative disorders: murderer or accomplice? Natu Med 1998; 7:755–757.
92. Khachaturian ZS. Diagnosis of Alzheimer's disease. Arch Neurol 1985; 42:1097–1105.
93. Clark AW, Manz HJ, White III CL, Lehmann J, Miller D, Coyle JT. Cortical degeneration with swollen chromatolytic neurons: its relationship to Pick's disease. J Neuropathol Exp Neurol 1986; 45:268–284.
94. Delacourte A, Robitaille Y, Sergeant N, Buée L, Hof PR, Wattez A, Laroche-Cholette A, Mathieu J, Chagnon P, Gauvreau D. Specific pathological tau protein variants characterize Pick's disease. J Neuropathol Exp Neurol 1996; 55:159–168.
95. Brion J-P. Neurofibrillary tangles and Alzheimer's disease. Eur Neurol 1998; 40:130–140.
96. Buée-Scherrer V, Hof PR, Buée L, Leveugle B, Vermersch P, Perl DP, Olanow CW, Delacourte A. Hyperphosphorylated tau proteins differentiate corticobasal degeneration and Pick's disease. Acta Neuropathol 1996; 91:351–359.
97. Williams HW. The peculiar cells of Pick's disease. Their pathogenesis and distribution in disease. Arch Neurol Psychiatry 1935; 34:508–519.
98. Dickson DW, Yen S-H, Suzuki KI, Davies P, Garcia JH, Hirano A. Ballooned neurons in select neurodegenerative diseases contain phosphorylated neurofilament epitopes. Acta Neuropathol 1986; 71:216–223.
99. Cooper PN, Jackson M, Lennox G, Lowe J, Mann DMA. τ, ubiquitin, and β-crystallin immunohistochemistry define the principal causes of degenerative frontotemporal dementia. Arch Neurol 1995; 52:1011–1015.
100. Wood BT, McKee AC. Case Records of the Massachusetts General Hospital. Case 6–1992. N Engl J Med 1992; 326:397–405.
101. Masters CL, Richardson EP, Jr. Subacute spongiform encephalopathy (Creutzfeldt-Jakob disease). The nature and progression of spongiform change. Brain 1978; 101:333–344.
102. Neumann MA. Pick's disease. J Neuropathol Exp Neurol 1949; 8:255–282.
103. Sjögren T, Sjögren H, Lindgren AGH. Morbus Alzheimer and morbus Pick: a genetic, clinical and patho-anatomical study. Acta Psychiatri Neurol Scand 1952; Suppl 82:1–152.
104. Gustafson L, Nilsson L. Differential diagnosis of presenile dementia on clinical grounds. Acta Psychiatr Scand 1982; 65:194–209.
105. The Lund and Manchester Groups. Clinical and neuropathological criteria for frontotemporal dementia. J Neurol Neurosurg Psychiatry 1994; 57:416–418.
106. Hansen LA, Crain B. Making the diagnosis of mixed and non-Alzheimer's disease. Arch Pathol Lab Med 1995; 119:1023–1031.
107. Schenk VWD. Maladie de Pick. Étude anatomo-clinique de 8 cas. Ann Med Psychol 1951; 109:574–587.
108. Baldwin B, Förstl H. "Pick's disease"—101 years on still there, but in need of reform. Br J Psychiatry 1993; 163:100–104.
109. Litvan I, Hauw JJ, Bartko JJ, Lantos PL, Daniel SE, Horoupian DS, Mc Kee A, Dickson D, Bancher C, Taabaton M, Jellinger K, Anderson DW. Validity and reliability of the preliminary NINDS neuropathologic criteria for progressive supranuclear palsy and related disorders. J Neuropathol Exp Neurol 1996; 55:97–105.
110. Litvan I, Agid Y, Sastrj N, Jankovic J, Wenning GK, Goetz CG, Verny M, Brandel JP, Jellinger K, Ray Chaudhuri K, McKee A, Lai EC, Pearce RKB, ABartko JJ. What are the obstacles for an accurate clinical diagnosis of Pick's disease? A clincopathologic study. Neurology 1997; 49:62–69.
111. Morrison JH, Hof PR. Life and death of neurons in the aging brain. Science 1997; 278:412–419.
112. Giannakopoulos P, Hof PR, Bouras C. Dementia lacking distinctive histopathology: clinicopathological evaluation of 32 cases. Acta Neuropathol 1995; 89:346–355.
113. Mann DMA, South PW, Snowden JS, Neary D. Dementia of frontal lobe type: neuropathology and immunohistochemistry. J Neurol Neurosurg Psychiatry 1993; 56:605–614.
114. Neary D. Non-Alzheimer's disease forms of cerebral atrophy. J Neurol Neurosurg Psychiatry 1990; 53:929–931.
115. Wightman G, Anderson VER, Martin J, Swash M, Aderton BH, Neary D, Mann D, Luthert P, Leigh PN. Hippocampal and neocortical ubiquitin-immunoreactive inclusions in amyotrophic lateral sclerosis with dementia. Neurosci Lett 1992; 139:269–274.
116. Lippa CF, Cohen R, Smith TW, Drachman DA. Primary progressive aphasia with focal neuronal achromasia. Neurology 1991; 41:882–886.
117. Mesulam MM, Weintraub S. Spectrum of primary progressive aphasia. In: Rossor MN, ed. Baillière's Clinical Neurology. International Practice and Research. Unusual Dementias. London: Baillière Tindall/W.B. Saunders, 1992:583–609.
118. Scheltens P, Ravid R, Kamphorst W. Pathologic findings in a case of primary progressive aphasia. Neurology 1994; 44:279–282.
119. Knopman DS, Mastri AR, Frey WH, Sung JH, Rustan T. Dementia lacking distinctive histologic features: a common non-Alzheimer degenerative dementia. Neurology 1990; 40:251–256.
120. Jackson M, Lowe J. The new neuropathology of degenerative frontotemporal dementias. Acta Neuropathol 1996; 91:127–134.
121. Turner RS, Kenyon LC, Trojanowski JQ, Gonatas N, Grossman M. Clinical, neuroimaging, and pathologic features of progressive non fluent aphasia. Ann Neurol 1996; 39:166–173.
121a. World Health Organization's International classification of diseases 10th Revision (ICD-10)
122. Rebeiz JJ, Kolodny EH, Richardson EP, Jr. Corticodentatonigral degeneration with neuronal achromasia. Arch Neurol 1968; 18:20–33.
123. Gibb RG, Luthert PJ, Marsden CD. Corticobasal degeneration. Brain 1989; 112:1171–1192.
124. Lippa CF, Smith TW, Fontneau N. Corticonigral degeneration with neuronal achromasia. A clinicopathologic study of two cases. J Neurol Sci 1990; 98:301–310.
125. Budka H, Aguzzi A, Brown P, Brucher J-M, Bugiani O, Gullotta F, Haltia M, Hauw J-J, Ironside J-W,

126. Feany MB, Dickson DW. Widespread cytoskeletal pathology characterizes corticobasal degeneration. Am J Pathol 1995; 146:1388–1396.
127. Mackenzie IRA, Hudson LP. Achromatic neurons in the cortex of progressive supranuclear palsy. Acta Neuropathol 1995; 90:615–619.
128. Pillon B, Blin J, Vidailhet M, Deweer B, Sirigu A, Dubois B, Agid Y. The neuropsychological pattern of corticobasal degeneration: comparison with progressive supranuclear palsy and Alzheimer's disease. Neurology 1995; 45:1477–1483.
129. Parchi P, Giese A, Capellari S, Brown P, Schulz-Schaeffer W, Windl O, Zerr I, Budka H, Knopp N, Piccardo P, Poser S, Rojiani A, Streichemberger N, Julien J, Vital C, Ghetti B, Gambetti P, Kretzschmar H. Classification of sporadic Creutzfeldt-Jakob disease based on molecular and phenotypic analysis of 300 subjects. Ann Neurol 1999; 46:224–233.
130. Dickson DW, Ksiezak-Reding H, Liu W-K, Davies P, Crowe A, Yen S-HC. Immunocytochemistry of neurofibrillary tangles with antibodies to subregions of tau protein: identification of hidden and cleaved tau epitopes and a new phosphorylation site. Acta Neuropathol 1992; 84:596–605.
131. Jendroska K, Rossor MN, Mathias CJ, Daniel SE. Morphological overlap between corticobasal degeneration and Pick's disease: a clinicopathological report. Mov Disord 1995; 10:111–114.
132. Feany MB, Dickson DW. Neurodegenerative disorders with extensive tau pathology: a comparative study and review. Ann Neurol 1996; 40:139–148.
133. Sparks DL, Danner FW, Davis DG, Hackney C, Landers T, Coyne CM. Neurochemical and histopathologic alterations characteristic of Pick's disease in a non-demented individual. J Neuropathol Exp Neurol 1994; 53:37–42.

Jellinger K, Kretzschmar HA, Lantos PL, Masullo C, Schlote W, Tateishi J, Weller RO. Neuropathological diagnostic criteria for Creutzfeldt-Jakob disease (CJD) and other human spongiform encephalopathies (Prion diseases). Brain Pathol 1995; 5:459–466.

8. Alzheimer's Disease

JEAN-JACQUES HAUW AND CHARLES DUYCKAERTS

Alzheimer's disease[1] (AD) is the most common cause of dementia in adults in the industrialized countries. It accounts for around 30%–50% of all demented people and contributes to another 15%–45% of cases in which it is combined with the consequences of cerebrovascular disease or other dementing conditions. In demented elderly women, the predominance of AD over other causes of dementia is even more striking. The prevalence of dementia increases dramatically with age, reaching 10% to 20% and more in the ninth decade,[2] and the incidence of both dementia and AD rises exponentially up to the age of 90 years, with no sign of this rate leveling off.[3] Consequently, the prevalence of the disease increases steadily in aging countries.[4-6] Signs and symptoms are a loss of memory and cognitive functions with insidious onset and slow progress, beginning usually with disturbance in recent memory and a loss of initiative in an otherwise alert patient. Affective disorders such as depression, and disorientation in time and place may occur early in the disease course. Since the same symptoms can be produced in a curable pathology, the first diagnostic consideration should be a search for treatable disorders.[7,8] The loss of intellectual abilities progresses steadily (although occasional plateaus and even momentary improvements are possible) to such a severity as to interfere with social and/or occupational function.[9] Focal neurological signs and symptoms are rare early in the course of the disease, but aphasia, apraxias, and agnosias become predominant in some cases, especially in early-onset AD. Seizures and myoclonus are seen only in some far-advanced instances. Behavioral symptoms are frequent.[10] The course of the disease is usually long (8 to 10 years on average) and has increased in the last few decades. Death in bed-ridden patients is usually due to infections such as inhalation pneumonia.

Clinical diagnosis of AD has improved in recent years with the wider use of diagnostic criteria, especially those from the National Institute of Neurological and Communicative Disorders and Stroke-Alzheimer's Disease and Related Disorder Association (NINCDS-ADRDA)[11] and the *Diagnostic and Statistical Manual of Mental Disorders* (DSM) III and IV.[9] In the early 1950s, autopsy studies had shown inaccuracy in the premortem diagnosis ranging from 18% to 45%.[12] In the last decades, however, the clinical diagnostic accuracy has increased to up to 90%, or even 100%, in cases in which clinical criteria such as those of primary degenerative dementia of DSM-II were met. In a series of 150 hemispheres from patients with clinically diagnosed AD received consecutively over a 3-year period from numerous sources as part of a research program, 87% of the cases fulfilled the histological criteria for AD, sometimes with additional findings such as Parkinson's disease or stroke.[13] In another prospective series of 26 consecutive postmortem examinations, AD was histologically proven in all subjects and was the primary dementing illness. Seventeen of these patients had been diagnosed when only mildly demented.[14] In more recent reports, this has proved essentially true for long-term studies of early-onset patients after use of the entire spectrum of modern neuroimaging and when the main diagnosis alone was considered. In addition, an "autopsy bias" has been described: in some cohort series, the range of clinical diagnoses was significantly different in the population who died from that of those patients who survived. There were more patients with fatal conditions in the necropsy group, resulting in an easier diagnosis. This artefactually raised the apparent diagnostic value of the clinical criteria.[15] In the first 108 autopsies of the Consortium to Establish a Register for Alzheimer's Disease (CERAD), the neuropathologists confirmed the diagnosis of possible or probable AD in 92 cases (87%). However, coexistent Parkinson's disease was present in 19 (21%) and vascular lesions of varying nature and size in 26 (28%) of them.[16] The results of two more recent studies are similar: the positive predictive value of the clinical diagnosis of AD was 81% after autopsy and fell to 44% when limited to pure cases.[15] The sensitivity of NINCDS-ADRDA "probable AD" was 83% (diagnosing AD correctly) and overall clinical diagnostic accuracy was 75%. However, there was a high rate of additional neuropathological findings. Only 34 of the 94 cases had pure AD on neuropathologic examination, whereas the remainder frequently had coexisting vascular or Parkinson's disease lesions.[17] These data emphasize the difficulty of diagnosing so-called mixed dementia.

Some authors distinguish AD from senile dementia of the Alzheimer type (SDAT) according to the age of onset: AD occurs before age 65,[18,19] or age 70.[20] Others make distinctions between forms beginning before and after age 80.[21] They may be characterized by different clinical patterns—for example, the higher frequency of aphasia in AD of early onset, an observation that has been challenged.[22] Perhaps because of historical circumstances,[23] the distinctions between senile and presenile variants of the disease are still regularly made in Europe whereas neurologists in North America tend to combine both diseases. Until now, epidemiological studies, whether clinical or pathological, have failed to determine two different peaks of incidence of AD—for example, that in the sixth decade and the other in the eighth to ninth decades. On the contrary, a continuous increase in the density of the lesions of AD has been found in very large series of autopsies.[24] Morphological lesions are qualitatively identical and there is little use in making two different sets of descriptions. Unless specified, we shall use the term "AD" for both AD and SDAT.

Pathological changes observed in AD are qualitatively similar to some of those seen in so-called normal aging, but normality of an aged brain is hard to define. It has been long debated whether the changes commonly seen in the elderly must be considered "physiological" or are the morphological counterpart of an actual disease occurring particularly frequently in the elderly. Part of the problem is semantic and depends on the definition of normality—whether it is statistical (included in confidence interval), descriptive (habitual), genetic (fittest), or clinical (innocuous, harmless).[25] The answer also depends on the data at hand: when clinical data alone are considered, normality of an aged person refers to his or her clinical abilities, whatever the state of the brain. When neuropathological data are considered, morphological alterations are usually thought to be abnormal, regardless of their clinical consequences. However, some of them (such as corpora amylacea or age-related lipofuscin storage) are not usually linked to clinical symptoms and signs. Moreover, clinical abnormalities are related to the density and/or the location of the morphological changes, such as neurofibrillary tangles, and the correlation between lesions and symptoms varies with respect to age.[24] Clinical and pathological data are obviously linked, but the linkage is complex and it has become quite clear that a number of spurious conclusions have been drawn from studies that were only clinical or only pathological. A clinico pathological point of view is adopted here: "dementia" is considered a clinical term. Alzheimer changes are microscopic; clinical examination is thus insufficient for recognizing senile plaques and neurofibrillary tangles and neuropathologic study insufficient for diagnosing dementia. However, since the mental decline and microscopic changes are linked, the diagnosis of AD and especially SDAT can be made with some degree of probability using only clinical or only histological means.[26] But to ascertain a diagnosis with the highest degree of probability, both clinical and pathological information must be used. Finally, the diagnosis of AD according to the usual clinical criteria has been restrictive. The present clinicopathological criteria have left some syndromes unlabeled:

e.g., memory decline without significant cognitive changes and with numerous Alzheimer's lesions in the hippocampus (called "presbyophrenia variant of AD" by the classic German and French authors). Isolated memory failure is insufficient for making the diagnosis of dementia and thus of AD. The use of two terms, one clinical and the other pathologic (e.g., amnesia of the Alzheimer's type) could help us describe these situations. The difficulties met in the diagnosis of cases with only mild dementia or with only a few lesions, and the absence of a clear-cut border between normal and diseased brain in the elderly have led us to consider and, if possible, to contrast SDAT and aging in this chapter.

The first neuropathological studies were cross-sectional and retrospective. Their conclusions were probably valid for the deeply demented patients. Questions arise, however, concerning the control group studies, which were probably contaminated by cases at the beginning of the disease (preclinical disease)[27–29] or with so-called pathological aging.[30] In the elderly, the frequency of SDAT is indeed very high in the general population, especially in institutions where anatomical cases are generally recruited and where it may be over 50%.[31] The first symptoms and signs can be moderate, however, and not easily recognized unless specifically looked for in a prospective way. Since the pioneer longitudinal study planned by Tomlinson et al.[32] the analysis of prospective clinicopathological series has provided new insight into the neuropathology of AD. They do not, however, fully discriminate AD from so-called normal aging. The data at hand must be carefully compared to those obtained by population studies, for the biases in any type of clinicopathological studies are numerous.

GROSS EXAMINATION OF THE BRAIN

Most findings are negative: there is no indication of vascular disease (infarcts, lacunes, or hemorrhages) or of other conditions that can induce or mimic dementia (such as frontal tumor or hydrocephalus). Those alterations do not preclude the diagnosis of mixed dementia; AD, being highly prevalent, is indeed often associated with other dementing disorders. But small lesions (such as lacunes or meningioma) alone are rarely a cause of dementia and associated AD is more common.[33,34] The substantia nigra is not depigmented unless Alzheimer pathology is associated with the presence of Lewy bodies. Faint pigmentation of the locus coeruleus can be found in advanced cases.[19]

Cerebral Atrophy

LOSS OF BRAIN WEIGHT AND VOLUME

Age-related decrease in normal adult brain weight[35] has been overestimated because of a cohort effect in cross-sectional studies: young brains came from patients born much later in the century.[36] Once the secular increase in adult body length and brain weight is taken into account, the volume of the cerebral hemispheres does not change significantly until age 50; from then on, it decreases 2% per decade.[37,38] In a series of 51 normal, carefully selected brains, the decline appeared to occur mostly after age 55.[39] Atrophy is best assessed by comparing the volume of a given brain to that of its own cranial capacity.[40] The brain fills about 92% of the cavity in the sixth decade, 83% in the ninth, and 81% in the tenth. The loss of brain weight is particularly severe in AD of early onset: 200 to 300 g, i.e., 15% to 25% in most studies. It is usually less severe in SDAT (10%), with a wide range and frequent overlaps with age-matched controls. Large series have shown clear differences between the mean weight of brains with microscopic changes of AD and those without, regardless of age, but these group differences cannot be safely used for the diagnosis of individual cases.[34,41,42] In a comparison of the weight of individual lobes in AD cases and controls, the decrease in weight was 41% for the temporal lobe, 30% for the parietal lobe, and 14% (not significant) for the frontal lobe.[43]

GYRAL ATROPHY

Tomlinson et al.[44] found no case with marked or generalized cortical atrophy in elderly normal individuals on neuropathological examination. Slight atrophy in the parasagittal gyri of the frontal and parietal lobes or generalized isolated frontal atrophy was sometimes observed, in contrast with the normal shape of the cerebellum. On computed tomography (CT) scans, gyral atrophy is first seen at about age 40 and increases later on.[45] Researchers have attempted to follow longitudinally the decrease in volume of the brain with age.[46,47] Using magnetic resonance imaging (MRI) the mean rate of decrease in hippocampal volume was found to be 1.55 +/- 1.38% per year in intellectually normal individuals aged 70 to 89. It reached 4% in AD cases. However, atrophy is lacking in some aged individuals, and some who do show atrophy have normal brain function. Finally, brains at autopsy sometimes fail to exhibit the atrophy that had been seen with CT. The volume of the brain in vivo is indeed highly dependent on the hydration status and can thus fluctuate.

Gyral atrophy is usually less marked in SDAT than in early-onset AD.[48] It is significant only on average. Recognizable atrophy is lacking in some patients with SDAT or AD

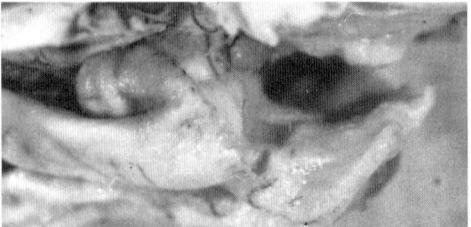
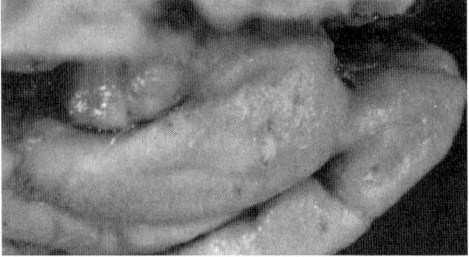

Figure 8–2. Marked atrophy of the amygdaloid body and of the anterior part of hippocampal formation in a case of severe Alzheimer's disease (top) compared with a control case (bottom).

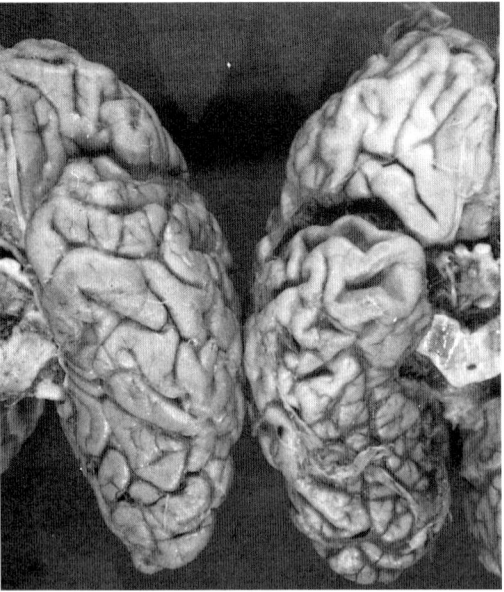

Figure 8–1. Inferior view of the brain showing atrophy prominent in the temporal lobe (right; severe Alzheimer's disease) as compared with a control brain (left). Gyral atrophy, enlargement of the sylvian fissure, and marked reduction in the anteroposterior size of the temporal lobe are evident.

(40% in Tomlinsou et al.'s study[32]). When present, gyral atrophy is prominent in the parasagittal areas and in the temporal lobes, more specifically, their poles[49] (Figs. 8–1 to 8–4). The frontal lobe has been said to be more atrophic than the parietal lobe. The occipital cortex is generally considered to be well preserved.[50] Gray and white matter appear to be affected equally,[49] but the white matter has been shown to be affected earlier in a small series of cases.[51] The most severely affected areas are usually the temporal pole, the anterior part of the hippocampal gyrus, and the amygdala, as discussed in the neuronal loss section. Occasionally, atrophy may be asymmetric or focal, mimicking primary lobar atrophies, including that of Pick's disease.[18,19,42] These focal atrophies may be associated with focal cognitive deficits such as progressive aphasia[52,53] or agnosia.[54]

THICKNESS AND LENGTH OF THE CORTICAL RIBBON

The thickness of the isocortex is only slightly affected by normal aging.[41] Terry et al.[39] showed a moderate but significant decrease with age in the midfrontal and superior temporal areas but not in inferior parietal areas. A decrease of 28% in the thickness of the subiculum has been observed in old individ-

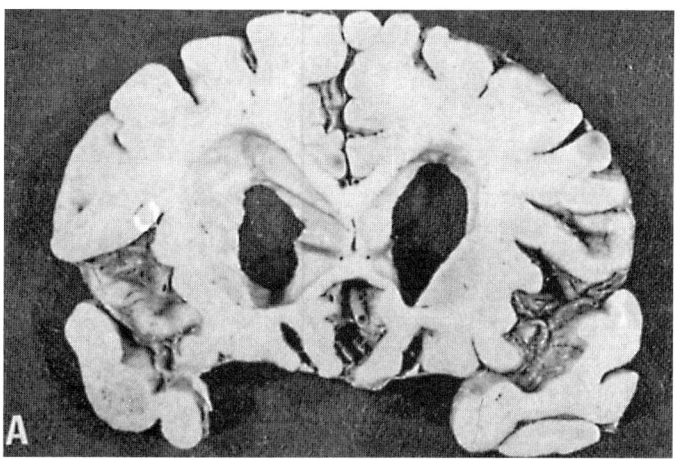
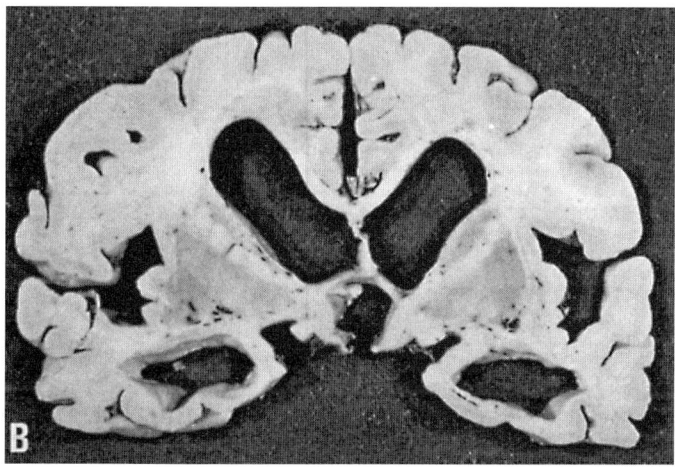
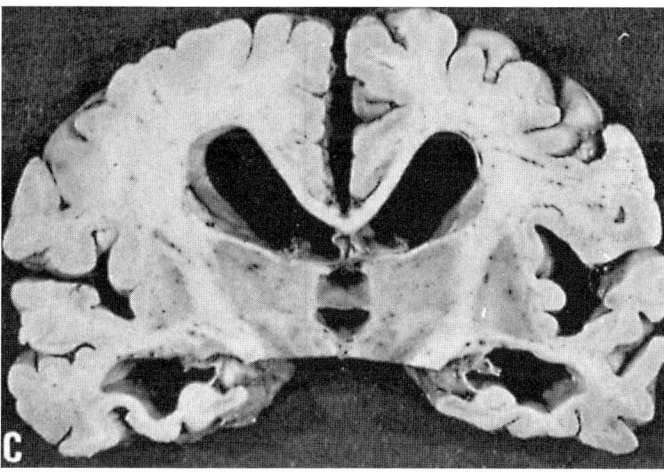

Figure 8–3. Gross appearance of coronal sections of the brain involving the prefrontal cortex (*A*), anterior part of the basal ganglia (*B*), and their posterior part (*C*) in a case of severe Alzheimer's disease. Gyral atrophy, enlargement of the sylvian fissure, and ventricular dilation are seen.

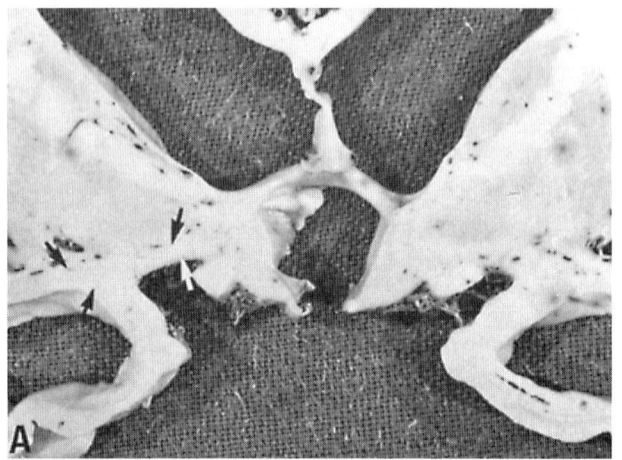
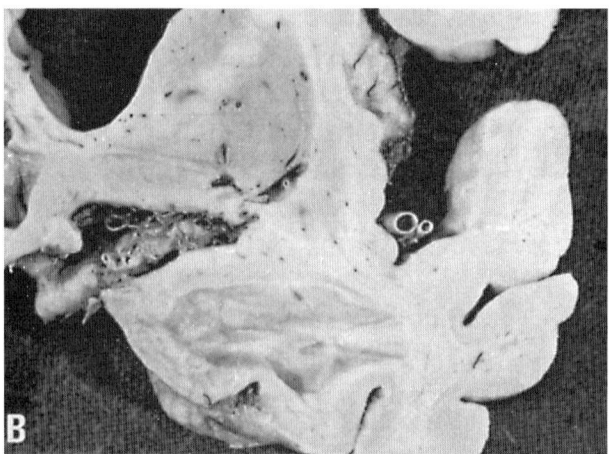
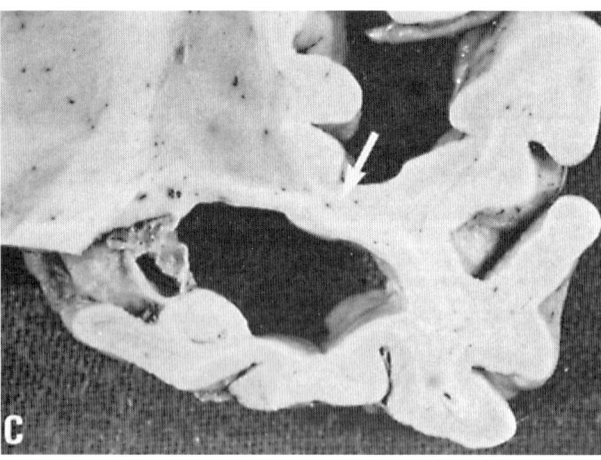

Figure 8–4. Gross appearance of coronal sections of the brain in a case of severe Alzheimer's disease demonstrating the topography of the sublenticular area where the nucleus basalis of Meynert is located (*A*, arrows), atrophy of the amygdaloid body and hippocampal uncus (*B*), and atrophy of the temporal stem (*C*, arrow).

uals (Shefer, 1972, quoted in Kemper[41]). In AD, by contrast the neocortical volume of all the cerebral lobes was significantly decreased in early-onset forms, whereas only the temporal lobe was atrophic in cases of SDAT in patients over age 80.[48] A decrease in the thickness of the isocortex is moderate in AD and SDAT, however[41,55] and not directly proportional to the atrophy.[56] It has been proposed that the decrease in the cortical area in sections of the brain (i.e., atrophy) could be due to a decrease in the length of the cortical ribbon, measured in coronal sections, whereas its thickness does not vary significantly in the early stages of the disease. A correlation was indeed found between the length—and not the thickness—of the cortical ribbon and the premortem mental score.[56] These data suggest a loss of columns of neurons or of fibers arranged perpendicularly to the surface of the cortex (Fig. 8–5). The loss of selective layers of the isocortex (laminar loss) would alter the thickness of the cortical ribbon (Fig. 8–3). The latter is detectable only in the most affected cases, where it can be seen on gross examination, especially in the temporal cortex.

VENTRICULAR DILATION

Ventricular size increases from about age 45 until about age 80 in men and age 85 in women.[57] Ventricles are larger on average in SDAT but their sizes are poorly correlated with intellectual status. Only 13 (57%) of the 23 demented patients showing the microscopic changes of SDAT had a ventricular volume above the upper limit of normal in the series of Hubbard and Anderson.[58] Ventricular enlargement as evaluated by CT scan or MRI appears to be a poorly sensitive sign of SDAT (the sensitivity has been rated at 46 +/− 20%), although it appears to be more specific (90 +/− 7%).[59] The yearly rate of enlargement of lateral ventricle volume, by contrast, was found to be both sensitive (100%) and specific (100%).[60]

NEURONAL LOSS, PERIKARYAL ATROPHY, AND APOPTOSIS

The bias introduced in the cell-counting procedure performed on sections has been recognized for a long time,[61,62] the probability of

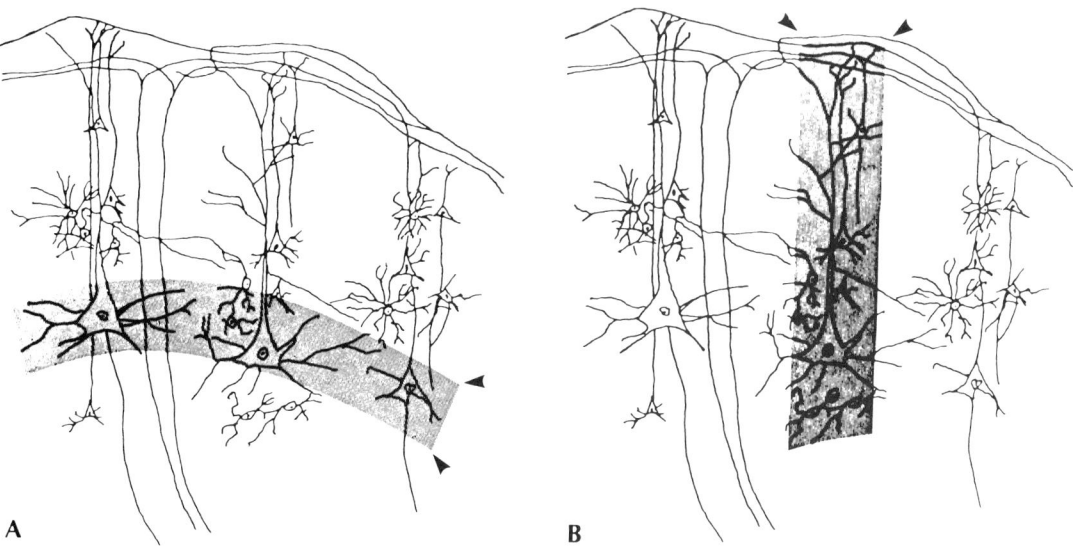

Figure 8–5. Models of cortical atrophy in aging and Alzheimer's disease. *A.* Laminar distribution of changes causing a decrease in thickness of the cortical ribbon. *B.* Columnar distribution of changes causing a decrease in length of the cortical ribbon without thinning. The latter seems to predominate at least in the early stages of Alzheimer's disease.

finding a cell profile on a section is higher when the cell is large. The number of small cells in the structure under study is thus underevaluated, a "stereological bias" that has prompted the development of new methods. The disector[63] necessitates the examination of two, real or optical, contiguous sections. Only those cells that are present in the first and absent from the second section are counted. This type of count is not biased. The disector is useful in obtaining an accurate count,[64] but previous results obtained in the literature are still to be considered since the bias introduced by the standard counting procedure is often small.[65] Therefore, we will not confine our discussion to the results obtained with the dissector method. The new sterological literature has also stressed the need for a "design-based" sampling scheme.[64,66] New emphasis has been placed on sampling the whole structure under study; it is important to evaluate the total number of neurons, rather than the packing density of neuronal profiles in a restricted region. The recommended systematic procedures have provided new data on the total number of neurons in many nuclei or areas of the brain.

Neuronal loss (amounting to 12% of the neuronal profiles) has been documented in the hippocampus during aging.[67,68] This loss involves mainly the hilar region and the subiculum. In AD, the CA1 region is mainly affected, as shown by studies using the disector method.[69,70]

The loss of isocortical neurons with aging has been discussed. Brody[71] found a high correlation between age and the number of neuronal profiles included in five strips of cortex, taken perpendicularly to the pial surface. The greatest changes were found in the superior temporal gyrus and the precentral gyrus, while postcentral gyrus and the area striata (visual cortex) were the least affected.[71] By contrast, Haug et al.[72] and Terry et al.[39] did not find any significant change in the density of neuronal profiles but observed a negative correlation between the size of the perikaryon and age. The ratio of large to small neurons was also found to decrease with age in other studies.[39,73] This atrophy of the cell body of neurons reduces their apparent number on sections (pseudo-loss).[74]

The total number of neurons in the neocortex in relation to aging has been studied more recently with the disector method[75]: the loss of neocortical neurons over the course of 20 to 90 years of age was considered to reach 10%. Such a decrease in neuronal number would cause an "average" loss of about 85,000 neurons per day. It is interesting to note that this figure was reached previously by other means.[76,77] In summary, the density of neuronal profiles in sections does not change much with age but the volume of the brain decreases slightly. The net effect is a relatively mild loss of neurons, in view of the individual variations (which can reach 200%).

In the brain stem, documented neuronal loss during aging appears to be heterogeneous. Some nuclei, such as the ventral cochlear, trochlear, and abducens nuclei or the inferior olive, show no cell loss with age.[78–81] But the number of neurons decreases in the locus ceruleus,[79,82] a finding that has recently been disputed,[83,84] and in the Purkinje cell layer.[85] In the substantia nigra, the neuronal loss involves mainly the medial and dorsal tier of the pars compacta, when the brunt of the pathology is located in the lateral tier in Parkinson's disease.[86–88] Neuronal loss has also been documented in the thalamus,[89] putamen,[90] medial central, medial, and cortical nuclei of the amygdala,[91] and nucleus basalis of Meynert.[92,93]

Numerous researchers have come to the conclusion that a severe neuronal loss occurs in AD and SDAT. In the hippocampus, the decrease in the density of neuronal profiles may reach 57%.[67] As already mentioned, the sensitive areas of the hippocampus are different in aging and in AD: whereas the hilus of the dentate gyrus and the subiculum are involved in "normal" aging, the CA1 is mainly affected in AD.[69,70] The loss has been found to be highly correlated with the number of tangle-bearing cells.[67,94] A marked neuronal loss, assessed by the dissector method, has also been documented in the entorhinal cortex;[95] in advanced cases it reaches 90%.

In the isocortex, the loss of large neurons is predominant[96] and is more severe in younger cases.[97–99] One study only,[100] which made use of the disector method to evaluate the total number of neurons in the cortex, found no global neuronal loss during SDAT. The coefficient of error of the measurement was high.

Several criticisms concerning the method used and the interpretation of the results were put forward in the discussion accompanying that study.[101–104] Using the same methodology but focusing on a specific cortical area, Gomez-Isla et al. found a 50% neuronal loss in the cortex of the superior temporal sulcus,[105] exceeding by many-fold the amount of neurofibrillary tangles accumulated. It was suggested that the formation of neurofibrillary tangles was not the only cause of neuronal death. It could also be that neurofibrillary tangles finally disappeared after the death of the cells that bear them; their number at a given time would then be lower than their total number during the full course of the disease. Grignon et al.[106] studied area 40 with a method devised to analyze local variation in neuronal density.[107] They also concluded that neuronal loss was severe, and linked it to the density of neurofibrillary tangles. An average difference of 98 million neurons per parietal lobe was found between the cases with <5 neurofibrillary tangles/mm² and those with more. Such a high density of neurofibrillary tangles is reached only in cases with severe involvement of that area, an observation that led to the conclusion that the neuronal loss was a late event in the pathogenetic cascade. The neuronal loss occurred predominantly in layers II and III (upper part). The neurons located in these layers are known to be involved in corticocortical connections.[108–110]

Neuronal loss has also been documented in the anterior olfactory nucleus.[111,112] In younger patients, the loss can reach 75% of the total number of neurons while the olfactory bulb is relatively spared. Data concerning neuronal loss in the supraoptic and paraventricular nuclei (secreting vasopressin and oxytocin) are contradictory.[113,114] Neuronal hypertrophy has been shown to occur in these nuclei in aging and AD brains[133,115] and involves principally the vasopressin cells. The suprachiasmatic nucleus, which contributes to the genesis of circadian rhythm, is altered in AD and these lesions (including a neuronal loss) could explain the disturbance of biological rhythms in SDAT.[116] The lateral tuberal nucleus, which is prone to accumulate Alz 50–positive material (see below) without true neurofibrillary tangle, shows no neuronal loss.[117] In summary, lesions in the hypothalamus are heterogeneous and, as will be shown later, include specific neurofibrillary alterations that are of a different nature and/or take a different course han those seen elsewhere in the brain.

All subdivisions of the amygdaloid complex, which is involved in affective behavior, appear to be affected to a varying degree (23% to 52% decrease in the packing density of neuronal profiles). Cell loss is most marked in the nuclei, that are known to be affected by aging (medial, medial central, and cortical).[91] Neuronal loss has been confirmed in another study using the disector method[118] and reached 56%. Several studies have emphasized the importance of the involvement of the nucleus basalis of Meynert in AD.[119–121] The nucleus basalis is part of the basal magnocellular complex, along with the medial septal nucleus and the nucleus of the diagonal band of Broca, which ensures cholinergic innervation of the cortex. Loss of this innervation has been thought to be responsible for a whole gamut of clinical signs, and has been the focus of therapeutic trials. This neuronal loss, however, is variable and may be mild[119] or absent.[122] The involvement of various subnuclei is heterogeneous in the least affected cases.[123,124] Careful stereological assessment showed an average loss of 15.5%, reaching 36% in the most caudal part of the nucleus.[125] The surviving neurons have small Golgi apparatus, compared to controls, a finding that suggests decreased activity.[126] A severe cell loss—50% on average in the cases meeting the diagnostic criteria of AD—has also been found in the noradrenergic locus coeruleus through the disector technique.[127] This loss affects mainly the rostral, cortical-projecting part of the nucleus and spares the caudal, noncortical-projecting cells.[128,129] The spared neurons show signs of increased activity.[130] The serotoninergic raphe nuclei are also affected.[131–133] A total loss of 40% has been found through the disector method.[131] The loss of aminergic neurons has been correlated with depression, which sometimes occurs in the course of AD,[134] a finding that has not been confirmed.[135] The medial subnuclei of the substantia nigra, projecting to the cortex, contain neurofibrillary tangles and are depleted in neurons.[136–138] Severe neuronal loss in the substantia nigra suggests an association with Lewy type pathology[136] (for review, see Mann).[139] In summary, lesions of the brain stem nuclei occur frequently in AD; they concern specific nuclei and subnuclei, most of which appear directly connected with the cerebral cortex.[140] A loss of ganglion cells in the retina has been described in AD,[141] both in the foveal region[142] and on the periphery,[143] but this finding has been debated.[144] This loss could be associated with axonal degeneration of the optic nerves,[145] and suggests that neurons can die in regions known to be devoid of neurofibrillary tangles.

Neuronal loss seen in AD thus appears to involve mainly the regions rich in neurofibrillary pathology: the entorhinal cortex, the hippocampus, and the isocortex. In the brain stem, the affected nuclei (mainly the raphe nuclei and the locus coeruleus) also contain neurofibrillary tangles. The selective vulnerability of the lesioned nuclei in the brain stem could be related to their connections with the cortex. The status of the hypothalamus is peculiar: the neurofibrillary pathology is not always related to neuronal loss and for some nuclei seems to be unrelated to the cortical lesions.[146,147]

Although neuronal loss has been documented in AD, the mechanism that leads to the death of the cell has yet to be determined. Apoptosis appeared, at one time, to be likely candidate, as several degenerative processes are thought to trigger the apoptotic cascade and the amyloid (Aβ) peptide has been found to exhibit some apoptotic effects in culture.[148] A twofold increase in the number of DNA breaks was found in Alzheimer's brains compared to controls.[149] Moreover, methods based on the use of terminal deoxynucleotidyl transferase (TdT) incorporating nucleotides at the free ends of the DNA strand (in situ end labeling) have shown the abundance of DNA breaks in neuronal and glial nuclei.[150–152] However, contradictory results have been obtained,[153] and, moreover, the nuclear lesions associated with apoptosis (fragmentation and condensation of the nucleus) are generally said to be either rare or absent. The expression of proteins associated with activation of the apoptotic cascade, such as the inducible transcription factor C-Jun, has been studied, with disputable results.[154,155] The conclusion has been drawn that the increase in DNA fragmentation was not associated with apoptosis[155] and was the consequence of abnormal sensitivity of the DNA to metabolic disturbances of the *premortem* period. According to another hypothesis, neuronal death in AD could be the consequence of uncontrolled re-entry of postmitotic neurons in the cell cycle.[156]

The pathology of AD involves a number of proteins, among which tau, Aβ, and presenilins are the best characterized. Discussed below are the lesions associated with these proteins.

TAU- AND Aβ-ASSOCIATED LESIONS (SENILE CHANGES)

Lesions seen in the elderly brain and in pathologic conditions such as AD and middle-age Down's syndrome include neurofibrillary tangles (NFTs) neuropil threads, and senile plaque (SPs). They may be divided into two groups: the lesions immunolabeled by the anti-tau antibody and those detected by the anti-Aβ antibody.

Tau-Associated Alterations (Neurofibrillary lesions) Neurofibrillary Tangles, Neuropil Threads, and Senile Plaque Crowns

MORPHOLOGY

Neurofibrillary tangles are torch-like or globose inclusions located in the neuronal soma (Fig. 8–6). Sometimes they are found free in the neuropil, especially in the hippocampus, left behind after neuronal death ("ghost tangles"). The frequency of the ghost tangles varies according to the region. They are common in the entorhinal cortex, hippocampus, and in the *nucleus basalis* of Meynert, and rare in the isocortex and hypothalamus. Neurofibrillary tangles are revealed by silver methods (such as Bodian's, Bielschowsky's, Campbell's Gavey's, Holmes', Gallyas', Palmgren's, or methenamine silver). Thioflavin S and, less regularly, Congo red also label tangle-bearing neurons, a finding suggesting that NFTs are *amyloid*, i.e., contain a high proportion of polypeptide chains with a β-pleated sheet secondary structure.[157] However, X-ray diffraction has not confirmed this suggestion,[158] and the

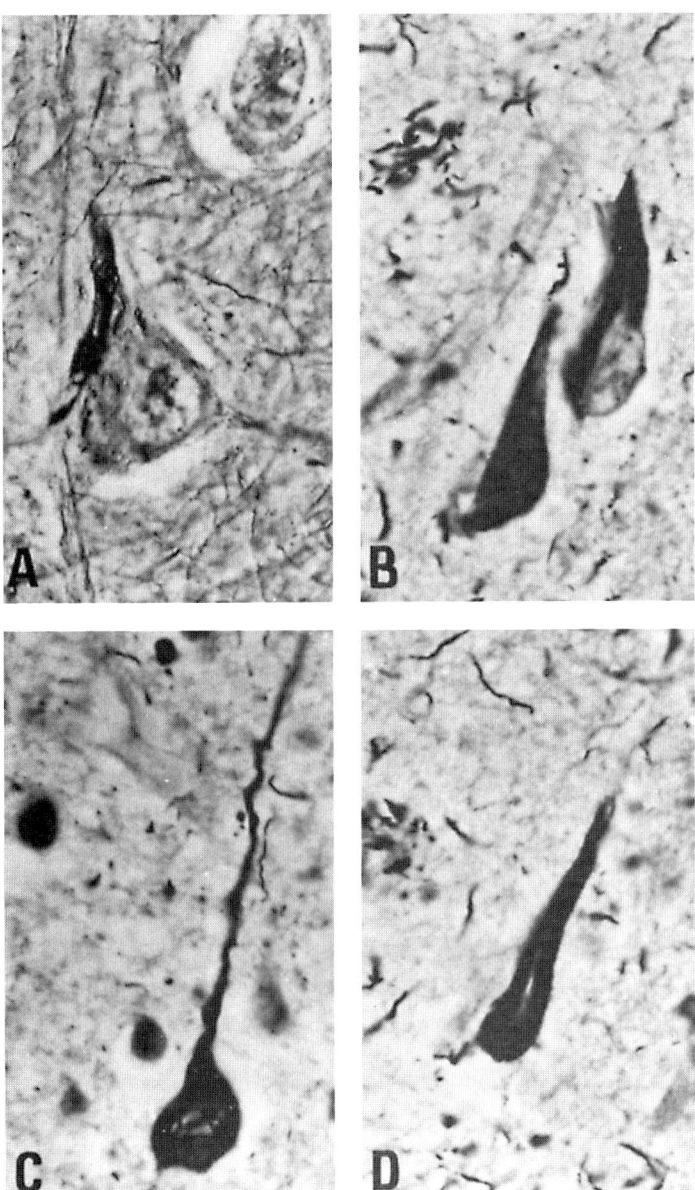

Figure 8–6. Neurofibrillary tangles. A. Palmgren method (Cross modification), showing discrete argyrophilic tangles in a pyramidal neuron. B. Torch-like. C. Plump. D. Extracellular neurofibrillary tangle. B to D: Bodian stain and luxol fast blue, ×100.

possibility that the amyloid tinctorial properties of some neurons are linked to deposition of Aβ peptide has been put forward.[159] At the ultrastructural level,[160] NFTs appear to be made of fibrillar structures with regular constrictions when viewed in longitudinal sections (Fig. 8–7). These are located at 79 nm intervals (range: 50–105 nm) on average.[161] At the constrictions, the fibrils are 10 nm wide. They are 20 to 25 nm wide midway between two constrictions. Various interpretations of this morphology have been given. Kidd[162,163] suggested that they were made up of two filaments 10 nm wide, twisted in a helical structure, or paired helical filaments (PHFs). Using tilt analysis, Wisniewski et al.[164] thought that they were made of four protofilaments 3–5 nm wide. Through image reconstruction Wischik et al.[165] concluded that a set of six spherical subunits (axial dimension 4 nm) overlapped to form a ribbon twisted in a left-handed helix. More recently, the PHFs were also considered

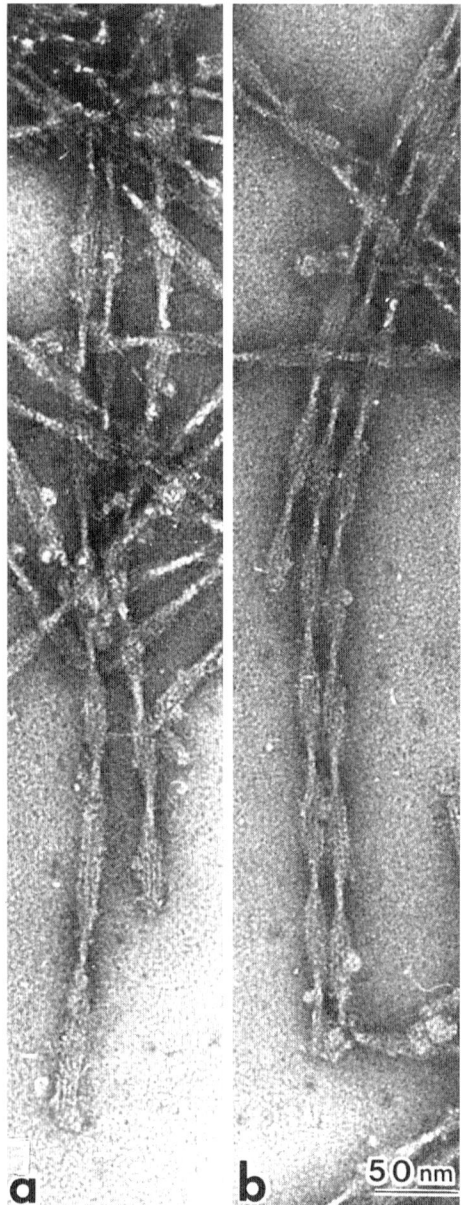

Figure 8–7. Isolated paired helical filament (PHF) negatively stained with phosphotungstic acid (*a*, *b*). These micrographs illustrate four protofilaments of a PHF along its length (× 215,000). [From Wisniewski et al., J. Neuropathol. Exp. Neurol. 1984; 43:643, with permission.]

to be, in fact, twisted ribbons.[166,167] In addition to PHFs, straight tubules of 15 nm in diameter have been identified, either constituting the entire tangle or coexisting with the PHF. Structures combining straight and helical segments have been observed.[168] The density of neurotubules is decreased in the tangle-bearing neurons,[169,170] as is the immunoreactivity to acetylated α-tubulin.[171] The sequestration of tau in NFTs (see Tau Proteins below) seems thus accompanied by changes in neurotubules to which they are functionally linked.

The neuropil threads[172] are short and tortuous[173] neurites loaded with PHF, particularly well shown by Gallyas method, which stains them electively. Most of them are probably dendrites, but up to 10% have been identified as myelinated axons on electron microscopy.[174,175]

The crown of the senile plaque contains processes that have many characteristics in common with the neuropil threads, principally the presence of PHFs. Other specificities (such as the presence of amyloid precursor protein) of senile plaque crown are discussed in the section Senile Plaques, below.

TAU PROTEINS

The nature of the PHF has been difficult to unravel. Their insolubility in most solvents was initially used to isolate them[176] but rendered protein sequencing difficult. Antibodies to neurofilament constituents have been repeatedly shown to label NFTs.[177,178] Some antibodies have been raised against enriched fractions of NFTs or against homogenates of brain tissue from patients with AD.[179–181] The density of tangles identified by the anti-NFT antibody is similar to that shown by silver impregnation.[182] These antibodies generally exhibit a high anti-tau activity.[183] Antibodies directed against the tau proteins regularly and strongly label the neurofibrillary tangles and the crown of the plaques[184] as well as the neuropil threads.[185] Further analysis has shown that tau is indeed the main constituent of the PHFs seen in those three lesions[186,187] (see review[188]). The gene of the tau proteins is located on the long arm of chromosome 17 (band 17q21). It is approximately 100 kb long and comprises 16 exons, 3 of which are not expressed in the human brain. The gene also includes three or four tandem repeats coding for a sequence of 31 amino acids (one of the tandem repeats is coded by exon 10). The repeat regions of tau belong to the microtubule-binding domain. Tau isoforms may contain exons 2 and 3, only exon 2, or neither exon 2 nor 3, each one of these three isoforms having four tandem repeats (with exon 10) or only three (without exon 10).[189–191] This makes a total of six isoforms. More than 30 phosphorylation sites have been identified on the tau protein, some of which appear specific to AD (for instance, serine 422). Antibodies directed against some of those phosphorylated sites are available (see review[189]). When a brain homogenate is analyzed immediately after sampling, tau is found to be heavily phosphorylated even in normal tissues.[192,193] When the analysis is performed after a delay (for example, a postmortem delay of several hours), persistant phosphatase activity dephosphorylates normal tau but is inefficient on tau sequestrated in NFTs. This explains why NFT tau appears hyperphosphorylated compared to normal tau,[194] with only a few phosphorylation sites (including serine 422) being truly specific to NFT.[195] The NFT found in AD contain all six tau isoforms in a state of hyperphosphorylation. Because of similarities in the molecular weight of some hyperphosporylated isoforms, only four bands are visible (three major ones at 55, 64, and 69 and one minor one at 74 kDa) on Western blot analysis of AD tissue, whereas six are present in normal tissue.[189] The location of the four bands differs slightly, depending on the study (60, 64, 68, and 72 kDa for Spillantini et al.[191]).

Abnormally phosphorylated tau may be found in the cell body and its processes (axons and dendrites).[196] The secondary detachment of dendrites filled by abnormally phosphorylated tau has been observed in the CA1 sector.[197] However, the continuity between the cell body and the axons innervating the senile plaque has never been fully demonstrated, although the continuity between neuropil threads and both tangle-free and tangle-bearing neurons has been documented.[198] The proportion of volume occupied by the tau neurofibrillary alterations in an AD brain is high, sometimes higher than the proportion of volume occupied by the Aβ peptide—up to 37% in some cases.[199]

OTHER CONSTITUENTS OF NEUROFIBRILLARY LESIONS

Some NFT and some of the neurites of the senile plaque are ubiquitinated.[200] Ubiquitination occurs secondarily to tau accumulation.[201] In a series of 27 cases, at the most 33% of the NFTs in the CA1 sector of the hippocampus were ubiquitinated and 53% in Brodmann area 22.[202] The neuropil threads are probably less ubiquitinated, but quantitative data to support this are lacking. Ghost tangles contain epitopes of the amyloid P component and some complement factors (C4d) that may trigger an inflammatory response.[203] Immunoreactivity to middle and high-molecular-weight neurofilament subunits has also been found in NFTs.[204,205] Cholinesterase activity within NFTs has been mentioned.[206] Covalent modifications are also present including ubiquitination, glycosilation, and glycation (see review[207]).

DISTRIBUTION OF NEUROFIBRILLARY TANGLES

Neurofibrillary tangles in the brain are probably long-lived as neuronal loss in the hippocampus was found to be grossly proportional to the density of ghost tangles.[94] Ghost tangles are present in the entorhinal cortex (the first area to be involved), even in the last stage of severe AD. From these observations, researchers have suggested that NFTs are not phagocyted, or only slowly, and remain in the brain even after the death of the neurons that bear them, probably for decades.[24,208] Because NFT accumulate over time, we are better able to understand their spread in the brain and can use this accumulation to assess the course of the disease and its severity.

The topography of NFTs is not random; they are present only in certain types of neurons and in selective areas. The neurons most frequently involved are medium-sized pyramidal neurons (layers III and V of the isocortex), which express an epitope of a nonphosphorylated neurofilament.[209] Granule cells (layer 4 of the isocortex; fascia dentata) are usually spared, as are the large Betz cells.[210] The cortical areas may be ranked hierarchically such that involvement of a given area is observed only if the areas of a lower rank are also involved.[26] Hippocampal NFTs are never seen in the absence of entorhinal involvement and isocortical neurofibrillary tangles are never seen in the absence of hippocampal involvement. This observation strongly suggests a progression of lesions from the entorhinal cortex to the hippocampus and from the hippocampus to the isocortex. This progression is helpful in evaluating the severity of disease (Braak and Braak staging).[211] The Braak and Braak staging[211] comprises six stages according to the topography of the affected areas: in stages I and II, the entorhinal cortex is involved, in stages III and IV, the hippocampus, and in staged V and VI, the isocortex. Large discrepancies from this hierarchical scheme appear to be rare.[213] The pathology in the hippocampus progresses in the following order: subiculum, H1 field, endplate, presubiculum, H2 field.[214] The topography of abnormal tau accumulation in the isocortex has also been studied by means of immunoblots on small samples from selected areas,[215] and through this technique, new insights into the progression of tau pathology have been gained. The isocortical phase of the disease was further analyzed, resulting in the following stages: S1 involves the transentorhinal cortex; S2, the entorhinal cortex; S3 the hippocampus; S4, the anterior temporal cortex; S5, the inferior temporal cortex; S6, the middle temporal cortex; S7, the polymodal association areas (prefrontal, parietal inferior, temporal superior); S8, the unimodal areas; S9, the primary areas; either motor (S9a) or sensory (S9b, S9c); and S10, all neocortical areas.[215] The parallel between the architectonic maps and the topography of the lesions is striking[216] ("Alzheimer's disease knows neuroanatomy"). Focal onset of AD (particularly progressive aphasia) is documented.[52] These cases are intriguing because they could present important exceptions to the hierarchical scheme. To the best of our knowledge, however, no case of AD with isocortical neurofibrillary tangles but without hippocampal involvement has ever been documented.

In the subcortical areas, the selectivity of neurofibrillary pathology is also striking. The NFTs are abundant in the limbic nuclei of the thalamus.[217] They are found in the magnocellular basal complex (medial septal nuclei, nucleus of the diagonal band of Broca, and nucleus basalis of Meynert). In the amygdala, the corticomedial nuclei are more severely involved than the laterobasal nuclei. The lesions predominate in the ventromedial region of those nuclei,[218–220] an area that receives the projection issued from the hippocampal formation.[218,219] In the brain stem the locus coeruleus, the raphe nuclei, and the medial part of the substantia nigra, all of them projecting directly to the cortex, are selectively involved.[140]

At least three hypotheses have been proposed to explain the selective distribution of NFTs:

1. The sensitivity hypothesis: Some areas are more prone to respond to the (still unknown) noxious agent. Various explanations have been proposed to explain those differences in sensitivity (e.g., differences in myelination,[221] in capacity of remodeling,[222] or in neurofilament characteristics[223]).

2. The inactivity hypothesis: Some neurons, when inactive, develop NFTs.[224]

3. The connectivity hypothesis: The neurofibrillary pathology propagates through connections[109,110,225,226] "invading" first the limbic, then the associative, and finally the primary sensory areas. A set of data supports this hypothesis: within involved cortical areas or nuclei, certain layers[227] or subnuclei[140,218] are selectively lesioned—generally those that are connected with already affected regions. In exceptional occasions, additional lesions might disturb the usual progression of the neurofibrillary pathology. In a disconnected piece of cortex, no neurofibrillary alteration could be seen, although numerous Aβ peptide deposits were present.[228]

PREVALENCE AND SIGNIFICANCE OF NEUROFIBRILLARY TANGLES

The cognitive deficits seen in AD are better correlated with the density of NFTs than with any other pathological alterations,[26,229–234] with the possible exception of synaptophysin immunoreactivity in midfrontal and inferior parietal gyri.[235] The spread of NFTs is significant, the number of affected regions being highly correlated with cognitive deficits.[26] When only a few areas (e.g., transentorhinal and entorhinal areas) are involved, patients are not demented, mildly impaired, or even normal upon formal testing.[27,229,236–239] Are these patients suffering from preclinical AD or are these alterations the mere consequence of aging? The question remains unresolved. It has been clearly established that the prevalence of NFTs is highly correlated with age. Braak and Braak[24] staged a series of 2661 unselected brains. The results of their investigation were plotted on actuarial curves,[240] which showed that half the population at the age of 47 had at least one NFT in the entorhinal region. It should be noted, however, that the involvement of the hippocampus is rarer and occurs at a later age: the age at which half the population could be categorized as stage III or higher (i.e., at least hippocampal involvement) in the study of Braak and Braak[24] was 86.[240] The prevalence of NFTs reached 100% in several studies involving elderly people.[236] NFTs were also constant in a nonselected series of institutionalized centenarians,[241] although the percentage of brains with a high density of NFTs has been reported to decrease from the ninth to the tenth decade in a few series (see review[41]). Three out of nine brains of nondemented individuals of the eleventh decade, whom we have studied,[241] had very few NFTs among the 11 samples examined. The NFT were constant in the hippocampus and the temporal cortex (parahippocampal gyrus and adjacent isocortex), less frequent in the cingulate cortex (4/9) and the prefrontal cortex (1/9), and were absent in the occipital cortex. They were seen in the *nucleus basalis* of Meynert in eight cases, in the septal nuclei in three, in the other basal ganglia in four and in the brain stem.[241] The density of tangles seen in demented cases could be distinguished from that seen in centenarians who were considered normal or mildly impaired intellectually. A similar conclusion was reached in another study analyzing the neuropathology of centenarians[242]: a clear-cut difference could be seen between the density of NFTs seen in normal aged people and that in Alzheimer cases. However, these observations also indicate that NFTs, particularly in the entorhinal area, are a constant accompaniment of old age. The NFT seen in normal old people cannot be morphologically distinguished from those seen in AD or in SDAT; they are qualitatively the same and occupy areas that are also involved in AD and SDAT.

Cases have been described with a predominant tangle pathology, in which no or but little Aβ deposits are present.[243-246] The patients are generally old and the Apo-E4 genotype (risk factor for AD) is generally underrepresented in this pathological group.[247] The neurofibrillary pathology in these cases is often limited to the limbic system. By contrast, isocortical NFT are seen only in patients with abundant amyloid. Comparisons of the prevalence curves for amyloid and neurofibrillary pathology indicate that the isocortical Aβ deposits occur between the transentorhinal and hippocampal neurofibrillary stages. These observations are compatible with a "two-variables" model: one is normal aging, to which entorhinal NFTs are linked; the other is the increase in Aβ synthesis, noxious only in the presence of NFTs and which would allow their diffusion to numerous brain areas. This would explain why AD develops relatively late in life, even in genetically determined cases.[240]

NEUROFIBRILLARY TANGLES IN CONDITIONS OTHER THAN ALZHEIMER'S DISEASE

Neurofibrillary tangles that are morphologically similar (on electron microscopy and immunocytochemistry) to those seen in AD have been reported in neurons of the upper cervical ganglia, i.e., in the peripheral nervous system,[248] but they are uncommon and probably unrelated to AD.[249] Although structures bearing some similarities to that of the PHF have been described in various animal species,[250] none were similar at the ultrastructural level.

Intracellular tau accumulation in NFTs or in other inclusions such as Pick bodies and glial fibrillary tangles are observed in various conditions. On Western blots of brain homogenates from Pick disease cases, tau appeared in two major bands (55 and 64 kDa), with a minor band at 69 kDa. Specific antibodies have shown that in that condition, tau lacks exon 10.[251] By contrast, in progressive supranuclear palsy (PSP) and corticobasal degeneration, tau is exclusively made of isoforms that include exon 10.[252] On Western blots, two major bands are seen at 64 and 69 kDa, with a minor band at 74 kDa The NFTs seen in PSP (and probably in postencephalitic Parkinson disease) are mainly composed of straight 15 nm tubule-like structures. The NFTs that are seen in Down syndrome, Parkinsonism–dementia complex of Guam, Niemann-Pick disease type C, and Gerstmann-Sträussler-Scheinker disease cannot be distinguished on Western blot from those seen in AD and aging brain. Recently, several mutations in the tau gene have been identified in familial cases of dementia and parkinsonism of various types. In these cases, grouped under the common heading 'frontotemporal dementia and parkinsonism linked to chromosome 17' (FTDP 17),[253,254] the accumulation of tau may occur not only in neurons but also in glial cells. The tangles are of different types—sometimes they are similar to the Alzheimer's-type tau (as, for example, in Seattle family 1), sometimes to the PSP type (exclusively with exon 10), as in Dutch family 1.[191]

Neurofibrillary tangles have also been found in subacute sclerosing panencephalitis, adult lipofuscinosis, sudanophilic leukodystrophy, tuberous sclerosis, juvenile dystonic lipidosis, advanced hydrocephalus, and lead encephalopathy.[234,255–258] The NFTs seen in experimental aluminum intoxication also contain tau protein[259] and are made of bundles of intermediate filaments 10 nm wide.

The specificity of tau accumulation seen in many different conditions, has been questioned, and the importance of senile plaques in the diagnosis of AD has been emphasized.[260] The variety of tau pathology, recently evidenced by the findings of tau mutations, has not yet been fully explained. The differences in the migration of tau on Western blots, which is related to the differential expression of various exons, could be related to the neurons in which the accumulation takes place. Different isoforms of tau are indeed expressed in different cell populations.[251]

Aβ-Associated Alterations: Senile Plaques and Other Deposits of Amyloid β, Including Amyloid Angiopathy

SENILE PLAQUES

The most characteristic senile plaques (SPs) are made up of two distinct components: a crown of argyrophilic fibers, some of which contain abnormal tau proteins similar to those found in NFTs and neuropil threads (see Tau proteins supra), and an extracellular amyloid core, the main constituent of which is the amyloid-β protein, or Aβ peptide (Fig. 8–7). Such plaques have been called "neuritic" by Wisniewski and Terry,[261] or "classical" or "mature" (synonyms include "amyloid" and "argyrophilic plaques"[34]). A large variety of lesions, however, have been classified under the term "senile plaques"[33,34,207,262] making this term quite imprecise. Some of these lesions lack the amyloid core, others, which are not associated with tau abnormalities, are principally recognized in sections stained by Aβ immunohistochemistry (some also being demonstrated by certain silver impregnations such as Bielschowsky's or Campbell-Switzer). When seen only with Aβ immunohistochemisty (and not with the amyloid-specific stains such as Congo red), the deposits are preamyloid.[263] According to their shape, they have been called "diffuse deposits" of Aβ peptide (sometimes called *diffuse plaques*) and "focal" (or "dense" or "cored") "deposits." In contrast to diffuse deposits, some focal deposits are stained by the dyes characteristic of amyloid. Lastly, the use of ubiquitin and amyloid precursor protein (APP) immunohistochemistry allows the identification of dystrophic neurites, some of which do not contain abnormal tau, in various types of SPs. Following is a discussion of the neuritic plaques, then of the other varieties.

Neuritic Senile Plaques (Neuritic Plaques)

Because of the composite nature of these plaques, they are stained by a great number of methods (Fig. 8–8). The amyloid core is seen better after hematoxylin-eosin (H&E) staining or with the periodic acid-schiff (PAS) method than with cresyl violet, but all these techniques fail to reveal a great number of neuritic SPs and cannot be used alone to establish a diagnosis of AD. Alcyan blue and Masson's trichromic method readily stain the core of the SP. Thioflavin S, which is used to reveal amyloid substances when other stains such as Congo red fail to do so, also shows many more SPs. Silver impregnations show either principally the neuritic component (Bodian's technique) or both the neuritic and amyloid lesions (methenamine silver, von Braunmühl's and Bielschowsky's techniques). The most sensitive techniques by far, however, are Bielschowsky's method and Aβ immunohistochemistry[264] (Fig. 8–9), although the high sensitivity of the nickel peroxidase method has also been reported.[265] Neuritic SPs appear as spherical lesions, including an extracellular core of amyloid substance. Evaluation of their mean diameter has produced

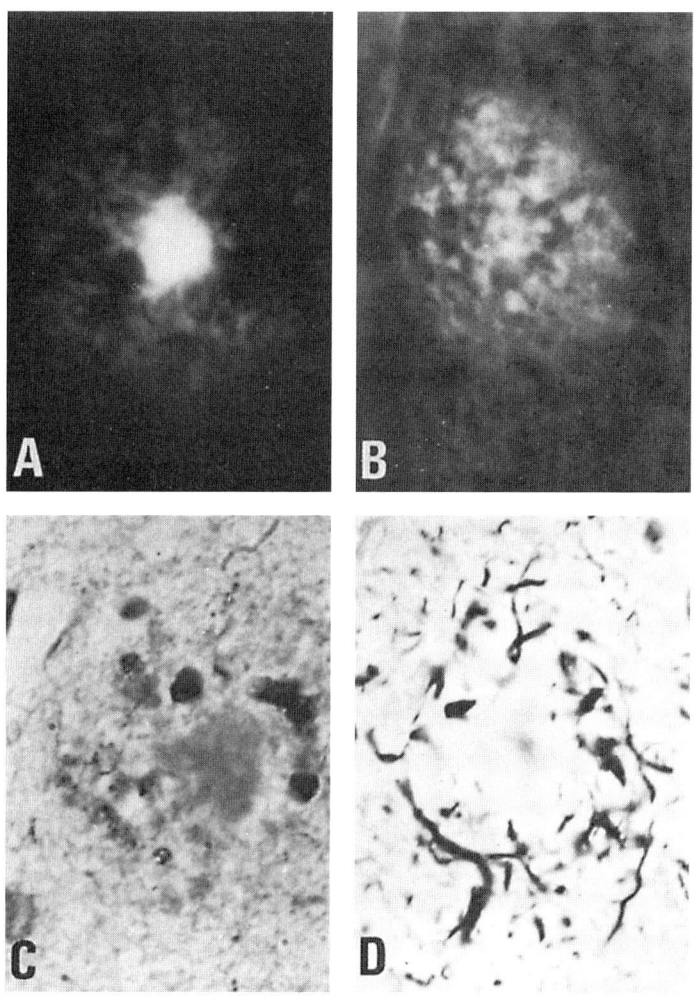

Figure 8–8. Senile plaques. *A.* Dense core of amyloid (thioflavin S). *B.* Amyloid wisp without dense core (thioflavin S). *C.* Anti-paired helical filament labeled processes surrounding a core of amyloid substances. *D.* Neurites impregnated by silver. Bodian stain and luxol fast blue, ×100.

various results 36–50 μm,[266] 42–49 μm,[267] up to 200 μm[19], depending on the technique used. Congo red and some silver impregnations such as Bodian's technique show smaller plaques than thioflavin stain, silver impregnations such as Gallyas' and Bielschowsky's and Aβ immunohistochemistry. The abnormal fibers surrounding SPs are stained by the various silver techniques that label NFTs.

The Processes

The crown of the SP can be labelled immunohistochemiscally with anti-NFT, anti-tau, and anti-ubiquitin. Most neurites are axonal processes,[268] identified by the presence of presynaptic vesicles, but some are dendritic,[261] as confirmed through Golgi stain.[269] Two classes of neuritic components can be recognized.[207] Dystrophic neurites, which are immunoreactive for amyloid precursor protein (APP) and ubiquitin, contain electron-dense lamellar and membranous cytoplasmic bodies, some of which show lysosomal enzyme activity. These neurites may differ in chromogranin and neurofilament content in the early and late stages of AD.[270] The PHF-type neurites are immunoreactive for PHF and tau and sometimes for ubiquitin. They are massively enlarged and contain PHFs identical to those found in NFTs, granular degenerating mitochondria, and many lysosomes.[19] Two classes of ubiquitin-labeled SPs can be identified: in the first variety, the processes are globular and weakly stained and are seen mainly in the aging process. In the second variety, the processes are

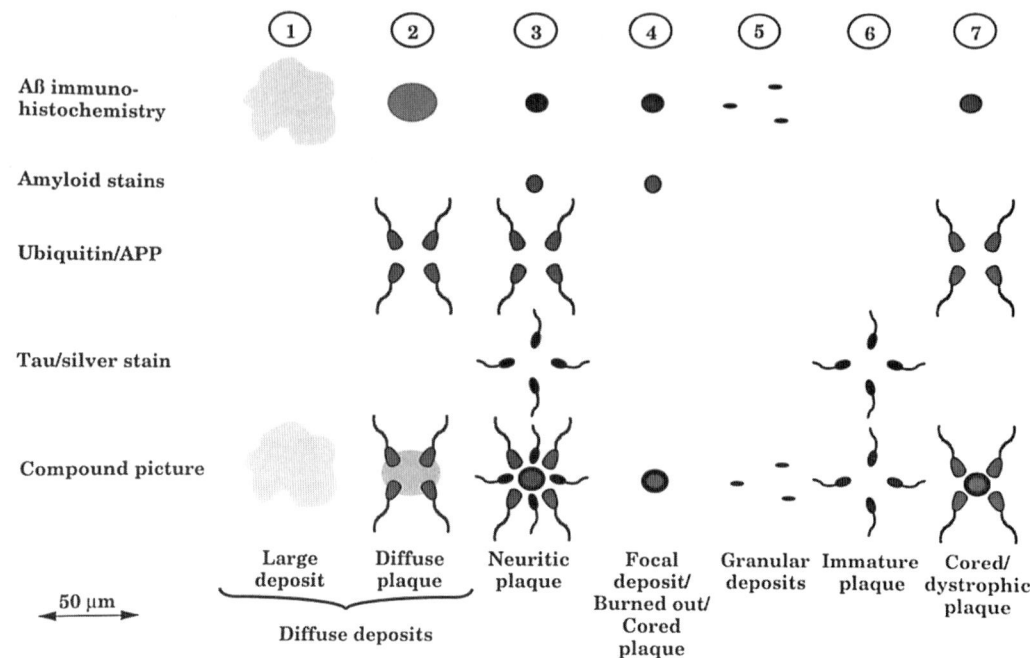

Figure 8–9. Schematic drawing of main lesions called senile plaques.

curly shaped and strongly immunostained, and are linked to cognitive impairment.[271]

Through histochemical analysis acetyl cholinesterase activity has been found in some of the fibers of the crown of the SP[272] and provides evidence for the presence of cholinergic fibers issuing from the *nucleus basalis* of Meynert. This innervation was used to support the cholinergic hypothesis which states that the main disturbances are located in the *nucleus basalis* of Meynert and in the cholinergic fibers arising from this nucleus.[120,273] Numerous other neurotransmitters have also been demonstrated in the SP: neuropeptide Y, substance P, neurotensin, cholecystokinin, catecholamine, and somatostatin.[274] The neuromediator content depends on the location of the SP; an antibody against tyrosine hydroxylase labeled most of the SPs seen in the amygdala (which is richly innervated by cholinergic fibers) but almost none of the SP located in the nearby isocortex (which, by contrast, is poorly innervated in normal cases).[275]

Enlarged processes from astrocytes[276–278] and microglial cells[261,279] also take part in the formation of the crown of the SP. Activated microglia occasionally contain intracytoplasmic non–membrane bound bundles of amyloid fibers, which could be either phagocytosed or secreted.[280] The microglial cell could thus play an important role in the processing of amyloid.[281] It could also be one of the agents that initiates the chronic inflammatory process seen in AD.[279,282]

The Core: the Aβ peptide

The core of the SP, as shown through electron microscopy, comprises abundant amyloid fibrils (7–10nm) intermingled with nonfibrillar deposits. Through confocal microscopy a porous, sponge-like pattern can be seen in essentially all plaques,[34] whereas the abnormal neurites appear to be more centrally located than previously thought.[285] The core of the senile plaque contains a hydrophobic peptide that has been sequenced,[286] called "Aβ" (amyloid β peptide, on account of the β-pleated structure that it can adopt), "βA4" (because its molecular mass is close to 4 kDa) or "β-amyloid." The Aβ peptide is secreted in normal cells in culture and is normally found in the cerebrospinal fluid (CSF) and plasma in humans and other mammals.[287–289] Although the Aβ peptide is also called the "amyloid peptide," Aβ deposits are not always amyloid in the strict sense: the term "amyloid" indeed designates deposits that are Congo red and thioflavin positive, with a filamentous aspect on electron microscopy, regardless of the protein or peptide that formed a precipitate. These characteristics are thought to be related to the presence of polypeptide chains rich in β-pleated sheet secondary structure. In AD, Aβ is the peptide that forms a precipitate. The amyloid core of SP can be seen by means of Aβ immunohistochemistry and amyloid stains. Aβ is the product of proteolysis of a large precursor, the amyloid β–protein precursor (APP), which comprises a group of polypeptides whose heterogeneity arises from both alternative splicing and post-translational processing.[290] Non-neuronal cells express 751–770 forms that contain a 56 amino acid motive homologous to the Kunitz type of serine protease inhibitor. Neurons express a 695-residue isoform that does not contain this motive. The functions of these different peptides are not known. In mice, APP deletion results in late and mild consequences. In vitro, APP has been shown to promote inhibition of some serine proteases, enhancement of cell–substrate adhesion neurite outgrowth, and neuroprotection.[283] Amyloid precursor protein enters at least two metabolic pathways: in the secretory pathway, an enzyme, the α-secretase, cleaves APP within the protein motive that corresponds to the Aβ peptide. The α-secretase activity thus precludes Aβ formation. Although the protein that is responsible for the α-secretase activity has not been identified, it has been shown that the metalloprotease desintegrins that are able to cast off the ectodomains of proteins such as tumor-necrosis factor alpha (TNF-α) can modulate the regulated cleavage of APP.[291,292] In most cell types, only a few APP molecules are involved in the α-secretory pathway.[283] At least another metabolic pathway, called the "endosomal pathway," produces intact fragments of APP long enough to contain the full-length Aβ sequence. β and γ-secretases cleave APP into a soluble form of Aβ (see review[283,293,295]). β-secretase has been recently cloned; it is a transmembrane aspartic protease termed "β-site APP cleaving enzyme" (BACE) which is predominantly localized in Golgi apparatus and endosomes.[296a] It has been recently suggested that presenilin itself was involved in the gamma-secretase activity.[296b,296c] A few families with missense mutations of the APP gene, located on the chromosome 21, have been recognized. The position of the AD-causing mutations frame the β-amyloid sequence at exactly the position that one would expect to influence processing.[297] In transgenic mice, the overexpression of a mutated human gene leads to amyloid deposits[298] with[299] or without[300] neuronal loss, but the full pathology of human AD has not been observed. The exact link between these mutations and Aβ pathology, and the reasons for the primary pathology being borne by brain tissue and brain vessels in most cases (hereditary AD) and by brain vessels in others (hereditary amyloid angiopathy) are not clear, however. A mutation may lead to inappropriate degradation of APP, perhaps by abnormal conformation, and thus to accumulation of an insoluble amyloid form of Aβ. In another hypothesis, several alternative pathways may be available for APP processing, and the mutation shifts the protein into an amyloidogenic pathway. These mutations are rare. Most families with AD are linked to other genes, located on other chromosomes (see presenilin section). In the absence of mutation, overexpression or up-regulation of the APP gene could overload the normal proteolysis process of APP. One possible candidate for this scenario is trisomy 21, which is associated with a 50% increase in gene dosage. A second possibility may occur in a number of tissue injuries such as trauma, ischemia, or any excitotoxic injury, all of which induce overexpression of cytokines that up-regulate the APP gene.

Two main varieties of Aβ have been recognized: the 40 amino acid form (Aβ 40, or Aβ 1–40) and the 42–43 amino acid form (Aβ 42, or Aβ 1–42/43);[283] Aβ 40 is normally produced in higher quantities (90%) than Aβ 42. Other varieties (such as Aβ 1–38, Aβ 1–36, and Aβ 2–40) have also been described.[301] The two main forms of Aβ, which are distinguished by the heterogeneity of their carboxyl terminus, are each recognizable by monoclonal antibodies.[302,303] Aβ 40, the major form of soluble Aβ and of the secreted pool, is found in the largest quantities in the cerebral fluid. Aβ 42, which can polymerize into amyloid fibers at a fast rate in vitro, is the major form of the non-secreted, intracellular pool, and appears to be the major component in brain tissue. Since this form shows a greater propensity to self-aggregate, it has been suggested that its deposition acts as a nidus for the formation of amyloid fibrils. N terminus of Aβ also exibits several different modifications, including ragged N termini, pyroglutamatation, racemization, and isomerization. AβN3 (pyroGlu)-42 and Aβ x42 (where x is a residue at position 2 or less in Aβ) are the predominant forms, deposited in parenchymal amyloid[283,305–307] Aβ varieties distinguished by heterogeneity of their carboxyl terminus may be generated early in the secretory processing, with Aβ 42 being the most abundant variety in the endoplasmic reticulum and Aβ 40 in the Golgi apparatus.[308] The posttranslational mechanism through which the apparently normal, soluble Aβ is changed into pathologic fibrillar amyloid (comprising β-pleated sheets) in the neuritic plaque remains to be elucidated. As already mentioned, the carboxyl-terminal heterogeneity of Aβ may be important for its aggregation. Aβ 42, which is normally produced in lower quantities than Aβ 40, can accumulate as diffuse deposits in some areas (for example, the cerebellum or the striatum) without changing further to amyloid deposits (fibrils in a β-pleated conformation). The deposits, when amyloid, contain the Aβ 40 epitope in addition to the Aβ 42 variety. The emergence of the Aβ 40 epitope seems thus to correspond with the transition from preamyloid to amyloid deposit. A role for the fragments of Aβ, truncated at the N terminus has also be suggested (see review[309–311]).

In vitro, Aβ exists as a monomer at physiological concentrations, and deposition of monomers, rather than of oligomeric Aβ assemblies, mediates the growth of existing amyloid in human brain preparations.[312] A disturbance of the chaperone protein system, i.e., those proteins that regulate the spatial conformation of other proteins (Apo E, α1-antichymotrypsin, glycosaminoglycans), has been suggested to handle amyloid deposition.[313] This might explain the increased risk of AD in Apo E-ε4 subjects. We examined a patient whose disease, however, did not support the chaperone hypothesis: an 87-year-old patient with an exceptionally large number of Aβ deposits without amyloid characteristics had an ε3/ε4 genotype.[314] The presence of the Apo E-ε4 allele had not promoted the conversion of soluble Aβ into amyloid deposits.

Other Constituents of Senile Plaques

Apo E is present in Aβ diffuse deposits, in the core of neuritic plaques, and in microglial cells.[315–318] Apo E may accumulate as punctuate deposits in the early stage of Aβ deposition or even before this.[319] Non-Aβ component (NAC) of amyloid was identified biochemically from brain tissue of AD patients. It is at least 35 amino acids long, although its amino terminus is not completely determined. It is derived from a 140 amino acid long precursor, a presynaptic protein called "NACP" or "α-synuclein." α-synuclein is also found in the Lewy bodies of Parkinson's disease and in some inclusions of multiple system atrophy. The aggregates of NAC, which have amyloid properties, are found in the core of plaques. Its role remains unknown.[320,321] A new antigen, AMY 117, has been found in plaques that were said to be Aβ negative.[322] A recent report, however, found this epitope to be co-localized with the Aβ peptide, mainly in the cored plaques.[323] α1-antichymotrypsin, a serine protease inhibitor synthesized in the liver, consistently co-localizes with amyloid deposits[324–326] and is associated with activated astrocytes.[327] Components of the extracellular matrix, such as heparan sulfate proteoglycan, thrombospondin, and ICAM-1, are also present in senile plaques.[328–332] They may act as chaperone proteins, and are involved in a chronic inflammatory process that may be related to the pro-inflammatory properties of Aβ.[333,334]

Inflammation

Although conventional histological techniques do not show in AD the lesions classically related to inflammation (fibrinoid necrosis, mononuclear cell infiltrates), immunohistochemical and immunochemical studies show that a weak inflammatory process is acting in the AD brain, and that it is principally located in the areas affected by neuropathological markers (senile plaques and neurofibrillary tangles) and neuronal death. Acute-phase response agents are indeed present in the plaque, some of them coming from the blood, others possibly produced in the brain. Serum and tissue proteins involved in the inflammatory process, such as the early and terminal components of the complement cascade (the latter also called the "membrane attack complex"), various types of interleukins and other cytokines,[335,336] chemokines, pentraxins and fibrinogen, serum amyloid P and some protease inhibitors are also found in senile plaques. The presence of these serum and tissue proteins indicates a chronic inflammatory process that shares some features with a chronic granulomatous-type lesion.[336–346] Evidence for operation of oxydative stress has been found.[347–350]

OTHER VARIANTS OF SENILE PLAQUES

Various names have been used for this class of lesions, and the terminology is often confusing (Fig. 8–9). The variable aspect of the plaque is due mainly to differences in the staining techniques used to reveal them. Some plaques are made only of a focal (compact) deposit of amyloid, without dystrophic nor PHF-type neurites. They are markedly stained by Aβ immunohistochemical methods, especially with anti-Aβ 40 antibodies. These non-neuritic plaques have been called "burned out"[351] or "cored"[207] plaques. We do not know whether they always occur at the last stages of plaque course. Plaques with compact amyloid and dystrophic neurites (ubiquitin or APP positive), lacking PHF-type neurites (tau positive), are seen in the aged brain.[207] Some lesions are only made of argyrophilic processes, which have been shown to be PHF-type neurites. The absence of amyloid core may be due to the plane of sectioning missing the amyloid core of a neuritic plaque, but the possibility that recognizable amyloid has not formed has also been proposed.[33] These neurite-only plaques have been called "immature" by von Braunmühl[352] and Wisniewski and Terry,[261] but this term is also used by some authors[353] for some nonamyloid Aβ deposits. A number of *nonamyloid deposits* of Aβ can be recognized, primarily by immunohistochemical means. Mainly made of Aβ 42 peptide, they are devoid of PHF-type neurites, but a few dystrophic neurites can be seen,[354] especially in the cerebellar molecular layer and in the striatum.[207]

Four categories of Aβ deposits can be schematically identified.[34,207,355–357] *Diffuse deposits* are weakly immunoreactive, faintly demarcated, and may be large (large diffuse deposits can reach many hundreds of micrometers in size).[33] When rounded and of intermediate size (20–40 mm) they are *"diffuse plaques,"* (sometimes called "primitive" or "immature"[33]), which are characterized by increased numbers of non-enlarged neurites. Although they are devoid of amyloid deposit when viewed with light microscopy, a few amyloid fibrils can be seen on electron microscopy. *Focal* (or dense) *deposits* are distinct, rounded, sharply limited lesions markedly stained using Aβ immunohistochemistry. They can be of amorphous or reticular appearance and they sometimes have radiating fibrils. Their size is usually similar to that of the cores of neuritic plaques (20–30 μ), to which they probably correspond in a great number of cases, a possibility that cannot be ascertained if only Aβ immunohistochemical staining has been used. The very immunoreactive *granular deposits* are a few micrometers in size. In addition, *fleecy deposits* are unusually large, ill-defined clouds of Aβ deposition that has been shown to occur in the internal entorhinal layers and are made of N-terminal truncated fragments of Aβ.[358] *Lake-like deposits* are similar lesions found in the presubicular area. They do not have the tinctorial characteristics of amyloid and are mainly made of Aβ 42, possibly of neuronal origin.[359]

DISTRIBUTION OF SENILE PLAQUES

The natural history of Aβ deposition in the brain is not known. Nonamyloid diffuse and focal deposits correspond to accumulation of primarily extracellular Aβ. They may be inaugural and they could lead in some instances to focal amyloid deposits and mature senile plaques. Granular deposits, by contrast, may be astrocytic in location and could be related to the resoption of other deposits.[357]

Aβ deposits are seen in the cerebral cortex, basal ganglia, and cerebellum.[360] Distribution of the SP is diffuse over the cortex, where they have a laminar distribution; they are more frequent in layers II and III,[227,361–363] the neuritic plaques tending to occur in the deep layers, and non-neuritic ones in the superficial layers.[34] In the isocortex, they are located between dendritic clusters, with pyramidal cell apical dendritic shafts excluded from the plaques.[364] They are seen in regions usually devoid of NFTs, such as the occipital lobe, the association cortices being more heavily involved than primary areas. Medial temporal lobe structures are generally less affected than is the isocortex. They are numerous, however, in the hippocampal formation and in the amygdala[91,220] and olfactory bulb.[111] They are also seen in the hypothalamus in the basal ganglia,[274] especially in the striatum and the reticular nucleus of the thalamus,[365] and in the *substantia innominata*.[366] They are rare in the brain stem,[367] where they affect mainly the upper areas.[34]

In rare cases, plaques are the only histological markers of an otherwise typical AD, the NFTs being absent from the isocortex. To our knowledge, tangles are always present in the entorhinal area and the hippocampus. This plaque-only AD may constitute a separate group of the disease,[368] to which one of Alzheimer's seminal cases may belong.[369] Dementia with Lewy body is frequently of the plaque-only type.[370]

In normal aging, neuritic plaques occur in small numbers, with increasing frequency from the fifth decade on, in the amygdala, the hippocampus, and the neocortex,[237] with a predilection for the parahippocampal and occipitotemporal (fusiform) gyri and for the prefrontal cortex.[266] The frequency of their distribution increases monotically after age 71 in a general autopsy population.[371,372] In centenarians, neuritic plaques were found in 8 of 9 nondemented individuals—mainly in the hippocampus (8/9), occipital cortex (6/9), parahippocampal gyrus, and prefrontal cortices (5/9), the cingular cortex being less affected (2/9).[241] Further studies confirmed that Aβ diffuse and focal deposits (usually studied together), can be seen in the isocortex early in the life of some individuals, and that their prevalence in the general population increases steadily until reaching 100% in centenarians.

Braak and Braak[24] used a silver-pyridine method for detection of amyloid deposits in 2661 nonselected brains obtained at autopsy from three departments of pathology and one department of forensic pathology. Using the amyloid stages that they had previously published,[211] they showed that Aβ pathology progressed with age, starting in poorly myelinated areas of the basal isocortex (stage A), then spreading into adjoining areas and into the hippocampus (stage B) and finally (stage C) involving all the isocortical areas. The first deposits were seen in some young individuals, but with a low prevalence (less than a few percentage points up to the age of 45). The peak value in the prevalence of stage A, calculated by interpolating a logistic curve,[240] was 22%; this was reached at age 72. The peak of prevalence for stage B was 31%, reached at age 82. In the 91–95 class, there were no deposits in 21% of the brains. Delaère et al.,[373] using Aβ immunohistochemical staining, showed that the deposits were constant in a series of 20 institutionalized centenarians.

SENILE PLAQUES AND INTELLECTUAL DEFICIT

The relationship between the density of plaques and cognitive deficit has been debated. The controversies are partly explained by the different meanings given to the term "senile plaque." Blessed et al.,[374] using a silver impregnation method to reveal the neuritic plaques, showed that there was a linear relationship between intellectual status, as measured by a simple clinical scale, and the number of neuritic plaques. This has been confirmed by other studies.[199,227,234] However, opposite results have also been found: a number of elderly patients living in a nursing home and considered intellectually normal were shown to exhibit a high density of SPs at postmortem examination, sometimes sufficient to have met Khatchaturian or CERAD criteria for AD.[375,376] The authors suggested that the density of SP was not the predictive variable for the intellectual status, but the density of large neurons that disappear in AD and SDAT. The measure of amyloid load or burden (the volume occupied by Aβ deposits in the brain) may be better linked to the severity of dementia than the actual count of plaques.[377,378] It should be stressed that thioflavin S or other stains (such as Bielschowsky's) labeling a certain number of SPs apparently devoid of abnormal neurites (diffuse deposits) were used to reveal SPs in most studies. The presence of abnormal neurites around the SPs could play an important role in their contribution to mental impairment,[267] and could at least be correlated with a high level of tau pathology. This hypothesis received support from the authors of a case report in which the cognitive level had been assessed a few weeks before the death of the patient, and was normal: numerous diffuse Aβ deposits were demonstrated by immunohistochemical staining in the temporal isocortex, but there were no neuritic plaques.[379] The relation between the number of lesions and intellectual status is undoubtedly complex.[232] The density of changes at the time of the examination is the result of the production and catabolism of the lesions.[280,350] A threshold in the density of SPs must be reached before clinical consequences occur (threshold effect). Recent studies have demonstrated that the brain of cognitively normal, relatively well-educated elderly individuals contain numerous degenerative changes, such as neuritic plaques and NFTs, that remain apparently silent (see review[351]). The differences in severely affected patients (ceiling effect) are also usually undetectable using a clinical scale.

AMYLOID β PLAQUES IN OTHER CONDITIONS AND OTHER TYPES OF PLAQUES

Amyloid β plaques have been described in disorders other than AD, Down syndrome, and cerebral amyloid angiopathy.[382] They could be due to coincidental AD or to so-called normal aging. For example, diffuse plaques lacking dystrophic neurites were observed in two-thirds of elderly Steele-Richardson-Olszewski's disease cases.[382] Plaques seen in prion diseases caused by unconventional agents (kuru, the Gerstmann-Sträussler-Scheinker syndrome, and some cases of Creutzfeldt-Jakob disease) frequently occur in the cerebellum and are often purely amyloid without a crown of neuronal processes. These plaques contain prion protein (PrP) amyloid, in contrast with those of normal aging, Down syndrome, and AD. They are thus different from neuritic or other varieties of SPs and in all likelihood have a different pathogenesis. In rare families of Gerstmann-Sträussler-Scheinker syndrome, however, Aβ, tau, and PrP pathologies appear to coexist.[383,384]

Astrocytic plaques[385] are distinct lesions that can be superficially mistaken for a neuritic plaque. They consist of tau-positive astrocytic processes[386] that surround a nonlabeled area devoid of Aβ. They are seen in corticobasal degeneration, and occasionally in progressive supranucleat palsy.[387,388]

AMYLOID ANGIOPATHY

Cerebral amyloid angiopathy (CAA) of AD and related disorders is characterized by the deposition of Aβ amyloid in the walls of the cerebral blood vessels, without involvement of extracerebral vessels (see review[389,390]). It affects small arteries and arterioles of the leptomeninges and penetrating arterioles of the cerebral cortex (Fig. 8–10). On light microscopic examination, small focal deposits can be seen between the muscle cells. As the lesion becomes more extensive, amyloid containing bands appear that become increasingly closer to one another as vascular bifurcations are approached. In severe amyloid involvement, continuous dense deposits are seen. The whole wall of the artery may be involved; the vessels walls appear thickened and very eosinophilic, the muscle cells have disappeared, and the lumen are usually wide open. In addition, deposits can be seen extending in radial spikes into the brain tissue. Not unfrequently, these amyloid deposits appear to participate to genuine neuritic plaques that seem centered by the vessel.[391] About 10% of the vessels show discrete aneurysmal dilatation (diameter of the vessel is 50% to 100% greater than elsewhere).[392] Other associated lesions in the vessel walls include frequent arteriolosclerosis[393] and rare cases of isolated cerebral vasculitis and granulomatous angeitis. The vasculitis has been compared to that of rheumatoid disease, for it is characterized by segmental fibrinoid necrosis, adventitial inflammatory infiltrate, and obliterative endarteritis.[394] In other cases, a granulomatous angeitis with prominent giant cells is seen.[392,395] The mechanism of such lesions has not been determined. They may be related to a chronic inflammatory process, which could be the cause or the consequence of the amyloid deposit. Amyloid angiopathy is more frequently seen in the occipital cortex, where it sometimes selectively affects area 17 of Brodmann—more precisely, layers 1V b and c.[396] In a study by Pantelakis[397] of 26 cases, distribution of this lesion was constant in the occipital cortex, found in the prefrontal cortex

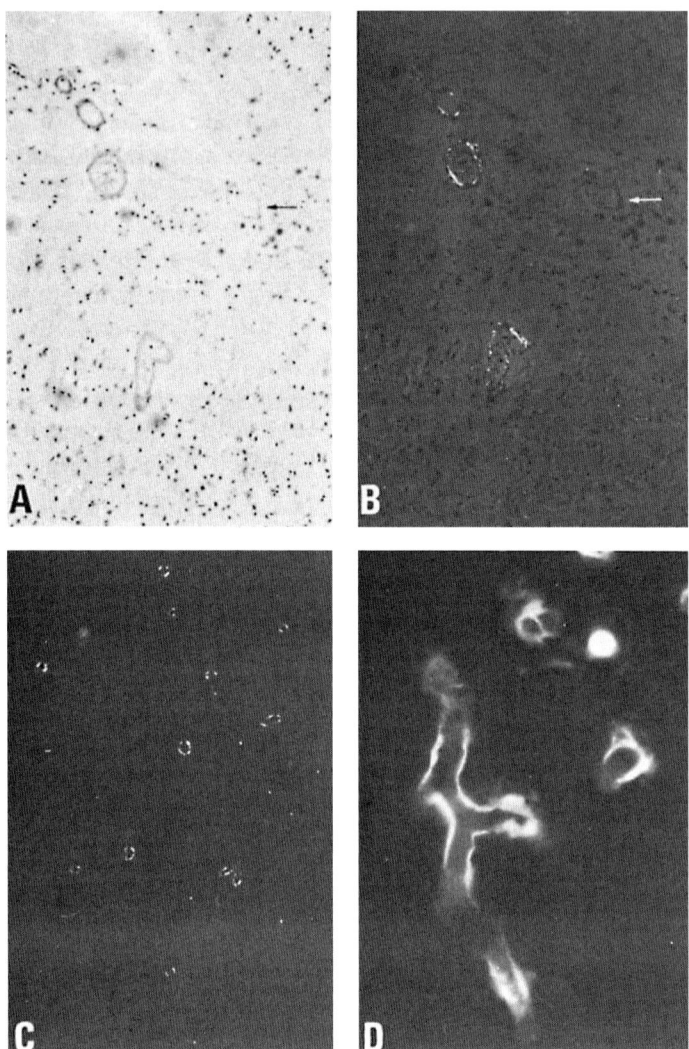

Figure 8–10. Amyloid angiopathy. *A, B*. Congo red staining before (*A*) and after (*B*) polarization. Note the absence of amyloid angiopathy in one vessel (arrow), ×10. *C, D*. Amyloid deposits in vessel walls (thioflavin S). When the amyloid deposit is present in large vessels, some European authors use the term "congophilic angiopathy" (*A* and *B*). The amyloid deposit in small vessels also involves the adjoining parenchyma (*D*); these same authors call this "dyshoric angiopathy." C, ×10; D, ×63.

in 15 cases (58%), in the central gyrus in 14 cases (54%), in the Ammon's horn and the cerebellar cortex in 11 (42%), where it involved the molecular layer, and it was not found in the white matter and spinal cord. Amyloid angiopathy may seldom involve the basal ganglia,[398] and has been rarely seen in the spinal cord.[399] Amyloid angiopathy is not restricted to AD; it can also be seen in Down's syndrome and in rare familial cases linked to mutations on the APP gene. Hereditary cerebral hemorrhage with amyloidosis-Dutch type (HCHWA-D) is caused by a mutation that changes an amino acid at codon 693.[400,401] A different disorder, early-onset Alzheimer's disease type dementia and cerebral hemorrhage with amyloidosis, is caused by a mutation that changes an amino acid at codon 692,[402] and has been identified in only one family (family 1302). The relationship of this disorder to HCHAWA-D and familial AD remains to be determined as only biopsy material has been studied.[403] The apo E-ε4[404] or E-ε2[405] alleles do not influence the clinical expression of the APP gene in mutations occuring at codons 693 or 692.

Amyloid angiopathy can also be found as the main lesion in sporadic cases with cerebral hemorrhages or other symptoms and signs such as recurrent transient neurologic symptoms or subacute dementia (see review[389]). In a review of 107 cases reported in 20 clinicopathological series of sporadic CAA, published from 1975 to 1985, Vinters,[399] found that a pathological diagnosis of AD had been made in 47 cases. Amyloid angiopathy is a frequent pathological finding in "normal" aged persons. The prevalence of amyloid deposits in the vessel walls has been estimated in some autopsy series concerning nonselected cases that may be considered population studies. In the "physiological series" (302 patients aged 80 or over from a general hospital) studied by Wildi and Dago-Akribi in Geneva, 30% of the patients had amyloid deposits of the cerebral vessel walls, and there was a significant preponderance in women: 36.7% versus 20.6% in men. These proportions increased with age: 36.2% in women and 21.1% in men between ages 80 and 85, and 40.6% in women and 20.5% in men between ages 86 and 91. Similar results were found in Japan: in 400 autopsies of patients age 40 years and older, amyloid deposits of the cerebral vessel walls were also more frequent in women (28%) than in men (18.3%), and the prevalence increased with age in both sexes up to 44% in the age group 90 years and older.[407] In another series, prevalence reached up to 74% in the group of patients over 90, but no difference in prevalence was found between men and women.[408] In centenarians at a geriatric hospital who had been enrolled in the study on account of their age, regardless of their clinical status, 8 of 12 patients had amyloid deposits in the vessel walls.[241] In AD, the prevalence of amyloid deposits in the vessel walls has been estimated to be from 50% to 100% of cases.[392,409,410] In Down syndrome, CAA rarely occurs before 40 years of age,[411] and its prevalence increases with age. In some series, it was found constant in patients over 42, without always being concomitant with neuritic SPs.[412]

Immunohistochemical analysis shows that the amyloid deposits consist mainly of Aβ and share most constituents with neuritic plaques. Although the proportion of Aβ 40 and Aβ 42 in vascular amyloid angiopathy and the chronological relationship of deposition of both varieties in the vessel walls have been debated,[307] it has been determined that a high tissue content of Aβ 40 is not linked to the abundance of neuritic plaques but is invariably associated with CAA.[301,413] Antibodies against cystatin C γ-trace also label the vessel walls, albeit less constantly.[414,415] The precise location of amyloid deposits in the vessel wall of AD affected patients can be ascertained by means of electron microscopic immunocytochemistry. In the leptomeningeal arteries, the smallest groups of Aβ fibrils, which may be the first to appear, are seen on the external side of the basal membrane of the muscle fibers located at the border of the adventitia; APP mRNA is expressed throughout the entire vessel wall.[416] In the smallest leptomeningeal arteries and the intracerebral arterioles, the small groups of Aβ fibrils are also the most dense at the external border of muscle fibers. They are less numerous near the basal lamina, which delineates endothelium from muscle cells. In the cerebral capillaries, by contrast, the small Aβ deposits are seen in the endothelial basal lamina itself.[417] The amyloid angiopathy of small arteries (which can occur in the leptomeningeal space) may be different from that of arterioles, capillaries, and veinules (usually seen in the brain tissue itself). The reasons for only occasional Aβ peptide deposition in vessel walls and selective involvement of some cerebral vessels are still unclear. The pathogenetic mechanism of the vascular deposits is likely distinct, at least for the deposits in the largest vessels, from that of SP. Constitutively secreted, soluble Aβ (mostly Aβ 40) could be the precursor of amyloid deposits seen in the vessel walls.[418] Because the Aβ transcript is distributed throughout both neural and nonneural tissue, it has been suggested that soluble Aβ may originate from the brain tissue,[419] from the blood,[420] or in the vessel wall itself.[421] Endothelial cells, pericytes, and muscle cells[422] of the cerebral vessel walls express the APP mRNA. In addition, a selective deposit of Aβ from the brain or blood on the proteoglycans of the vessel wall, the structure of which is different in the brain and other organs,[423] may occur.[424] Either the matrix proteins secreted by activated or degenerating muscle cells or protease inhibitors such as α 1-antichymotrypsin and cystatin C (specifically found in the vessel wall) may promote amyloidogenesis.[425] Another possibility is a coincidental occurrence, in which only affinity to the amyloid structure would be expressed. The degeneration of vascular muscle cells of the brain in amyloid angiopathy associated with AD, the close association of Aβ and smooth muscle cells of vessels walls in this disease, and the production of Aβ in smooth muscle cells in vitro, isolated from similar vessels in aging dogs (myocytes cultured from young animals do not produce Aβ)[426] all favor the hypothesis of the proliferation and degeneration of smooth muscle cells of cerebral vessels producing Aβ *in vivo*, as they do *in vitro*.

Some of the data discussed above are conflicting. The discrepancies in findings can be explained by a leakage of plasma components through the altered blood–brain barrier in vivo or in the postmortem material used for most studies. Other differences may be due to inter-individual variations, the heterogeneity of the diseases, or to the different properties of Aβ amyloid in small capillaries and larger vessels. The amyloid angiopathy of small arteries (which may occur in the leptomeningeal space) may be different from that of arterioles, capillaries, and veinules (usually seen in the brain tissue itself). This discrepancy parallels the distinction made by the German and Swiss neuropathologists of the mid-century between congophilic angiopathy (involving large arteries) and dyshoric angiopathy (of small vessels). That terminology was confusing, but it may still be useful for distinguishing the amyloid angiopathy of small arteries from that of the more distal microcirculation.[389]

Presenilins

Pathogenic mutations have shown the importance of presenilins 1 and 2 (PS-1 and PS-2) in the mechanism of AD. Their genes are located on chromosomes 14 and 1, respectively (see review[290,427–432]). These polytopic membrane proteins are localized to the endoplasmic reticulum and the Golgi apparatus. They are believed to have several transmembrane domains. Their activities are not known, but in *C elegans*, a member of the presenilin family is a facilitator of Notch signaling during development. In addition, PS-1 may interact with members of the Armadillo family of proteins that serve in cell–cell adhesion complexes (see review[283]). Presenilins are expressed in most cell types, including neurons, in both normal controls and in AD;[433] the full-length proteins are at low levels on account of consistent endoproteolysis. An epitope of PS-1, located at the carboxy-terminal of the protein and associated with Aβ, is found in the core of neuritic plaque.[434] With other antibodies, the plaques are not labeled.[433,435] Presenilin-1-positive neurons have been said to be protected against apoptosis,[436] but this remains controversial; in another study the PS-1-positive neurons appeared specifically lost in some cortical layers.[437]

DENDRITIC CHANGES AND SYNAPTIC LOSS

The Golgi method has been used to study dendritic morphology in aging, AD, and SDAT. Postmortem delay has been shown to alter unavoidably dendritic shape.[438,439] Some aspects once thought to be typical of aging are now considered mere artifacts. Carefully controlled studies have suggested that dendritic spatial extension increases with age in pyramidal cells of the parahippocampal gyrus, granule cells of the dentate gyrus, and reticular neurons of the basal magnocellular complex.[440–442] In normal aging, the size of the dendritic tree increases (extensive growth) whereas in AD, there is an increase in dendritic density (intensive growth). Some abnormal processes (filopodia) have sometimes been observed on reticular neurons.[443] A meshwork of abnormal dendrites was also described in a case of early-onset AD.[444] The distribution of receptors for kainic acid and of acetylcholinesterase in early cases of AD also indicate the persistence of some plasticity in the hippocampus;[445] this was not seen in late-onset cases.[446]

The concentration of synaptophysin, located within small presynaptic vesicles, is decreased in the cerebral cortex in correlation with intellectual status.[235,447–450] The concentration of chromogranin A located in large, dense core vesicles appears, on the contrary, to increase.[451] Observations with electron microscopy have shown that the synapses decrease in number but are enlarged, the total apposition length remaining unchanged.[452–455] More recently it has been shown that presynaptic *membrane* components (synaptotagmin, SNAP-25, and syntaxin 1/HPC-1) are little affected (−10% the value of the controls) compared to the vesicular components (synaptobrevin and synaptophysin = −30% of the controls).[456] Results obtained with SNAP 25 immunohistochemistry tend to show a much smaller synaptic loss than that of synaptophysin.[457,458] All of these synaptic markers are presynaptic and depend on the metabolism of cell bodies that are sometimes located far away, thus it is difficult to determine if the presynaptic alterations appear early[459] or late[460] in the cascade of pathological events, and whether these are a major[235] or a minor correlate[231] of dementia. It has been shown that the decrease in synaptophysin immunoreactivity is not linked to the presence of Aβ deposits,[461] and in the entorhinal–dentate gyrus system it could be related to the density of NFTs in the entorhinal cortex.[448]

OTHER CHANGES IN GRAY MATTER

Granulovacuolar Degeneration

Granulovacuolar degeneration is a neuronal intracytoplasmic vesicle containing a central granule that is eosinophilic with standard hematein-eosin staining and can be impregnated through usual silver staining methods (Fig. 8–11). On electron microscopy, it is bound by a unit membrane; a dense, finely granular mass makes up the granule. It is immunolabeled by anti-tubulin,[462] and some anti-neurofilament.[463] Its content of tau protein has been debated.[194,464–467] In the aging brain, granulovacuolar degeneration is usually seen in a few hippocampal pyramidal cells, especially in the CA1–2 fields, in association with NFTs. Granulovacuolar degeneration was seen in every case of a series of 12 centenarians.[241] In Guam-amyotrophic lateral sclerosis (ALS)–Parkinsonism dementia complex, Pick's disease, Down syndrome, and in AD, the density of affected cells is markedly increased and it spreads to other fields of the hippocampus, particularly the subiculum. Granulovacuolar degeneration is rare in the isocortex, amygdala, hypothalamus, and paramedian nuclei of the midbrain. Other areas of the brain are usually spared (see review[34,360]).

Hirano Bodies

Hirano bodies are eosinophilic, rod-like structures that are located almost exclusively in the Sommer's sector of the hippocampal pyramidal layer, adjacent to neuronal cell bodies,

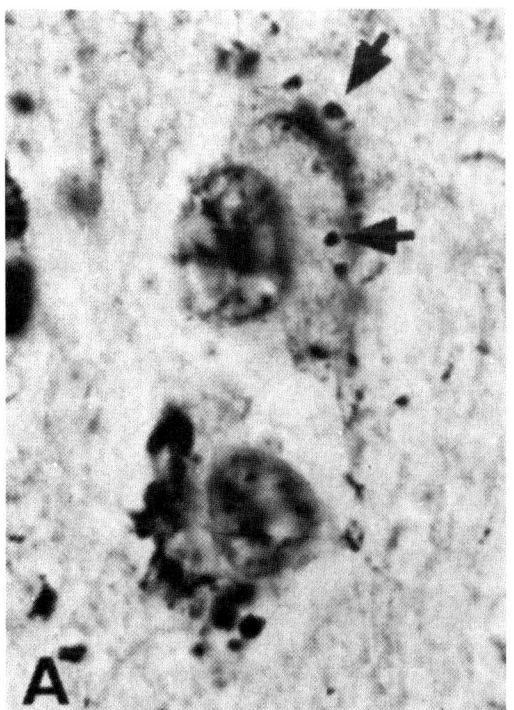
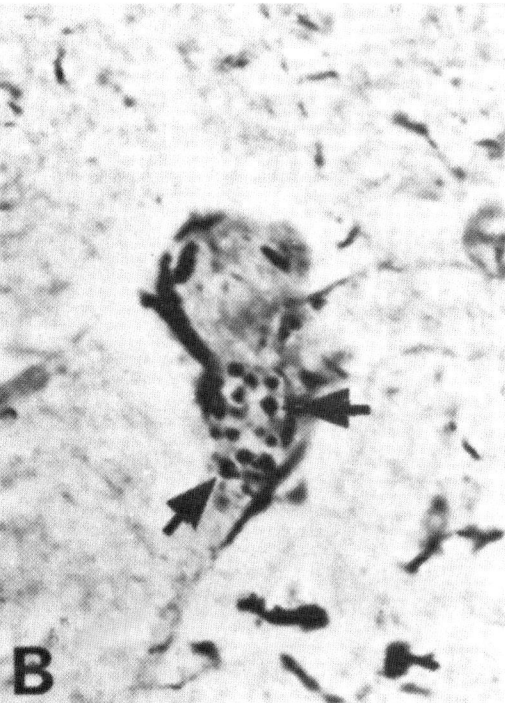

Figure 8–11. *A, B.* Granulovacuolar degeneration (arrows) Bielschowsky's method, ×100.

and occasionally within them. They have a paracrystalline appearance on electron microscopy. They contain epitopes of actin and actin-associated proteins,[468] tau,[469] middle-molecular-weight neurofilament subunit,[470] and a C-terminal fragment of APP[471] (see review[472]). The presence of antigens of advanced glycation end products suggests that these inclusion bodies are subjected to post-translational modifications.[473] When compared to age-matched controls, AD brains show a higher concentration of Hirano bodies with a broad overlap with controls.[474] Hirano bodies are found in other conditions, especially Pick's disease and Guam–Parkinson–dementia complex.

Lewy bodies, considered to be essential for the diagnosis of idiopathic Parkinson's disease,[475] are seen in some cases of AD, with or without parkinsonism. The significance of this association is discussed in Alzheimer's Disease, Parkinson's Disease with Dementia, and Dementia with Lewy Bodies, below.

Decrease in Volume of Nucleolus and Fragmentation of Golgi Apparatus

Reduction in the size of the nucleus and nucleolus and the decrease in content of cytoplasmic RNA in AD and normal aging have been extensively studied by Mann et al.[139] These alterations suggest a decrease in protein synthesis; they are early consequences of the disease process, as they have been found in cortical biopsy specimens of little-affected cases.[266] The decrease in volume of the Golgi apparatus has also been documented in neurons with or without NFTs. No relationship was found between the volume of the Golgi apparatus and the density of SPs.[126,476]

Accumulation of lipofuscin pigment within nerve cells in aging is usual. In AD, it has never been demonstrated to be linked to the level of dementia.[477] However, NFT-bearing neurons appear to contain more lipofuscin pigment than the other nerve populations. This could be due to either more selective storage in these degenerating cells or to a reduction in the volume of free cytoplasm because of cell atrophy and the presence of NFT material.[478]

Spongiform Changes

A spongiform or vacuolar change is frequently seen in the upper layers of the isocortex, rarely in the deeper layers, especially in the most severe cases of AD.[169,479,480] When this pattern occurs, it may be difficult to distinguish AD lesions from the more intense and diffuse lesions of Creutzfeldt-Jakob disease. In the hippocampus of AD cases, a band of spongiosis located in the outer molecular layer of the dentate gyrus is present when the neuronal loss is severe in the entorhinal cortex. In that location, the status spongiosus is most likely due to de-afferentation.[481]

Astrocytosis

Astrocytic hypertrophy has been documented by immunohistochemical means with antibodies directed against glial fibrillary acid protein (GFAP). A marked increase in the number of fibrous astrocytes in layers 2 to 6, without change in the total number of glial cells, was found in the cortex of the frontal, temporal, and parietal lobes.[277] This increase has been confirmed immunochemically on brain extracts.[482] The increase in density of small cellular profiles found in the patient group of several clinicopathological series has been interpreted as evidence of an increase in the density of astroglial cells.[483,484] Astrocytes surround SP, as shown on electron microscopy[261] and immunohistochemistry,[277] and they are able to circumvent and penetrate the NFTs after neuronal death.[485] In tissue culture, the presence of astrocytes prevents phagocytosis of the amyloid core of plaque by macrophages.[486] Astrocytes may regulate amyloid deposition and resorption in SP.[280]

CHANGES IN WHITE MATTER

Neuronal loss observed in AD and aging involves neurons that project onto distant areas. The effects of the loss of cortical neurons with long axons on the morphological characteristics of the centrum semi-ovale are partly unknown. This type of loss could lead to (1) a decrease in fiber density, causing myelin pallor on histological sections—the total volume of white matter must remain relatively stable if a drop in the density of fibers is to be expected; (2) a decrease in the volume of white matter, which, if severe, could prevent the decrease in fiber density expected after fiber loss; or (3) both.

Volume of White Matter

The ratio of gray to white matter volume was found to be 1.28 in individuals born 20 years ago, 1.13 in those born 50 years ago, and 1.55 in centenarians. These results suggest a preferential loss of gray matter at around 50 years of age and of white matter later on, given that the fiber density of white matter remains constant during aging. In SDAT the ratio of gray to white matter remains unchanged.[38]

Density of White Matter

Rarefaction of white matter has long been known from gross examination of the brain in the elderly.[487,488] Kemper[41] considered on qualitative grounds that the older normal brains of the Yakovlev collection showed a pallor of myelin staining on the forebrain that appeared to be confined to the corona radiata and stratum sagitalle interna. This observation suggests that fiber density decreased with age but awaits quantitative confirmation. A primary, age-related demyelination has been postulated for these changes that principally occur in late-myelinated areas.[41] Loss of fibers secondary to neuronal degeneration seems also plausible, given our current knowledge. Rarefaction of fibers and oligodendroglia in the white matter during SDAT has been described by Brun and Englund,[488] who thought this could be the consequence of vascular disturbances responsible for the hyalinosis of vessel walls. These changes have been called "selective incomplete white matter infarction." To our knowledge, the fiber loss in white matter has never been quantified during the course of AD and compared to that in a control group. These data are required for confirmation of the hypothesis that SDAT is a primary disease of the white matter.[51] For most authors, the brunt of the disease (at least morphologically) is visible in the gray matter and the white matter changes are less conspicuous and considered secondary.

Leukoaraiosis and Magnetic Resonance Imaging Hypersignals

Areas of hypodensity in the white matter without any demonstrable cause are sometimes evident on CT scans, and MRI hypersignals are seen in the same areas. The word "leukoaraiosis," a purely radiological term, was coined to describe these changes seen on CT scans.[487] The pathology of this condition remains largely unsettled, although it is likely nonspecific. Vascular disorders such as a lacunes, degeneration of myelinated fibers as seen in subcortical arteriosclerotic encephalopathy (Binswanger's disease), and, above all, état criblé (dilatation of the perivascular space), described by Durand-Fardel,[489] are responsible in a number of cases. The latter could be the sequela of hypertensive cerebral edema, the consequence of vascular ectasia and tortuosity associated with age and hypertension, or, more frequently, the mere consequence of cerebral atrophy. Interestingly, Durand-Fardell reported a "brain interstitial atrophy" associated with état criblé, and described leukoaraiosis from gross examination of the brain more than 130 years before it was recognized on CT scan.[490] MRI hypersignals in T2-weighed sequences have been reported in the elderly and were associated at postmortem examination with enlarged perivascular spaces, characteristic of état criblé.[491] Leukoaraiosis is visible in some apparently normal old individuals, but it seems to be statistically correlated with intellectual impairment, mild neurologic signs and symptoms, and vascular risk factors.[492,493] In AD, leukoaraiosis affects neither the age of onset nor the rate of progression.[494]

DIAGNOSTIC CRITERIA

Because of the high prevalence of SP and NFT in aged people, it is difficult to draw a clear boundary between "normal" aging and AD, thus conventional limits are needed to outline the significant pathology. The first attempt to reach a consensus was strongly biased toward the diagnostic meaning of SPs. As a final report of a consensus meeting, Khachaturian[495] proposed that the density of SPs ensures the diagnosis when it reaches a given threshold adapted for age. Two staining methods were recommended: thioflavin S and Bielschowsky; one was discouraged (Bodian silver technique). The counting procedure was not described. A significant improvement in these criteria was made by the CERAD[496] that was also heavily based on SP count. Assessment of SP density, however, relied on a comparison of the examined microscopical field with pictures that enabled recognition of four stages (absence, sparse, moderate, frequent) in the severity of lesions. The tangles had to be reported but were not taken into account for the final diagnosis. Mention was also made of the Lewy bodies. Meanwhile, Braak and Braak[211] had also proposed a procedure that did not aim at reaching a diagnosis but rather that intended to stage the cases. The presence of one single NFT was considered evidence of AD, even if at a preclinical stage. Although staging for amyloid deposition was also proposed, it was the staging of neurofibrillary pathology that rapidly met general agreement and is currently widely used. It recognizes six stages, grouped by pairs in so-called transentorhinal, limbic, and isocortical stages. The criteria proposed by a working group at the National Institute on Aging, and Reagan Institute[497] include both the CERAD and Khachaturian emphasis on the SP, and the neurofibrillary Braak stages.

NEUROCHEMICAL DEFICITS

The Cholinergic Hypothesis

The search for a specific neurochemical deficit in AD and SDAT seemed to have met success when a consistent decrease in the choline acetyltransferase (ChAT) activity of the cerebral cortex was discovered in autopsy AD brains.[498–504] This deficit is more severe in AD of early onset than in SDAT.[97] Choline acetyltransferase is not the only cholinergic marker shown to be depressed in the cortex of AD: synaptosomal choline uptake is reduced,[505] acetylcholine synthesis and release from biopsy specimens are decreased,[506] and synthesis and release of acetylcholine from nerve terminals are depressed.[507] These data demonstrate that the decrease in ChAT activity is not purely an enzymatic deficit but is probably the direct consequence of the loss of cholinergic fibers. Most authors agree that the number of postsynaptic cholinergic receptors (especially muscarinic binding sites) is normal or increased.[119,508–511]

The finding of a cholinergic deficit in AD prompted a great number of studies of cholinergic pathways and function in animals and humans. The basal forebrain cholinergic neurons in the monkey belong to a group of cells spreading at the ventral surface of the brain including the nucleus basalis of Meynert, the nucleus of the diagonal band, and the medial septal nucleus. Neurons in a similar topography, known as the "basal magnocellular complex," had been found in the human brain. It has been shown in humans that 90% of the large neurons in the nucleus basalis of Meynert (NBM) are cholinergic, as are 70% in the nucleus of the diagonal band (NDB) and 40% in the medial septal nucleus. Tracing studies in animals have shown that the septal area and the NDB are the major sources of cholinergic innervation of the hippocampus, whereas the isocortex is mainly innervated by the adjacent nucleus basalis of Meynert.[501] The possibility of intrinsic cortical neurons being cholinergic has been suggested by authors who performed lesions in the rat[512] and has not been ruled out, although intrinsic cholinergic cortical neurons have never been visualized (neither in animals nor in humans) using ChAT immunohistochemistry. The electrophysiological effects of acetylcholine on sensitive neurons of the cortex and of the stimulation of basal forebrain neurons have been thoroughly studied in the rat[513] and seem to be mainly excitatory. The behavioral correlates of cholinergic blockade have been described in young volunteers and were found to mimic some clinical aspects of AD.[514] A significant negative correlation has also been reported between cortical ChAT activity and the degree of dementia (see review[515]). Finally, neuronal loss has been found in the basal forebrain of AD.[119,120] It has been suggested that the cholinergic fibers initiate SP formation, since some SPs are innervated by cholinergic fibers and there is a relationship between the topography of the changes in nucleus basalis of Meynert and the number of SPs in some cortical areas.[516,517] An association has also been found between cholinergic fiber loss and diffuse plaques in nondemented elderly subjects. The authors hypothesized that these alterations could represent a preclinical stage of AD.[518] This set of data on the correlation of neuronal loss in the basal forebrain and cortical cholinergic denervation with the behavioral deficit became known in the literature as the cholinergic hypothesis.[519] It is now widely accepted that the cholinergic hypothesis in its most radical version (i.e., AD results exclusively from a cholinergic defect) is not valid for the following reasons: a number of other neurotransmitters are affected; NFT are spread over much wider regions than the basal forebrain innervaton and microscopical changes in the cortex cannot be explained by cholinergic denervation; SPs contain neurites belonging to several neurotransmitter systems; and the behavioral deficit is larger than that obtained through cholinergic blockade.

The postulate of a connection between some cognitive impairments and a disturbance in cholinergic neurotransmission has nonetheless been refined.[520] First, it was admitted that AD and SDAT are not neurotransmitter diseases per se but diseases disturbing neurotransmission through cellular loss and dysfunction. In this respect, Perry's[520] observation that extensive loss of ChAT activity is not reflected by neuronal loss in the NBM in AD is important because it demonstrates that neuronal dysfunction may long precede cellular loss. The cholinergic deficit in the cerebral cortex is only one of the neurochemical disturbances of AD, and even if it is the most constant,[498] it is not a necessary correlate of the disease. Palmer et al. isolated a group of elderly patients (with histologically assessed SDAT) who had no significant loss of ChAT in the neocortex and hippocampus. In these patients, ChAT decrease was confined to the amygdala.[521] In addition, no correlation was found between neuronal loss in the NBM and cortical histopathology.[522] It should be also noted that more recent studies have failed to show a correlation between loss of cortical cholinergic fibers and density of Aβ deposits, regardless of type, while a significant correlation was often found with the density of NFT's.[523] A third refinement of the cholinergic hypothesis was achieved when it was shown that factors associated with the cholinergic system influence the processing and metabolism of APP and tau. They induced an increase in secretory APP processing via stimulation of G protein–coupled receptors and an increase in α-secretase processing by muscarinic m1 receptors (see review[499,501]).

The Noradrenergic System

Animal studies have shown that noradrenergic fibers stem mainly from the locus ceruleus, a pigmented nucleus located in the dorsal and upper pons; this is also the case in humans but pathways are not known as precisely (for review of the noradrenergic system see Francis et al.[524] and Saura et al.[525]). Although a decrease in the number of neurons in this nucleus during aging has been debated, its involvement in AD is fully documented.[129,526–528] Reduced concentration of norepinephrine in the cortex has been reported by some authors, with differences between normal levels and those in patients with AD being much less significant in older patients.[529] The activity of dopamine-β-hydroxylase, the enzyme that converts dopamine to noradrenaline, was found reduced in some but not all patients.[530] Berger et al.,[531,532] using catecholamine fluorescence histochemistry on neurosurgical samples of the frontal cortex, showed that the number of fluorescent fibers was reduced in AD and that the remaining fluorescent axons were paler and shorter than those in non-AD patients. Some fluorescent fibers were observed within SPs. Cross et al.[530] found that postsynaptic adrenergic receptors were spared.

The alterations in noradrenergic content of the cortex are thought to be the consequences of neuronal loss or dysfunction in the locus ceruleus. Neuronal loss has been found in a high percentage of AD cases in several studies[527,528,533] and concerns principally the dorsal areas of the nucleus.[129] Neurofibrillary tangles have been seen in the locus ceruleus,[367] where they affect mainly the dorsal and medial regions, and could be the cause of the neuronal loss.[127] In some cases, generally with late onset, neuronal loss is lacking.

The Serotoninergic System

Animal tracing studies have shown that serotonin (5-HT)–containing fibers originate from the raphe nuclei dorsalis and centralis superior[534] (see review of serotoninergic system, in relation to AD[500,535,536]). Neurofibrillary tangles are often numerous in these nuclei.[132] The decrease in 5-HT and 5-HIAA concentrations in the cortex is generally agreed upon. The density of both S1 and S2 receptors is decreased. The location of these receptors remains unknown. It has been suggested that they could be located on vulnerable, cortical neurons.[139]

The Dopaminergic System

Changes in dopamine concentration are generally considered minimal or secondary[139] in pure AD, in parallel with the scarcity of NFTs in the parent neurons of the substantia nigra.[367,537,538] It should be noted, however, that the cortical dopaminergic innervation of primates arises from the ventral tegmental area.[273] In humans, NFTs are frequently seen in this area.[539] The sparing of the substantia nigra projecting to the basal nuclei and the alterations of the ventral tegmental area projecting to the cortex favors the hypothesis in which the changes in the brain stem are secondary to the lesions of the cortex and affect the connected nuclei in a retrograde manner.[140]

Neuropeptides

The distribution of neuropeptides in relation to the occurrence of AD has been widely studied (see reviews[509,524,540,541]). Somatostatin has a widespread distribution in human brain, where it is seen in neurons, with high concentrations in the isocortex, amygdala, and striatum.[542–544] It has been found to be regularly and sometimes massively affected (up to 80% in some series,[545] especially in patients carrying the apolipoprotein ε4 allele[546]). The distribution of the deficit did not correlate with that of ChAT.[547] Neurofibrillary tangles are localized in somatostatin neurons among middle-sized nonpyramidal neurons of layers II–III and VI.[548]

Neuropeptide Y is present at high concentrations in the human brain in the basal ganglia, the limbic system, and the isocortex.[549] In some cortical neurons, neuropeptide Y is colocalized with somatostatin.[550] Somatostatin concentration is reduced in AD and lesions of NPY-containing neurons have been seen with immunohistochemistry,[551,552] The decrease in colocalized NPY was expected, but this could not be confirmed.[553–555] This suggests that among the somatostatin—containing neurons, those that also contain neuropeptide Y are resistant to the disease process.[556]

Most studies emphasize the relative sparing of the other neuropeptides that have been studied in relation to AD: thyroid-releasing hormone (TRH), Met-enkephalin, lunteinizing hormone–releasing hormone (LHRH), and neurotensin. Cholecystokinin and substance P were found to be decreased in some cases,[557,558] whereas no modifications were detected by other authors.[509,559,560] Vasoactive intestinal polypeptide (*VIP*) concentration remains unchanged in the cerebral cortex,[558] but Swaab et al. found a marked decrease in the total number of VIP neurons in the suprachiasmatic nucleus of the hypothalamus.[116] Corticotrophin-releasing factor (*CRF*)–like immunoreactivity is also reduced in the cerebral cortex. The number of receptors increases, suggesting a hypersensitivity due to denervation.[561,562] Galanin has widespread distribution throughout the human cortex. Galanin receptors are present in the substantia innominata, hypothalamus, the bed nucleus of the stria terminalis, and the entorhinal cortex.[563] Galanin-like immunoreactivity is increased in the postmortem cerebral cortex from patients with AD.[564] I-125-Galanin binding sites are increased in hippocampal subfields and decreased in the caudate nucleus.[565] As for the classical neurotransmitters, it has been suggested that neuropeptide systems may influence the processing and metabolism of APP. Vasopressin and bradykinin may regulate secretory processing of the APP,[566] and APP may be a key sorting and targeting receptor for neuropeptidases.[567]

Amino Acids

Gamma-aminobutyric acid (GABA) and glutamic acid are thought to be cortical transmitters used by interneurons and have been studied in relation to AD (see reviews[524,568,569]). Glutamic acid decarboxylase activity has been used as a marker of GABA neurons but is highly influenced at postmortem examination by the length of terminal coma and postmortem delay before assay.[502] In AD, GABA concentration was decreased by about 30% in the temporal cortex and in younger patients in the study by Rossor et al. The deficit occurred in areas with severe pathological changes.[570] Lowe et al.[571] measured the concentration of GABA in samples obtained at cortical biopsy or at necropsy. They found a decrease in GABA concentration mainly in the *postmortem* material. They thought that those differences were not artefactual, or on account of postmortem delay, but reflected the stages of the disease. The patients who underwent biopsies had an average disease duration of 3 years, whereas in the necropsy series the average duration was 8 years.[571] Presynaptic glutamate uptake sites are reduced in AD,[572] while postsynaptic NMDA receptor levels are unchanged.[573] The normal release of glutamate and aspartate from biopsy samples of cortex in AD[574] suggests a sparing of intrinsic cortical perikarya, which contrasts with the loss of glutamatergic nerve terminals. This could indicate a loss of corticocortical association fibers using GABA (intrinsic cells) or glutamate (projecting pyramidal neurons of layer III). In addition, there is indirect evidence of a deficiency in the descending corticostriatal pathways, which are presumed to use glutamate and/or aspartate as a transmitter (see review[139]). The dementia score correlates with ChAT activity in the temporal cortex, but not with GABA levels.[509] As emphasized by Bowen et al.[575] and by Mann,[139] when interpreting these studies, one must bear in mind that the variable atrophy of the cerebral cortex that occurs in AD, especially in the early stages of the disease, may mask an actual loss of biochemical markers.

In summary, deficits of acetylcholine, noradrenalin, serotonin, and less clearly, dopamine are established in AD. Somatostatin levels have also been shown to be be decreased. Deficits in other neuromediators are not as well documented.

MIXED DEMENTIA (COMBINED VASCULAR DEMENTIA AND ALZHEIMER'S DISEASE)

Since the description by Delay and Brion[18] of cases in which both pathologies coexist in the same patient (mixed dementia) the distinction between mixed dementia, isolated AD and vascular dementia (VaD) remains a controversial issue and one of the most difficult diagnostic challenges.[576] It may be recalled that clinicopathologic correlations showed that among the first 100 cases of clinically diagnosed AD evaluated following the CERAD criteria, 26 had AD associated with vascular lesions of the brain.[16] More recently, two different prospective studies produced similar results: 16% and 42% of the cases clinically classified as AD were found to be AD associated with vascular disorders of the brain.[15,17] The large diagnostic range for mixed dementia on neuropathological examination is evident from the diversity of prevalence values reported in postmortem studies (from 2% to 38%). This is likely related in part to differences in diagnostic criteria. For some authors, the diagnosis can be made only if there are enough vascular and degenerative lesions to perform each diagnosis independently.[496,577–579] For other authors, this diagnosis necessitates only AD diagnosis, with associated ischemic lesions.[580,581] Lastly, some authors believe that degenerative and vascular lesions, each alone being insufficient to account for dementia, can potentiate each other and explain dementia when associated.[409,582] In other words, the contribution of the degenerative and vascular lesions to the dementing process is different (incidental, contributory, or causal) according to the explicit or implicit criteria used. As far as the diagnostic criteria of AD are concerned, for the CERAD, the presence or absence of other pathological lesions likely to cause dementia does not interfere with the diagnosis of definite, possible or probable AD.[496] According to the (state of California's) Alzheimer's Disease Diagnostic and Treatment Centers' (ADDTC) criteria,[583] a second systemic or brain disorder in addition to AD must be causally related to dementia for a mixed dementia to occur. For the NINDS-AIREN,[584] "AD with cerebrovascular disease" is used to classify patients fulfilling the clinical criteria for possible AD and who present with clinical or brain imaging evidence of relevant cerebrovascular disease, the term "mixed dementia" being avoided. Recently, some authors have recommended that this terminology be reevaluated and refined.[585,586] Three recent studies, however, argue for an additive effect of degenerative and vascular lesions of the brain on the process of dementia. The so-called nun study indicated that brain infarction may participate in the clinical expression of AD.[587] Nagy et al. showed that, for any given level of cognitive defect, the densities of either all plaques or neuritic plaques alone in the neocortex were significantly lower in cases of AD occurring with other pathologies of the central nervous system than in cases of AD with no other pathology.[588] This was confirmed through morphometric analysis of a group of 27 demented patients with AD pathology and/or vascular lesions of the brain in whom the age, sex ratio, mean education level, and severity of dementia were similar. The mean volume of vascular lesions was significantly lower in mixed dementia than in vascular dementia. The density of Aβ focal deposits, NFT, and neuritic plaques in frontal and temporal isocortex was significantly lower when there were bilateral infarcts, or unilateral infarcts involving the territory of either the posterior cerebral artery or the anterior cerebral artery than in AD alone. This indicates that degenerative and vascular lesions had additive effects on the mechanism of dementia.[589] Also, recent epidemiological studies have shown that vascular risk factors (mainly high blood pressure) are associated with AD.[590] These data have been used to argue that AD may be due to general arterial diseases and chronic ischemia of the brain, or that vascular factors are important in the cascade of AD lesions.[591,592] According to a simpler hypothesis, any cerebral lesion of vascular etiology (infarct, lacune, hemorrhage) leads to the earlier recognition and a shorter course of AD, and increases the proportion of AD associated with vascular risk factors in comparison to control cases.

DOWN SYNDROME AND ALZHEIMER'S DISEASE

Large densities of SPs and NFTs occur in the brain of almost all middle-aged patients with Down syndrome (trisomy 21).[593–598] This is very likely related to the presence of three copies of the APP genes: in one case of partial trisomy 21 where the gene sequence for APP was present in only two copies, there was no evidence of Alzheimer's pathology at the age of 78.[599] Trisomy 21 patients dying in their 30s, and occasionally earlier, develop SPs, and later on (10–20 years) develop NFTs. Diffuse Aβ plaques can be found earlier than other lesions,[600] as early as the age of 10.[601] These changes have been reported to be constant after age 50. In addition, Lewy bodies are frequent in the cerebral cortex of aged Down syndrome patients.[305,602] The selective reduction in neurons in the hippocampus and cholinergic and noradrenergic neuronal systems seen in usual Alzheimer's cases is also found in Down syndrome.[593,598] Although the similarity of SPs and NFTs seen in AD and trisomy 21 has been stessed, SPs in trisomy 21 may be mostly of the amyloid type[603] and may contain more sugar residues than those observed in AD.[604] In some patients, the clinical picture of AD appears early. However, half or two-thirds of elderly people with trisomy 21 (and especially with mosaicism) have been reported not to develop dementia, although they should on account of their brain pathology.[598] Neuropathology could thus antedate the appearance of clinical signs by a considerable margin of time.[598,605] Using a modified version of the informant interview of the Cambridge Examination for Mental Disorders of the Elderly, in a population-based study, Holland et al showed that the prevalence rates of dementia for patients with trisomy 21 were similar to those for patients with AD, only the dementia occurred 30–40 years earlier in life.[606] This means that the effects of NFTs on mental performance are not different in Down syndrome and in AD, given the difficulties in assessing a cognitive decline in Down syndrome.

ALZHEIMER'S DISEASE, PARKINSON'S DISEASE WITH DEMENTIA, AND DEMENTIA WITH LEWY BODIES

Lewy bodies, the markers of Parkinson's disease, are round, eosinophilic, intraneuronal inclusions surrounded by a clear halo that are found in the cell bodies of neurons of the *substantia nigra, locus coeruleus*, and dorsal vagal nucleus. They exhibit neurofilament and ubiquitin epitopes. Recently it has been shown that they contain α-synuclein in high concentrations. Lewy bodies have also been found in the cerebral cortex in cases of dementia.[607–610] They involve predominantly the entorhinal cortex, insula, and cingulate gyri. The aspect of the cortical and brainstem Lewy body is different: in the cortex, the cortical halo is lacking. Several groups have mentioned the presence of cortical Lewy bodies in cases in which plaques and tangles are also present. Sometimes, a prominent spongiosis is also seen. Lesions of the *substantia nigra* and *locus coeruleus* have been noticed in association with cortical pathology. Different terms have been proposed to describe this apparently new entity, such as "senile dementia of Lewy body type"[611] or "Lewy body variant of Alzheimer's disease."[612] Other terms have emphasized the importance of the Lewy body ("diffuse Lewy body disease"[610,613]). Some clinical pecularities have been observed in these patients: visual hallucinations are frequent, clinical fluctuations are often marked, and neuroleptics produce severe adverse effects. Diagnostic criteria have been proposed,[614] taking these clinical characteristics into account. However, various questions have remained unsolved, including the role of Lewy bodies in dementia and their relation to Alzheimer's and Parkinson's disease. At autopsy, Lewy bodies are present in the cortex of almost all cases of common Parkinson's disease.[615] The risk of developing dementia with Lewy bodies is increased by the presence of apolipoprotein (Apo E) ε4 allele when Alzheimer pathology is associated.[616] In several cases of familial Alzheimer disease, Lewy bodies have been found in addition to plaques and tangles.[617,618] It has now been established that, even when the intellectual deficit is partly explained by Alzheimer changes, the density of Lewy bodies has a deleterious effect on cognition.[619] Because of these findings, some authors suggest that the presence of dementia associated with Lewy bodies is the mark of a specific disease entity,[620,621] whereas others argue for the possibility of a synergy between two initially independent diseases (Alzheimer's and Parkinson's).[622] A more recent consensus conference left open the interpretation of the data by proposing the term "dementia with Lewy bodies."[623]

HYPOTHESES ABOUT ALZHEIMER'S DISEASE ETIOLOGY

Until recently, age was the only defined risk factor for AD. The annual incidence rate increases from 2.4 cases per 100,000 for ages 40 to 60, to 127 cases per 100,000 after age 60; the prevalence is estimated at 2%–3% in the age-groups over 65, doubles approximately every 5 years for those between the ages of 65 and 85, and increases to up to 45% after age 85 in some studies.[2,6,624–627]

A number of other risk factors have recently been demonstrated or suggested (see also Chapter 6).[6,628] A genetic factor in the etiology of AD has received confirmation in the past decade.[33,629–632] The overall relative risk for AD in a given individual is 3.5 if one first-degree relative has AD, and is higher (7.5) if more first-degree relatives are diseased. The relative risk is higher in those cases with early onset. The familial forms of AD with multiple affected individuals are, on the whole, rare. The disease segregates as an autosomal dominant disorder. Mutations in three genes coding for APP (located on chromosome 21) and presenilins 1 and 2 (PS-1, PS-2; located on chromosomes 14 and 1, respectively) have been identified. In these families, the age of onset is usually early (45–60) and constant within the kinship. The frequency of this kind of transmission is difficult to assess. Genetic cases may appear sporadic if other members of the family died before they developed the disease. On the contrary, familial cases may appear genetic if they cluster for other reasons, for example, because of environmental factors. Because of their rarity, the affected families represent a biased sample of AD. Chromosome 21 mutations occur on three different sites (codons 670–671, 692–693, and 717). In pedigrees with codon 692 mutation (near the α-secretase site, within the Aβ domain), patients present with dementia and cerebral hemorrhages due to Aβ amyloid angiopathy and the diagnosis of familial AD has been made. Mutation at the next codon (693) is also associated with hereditary cerebral hemorrhage with amyloidosis. In these families, the diagnosis of hereditary cerebral hemorrhage with amyloidosis-Dutch type (HCHWA-D) has been made.[389] In some clinicopathologic reports on PS-1 and PS-2 gene mutation–associated AD, Lewy bodies and amyloid angiopathy were present[428,633–636]

The most potent genetic risk factor is the Apo E genotype ε4, which has been implicated in early and late-onset, sporadic, and familial AD.[637,638] This glycosylated protein of 299 amino acids is a constituent of several plasma lipoproteins playing a rôle in cholesterol transport and interacting with specific receptors. Apo E epitopes have also been found in cerebral amyloid deposits and NFTs.[317,318,639] Apo E is coded by a gene located on chromosome 19. Three major isoforms (Apo E2, Apo E3, and Apo E4) that differ by only two amino acids are produced by the three homologous alleles (Apo E ε2, ε3, and ε4). Apo E4, present in SPs and amyloid angiopathy,[639] is more frequent in both familial and sporadic AD than in the general population.[640,641] The number of plaques and of NFTs is increased in Apo E-ε4 cases. This holds true for diffuse deposits of Aβ,[642] even in nondemented patients.[314] An increased frequency of the Apo E4 allele has also been found in some studies of vascular dementia and in Lewy body–associated dementia, where it is seen only in those cases with predominant AD pathology.[643] Apo E2 may have a protective effect.[644-646] Recently, it has been reported that over-representation of Apo E-ε2 in cerebral amyloid angiopathy may result from its association with fibrinoid necrosis, which would increase the prevalence of cases revealed by a cerebral hemorrhage.[647]

Other yet unidentified mutations or genetic risk factors are likely. A genomic screen in families affected with late-onset AD identified four regions of interest. Chromosome 12 gave the strongest and most consistent results, suggesting that this region contains a new susceptibility gene for AD.[648]

Twin studies suggest that environmental factors play a role in AD. In 22 twin pairs (in 4 cases, the diagnosis was confirmed at autopsy), 7 monozygotic pairs were concordant for AD and 3 were discordant (concordance rate: 40%). Although the difficulties mentioned for the other genetic studies must be kept in mind, this study supports the belief that, etiologically, AD cannot be entirely accounted for by a genetic mechanism.[649]

Some authors suggest that the accumulation of aluminum in the brain is the cause of NFTs and dementia.[650,651] The data concerning the presence of aluminum in the brain of AD cases are conflicting.[652-654] In addition, the cytoskeleton lesions in the neurons of aluminum-intoxicated animals contain abnormal tau proteins,[259] but the neurofibrillary changes are composed of 10 nm–diameter filaments, which ultrastructurally resemble normal neurofilaments and thus are different from the PHFs of AD. Other agents have also been incriminated, including exposure to solvent that is strongly associated with dementia,[655] or electrical occupation and magnetic field exposure, for which the associations are modest.[656] Whether these are risk factors for AD or for dementia of another cause remains to be elucidated. Other hypotheses, such as the role of chronic low-level exposure to lead in early life[657] or that of combined aluminum intoxication with Ca-Mg deficiencies,[658] have yet to be demonstrated. *Head injury* has been repeatedly reported to be a risk factor for AD, but this remains debated.[6] Although some studies indicate an association with Apo E-ε4,[659] others suggest that these risk factors are independent.[660] *Vascular risk factors* and decreased cerebral blood flow have recently been emphasized (see Mixed Dementia, above and Chapter 6). An *infectious agent*, possibly an unconventional agent or Prion, has also been suspected as participating in the mechanism of AD because the features bear some resemblance in both pathologies. This seems unlikely, since scrapie-associated fibers (characteristic of unconventional infections, kuru, Creutzfeldt-Jakob disease, the Gerstmann-Sträussler-Scheinker syndrome in human and of scrapie in animal) have not been seen in AD. In addition, the Prion protein (PrP) making the amyloid fibers seen in these disorders is different from the Aβ protein found in AD. Lastly, none of the many transmission studies has been positive in AD.[661] Interestingly, however, in some Gerstmann-Sträussler-Scheinker cases, the density of NFTs is higher than would be expected from the age of the patient, and labeling of some plaques or amyloid angiopathies by antibodies against both Aβ and PrP can be seen.[383,384]

The protective influence of a few environmental factors has been demonstrated, especially estrogen therapy (see review,[5,662-664]), nonsteroidal anti-inflammatory drugs,[662,664a] and antioxydants, including vitamin E and selegiline therapy.[5,662] Other reported protective factors remain debated—for example, smoking,[6,665,666] and high educational level,[6,667,668]—or have yet to be confirmed, for example, low-dose alcohol consumption, especially of red wine,[669,670] or treatment by benzodiazepine.[671]

Could AD be due to an accelerated aging process alone? Age is the highest risk factor for AD. However in a few studies, the prevalence of dementia in the oldest-old (over 90) seems to reach a plateau.[627] In addition, neuronal atrophy and loss, plaques, tangles, amyloid angiopathy, granulovacuolar degeneration, and Hirano bodies are found with a density that increases with age in the brain of nondemented old people. However, they do not reach the density found in AD and cases difficult to identify as AD or normal aging are, on the whole, rare. Despite the fact that the severity of lesions is usually less marked among the elderly with SDAT than in younger cases, significant differences in the density of lesions are detectable between that found in very old AD brain and that in age-matched controls.[97,672] This is still the case in centenarians.[241,242,673,674] It has been proposed that a threshold value for these changes[675] or for some of them, such as neuronal atrophy and loss, must be exceeded before dementia appears. This would explain why easily recognizable lesions (positive changes such as plaques and tangles) are usually less marked in late-onset AD than in early-onset cases. Since most elderly people, even the very old, do not reach these threshold values,[241] aging alone is not likely the cause of AD. Some changes due to age, such as lipofuscin storage, are not linked to dementia. Some constituents of the aging process may thus contribute to the development of dementia of the Alzheimer type, but other factors (genetic and/or environmental) would be needed to develop the disease.

We thank Dr. A. Alpérovitch for valuable suggestions.

REFERENCES

1. Alzheimer A. Uber eine eigenartige Erkrankung der Hirnrinde. Allgemeine Zeitschr Psychiatr Gericht Med 1907; 64:146–148.
2. Evans DA, Funkenstein HH, Albert MS, et al. Prevalence of Alzheimer's disease in a community population of older persons; higher than previously reported. JAMA 1989; 262:2251–2556.
3. Jorm A, Jolley D. The incidence of dementia: a meta-analysis. Neurology 1998; 51:728–733.
4. Katzman R, Kawas CH. The epidemiology of dementia and Alzheimer disease. In: Terry RD, Katzman R, Bick KL, eds. Alzheimer Disease. New York: Raven Press, 1993; pp. 105–122.
5. Hendrie H. Epidemiology of dementia and Alzheimer's disease. Am J Geriatr Psychiatry 1998; 6(Suppl 1):S3–S18.
6. Launer L, Andersen K, Deweyn M, et al. Rates and risk factors for dementia and Alzheimer's disease: results from EURODEM pooled analyses. EURODEM Incidence Research Group and Work Groups. European Studies of Dementia. Neurology 1999; 52:78–84.
7. Berg L, Morris J. Diagnosis. In Terry RD, Katzman R, Bick KL eds. Alzheimer Disease. New York: Raven Press, 1994; pp. 7–25.
8. Cummings J, Vinters H, Cole G, et al. Alzheimer's disease: etiologies, pathophysiology, cognitive reserve, and treatment opportunities. Neurology 1998; 51:S2–S17.
9. American Association of Psychiatry. Diagnostic and Statistical Manual of Mental Disorders IV. Washington, DC: American Association of Psychiatry, 1994.
10. Mega MS, Cummings JL, Fiorello T, et al. The spectrum of behavioral changes in Alzheimer's disease. Neurology 1996; 46:130–135.
11. McKhann G, Drachman D, Folstein M, et al. Clinical diagnosis of Alzheimer's disease: report of the NINCDS-ADRDA work group under the auspices of Department of Health and Human Services Task Force on Alzheimer's disease. Neurology 1984; 19:939–944.
12. Katzman R, Lasker B, Berstein N. Advances in the diagnosis of dementia: accuracy of diagnosis and consequences of misdiagnosis of disorders causing dementia. In: Terry RD, ed. Aging and the Brain. New York: Raven Press, 1988; pp. 17–62.
13. Joachim CL, Morris JH, Selkoe DJ. Clinically diagnosed Alzheimer's disease: autopsy results in 150 cases. Ann Neurol 1988; 24:50–56.
14. Morris JC, McKeel DW, Fulling K, et al. Validation of clinical diagnostic criteria for Alzheimer's disease. Ann Neurol 1988; 24:17–22.
15. Bowler J, Munoz D, Merskey H, et al. Fallacies in the pathological confirmation of the diagnosis of Alzheimer's disease. J. Neurol Neurosurg Psychiatry 1998; 64:18–24.
16. Gearing M, Mirra S, Hedreen J, et al. The consortium to establish a registry for Alzheimer's disease (CERAD), Part X: neuropathology confirmation of the clinical diagnosis of Alzheimer's disease. Neurology 1995; 45:461–466.
17. Lim A, Tsuang D, Kukull W, et al. Clinico-neuropathological correlation of Alzheimer's disease in a community-based case series. J Am Geriatr Soc 1999; 47:564–569.
18. Delay J. Brion S. Les Démences Tardives. Paris: Masson, 1962.
19. Terry RD. Alzheimer's disease. In: Davis L, Robertson DM, eds. Neuropathology. Baltimore: Williams & Wilkins, 1985; pp. 824–841.
20. Constantinidis J. Is Alzheimer's disease a major form of senile dementia? Clinical, anatomical and genetic data. In: Katzman R, Terry RD, Bick KL, eds. Alzheimer's Disease: Senile Dementia and Related Disorders. New York: Raven Press, 1978; pp. 15–25.
21. Roth M, Wischik CM. The heterogeneity of Alzheimer's disease and its implications for scientific investigations of the disorder. In: Arie T, ed. Recent Advances in Psychogeriatrics. Edinburgh: Churchill Livingstone, 1985; pp. 71–92.
22. Selnes OA, Carson K, Rovner B, et al. Language dysfunction in early- and late-onset possible Alzheimer's disease. Neurology 1988; 38:1053–1056.
23. Amaducci LA, Rocca WA, Schoenberg BS. Origin of the distinction between Alzheimer's disease and senile

dementia: how history can clarify nosology. Neurology 1986; 36:1497–1499.
24. Braak H, Braak E. Frequency of stages of Alzheimer-related lesions in different age categories. Neurobiol Aging 1997; 18:351–357.
25. Galen RS, Gambino SR. Beyond Normality: the Predictive Value and Efficiency of Medical Diagnoses. New York: Churchill Livingstone, 1975; 237.
26. Duyckaerts C, Bennecib M, Grignon Y, et al. Modeling the relation between neurofibrillary tangles and intellectual status. Neurobiol Aging 1997; 18:267–273.
27. Price JL, Morris JC. Tangles and plaques in nondemented aging and "preclinical" Alzheimer's disease. Ann Neurol 1999; 45:358–368.
28. Troncoso JC, Cataldo AM, Nixon RA, et al. Neuropathology of preclinical and clinical late-onset Alzheimer's disease. Ann Neurol 1998; 43:673–676.
29. Almkvist O, Basun H, Backman L, et al. Mild cognitive impairment-an early stage of Alzheimer's disease? J Neural Transm Suppl 1998; 54:21–29.
30. Dickson DW, Crystal HA, Mattiace LA, et al. Identification of normal and pathological aging in prospectively studied nondemented elderly humans. Neurobiol Aging 1991; 13:179–189.
31. Adolfsson R, Gottfries CG, Nyström L, et al. Prevalence of dementia disorders in institutionalized Swedish old people. Acta Psychiatr Scand 1981; 631:225–244.
32. Tomlinson BE, Blessed G, Roth M. Observation on the brains of demented old people. J. Neurol Med 1970; 11:205–242.
33. DeArmond S, Dickson D, DeArmond B. Degenerative diseases of the central nervous system. In: Davis R, Robertson D, eds. Textbook of Neuropathology. Baltimore: Williams & Wilkins, 1997: pp. 1063–1178.
34. Esiri MM, Hyman BT, Beyreuther K, et al. Ageing and dementia. In: Graham DI, Lantos P, eds. Greenfield's Neuropathology. London: Arnold, 1997: pp. 153–234.
35. Pakkenberg H, Voigt J. Brain weight of the Danes. A forensic material. Acta Anat 1964; 56:297–307.
36. Miller AKH, Corsellis JAN. Evidence for a secular increase in human brain weight during the past century. Ann Hum Biol 1977; 253–257.
37. Dekaban AS, Sadowsky D. Changes in brain weight during the span of human life: relation of brain weight to body height and body weight. Ann Neurol 1978; 4: 345–356.
38. Miller AKH, Alston RL, Corsellis JAN. Variations with age in the volumes of gray and white matter in the cerebral hemispheres of man: measurements with an image analyser. Neuropathol Appl Neurobiol 1980; 6:119–132.
39. Terry RD, DeTeresa R, Hansen LA. Neocortical cell counts in normal human adult aging. Ann Neurol 1987; 21:530–539.
40. Davis PJM, Wright EA. A new method for measuring cranial capacity volume and its application to the assessment of cerebral atrophy at autopsy. Neuropathol Appl Neurobiol 1977; 3:341–358.
41. Kemper T. Neuroanatomical and neuropathological changes in normal aging and dementia. In: Albert LM, ed. Clinical Neurology of Aging. New York: Oxford University Press, 1984 pp. g–52.
42. Tomlinson BE. Ageing and the dementias. In: Hume Adams J, Duchen LW, eds. Greenfied's Neuropathology, 5th ed. London: Edward Arnold, 1992; pp. 1284–1410.
43. Najlerahim A, Bowen DM. Regional weight loss in the cerebral cortex and some subcortical nuclei in senile dementia of the Alzheimer type. Acta Neuropathol (Berl) 1989; 75:509–512.
44. Tomlinson BE, Blessed G, Roth M. Observation on the brains of non-demented old people. J Neurol Sci 1968; 7:331–356.
45. Jacoby RJ, Levy R. Computed tomography in the elderly II: senile dementia: diagnosis and functional impairment. Br J Psychiatry 1980; 136:256–269.
46. Jack CJ, Petersen R, Xu Y, et al. Prediction of AD with MRI-based hippocampal volume in mild cognitive impairment. Neurology 1999; 52:1397–1403.
47. Jack CJ, Petersen R, Xu Y, et al. Rate of medial temporal lobe atrophy in typical aging and Alzheimer's disease. Neurology 1998; 51:993–999.
48. Hubbard BM, Anderson JM. A quantitative study of cerebral atrophy in old age and senile dementia. J Neurol Sci 1981; 50:135–145.
49. Mann DMA. The topographic distribution of brain atrophy in Alzheimer's disease. Acta Neuropathol (Berl) 1991; 83:81–86.
50. Poppe W, Tennstedt A. Studie über hirnatrophische Prozesse unter besondere Berücksichtigung des Morbus Pick und des Morbus Alzheimer. Jena: Fischer, 1969.
51. De La Monte S. Quantitation of cerebral atrophy in preclinical and end-stage Alzheimer's disease. Ann Neurol 1989; 25:450–459.
52. Pogacar S, Williams RS. Alzheimer's disease presenting as slowly progressive aphasia. RI Med J 1984; 67: 181–185.
53. Mesulam MM. Primary progressive aphasia: differentiation from Alzheimer's disease. Ann Neurol 1987; 22:533–534.
54. Benson DF. Posterior cortical atrophy: a new entity or Alzheimer's disease? Arch Neurol 1989; 46:843–844.
55. Tomlinson BE, Corsellis JAN. Ageing and the dementias. In: Humes Adams J, Corsellis JAN, Duchen, LW, eds. Greenfield's Neuropathology. London: Edward Arnold, 1984: pp. 951–1025.
56. Duyckaerts C, Hauw J-J, Piette F, et al. Cortical atrophy in senile dementia of the Alzheimer type is mainly due to a decrease in cortical length. Acta Neuropathol (Berl) 1985; 66:72–74.
57. Morel F, Wildi E. Contribution à la connaissance des différentes altérations cérébrales du grand âge. Arch Suisse Neurol Psychiatrie 1955; 76:174–222.
58. Hubbard BM, Anderson JM. Age, senile dementia and ventricular enlargement. J Neurol Neurosurg Psychiatry 1981; 44:631–635.
59. DeCarli C, Kaye JA, Horwitz B, et al. Critical analysis of the use of computer-assisted transverse axial tomography to study human brain in aging and dementia of the Alzheimer type. Neurology 1990; 40:872–883.
60. Luxenberg JS, Haxby JV, Creasey H, et al. Rate of ventricular enlargement in dementia of the Alzheimer type correlates with rate of neuropsychological deterioration. Neurology 1987; 37:1135–1140.
61. Agduhr E. A contribution to the technique of determining the number of nerve cells per volume unit of tissue. Anat Rec 1941; 80:191–202.

62. Abercrombie M. Estimation of nuclear populations from microtome sections. Anat Rec 1946; 94:239–247.
63. Sterio DC. The unbiased estimation of number and sizes of arbitrary particles using the disector. J Microsc 1984; 134:127–136.
64. West MJ. Stereological methods for estimating the total number of neurons and synapses: issues of precision and bias. Trends Neurosci 1999; 22:51–61.
65. Duyckaerts C, Delaère P, Costa C, et al. Factors influencing neuronal density on sections: quantitative data obtained by computer simulation. In: Conn, PM, ed. Computers and Computations in the Neurosciences. San Diego: Academic Press, 1993: pp. 526–548.
66. Gundersen HJG, Jensen EB. The efficiency of systematic sampling in stereology and its prediction. J Microsc 1987; 147:229–263.
67. Ball MJ. Neuronal loss, neurofibrillary tangles and granulovascuolar degeneration in the hippocampus with ageing and dementia. Acta Neuropathol (Berl) 1977; 37:111–118.
68. Dam AM. The density of neurons in the human hippocampus. Neuropathol Appl Neurobiol 1979; 5:249–264.
69. West MJ, Coleman PD, Flood DG, et al. Differences in the pattern of hippocampal neuronal loss in normal aging and Alzheimer disease. Lancet 1994; 344:769–772.
70. West MJ. Regionally specific loss of neurons in the aging human hippocampus. Neurobiol Aging 1993; 14:287–293.
71. Brody H. Organization of cerebral cortex. III. A study of aging in the human cerebral cortex. J Comp Neurol 1955; 102:511–556.
72. Haug H, Barmwater U, Eggers R, et al. Anatomical changes in aging brain: morphometric analysis of the human prosencephalon. In: Cervos-Navarro J, Sarkander H-I, eds. Brain Aging: Neuropathology and Neuropharmacology (Aging, Vol. 21). New York: Raven Press, 1983: pp. 1–12.
73. Henderson G. Tomlinson BE, Gibson PH. Cell counts in human cerebral cortex in normal adults throughout life using an image analysing machine. Neurol Sci 1980; 46:113–136.
74. Duyckaerts C, Llamas E, Delaère P, et al. Neuronal loss and neuronal atrophy. Computer simulation in connection with Alzheimer's disease. Brain Res 1989; 504:94–100.
75. Pakkenberg B, Gundersen HJG. Neocortical neuron number in humans: effect of sex and age. J Comp Neurol 1997; 384:312–320.
76. Brody H. Cell counts in cerebral cortex and brainstem in Alzheimer's disease. In: Katzman R, Terry RD, Bick KL, eds. Senile Dementia and Related Disorders. New York: Raven Press, 1978: pp. 345–351.
77. Burns BD. The Mammalian Cerebral Cortex. London: Edward Arnold, 1958.
78. Vijayashankar N, Brody H. A study of aging in the human abducens nucleus. J Comp Neurol 1977; 173:433–438.
79. Vijayashankar N, Brody H. The neuronal population of the nuclei of the trochlear nerve and the locus coeruleus in the human. Anat Rec 1973;172:421–422.
80. Konigsmark BW, Murphy EA. Volume of ventral cochlear nucleus in man: its relationship to neuronal population and age. J Neuropathol Exp Neurol 1972; 31:304–316.
81. Monagle RD, Brody H. The effects of age upon the main nucleus of the inferior olive in the human. J Comp Neurol 1974; 155:61–66.
82. Vijayashankar N, Brody H. A quantitative study of the pigmented neurons in the nuclei coeruleus and subcoeruleus in man as related to aging. J Neuropathol Exp Neurol 1979; 38:490–497.
83. Mouton PR, Pakkenberg B, Gundersen HJ, et al. Absolute number and size of pigmented locus coeruleus neurons in young and aged individuals. J Chem Neuroanat 1994; 7:185–190.
84. Ohm TGB, H Busch C, Bohl J. Unbiased estimation of neuronal numbers in the human nucleus coeruleus during aging. Neurobiol Aging 1997; 18:393–399.
85. Hall TC, Miller AKH, Corsellis JAN. Variation in human Purkinje cell population according to age and sex. Neuropathol Appl Neurobiol 1975; 1:267–292.
86. Fearnley JM, Lees AJ. Ageing and Parkinson's disease: substantia nigra regional selectivity. Brain 1991; 114:2283–2301.
87. Mann DMA, Yates PO. The effects of ageing on the pigmented nerve cells of the human locus coeruleus and substantia nigra. Acta Neuropathol (Berl) 1979; 47:93–97.
88. McGeer PL, McGeer EG, Suzuki PS. Aging and extrapyramidal function. Arch Neurol 1977; 34:33–35.
89. Brody H, Vijayashankar N. Anatomical changes in the nervous system. In: Finch, CE, Hayflick, L, eds. Handbook of the Biology of Aging. New York: Van Nostrand, 1977. pp. 241–261.
90. Bugiani O, Salvarani S, Perdelli F, et al. Nerve cell loss with aging in the putamen. Eur Neurol 1978; 17:286–291.
91. Herzog AG, Kemper TL. Amygdaloid changes in aging and dementia. Arch Neurol 1980; 37:625–629.
92. de Lacalle S, Iraizoz I, Ma Gonzalo L. Differential changes in cell size and number in topographic subdivisions of human basal nucleus in normal aging. Neuroscience 1991; 43:445–456.
93. Szenborn M. Neuropathological study on the nucleus basalis of Meynert in mature and old age. Patol Pol 1993; 44:211–216.
94. Cras P, Smith MA, Richey PL, et al. Extracellular neurofibrillary tangles reflect neuronal loss and provide further evidence of extensive protein cross-linking in Alzheimer disease. Acta Neuropathol (Berl) 1995; 89:291–295.
95. Gomez-Isla T, Price JL, McKeel DW, et al. Profound loss of layer II entorhinal cortex neurons occurs in very mild Alzheimer's disease. J Neurosci 1996; 16:4491–4500.
96. Terry RD, Peck A, DeTeresa R, et al. Some morphometric aspects of the brain in senile dementia of the Alzheimer type. Ann Neurol 1981; 10:184–192.
97. Hansen LA, DeTeresa R, Davies P, et al. Neocortical morphometry, lesion counts, and choline acetyltransferase levels in the age spectrum of Alzheimer's disease. Neurology 1988; 38:48–54.
98. Mann DMA, Yates PO, Marcyniuk B. Some morphometric observations on the cerebral cortex and hippocampus in presenile Alzheimer's disease, senile dementia of Alzheimer type and Down's syndrome in middle age. J Neurol Sci 1985; 69:139–159.
99. Mountjoy CQ. Correlations between neuropathologi-

cal and neurochemical changes. Br Med Bull 1986; 42:81–85.
100. Regeur L, Badsberg Jensen G, Pakkenberg H, et al. No global neocortical nerve cell loss in brains from patients with senile dementia of Alzheimer's type. Neurobiol Aging 1994; 15:347–352.
101. Flood DG. Thoughts on no neocortical neuronal loss but loss of volume in AD. Neurobiol Aging 1994; 15:363–365.
102. Hyman BT, Gomez-Isla T. Alzheimer disease is a laminar, regional, and neural system specific disease, not a global brain disease. Neurobiol Aging 1994; 15:353–354.
103. Mann DMA. Pathological correlates of dementia in Alzheimer's disease. Neurobiol Aging 1944; 15:357–360.
104. Mufson EJ, Benzing WC. Lack of neocortical nerve cell loss in Alzheimer's disease: reality or methodological artifact. Neurobiol Aging 1994; 15:379–380.
105. Gomez-Isla T, Hollister R, West H, et al. Neuronal loss correlates with but exceeds neurofibrillary tangles in Alzheimer's disease. Ann Neurol 1997; 41:17–24.
106. Grignon Y, Duyckaerts C, Bennecib M, et al. Cytoarchitectonic alterations in supramarginal gyrus of late onset Alzheimer's disease. Acta Neuropathol (Berl) 1998; 95:395–406.
107. Duyckaerts C, Godefroy G, Hauw J-J. Evaluation of neuronal numerical density by Dirichlet tessellation. J Neurosci Methods 1994; 51:47–69.
108. Hyman BT, Van Hoesen GW, Damasio AR, et al. Alzheimer's disease: cell-specific pathology isolates the hippocampal formation. Science 1984; 225:1168–1170.
109. Duyckaerts C, Delaère P, Hauw J-J. Alzheimer's disease and neuroanatomy: hypotheses and proposals. In: Boller F, Forette F, Khachaturian Z, Poncet M, Christen Y, eds. Heterogeneity of Alzheimer's Disease. Berlin: Springer-Verlag, 1992: pp. 144–155.
110. Delacoste MC, White CL. The role of connectivity in Alzheimer's disease pathogenesis. A review and model system. Neurobiol Aging 1993; 14:1–16.
111. Esiri MM, Wilcock GK. The olfactory bulb in Alzheimer's disease. J Neurol Neurosurg Psychiatry 1984; 47:56–60.
112. ter Laak HJ, Renkawek K, van Workum FP. The olfactory bulb in Alzheimer disease: a morphologic study of neuron loss, tangles, and senile plaques in relation to olfaction. Alzheimer Dis Assoc Disord 1994; 8:38–48.
113. Vogels OJ, Broere CA, Nieuwenhuys R. Neuronal hypertrophy in the human supraoptic and paraventricular nucleus in aging and Alzheimer's disease. Neurosci Lett 1990; 109:62–67.
114. Mann DMA, Yates PO, Marcyniuk B. Changes in Alzheimer's disease in the magnocellular neurones of the supraoptic and paraventricular nuclei of the hypothalamus and their relationship to the noradrenergic deficit. Clin Neuropathol 1985; 4:127–134.
115. Fliers E, Swaab DF, Pool CW, et al. The vasopressin and oxytocin neurons in the human supraoptic and paraventricular nucleus; changes with aging and in senile dementia. Brain Res 1985; 342:45–53.
116. Swaab DF, Fliers E, Partiman TS. The suprachiasmatic nucleus of the human brain in relation to sex, age and senile dementia. Brain Res 1985; 342:37–44.
117. Kremer B, Swaab D, Bots G, et al. The hypothalamic lateral tuberal nucleus in Alzheimer's disease. Ann Neurol 1991; 29:279–284.
118. Vereecken TH, Vogels OJ, Nieuwenhuys R. Neuron loss and shrinkage in the amygdala in Alzheimer's disease. Neurobiol Aging 1994; 15:45–54.
119. Höhman C, Antuono P, Coyle JT. Basal forebrain cholinergic neurons and Alzheimer's disease. In: Iversen LL, Iversen SD, Snyder SH, eds. Psychopharmacology of the Aging Nervous System. New York: Plenum Press, 1988: pp. 69–106.
120. Whitehouse PJ, Price DL, Clark AW, et al. Alzheimer disease: evidence for selective loss of cholinergic neurons in the nucleus basalis. Ann Neurol 1981; 10:122–126.
121. Whitehouse PJ, Hedreen JC, White CL, et al. Basal forebrain neurons in the dementia of Parkinson disease. Ann Neurol 1983; 13:243–248.
122. Gilmor ML, Erickson JD, Varoqui H, et al. Preservation of nucleus basalis neurons containing choline acetyltransferase and the vesicular acetylcholine transporter in the elderly with mild cognitive impairment and early Alzheimer's disease. J Comp Neurol 1999; 411:693–704.
123. Doucette R, Fishman M, Hachinski VC, et al. Cell loss from the nucleus basalis of Meynert in Alzheimer's disease. Can J Neurol Sci 1986; 13:435–440.
124. Lehericy S, Hirsch EC, Cervera-Pierot P, et al. Heterogeneity and selectivity of the degeneration of cholinergic neurons in the basal forebrain of patients with Alzheimer's disease. J Comp Neurol 1993; 330:15–31.
125. Vogels OJ, Broere CA, ter Laak HJ, et al. Cell loss and shrinkage in the nucleus basalis Meynert complex in Alzheimer's disease. Neurobiol Aging 1990; 11:3–13.
126 Salehi A, Lucassen PJ, Pool CW, et al. Decreased neuronal activity in the nucleus basalis of Meynert in Alzheimer's disease as suggested by the size of the Golgi apparatus. Neuroscience 1994; 59:871–880.
127. Busch C, Bohl J, Ohm TG. Spatial, temporal and numeric analysis of Alzheimer changes in the nucleus coeruleus. Neurobiol Aging 1997; 18:401–416.
128. German DC, Manaye KF, White CLD, et al. Disease-specific patterns of locus coeruleus cell loss. Ann Neurol 1992; 32:667–676.
129. Marcyniuk B, Mann DMA, Yates PO. The topography of cell loss from locus coeruleus in Alzheimer's disease. J Neurol Sci 1986; 76:335–345.
130. Hoogendijk WJ, Feenstra MG, Botterblom MH, et al. Increased activity of surviving locus ceruleus neurons in Alzheimer's disease. Ann Neurol 1999; 45:82–91.
131. Aletrino MA, Vogels OJ, Van Domburg PH, et al. Cell loss in the nucleus raphes dorsalis in Alzheimer's disease. Neurobiol Aging 1992; 13:461–468.
132. Curcio CA, Kemper T. Nucleus raphe dorsalis in dementia of the Alzheimer type: neuronal changes and neuronal packing density. J Neuropathol Exp Neurol 1984; 43:359–368.
133. Yamamoto T, Hirano A. Nucleus raphe dorsalis in Alzheimer's disease: neurofibrillary tangles and loss of large neurons. Ann Neurol 1985; 17:573–577.
134. Zweig RM, Ross CA, Hedreen JC, et al. The neu-

ropathology of aminergic nuclei in Alzheimer's disease. Ann Neurol 1988; 24:233–242.
135. Hoogendijk WJ, Sommer IE, Pool CW, et al. Lack of association between depression and loss of neurons in the locus coeruleus in Alzheimer disease. Arch Gen Psychiatry 1999; 56:45–51.
136. Gibb WR, Mountjoy CQ, Mann DM, et al. The substantia nigra and ventral tegmental area in Alzheimer's disease and Down's syndrome. J Neurol Neurosurg Psychiatry 1989; 52:193–200.
137. Uchihara T, Kondo H, Ikeda K, et al. Alzheimer-type pathology in melanin-bleached sections of substantia nigra. J Neurol 1995; 242:485–489.
138. Uchihara T, Kondo H, Kosaka K, et al. Selective loss of nigral neurons in Alzheimer's disease: a morphometric study. Acta Neuropathol (Berl) 1992; 83:271–276.
139. Mann DMA. Neuropathology and neurochemical aspects of Alzheimer's disease. In: Iversen LL, Iversen SD, Snyder SH, eds. Psychopharmacology of the Aging Nervous System, Handbook of Psychopharmacology. New York: Plenum Press, 1988: pp. 1–67.
140. German DC, White CL, Sparkman DR. Alzheimer's disease: neurofibrillary changes in nuclei that project to the cerebral cortex. Neuroscience 1987; 21:305–312.
141. Blanks JC, Hinton DR, Sadun AA, et al. Retinal ganglion cell degeneration in Alzheimer's disease. Brain Res 1989; 501:364–372.
142. Blanks JC, Torigoe Y, Hinton DR, et al. Retinal pathology in Alzheimer's disease. I. Ganglion cell loss in foveal/parafoveal retina. Neurobiol Aging 1996; 17:377–384.
143. Blanks JC, Schmidt SY, Torigoe Y, et al. Retinal pathology in Alzheimer's disease. II. Regional neuron loss and glial changes in GCL. Neurobiol Aging 1996; 17:385–395.
144. Curcio CA, Drucker DN. Retinal ganglion cells in Azheimer disease and aging. Ann Neurol 1993; 33:248–257.
145. Hinton DR, Sadum AA, Blanks JC, et al. Optic-nerve degeneration in Alzheimer's disease. N Engl J Med 1986; 315:485–487.
146. Schultz C, Braak H, Braak E. A sex difference in neurodegeneration of the human hypothalamus. Neurosci Lett 1996; 212:103–106.
147. Schultz C, Ghebremedhin E, Braak H, et al. Neurofibrillary pathology in the human paraventricular and supraoptic nuclei. Acta Neuropathol (Berl) 1997; 94:99–102.
148. Cotman CW, Anderson AJ. A potential role for apoptosis in neurodegeneration and Alzheimer's disease. Mol Neurobiol 1995; 10:19–45.
149. Mullaart E, Boerrigter ME, Ravid R, et al. Increased levels of DNA breaks in cerebral cortex of Alzheimer's disease patients. Neurobiol Aging 1990; 11:169–173.
150. Dragunow M, Faull RL, Lawlor P, et al. In situ evidence for DNA fragmentation in Huntington's disease striatum and Alzheimer's disease temporal lobes. NeuroReport 1995; 6:1053–1057.
151. Lassmann H, Bancher C, Breitschopf H, et al. Cell death in Alzheimer's disease evaluated by DNA fragmentation in situ. Acta Neuropathol (Berl) 1995; 89:35–41.
152. Lucassen PJ, Chung WC, Kamphorst W, et al. DNA damage distribution in the human brain as shown by in situ end labeling; area-specific differences in aging and Alzheimer disease in the absence of apoptotic morphology. J Neuropathol Exp Neurol 1997; 56:887–900.
153. Migheli A, Cavalla P, Marino S, et al. A study of apoptosis in normal and pathologic nervous tissue after in situ end-labeling of DNA strand breaks. J Neuropathol Exp Neurol 1994; 53:606–616.
154. MacGibbon GA, Lawlor PA, Walton M, et al. Expression of Fos, Jun, and Krox family proteins in Alzheimer's disease. Exp Neurol 1997; 147:316–332.
155. Stadelmann C, Bruck W, Bancher C, et al. Alzheimer disease: DNA fragmentation indicates increased neuronal vulnerability, but not apoptosis. J Neuropathol Exp Neurol 1998; 57:456–464.
156. Nagy Z, Esiri MM, Smith AD. The cell division cycle and the pathophysiology of Alzheimer's disease. Neuroscience 1998; 87:731–739.
157. Glenner GG. Amyloid deposits and amyloidosis. The β-fibrilloses. N Engl J Med 1980; 302:1283–1292.
158. Schweers O, Schonbrunn-Hanebeck E, Marx A, et al. Structural studies of tau protein and Alzheimer paired helical filaments show no evidence for beta-structure. J Biol Chem 1994; 269:24290–24297.
159. Rosenblum WI. The presence, origin, and significance of A beta peptide in the cell bodies of neurons. J Neuropathol Exp Neurol 1999; 58:575–581.
160. Itoh Y, Amano N, Inoue M, et al. Scanning electron microscopical study of the neurofibrillary tangles of Alzheimer's disease. Acta Neuropathol (Berl) 1997; 94:78–86.
161. Crowther RA, Wishik CM. Image reconstruction of the Alzheimer's paired helical filament. EMBO J 1985; 4:3661–3665.
162. Kidd M. Paired helical filaments in electron microscopy in Alzheimer's disease. Nature 1963; 197:262–268.
163. Kidd M. Alzheimer's disease. An electron microscopic study. Brain 1964; 87:307–320.
164. Wisniewski HM, Narang NK, Corsellis JAN, et al. Ultrastructural studies of the neuropil and neurofibrillary tangles in Alzheimer's disease and posttraumatic dementia. J Neuropathol Exp Neurol 1976; 35:367 (abstr).
165. Wischik CM, Crowther RA, Stewart M, et al. Subunit structure of paired helical filaments in Alzheimer's disease. J Cell Biol 1985; 100:1905–1912.
166. Pollanen MS, Markiewicz P, Goh MC. Paired helical filaments are twisted ribbons composed of two parallel and aligned components: image reconstruction and modeling of filament structure using atomic force microscopy. J Neuropathol Exp Neurol 1997; 56:79–85.
167. Ruben GC, Iqbal K, Grundke-Iqbal I. Helical ribbon morphology in neurofibrillary tangles of paired helical filaments. In: Iqbal K, Mortimer JA, Winblad B, Wisniewski HM, eds. Research Advances in Alzheimer's Disease and Related Disorders. Chichester: John Wiley & Sons, 1995: pp. 477–485.
168. Miyakawa T, Katsuragi S, Yamashita K, et al. Morphological investigation of neurofibrillary tangles in Alzheimer's disease. Jpn J Psychiatr Neurol 1994; 48:43–47.
169. Flament-Durand J, Couck AM. Spongiform altera-

tions in brain biopsies of presenile dementia. Acta Neuropathol (Berl) 1979; 46:159–162.
170. Gray EG. Spongiform encephalopathy: a neurocytologist's viewpoint with a note on Alzheimer's disease. Neuropathol Appl Neurobiol 1986; 12:149–172.
171. Hempen B, Brion JP. Reduction of acetylated alpha-tubulin immunoreactivity in neurofibrillary tangle-bearing neurons in Alzheimer's disease. J Neuropathol Exp Neurol 1996; 55:964–972.
172. Braak H, Braak E, Grundke-Iqbal I, et al. Occurrence of neuropil threads in the senile human brain and in Alzheimer's disease. A 3rd location of paired helical filaments outside of neurofilament tangles and neuritic plaques. Neurosci Lett 1986; 65:351–355.
173. Duyckaerts C, Kawasaki H, Delaère P, et al. Fiber disorganization in the neocortex of patients with senile dementia of the Alzheimer type. Neuropathol Appl Neurobiol 1989; 15:233–247.
174. Ohtsubo K, Izumiyama N, Kuzuhara S, et al. Curly fibers are tau-positive strands in the pre- and post-synaptic neurites, consisting of paired helical filaments: observations by the freeze-etch and replica method. Acta Neuropathol (Berl) 1990; 81:111–115.
175. Perry G, Kawai M, Tabaton M, et al. Neuropil threads of Alzheimer's disease show a marked alteration of the normal cytoskeleton. J Neurosci 1991; 11:1748–1755.
176. Selkoe DJ, Ihara Y, Salazar FJ. Alzheimer's disease: insolubility of partially purified paired helical filaments in sodium dodecyl sulfate and urea. Science 1982; 215:1243–1245.
177. Anderton BH, Breinburg D, Downes MJ, et al. Monoclonal antibodies show that neurofibrillary tangles and neurofilaments share antigenic determinants. Nature 1982; 298:84–86.
178. Perry G, Rizzuto N, Autilio-Gambetti L, et al. Paired helical filaments from Alzheimer disease patients contain cytoskeletal components. Proc Natl Acad Sci USA 1986; 82:3916–3920.
179. Brion JP, Couck AM, Passeirero E, et al. Neurofibrillary tangles in Alzheimer's disease: an immunohistochemical study. J Submicrosc Cytol 1985; 17:89–96.
180. Wolozin BL, Pruchnicki A, Dickson DW, et al. A neuronal antigen in the brain of Alzheimer patients. Science 1986; 232:648–652.
181. Wolozin B, Davies P. Alzheimer-related neuronal protein A68: specificity and distribution. Ann Neurol 1987; 22:521–526.
182. Duyckaerts C, Brion J-P, Hauw J-J, et al. Quantitative assessment of the density of neurofibrillary tangles and senile plaques in senile dementia of the Alzheimer type. Comparison of immunocytochemistry with a specific antibody and Bodian's protargol method. Acta Neuropathol (Berl) 1987; 73:167–170.
183. Brion JP, Hanger DP, Couck AM, et al. A68 proteins in Alzheimer's disease are composed of several tau isoforms in a phosphorylated state which affects their electrophoretic mobilities. Biochemistry 1991; 279:831–836.
184. Brion JP, Passareiro H, Nunez J, et al. Mise en évidence immunologique de la protéine tau au niveau des lésions de dégénérescence neurofibrillaire de la maladie d'Alzheimer. Arch Biol (Brux) 1985; 95:229–235.
185. Kowall NW, Kosik KS. Axonal disruption and aberrant localization of tau protein characterize the neuropil pathology of Alzheimer's disease. Ann Neurol 1987; 22:639–643.
186. Delacourte A, Defossez A. Alzheimer's disease: tau proteins, the promoting factors of microtubule assembly are major components of paired helical filaments. J Neurol Sci 1986; 76:173–186.
187. Kosik KS, Joachim CL, Selkoe DJ. Microtubule-associated protein tau is a major component of paired helical filaments in Alzheimer disease. Proc Natl Acad Sci USA 1986; 83:4044–4048.
188. Mandelkow EM, Mandelkow E. Tau in Alzheimer's disease. Trends Cell Biol 1998; 8:425–427.
189. Delacourte A. Tau pathology in aging and neurodegenerative disorders. Curr Res Alzheimer's Dis 1998; 3:228–235.
190. Goedert M, Trojanowski JQ, Lee VMY. Tau protein and the neurofibrillary pathology of Alzheimer's disease. In: Wasco W, Tanzi RE, eds. Molecular Mechanisms of Dementia. Totowa, NJ: Humana Press, 1996: pp. 199–21.
191. Spillantini MG, Goedert M. Tau protein pathology in neurodegenerative diseases. Trends Neurosci 1998; 21:428–433.
192. Matsuo ES, Shin RW, Billingsley ML, et al. Biopsy-derived adult human tau is phosphorylated at many of the same sites as Alzheimer's disease paired helical filament tau. Neuron 1994; 13:989–1002.
193. Sergeant N, Bussière T, Vermersch P, et al. Isoelectric point differentiates PHF-tau from biopsy-derived human brain tau proteins. NeuroReport 1995; 6:2217–2220.
194. Grundke-Iqbal I, Iqbal K, Tung YC, et al. Abnormal phosphorylation of the microtubule associated protein (tau) in Alzheimer cytoskeletal pathology. Proc Natl Acad Sci USA 1986; 83:4913–4917.
195. Bussiere T, Hof PR, Mailliot C, et al. Phosphorylated serine422 on tau proteins is a pathological epitope found in several diseases with neurofibrillary degeneration. Acta Neuropathol (Berl) 1999; 97:221–230.
196. Braak E, Braak H, Mandelkow EM. A sequence of cytoskeleton changes related to the formation of neurofibrillary tangles and neuropil threads. Acta Neuropathol (Berl) 1994; 87:554–567.
197. Braak E, Braak H. Alzheimer's disease: transiently developing dendritic changes in pyramidal cells of sector CA1 of the Ammon's horn. Acta Neuropathol (Berl) 1997; 93:323–325.
198. Schmidt ML, Murray JM, Trojanowski JQ. Continuity of neuropil threads with tangle-bearing and tangle-free neurons in Alzheimer disease cortex. Mol Chem Neuropathol 1993; 18:299–312.
199. Cummings BJ, Pike CJ, Shankle R, et al. β-amyloid deposition and other measures of neuropathology predict cognitive status in Alzheimer's disease. Neurobiol Aging. 1996; 17:921–933.
200. Lowe J, Blanchard A, Morrell K, et al. Ubiquitin is common factor in intermediate filament inclusion bodies of diverse type in man, including those of Parkinson's disease, Pick's disease, and Alzheimer's disease, as well as Rosenthal fibres in cerebellar astrocytomas, cytoplasmic bodies in muscle, and Mal-

lory bodies in alcoholic liver disease. J Pathol 1988; 155:9–15.
201. Bancher C, Grundke-Iqbal I, Iqbal K, et al. Abnormal phosphorylation of tau precedes ubiquitination in neurofibrillary pathology of Alzheimer disease. Brain Res 1991; 539:11–18.
202. Duyckaerts C, Colle M-A, Hauw J-J. A sketch of Alzheimer's disease histopathology. In: Iqbal K, Swaab DF, Winblad B, Wisniewski H, eds. Alzheimer's Disease and Related Disorders. Chichester: John Wiley & Sons, 1999: pp. 137–51.
203. Schwab C, Steele JC, McGeer EG, et al. Amyloid P immunoreactivity precedes C4d deposition on extracellular neurofibrillary tangles. Acta Neuropathol (Berl) 1997; 93:87–92.
204. de la Monte SM, Wands JR. Diagnostic utility of quantitating neurofilament-immunoreactive Alzheimer's disease lesions. J Histochem Cytochem 1994; 42:1625–1634.
205. Vickers JC, Riederer BM, Marugg RA, et al. Alterations in neurofilament protein immunoreactivity in human hippocampal neurons related to normal aging and Alzheimer's disease. Neuroscience 1994; 62:1–13.
206. Mesulam MM, Moran MA. Cholinesterases within neurofibrillary tangles related to age and Alzheimer's disease. Ann Neurol 1987; 22:223–228.
207. Dickson DW. The pathogenesis of senile plaques. J Neuropathol Exp Neurol 1997; 56:321–339.
208. Morsch R, Simon W, Coleman PD. Neurons may live for decades with neurofibrillary tangles. J Neuropathol Exp Neurol 1999; 58:188–197.
209. Morrison JH, Lewis DA, Campbell MJ et al. A monoclonal antibody to non-phosphorylated neurofilament protein marks the vulnerable cortical neurons in Alzheimer's disease. Brain Res 1987; 416:331–336.
210. Delaère P, Duyckaerts C, Brion JP, et al. Tau, paired helical filaments and amyloid in the neocortex: a morphometric study of 15 cases with graded intellectual status in aging and senile dementia of Alzheimer type. Acta Neuropathol (Berl) 1989; 77:645–753.
211. Braak H, Braak E. Neuropathological staging of Alzheimer-related changes. Acta Neuropathol (Berl) 1991; 82:239–259.
212. Nagy Z, Vatter-Bittner B, Braak H, et al. Staging of Alzheimer-type pathology: an interrater-intrarater study. Dement Geriatr Cogn Disord 1997; 8:248–251.
213. Gertz HJ, Xuereb J, Huppert F, et al. Examination of the validity of the hierarchical model of neuropathological staging in normal aging and Alzheimer's disease. Acta Neuropathol (Berl) 1998; 95:154–158.
214. Ball MJ, Nutall K. Topographic distribution of neurofibrillary tangles and granulo-vacuolar degeneration in hippocampal cortex of aging and demented patients. A quantitative study. Acta Neuropathol (Berl) 1978; 42:73–80.
215. Delacourte A, David JP, Sergeant N, et al. The biochemical pathway of neurofibrillary degeneration in aging and Alzheimer's disease. Neurology 1999; 52:1158–1165.
216. Arnold SE, Hyman BT, Flory J, et al. The topographical and neuroanatomical distribution of neurofibrillary tangles and neuritic plaques in the cerebral cortex of patients with Alzheimer's disease. Cereb Cortex 1991; 1:103–116.
217. Braak H, Braak E. Alzheimer's disease affects limbic nuclei of the thalamus. Acta Neuropathol (Berl) 1991; 81:261–268.
218. Hyman BT, van Hoesen GW, Damasio AR. Memory-related neural systems in Alzheimer's disease: an anatomical study. Neurology 1990; 40:1721–1730.
219. Unger JW, Lapham LW, McNeil TH, et al. The amygdala in Alzheimer's disease: neuropathology and Alz 50 immunoreactivity. Neurobiol Aging 1991; 12:389–399.
220. Tsuchiya K, Kosaka K. Neuropathological study of the amygdala in presenile Alzheimer's disease. J Neurol Sci 1990; 100:165–173.
221. Braak H, Braak E. Development of Alzheimer-related neurofibrillary changes in the neocortex inversely recapitulates cortical myelogenesis. Acta Neuropathol (Berl) 1996; 92:197–201.
222. Arendt T, Bruckner MK, Gertz HJ, et al. Cortical distribution of neurofibrillary tangles in Alzheimer's disease matches the pattern of neurons that retain their capacity of plastic remodelling in the adult brain. Neuroscience 1998; 83:991–1002.
223. Hof PR, Cox K, Morrison JH. Quantitative analysis of a vulnerable subset of pyramidal neurons in Alzheimer's disease: I. Superior frontal and inferior temporal cortex. J Comp Neurol 1990; 301:44–54.
224. Swaab DF, Salehi A. The pathogenesis of Alzheimer disease: an alternative to the amyloid hypothesis. J Neuropathol Exp Neurol 1997; 56:216–.
225. Hyman BT, Duyckaerts CD, Christen Y. Connections, Cognition and Alzheimer Disease. Berlin: Springer-Verlag, 1997.
226. Su JH, Deng G, Cotman CW. Transneuronal degeneration in the spread of Alzheimer's disease pathology: immunohistochemical evidence for the transmission of tau hyperphosphorylation. Neurobiol Dis 1997; 4:365–375.
227. Duyckaerts C, Hauw J-J, Bastenaire F, et al. Laminar distribution of neocortical plaques in senile dementia of the Alzheimer type. Acta Neuropathol (Berl) 1986; 70:249–256.
228. Duyckaerts C, Uchihara T, Seilhean D, et al. Dissociation of Alzheimer type pathology in a disconnected piece of cortex. Acta Neuropathol (Berl) 1997; 93:501–507.
229. Berg L, McKeel DWJ, Miller JP, et al. Clinicopathologic studies in cognitively healthy aging and Alzheimer's disease: relation of histologic markers to dementia severity, age, sex, and apolipoprotein E genotype. Arch Neurol 1998; 55:326–335.
230. Braak H, Duyckaerts C, Braak E, et al. Neuropathological staging of Alzheimer-related changes correlates with psychometrically assessed intellectual status. In: Corain B, Iqbal K, Nicolini M, Winblad B, Wisniewski H, Zatta P, eds. Alzheimer's Disease: Advances in Clinical and Basic Research. Chichester: John Wiley & Sons, 1993: pp. 131–137.
231. Dickson DW, Crystal HA, Bevona C, et al. Correlations of synaptic and pathological markers with cognition of the elderly. Neurobiol Aging 1995; 16:285–304.
232. Duyckaerts C, Hauw J-J. Diagnosis and staging of

Alzheimer disease. Neurobiol Aging 1997; 18:S4: S33–S42.
233. Nagy Z, Esiri MM, Jobst KA, et al. Relative roles of plaques and tangles in the dementia of Alzheimer's disease: correlations using three sets of neuropathological criteria. Dementia 1995; 6:21–31.
234. Wilcock GK, Esiri MM. Plaques, tangles and dementia. A quantitative study. J Neurol Sci 1982; 56: 343–356.
235. Terry RD, Masliah E, Salmon DP, et al. Physical basis of cognitive alterations in Alzheimer's disease: synapse loss is the major correlate of cognitive impairment. Ann Neurol 1991; 30:572–580.
236. Haroutunian V, Purohit DP, Perl DP, et al. Neurofibrillary tangles in nondemented elderly subjects and mild Alzheimer disease. Arch Neurol 1999; 56: 713–718.
237. Mann DM, TC, Yates PE. The topographic distribution of senile plaques and neurofibrillary tangles in the brain of non-demented persons of different ages. Neuropathol Appl Neurobiol 1987; 13:123–139.
238. Ulrich J. Senile plaques and neurofibrillary tangles of the Alzheimer type in non demented individuals at presenile age. Gerontology 1982; 28:86–90.
239. Ulrich J. Alzheimer changes in nondemented patients younger than sixty-five: possible early stages of Alzheimer's disease and senile dementia of Alzheimer disease. Ann Neurol 1985; 17:273–277.
240. Duyckaerts C, Hauw J-J. Prevalence, incidence and duration of Braak's stages in the general population: can we know? Neurobiol Aging 1997; 18:362–369.
241. Hauw J-J, Vignolo P, Duyckaerts C, et al. Etude neuropathologique de 12 centenaires: la fréquence de la démence sénile de type Alzheimer n'est pas particulièrement élevée dans ce groupe de personnes très agées. Rev Neurol (Paris) 1986; 142:107–115.
242. Itoh Y, Yamada M, Suematsu N, et al. An immunohistochemical study of centenarian brains: a comparison. J Neurol Sci 1998; 157:73–81.
243. Bancher C, Jellinger KA. Neurofibrillary predominant form of Alzheimer's disease: a rare subtype in very old subjects. Acta Neuropathol (Berl) 1994; 84: 565–570.
244. Jellinger KA, Bancher C. H Senile dementia with tangles (tangle predominant form of senile dementia). Brain Pathol 1998; 8:367–376.
245. Ikeda K, Akiyama H, Arai T, et al. Clinical aspects of 'senile dementia of the tangle type'—a subset of dementia in the senium separable from late-onset Alzheimer's disease. Dementia Geriatr Cogn Dis 1999; 10:6–11.
246. Jellinger KA, Bancher C. Senile dementia with tangles (tangle predominant form of senile dementia). Brain Pathol 1998; 8:367–376.
247. Bancher C, Egensperger R, Kosel S, et al. Low prevalence of apolipoprotein E epsilon 4 allele in the neurofibrillary tangle predominant form of senile dementia. Acta Neuropathol (Berl) 1997; 94:403–409.
248. Kawasaki H, Murayama S, Tomonaga M, et al. Neurofibrillary tangles in human upper cervical ganglia. Morphological study with immunohistochemistry and electron microscopy. Acta Neuropathol (Berl) 1987; 75:156–159.
249. Wakabayashi K, Hayashi S, Morita T, et al. Neurofibrillary tangles in the peripheral sympathetic ganglia of non-Alzheimer elderly individuals. Clin Neuropathol 1999; 18:171–175.
250. Van den Bosch de Aguilar P, Goemaere-Vanneste J. Paired helical filaments in spinal ganglion neurons of elderly rats. Virchows Arch Cell Pathol 1984; 47: 217–222.
251. Delacourte A, Sergeant N, Wattez A, et al. Vulnerable neuronal subsets in Alzheimer's and Pick's disease are distinguished by their isoform distribution and phosphorylation. Ann Neurol 1998; 43:193–204.
252. Sergeant N, Wattez A, Delacourte A. Neurofibrillary degeneration in progressive supranuclear palsy and corticobasal degeneration: tau pathologies with exclusively "exon 10" isoforms. J Neurochem 1999; 72: 1243–1249.
253. Foster NL, Wilhelmsen K, Sima AA, et al. Frontotemporal dementia and parkinsonism linked to chromosome 17: a consensus conference. Ann Neurol 1997; 41:706–715.
254. Spillantini MG, Bird TD, Ghetti B. Frontotemporal dementia and parkinsonism linked to chromosome 17: a new group of tauopathies. Brain Pathol 1998; 8:387–402.
255. Wisniewski K, Jervis GA, Moretz RC, et al. Alzheimer neurofibrillary tangles in diseases other than senile and presenile dementia. Ann Neurol 1979; 5: 288–294.
256. Wisniewski HM, Popovitch ER, Kaufman MA, et al. Neurofibrillary changes in advanced hydrocephalus: a clinicopathological study. J Neuropathol Exp Neurol 1987; 46:340 (abstr).
257. Nicklowitz WJ, Mandybur TI. Neurofibrillary changes following childhood lead encephalopathy. J Neuropathol Exp Neurol 1975; 34:445–455.
258. Harada K, Krucke W, Mancardi JL, et al. Alzheimer's tangles in sudanophilic leukodystrophy. Neurology 1988; 38:55–59.
259. Singer SM, Chambers CB, Newfry GA, et al. Tau in aluminum-induced neurofibrillary tangles. Neurotoxicology 1997; 18:63–76.
260. Wisniewski HM, Currie JR, Barcikowska M, et al. Alzheimer's disease, a cerebral form of amyloidosis. In: Poupland-Barthelaix A, Emile J, Christen Y, eds. Immunology and Alzheimer's Disease. Berlin: Springer-Verlag, 1988 1–6.
261. Wisniewski HM, Terry RD. Reexamination of the pathogenesis of the senile plaques. In: Zimmerman HM, ed. Progress in Neuropathology. New York: Grune & Straton, 1973:1–15.
262. Wisniewski HM, Wegiel J, Kotula L. Some neuropathological aspects of Alzheimer's disease and its relevance to other disciplines. Neuropathol Appl Neurobiol 1996; 22:3–11.
263. Bugiani O, Tagliavini F, Giaccone G. Preamyloid deposits, amyloid deposits, and senile plaques in Alzheimer's disease, Down syndrome, and aging. Ann N Y Acad Sci 1991; 640:122–128.
264. Lamy C, Duyckaerts C, Delaère P, et al. Comparison of seven staining methods for senile plaques and neurofibrillary tangles in a prospective study of 15 elderly patients. Neuropathol Appl Neurobiol 1989; 15:563–578.
265. Cullen KM, Halliday GM, Cartwright H, et al. Improved selectivity and sensitivity in the visualization of neurofibrillary tangles, plaques and neuropil threads. Neurodegeneration 1996; 5:177–187.

266. Mann DMA, Marcyniuk B, Yates PO, et al. The progression of the pathological changes of Alzheimer's disease in frontal and temporal neocortex both at biopsy and autopsy. Neuropathol Appl Neurobiol 1988; 14:177–195.
267. Duyckaerts C, Delaère P, Poulain V, et al. Does amyloid precede paired helical filaments in the senile plaque? A study of 15 cases with graded intellectual status in aging and Alzheimer disease. Neurosci Lett 1988; 91:354–359.
268. Schmidt M, Lee V, Trojanowski J. Comparative epitope analysis of neuronal cytoskeletal proteins in Alzheimer's disease senile plaque, neurites and neuropil threads. Lab Invest 1991; 64:352–357.
269. Probst A, Basler V, Bron B, et al. Neuritic plaques in senile dementia of the Alzheimer type: a Golgi analysis in the hippocampal region. Brain Res 1983; 268:249–254.
270. Dickson TC, King CE, McCormack GH, et al. Neurochemical diversity of dystrophic neurites in the early and late stages of Alzheimer's disease. Exp Neurol 1999; 156:100–110.
271. He Y, Delaère P, Duyckaerts C, et al. Two distinct ubiquitin immunoreactive senile plaques in Alzheimer's disease: relationship with the intellectual status in 29 cases. Acta Neuropathol (Berl) 1993; 86:109–116.
272. Struble RG, Cork LC, Whitehouse PJ, et al. Cholinergic innervation in neuritic plaques. Science 1982; 216:413–415.
273. Geula C, Mesulam MM. Cholinergic systems and related neuropathological prediction patterns in Alzheimer disease. In:Terry RD, Katzman R, Bick KL, eds. Alzheimer Disease. New York: Raven Press, 1994 pp. 263–291.
274. Walker LC, Kitt CA, Cork LC, et al. Multiple transmitter systems contribute neurites to individual senile plaques. J Neuropathol Exp Neurol 1988; 47:138–144.
275. Cervera P, Duyckaerts C, Ruberg M, et al. Tyrosine hydroxylase-positive fibers in patients with Alzheimer's disease. Neurosci Lett 1990; 110:210–215.
276. Braunmühl von A. Alterskrankung des Zentralnervensystems. Senile Involution. Senile Demenz. Alzheimersche Krankheit. In: Scholtz W, ed. Handbuch der Speziellen Pathologischen Anatomie und Histologie. Berlin: Springer-Verlag, 1957:pp. 337–539.
277. Schechter R, Yen SH, Terry RD. Fibrous astrocytes in senile dementia of the Alzheimer type. J Neuropathol Exp Neurol 1981; 40:95–101.
278. Brion JP, van den Bosch de Aguilar F-DJ. Senile dementia of the Alzheimer type: morphological and immunocytochemical studies. In: Joynt JR Weindl A, eds. Senile Dementia of the Alzheimer Type: Early Diagnosis, Neuropathology and Animal Models. Berlin: Springer-Verlag, 1985: pp. 164–174.
279. Dickson DW. Microglia in Alzheimer's disease and transgenic models—how close the fit? Am J Pathol 1999; 154:1627–1631.
280. Hauw J-J, Duyckaerts C, Delaère P, et al. Maladie d'Alzheimer, amyloïde, microglie et astrocytes. Rev Neurol (Paris) 1988; 144:155–157.
281. Frackowiak J, Wisniewski HM, Wegiel J, et al. Ultrastructure of the microglia that phagocytes amyloid and the microglia that produces beta-amyloid fibrils. Acta Neuropathol (Berl) 1992; 84:225–232.
282. Combs CK, Johnson DE, Cannady SB, et al. Identification of microglial signal transduction pathways mediating a neurotoxic response to amyloidogenic fragments of beta-amyloid and prion proteins. J Neurosci 1999; 19:928–93g.
283. Selkoe D. Translating cell biology into therapeutic advances in Alzheimer's disease. Nature 1999;399 (Suppl):A23–A31.
284. Younkin S. The role of Aβ42 in Alzheimer's disease. J Physiol (Paris) 1998; 92:289–292.
285. Masliah E, Mallory M, Deerinck T, et al. Re-evaluation of the structural organization of neuritic plaques in Alzheimer's disease. J Neuropathol Exp Neurol 1993; 52:619–632.
286. Glenner GG, Wong CW. Alzheimer's disease: initial report of the purification and characterization of a novel cerebrovascular amyloid protein. Biochem Biophys Res Commun 1984; 120:885–890.
287. Haass C, Schlossmacher MG, Hung AY, et al. Amyloid β-peptide is produced by cultured cells during normal metabolism. Nature 1992; 359:322–325.
288. Seubert P, Vigo-Pelfrey C, Esch F, et al. Isolation and quantification of soluble Alzheimer's β-peptide from biological fluids. Nature 1992; 359:325–327.
289. Busciglio J, Gabuzda D, Matsudaira P, et al. Generation of β-amyloid in the secretoty pathway in neuronal and nonneuronal cells. Proc Natl Acad Sci USA 1993; 90:2092–2096.
290. Selkoe DJ. The cell biology of beta-amyloid precursor protein and presenilin in Alzheimer's disease. Trends Cell Biol 1998; 8:447–453.
291. Black RA, Rauch CT, Kozlosky CJ, et al. A metalloproteinase disintegrin that releases tumour-necrosis factor-alpha from cells. Nature 1997;385: 729–733.
292. Buxbaum JD, Liu KN, Luo Y, et al. Evidence that tumour necrosis factor alpha converting enzyme is involved in regulated alpha-secretase cleavage of the Alzheimer amyloid protein precursor. J Biol Chem 1998; 273:27765–27767.
293. Beyreuther K, Masters C. Alzheimer's disease—the ins and outs of amyloid-beta. Nature 1997; 389:677–678.
294. Checler F. Processing of the β-amyloid precursor protein and its regulation in Alzheimer's disease. J Neurochem 1995; 65:1431–1444.
295. Octave JN. The amyloid peptide and its precursor in Alzheimer's disease. Rev Neurosci 1995; 6:287–316.
296a. Vassar R, Bennett BD, Babu-Khan S, et al. Beta-secretase cleavage of Alzheimer's amyloid precursor protein by the transmembrane aspartic protease BACE. Science 1999; 286:735–741.
296b. Selkoe DJ, Wolfe MS. In search of gamma-secretase: Presenilin at the cutting edge. Proc Nat Acad Sci USA, 2000; 97:5690–5692.
296c. Wolfe, M. S. and Haass, C.: The role of presenilins in gamma-secretase activity. J Biol Chem 2001; in press.
297. Hardy J. Alzheimer's disease: the present situation and our tasks. Neurobiol Aging 1994; 15:5111–5112.
298. Hsiao K, Chapman P, Nilsen S, et al. Correlative memory deficits, Abeta elevation, and amyloid plaques in trangenic mice. Science 1996; 274:99–102.
299. Staufenbiel M, Sommer B, Jucker M. Neuron loss in APP transgenic mice. Nature 1998; 395:755–756.
300. Irizarry MC, Soriano F, McNamara M, et al. Abeta deposition is associated with neuropil changes, but

not with overt neuronal loss in the human amyloid precursor protein V717F (PDAPP) transgenic mouse. J Neurosci 1997; 17:7053–7059.
301. Castano EM, Prelli F, Soto C, et al. The length of amyloid-beta in hereditary cerebral hemorrhage with amyloidosis, Dutch type. Implication for the role of amyloid beta 1-42 in Alzheimer's disease. J Biol Chem 1996; 271:32185–32191.
302. Iwatsubo T, Odaka A, Suzuki N, et al. Visualization of Aβ42(43) and Aβ40 in senile plaques with end-specific Aβ monoclonals: evidence that an initially deposited species is Aβ42(43). Neuron 1994; 13:45–53.
303. Barelli H, Lebeau A, Vizzavona J, et al. Characterization of new polyclonal antibodies specific for 40 and 42 amino acid-long amyloid beta peptides: their use to examine the cell biology of presenilins and the immunohistochemistry of sporadic Alzheimer's disease and cerebral amyloid angiopathy cases. Mol Med 1997; 3:695–707.
304. Jarrett J, Lansbury P. Seeding "one dimensional crystallization" of amyloid: a pathogenic mechanism in Alzheimer's disease and scrapie? Cell 1993; 73:1055–1058.
305. Hosoda R, Saido TC, Otvos L, et al. Quantification of modified amyloid beta peptides in Alzheimer disease and Down syndrome brains. J Neuropathol Exp Neurol 1998; 57:1089–1095.
306. Mori H, Takio K, Ogawara M, et al. Mass spectrometry of purified amyloid β protein in Alzheimer's disease. J Biol Chem 1992; 267:17082–17086.
307. Roher AE, Lowenson JD, Clarke S, et al. β-Amyloid-(1-42) is a major component of cerebrovascular amyloid deposits: implications for the pathology of Alzheimer disease. Proc Natl Acad Sci USA 1883; 90:10836–10840.
308. Wilson CA, Doms RW, Lee VM-Y. Intracellular processing and Aβ production in Alzheimer's disease. J Neuropathol Exp Neurol 1999; 58:787–794.
309. Larner A. Hypothesis: amyloid β-peptides truncated at the N-terminus contribute to the pathogenesis of Alzheimer's disease. Neurobiol Aging 1999; 20:65–69.
310. Teplow D. Truncating the amyloid cascade hypothesis: the role of C-terminal Aβ peptides in Alzheimer's disease. Neurobiol Aging 1999; 20:71–73.
311. Geddes J, Tekirian T, Mattson M. N-terminus truncated β-amyloid peptides and C-terminus truncated secreted forms of amyloid precursor protein: distinct roles in the pathogenesis of Alzheimer's disease. Neurobiol Aging 1999; 20:75–79.
312. Tseng B, Esler W, Clish C, et al. Deposition of monomeric, not oligomeric, abeta mediates growth of Alzheimer's disease amyloid plaques in human brain preparations. Biochemistry 1999; 38:10424–10431.
313. Wisniewski T, Frangione B. Apolipoprotein E. A pathological chaperone protein in patients with cerebral and systemic amyloid. Neurosci Lett 1992; 135:235–238.
314. Berr C, Hauw J-J, Delaère P, et al. Apolipoprotein E allele e4 is linked to increased deposition of the amyloid b peptide (A-b) in cases with or without Alzheimer's disease. Neurosci Lett 1994; 178:221–224.
315. Dickson TC, Saunders HL, Vickers JC. Relationship between apolipoprotein E and the amyloid deposits and dystrophic neurites of Alzheimer's disease. Neuropathol Appl Neurobiol 1997; 23:483–491.
316. Namba Y, Tomonaga M, Kawasaki H, et al. Apolipoprotein E immunoreactivity in cerebral amyloid deposits and neurofibrillary tangles in Alzheimer's disease and kuru plaque amyloid in Creutzfeldt-Jakob disease. Brain Res 1991; 541:163–166.
317. Uchihara T, Duyckaerts C, He Y, et al. ApoE immunoreactivity and microglial cells in Alzheimer's disease brain. Neurosci Lett 1995; 195:5–8.
318. Uchihara T, Duyckaerts C, Lazarini F, et al. Inconstant apolipoprotein E (ApoE)-like immunoreactivity in amyloid beta protein deposits: relationship with APOE genotype in aging brain and Alzheimer's disease. Acta Neuropathol (Berl) 1996; 92:180–185.
319. Yamaguchi H, Ishiguro K, Sugihara S, et al. Presence of apolipoprotein E on extracellular neurofibrillary tangles and on meningeal blood vessels precedes the Alzheimer β-amyloid deposition. Acta Neuropathol (Berl) 1994; 88:413–419.
320. Iwai A, Yoshimoto M, Masliah E, et al. Non-A beta component of Alzheimer's disease amyloid (NAC) is amyloidogenic. Biochemistry 1995; 34:10139–10145.
321. Masliah E, Iwai A, Mallory M, et al. Altered presynaptic protein NACP is associated with plaque formation and neurodegeneration in Alzheimer's disease. Am J Pathol 1996; 148:201–210.
322. Schmidt ML, Lee VM, Forman M, et al. Monoclonal antibodies to a 100-kd protein reveal abundant A beta-negative plaques throughout gray matter of Alzheimer's disease brains. Am J Pathol 1997; 151:69–80.
323. Lemere CA, Grenfell TJ, Selkoe DJ. The AMY antigen co-occurs with abeta and follows its deposition in the amyloid plaques of Alzheimer's disease and down syndrome. Am J Pathol 1999; 155:29–37.
324. Abraham CR, Selkoe DJ, Potter H. Immunochemical identification of the serine protease inhibitor α-1 antichymotrypsin in the brain amyloid deposits of Alzheimer's disease. Cell 1988; 52:487–501.
325. Ishiguro K, Shoji M, Yamaguchi H, et al. Differential expression of α1-antichymotrypsin in the aged human brain. Virchows Arch B Cell Pathol 1993; 64:221–227.
326. Gollin PA, Kalaria RN, Eikelenboom P, et al. Alpha 1-antitrypsin and alpha 1-antichymotrypsin are in the lesions of Alzheimer's disease. NeuroReport 1992; 3:201–204.
327. Licastro F, Mallory M, Lawrence AH, et al. Increased levels of alpha-1-antichymotrypsin in brains of patients with Alzheimer's disease correlate with activated astrocytes and are affected by APOE 4 genotype. J Neuroimmunol 1998; 88:105–110.
328. Buée L, Hof PR, Roberts DD, et al. Immunohistochemical identification of thrombospondin in normal brain and in Alzheimer's disease. Am J Pathol 1992; 141:783–788.
329. Snow AD, Wight TN. Proteoglycans in the pathogenesis of Alzheimer's disease and other amyloidoses. Neurobiol Aging 1989; 10:481–497.
330. Verbeek MM, Otte-Höller I, Westphal JR, et al. Accumulation of intercellular adhesion molecule-1 in senile plaques in brain tissue of patients with Alzheimer's disease. Am J Pathol 1994; 144:104–116.
331. Verbeek MM, OtteHoller I, Veerhuis R, et al. Distribution of A beta-associated proteins in cerebro-

331. vascular amyloid of Alzheimer's disease. Acta Neuropathol (Berl) 1998; 96:628–636.
332. Zambenedetti P, Giordano R, Zatta P. Histochemical localization of gylcoconjugates on microglial cells in Alzheimer's disease brain samples by using *Abrus precatorius, Maackia amurensis, Momordica charantia,* and *Sambucus nigra* lectins. Exp Neurol 1998; 153:167–171.
333. Bradt BM, Kolb WP, Cooper NR. Complement-dependent proinflammatory properties of the Alzheimer's disease beta-peptide. J Exp Med 1998; 188:431–438.
334. McDonald DR, Bamberger ME, Combs CK, et al. Beta-amyloid fibrils activate parallel mitogen-activated protein kinase pathways in microglia and THP1 monocytes. J Neurosci 1998; 18:4451–4460.
335. Wyss-Coray T, Masliah E, Mallory M, et al. Amyloidogenic role of cytokine TGF-beta1 in transgenic mice and Alzheimer's disease. Nature 1997; 389: 603–606.
336. Zhao BY, Schwartz JP. Involvement of cytokines in normal CNS development and neurological diseases: recent progress and perspectives. J Neurosci Res 1998; 52:7–16.
337. Dickson DW, Lee SC, Mattiace LA, et al. Microglia and cytokines in neurological disease, with special reference to AIDS and Alzheimer's disease. Glia 1993; 7:75–83.
338. Eikelenboom P, Rozemuller JM, van Muiswinkel FL. Inflammation and Alzheimer's disease: relationships between pathogenic mechanisms and clinical expression. Exp Neurol 1998; 154:89–98.
339. Ishii T, Haga S. Identification of components of immunoglobulins in senile plaques by means of fluorescent antibody technique. Acta Neuropathol (Berl) 1975; 32:157–162.
340. Goust JM, Mangum M, Powers JM. An immunologic assessment of brain-associated IgG in senile cerebral amyloidosis. J Neuropathol Exp Neurol 1984; 43: 481–488.
341. Kalaria R, Harshbargerkelly M, Cohen D, et al. Molecular aspects of inflammatory and immune responses in Alzheimer's disease. Neurobiol Aging 1996; 17:687–693.
342. Marx F, Blasko I, Pavelka M, et al. The possible role of the immune system in Alzheimer's disease. Exp Gerontol 1998; 33:871–881.
343. McGeer EG, McGeer PL. The importance of inflammatory mechanisms in Alzheimer disease. Exp Gerontol 1998; 33:371–378.
344. McRae A, Dahlström A, Ling E.A. Microglia in neurodegenerative disorders: emphasis on Alzheimer's disease. Gerontology 1997; 43:95–108.
345. Torack RM, Lynch RG. Cytochemistry of brain amyloid in adult dementia. Acta Neuropathol (Berl) 1981; 53:189–196.
346. Webster S, Lue LF, Brachova L, et al. Molecular and cellular characterization of the membrane attack complex, C5b-9, in Alzheimer's disease. Neurobiol Aging 1997; 18:415–421.
347. Hensley K, Floyd RA, Zheng NY, et al. p38 kinase is activated in the Alzheimer's disease brain. J Neurochem 1999; 72:2053–2058.
348. Klegeris A, McGeer PL. Beta-amyloid protein enhances macrophage production of oxygen free radicals and glutamate. J Neurosci Res 1997; 49:229–235.
349. Pasinetti GM. Cyclooxygenase and inflammation in Alzheimer's disease: experimental approaches and clinical interventions. J Neurosci Res 1998; 49:229–235.
350. Rottkamp CA, Nunomura A, Raina AK, et al. Oxidative stress, antioxidants, and Alzheimer disease. Alzheimer Dis Assoc Disord 2000;14 Suppl 1:S62–66.
351. Terry RD, Gonatas JK, Weiss M. Ultrastructural studies in Alzheimer presenile dementia. Am J Pathol 1964; 44:269–297.
352. Braunmühl von A. Alterserkrankungen des Zentralnervensystems. Senile Involution. Senile Demex. Alzheimersche Krankeit. In: Lubarsch O, Henke F, Rössle R, eds. Handbuch der Speziellen Pathologischen Anatomie und Histologie. Berlin: Springer-Verlag, 1957: pp. 337–539.
353. Tamaoka A, Sawamura N, Odaka A, et al. Amyloid beta protein 1-42/43 (A beta 1-42/43) in cerebellar diffuse plaques: enzyme-linked immunosorbent assay and immunocytochemical study. Brain Res 1995; 679:151–156.
354. Price JL, Davis PB, Morris JC, et al. The distribution of tangles, plaques and related immunohistochemical markers in healthy aging and Alzheimer's disease. Neurobiol Aging 1991; 12:295–312.
355. Delaère P, Duyckaerts C, He Y, et al. Subtypes and differential laminar distributions of βA4 deposits in Alzheimer's disease: relationship with the intellectual status of 26 cases. Acta Neuropathol (Berl) 1991; 81: 328–335.
356. Hauw J, Seilhean D, Colle M-A, et al. Les marqueurs neuropathologiques des démences dégénératives. Rev Neurol 1998; H154 suppl 2:350–64.
357. Yamaguchi H, Sugihara S, Ogawa A, et al. Diffuse plaques associated with astroglial amyloid beta protein, possibly showing a disappearing stage of senile plaques. Acta Neuropathol (Berl) 1998; 95:217–222.
358. Thal DR, Sassin, I, Schultz C, et al. Fleecy amyloid deposits in the internal layers of the human entorhinal cortex are comprised of N-terminal truncated fragments of Abeta. Neuropathol Exp Neurol 1999; 58:210–216.
359. Wisniewski HM, Sadowski M, Jakubowska-Sadowska K, et al. Diffuse, lake-like amyloid-beta deposits in the paravopyramidal layer of the presubiculum in Alzheimer disease. J Neuropathol Exp Neurol 1998; 57:674–683.
360. Terry D, Masliah E, Hansen LA. Structural basis of the cognitive alterations in Alzheimer disease. In: Terry RD, Katzman R, Bick KL, eds. Alzheimer Disease. New York: Raven Press, 1994 pp. 179–196.
361. Pearson RCA, Esiri MM, Hiorns RW, et al. Anatomical correlates of the distribution of the pathological changes in the neocortex in Alzheimer disease. Proc Natl Acad Sci USA 1985; 82:4531–4534.
362. Rogers J, Morrison JH. Quantitative morphology and regional and laminar distribution of senile plaques in Alzheimer's disease. J Neurosci 1985; 5: 2801–2808.
363. Lewis DA, Campbell MJ, Terry RD, et al. Laminar and regional distribution of neurofibrillary tangles and neuritic plaques in Alzheimer's disease. A quantitative study of visual and auditory cortices. J Neurosci 1987; 7:1799–1808.
364. Kosik KS, Rogers J, Kowall NW. Senile plaques are located between apical dendritic clusters. J Neuropathol Exp Neurol 1987; 46:1–11.

365. Mann DMA. Neuropathological and neurochemical aspects of Alzheimer's disease. In: Iversen LL, Iversen SD, Snyder SH, eds. Psychopharmacology of the Aging Nervous System, Handbook of Psychopharmacology. New York: Plenum Press, 1988 pp. 2–67.
366. Arendt T, Taubert G, Bigl V, et al. Amyloid deposition in the nucleus basalis of Meynert complex: a topographic marker for degenerating cell clusters in Alzheimer's disease. Acta Neuropathol (Berl) 1988; 75:226–232.
367. Ishii T. Distribution of Alzheimer's neurofibrillary changes in the brain stem and hypothalamus of senile dementia. Acta Neuropathol (Berl) 1966; 6:181–187.
368. Terry RD, Hansen LA, DeTeresa R, et al. Senile dementia of the Alzheimer type without neocortical neurofibrillary tangles. J Neuropathol Exp Neurol 1987; 46:262–268.
369. Möller HJ, Graeber MB. The case described by Alois Alzheimer in 1911. Eur Arch Psychiatry Clin Neurosci 1998; 248:111–122.
370. Hansen LA, Masliah E, Galasko D, et al. Plaque only Alzheimer disease is usually the Lewy body variant and vice versa. J Neuropathol Exp Neurol 1993; 52: 648–654.
371. Matsuyama H, Nakamura S. Senile changes in the brain in the Japanese: incidence of Alzheimer's neurofibrillary changes and senile plaque. In: Katzman R, Terry RD, Bick KL, eds. Alzheimer's Disease: Senile Dementia and Related Disorders. New York: Raven Press, 1978:pp. 287–97.
372. Miller FD, Hicks SP, D'Amato CJ, et al. A descriptive study of neuritic plaques and neurofibrillary tangles in an autopsy population. Am J Epidemiol 1984; 120:331–341.
373. Delaère P, He Y, Fayet G, et al, βA4 deposits are constant in the brain of the oldest old: an immunocytochemical study of 20 French centenarians. Neurobiol Aging 1993; 14:191–194.
374. Blessed G, Tomlinson BE, Roth M. The association between quantitative measures of dementia and of senile change in the cerebral grey matter of elderly subjects. Br J Psychiatry 1968; 114:797–811.
375. Crystal H, Dickson D, Fuld P, et al. Clinicopathologic studies in dementia: non-demented subjects with pathologically confirmed Alzheimer's disease. Neurology 1988; 38:1682–1687.
376. Katzman R, Terry R, DeTeresa, et al. Clinical, pathological, and neurochemical changes in dementia: a subgroup with preserved mental status and numerous neocortical plaques. Ann Neurol 1988; 23:138–144.
377. Cummings B, Pike C, Shankle R, et al. Beta-amyloid deposition and other measures of neuropathology predict cognitive status in Alzheimer's disease. Neurobiol Aging 1996; 17:921–933.
378. Hanzel D, Trojanowski J, Johnston R, et al. High-throughput quantitative histological analysis of Alzheimer's disease pathology using a confocal digital microscanner. Nat Biotechnol 1999; 17:53–57.
379. Delaère P, Duyckaerts C, Masters C, et al. Large amounts of neocortical βA4 deposits without Alzheimer changes in a nondemented case. Neurosci Lett 1990; 116:87–93.
380. Greenberg BD. Alzheimer's disease pathogenesis; the challenge of establishing dynamic biological processes from static measurements. Neurobiol Aging 1996; 17:936–939.
381. Davis DG, Schmidt FA, Wekstein DR, et al. Alzheimer neuropathologic alterations in aged cognitively normal subjects. J Neuropathol Exp Neurol 1999; 58:376–388.
382. Mann DMA, Jones D. Deposition of amyloid (βA4) protein within the brains of persons with dementing disorders other than Alzheimer's disease and Down's syndrome. Neurosci Lett 1990; 109:68–75.
383. Bugiani O, Giaccone G, Verga L, et al βPP participates in PrP-amyloid plaques of Gerstmann-Sträussler-Scheinker disease, Indiana kindred. J Neuropathol Exp Neurol 1993; 52:64–70.
384. Ghetti T, Piccardo P, Spillanti MG, et al. Vascular variant of prion protein cerebral amyloidosis with t-positive neurofibrillary tangles: the phenotype of the stop codon 145 mutation in PRNP. Proc Natl Acad Sci USA 1997; 93:744–748.
385. Feany MB, Dickson DW. Widespread cytoskeletal pathology characterizes cortico-basal degeneration. Am J Pathol 1995; 90:37–43.
386. Hauw J-J, Verny M, Delaère P, et al. Constant neurofibrillary changes in the neocortex in progressive supranuclear palsy. Basic with aging and aging. Neurosci Lett 1990; 119:182–186.
387. Ikeda K, Akiyama H, Aral T, et al. Glial tau pathology in neurodegenerative diseases; their nature and comparison with neuronal tangles. Neurobiol Aging 1998; 19:S85–S91.
388. Nishimura T, Ikeda K, Akiyama H, et al. Immunohistochemical investigation of t-positive structures of cerebral cortex in patients with progressive supranuclear palsy. Neurosci Lett 1995; 201:123–126.
389. Hauw J-J, Seilhean D, Duyckaerts C. Cerebral amyloid angiopathy. In: Ginsberg MD, Bogousslavsky J, eds. Cerebrovascular Disease. Pathophysiology, Diagnosis and Management. Cambridge: Blackwell Scientific Publications, 1998: pp. 1772–1795.
390. Vinters H, Wang Z, Secor D. Brain parenchymal and microvascular amyloid in Alzheimer's disease. Brain Pathol 1996; 6:179–195.
391. Peers MC, Lenders MB, Defossez A, et al. Cortical angiopathy in Alzheimer's disease: the formation of dystrophic prtivascular neurites is related to the exudation of amyloid fibrills from the pathological vessels. Virchow Arch A Pathol Anat 1988; 414:15–20.
392. Vonsattel JP, Myers RH, Hedley-White ET, et al. Cerebral amyloid angiopathy without and with cerebral hemorrhage: a comparative histologic study. Ann Neurol 1991; 30:637–649.
393. Jellinger K. Cerebral hemorrhage in amyloid angiopathy (letter). Ann Neurol 1977; 1:604.
394. Mandybur TI. Cerebral amyloid angiopathy:Possible relationship to rheumatoid vasculitis. Neurology 1979; 29:1336–1340.
395. Mandybur TI, Balko G. Cerebral amyloid angiopathy with granulomatous angeitis ameliorated by steroid-cytoxan treatment. Clin Neuropharmacol 1992; 15: 241–247.
396. Morel F, Wildi E. General and cellular pathochemistry of senile and presenile alterations of the brain. In: Torino ?, Rosenberg ?, Sellien ?, eds. Proceedings of the First International Congress of Neuropathology. 1952:pp. 347–374.

397. Pantelakis S. Un type particulier d'angiopathie sénile du système nerveux central: L'angiopathie congophile. Topographie et fréquence. Monatsschr Psychiatr Neurol 1954; 128:219–256.
398. Mandybur TI, Bates SRD. Fatal massive intracerebral hemorrhage complicating cerebral amyloid angiopathy. Arch Neurol 1978; 35:246–248.
399. Vinters HV. Cerebral amyloid angiopathy: a critical review. Stroke 1987; 18:311–324.
400. Bakker E, Van Broeckhoven C, Haan J, et al. DNA-diagnosis for hereditary cerebral haemorrhage with amyloidosis (Dutch type). Am J Hum Genet 1991; 49:518–521.
401. Levy E, Carman MD, Fernandez-Madrid IJ, et al. Mutation of the Alzheimer's disease amyloid gene in hereditary hemorrhage, Dutch type. Science 1990; 248:1124–1126.
402. Hendricks L, van Duijn CM, Cras P, et al. Presenile dementia and cerebral haemorrhage linked to a mutation at codon 692 of the β-amyloid precursor protein gene. Nat Genet 1992; 1:218–221.
403. Schellenberg GD. Molecular genetics of familial Alzheimer's disease. Arzneimittelforschung Drug Res 1995; 45:418–424.
404. Haan J, Van Broeckhoven C, van Duijn CM, et al. The apolipoprotein E epsilon 4 allele does not influence the clinical expression of the amyloid precursor protein gene codon 693 or 692 mutations. Ann Neurol 1994; 36:434–437.
405. Haan J, Roos RAC, Bakker E. No protective effect of apoprotein Eε2 allele in Dutch hereditary cerebral amyloid angiopathy. Ann Neurol 1995; 37:282.
406. Wildi E, Dago-Akribi A. Alération cérébrales chez l'homme agé. Bull Suisse Acad Med Sci 1968; 24:107–132.
407. Masuda J, Tanaka K, Ueda K, et al. Autopsy study of incidence and distribution of cerebral amyloid angiopathy in Hisayama, Japan. Stroke 1988; 19:205–210.
408. Yamada M, Tsukagoshi H, Otomo E, et al. Cerebral amyloid angiopathy in the aged. J Neurol 1987; 234:371–376.
409. Esiri MM, Wilcock GK. Cerebral amyloid angiopathy in dementia and old age. J Neurol Neurosurg Psychiatry 1986; 46:1221–1226.
410. Joachim CL, Morris JH, Selkoe DJ. Amyloid angiopathy in 100 cases of Alzheimer's disease. Neurology 1987; 37 (Suppl 1):225 (abstr).
411. Mann DMA. Cerebral amyloidosis, ageing and Alzheimer's disease: a contribution from studies on Down's syndrome. Neurobiol Aging 1989; 10:397–399.
412. Iwatsubo T, Mann DMA, Odaka A, et al. Amyloid β protein (Aβ) deposition: Aβ43(43) precedes Aβ40 in Down syndrome. Ann Neurol 1995; 37:294–299.
413. Suzuki N, Iwatsubo T, Odaka A, et al. High tissue content of soluble β1–40 is linked to cerebral amyloid angiopathy. Am J Pathol 1994; 145:452–460.
414. Maruyama K, Ikeda S, Ischihara T, et al. Immunohistochemical characterization of cerebrovascular amyloid in 46 autopsied cases using antibodies to β protein and cystatin C. Stroke 1990; 21:397–403.
415. Yong WH, Robert ME, Secor DL, et al. Cerebral hemorrhage with biopsy-proved amyloid angiopathy. Arch Neurol 1992; 49:51–59.
416. Natte R, de Boer WI, Maat-Schieman ML, et al. Amyloid beta precursor protein-mRNA is expressed throughout cerebral vessel walls. Brain Res 1999; 828:179–183.
417. Yamaguchi H, Yamazaki T, Lemere CA, et al. Beta amyloid is focally deposited within the outer basement membrane in the amyloid angiopathy of Alzheimer's disease. Am J Pathol 1992; 141:249–259.
418. Armstrong RA, Myers D, Smith CUM. The ratio of diffuse to mature beta/A4 deposits in Alheimer's disease varies in case with and without pronounced congophilic angiopathy. Dementia 1993; 4:251–255.
419. Neve RL, Finch EA, Dawes LR. Expression of the Alzheimer amyloid precursor gene transcript in the human brain. Neuron 1988; 1:669–677.
420. Selkoe DJ. Molecular pathology of amyloidogenic proteins and the role of vascular amyloidosis in Alzheimer's disease. Neurobiol Aging 1989; 10:387–395.
421. Wisniewski HM, Wegiel J. β-amyloid formation by myocytes of leptomeningeal vessels. Acta Neuropathol (Berl) 1994; 87:233–241.
422. Frackowiak J, Zoltowska A, Wisniewski HM. Nonfibrillar β-amyloid protein is associated with smooth muscle cells of vessel walls in Alzheimer disease. J Neuropathol Exp Neurol 1994; 53:637–645.
423. Lindahl B, Eriksson L, Lindahl U. Structure of heparan sulfate from human brain, with special regard to Alzheimer's disease. Biochem J 1995; 306:117–184.
424. Buce L, Ding WH, Anderson JP, et al. Binding of vascular heparan sulfate proteoglycan to Alzheimer's amyloid precursor protein is mediated in part by the N-terminal region of A4 peptide. Brain Res 1994; 627:199–204.
425. Narindrasorasak S, Lowery D, Gonzales-De Whitt P, et al. High affinity interactions between the Alzheimer's β-amyloid precursor proteins and the basement membrane form of heparan sulfate proteoglycan. J Biol Chem 1991; 266:12878–12883.
426. Frackowiak J, Mazur-Kolecka B, Wisniewski HM, et al. Secretion and accumulation of Alzheimer's β-protein by cultured vascular smooth muscle cells from old and young dogs. Brain Res 1995; 676:225–230.
427. Campion D, Flaman J-M, Brice A, et al. Mutations of the presenilin I gene in families with early-onset Alzheimer's disease. Hum Mol Genet 1995; 4:2373–2377.
428. Gomez-Isla T, Growdon W, McNamara M, et al. The impact of different presenilin 1 and presenilin 2 mutations on amyloid deposition, neurofibrillary changes and neuronal loss in the familial Alzheimer's disease brain: evidence for other phenotype-modifying factors. Brain 1999; 122:1709–1719.
429. Hardy J. Amyloids, the presenilins and Alzheimer's disease. Trends Neurosci 1997; 20:154–159.
430. Huynh D, Vinters H, Ho D, et al. Neuronal expression and intracellular localization of presenilins in normal and Alzheimer disease brains. J Neuropathol Exp Neurol 1997; 56:1009–1017.
431. Kovacs DM, Fausett HJ, Page KJ, et al. Alzheimer-associated presenilins 1 and 2: neuronal expression in brain and localization to intracellular membranes in mammalian cells. Nat Med 1996; 2:224–229.
432. Mattson M, Guo Q. Cell and molecular neurobiology of presenilins: a role for the endoplasmic retic-

ulum in the pathogenesis of Alzheimer's disease. J Neurosci Res 1997; 50:505–513.
433. Uchihara T, Elhachimi HK, Duyckaerts C, et al. Widespread immunoreactivity of presenilin in neurons of normal and Alzheimer's disease brains: double-labeling immunohistochemical study. Acta Neuropathol (Berl) 1996; 92:325–330.
434. Wisniewski T, Dowjat WK, Permanne B, et al. Presinilin-1 is associated with Alzheimer's disease amyloid. Am J. Pathol 1997; 151:601–610.
435. Hendriks L, De Jonghe C, Lubke U, et al. Immunoreactivity of presenilin-1 and tau in Alzheimer's disease brain. Exp Neurol 1998; 149:341–348.
436. Giannakopoulos P, Bouras C, Kovari E, et al. Presenilin-1-immunoreactive neurons are preserved in late-onset Alzheimer's disease. Am J Pathol 1997; 150:429–436.
437. Colle M-A, Duyckaerts C, Laquerrière C, et al. Laminar specific loss of isocortical presenilin 1 immunoreactivity in Alzheimer disease. Correlations with the amyloid load and density of tau positive neurofibrillary tangles. Neuropathol Appl Neurobiol 2000; 26:117–123.
438. Braak H, Braak E. Golgi preparation as a tool in Neuropathology with particular reference to investigations of the human telencephalic cortex. Prog Neurobiol 1985; 25:93–139.
439. Williams RS, Ferrante RJ, Caviness VS. The Golgi rapid method in clinical neuropathology: the morphologic consequences of suboptimal fixation. J Neuropathol Exp Neurol 1978; 37:13–33.
440. Arendt T, Bruckner MK, Bigl V, et al. Dendritic reorganisation in the basal forebrain under degenerative conditions and its defects in Alzheimer's disease. II. Ageing, Korsakoff's disease, Parkinson's disease, and Alzheimer's disease. J Comp Neurol 1995; 351:189–222.
441. Buell SJ, Coleman PD. Quantitative evidence for selective dendritic growth in normal human aging but not in senile dementia. Brain Res 1981; 214:23–41.
442. Flood DG, Buell SJ, Horvitz GJ, et al. Dendritic extent in human dentate gyrus granule cells in normal aging and senile dementia. Brain Res 1987; 402:205–216.
443. Arendt T, Zvegintseva HG, Leontovich TA. Dendritic changes in the basal nucleus of Meynert and in the diagonal band in Alzheimer disease. A quantitative Golgi investigation. Neuroscience 1986; 19:1265–1278.
444. Ferrer I, Aymami A, Rovira A, et al. Growth of abnormal neurites in atypical Alzheimer's disease. A study with the Golgi method. Acta Neuropathol (Berl) 1983; 59:167–170.
445. Geddes JW, Monaghan DT, Cotman CW, et al. Plasticity of hippocampal circuitry in Alzheimer's disease. Science 1985; 230:1179–1181.
446. Represa A, Duyckaerts C, Tremblay E, et al. Is senile dementia of the Alzheimer associated with hippocampal plasticity? Brain Res 1988; 457:355–359.
447. Masliah E, Terry RD, DeTeresa RM, et al. Immunohistochemical quantification of the synapse-related protein synaptophysin in Alzheimer disease. Neurosci Lett 1989; 103:234–239.
448. Hamos JE, DeGennaro LJ, Drachman DA. Synaptic loss in Alzheimer's disease and other dementias. Neurology 1989; 39:355–361.
449. Zhan SS, Beyreuther K, Schmitt HP. Quantitative assessment of the synaptophysin immuno-reactivity of the cortical neuropil in various neurodegenerative disorders with dementia. Dementia 1993; 4:66–74.
450. Bancher C, Jellinger K, Lassmann H, et al. Correlations between mental state and quantitative neuropathology in the Vienna Longitudinal Study on Dementia. Eur Arch Psychiatr Clin Neurosci 1996; 246:137–146.
451. Lassmann H, Weiler R, Fischer P, et al. Synaptic pathology in Alzheimer's disease: immunological data for markers of synaptic and large dense-core vesicles. Neuroscience 1992;46:1–8.
452. Bertoni-Freddari C, Fattoretti P, Casoli T, et al. Deterioration threshold of synaptic morphology in aging and senile dementia of Alzheimer's type. Anal Quant Cytol Histol 1996; 18:209–213.
453. DeKosky ST, Scheff W. Synapse loss in frontal cortex biopsies in Alzheimer's disease: correlation with cognitive severity. Ann Neurol 1990; 27:457–464.
454. Scheff SW, DeKosky ST, Price DA. Quantitative assessment of cortical synaptic density in Alzheimer's disease. Neurobiol Aging 1990; 11:29–37.
455. Scheff SW, Price DA. Synapse loss in the temporal lobe in Alzheimer's disease. Ann Neurol 1993; 33: 190–199.
456. Shimohama S, Kamiya S, Taniguchi T, et al. Differential involvement of synaptic vesicle and presynaptic plasma membrane proteins in Alzheimer's disease. Biochem Biophys Res Commun 1997; 236: 239–242.
457. Clinton J, Blackman SE, Royston MC, et al. Differential synaptic loss in the cortex in Alzheimer's disease: a study using archival material. NeuroReport 1994; 5:497–500.
458. Dessi F, Colle MA, Hauw J-J, et al. Accumulation of SNAP-25 immunoreactive material in axons of Alzheimer's disease. Neuroreport 1997; 8:3685–3689.
459. Heinonen O, Soininen H, Sorvari H, et al. Loss of synaptophysin-like immunoreactivity in the hippocampal formation is an early phenomenon in Alzheimer's disease. Neuroscience 1995; 64:375–384.
460. Lassmann H. Patterns of synaptic and nerve cell pathology in Alzheimer's disease. Behav Brain Res 1996; 78:9–14.
461. Masliah E, Terry RD, Mallory M, et al. Diffuse plaques do not accentuate synapse loss in Alzheimer's disease. Am J Pathol 1990; 137:1293–1297.
462. Price DL, Altschuler RJ, Struble RG, et al. Sequestration of tubulin in neurons in Alzheimer's disease. Brain Res 1986; 385:305–310.
463. Kahn J, Anderton BH, Probst A, et al. Immunologic studies of granulovacuolar degeneration using monoclonal antibodies to neurofilaments. J Neurol Neurosurg Psychiatry 1985; 48:926–927.
464. Dickson DW, Ksiezak-Reding H, Davies P, et al. A monoclonal antibody that recognizes a phosphorylated epitope in Alzheimer's neurofibrillary tangles, neurofilaments and tau proteins immunostains granulo-vacuolar degeneration. Acta Neuropathol (Berl) 1987; 73:254–258.
465. Dickson DW, Liu WK, Kress Y, et al. Phosphorylated tau immunoreactivity of granulovacuolar bodies (GVB) of Alzheimer's disease: localization of two amino terminal tau epitopes in GVB. Acta Neuropathol (Berl) 1993; 85:463–470.

466. Joachim CL, Morris JH, Selkoe DJ, et al. Tau epitopes are incorporated into a range of lesions in Alzheimer's disease. J Neuropathol Exp Neurol 1987; 46:611–622.
467. Mukaetova-Ladinska EB, Harrington CR, Roth M, et al. Biochemical and anatomical redistribution of tau protein in Alzheimer's disease. Am J Pathol 1993; 143:565–578.
468. Galloway PG, Perry G, Gambetti P. A study of actin binding proteins in Hirano bodies. J Neuropathol Exp Neurol 1986; 45:335 (abstr).
469. Galloway PG, Perry G, Kosik KS, et al. Hirano bodies contain tau protein. Brain Res 1987; 403:337–340.
470. Schmidt ML, Lee VM-Y, Trojanowski JQ. Analysis of epitopes shared by Hirano bodies and neurofilament protein in normal and Alzheimer's disease hippocampus. Lab Invest 1989; 60:513–522.
471. Munoz DG, Wang D, Greenberg BD. Hirano bodies accumulate C-terminal sequence of beta-amyloid precursor protein (beta-APP) epitopes. J Neuropathol Exp Neurol 1993; 52:14–21.
472. Hirano A. Hirano bodies and related neuronal inclusions. Neuropathol Appl Neurobiol 1994; 20:3–11.
473. Munch G, Cunningham AM, Riederer P, et al. Advanced glycation endproducts are associated with Hirano bodies in Alzheimer's disease. Brain Res 1998; 796:307–310.
474. Gibson PH, Tomlinson BE. Numbers of Hirano bodies in the hippocampus of normal and demented people with Alzheimer's disease. J Neurol Sci 1977; 33:199–206.
475. Hughes AJ, Daniel SE, Kilford L, et al. Accuracy of clinical diagnosis of idiopathic Parkinson's disease: a clinico-pathological study of 100 cases. J Neurol Neurosurg Psychiatry 1992; 55:181–184.
476. Salehi A, Ravid R, Gonatas NK, et al. Decreased activity of hippocampal neurons in Alzheimer's disease is not related to the presence of neurofibrillary tangles. J Neuropathol Exp Neurol 1995; 54:704–709.
477. Drach LM, Bohl J, Goebel HH. The lipofuscin content of nerve cells of the inferior olivary nucleus in Alzheimer's disease. Dementia 1994; 5:234–239.
478. Sumpter PQ, Mann DMA, Davies CA, et al. An ultrastructural analysis of the effects of accumulation of neurofibrillary tangles in pyramidal cells of the cerebral cortex in Alzheimer's disease. Neuropathol Appl Neurobiol 1986; 12:305–319.
479. Brion S, Masse G, Plas J. Histopathologie de la spongiose dans la maladie de Creutzfeldt-Jakob et dans les démences séniles et préséniles. In: Court LA, Cathala F, eds. Virus Non Conventionnels et Affections du Système Nerveux Central. Paris: Masson, 1983:227–234.
480. Smith TW, Anwer U, DeGirolami U, et al. Vacuolar change in Alzheimer's disease. Arch Neurol 1987; 44:1225–1228.
481. Duyckaerts C, Colle MA, Seilhean D, et al. Laminar spongiosis of the dentate gyrus: a sign of disconnection, present in cases of Alzheimer disease. Acta Neuropathol (Berl) 1998; 95:413–420.
482. Delacourte A. General and dramatic glial reaction in Alzheimer brains. Neurology 1990; 40:33–37.
483. Mountjoy CQ, Roth M, Evans NJR, et al. Cortical neuronal counts in normal elderly. Neurobiol Aging 1983; 4:1–11.
484. Terry RD, Hansen LA. Some morphometric aspects of Alzheimer disease and of normal aging. In: Terry RD, ed. Aging and the Brain. New York: Raven Press, 1988:109–114.
485. Probst A, Ulrich J, Heiz, PU. Senile dementia of the Alzheimer type: astroglial reaction to extracellular neurofibrillary tangles in the hippocampus. Acta Neuropathol (Berl) 1982; 57:75–79.
486. DeWitt DA, Perry G, Cohen M, et al. Astrocytes regulate miocroglial phagocytosis of senile plaque cores of Alzheimer's disease. Exp Neurol 1998; 149:329–340.
487. Hachinski VC, Potter P, Merskey H. Leuko-araiosis. Arch Neurol 1987; 44:21–23.
488. Brun A, Englund E. A white matter disorder in dementia of the Alzheimer type: a pathoanatomical study. Ann Neurol 1986; 19:253–262.
489. Durand-Fardel M. Traité Clinique et Pratique des Maladies des Vieillards. Paris: Germer Baillière, 1854.
490. Hauw J-J. Leukoaraiosis: the brain interstitial atrophy ("l'atrophie interstitielle du cerveau") of Durand-Fardel. Arch Neurol 1988; 45:140–141.
491. Awad IA, Johnson PC, Spetzler RF, et al. Incidental subcortical lesions identified on magnetic resonance imaging in the elderly. II. Postmortem pathological correlations. Stroke 1986; 17:1090–1097.
492. Inzitari D, Diaz F, Fox A, et al. Vascular risk factors and leukoaraiosis. Arch Neurol 1987; 44:42–47.
493. Verny M, Duyckaerts C, Pierot L, et al. Leukoaraiosis. Dev Neurosci 1991; 13:245–250.
494. Bowler J, Munoz D, Merskey H, et al. Factors affecting the age of onset and rate of progression of Alzheimer's disease. J Neurol Neurosurg Psychiatry 1998; 65:184–190.
495. Khachaturian ZS. Diagnosis of Alzheimer's disease. Arch Neurol 1985; 42:1097–1105.
496. Mirra SS, Heyman A, McKeel D, et al. The consortium to establish a registry for Alzheimer's disease (CERAD). Part II. Standardization of the neuropathological assessment of Alzheimer's disease. Neurology 1991; 41:479–486.
497. The National Institute on Aging, and Reagan Institute Working Group on Diagnostic Criteria for the Neuropathological Assessment of Alzheimer's Disease. Consensus recommendations for the postmortem diagnosis of Alzheimer's disease. Neurobiol Aging 1997; 18(4 Suppl):S1–S2.
498. Bierer L, Haroutunian V, Gabriel S, et al. Neurochemical correlates of dementia severity in Alzheimer's disease: Relative importance of the cholinergic deficits. J Neurochem 1995; 64:749–760.
499. Nitsch R. From acetylcholine to amyloid: neurotransmitters and the pathology of Alzheimer's disease. Neurodegeneration 1996; 5:477–482.
500. Procter A. The neurochemical correlates of dementia. Neurodegeneration 1996; 5:403–407.
501. Roberson M, Harrel L. Cholinergic activity and amyloid precursor protein metabolism. Brain Res Rev 1997; 25:50–69.
502. Bowen DM, Smith CB, White P, et al. Neurotransmitter enzymes and indices of hypoxia in senile dementia and other abiotrophies. Brain 1976; 99:459–496.

503. Davies P, Maloney AJF. Selective loss of cholinergic neurons in Alzheimer's disease. Lancet 1976; 2: 1403– .
504. Perry EK, Perry RH, Blessed G, et al. Necropsy evidence of central cholinergic deficits in senile dementia. Lancet 1977; 1:189– .
505. Rylett EG, Ball MJ, Colhoun EH. Evidence for high affinity choline transport in synaptosomes prepared from hippocampus and neocortex of patients with Alzheimer's disease. Brain Res 1983; 289:169–175.
506. Sims NR, Bowen DM, Allen SJ, et al. Presynaptic cholinergic dysfunction in patients with dementia. J Neurochem 1983; 40:503–509.
507. Neary D, Snowden JS, Mann DMA, et al. Alzheimer's disease: a correlative study. J Neurol Neurourg Psychiatry 1986; 49:229–237.
508. Nordberg A, Adem A, Hardy J, et al. Change in nicotinic receptor subtypes in temporal cortex of Alzheimer brains. Neurosci Lett 1988; 86:317–321.
509. Rossor M. Neurochemical studies in dementia. In: Iversen, LL, Iversen SD, Snyder SH, eds. Psychopharmacology of the Aging Nervous System, Handbook of Psychopharmacology. New York: Plenum Press, 1988 pp. 107–130.
510. Whitehouse PJ, Martino AM, Wagster MV, et al. Reductions in 3H nicotinic acetylcholine binding in Alzheimer's disease and Parkinson's disease: an autoradiographic study. Neurology 1988; 38:720–723.
511. Geula C, Mesulam M-M. Cholinergic systems and related neuropathological predilection patterns in Alzheimer's disease. In: Terry RD, Katzman R, Bick KL, eds. Alzheimer Disease. New York: Raven Press, 1994 pp. 263–291.
512. Johnston MV, McKinney M, Coyle JT. Neocortical cholinergic innervation: a description of extrinsic and intrinsic components in the rat. Exp Brain Res 1981; 43:159–172.
513. Lamour Y, Dutar P, Rascol O, et al. Basal forebrain neurons projecting to the rat frontoparietal cortex: electrophysiological and pharmacological properties. Brain Res 1986; 362:122–131.
514. Drachman DA, Leavitt J. Human memory and the cholinergic system: a relationship to aging? Arch Neurol 1974; 30:113–121.
515. Dekosky S, Harbaugh R, Schmidt F, et al. Cortical biopsy in Alzheimer's disease: diagnostic accuracy and neurochemical, neuropathological, and cognitive correlates. Ann Neurol 1992; ??:625–632.
516. Arendt T, Bigl V. Alzheimer plaques and cortical cholinergic innervation. Neuroscience 1986; 17:277–279.
517. Price DL, Cork LC, Struble Rg, et al. Neuropathological, neurochemical, and behavioral studies of the aging non-human primate. In: Davis RT, Leathers CW, eds. Behavior and Pathology of Aging in Rhesus Monkeys. New York: Alan R. Liss, 1985: pp. 113–135.
518. Beach TG, Honer WG, Hughes LH. Cholinergic fibre loss associated with diffuse plaques in the nondemented elderly: the preclinical stage of Alzheimer's disease? Acta Neuropathol (Berl) 1997; 93: 146–153.
519. Bartus R, Dean R, Beer D, et al. The cholinergic hypothesis of geriatric memory dysfunction. Science 1982; 217:408–417.
520. Perry EK. The cholinergic hypothesis—ten years on. Br Med Bull 1986; 42:63–69.
521. Palmer A, Proctor AW, Stratmann G, et al. Excitatory aminoacid-releasing and cholinergic neurones in Alzheimer's disease. Neurosci Lett 1986; 66:199–204.
522. Culen K, Halliday G, Double K, et al. Cell loss in the nucleus basalis is related to regional cortical atrophy in Alzheimer's disease. Neuroscience 1997; 78:641–652.
523. Gieula C, Mesulam M, Saroff D, et al. Relationship between plaques, tangles, and loss of cortical cholinergic fibers in Alzheimer disease. J Neuropathol Exp Neurol 1998; 57:63–75.
524. Francis PT, Cross AJ, Bowen DM. Neurotransmitters and neuropeptides. In: Terry RD, Katzman R, Bick KL, eds. Alzheimer Disease. New York: Raven Press, 1994; p247–261.
525. Saura J, Bleuel Z, Ulrich J, et al. Molecular neuroanatomy of human monoamine oxidases A and B revealed by quantitative enzyme radioautography and in situ hybridization histochemistry. Neuroscience 1996; 70:755–774.
526. Forno LS. The locus ceruleus in Alzheimer's disease. J Neuropathol Exp Neurol 1978; 37:614 (abstr)
527. Mann DMA, Yates PO, Marcyniuk B. A comparison of changes in the nucleus basalis and locus caeruleus in Alzheimer's disease. J Neurol Psychiatry 1984; 47: 201–203.
528. Tomlinson BE, Irvin D, Blessed G. Cells loss in the locus coeruleus in senile dementia of Alzheimer type. J Neurol Sci 1981; 49:419–428.
529. Rossor MN, Iversen LL, Reynolds GP, et al. Neurochemical characteristics of early and late onset types of Alzheimer's disease. BMJ 1984; 288:961–964.
530. Cross AJ, Crow TJ, Johnson JA, et al. Studies on neurotransmitter receptor systems in neocortex and hippocampus in senile dementia of the Alzheimer type. J Neurol Sci 1984; 74:109–117.
531. Berger B, Escourolle R, Moyne MA. Axones catécholaminergiques du cortex cérébral humain. Observation, en histofluorescence, de biopsies cérébrales dont 2 cas de maladie d'Alzheimer. Rev Neurol (Paris) 1976; 132:183–194.
532. Berger B, Tassin JP, Rancurel G, et al. Catecholaminergic innervation of the human cerebral cortex in presenile and senile dementia: histochemical and biochemical studies. In: Usdin E, Sourkes TL, Youdim MBH, eds. Enzymes and Neurotransmitters in Mental Disease. Chichester: John Wiley & Sons, 1980 pp. 317–328.
533. Iversen LL, Rossor MN, Reynolds GP, et al. Loss of pigmented dopamine β hydroxylase positive cells from locus caeruleus in senile dementia of Alzheimer type. Neurosci Lett 1983; 39:95–100.
534. Felten DL, Sladek JR. Monoamine distribution in primate brain. V. Monoaminergic nuclei: anatomy, pathways and local organization. Brain Res Bull 1983; 10:171–284.
535. Chen C, Alder J, Bowen D, et al. Presynaptic serotonergic markers in community-acquired cases of Alzheimer's disease: correlations with depression and neuroleptic medication. J Neurochem 1996; 66: 1592–1598.

536. Meltzer CC, Smith G, DeKosky ST, et al. Serotonin in aging, late-life depression, and Alzheimer's disease: the emerging role of functional imaging. Neuropsychopharmacology 1998; 18:407–430.
537. Hirano A, Zimmerman HM. Alzheimer's neurofibrillary changes. A topographical study. Arch Neurol 1962; 7:227–242.
538. Mann DMA, Yates PO, Marcyniuk B. Dopaminergic neurotransmitter systems in Alzheimer's disease and in Down's syndrome at middle age. J Neurol Neurosurg Psychiatry 1987; 50:341–344.
539. Porrino LJ, Goldman-Rakic PS. Brainstem innervation of prefrontal and anterior cingulate cortex in the rhesus monkey revealed by retrograde transport of HRP. J Comp Neurol 1982; 205:63–76.
540. Gottfries CG, Frederiksen SO, Heilig M. Neuropeptides and Alzheimer's disease. Eur Neuropsychopharmacol 1995; 5:491–500.
541. Valenti G. Neuropeptide changes in dementia: pathogenetic implications and diagnostic value. Gerontology 1996; 42:241–256.
542. Beal MF, Mazurek MF, Svendsen CN, et al. Widespread reduction of somatostatin-like immunoreactivity in the cerebral cortex in Alzheimer's disease. Ann Neurol 1986; 20:489–495.
543. Cervera-Pierrot P, Hirsch EC, Javoy-Agid F, et al. Hippocampal and parahippocampal somatostatin 28 and neuropeptide Y containing neurons in Alzheimer's disease. Dementia 1992; 3:282–298.
544. Epelbaum J. Somatostatin in the central nervous system: physiology and pathological modifications. Prog Neurobiol 1986; 6:755–768.
545. Davies P, Katzman R, Terry RD. Reduced somatostatin immunoreactivity in cases of Alzheimer's disease and Alzheimer senile dementia. Nature 1980; 288:279–280.
546. Grouselle D, Winsky Sommerer R, David JP, et al. Loss of somatostatin-like immunoreactivity in the frontal cortex of Alzheimer patients carrying the apolipoprotein epsilon 4 allele. Neurosci Lett 1988; 255:21–24.
547. Dournaud P, Delaère P, Hauw J, et al. Somatostatin and choline acetyltransferase deficits in Alzheimer's disease; differential correlation with the neuropathology and the cognitive state. Neurobiol Aging 1995; 16:817–823.
548. Roberts GW, Crow TJ, Polak JM. Localization of neuronal tangles in somatostatin neurones in Alzheimer's disease. Nature 1985; 314:92–392.
549. Adrian TE, Allen JM, Bloom SR, et al. Neuropeptide Y distribution in human brain. Nature 1983; 306:584–586.
550. Vincent SR, Johansson O, Hokfelt T, et al. Neuropeptide coexistence in human cortical neurones. Nature 1982; 298:65–67.
551. Chan-Palay V, Lang W, Haesler U, et al. Distribution of altered hippocampal neurones and axons immunoreactive with antisera against neuropeptide Y in Alzheimer type dementia. J Comp Neurol 1986; 248:376–394.
552. Nakamura S, Vincent SR. Somatostatin and neuropeptide Y immunoreactive neurons in the neocortex in senile dementia of Alzheimer type. Brain Res 1986; 370:11–20.
553. Allen JM, Ferrier IN, Roberts GW, et al. Elevation of neuropeptide Y (NPY) in substantia innominata in Alzheimer's type dementia. J Neurol Sci 1984; 64:325–331.
554. Dawbarn D, Rossor MN, Mountjoy CQ, et al. Decreased somatostatin immunoreactivity but not neuropeptide Y immunoreactivity in cerebral cortex in senile dementia of Alzheimer type. Neurosci Lett 1986; 70:154–159.
555. Foster NL, Tamminga CA, O'Donohue TL, et al. Brain choline acetyltransferase activity and neuropeptide Y concentrations in Alzheimer's disease. Neurosci Lett 1986; 63:71–75.
556. Gaspar P, Duyckaerts C, Febvret A, et al. Subpopulations of somatostatin 28-immunoreactive neurons display different vulnerability in senile dementia of the Alzheimer type. Brain Res 1989; 490:1–13.
557. Crystal HA, Davies P. Cortical substance P-like immunoreactivity in cases of Alzheimer's disease and senile dementia of the Alzheimer type. J Neurochem 1982; 38:1781–1784.
558. Perry RH, Dockray GJ, Dimaline R, et al. Neuropeptides in Alzheimer's disease, depression and schizophrenia. A postmortem analysis of vasoactive intestinal polypeptide and cholecystokinin in cerebral cortex. J Neurol Sci 1981; 51:465–472.
559. Ferrier IN, Cross AJ, Johnson JA, et al. Neuropeptides in Alzheimer type dementia. J Neurol Sci 1983; 62:159–170.
560. Yates CM, H Harmar AJ, Rosie R et al. Thyrotropin releasing hormone, luteinizing hormone-releasing hormone and substance P immunoreactivity in postmortem brain from cases of Alzheimer type dementia and Down's syndrome. Brain Res 1983; 258:45–52.
561. Bissette G, Reynolds GP, Kilts CD, et al. Corticotropin-releasing factor-like immunoreactivity in senile dementia of the Alzheimer type. JAMA 1985; 254:3067–3069.
562. De Souza EB, Whitehouse PJ, Kuhar MJ, et al. Reciprocal changes in corticotropin-releasing factor (CRF)-like immunoreactivity and CRF receptors in cerebral cortex of Alzheimer's disease. Nature 1986; 319:593–595.
563. Deecher DC, Mash DC, Staley JK, et al. Characterization and localization of galanin receptors in human entorhinal cortex. Regul Peptides 1998; 73:149–159.
564. Gabriel SM, Bierer LM, Davidson M, et al. Galanin-like immunoreactivity is increased in the postmortem cerebral cortex from patients with Alzheimer's disease. J Neurochem 1994; 62:1516–1523.
565. Rodriguez Puertas R, Nilsson S, Pascual J, et al. I-125-Galanin binding sites in Alzheimer's disease: increases in hippocampal subfields and a decrease in the caudate nucleus. J Neurochem 1997; 68:1106–1113.
566. Nitsch RM, Kim C, Growdon JH. Vasopressin and bradykinin regulate secretory processing of the amyloid protein precursor of Alzheimer's disease. Neurochem Res 1998; 23:807–814.
567. Fine RE, Abraham CR. Hypothesis: beta amyloid precursor protein is a key sorting and targeting receptor for neuropeptidases. Amyloid Int J Exp Clin Invest 1997; 4:233–239.
568. Marczynski TJ. GABAergic deafferentation hypoth-

esis of brain aging and Alzheimer's disease revisited. Brain Res Bull 1998; 45:341–379.
569. Pakaski M, Farkas Z, Kasa P, et al. Vulnerability of small GABAergic neurons to human beta-amyloid pentapeptide. Brain Res 1998; 239–246.
570. Rossor MN, Garrett NJ, Johnson AL, et al. A postmortem study of the cholinergic and GABA systems in senile dementia. Brain 1982; 105:313–330.
571. Lowe SL, Francis PT, Procter AW, et al. Gamma-aminobutyric acid concentration in brain tissue at two stages of Alzheimer's disease. Brain 1988; 111–785–799.
572. Hardy J, Cowburn R, Barton A, et al. Region specific loss of glutamate innervation in Alzheimer's disease. Neurosci Lett 1987; 73:77–80.
573. Cowburn R, Hardy J, Roberts P, et al. Presynaptic and postsynaptic glutaminergic function in Alzheimer's disease. Neurosci Lett 1988; 66:109–115.
574. Smith CC, Bowen DM, Sims NR, et al. Aminoacid release from biopsy samples of temporal neocortex from patients with Alzheimer's disease. Brain Res 1983; 264:138–141.
575. Bowen DM, Palmer AM, Francis PT, et al. "Classical" neurotransmitters in Alzheimer disease. In: Terry RD, ed. Aging and the Brain. New York: Raven Press, 1988 pp. 115–128.
576. Kaye JA. Diagnostic challenges in dementia. Neurology 1998; 5:S45–S52.
577. Boller F, Lopez OL, Moossy J. Diagnosis of dementia: clinicopathologic correlations. Neurology 1989; 39:76–79.
578. Jellinger K, Danielczyk W, Fischer P, et al. Clinicopathological analysis of dementia disorders in the elderly. J Neurol Sci 1990; 95:239–258.
579. Kokmen E, Offord K, Okasaki H. A clinical and autopsy study of dementia in Olmsted Country, Minnesota, 1980–1981. Neurology 1987; 37:426–430.
580. Buhl L, Bojsen-Moller M. Frequency of Alzheimer's disease in a post-mortem study of psychiatric patients. Dan Med Bull 1988; 35:288–290.
581. Mendez MF, Mastri AR, Sung JH, et al. Clinically diagnosed Alzheimer disease: neuropathologic findings in 650 cases. Alzheimer Dis Assoc Disord 1992; 6:35–43.
582. Cummings JL, Benson DF. Dementia. A Clinical Approach. Boston: Butterworths, 1983.
583. Chui HC, Victoroff JI, Margolin D, et al. Criteria for the diagnosis of ischemic vascular dementia proposed by the state of California Alzheimer's disease diagnostic and treatment centers. Neurology 1992; 42:473–480.
584. Roman GC, Tatemichi TK, Erkinjuntti T, et al. Vascular dementia: diagnostic criteria for research studies Report of the NINDS-AIREN International Workshop. Neurology 1993; 43:250–260.
585. Cohen CI, Araujo L, Guerrier R, et al. "Mixed dementia": adequate or antiquated? A critical review. Am J Geriatr Psychiatry 1997 5:279–283.
586. Rockwood K. Lessons from mixed dementia. Int Psychogeriatr 1997; 9:245–249.
587. Snowdon DA, Greiner LH, Mortimer JA, et al. Brain infarction and the clinical expression of Alzheimer's disease: the nun study. JAMA 1997; 277:813–817.
588. Nagy Z, Esiri M, Jobst KA, et al. The effects of additional pathology on the cognitive deficit in Alzheimer disease. J Neuropathol Exp Neurol 1997; 56:165–170.
589. Zekri D, Duyckaerts C, Belmin J, et al. Vascular, degenerative and mixed dementia. A clinicopathological study in 33 cases. Brain Pathol 1997; 7:1213– (abstr)
590. Ott A, Breteler M, van Harskamp F, et al. Incidence and risk of dementia. The Rotterdam Study. Am J Epidemiol 1998; 147:574–580.
591. Crawford J. Alzheimer's disease risk factors as related to cerebral blood flow: additional evidence. Med Hypotheses 1998; 50:25–36.
592. de la Torre JC. Critical threshold cerebral hypoperfusion causes Alzheimer's disease. Acta Neuropathol (Berl) 1999; 98:1–8.
593. Ball MJ, Schapiro MB, Rapaport SI. Neuropathological relationship between Down Syndrome and senile dementia of the Alzheimer type. In: Epstein CJ, ed. The Neurobiology of Down Syndrome. New York: Raven Press, 1986: pp. 45–58.
594. Bertrand I, Koffas D. Cas d'idiotie mongolienne adulte avec nombreuses plaques séniles et concrétions calcaires pallidales. Rev Neurol (Paris) 1946; 78: 338–.
595. Leverenz JB, Raskind MA. Early amyloid deposition in the medial temporal lobe of young Down syndrome patients: a regional quantitative analysis. Exp Neurol 1998; 150:296–304.
596. Sadowski R, Wisniewski HM, Tarnawski M, et al. Entorhinal cortex of aged subjects with Down's syndrome shows severe-neuronal loss caused by neurofibrillary pathology. Acta Neuropathol (Berl) 1999; 97:156–164.
597. Solitaire GB, Lamarche JB. Alzheimer's disease and senile dementia as seen in mongoloids. Am J Ment Defic 1966; 70:840–848.
598. Wisniewski HM, Rabe A, Wisniewski E. Neuropathology and dementia in people with Down's syndrome. In: Davies P, Finch CE, eds. Molecular Neuropathology of Aging. Cold Spring Harbor, NY: Cold Spring Harbor Laboratory Press, 1987 pp. 399–413.
599. Prasher VP, Farrer MJ, Kessling AM, et al. Molecular mapping of Alzheimer-type dementia in Down's syndrome. Ann Neurol 1998; 43:380–383.
600. Mann DMA, Esiri MM. The pattern of acquisition of plaques and tangles in the brains of patients under 50 years of age with Down's syndrome. J Neurol Sci 1989; 89:169–179.
601. Rumble B, Retallack R, Hilbich C, et al. Amyloid A4 protein and its precursor in Down's syndrome and Alzheimer's disease. N Engl J Med 1989; 320:1446–1452.
602. Lippa CF, Schmidt L, Lee VM-Y, et al. Antibodies to a-synuclein detect Lewy bodies in many Down's syndrome brain's with Alzheimer's disease. Ann Neurol 1999; 45:353–357.
603. Allsop D, Kidd M, Landon M, et al. Isolated senile plaque cores in Alzheimer's disease and Down's syndrome show differences in morphology. J Neurol Neurosurg Psychiatry 1986; 49:886–890.
604. Szumanska G, Vorbrodt AW, Mandybur TI, et al. Lectin histochemistry of plaques and tangles in Alzheimer disease. Acta Neuropathol (Berl) 1987; 73: 1–11.
605. Sylvester PE. Ageing in the mentally retarded. In:

605. First European Symposium on Scientific Studies in Mental Retardation. London: Royal Society of Medicine, 1983: pp. 259.
606. Holland A, Hon J, Huppert F, et al. Population-based study of the prevalence and presentation of dementia in adults with Down's syndrome. Br J Psychiatry 1998; 172:493–498.
607. Okazaki H, Lipkin LE, Aronson SM. Diffuse intracytoplasmic inclusions (Lewy type) associated with progressive dementia and quadriparesis in flexion. J Neuropathol Exp Neurol 1967; 20:237–244.
608. Kosaka K, Oyanagi S, Matsushita M, et al. Presenile dementia with Alzheimer-, Pick- and Lewy-body changes. Acta Neuropathol (Berl) 1976; 36:221–233.
609. Kosaka K. Lewy bodies in cerebral cortex. Report of three cases. Acta Neuropathol (Berl) 1978; 42:127–134.
610. Kosaka K. Diffuse Lewy body disease in Japan. J Neurol 1990;237:197–204.
611. Perry RH, Irving D, Blessed G, et al. Senile dementia of Lewy body type. A clinically and neuropathologically distinct form of Lewy body dementia in elderly. J Neurol Sci 1990; 95:119–139.
612. Hansen L, Salmon D, Galasko D, et al. The Lewy body variant of Alzheimer's disease: a clinical and pathological entity. Neurology 1990; 40:1–8.
613. Lennox G, Lowe J, Byrne EJ, et al. Diffuse Lewy body disease. Lancet 1989; i:323–324.
614. McKeith IG, Perry RH, Fairbairn AF, et al. Operational criteria for senile dementia of Lewy body type (SDLT). Psychiatr Med 1992; 22:911–922.
615. Hughes AJ, Daniel SE, Blankson S, et al. A clinicopathologic study of 100 cases of Parkinson's disease. Arch Neurol 1993; 50:140–148.
616. Mattila PM, Koskela T, Roytta M, et al. Apolipoprotein E epsilon4 allele frequency is increased in Parkinson's disease only with co-existing Alzheimer pathology. Acta Neuropathol (Berl) 1998; 96:417–420.
617. Lantos PL, Ovenstone IM, Johnson J, et al. Lewy bodies in the brain of two members of a family with the 717 (Val to Ile) mutation of the amyloid precursor protein gene. Neurosci Lett 1994; 172:77–79.
618. Revesz T, McLaughlin JL, Rossor MN, et al. Pathology of familial Alzheimer's disease with Lewy bodies. J Neural Transm 1997; 51 (Suppl):121–135.
619. Mattila PM, Roytta M, Torikka H, et al. Cortical Lewy bodies and Alzheimer-type changes in patients with Parkinson's disease. Acta Neuropathol (Berl) 1998; 95:576–582.
620. Ince PG, Perry EK, Morris, CM. Dementia with Lewy bodies. A distinct non-Alzheimer dementia syndrome? Brain Pathol 1998; 8:299–324.
621. McKeith IG, Ince P, Jaros EB, et al. What are the relations between Lewy body disease and AD? J Neural Transm 1998; 54 (Suppl):107–116.
622. Brown DF, Dababo MA, Bigio EH, et al. Neuropathologic evidence that the Lewy body variant of Alzheimer disease represents coexistence of Alzheimer disease and idiopathic Parkinson disease. J Neuropathol Exp Neurol 1998; 57:39–46.
623. McKeith IG, Galasko D, Kosaka K, et al. Consensus guidelines for the clinical and pathologic diagnosis of dementia with Lewy bodies (DLB): report of the consortium on DLB international workshop. Neurology 1996; 47:1113–1124.
624. Ewbank D. Deaths attributable to Alzheimer's disease in the United States. Am J Public Health 1999; 89:90–92.
625. Katzman R, Kawas C. The epidemiology of dementia and Alzheimer's disease. In: Terry RD, Katzman R, Bick KL, eds. Alzheimer Disease. New York: Raven Press, 1994; pp. 105–122.
626. Launer LJ, Fratiglioni L, Andersen K, et al. Regional differences in the incidence of dementia in Europe: EURODEM collaborative analyses. In: Iqbal K, Swaab DF, Winblad B, Wisniewski HM, eds. Alzheimer's Disease and Related Disorders. Etiology, Pathogenesis and Therapeutics. Chichester: John Wiley & Sons, 1999; pp. 9–15.
627. Ritchie K, Kildea D, Robine JM. The relationship between age and the prevalence of senile dementia: a meta-analysis of recent data. Int J Epidemiol 1992; 21:763–769.
628. Zubenko G, Winwood E, Jacobs B, et al. Prospective study of risk factors for Alzheimer's disease: results at 7.5 years. Am J Psychiatry 1999; 156:50–57.
629. Hardy J, Gwinn Hardy K. Genetic classification of primary neurodegenerative disease. Science 1998; 282:1075–1079.
630. Katzman R, Kang D, Thomas R. Interaction of apolipoprotein E epsilon 4 with other genetic and nongenetic risk factors in late onset Alzheimer disease: problems pacing the investigator. Neurochem Res 1988; 23:369–376.
631. Shastry BS. Molecular genetics of familial Alzheimer disease. Am J Med Sci 1998; 315:266–272.
632. Slooter AJC, van Duijn CM. Genetic epidemiology of Alzheimer disease. Epidemiol Rev 1997; 19:107–119.
633. Fox NC, Kennedy AM, Harvey RJ, et al. Clinicopathological features of familial Alzheimer's disease associated with the M139V mutation in the presenilin 1 gene. Pedigree but not mutation specific age at onset provides evidence for a further genetic factor. Brain 1997; 120:491–501.
634. Harvey RJ, Ellison D, Hardy J, et al. Chromosome 14 familial Alzheimer's disease: the clinical and neuropathological characteristics of a family with a leucine->serine (L250S) substitution at codon 250 of the presenilin 1 gene. J Neurol Neurosurg Psychiatry 1998; 64:44–49.
635. Lippa CF, Fujiwara H, Mann DMA, et al. Lewy bodies contain altered alpha-synuclein in brains of many familial Alzheimer's disease patients with mutations in presenilin and amyloid precursor protein genes. Am J Pathol 1998; 153:1365–1370.
636. Nochlin D, Bird TD, Nemens EJ, et al. Amyloid angiopathy in a Volga German family with Alzheimer's disease and a presenilin-2 mutation ((NI)-I-141). Ann Neurol 1998; 43:131–135.
637. Gomez-Isla T, West HL, Rebeck GW, et al. Clinical and pathological correlates of apolipoprotein E epsilon 4 in Alzheimer's disease. Ann Neurol 1996; 39:62–570.
638. Myers RH, Schaefer EJ, Wilson PWF, et al. Apolipoprotein E ε4 association with dementia in a population-based study: the Framingham study. Neurology 1996; 46:673–677.
639. Namba Y, Tomonoga M, Kawasaki H, et al. Apolipoprotein E immunoreactivity in cerebral amyloid deposits and neurofibrillary tangles in Alzheimer's

disease and kuru plaque amyloid in Creutzfeldt-Jakob disease. Brain Res 1991; 541:163–166.
640. Poirier J, Davignon J, Bouthillier D, et al. Apolipoprotein E polymorphism and Alzheimer's disease. Lancet 1993; 342:697–699.
641. Saunders AM, Strittmatter WJ, Schmechel D, et al. Association of apolipoprotein E allele ε4 with late-onset familial and sporadic Alzheimer's disease. Neurology 1993; 43:1467–1472.
642. Schmechel DE, Saunders AE, Strittmatter WJ, et al. Increased amyloid β-peptide deposition in cerebral cortex as a consequence of apolipoprotein E genotype in late-onset Alzheimer disease. Proc Natl Acad Sci USA 1993; 90:9649–9653.
643. Galasko D, Saitoh T, Xia Y, et al. The apolipoprotein E allele ε4 is overrepresented in patients with the Lewy body variant of Alzheimer's disease. Neurology 1994; 44:1950–1951.
644. Drigalenko E, Poduslo S, Elston, R. Interaction of the apolipoprotein E and CI loci in predisposing to late-onset Alzheimer's disease. Neurology 1998; 51:131–135.
645. Breitner J, Jarvik G, Plassman B, et al. Risk of Alzheimer disease with the epsilon4 allele for apolipoprotein E in a population-based study of men aged 62–73 years. Alzheimer Dis Assoc Disord 1998; 12:40–44.
646. Strittmater WJ, Roses AD. Apolipoprotein E and Alzheimer's disease. Annu Rev Neurosci 1996; 19:53–77.
647. McCarron M, Nicoll J, Stewart J, et al. The apolipoprotein E epsilon2 allele and the pathological features in cerebral amyloid angiopathy-related hemorrhage. J Neuropathol Exp Neurol 1999; 58:711–718.
648. Pericak-Vance M, Bass M, Yamaoka L, et al. Complete genomic screen in late-onset familial Alzheimer disease. Evidence for a new locus on chromosome 12. JAMA 1997; 278:1237–1241.
649. Alpérovitch A, Berr C. Familial aggregation of dementia of Alzheimer type: analysis from an epidemiological point of view. In: Sinet PM, Lamour Y, Christen Y, eds. Genetics and Alzheimer's Disease. Berlin: Springer-Verlag, 1988; 31–39.
650. Forbes W, Hill G. Is exposure to aluminum a risk factor for the development of Alzheimer disease?—Yes. Arch Neurol 1998; 55:740–741.
651. Munoz D. Is exposure to aluminum a risk factor for the development of Alzheimer disease?—No. Arch Neurol 1998; 55:737–739.
652. Candy JM, et al. Aluminosilicates and senile plaques formation in Alzheimer's disease. Lancet 1986; 1:354–357.
653. Chafi AH, Hauw J-J, Rancurel G, et al. Absence of aluminium in Alzheimer's disease brain tissue: electron microprobe and ion micropobe studies. Neurosci Lett 1991; 123:61–64.
654. Bjertness E, Candy JM, Torvik A, et al. Content of brain aluminium is not elevated in Alzheimer's disease. Alzheimer Dis Assoc Disord 1996; 10:171–174.
655. Kukull WA, Larson EB, Bowen JD, et al. Solvent exposure as a risk factor for Alzheimer disease: a case-control study. Am J Epidemiol 1995; 141:1059–1071.
656. Savitz D, Checkoway H, Loomis, D. Magnetic field exposure and neurodegenerative disease mortality among electric utility workers. Epidemiology 1998; 9:398–404.
657. Prince M. Is chronic low-level lead exposure in early life an etiologic factor in Alzheimer's disease? Epidemiology 1998; 9:618–621.
658. Durlach J, Bac P, Durlach V, et al. Are age-related neurodegenerative diseases linked with various types of magnesium depletion? Magnes Res 1997; 10:339–353.
659. Graham D, Gentleman S, Nicoll J, et al. Is there a genetic basis for the deposition of beta-amyloid after fatal head injury? Cell Mol Neurobiol 1999; 19:19–30.
660. O'Meara E, Kukull W, Sheppard L, et al. Head injury and risk of Alzheimer's disease by apolipoprotein E genotype. Am J Epidemiol 1997; 146:373–384.
661. Brown P, Gibbs CJJ, Rodgers-Johnson P, et al. Human spongiform encephalopathy: the National Institutes of Health series of 300 cases of experimentally transmitted disease. Ann Neurol 1994; 35:513–529.
662. Brinton RD, Yamazaki RS. Advances and challenges in the prevention and treatment of Alzheimer's disease. Pharm Res 1998; 15:386–398.
663. Henderson VW. Estrogen, cognition, and a woman risk of Alzheimer's disease. Am J Med 1997; 103:11S–18S.
664. Inestrosa N, Marzolo M, Bonnefont A. Cellular and molecular basis of estrogen's neuroprotection. Potential relevance for Alzheimer's disease. Mol Neurobiol 1998; 17:73–86.
664a. In't Veld BA, Launer LJ, Hoes AW, Ott A, Hofman A, Breteler MM, Stricker BH. NSAIDs and incident Alzheimer's disease. The Rotterdam Study. Neurobiol Aging. 1998; 19:607–611.
665. Ulrich J, Johannson-Locher G, Seiler WO, et al. Does smoking protect from Alzheimer's disease? Alzheimer-type changes in 301 unselected brains from patients with known smoking history. Acta Neuropathol (Berl) 1997; 94:450–454.
666. Wang H, Fratiglioni L, Frisoni G, et al. Smoking and the occurrence of Alzheimer's disease: cross-sectional and longitudinal data in a population-based study. Am J Epidemiol 1999; 149:640–644.
667. Evans D, Hebert L, Beckett L, et al. Education and other measures of socioeconomic status and risk of incident Alzheimer disease in a defined population of older persons. Arch Neurol 1997; 54:1399–1405.
668. Geerlings M, Schmand B, Jonker C, et al. Education and incident Alzheimer's disease: a biased association due to selective attrition and use of a two-step diagnostic procedure? Int J Epidemiol 1999; 28:492–497.
669. Lemeshow S, Letenneur L, Dartigues J, et al. Illustration of analysis taking into account complex survey considerations: the association between wine consumption and dementia in the PAQUID study. Personnes Agées Quid. Am J Epidemiol 1998; 148:298–306.
670. Orgozozo J-M, Dartigues JF, Lafont S, et al. Wine consumption and dementia in the elderly: a prospective community study in the Bordeaux area. Rev Neurol 1997; 153:185–192.
671. Fastbom J, Forsell Y, Winblad, B. Benzodiazepines may have protective effects against Alzheimer disease. Alzheimer Dis Assoc Disord 1998; 12:14–17.

672. Giannakopoulos P, Hof PR, Kövari E, et al. Distinct patterns of neuronal loss and Alzheimer's disease lesion distribution in elderly individuals older than 90 years. J Neuropathol Exp Neurol 1996; 55:1210–1220.
673. Hauw J-J, Delaère P, He Y, et al. The centenarian's brain. Adv Biosci 1993; 87:127–135.
674. Mizutani T, Shimada H. Neuropathological background of twenty-seven centenarian brains. J Neurol Sci 1992; 108:168–177.
675. Roth M. The association of clinical and neurological findings and its bearing on the classification and aetiology of Alzheimer's disease. Br Med Bull 1986; 42:42–50.

9. Parkinson's Disease

TAMAS REVESZ, FRANCOISE GRAY, AND
FRANCESCO SCARAVILLI

Parkinsonism is characterized clinically by the development of extrapyramidal movement disturbance manifested by a combination of rigidity and bradykinesia with or without resting tremor. These signs have been correlated with a lesion of the nigrostriatal dopaminergic system, in particular with depletion of dopamine in the striatum, which, in most cases, is secondary to severe nerve cell loss in the substantia nigra.[1]

In addition to the idiopathic form (Parkinson's disease, paralysis agitans), the prototype Lewy body (LB) disorder, clinically similar syndromes may be secondary to lesions of the substantia nigra due to other causes. Involvement of the substantia nigra and parkinsonism may also occur in other neurodegenerative diseases involving predominantly the basal ganglia, the cerebral cortex, or the spinocerebellar system.

PARKINSON'S DISEASE

Parkinson's disease (PD) affects both sexes. Its incidence increases with age and the mean age at onset is around 61 years and average disease duration is around 13 years.[2] The disease is most prevalent in octogenerians—75% to 88% are in their seventh or eighth decade of life,[3]—however, young-onset parkinsonism with onset between 21 and 40 years may be associated with the same pathology as late-onset PD.[4] Establishing the precise incidence and prevalence of PD is very difficult because of a high rate of clinical misdiagnosis,[5] therefore estimates vary in the different studies: between 30 to 190 per 100,000 population for prevalence and 7 to 19 per 100,000 population for annual incidence.[6] Because of the limitation of the lesions to specific brain stem nuclei, the predominant involvement of nerve cells, and its possible occurrence in families, PD is included in the group of neurodegenerative illnesses. No causative agents are known; however, three factors have been proposed to explain the pathogenesis of PD: an environmental agent, genetic susceptibility, and accelerated aging. On the one hand, several families have been documented as having either autosomal dominant or recessive parkinsonism, some but not all with LB pathology.[7-10] On the other hand, there is increasing evidence that oxidative stress may be an important factor in the pathogenesis of neuronal death in PD, possibly by inducing apoptosis of dopaminergic neurons.[11-14] Finally, it is likely that PD will be explained by genetic susceptibility to environmental agents predisposing to oxidative stress and free radical–mediated damage in a neuronal population that is already under oxidative stress as part of a normal metabolic requirement in producing dopamine.[15]

History

The evolution of our knowledge of the pathologic changes in this disease developed over several stages. In his *Essay on the Shaking Palsy* (Fig. 9–1), Parkinson[6] suggested that the lesion is localized to the upper cervical cord and lower medulla. Subsequently, other au-

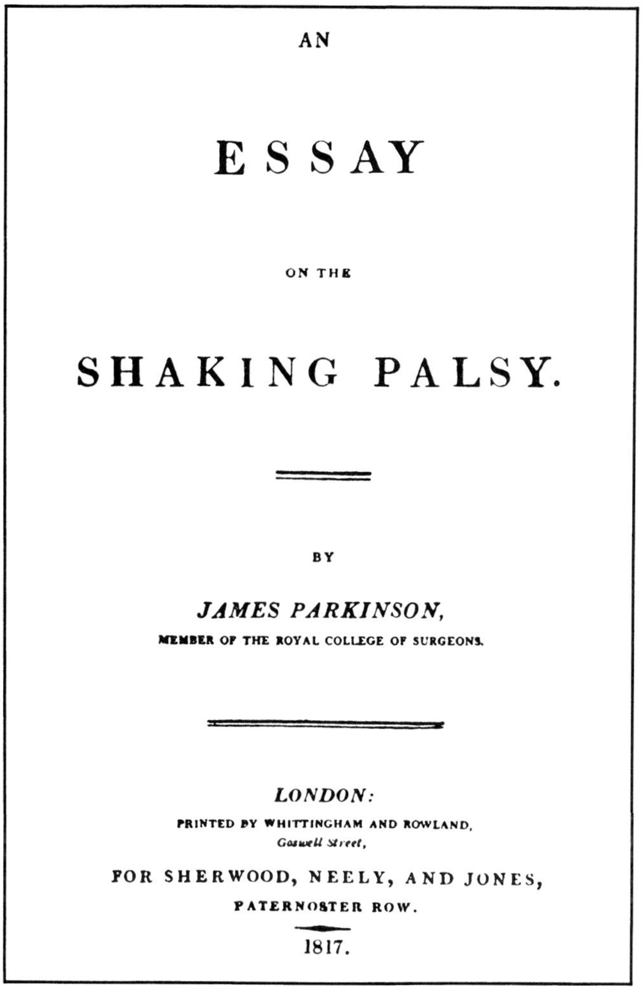
AN

ESSAY

ON THE

SHAKING PALSY.

BY

JAMES PARKINSON,

MEMBER OF THE ROYAL COLLEGE OF SURGEONS.

LONDON:

PRINTED BY WHITTINGHAM AND ROWLAND,

Goswell Street,

FOR SHERWOOD, NEELY, AND JONES,

PATERNOSTER ROW.

1817.

Figure 9–1. Title page of the initial description of the disease by Sir James Parkinson.

thors suggested the possibility of involvement of the basal ganglia and, in particular, of the pallidum.[17–21] Finally, the characteristic lesions of the substantia nigra were recognized (Figs. 9–2 and 9–3).[22–31] The essential role of the changes in the substantia nigra (Fig. 9–4) and, in particular, of the degeneration of the dopaminergic cells in the production of the extrapyramidal symptoms has been proven by the demonstration of low levels of dopamine in the striatum of patients with PD[11] by the improvement of motor symptoms after treatment with L-dopa, and by the appearance of a parkinsonian syndrome after intoxication with 1-methyl-4-phenyl-1,2,3,4,6-tetrahydropyridine (MPTP), which is known to produce degeneration of the dopaminergic neurons of the nigrostriatal pathway.[32]

Lewy Body

The pathological hallmark of idiopathic PD is a loss of dopaminergic neurons in the substantia nigra associated with the presence of intraneuronal inclusions, LBs (Fig. 9–5A). These were initially described by Lewy in the substantia innominata and dorsal motor vagal nucleus,[8] but they were called "corps de Lewy" by Tretiakoff when seen in the substantia nigra.[23] The fact that pathologic changes are not limited exclusively to the substantia nigra is in keeping with the existence of symptoms other than extrapyramidal ones, in particular with those due to autonomic failure or with a disorder of higher cerebral functions, which, on occasion, may be severe. It is now widely accepted that idiopathic PD is only one subtype

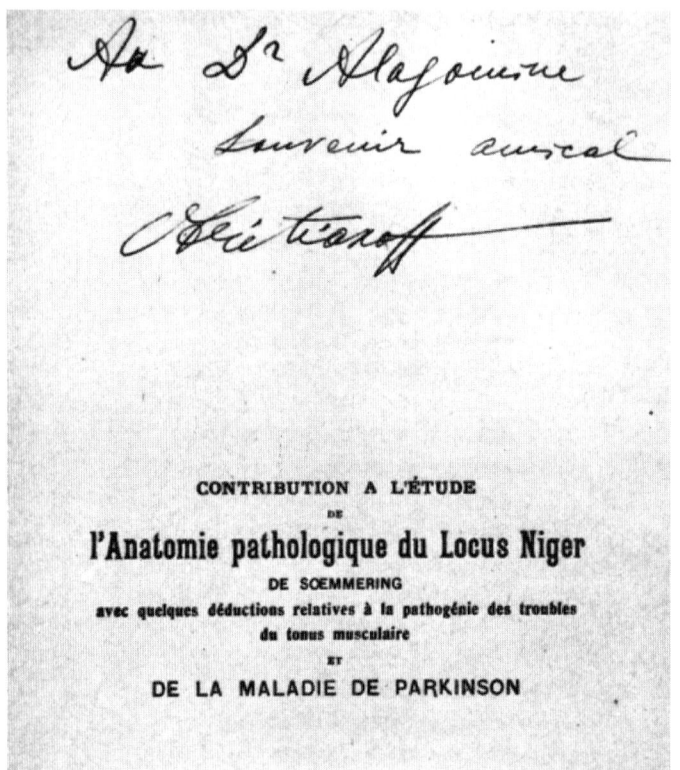

Figure 9–2. Title page of the thesis of Tretiakoff dedicated to Professor Alajouanine.

of a wider group of LB disorders that show considerable clinical and pathological overlap and also include autonomic failure, LB dysphagia, and dementia with Lewy bodies (DLB).[15] Lewy bodies may be observed in other conditions as well as in the brains of some aged individuals without any clinical evidence of disease.[33] On the basis of autopsy studies it has been suggested that 2%–10% of such neurologically unaffected individuals may have incidental brain stem LBs[34,35] when incidental LBs may represent preclinical or subclinical PD. It has been, suggested, however, that, in contrast to brain stem LBs, cortical LBs are not features of normal aging.[36] The presence of LBs in other pathologic conditions involving the substantia nigra, such as postencephalitic parkinsonism (PEP),[33,37] olivopontocerebellar atrophy (OPCA)[38] and progressive supranuclear palsy (PSP)[39–41] represent a coexistence of two neurodegenerative diseases.

The classical or brain stem LBs are found in the perikarya of the affected neurons, and the nucleus and melanin pigment of a typical affected nigral neuron are displaced toward the cell border.[15] Classical LBs are round or oval in shape, measure 7–25 μm in diameter, and consist of an intensely eosinophilic, hyaline core surrounded by a peripheral halo (Fig. 9–5A).[42] The central core is usually homogeneous, but less commonly it may contain a darker, more densely stained center or may have concentric, darker layers, making LBs resemble a target. Their numbers vary: they may be single in an affected neuron, but multiple LBs are commonly observed. Pale bodies are seen in the pigmented neurons of the substantia nigra and locus ceruleus, where they appear as rounded, pale eosinophilic intracytoplasmic masses displacing neuromelanin (Fig. 9–5B). These inclusions, which presumably are precursors of LBs, have a similar immunohistochemical profile, including positivity for α-synuclein, to that of LBs.[43–45] In the nucleus basalis of Meynert and dorsal nucleus of the vagus, locus ceruleus, hypothalamus, and, above all, in the sympathetic ganglia, in addition to typical intracytoplasmic bodies, the cell processes of some neurons may be the site of hyaline and acidophilic inclusions that are

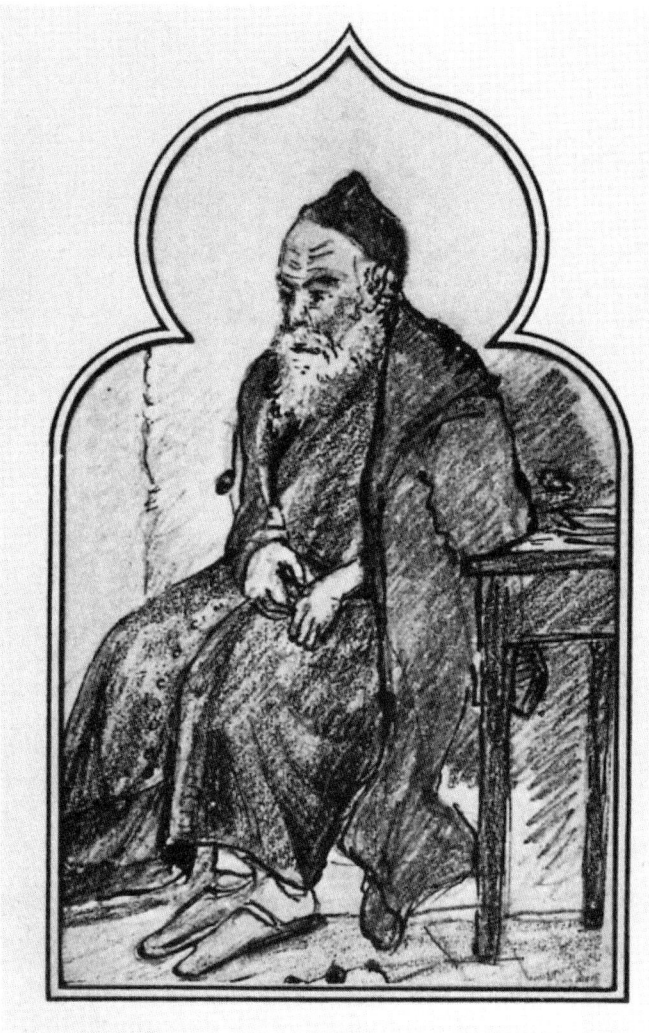

Figure 9–3. Drawing representing "a Jew from Tetouan with Parkinson's disease" made by Charcot during a travel to Morocco.

more elongated or more complex in shape and are also known as "intraneuritic LBs" (Fig. 9–5F).

Ultrastructurally, LBs consist of 8 to 10 nm–wide filaments, intermingled with granular material and dense core vesicles. The filaments are haphazardly arranged in the core and are radially oriented in the outer zone.[46–48]

Molecular Biology of Lewy Bodies and Genetics of Parkinson's Disease

The genetics of PD and the molecular understanding of LBs in PD as well as DLB was limited up until the mid-1990s, although it was known that LBs contain neurofilaments, synaptic proteins, ubiquitin, and proteins involved in the ubiquitin pathway.[49–53] The discovery of a rare association of familial, autosomal dominant forms of PD with mutations of the α-synuclein gene[54–56] facilitated further investigations, which have shown that α-synuclein is a prominent constituent of LBs and Lewy neurites (see below) in both idiopathic PD and DLB (Fig. 9–5E–G).[57–59] α-Synuclein, encoded by a gene located on chromosome 4q, is a 140 amino acid–long protein with little or no secondary structure.[60] Little is known about the normal function of α-synuclein, although it is regarded as a presynaptic protein and pre-

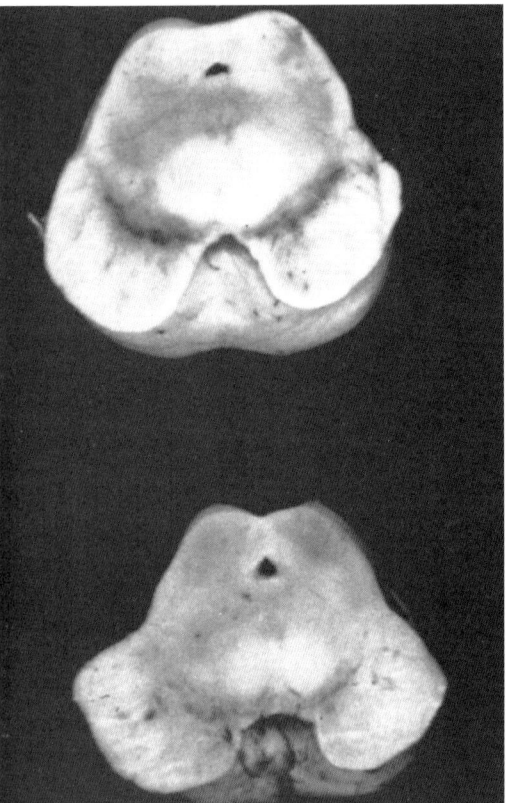

Figure 9–4. Parkinson's disease; macroscopic aspect. Horizontal section of the cerebral peduncle through the decussation of the superior cerebellar peduncles shows depigmentation of the substantia nigra (*below*), compared with a normal substantia nigra (*top*).

sumed to have a role in neuronal plasticity.[61] Aggregation of α-synuclein into insoluble fibrils, which is an important step in LB formation, presumably is facilitated by abnormal folding of the protein because of a mutation in the familial form of the disease or damage to the protein by oxidation or free radical attack in the sporadic cases.[59] The importance of oxidative stress and mitochondrial dysfunction in PD has been emphasized by several investigators for several years.[62–64]

A second gene, named "parkin," located on chromosome 6q, has also been identified in families with early-onset parkinsonism inherited in an autosomal recessive manner.[65–67] The novel protein parkin is expressed in several tissue types, including brain, and shows an interesting homology to ubiquitin. Another locus for familial PD has also been found in a large family with levodopa-responsive, LB parkinsonism in which a chromosome 4p haplotype segregates with the disease.[68] There is also linkage to chromosome 2p in an autosomal dominant form of familial PD, in which the clinical picture resembles that of sporadic PD.[69] In a single small kindred with PD, the heterozygous missense mutation in the ubiquitin carboxy-terminal hydrolase L1 (*UCH-L1*) gene, also located on chromosome 4, has been described, although the pathogenetic importance of this mutation has yet to be proven.[70,71]

Neuropathology of Idiopathic Parkinson's Disease

Parkinson's disease is characterized by the involvement of a selected group of nuclei in which neuronal loss of variable severity and specific inclusions are observed. Histologic examination has confirmed the presence of lesions morphologically similar to those of the substantia nigra in pigmented and nonpigmented nuclei in the brain stem.[30,31,72] Moreover, biochemical investigations[73] have shown that, in addition to the striatum, other dopaminergic as well as nondopaminergic pathways are affected by the disease.

The lesions of the pigmented nuclei of the brain stem represent a constant feature. On macroscopic examination, the substantia nigra appears pale in all cases (Fig. 9–4); the loss of pigment is usually bilateral and symmetrical and is most severe in the middle part of the zona compacta, while the medial and lateral areas are relatively spared. The pathologic condition consists of selective nerve cell loss of variable intensity, while residual melanin pigment may be seen in the neuropil or contained in macrophages. Astrocytic and microglial proliferation is also present but is usually mild. Lewy bodies are observed in most cases (Fig. 9–5A,B,E,F). A most discrete cell loss and the presence of LBs are also observed in the nucleus paranigralis. Similar lesions may also be found in the locus ceruleus, the principal source of noradrenergic innervation of the central nervous system (CNS), and in the dorsal nucleus of the vagus.[31] In addition, LBs have been frequently observed in the nucleus parabranchialis pigmentosus, nucleus tegmenti pedunculopontinus, and nucleus sub-

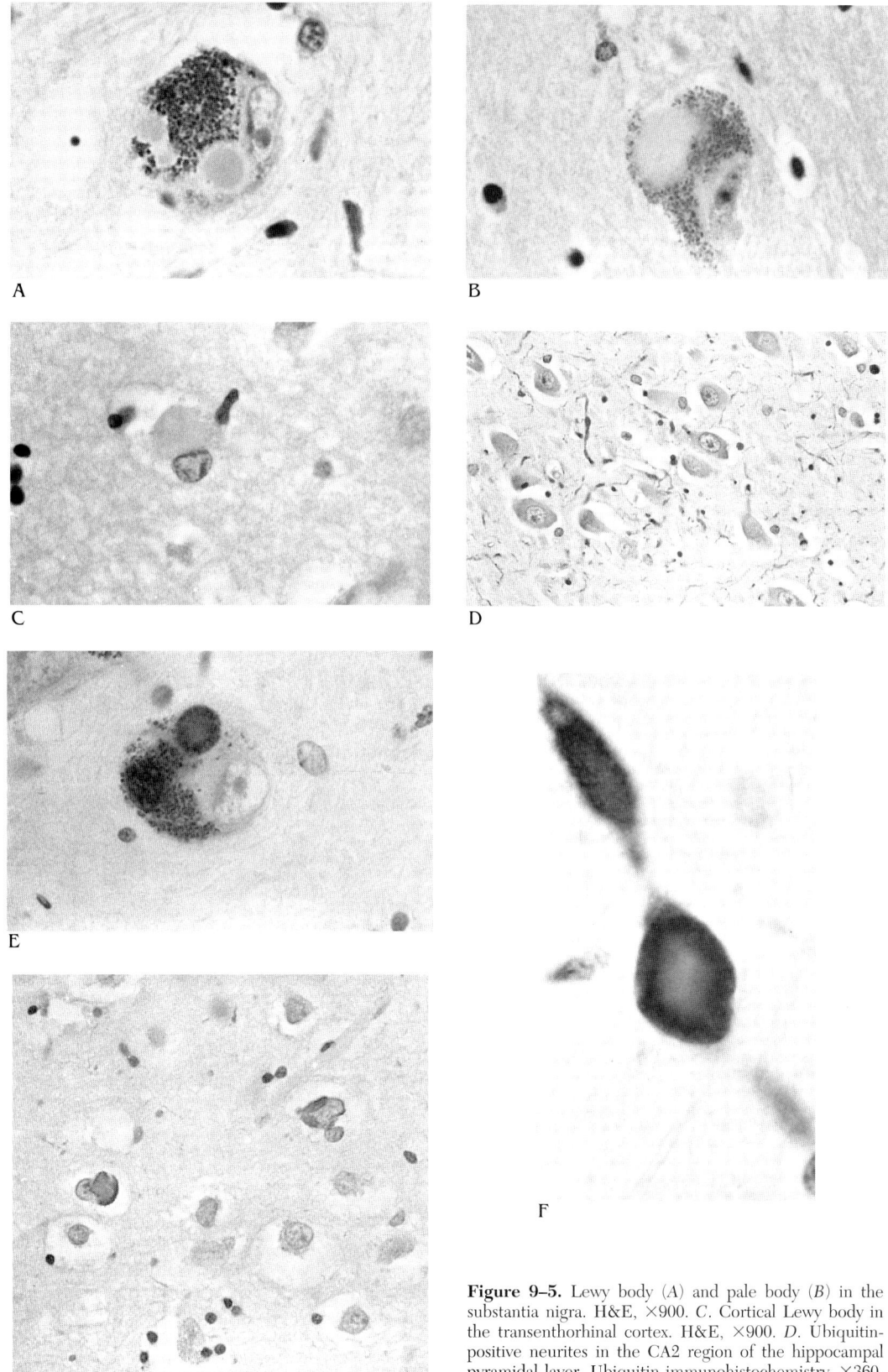

Figure 9–5. Lewy body (A) and pale body (B) in the substantia nigra. H&E, ×900. C. Cortical Lewy body in the transenthorhinal cortex. H&E, ×900. D. Ubiquitin-positive neurites in the CA2 region of the hippocampal pyramidal layer. Ubiquitin immunohistochemistry, ×360. Lewy body (E), intraneuritic Lewy body in the substantia nigra (F) and cortical Lewy bodies (G) are α-synuclein positive. α-Synuclein immunohistochemistry, E,F: ×900, G: ×600.

ceruleus.[72,74,75] Lewy bodies associated with cell loss and the presence of nodules of Nageotte are also found in the neurons of the sympathetic ganglia, which are known to contain neuromelanin.[46,72]

Nonpigmented nuclei in various regions of the CNS may also be involved in the disease. Abnormalities of the nucleus basalis of Meynert, the principal site of origin of neocortical cholinergic innervation, have been known for a long time.[18,24,28,76] Neuronal loss is present in nearly all cases; it varies in severity and is associated with a glial reaction and, in numerous instances, with LBs.[77-82] Lewy bodies have been consistently observed in the posterolateral hypothalamus and the limbic system.[83,84] The lesions have also been described in the reticular substance of the mesencephalon and pons, in particular in the griseum centrale mesencephali, nucleus supratrochlearis, centralis superior and processus griseus pontis supralemniscalis, in the nucleus of Darkschewitsch, in the dorsal nucleus of the raphe, and in the nucleus of Edinger-Westphal.[72,85,86] Lewy bodies and nerve cell loss have been frequently observed in the intermediolateral tract of the thoracic cord,[31] usually associated with dysautonomia,[87] and, on rare occasions, in the anterior horn of the spinal cord.

Changes in cerebral cortex are variable but usually mild in PD. Cortical LBs morphologically are eosinophilic in the hematoxylin and eosin (H&E)–stained sections and, compared with the brain stem LBs, are poorly defined and mostly lack an obvious halo. Some are rounded, but others may be angular or reniform in shape (Fig. 9–5C, G).[88-91] Cortical LBs are hallmarks of DLB (see also Dementia with Lewy bodies, below), but some degree of cortical involvement, predominantly in the amygdaloparahippocampal region, is also found in PD irrespective of whether the patient had dementia in life or not[2] (see also Dementia with Lewy Bodies, below). Senile plaques and neurofibrillary tangles, in variable amounts, may be observed.

Using ubiquitin immunocytochemistry a distinctive neuritic degeneration has been demonstrated in the CA2–CA3 region of the hippocampus (Fig. 9–5D), which is also seen in the amygdala, basal forebrain, substantia nigra, pedunculopontine nucleus, raphe nuclei, dorsal vagal nuclei, and neocortex (see also Dementia with Lewy Bodies, below)[92-96] (Fig. 9–5). These abnormal neurites are invisible with H&E staining, but are immunoreactive for α-synuclein. They are sometimes associated with other linear hyaline structures that can be considered intraneuritic LBs. The abnormal neurites, also called "Lewy neurites" or "Lewy-related neurites" (LNs), occur in both PD and DLB.

A number of pathologic changes have been described in the nucleus lenticularis in PD. Bugiani et al.[97] observed nerve cell loss in the striatum, involving predominantly large neurons. However, it was shown that these changes are nonspecific and can be attributed to either aging or vascular pathologic condition and a morphometric study has shown that the density of nerve and glial cells and the nerve/glia ratio in parkinsonian patients are similar to those in normal controls of the same age.[98,99]

Treatment of PD, in addition to levodopa substitution and other drugs, has been attempted by transplantation of either embryonic mesencephalic cells or adrenal medulla into the basal ganglia to provide dopaminergic innervation.[100,101] In one patient who died 18 months after grafting with fetal cells, autopsy showed that the graft was viable and had integrated into the striatum with dopaminergic re-innervation in a patch matrix pattern.[102] Subsequently, treatment by long-term electrical neurostimulation of the nuclei has proved to be efficient against bradykinesia and rigidity.[103] In a recent study of eight patients (four with bilateral and four with unilateral electrode implantation), histopathologic analysis showed that therapeutic long-term neurostimulation does not cause damage to adjacent neural parenchyma.[104]

NEURODEGENERATIVE DISEASES WITH PARKINSONIAN SYMPTOMS

Under the term "neurodegenerative diseases" are described illnesses of the CNS that are due to nerve cell degeneration and are not produced by any known inflammatory, toxic metabolic, or vascular factor. Such diseases have common features that justify their grouping in as much as they appear in families and have a genetic basis.

NEURODEGENERATIVE DISEASES INVOLVING PREDOMINANTLY THE BASAL GANGLIA

Multisystem Atrophy

This term encompasses a group of neurodegenerative disorders characterized by sporadic appearance, progressive course, clinical symptoms including parkinsonism, cerebellar, pyramidal, and autonomic disturbances, and by well-defined pathological features. The entities, which were previously considered separate clinicopathological disorders are: (1) olivopontocerebellar atrophy (OPCA); (2) striatonigral degeneration; and (3) Shy-Drager syndrome.

Olivopontocerebellar atrophy was first described by Déjérine and Thomas in 1900 in a 52 year-old woman and a 42-year-old man.[105] In 1960 and 1961, van der Eeken et al.[106,107] reported three patients with pathological changes localized in the nigrostriatal axis. The third disorder, characterized by orthostatic hypotension, was described by Shy and Drager in 1960.[108] In 1969 Graham and Oppenheimer proposed to unify the three diseases, in view of shared clinical and pathological features, and suggested the name "multiple system atrophy" (MSA).[109] In 1998, a Consensus Conference on MSA[110] agreed on four clinical domains defining the disorder. These are (1) autonomic and urinary dysfunction; (2) parkinsonism; (3) cerebellar disorder; and (4) corticospinal dysfunction. The Conference also established diagnostic criteria to define cases as possible, probable, or definite MSA and stated that a definite diagnosis requires neuropathological confirmation by the presence of glial cytoplasmic inclusions (see below).

The incidence of MSA is difficult to establish; an annual incidence of 3 new cases per 100,000 individuals aged between 50 and 99 was reported by Bower et al.[111] The mean age of the patients is 54.3, with a range from 33 to 78 years[112] and males are more affected than females, a trend confirmed by a neuropathological study of 203 cases.[112] In a series of 100 patients studied by Wenning et al.,[113] the presenting symptoms were orthostatic hypotension in 68%, parkinsonism in 46%, autonomic symptoms in 41%, and cerebellar symptoms in 5%. Parkinsonian symptoms include bradykinesia, rigidity, and postural instability. Tremor is often present; it is irregular and postural, often includes myoclonus, but the classic pill-rolling rest tremor, typical of Parkinson's disease, is uncommon. Symptoms respond poorly to levodopa. Cerebellar dysfunction appears most commonly as ataxia of gait and is often accompanied by dysarthria, limb ataxia, and sometimes by gaze-evoked nystagmus and ocular dysmetria. Autonomic symptoms include, in addition to orthostatic hypotension, impotence or male erectile dysfunction, increased urinary frequency, urgency, and incontinence. Extensor plantar reflexes and hyperreflexia can be present in 50% of the patients.

Macroscopic examination of the brain shows changes localized predominantly to the striatonigral or olivopontocerebellar domains. In the former instance, the putamen is shrunken (Fig. 9–6A) and shows brown discoloration, whereas the substantia nigra (Fig. 9–6B) and locus ceruleus are pale. In OPCA severe atrophy is seen in the cerebellum (Fig. 9–7A), middle cerebellar peduncles, basis pontis (Fig. 9–7B), and olives (Fig. 9–7C). The superior cerebellar peduncle and dentate nuclei are spared. With regard to the cerebral hemispheres, cortical atrophy has been described, involving particularly motor and premotor cortex.

Histological examination reveals cell and myelin loss and reactive gliosis, whose localization and severity depend on the duration of the illness and clinical subtype. In striatonigral degeneration, changes are most severe in the dorsolateral part of the putamen (Fig. 9–8A), substantia nigra (Fig. 9–8B), and locus ceruleus. In OPCA, Purkinje cells (Fig. 9–9) are more severely affected in the vermis than in the hemispheres and the accessory olivary nucleus is more damaged than the inferior nucleus. In addition, Nakamura et al.[114] and Ozawa et al.[115] described loss of large histaminergic neurons in the tuberomammillary nucleus and of arginine vasopressin–positive neurons in the suprachiasmatic nucleus of the hypothalamus, respectively. In the spinal cord, neuronal loss involves motor neurons[116] and the intermediolateral column.[117] The peripheral nervous system may also take place in the pathological process, showing reduction of nonmyelinated fibers.[118] With regard to the

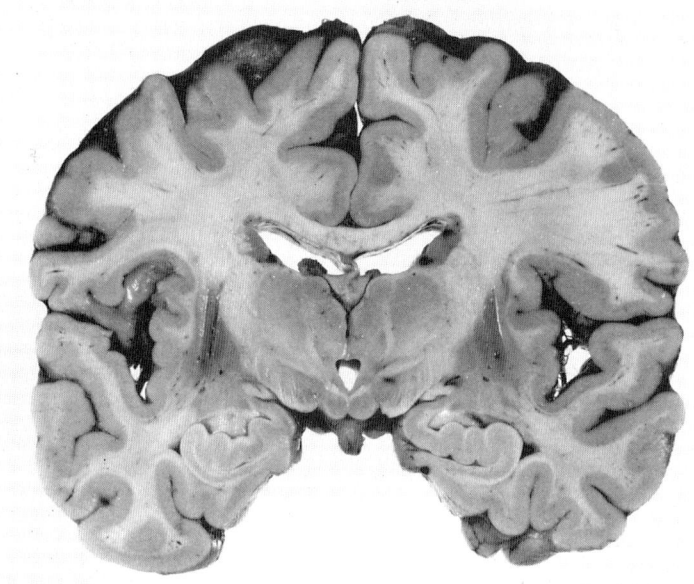

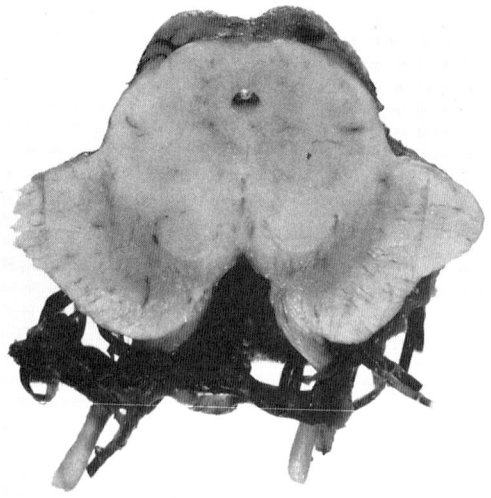

Figure 9–6. In the striatonigral type of multisystem atrophy the putamen appears shrunken (A), whereas the substantia nigra (B) has lost most of its normal pigmentation.

pathogenesis of nerve cells loss, Probst-Cousin et al.[119] opt for a nonapoptotic pathway, whereas de la Monte et al.[120] suggest apoptosis as the mechanism for neuronal death.

The discovery of glial cytoplasmic inclusions (GCI) within oligodendrocytes.[121] has changed the approach to multisystem atrophy by providing a specific pathological marker and possible pathogenetic clues. In addition, inclusions have been described in the nuclei of neurons and oligodendrocytes, in the cytoplasm of the former,[122] although only GCI are found consistently and in large numbers. They are not obvious in H&E preparations, in

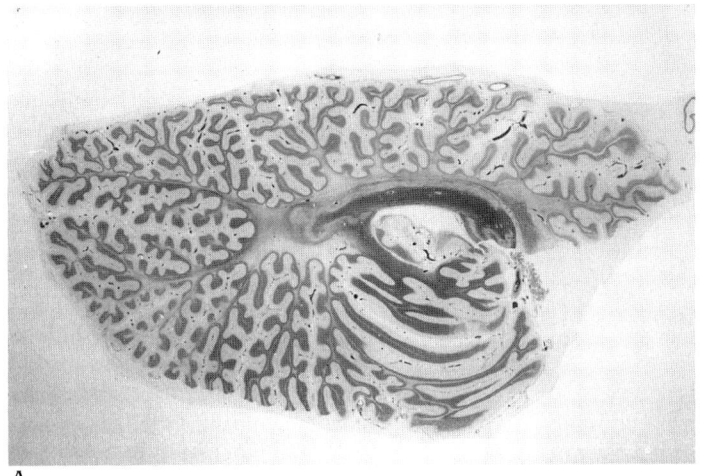

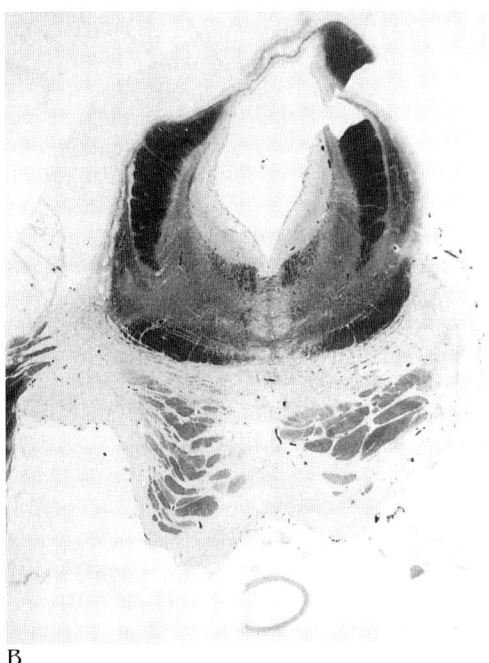

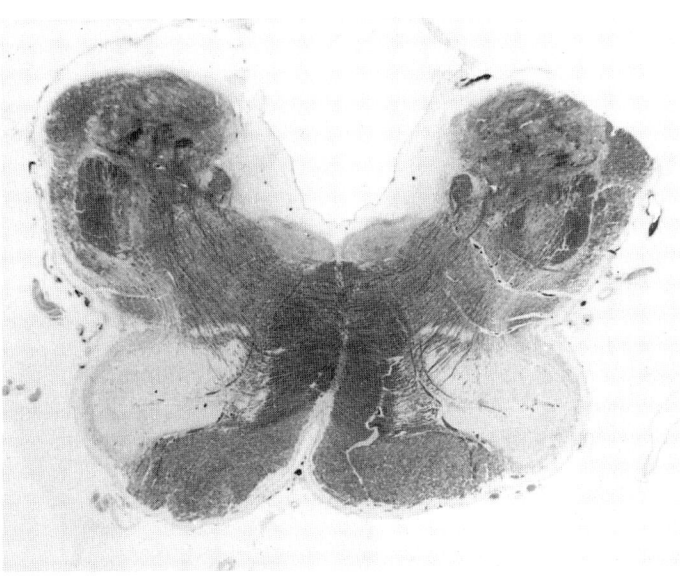

Figure 9–7. In olivopontocerebellar atrophy the main pathological features consist of cerebellar atrophy with severe loss of the myelin (*A*), extreme reduction in bulk of the basis of the pons (*B*), and atrophy of the olive with loss of the efferent myelinated fibers (*C*). Loyez myelin staining.

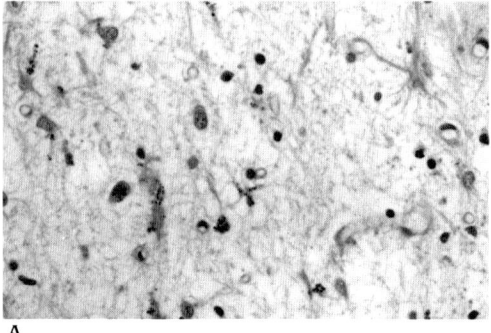

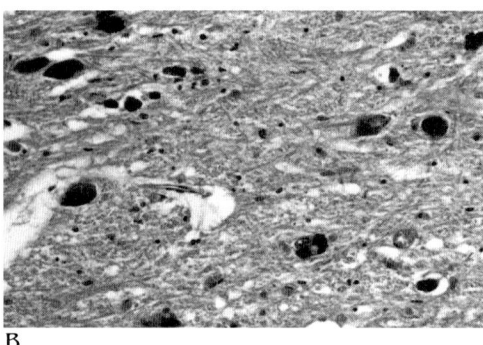

Figure 9–8. Photomicrographs of the posterior caudate nucleus (A) and substantia nigra (B) in a patient with striatonigral degeneration showing virtually complete neuronal loss and reactive gliosis in the former (A) and severe reduction in number of pigmented cells in the latter (B), with residual pigment free in the tissue. H&E, A: ×360; (A); B: ×225.

which they may be seen as faintly basophilic cytoplasmic material. Moreover, they are silver positive and best shown using the Gallyas method (Fig. 9–10), with which they appear as flame- or crescent-shaped formations, vaguely resembling neurofibrillary tangles (NFTs). On immunohistochemical analysis, GCI are positive for phosphorylation-independent tau, ubiquitin, α- and β-tubulin, and αB-crystallin antibodies. Neuronal cytoplasmic inclusions are found in the pons, putamen, subthalamic and cuneate nuclei, subiculum, amygdala, hippocampus, substantia nigra, inferior olive, and reticular formation of the brain stem. They appear as filamentous structures that are argyrophilic and ubiquitin positive. Nuclear inclusions in nerve and glial cells have also been described. In neurons they appear as a loose network of fine fibrils and are argyrophilic. The argyrophilic neuritic abnormalities described in MSA resemble neuritic threads in Alzheimer's disease; however, in MSA they are ubiquitin positive but tau negative.

Glial inclusions have been described in disorders other than MSA. In Alzheimer's and Pick disease and in argyrophilic grain dementia, the inclusions (coiled bodies) have a different morphology and react with phosphorylation-dependent tau antibodies. In PSP

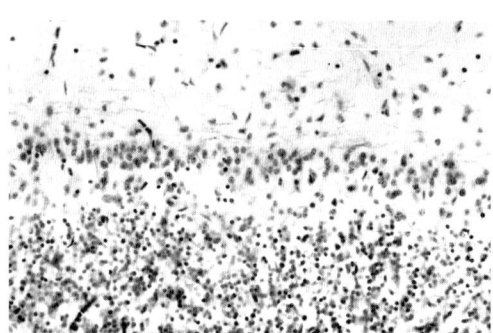

Figure 9–9. Photomicrograph of the cerebellar cortex in a patient affected by olivopontocerebellar atrophy. Note the complete disappearance of Purkinje cells and their replacement with reactive (Bergmann) glia. Loyez myelin stain, ×225.

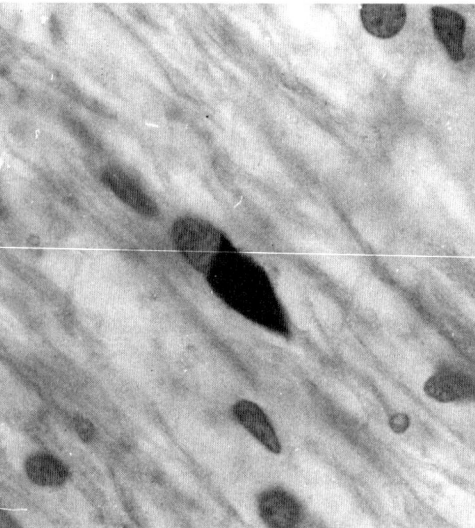

Figure 9–10. Photomicrograph of one glial cytoplasmic inclusion in the pons of a patient affected by multisystem atrophy. Note the flame-shaped appearance and the displacement of the nucleus to one pole of the cell. Gallyas silver method, ×900.

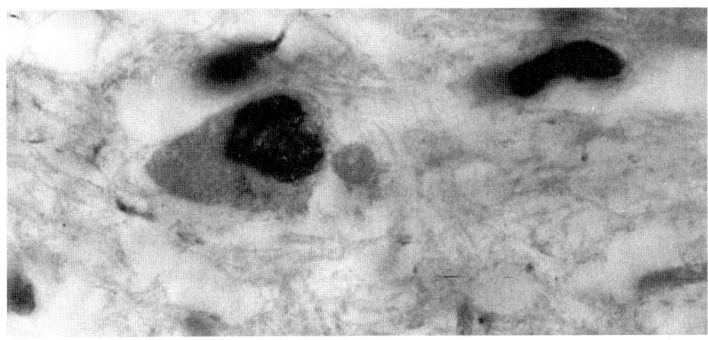

Figure 9–11. The pontine neuronal nucleus and an axonal process in a patient with multisystem atrophy are immunostained with α-synuclein antibody, ×900.

and corticobasal degeneration (CBD), the pathology is seen within astrocytes (tangles and thorn-shaped cells in PSP and astrocytic plaques in CBD), whereas coiled bodies are seen in oligodendrocytes.[123,124] The recent finding of α-synuclein in a number of disorders, including MSA, has provided a further tool: this protein has been described in GCI, neuronal cytoplasmic inclusions, abnormal neurites, and in the nucleus (Fig. 9–11). In addition it has been reported in LBs, both in PD and DLB,[57] in amyotrophic lateral sclerosis (ALS),[59] and in the neuropil thread of Alzheimer's disease (AD),[59] but not in other neurodegenerative disorders, including PSP and CBD.[125]

Although the diagnostic value of GCI is undisputed, their pathogenetic role is still a matter of discussion. It appears, however, that MSA is the only degenerative disease in which oligodendroglial pathology is the main and specific lesion.[126] Therefore, it could be suggested that damage and loss of nerve cells could be the effect of an abnormality triggered by a cell, the oligodendrocyte, which plays an essential role in the functioning and survival of both nerve cells and myelin sheath.

Progressive Supranuclear Palsy

Progressive supranuclear palsy (PSP), or the Steele-Richardson-Olszewski syndrome, is a late-onset neurodegenerative condition affecting the brain stem, basal ganglia, cerebral cortex, and cerebellum. This disorder is a rare condition and epidemiological data are scarce. In central New Jersey the age-adjusted prevalence was estimated to be 1.5 cases per 100,000 population (1.5 for men and 1.2 for women), about 1% of that of PD. The incidence of PSP is estimated at between 3 and 5 per 1,000,000 population per year.[127] No ethnic group or geographical area is favored for acquiring PSP, but males are more often affected than females.[128,129] The mean age at onset is around 62 years,[130,131] and the median survival around 6 years.[127] Most cases are sporadic, but families with PSP have also been well documented.[132–134] The pattern of inheritance according to one recent, large study is autosomal dominant with reduced penetrance.[134] Although no mutation of the tau gene has thus far been identified in familial PSP, an important association of a polymorphism in this gene has been linked to sporadic PSP, which occurs in the number of TG repeats in the intronic region between exons 9 and 10.[135–137]

The clinical diagnosis of PSP rests upon the presence of parkinsonism with bradykinesia, axial rigidity, neck dystonia, and gait disorder with falls, but without tremor or response to levodopa therapy. Supranuclear palsy of the vertical gaze is characteristic and the clinical presentation also includes dysarthria and dysphasia as well as cognitive decline.[138] Although the diagnosis of the disease may be straightforward in typical cases, in recent years it has become evident that PSP is a clinically heterogeneous condition and atypical cases without supranuclear gaze palsy, others with pure akinesia or severe dementia, have been described.[139–141] It has also been suggested that patients presenting without supranuclear gaze palsy tend to be older at the onset of disease and have a longer disease duration.[142,143] Furthermore it may also be difficult to clinically differentiate PSP from other parkinsonian and dementing disorders. In such cases, supranuclear gaze palsy and moderate or severe postural instability with falls during the first year after onset of symptoms appear to be the signs that best differentiate PSP from non-PSP patients.[144] An international panel of scientists involved in the clinical research of PSP recommended the use of the diagnostic categories of possible, probable, and definite PSP. The diagnosis of definite PSP requires histological evidence of typical PSP.[145]

Macroscopic changes, when present, characteristically affect the diencephalon, brain stem, and cerebellum. The brain weight may be slightly decreased or normal. Posterior frontal, anterior parietal, or diffuse cortical atrophy may be seen and this may be of considerable degree in some cases.[143] Other structures including the pallidum, thalamus, subthalamus, and brain stem tegmentum as well as the superior cerebellar peduncle and dentate nucleus are reduced in size in typical cases. Pallor, often severe, of the substantia nigra and loci coerulei as well as dilatation of the third and fourth ventricles and the cerebral aqueduct are also characteristic.[138,146–148]

The histological hallmarks of PSP include loss of neurons, gliosis, and the presence of tau-positive filamentous inclusions in both neurons (NFTs) and glia.[40,41,138,148] The severity of nerve cell loss seems to be related to NFT formation in that areas showing the largest numbers of tangles are usually most affected by depletion of nerve cells,[40,149] although exceptions to this rule may be observed. The NFTs are found in a widespread distribution and, in one large study, they were always present in the striatum, pallidum, subthalamus, substantia nigra, hippocampus, and parahippocampus. Furthermore, they almost always occurred in the frontal cortex, insular region, colliculi, periaqueductal gray, red nucleus, nucleus pontis, inferior olive, and dentate nucleus.[148] In contrast to the original description of PSP, in recent years a number of studies have shown that NFTs, glial/astrocytic tangles, and oligodendroglial inclusions are constant findings in the cerebral cortex, and it has also been suggested that the pedunculopontine nucleus may have a role in the spread of the cortical neurofibrillary lesions.[148,150,151] The NFTs in the substantia nigra and in other brain stem and subcortical nuclei usually have a globose appearance (Fig. 9–12A,B) whereas in the cerebral cortex they are flame shaped or coiled (Fig. 9–12C,D). The NFTs and glial inclusions are positive for both phosphorylation-dependent and -independent tau antibodies and their immunohistochemical profile is indistinguishable from that seen in AD.[152] In contrast to NFTSs in AD, the NFTs in PSP are poorly immunoreactive for ubiquitin.[153]

At sites most affected by NFT formation neuropil threads (NTs) are also characteristic. In addition to involvement of neurons, which was emphasized in the initial descriptions of PSP, glial pathology is also prominent, and the presence of both astrocytic and oligodendroglial inclusion have been documented.[148] Argyrophilic and tau-positive astrocytic inclusions are present in affected cortical regions, basal ganglia, thalamus, and to a lesser extent in the brain stem. One type has been described under several terms, including "tuft-shaped astrocytes" or 'glial fibrillary tangles' (Fig. 9–12E)[149,154,155] and another as "thorn-shaped astrocytes."[156,157] The tuft-shaped astrocytes have been shown to be prominent in the precentral and premotor cortices but scarce in the temporal lobe and limbic area. In the subcortical nuclei, they appear preferentially in the putamen and some examples are also found in other degenerating regions.[158] The presence of argyrophilic and tau-positive, coiled intracytoplasmic oligodendroglial inclusions are found in cortex and underlying white matter as well as in a number of subcortical structures including the subthalamic nucleus, pallidum, thalamus, substantia nigra, pons, and red nucleus (Fig. 9–12F).[148,155] The oligodendroglial inclusions in PSP and CBD are, however, different from GCIs in MSA morphologically and in their immunohistochemical profile, (see Multisystem Atrophy above).

As histological heterogeneity of PSP has also been recognized, a new classification, based on semiquantitative assessment of the neurofibrillary tangle pathology, has been recommended.[40,41] According to the criteria of this classification, in typical PSP the histological findings correspond to the original description whereas in the atypical form there is deviation from this in either the severity or the distribution of changes. In the combined form of PSP the typical histological changes of PSP are seen in association with another neurodegenerative condition.

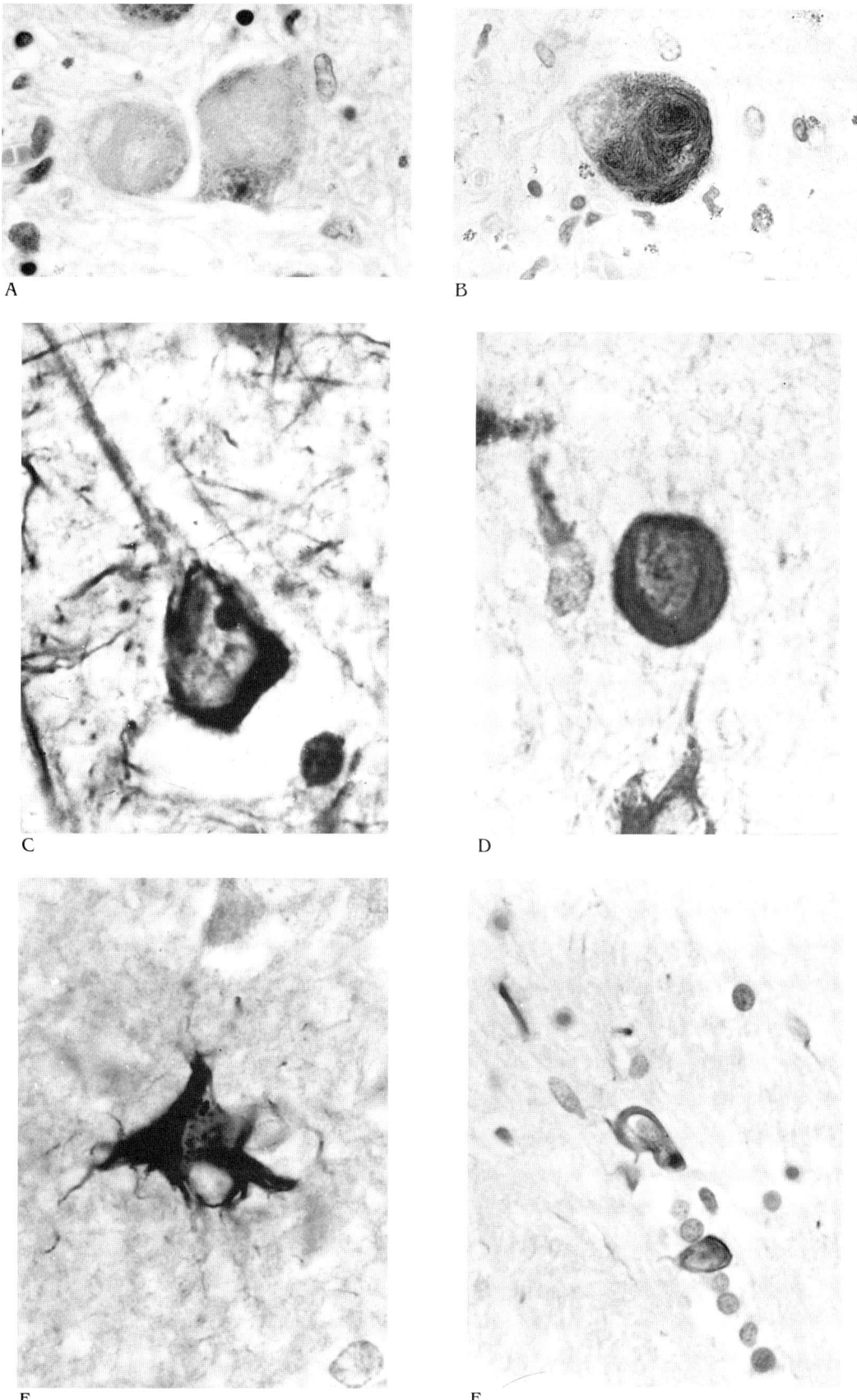

Figure 9–12. Globose neurofibrillary tangles in the substantia nigra stained with H&E (*A*) and an antibody to tau (*B*), ×900. *C,D.* Cortcial neurofibrillary tangles in the premotor cortex. C: Bielschowsky's silver impregnation, ×600; D: tau immunohistochemistry, ×600. *E.* Tuft-shaped astrocyte in the putament. Gallyas silver impregnation, ×900. *F.* Tau-positive coiled oligodendroglial inclusion in the internal capsule. Tau immunohistochemistry, ×600.

Corticobasal Degeneration

Corticobasal degeneration (CBD), also known as "corticodentatonigral degeneration with neuronal achromasia"[159,160] and "cortical-basal ganglionic degeneration,"[161] is a rare neurodegenerative condition. The mean age of disease onset is around 60 years, with age of onset ranging from 40 to 76 years.[162] There is no apparent sex predilection and a familial occurrence remains to be proven.[163]

The presenting, often asymmetrical, clinical signs include motor disabilities of an arm or a hand with akinesia, clumsiness, apraxia and dystonic posturing, cortical sensory loss, and action tremor.[162,164] The disease is slowly progressive and may remain unilateral for years. Focal reflex myoclonus is a distinct feature of the disease and the alien limb phenomenon is found in over 50% of patients.[164,165] When supranuclear gaze palsy is present it raises the possibility of PSP. With progression of the disease, the clinical signs become bilateral and the patients also develop dysarthria, dysphasia, severe rigidity, hyperreflexia, and Babinski sign. Dementia usually is not prominent until late, although cases presenting with cognitive decline are well documented.[166,167] The clinical picture outlined above, however, is not entirely specific for CBD, as cases with a similar clinical presentation but different underlying pathological processes have been described.[168]

Macroscopic examination reveals an often asymmetrical and severe cerebral atrophy predominantly affecting the posterior frontal and parietal cortices. This may be severe, although not of the "knife-edge" type seen in Pick disease. Atrophy of the striatum occurs in some cases. The substantia nigra is invariably pale, but brain stem atrophy characteristic of PSP is usually absent.[169]

Histologically there is a depletion of neurons in combination with astrocytosis and rarefaction as well as a spongy appearance of the neuropil in the affected cortical areas.[170–172] The underlying white matter is also affected. The presence of swollen, achromasic neurons, predominantly occurring in the deeper cortical laminae, is also a feature (Fig. 9–13A).[160,170,173] The perikarya of such swollen neurons are positive for phosphorylated neurofilament epitopes,[173,174] which normally are present only in axons, αB-crystallin,[175] and tau,[173,176] but the significance of ubiquitin immunohistochemistry is more controversial.[171,173,176–178] Such neurons have been found, usually in association with variable loss of neurons and gliosis, in a number of sites other than cerebral cortex and substantia nigra, and these include striatum, globus pallidus, thalamus, subthalamus, claustrum, amygdala, Meynert nucleus, red nucleus, and a number of other brain stem nuclei.[160,170] Achromasic, ballooned neurons are far from specific, as they occur in a number of pathological conditions other than CBD. The degeneration of the substantia nigra is prominent, with depletion of the pigmented neurons, pigment incontinence, and astrogliosis. Filamentous inclusions (see below) are also present in some of the remaining pigmented neurons.

Several types of intraneuronal and glial inclusions have been described in CBD. There are neocortical intraneuronal tau-positive inclusions, which are usually small, globular, or crescent shaped, and argyrophilic when the Gallyas silver impregnation method is used (Fig. 9–13B–D).[172,173,179] Electron microscopic examination shows them to consist of 15 nm– wide, smooth-surfaced tubules, which also show long periodicity at 120–150 nm.[180] The basophilic or corticobasal inclusions of the substantia nigra (Fig. 9–13E,F),[170] resemble the globose neurofibrillary tangles of PSP, and such inclusions may be found in a number of subcortical gray and brain stem nuclei including the striatum, globus pallidus, subthalamus, hypothalamus, septal nucleus, nucleus basalis of Meynert, superior colliculus, oculomotor nucleus, locus ceruleus, pontine raphe, brain stem reticular formation, inferior olive, dentate nucleus, and spinal gray matter (Fig. 9–13E,F).[169] The basophilic inclusions are argyrophilic and immunoreactive with antibodies to tau, (Fig. 9–13G),[171,173,178] but usually are negative for ubiquitin.[173,181] Ultrastructurally, such inclusions consist of 15 nm–wide, straight tubular structures.[173] In CBD both the astroglia and oligodendroglia contain filamentous tau-positive inclusions. The oligodendroglial inclusions are similar to the coiled bodies described in association with PSP, and although such inclusions may show a rather wide distribution, they appear more frequent in the frontal cortex, pre- and postcentral gyri, and the underlying white matter (Fig. 9–13H).[148,173,179,182] Ultrastructurally the oligodendroglial inclusions consist of 15 nm straight tubules that are seen in both the cell bodies and processes of the affected cells.[173] The astrocytic pathology in CBD is characteristic in that "astrocytic plaques" are seen in the affected cerebral cortices (Fig. 9–13I). It has been shown that these annular filamentous structures are due to accumulation of tau in focal dilatations of distal astrocytic cell processes.[179] In CBD, tau- and silver-positive neuropil threads are found in neocortex and subcortical gray and white matter.[177,179,183]

The major differential diagnosis of CBD typically includes PSP, Pick disease, chromosome 17q–related inherited tauopathies, and the tangle-predominant form of Alzheimer's disease.[184] The striking microscopic similarity between the basophilic/corticobasal inclusions in CBD and the globose tangles in PSP has been emphasized by numerous investigators.[171,173,176,181,183,185] The presence of achromasic, ballooned neurons in CBD and of frequent cortical NFTs in PSP is of considerable help in the differential diagnosis of these two conditions,[150] as there is a greater proportion of tau-positive glial inclusions as well as neuronal and glial processes in CBD than in PSP.[181] The astrocytic morphology appears also to be strikingly different in these two conditions in that astrocytic plaques have been reported to be a particular feature of CBD.[179,186] On histological grounds, Pick disease may be difficult to differentiate from CBD, as achromasic neurons occur in large numbers in both conditions. Furthermore, the cortical inclusions in CBD may resemble Pick bodies.[181,186–188] The distribution of the lobar atrophy in Pick disease as well as the overall histological features of Pick disease are usually different from those seen in CBD, although there are well-documented cases of Pick disease showing a marked parietal involvement.[189,190] It is of considerable help that Western blot analysis of the insoluble fraction of the abnormal tau highlights important biochemical differences between CBD and Pick disease (see below). Familial tauopathies with mutations of the tau gene in the region of exon 10 or the intronic region following exon 10 show histological and biochemical features resembling both PSP and CBD.[191,192] From the differential diagnosis point of view, it is noteworthy that cases with the P301L mutation of the tau gene show not only widespread neuronal and glial tau-positive inclusions and neuropil threads but also astrocytic plaque-like structures (see also below).[192]

Biochemical Characteristics of Tau in Corticobasal Degeneration and Progressive Supranuclear Palsy

The presence of filamentous tau-positive, neuronal, and, in some diseases, glial inclusions as well is a characteristic feature of a number of neurodegenerative conditions.[193] In conditions such as AD, postencephalitic parkinsonism, (PEP), the Guamanian Parkinson–dementia complex, and some other conditions (see Frontotemporal Dementias, below) the abnormal filaments, appearing as paired helical filaments and straight filaments ultrastructurally, are composed of all six tau isoforms that are normally present in adult, human brain. In these conditions, immunoblotting of the insoluble fraction of the abnormal tau shows them to aggregate into three strong bands of 68, 64, and 60 kDa, in addition to a weak minor band at 72 kDa.[194,195] The insoluble fraction of tau in both PSP and CBD shows a characteristic 68 and 64 kDa doublet electrophoretic migration pattern, in addition to a third weak band at 72 kDa.[182,196,197] Further analysis of tau in these conditions has shown that only the four-repeat isoforms are incorporated into the filaments,[198] in contrast to Pick disease, in which the 64 and 60 kDa doublet is exclusively composed of the three-repeat isoforms[199] (see Frontotemporal Dementias, below).

NEURODEGENERATIVE DISEASES INVOLVING PREDOMINANTLY THE CEREBRAL CORTEX AND CAUSING DEMENTIA

Dementia with Lewy Bodies

Cases clinically presenting with dementia and parkinsonism and pathologically characterized with cortical Lewy bodies were first reported

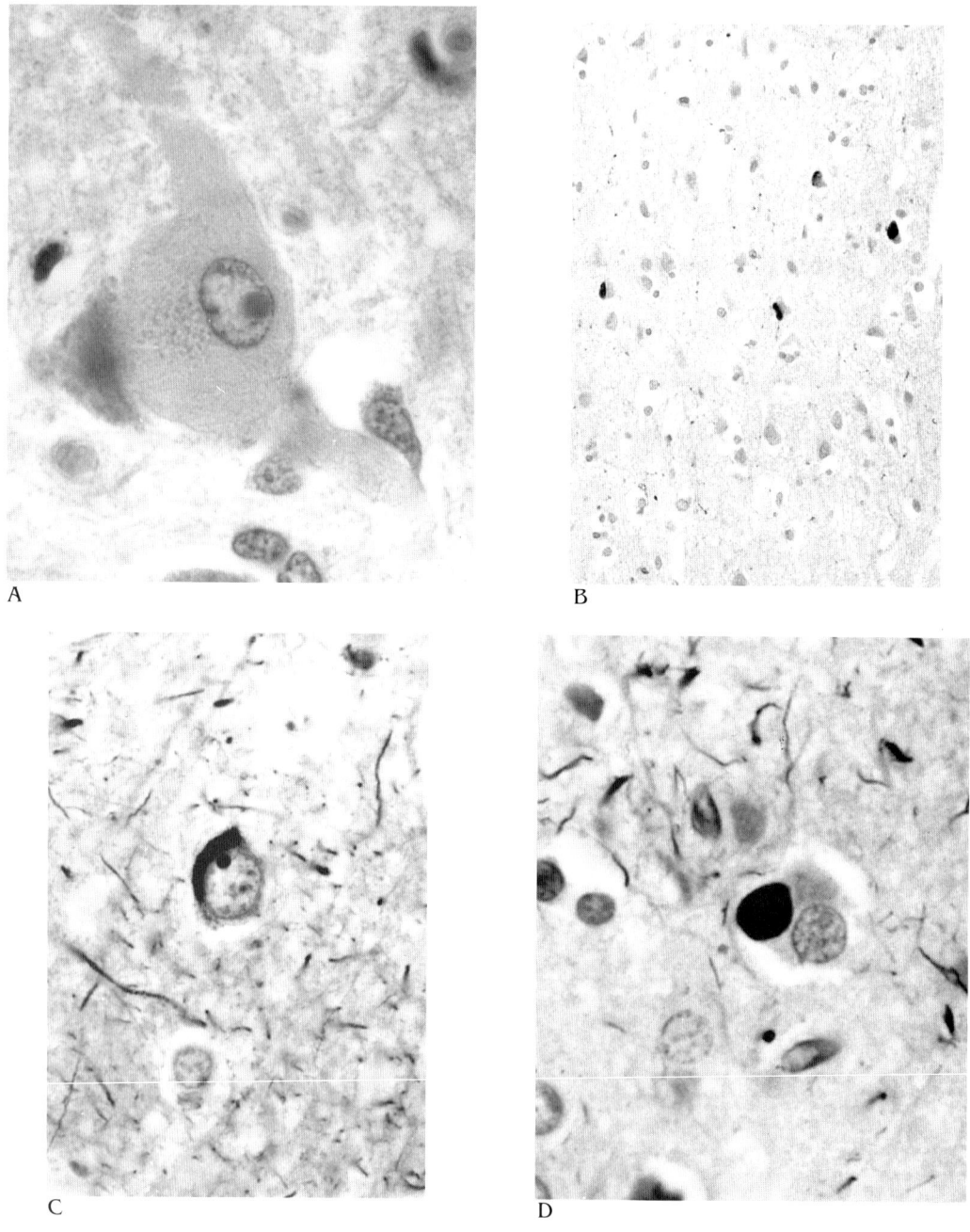

in the early 1960s.[200] After the first reports, several different terms were coined, which include "cortical Lewy body disease," "diffuse Lewy body disease," "senile dementia of the Lewy body type," or "Lewy body variant of Alzheimer's disease" (for review see Ince et al.,[201]). The now accepted and widely used name "dementia with Lewy bodies" (DLB) describes a common neurodegenerative disorder, that probably represents the second most frequent degenerative cause of dementia in several hospital-based series.[201–203]

The clinical presentation is characterized by a progressive dementing illness and the initial

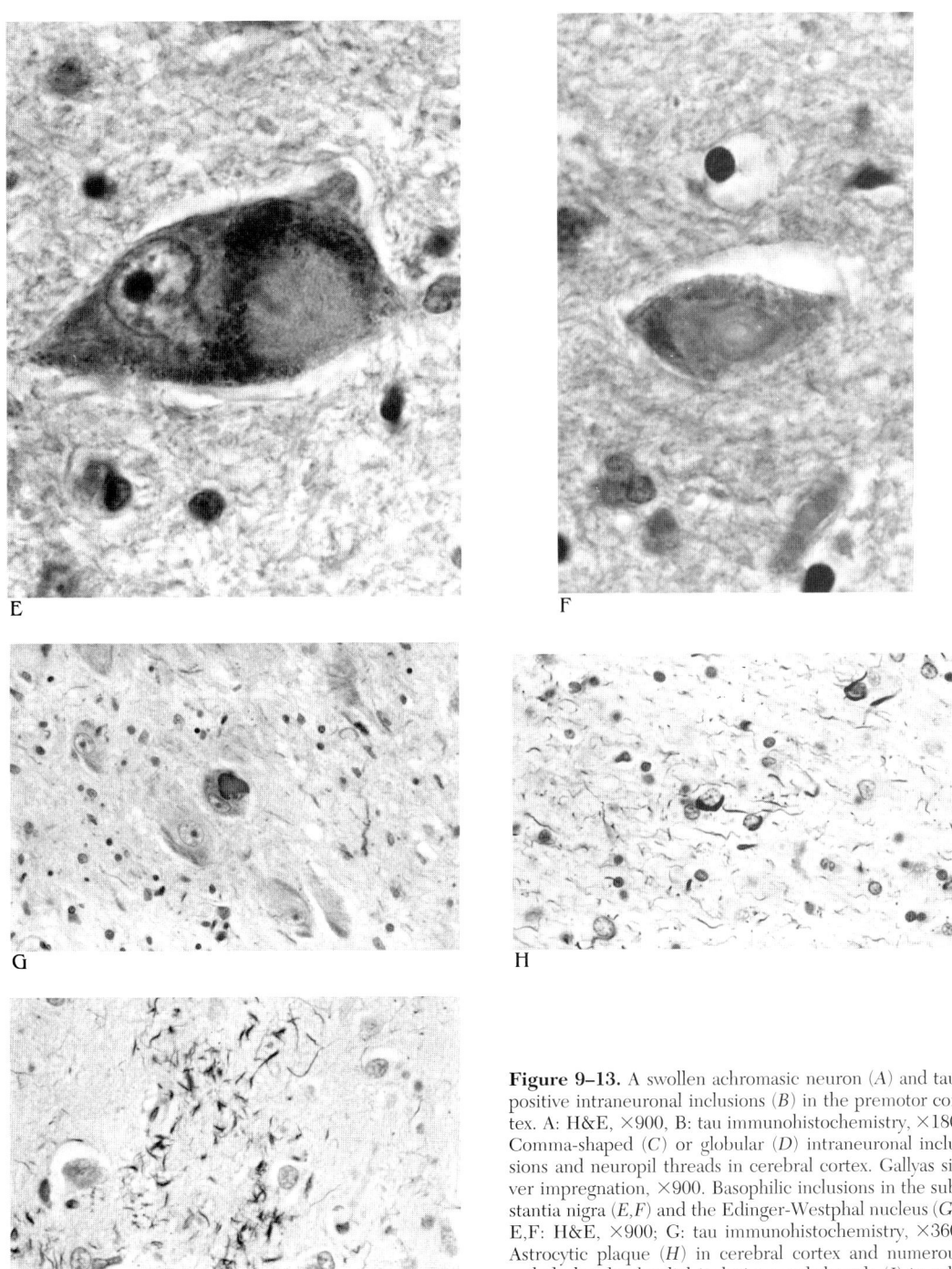

Figure 9–13. A swollen achromasic neuron (*A*) and tau-positive intraneuronal inclusions (*B*) in the premotor cortex. A: H&E, ×900, B: tau immunohistochemistry, ×180. Comma-shaped (*C*) or globular (*D*) intraneuronal inclusions and neuropil threads in cerebral cortex. Gallyas silver impregnation, ×900. Basophilic inclusions in the substantia nigra (*E,F*) and the Edinger-Westphal nucleus (*G*). E,F: H&E, ×900; G: tau immunohistochemistry, ×360. Astrocytic plaque (*H*) in cerebral cortex and numerous coiled oligodendroglial inclusions and threads (*I*) in subcortical white matter. Gallyas silver impregnation, ×600.

symptoms may include impairment of recent memory, word-finding difficulties, problems with visual tasks, and frontal features. Fluctuations between periods of lucidity and confusion, at least in the initial periods of the disease, the presence of complex, detailed visual hallucinations, the unreal nature of which may be recognized by patients; and delusions are also characteristic features.[203] The clinical presentation also includes symptoms and signs of parkinsonism, but these may be relatively mild. Myoclonus, usually mild, is also common. Another characteristic feature is an abnormal sensitivity of patients to neuroleptic therapy.[204] Although the clinical phenotype in DLB is distinct, it may be difficult to differentiate clinically this disease from AD when some of the established clinical criteria[205] are used for the diagnosis of the latter.[201] After a mean disease duration of 7 years, death usually occurs as a result of intercurrent disease.

The brains of patients with DLB usually show generalized cerebral atrophy, but an accentuation of the cortical atrophy in the frontal or frontotemporal regions may be noted. The most characteristic microscopic feature of DLB is the presence of cortical LBs, which are usually most numerous in the limbic areas of the mesial temporal region including the parahippocampal and periamygdaloid areas (Fig. 9–5C,G). They are also numerous in the anterior cingulate and insular gyri, but less frequent in the superior and middle temporal, frontal, and superior parietal cortices. However, LBs are, rare in the primary motor, sensory, and visual cortical areas. In the affected regions, LBs are most frequently found in the small and medium-sized pyramidal neurons of the deeper cortical layers, especially in laminae IV, V, and VI, which are also reduced in number.[90,26,206,207] The GABA-ergic, parvalbumin-positive interneurons show cell loss of a lesser degree.[207] Spongiform change in the temporal cortex is also a well-described feature of DLB.[208]

In addition to involvement of cortical areas, LBs are present in both subcortical structures, such as amygdala and Meynert nucleus, and brain stem nuclei. Of the latter the substantia nigra is invariably affected with some degree of cell loss, pigment incontinence, classical LBs, and LNs (Fig. 9–5A–C,F). The involvement of the nigra is usually intermediate in severity between that seen in idiopathic PD and normal aged-matched controls.[203] Other structures such as the ventral tegmental area, midbrain oculomotor nuclei, and dorsal vagal nuclei are also frequently involved.[201,209] Initially, the neuritic pathology that may be seen in the CA2–3 subregions of the hippocampal pyramidal layer was suggested to be a specific feature of DLB. (Fig. 9–5D).[92,93] Although the extent of CA2–3 neurites appear to correlate with the density of cortical LBs,[210] the CA2–3 neurites are not specific for DLB as they may be found in PD without any clinical evidence of dementia.[209] However, they are not features of the hippocampal pathology in AD, which is one of the major differential diagnoses of DLB. Lewy-related neurites are also found in a number of other structures in DLB (see above). Although in the past, ubiquitin immunohistochemistry or silver stains were used for the visualization of cortical LBs and LNs, as for that of brain stem LBs and LNs,[91,202,211] α-synuclein immunohistochemistry has become the method of choice for this purpose.[57]

A considerable proportion of DLB cases are associated with AD-type pathology and especially senile plaques, which is reflected by the terms "senile dementia of the Lewy body type" and "Lewy body variant of AD."[203,212,213] There are, however, strong scientific arguments in favor of DLB being distinct from AD, although the relationship between AD and DLB is still not fully understood.[201] Another association between these two pathologies is the relatively common finding of LB pathology in AD, especially in its familial form, and in Down's syndrome.[214–217] Furthermore the non-amyloidogenic component (NAC), which is an amyloid-associated molecule found in senile plaques of AD, corresponds to the middle part of the a-synuclein molecule, from amino acid 61 to 95.[218]

For the histological diagnosis of DLB the Consortium for Dementia with Lewy Bodies recommended guidelines for histological examination of different cerebral areas and also established quantitative criteria of the diagnosis.[219] The cortical areas to be sampled include the frontal, temporal, and parietal cortices, anterior cingulate gyrus, and the transentorhinal cortex. Brain stem structures including the substantia nigra, locus ceruleus, and dorsal vasal nucleus are also examined histologically. The density of cortical LBs is estimated by using a semiquantitative approach, which, having taken into account the distribution of LBs, finally results in establishing one of three types of the disease (predominantly brain stem, transitional, or neocortical).[219]

Alzheimer's Disease

For a complete discussion of Alzheimer's disease see Chapter 8.

Pick Disease

For a complete discussion of Pick disease see Chapter 7.

Frontotemporal Dementias

About 3% to 10% of cases with dementia in later life are lacking the neuropathological features of either AD or other common diseases. There have been several attempts at the categorization of this rather heterogeneous group of dementias and the terms recommended include "dementia lacking distinctive histopathology," "Pick disease without Pick bodies," "frontotemporal dementia," (FTD) or "dementia of frontal type."[220–222] The FTDs occur mostly in the presenium and affect predominantly the frontal and anterior temporal lobes.[223,224] Such cases are characterized clinically by behavioral and personality changes, deterioration of memory, progressive impairment of speech and executive functions, stereotypical behavior, and sometimes by a parkinsonian syndrome.[224] To improve recognition and provide research criteria, a consensus conference determined the diagnostic clinical criteria of FTD, which now include core and supportive features.[225]

A clinical presentation with a predominance of frontal lobe signs can, however, be associated with a number of other neurodegenerative disorders, including AD, corticobasal degeneration, Pick disease, motor neuron disease–inclusion dementia, and other familial and sporadic FTDs.[226–228]

In the FTD cases the major macroscopic findings include brain atrophy with a predominance in the anterior cerebral hemispheres involving frontal, anterior temporal, and anterior parietal lobes, which only in the most severe cases is of the "knife-edge" type.[229] Coronal sections also confirm the involvement of the anterior medial temporal structures, including amygdala, and a relative preservation of the more posterior temporal lobe, where the superior temporal gyrus and hippocampus are spared. Involvement of the caudate nucleus is also prominent; the changes in the substantia nigra are variable.

Up to 60% of patients with FTD may have a familial disease and it has also been recognized that a proportion of the hereditary cases have a genetic linkage to chromosome 17q21–22, which includes the region of the tau gene.[230–232] In the affected families the diversity of clinical presentation is well reflected by the number of different titles under which the different syndromes appear in the literature, such as "disinhibition dementia parkinsonism complex with amyotrophy,"[233] "rapidly progressive autosomal dominant parkinsonism and dementia with pallidopontonigral degeneration,"[234] "familial multiple system tauopathy with presenile dementia,"[57] "dementia lacking distinctive histology,"[235] and "familial progressive subcortical gliosis."[236] More recently, the use of "frontotemporal dementia and parkinsonism linked to chromosome 17" has been recommended as a unifying term by a consensus conference.[230] The neuropathological features of many of the familial FTD cases are those of tau-positive filamentous inclusions.[231] In some of these families inclusions are found in both neurons and glia (mainly oligodendroglia),[57,154,192,237–239] while in others the tau pathology is mainly neuronal.[240] Missense mutations of exons 9 (G272V),[241] 12 (V337M),[232] and 13 (R406W),[241] affecting all six brain tau isoforms, result mainly in neuronal pathology. In such cases, exemplified by those of Seattle family A, NFTs are flame shaped and the abnormal filaments are not only present in the neuronal cell soma but also extend into the apical dendrite.[238] At the ultrastructural level such NFTs are composed of typical paired helical filaments, as well as straight filaments and the electrophoretic migrating pattern of the insoluble tau is also indistinguishable from the triplet pattern seen in AD.[238] In contrast, cases with either a missense mutation of exon 10 (N279K and P301L) affecting only four-repeat tau isoforms[192,238,242] or those with intronic mutations in the region of the exon 10 splice-donor site,[241,243] have a different neuropathological phenotype in that they present with both neuronal and glial, mainly oligodendroglial, tau pathology. Furthermore, in cases with P301L mutation, astrocytic plaques similar to those in CBD have also been described. In both the exon 10 and exon 10 splice-donor site mutation cases, the neuronal tau inclusions are predominantly in the cell soma and appear either as globose tangles or pretangles.[243] Neuropil threads are also numerous and ultrastructurally the filaments appear as twisted ribbons. Immunoblotting of the insoluble tau shows that it aggregates into two strong bands at 68 and 64 kDa, in addition to a weaker third band at 72 kDa.[191,192] There are, however, fine biochemical differences within this group. In cases with intronic mutations the abnormal tau is composed of four-repeat tau isoforms, which are overproduced,[191,241,243] whereas in cases with mutations of exon 10, although the filaments consist predominantly of four-repeat tau, a small amount of the normally abundant three-repeat tau isoforms are also present, at least in cases with the P301L mutation.[192] It is also of interest that in cases with this latter type of mutation, the ultrastructural appearance of the filaments is also slightly different in that the twisted ribbons are narrower than those in familial multiple system tauopathy with presenile dementia, in which there is a G-to-A transition in the nucleotide adjacent to the splice-donor site of the intron following exon 10.[244] The precise prevalence of tau mutations in FTDs is difficult to assess, as this seems to be associated with the sensitivity of the diagnostic criteria used in the different patient series.

In a considerable proportion of cases of FTD, no neuronal and/or glial inclusions can be visualized with immunohistochemical staining for tau and ubiquitin,[227] and in such cases the major histological changes include microvacuolation of cortical layer II and the upper part of layer III of the affected frontal and temporal cortices, associated with neuronal loss, and, in some cases, swollen achromasic neurons. The astrogliosis is usually mild and restricted to the subpial area. In a proportion of cases, the substantia nigra shows marked cell loss with pigment incontinence.

Dementia of the frontotemporal type occurs in about 2–6% of patients with motor neuron disease (MND).[247] Neuropathologically, such cases, in addition to changes associated with MND, are characterized by neuronal loss and spongy degeneration, predominantly involving layers II and III of the affected frontal and temporal cortices (Fig. 9–14A). Reactive gliosis is present in these cortical areas and white matter. Degeneration of the substantia nigra and striatum may also be found. A characteristic diagnostic feature of such cases is the presence of ubiquitin-positive and tau-negative inclusions in neurons of the superficial cortical laminae (Fig. 9–14B) and in those of the granule cells of the hippocampal dentate fascia (Fig. 9–14C).[226,248–250] Ubiquitin-positive neurites are also noted in the affected cortices (Fig. 9–14D).

In 1996 Jackson et al.[251] described nine cases with a clinical history of FTD, but not with MND, in which the characteristic extramotor pathology, seen in MND with dementia, was found. For such cases, the term "motor neuron disease–inclusion dementia" (MND-ID) was recommended. Although it seems plausible to suggest that MND and MND-ID are likely to represent a disease spectrum, it is noteworthy that in some cases the involvement of the motor system, including those of spinal motor neurons, may be absent.[252,253]

Parkinsonism–Dementia Complex of Guam

The disease was endemic among the Chamorro population in Guam, one of the Mariana islands. It develops insidiously during the fifth or sixth decade and has a progressive evolution leading to death after approximately 4 years. The most typical clinical features are dementia, parkinsonian syndrome, and involvement of the lower motor neurons.[254] In recent years the prevalence of ALS of Guam disease has declined markedly, although parkinsonism and dementia remain common.[255] Similar neurodegenerative disease has also been described in Japan[256] and in New Guinea.[257]

The neuropathology of Guam disease was described by Hirano et al.[258,259] and Malamud et al.[260] and consists of cortical atrophy, particularly in the frontotemporal lobes, associated with loss of pigmentation of the substantia nigra and locus ceruleus. On histologic

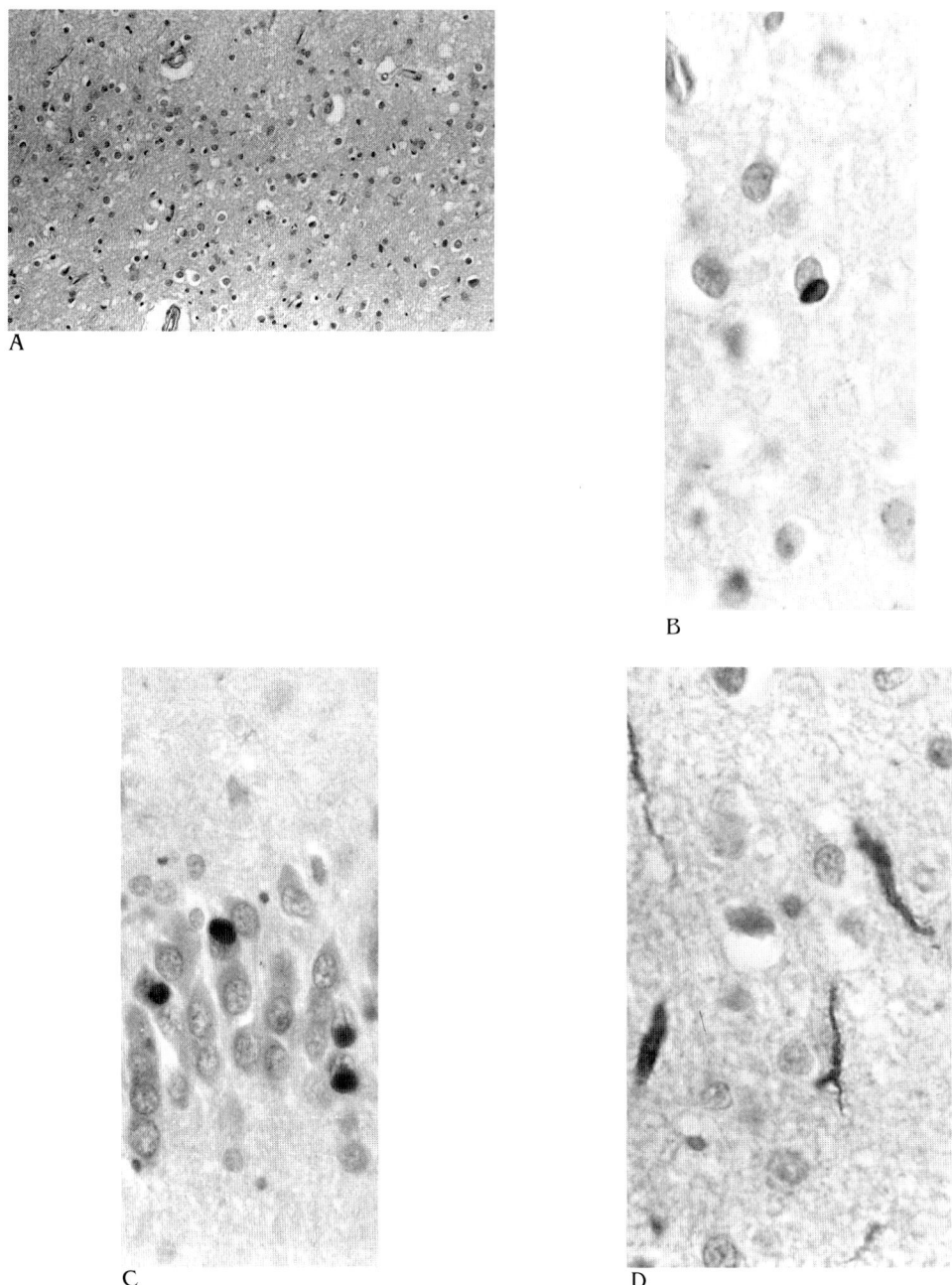

Figure 9–14. *A*. Neuronal loss and vacuolation of the neuropil in the superficial cortical laminae, H&E ×180. Ubiquitin-positive inclusions in cortical neurons (*B*), granule cells of the hippocampal dentate fascia (*C*), and ubiquitin-positive cortical neurites (*D*), ubiquitin immunohistochemistry ×600.

examination, changes are more widespread and extend to the cerebral cortex, hippocampus, amygdala, hypothalamus, globus pallidus, thalamus, substantia nigra and tegmentum. They consist of nerve cell loss, glial proliferation, presence of neurofibrillary tangles, and granulovacuolar degeneration (GVD). Similar alterations, but without GVD, are also described in the anterior horns of the spinal cord, particularly in the corticospinal tract degeneration, and in the nucleus of the hypoglossus. Ultrastructurally, the tangles resemble those in Alzheimer's disease,[261] but amyloid deposits are almost invariably absent.

The cause of this disease remains unclear. Genetic factors were initially suspected but this hypothesis was supported by neither epidemiological studies[262,263] nor by the change in the clinical characteristics of the disease over the last 20 years. Environmental factors seem more likely, however, studies demonstrating the causative role of diatery neurotoxin or metal intoxication by aluminium or iron have not been conclusive.

CEREBELLAR AND SPINOCEREBELLAR DEGENERATION

The definition of cytosine-adenine-guanine (CAG) polyglutamine tract expansion diseases encompasses a number of disorders previously considered completely separate entities. They are induced by a genetic mutation (an expansion) of the trinucleotide repeats as it was first identified in 1991 in spinal and bulbar muscular atrophy[264] The mutations are the consequence of a heritable unstable DNA and are called "dynamic" because the number of repeat units inherited changes from generation to generation.

At present, four types of trinucleotide repeat expansions are known:
1. long cytosine-guanine-guanine (CGG) repeats in the two fragile X syndromes (FRAXA and FRAXE)
2. long cytosine-thymine-guanine (CTG) repeat expansions in myotonic dystrophy
3. long guanine-adenine-adenine (CAA) repeat expansion, the mutation found in Friedreich's ataxia
4. short cytosine-adenine-guanine (CAG) repeat expansions responsible for eight neurodegenerative disorders.

Disorders produced by trinucleotide repeat expansion share the phenomenon of *anticipation*, i.e., an increased severity and younger age of presentation in successive generations.[265] Subsequent studies have revealed that in CAG-related disorders, anticipation is brought forward when the mutation is paternally inherited and that the severity and age at onset of the disorder are correlated with the larger size of the repeats.[266] In the eight disorders resulting from short CAG repeat expansions, the repeat is translated into a stretch of polyglutamines in the respective proteins. There is agreement that the presence of expanded polyglutamine results in a gain of function by the involved protein. However, despite the fact that the abnormal protein is ubiquitously expressed in the central and peripheral nervous system, only nerve cells in a number of locations degenerate and die as the result of expanded CAG repeat. The eight diseases in the CAG repeat expansion group are (*1*) X-linked spinal and bulbar muscular atrophy, (*2*) Huntington disease (HD); (*3*) spinocerebellar ataxia type 1 (SCA) (*4*) dentatorubral pallidoluysian atrophy (DRPLA); (*5*) SCA2, (*6*) SCA3/Machado-Joseph disease, (*7*) SCA6, and (*8*) SCA7.

Spinocerebellar atrophies are described further here because of the overlapping of pathological features of some of them with those seen in MSA, (disorders such as spinal and bulbar muscular atrophy, Huntington disease, and DRPLA are dealt with in Chapters 13). The classification of these disorders has been fraught with difficulties for decades. Within them a group has been labeled "olivopontocerebellar atrophy" (OPCA) and further subdivided by Berciano[267] into sporadic and inherited. In the same year, Harding[268] came to the conclusion that OPCA was not a useful label for the following reasons: (*1*) it was only a pathological description, (*2*) it does not take into account the lesions in the basal ganglia and spinal cord, frequently found to be associated with OPCA, and (*3*) there are patients with pathologically different changes but clinically similar presentation. In the same study, Harding labeled these disorders, including OPCA, as autosomal dominant cerebellar atax-

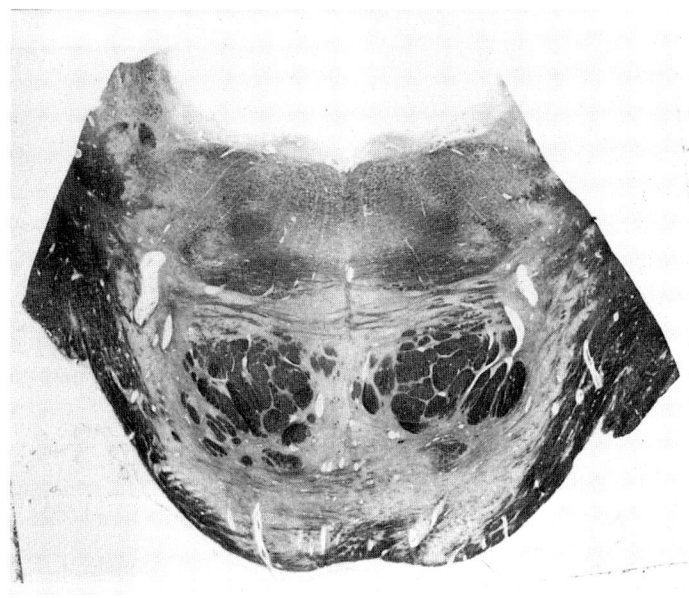

Figure 9–15. Transverse section of the pons of a patient with spinocerebellar ataxia type 1 (SCA1). Note the severe reduction in volume of the basis pontis. Luxol fast blue/cresyl violet.

ias (ADCA) of late onset and classified them into the following subgroups:
1. those presenting with ophthalmoplegia, optic atrophy, dementia, extrapyramidal features, and amyotrophy (ADCA1)
2. those presenting with pigmental retinal degeneration with or without ophthalmoplegia, dementia, or extrapyramidal features (ADCA2)
3. pure cerebellar syndrome without ocular or extrapyramidal features or dementia and late onset (60 or over) (ADCA3)
4. those presenting with myoclonus and deafness (ADCA4).

Subsequent genetic studies have improved our understanding of these diseases and have led to a more accurate classification.

The group labeled ADCA1 by Harding[268] includes SCA1, SCA2, SCA3, SCA4 and SCA5. SCA1–3 can be distinguished on a genetic basis; moreover, using genetic criteria, it was possible to identify patterns of preferential histological damage according to three types: (1) progressive and dominantly inherited ataxia of Menzel; (2) spinocerebellar atrophy, Cuban type; and (3) Machado-Joseph disease.

Spinocerebellar ataxia type 1 corresponds to OPCA 1 or the progressive and dominantly inherited ataxia of Menzel.[269] Its onset is in the third or fourth decades, although onset in childhood has been described.[270,271] During the early stages, the disorder is characterized clinically by gait ataxia, dysarthria, hypermetric saccades, and nystagmus. In the final stages there are also bulbar signs such as dysarthria and amyotrophy.

The neuropathology of SCA1 has been described by Robitaille et al.[272] Brains show mild to moderate atrophy, which includes the brain stem, particularly the pons (Fig. 9–15). The spinal cord takes part in this process by showing reduction in size of the enlargements. Coronal slices show basal ganglia of normal size; the substantia nigra is normally pigmented, but the basis pontis and the middle cerebellar peduncles are considerably atrophic. The inferior olives are also reduced in bulk, while the dentate nuclei are almost unidentifiable and the cerebellar cortex is atrophic.

Microscopic changes are particularly severe in the brain stem and spinal cord. In particular, there is severe neuronal loss in the nuclei pontis, inferior olive, and oculomotor and hypoglossal nuclei. The loss of motor and Clarke's neurons in the cord is extensive, with sparing of the nucleus of Onufrowicz and posterior columns. Sensory ganglia however appear normal. Severe involvement of Purkinje cells (Fig. 9–16A) is also seen, with preserva-

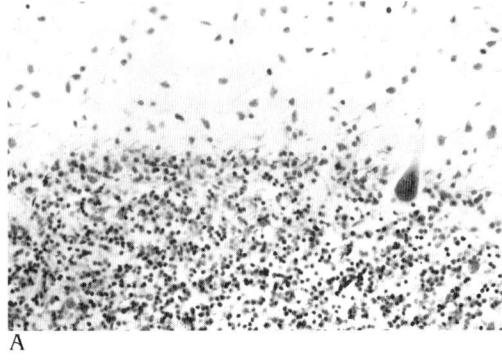

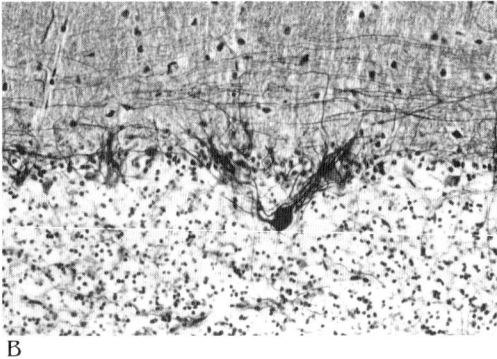

Figure 9–16. Photomicrographs of the cerebellar cortex in a patient with SCA1 showing almost complete loss of Purkinje and hyperplasia of the Bergmann glia (A) and preservation of basket cells (B). In B the axon of one surviving Purkinje cell is swollen, resulting in the formation of a torpedo. A: Luxol fast blue/cresyl violet, ×225; B: Bielschowsky's silver impregnation, ×360.

tion of basket cells (Fig. 9–16B) and marked Bergmann glial hypertrophy, as well as of the dentate nuclei. Consequently, all three cerebellar peduncles are atrophic. The substantia nigra shows slight to mild cell loss, but there is evidence of involvement of the nigrostriatal pathway. Unlike in sporadic cases of OPCA, in SCA1 no ubiquitin-positive glial cytoplasmic inclusions are seen, although Gilman et al.[273] described these inclusions and changes typical of multiple-system degeneration in one member of a family. It appears that in SCA1, cell death takes place via the mechanism of apoptosis.[274]

The chromosomal abnormality in SCA1 has been identified in the short arm of chromosome 6;[275] whereas the length of the normal CAG repeat in a normal allele is 19–38, it is 40–81 in affected individuals.[276] The gene product in SCA1 is a protein called "ataxin-1," which, in Purkinje cells, has been found both in the nucleus and the cytoplasm.[266] Whereas presence of ataxin-1,[277] as well as ataxin-3[278] in the cytoplasm may be a normal event, its aggregation inside the nucleus may be abnormal and lead to cell damage.[279]

Another disorder belonging to ADCA1, SCA2,[268] corresponds to OPCA2 or spinocerebellar atrophy, Cuban type.[280] This autosomal dominant disorder has been described in Japan,[281] Martinique,[282,283] Europe,[284] and in the United States.[285] Patients with this disorder present with ataxia, dysarthria, tremor, and extremely low saccades. Over half of them manifest hyporeflexia of the upper limbs and ophthalmoparesis, whereas retinopathy and optic atrophy are not features. Occasionally dementia appears, but it is not a characteristic symptom of SCA2.[282]

In patients with SCA2, the cerebellum and brain stem (in particular the basis pontis) are severely atrophic and Purkinje cells are dramatically reduced in number; the dentate nucleus is less involved. The nuclei of the pontine tegmentum and their fibers all but disappear, resulting in degeneration of the middle cerebellar peduncles. The white matter of the cerebellum is devastated because of the concomitant absence of fibers of Purkinje cells. The inferior cerebellar peduncle is also atrophic as there is severe loss of olivary neurons. In most cases, the substantia nigra shows considerable neuronal loss, which contrasts with the absence of parkinsonian symptoms; the locus ceruleus, however, is preserved.[280] In the spinal cord, fiber loss has been described in both motor and sensory pathways. In the latter, the gracile tract is more affected than the cuneate. The reduction in number of cells of the Clarke's column leads to pallor of the spinocerebellar tracts. Orozco et al.[280] have described reduction in number of motor neurons in lamina IX. Atrophy of the cerebral hemispheres has been described only in demented patients.[282]

The chromosomal abnormality responsible for SCA2 has been mapped to chromosome 12q24.[286] The abnormal allele has 36–51 repeats instead of the normal 22–23. The gene product is ataxin-2. This has been recognized in neuronal cytoplasm by a specific monoclonal antibody[287] raised against the polyglutamine expansion.

Spinocereballar ataxia type 3, also a mem-

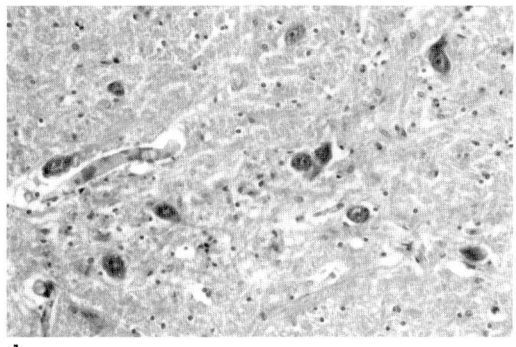

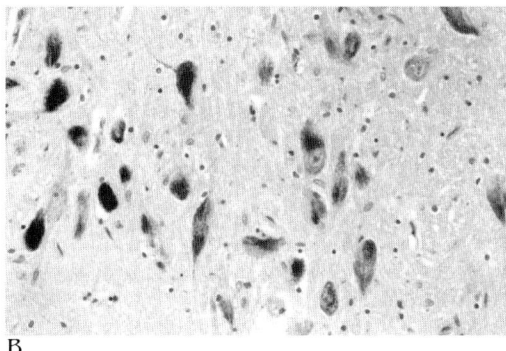

Figure 9–17. In patients affected by SCA3 the substantia nigra shows severe loss of pigmented cells (A). An age-matched normal specimen, (B) is shown for comparison. H&E, ×225.

gard to the cranial nerves, abnormalities have been reported in the three oculomotor, facial, vestibular nuclei, dorsal nucleus of the vagus, and hypoglossal. In one patient in whom the disease had appeared at the age of 8 and lasted 7 years, Coutinho et al.[292] also described involvement of sensory ganglia, intermediolateral columns, and gracile and cuneate nuclei. As both parents of the child were affected, he was considered to be homozygous for the mutation.

The gene responsible for SCA3/MJD has been mapped to the long arm of chromosome 14 (14q24.3-q32).[293,294] The repeat size of this locus is normally 13–40 CAG repeats, but is 68–82 in sufferers from the disease. Its protein is called "ataxin-3." It appears that whereas SCA3/MJD can be distinguished from SCA2, but not from SCA1 on clinical grounds, SCA3 and SCA1 have distinct pathological features.[295]

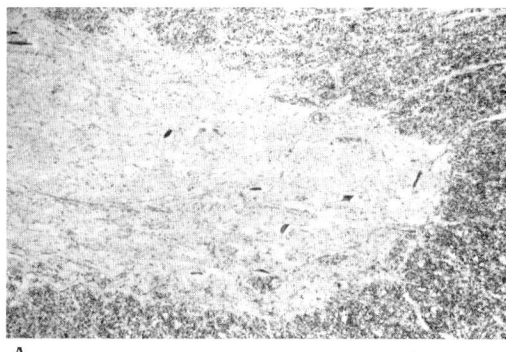

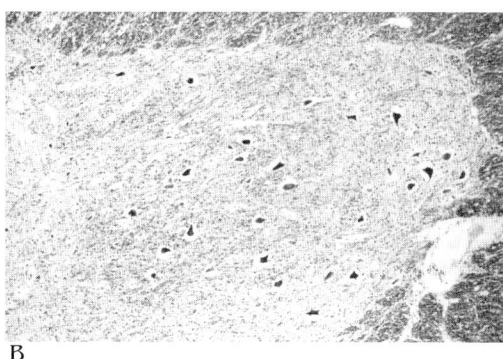

Figure 9–18. Photomicrographs of the anterior horn at the cervical enlargement in a patient with SCA3 (A) and in an age-matched normal individual (B). In the patient, the horn is smaller and its number of nerve cells is severely reduced compared to the control case. Luxol fast blue/cresyl violet ×48.

ber of ADCA1, corresponds to Machado-Joseph disease (MJD) a dominantly inherited spinocerebellar ataxia, originally described by Coutinho and Andrade[288] and Lima and Coutinho[289] in Portuguese families and by Nakano et al.[290] and Woods and Schaumburg[291] in American families of Portuguese origin. It is characterized by progressive cerebellar ataxia, pyramidal signs, and progressive external ophthalmoplegia with variable degree of extrapyramidal and peripheral signs. Other features of the disease include dystonia and prominent eye and facial twitching. The first symptoms usually appear during the fourth or fifth decades and the mean time of evolution is 15 years. Pathological findings include nerve cell loss and gliosis in the substantia nigra (Fig. 9–17A,B), dentate, and pontine nuclei, anterior horn cells (Fig. 9–18A,B), and Clarke's columns in the spinal cord, with consequent loss of fibers in the superior and middle cerebellar peduncles and spinocerebellar tracts. With re-

Using polymorphic CAG repeats to screen DNA in patients with late forms of neurodegenerative diseases, the disorder SCA6 (ADCA III according to Herding-1982) was identified as a separate entity. Affected individuals present with slowly progressive (over 20–30 years) cerebellar ataxia, dysarthria, and nystagmus, together with proprioceptive sensory loss and hypo- or areflexia. Macroscopic findings in the few patients examined to date[274] include cerebellar and brain stem atrophy. The main microscopic finding is the severe loss of Purkinje cells, with more discrete loss of granule and dentate nucleus and olivary neurons. The nuclei pontis and neurons in the spinal cord are not primarily affected.[296] A number of surviving Purkinje cells show poorly defined cell membrane, decreased number of dendritic arborizations, disorganized axons. In addition there are heterotopic Purkinje cells and others with two nuclei.

The gene responsible for the disease has been mapped to chromosome 19q13;[297] it encodes the human α1A voltage-dependent calcium channel subunit,[298] which is expressed in Purkinje cells. In normal individuals the repeat size is 4–6, whereas in affected individuals it reaches 21–37.

The disorder SCA7 (autosomal dominant cerebellar ataxia with retinal degeneration or ADCA II) is characterized by an association between cerebellar ataxia and progressive pigmentary macular dystrophy.[299] The neuropathology has been reported by Holmberg et al.[300] The brain they describe was small and showed reduction in size of the inferior olives and atrophy of the cerebellar vermis and dentate nucleus (Fig. 9–19A,B). Histological examination revealed severe Purkinje cell loss as well as loss of neurons of the dentate nucleus. Moderate nerve cell loss was also observed in the XII nerve nucleus, whereas the substantia nigra and the locus ceruleus were pale and showed moderate neuronal loss. The white matter was reduced accordingly but the corticospinal tracts were reported to be normal.

This disorder is caused by expansion of a highly unstable CAG repeat situated in the coding region of a gene on chromosome 3p14–21.1.[301,302] Normal SCA7 alleles carry between 4 and 35 CAG repeats, whereas the pathological ones have between 77 and approximately 200.[303] Intermediate alleles (IAs), including 28–35 repeats, are not associated with the SCA7 phenotype.

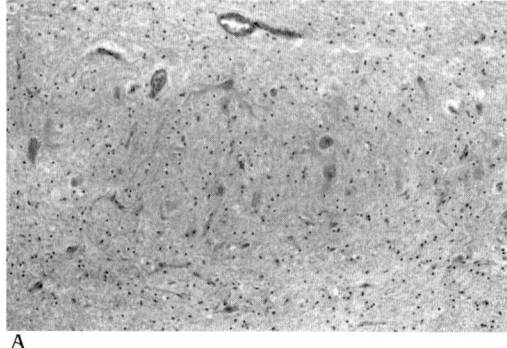

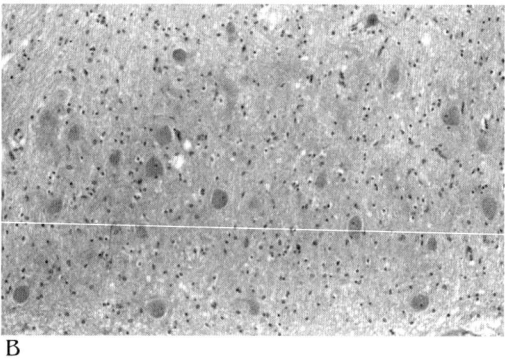

Figure 9–19. Cerebellar dentate nucleus in a patient with SCA7 (A) and in a control individual (B). Note the reduction in thickness and nerve cell content in A compared to in B. H&E ×90.

Three additional loci, have been identified that are associated with inherited ataxias, SCA4, SCA5, and SCA8, but these loci do not show any CAG repeat expansion sites. Spinocerebellar ataxia type 4, which has been mapped on chromosome 16q22.1, is a late-onset ataxia with a proximal sensory axonopathy. In SCA5, affected members have dysarthria, gait and limb ataxia, and nystagmus.[304] Disease onset varies from 10 to 68 years and anticipation is evident.[305] The disease maps to chromosome 11.[306] Spinocerebellar ataxia type 8 is a progressive SCA with infantile onset. This disorder has been described in 19 Finnish patients[307] who presented with slowly progressive clinical symptoms at between 1 and 2 years of age. At first, children appear clumsy and lose their ability to walk. Ataxia, athetosis, and muscle hypotonia with loss of deep tendon reflexes are also seen. Later on, affected children manifest ophthalmoplegia and hearing loss with sensory neuropathy appearing in adolescence; status epilepticus is a late manifestation. The abnormality has been mapped to chromosome 10q.[308]

A number of spinocerebellar degenerations, as well as HD and DRPLA, are characterized by the presence of intranuclear inclusions within selected groups of neurons. Inclusions are 0.5–6 μm in diameter and some nuclei may contain up to three, although most of them have only one.[309] On routine stains, inclusions are round and eosinophilic (Fig. 9–20A). Their appearance is in sharp contrast to that of the hematoxylinophilic nucleolus which is often seen adjacent to the inclusion. They are also reactive with ubiquitin (Fig. 9–20B) and to a polyglutamine-specific antibody, IC2 (Fig. 9–20C), which has been used to recog-

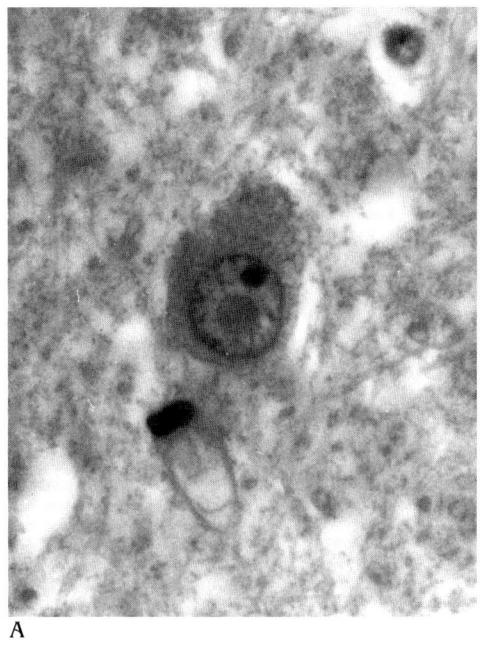
A

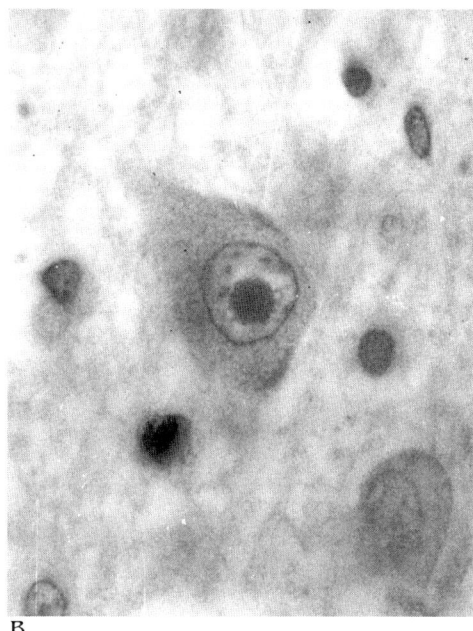
B

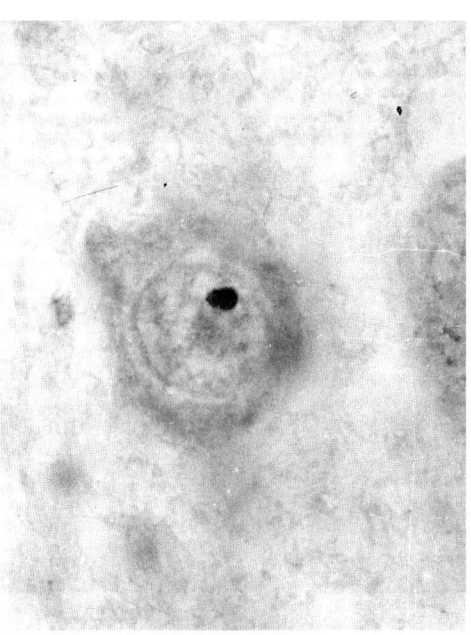
C

Figure 9–20. Intranuclear neuronal inclusions in SCA1 are well recognizable in H&E preparations (*A*). They are ubiquitin (*B*) and IC2 (*C*) positive ×900.

nize polyglutamines of pathological size.[287] Paulson et al.,[279] reported them in SCA3/MJD, Di Figlia et al.[310] described them in HD, Becher et al.[311] found them in DRPLA, Skinner et al.[312] in SCA1. Similar inclusions were found by Davies et al.[313] in transgenic animals overexpressing the short exon 1 N-terminal fragment of the huntingtin protein with a very long glutamine repeat.

Various questions have arisen following the discovery of these inclusions:

1. Their intranuclear location. Small proteins (up to 48 kDa) may enter the nucleus by diffusion from the cytoplasm, but both huntingtin in HD and atrophin 1 in DRPLA are large proteins. With regard to huntingtin, there is evidence of proteolysis by caspase 3.[314] It is possible that similar cleavage takes place with other glutamine-repeat proteins.

2. Their relation to cell loss. The presence of intranuclear inclusions in medium-sized neurons in the striatum and in cortical layers 3, 5, and 6, which are the most vulnerable in HD,[309] as well as in DRPLA,[311] SCA1,[312] and SCA3/MJD[279] suggests a role for these structures in cell death. Although there is no firm evidence for a correlation between inclusions and cell death, this is a plausible hypothesis.[309]

3. The selective vulnerability of nerve cells to a ubiquitous protein. One possibility is that this protein exerts its pathological effects after linking to other proteins present only in cells that are going to die; the second is that the cleavage of the protein is a cell-specific event.[309]

Similar intranuclear inclusions have been described in the so-called familial neuronal intranuclear hyaline inclusion disease (NIHID). This term was introduced by Sung et al. in 1980[315] to designate a disorder characterized by widespread neuronal degeneration with intranuclear hyaline inclusions. Clinical presentation includes psychomotor retardation, tonic-clonic seizures and myoclonus, dysarthria, dysphagia, ataxia, and signs of upper and lower motor neuron disease. A genetic basis for the disease has been reported in a number of patients and occurrence in identical twins[316,317] in siblings[318] is documented. Although the usual age at presentation is during childhood, adult-onset patients have been described.[319-321] On pathological examination cell loss involving particularly the cerebellum (Purkinje and granule cells), the inferior olives, anterior horn cells, and Clarke's nuclei are found. Intranuclear inclusions are ubiquitous and involve not only neuronal and glial cells but also other organs (see review[317]). Inclusions vary in size, are eosinophilic (Fig. 9–21A), and react with ubiquitin (Fig. 9–21B) but are IC2 negative. The only exception is the case reported by Lieberman et al.,[322] in

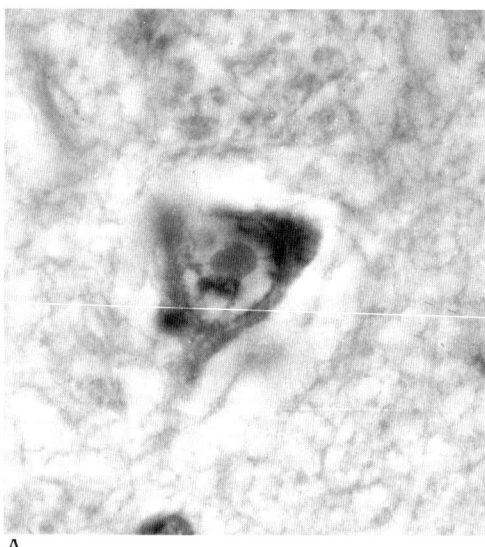

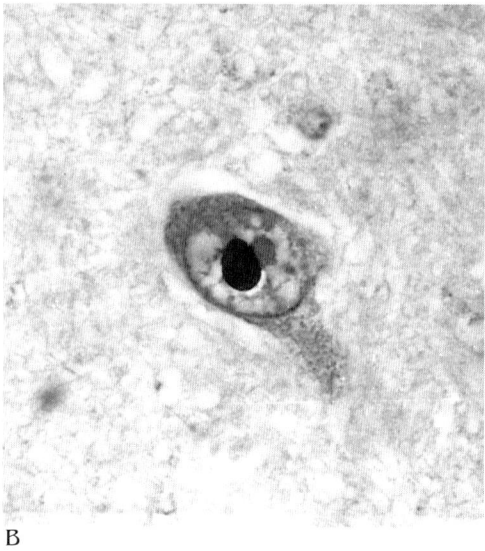

Figure 9–21. Intranuclear neuronal inclusions in neuronal intranuclear hyaline inclusion disease are undistinguishable from those seen in spinocerebellar ataxias in H&E (A) and ubiquitin (B) preparations, but are IC2 negative. ×900.

which about 1% of the inclusions were positive.

OTHER PARKINSONIAN SYNDROMES

Drug-Induced Parkinsonism

A common cause of secondary parkinsonism is drug intoxication, which is responsible for 90% of the cases.[3] Treatment with neuroleptic drugs produces extrapyramidal syndromes that disappear after either the drug is withdrawn or its dosage is reduced. As for the pathogenetic mechanisms producing the syndrome, central depletion of catecholamines (reserpine, tetrabenzamine) or a block of the postsynaptic dopaminergic receptors of the striatum (phenothiazines, butyrophenones) seem to be the most likely possibilities. The morphologic basis is poorly understood and the neuropathologic reports give conflicting descriptions. In most cases, cerebral abnormalities, observed after prolonged periods or treatment, are nonspecific and seem to be related to the age of the patients or to the events immediately preceding death.[323] It has been suggested that in patients over the age of 60 with presymptomatic PD, the disease may be unmasked by neuroleptic therapy and lead to drug-induced parkinsonism.[324] Cases of irreversible parkinsonian syndromes have been observed after intoxication with MPTP, derived from meperidine[32,325] in these cases, neuropathologic examination has revealed a selective neuronal loss in the substantia nigra with one occasional eosinophilic inclusion in the cytoplasm of nerve cells resembling Lewy bodies. Similar lesions have been produced in animals.[326]

Postencephalitic Parkinsonism

Cases of parkinsonian syndromes, often having oculocephalogyric crises, have appeared several years after an attack of encephalitis lethargica.[327] The encephalitis was observed in an epidemic form in Europe between 1915 and 1926, but sporadic cases were reported as late as 1935. Rare cases described after 1940 have also been described.[328] The organism responsible for the illness, most probably a virus, has not been isolated with the limited techniques available at the time of the epidemic and recent molecular investigation of archival material has failed to reveal a viral infection.[329] Parkinsonian syndromes, usually of short duration, may occur during an encephalitic episode of known etiology. Irreversible syndromes, appearing at variable times after such an episode, are rare and differ clinically from the PEP that follows encephalitis lethargica. There are no pathologic descriptions of the acute phases, but the possibility of a simultaneous occurrence of encephalitis and idiopathic PD cannot be ruled out.[330]

Pathologically proven PEP cases still occur, but the accuracy of the clinical diagnosis in the absence of a neuropathological examination is difficult to assess. A recent large, clinicopathological study found that the best clinical predictors of the diagnosis of PEP included age at onset below middle age, symptom duration lasting more than 10 years, and the presence of oculogyric crisis. History of encephalitis lethargica, present in most PEP cases, was also found to be an important individual diagnostic predictor.[331]

Unlike in idiopathic parkinsonism, morphologic lesions, although ubiquitous, are not localized in functionally related areas and predominate in the upper part of the brain stem. The original reports of lesions of the substantia nigra in PEP have been known since von Economo.[18,25,26,30,332] Although in most cases the whole substantia nigra appears uniformly pale, on occasion its involvement may be asymmetrical. Nerve cell loss is usually severe and sometimes complete, and reactive glial proliferation is usually proportional to the cell loss. Extracellular melanin pigment may be observed, although it may not be present in severe and/or old cases. The number of neurofibrillary tangles varies considerably, but they are nearly always found in these cases, while perivascular infiltrates of mononuclear cells are only occasionally seen. The reticular formation of the midbrain may be so severely affected by the pathologic process that the resulting atrophy of the tegmentum may become macroscopically evident. Severe neuronal loss and intense gliosis are observed; numerous intraneuronal NFTs are also seen, mainly in the midline structures. The abnormalities described in the midbrain may be present, although irregularly, in other nuclei of the brain stem[333] their severity and localization vary from case to case, and they may be asymmetrical. The locus ceruleus and, to lesser extent, the dorsal nucleus of the vagus may show neuronal loss with presence of free melanin, reactive gliosis, and presence of NFTs. The reticular formation of the pons and medulla, and the nuclei of the cranial nerves (oculomotor, XII) may be especially involved, whereas the cerebellum and spinal cord are usually unaffected. Morphologic changes may also be seen more cranially: numerous NFTs have been observed in the hypothalamus, where they are associated with moderate nerve cell loss and reactive gliosis.[333] The basal ganglia, in particular, the globus pallidus, may be normal or be the site of either non-specific changes or, in some cases, NFTs, which are typical of the disease. The NFTs are sometimes seen in the nucleus basalis of Meynert. When they are numerous, their presence is usually associated with moderate nerve cell loss, foci of gliosis, and an occasional inflammatory infiltrate in the Ammon's horn.[334]

Neurofibrillary changes in PEP were described in the original studies.[25,26] On light microscopy, they consist of interweaving bundles of abnormal filaments within the nerve cell cytoplasm. In the brain stem, the cells that show these changes are ballooned with displacement by the filaments of the normal components of the cell; cells in the cortex tend to assume a more fusiform shape, which is underlined by the bundles of fibrils. In both cases, at a later stage the fibrillary material may be the only remaining component of the cell. Ultrastructurally, the abnormal fibrillary material consists of paired helical filaments 10 nm wide arranged in bundles.[335] Straight filaments 15 nm in width that are similar to those present in PSP have been described in PEP, but only in the locus ceruleus.[333] Glial fibrillary tangles occurring in heavily affected brain regions have also been described in PEP. Such glial inclusions are described to have the appearance of tufts of spider-like radiating fibers or small thorn-like feature on Gallyas impregnation or tau immunohistochemistry.[336] The NFTs are tau and ubiquitin positive in PEP.[337,338] Furthermore, the immunohistochemical profile of the NFTs and the triplet electrophoretic migrating pattern that has been described are similar to those seen in AD.[339,340]

Parkinsonian Syndrome in Creutzfeldt-Jakob Disease

Although extrapyramidal signs are frequently observed during the dementing stage of Creutzfeldt-Jakob disease (CJD), a true parkinsonian syndrome develops only rarely. In 1978, Van Rossum[341] described three cases of CJD with slow evolution in which the substantia nigra was the most common site of lesions. Each patient presented with hypokinesia, rigidity, and, on occasion, tremor and dysarthria. Neuropathological features include loss of nerve cells, free pigment, gliosis, and spongiform changes. A PSP-like presentation has also been documented in CJD.[342]

Parkinsonian Syndromes Secondary to Carbon Monoxide Poisoning

Parkinsonian syndromes[343] are among the variety of extrapyramidal manifestations of carbon monoxide poisoning and are characterized by the severity of hypertonia, akinesia, tremor, and abnormal movements. Necrotic lesions result from anemia and involve most frequently the anterodorsal regions of the medial globus pallidus and the adjacent areas of the internal capsule. Their localization, whether in isolation or in association with lesions of the white matter, correlates with the extrapyramidal symptoms. Changes have also been described, though infrequently, in the substantia nigra and consist of mild nerve cell loss, presence of free pigment, and reactive glial proliferation. In a study of 22 cases of carbon monoxide poisoning, Lapresle and Fardeau[344] found changes of the globus pallidus in 17 instances, while only 1 case showed a circumscribed area of necrosis in the substantia nigra.

Parkinsonian Syndromes Following Manganese Poisoning

These cases were described initially by Edsall and Drinker in 1919.[345] Pathologic reports note severe neuronal loss and glial proliferation in the globus pallidus, which is most marked in its medial part.[346,347] In the cases descried by Canavan et al.,[348] the changes in the globus pallidus were associated with more widespread lesions, mainly in the cortex. In all the cases in which the substantia nigra has been examined, it has been reported to be normal. Experimental studies on monkeys of the effect of manganese[349] have confirmed the predominant involvement of the globus pallidus and the absence of abnormalities in the substantia nigra.

Arteriosclerotic Parkinsonism

In the past, stress has been often laid on vascular lesions as a cause of parkinsonism.[350] Following comprehensive review of the arteriosclerotic parkinsonian syndromes,[351] vascular pathology has been widely considered to be one of the causes of parkinsonism or, by some authors, even the cause of PD. This view has subsequently been criticized,[31,352,353] and at present, the role of vascular lesions in the etiology of parkinsonian syndromes is considered with skepticism.[354] While in rare instances unilateral infarction of the substantia nigra is followed by a parkinsonian syndrome,[353,355] in many cases the presence of "etat crible" or areas of disintegration of the basal ganglia in aged subjects is not associated with signs of parkinsonism. Indeed, numerous patients considered to be suffering from arteriosclerotic parkinsonism have the clinical features of pseudobulbar palsy and show morphologic appearances of lacunar lesions in the deep gray nuclei. Furthermore, the frequent association in the same brain of degenerative changes of the substantia nigra and Lewy bodies and variously distributed areas of ischemia or hemorrhage suggests that the two types of lesion may often coexist in the same aged individual.[2,31]

Parkinsonian Syndromes and Tumors

The occurrence of various types of parkinsonian syndromes in patients with cerebral tumors is a well-known, though rare, event. Extrapyramidal signs have been reported in 10 of 474 cases by Sciarra and Sprofkin[356] and 21 of the 1500 patients described by Tolosa et al.[357] presented with parkinsonian syndrome. Direct involvement of the substantia nigra by a space-occupying lesion, tuberculoma,[358] or lymphoma[359] localized in the cerebral peduncle has been only occasionally observed. Supratentorial tumors may produce a parkinsonian syndrome,[360,361] although tumors that infiltrate extensively the gray nuclei usually fail to produce it. In the great majority of cases, symptoms are produced by tumors of the midline (parasagittal meningiomas, frontal, septal, intraventricular, or suprasellar tumors) or by temporal tumors not infiltrating the gray nuclei. The pathogenetic mechanism of these syndromes is poorly understood and is probably not the same in every case. Destruction of the nerve cells of the substantia nigra by the tumor is observed only on rare occasions.[359] The disappearance of the syndrome following removal of the tumor indicates that either indirect compression or stretching of the gray nuclei (by the mass or by the intermediary of the temporal herniation) is the cause of the symptoms. A specific involvement of the nerve cells of the substantia nigra or their dopaminergic fibers directed to the striatum was suggested through biochemical studies in a case of craniopharyngioma[362] and by the improvement obtained through treatment with l-dopa in another case.[363] Other possible mechanisms have been proposed, such as changes in the extrapyramidal centers in the frontal cortex[363] or an association with a parkinsonian syndrome due to another cause.[364,365]

Post-traumatic Parkinsonian Syndromes

Once cases of PD following head injury or cerebral herniation have been excluded, parkinsonian syndromes directly related to brain trauma are rare.[366] Morphologic studies of three cases revealed hemorrhagic lesions within the substantia nigra secondary to uncal herniation.[367] Parkinsonian syndromes, uncomplicated or associated with progressive dementia (dementia pugilistica), have been described after repeated head injuries. This condition may occur years after the last trauma and affects amateur as well as professional boxers who have been dazed or knocked out on many occasions. Neuropathologic examination by Corsellis et al.[368] has shown nerve cell loss and free pigment in the substantia nigra, scarring and neuronal loss in the cerebellum, and changes in the midline structures, such as enlargement of the cavum and fenestration of the leaves of the intraventricular septum pellucidum and atrophy of the fornix or the corpus callosum. Although this study described numerous NFTs without senile plaques throughout the cerebral cortex (particularly the medial temporal regions) and the brain stem, subsequent re-examination of the same cases by immunohistochemical means showed that there is βA4-protein deposition comparable to that seen in AD in such cases. Although these findings may suggest similarities between dementia pugilistica and AD, there are also striking differences; in dementia pugilistica the βA4-positive plaques are of the diffuse type and are not visible with Congo red or standard silver stains, and the regional topography of NFTs is also different from that seen in AD.[369,370] The early histological changes that occur in association with repetitive head injury, eventually leading to dementia pugilistica, are those of neocortical NFTs and NTs with an immunohistochemical profile similar to that seen in AD. The neurofibrillary pathology is consistently situated around blood vessels, which suggests that the early cytoskeletal changes may involve damage to blood vessels.[371]

REFERENCES

1. Hornykiewicz O. Dopamine and extrapyramidal motor function and dysfunction. Res Publ Assoc Res Nerv Ment Dis 1972; 50:390–415.
2. Hughes AJ, Daniel SE, Blankson S, Lees AJ. A clinicopathologic study of 100 cases of Parkinson's disease. Arch Neurol 1993; 50:140–148.
3. Derouesne C. Mouvements involontaires. In: Practique Neurologique Paris: Flammarion, 1982:74–99.
4. Golbe LI. Young-onset Parkinson's disease: a clinical review. Neurology 1991; 41:168–173.
5. Rajput DR. Accuracy of clinical diagnosis of idiopathic Parkinsons disease. J Neurol Neurosurg Psychiatry, 1993; 56:938–939.
6. Schoenberg BS. Environmental risk factors for Parkinson's disease: the epidemiologic evidence. Can J Neurol Sci, 1987; 14:407–413.
7. Duvoisin RC, Johnson WG. Hereditary Lewy-body parkinsonism and evidence for a genetic etiology of Parkinson's disease. Brain Pathol, 1992; 2:309–320.
8. Duvoisin RC. The genetics of Parkinson's disease. A review. Adv Neurol 1993; 60:306–315.
9. Golbe LI, Lazzarini AM, Schwarz KO, Mark MH, Dickson DW, Duvoisin RC. Autosomal-dominant parkinsonism with benign course and typical Lewy-body pathology. Neurology 1993; 43:2222–2227.
10. Waters CH, Miller CA. Autosomal-dominant Lewy-body parkinsonism in a 4-generation family. Ann Neurol 1994; 35:59–64.
11. Ruberg M, France-Lanord V, Brugg B, Lambeng N, Michel PP, Anglade P, Hunot S, Damier P, Francheux B, Hirscht, Agid Y. (1997) Neuronal death caused by apoptosis in Parkinson disease Rev Neurol (Paris) 1997; 153:499–508.
12. France-Lanord V, Brugg B, Michel PP, Agid Y, Ruberg M. Mitochondrial free radical signal in ceramide-dependent apoptosis: a putative mechanism for neuronal death in Parkinson's disease. J Neurochem, 1997; 69:1612–1621.
13. Luo Y, Umegaki H, Wang X, Abe R, Roth GS. Dopamine induces apoptosis through an oxidation-involved SAPK/JNK activation pathway. J Biol Chem 1998; 273:3756–3764.
14. Zhang J, Perry G, Smith MA, Robertson D, Olson SJ, Graham DG, Montine TJ. Parkinson's disease is associated with oxidative damage to cytoplasmic DNA and RNA in substantia nigra neurons. Am J Pathol, 1999; 154:1423–1429.
15. Lowe J, Lennox G, Leigh PN. Disorders of movement and system degenerations. In: Graham DI, Lantos PL, eds. Greenfield's Neuropathology. London: Arnold, 1997:281–366.
16. Parkinson J. Essay on the Shaking Palsy. London: Willingham and Rowland, 1817.
17. Jelgersma G. Neue anatomosche Befunde bei Paralysis agitans und bei chronischer Chorea. Neurol Zentralbl 1908; 27:995–996.
18. Lewy FH. Paralysis agitans. I. Pathologische Anatomie. In: Lewandowsky M, ed. Handbuch des Neurologie, Band III. Berlin: Springer-Vetlag, 1912:920–933.
19. Vogt C, Vogt O. Zur Lehre der Erkrankungen des striaren Systems. J Psychol Neurol, 1920; 25 (Suppl 3):627–846.
20. Lhermitte J, Cornil L. Recherches antomiques sur la maladie de Parkinson. Rev Neurol (Paris) 1921; 28: 625–629.
21. Bielschowsky M. Weitere Bemerkungen zur normalen und pathologischen Histologie des striaren Systems. J Psychol Neurol 1922; 27:233–280.
22. Brissaud E. Lecons sur les Maladies Nerveuses (23ème leçon: Nature et Pathogenie de la Maladie de Parkinson). Paris: Masson, 1895:488–501.
23. Tretiakoff C. Contribution à l'etude de l'anatomie pathologique du locus niger de Soemmering avec quelques deductions relatives à la pathogénie des troubles du tonus musculaire et de la maladie de Parkinson. Thèse Medicine. Paris: University of Paris, 1919.
24. Foix C, Nicolesco J. Les Noyaux Gris Centraux et la Region Mesencephalo-sous-optique. Paris: Masson, 1925.
25. Hallervorden J. Zur Pathogenese des postencephalitischen Parkinsonismus. Klin Wochenschr 1933; 12:692–695.

26. Hallervorden J. Anatomische Untersuchungen zur Pathogenese des post-encephalitischen Parkinsonismus. Dtsch Z Nervenheilkd, 1935; 136:68–77.
27. Hallervorden J. Paralysis agitans. In: Cholz W, ed. Handbuch der speziellen Pathologischen Anatomie und Histologie des Nervensystems. Berlin: Springer-Verlag, 1957: XIII/1:900–924.
28. Hassler R. Paralysis agitans. In: Handbuch der speziellen Pathologischen Anatomie und Histologie des Nervensystems. J Psychol Neurol Leipzig 1938; 48: 387–476.
29. Klaue R. Parkinsonische Krankheit (Paralysis agitans, usw). Arch Psychiatr Nervenkrank, 1940; 140:251–321.
30. Greenfield JG, Bosanquet FD. The brainstem lesions in parkinsonism. J Neurol Neurosurg Psychiatry, 1953; 16:213–226.
31. Escourolle R, De Recondo J, Gray F. Etude anatomo-pathologique des syndromes parkinsoniens. In: Ajuriaguerra J, Gauthier G, eds. Monamines, Noyaux Gris Centraux et Syndrome de Parkinson. Geneva: George et Cie. S.A. 1971:173–229.
32. Davis GC, Williams AC, Markey SP, Ebert MH, Caine ED, Reichert CM, Kopin IJ. Chronic parkinsonism secondary to intravenous injection of meperidine analogues. Psychiatry Res 1979; 1:249–254.
33. Lipkin LE. Cytoplasmic inclusions in ganglion cells, associated with parkinsonian states. Am J Pathol, 1979; 35:1117–1133.
34. Forno LS. Concentric hyalin intraneuronal inclusions of Lewy type in the brains of elderly persons (50 incidental cases): relationship to parkinsonism. J Am Geriatr Soc, 1969; 17:557–575.
35. Gibb WR. Idiopathic Parkinson's disease and the Lewy body disorders. Neuropathol Appl Neurobiol, 1986; 12:223–234.
36. Dickson DW. Aging in the central nervous system. In: Markesbery WR, ed. Neuropathology of Dementing Disorders. London: Arnold, 1998:56–88.
37. Denny-Brown D. The Basal Ganglia and Their Relation to Disorders of Movements. Oxford: Oxford University Press, 1962.
38. Jellinger K, Danielczyk W. Striato-nigral degeneration. [in German]. Acta Neuropathol (Berl) 1968; 10: 242–257.
39. Mori H, Yoshimura M, Tomonaga M, Yamanouchi H. Progressive supranuclear palsy with Lewy bodies. Acta Neuropathol (Berl) 1986; 71:344–346.
40. Lantos PL. The neuropathology of progressive supranuclear palsy. J Neural Transm suppl, 1994; 42: 137–152.
41. Hauw JJ, Daniel SE, Dickson D, Horoupian DS, Jellinger K, Lantos PL, Mckee A, Tabaton M, Litvan I. Preliminary NINDS neuropathologic criteria for Steele-Richardson-Olszewski syndrome (progressive supranuclear palsy). Neurology 1994; 44:2015–2019.
42. Gibb WR, Lees AJ. The relevance of the Lewy body to the pathogenesis of idiopathic Parkinson's disease. J Neurol Neurosurg Psychiatry, 1988; 51:745–752.
43. Dale GE, Probst A, Luthert P, Martin J, Anderton BH, Leigh PN. Relationships between Lewy bodies and pale bodies in Parkinson's disease. Acta Neuropathol (Berl) 1992; 83:525–529.
44. Hayashida K, Oyanagi S, Mizutani Y, Yokochi M. An early cytoplasmic change before Lewy body maturation: an ultrastructual study of the substantia nigra from an autopsy case of juvenile parkinsonism. Acta Neuropathol (Berl) 1993; 85:445–448.
45. Irizarry MC, Growdon W, Gomezisla T, Newell K, George JM, Clayton DF, Hyman BT. Nigral and cortical Lewy bodies and dystrophic nigral neurites in Parkinson's disease and cortical Lewy body disease contain alpha-synuclein immunoractivity. J Neuropathol Exp Neurol, 1998; 57:334–337.
46. Forno LS, Norville RL. Ultrastructure of Lewy bodies in the stellate ganglion. Acta Neuropathol (Berl) 1976; 34:183–197.
47. Roy S, Wolman L. Ultrastructural observations in parkinsonism. J Pathol 1969; 99:39–44.
48. Forno LS. Neuropathology of Parkinson's disease. J Neuropathol Exp Neurol 1996; 55:259–272.
49. Goldman JE, Yen SH, Chiu FC, Peress NS. Lewy bodies of Parkinson's disease contain neurofilament antigens. Science 1983; 221:1082–1084.
50. Lowe J, Blanchard A, Morrell K, Lennox G, Reynolds L, Billett M, Landon M, Mayer RJ. Ubiquitin is a common factor in intermediate filament inclusion bodies of diverse type in man, including those of Parkinson's disease, Pick's disease, and Alzheimer's disease, as well as Rosenthal fibres in cerebellar astrocytomas, cytoplasmic bodies in muscle, and mallory bodies in alcoholic liver disease. J Pathol, 1988; 155: 9–15.
51. Lowe J, McDermott H, Landon M, Mayer RJ, Wilkinson KD. Ubiquitin carboxyl-terminal hydrolase (PGP 9.5) is selectively present in ubiquitinated inclusion-bodies characteristic of human neurodegenerative diseases. J Pathol 1990; 161:153–160.
52. Nishimura M, Tomimoto H, Suenaga T, Nakamura S, Namba Y, Ikeda K, Akiguchi I, Kimura J. Synaptophysin and chromogranin A immunoreactivities of Lewy bodies in Parkinson's disease brains. Brain Res 1994; 634:339–344.
53. Li K, Ito H, Tanaka K, Hirano A. Immunocytochemical co-localization of the proteasome in ubiquitinated structures in neurodegenerative diseases and the elderly. J Neuropathol Exp Neurol 1997; 56:125–131.
54. Polymeropoulos MH, Higgins JJ, Golbe LI, Johnson WG, Ide SE, Di Iorio G, Sanges G, Stenroos ES, Pho LT, Schaffer AA, Lazzarini AM, Nussbaum RL, Duvoisin RC. Mapping of a gene for Parkinson's disease to chromosome 4q21-q23 [see comments]. Science 1996; 274:1197–1199.
55. Polymeropoulos MH, Lavedan C, Leroy E, Ide SE, Dehejia A, Dutra A, Pike B, Root H, Rubenstein J, Boyer R, Stenroos ES, Chandrasekharappa S, Athanassiadou A, Papapetropoulos T, Johnson WG, Lazzarini AM, Duvoisin RC, Di Iorio G, Golbe LI, Nussbaum RL. Mutation in the alpha-synuclein gene identified in families with Parkinson's disease. Science 1997; 276:2045–2047.
56. Kruger R, Kuhn W, Muller T, Woitalla D, Graeber M, Kosel S, Przuntek H, Epplen JT, Schols L, Riess O. Ala30Pro mutation in the gene encoding alpha-synuclein in Parkinson's disease. Nat Genet 1998; 18: 106–108.
57. Spillantini MG, Schmidt ML, Lee VMY, Trojanowski JQ, Jakes R, Goedert M Alpha-synuclein in Lewy bodies. Nature 1997; 388:839–840.
58. Baba M, Nakajo S, Tu PH, Tomita T, Nakaya K, Lee VMY, Trojanowski JQ, Iwatsubo T. Aggregation of alpha-synuclein in Lewy bodies of sporadic Parkin-

59. Mezey E, Dehejia A, Harta G, Papp MI, Polymeropoulos MH, Brownstein MJ. Alpla-synuclein in neurodegenerative disorders: murderer or accomplice? Nat Med 1998;4:755–757.
60. Weinreb PH, Zhen W, Poon AW, Conway KA, Lansbury PTJ. NACP, a protein implicated in Alzheimer's disease and learning, is natively unfolded. Biochemistry 1996; 35:13709–13715.
61. George JM, Jin H, Woods WS, Clayton DF. Characterization of a novel protein regulated during the critical period for song learning in the zebra finch. Neuron 1995; 15:361–372.
62. Jenner P, Olanow CW. Oxidative stress and the pathogenesis of Parkinson's disease. Neurology, 1996; 47: S161–S170.
63. Schapira AH. Pathogenesis of Parkinson's disease. Baillieres Clin Neurol 1997; 6:15–36.
64. Schapira AH, Gu M, Taanman JW, Tabrizi SJ, Seaton T, Cleeter M, Cooper JM. Mitochondria in the etiology and pathogenesis of Parkinson's disease. Ann Neurol 1998; 44:S89–S98.
65. Kitada T. Asakawa S, Hattori N, Matsumine H, Yamamura Y, Minoshima S, Yokochi M, Mizuno Y, Shimizu N. Mutations in the parkin gene cause autosomal recessive juvenile parkinsonism [see comments]. Nature 1998; 392:605–608.
66. Tassin J, Durr A, De Broucker T, Abbas N, Bonifati V, De Michele G, De Michele G, Bonnet AM, Broussolle E, Pollak P, Vidailhet M, De Mari M, Marconi R, Medjbeur S, Filla A, Meco G, Agid Y, Brice A. Chromosome 6-linked autosomal recessive early-onset parkinsonism: linkage in European and Algerian families, extension of the clinical spectrum, and evidence of a small homozygous deletion in one family. The French Parkinson's Disease Genetics Study Group, and the European Consortium on Genetic Susceptibility in Parkinson's Disease. Am J Hum Genet 1998; 63:88–94.
67. Abbas N, Lucking CB, Ricard S, Durr A, Bonifati V, Demichele G, Bouley S, Vaughan JR, Gasser T, Marconi R, Broussolle E, Brefel-Courbon C, Harhangi BS, Oostra BA, Fabrizio E, Bohme GA, Pradier L, Wood NW, Filla A, Meco G, Denefle P, Agid Y, Brice A. A wide variety of mutations in the parkin gene are responsible for autosomal recessive parkinsonism in Europe. Hum Mol Genet 1999; 8:567–574.
68. Farrer M, Gwinn-Hardy K, Muenter M, Devrieze FW, Crook R, Perez-Tur J, Lincoln S, Maraganore D, Adler C, Newmann S, MacElwee K, McCarthy P, Miller C, Waters C, Hardy J. A chromosome 4p haplotype segregating with Parkinson's disease and postural tremor. Hum Mol Genet 1999; 8:81–85.
69. Gasser T, Muller-Myhsok B, Wszolek ZK, Oehlmann R, Calne DB, Bonifati V, Bereznai B, Fabrizio E, Vieregge P, Horstmann RD. A susceptibility locus for Parkinson's disease maps to chromosome 2p13. Nat Genet 1998; 18:262–265.
70. Leroy E, Boyer R, Auburger G, Leube B, Ulm G, Mezey E, Harta G, Brownstein MJ, Jonnalagada S, Chernova T, Dehejia A, Lavedan C, Gasser T, Steinbach PJ, Wilkinson KD, Polymeropoulos MH. The ubiquitin pathway in Parkinson's disease. Nature 1998; 395:451–452.
71. Harhangi BS, Farrer MJ, Lincoln S, Bonifati V, Meco G, De Michelle G, Brice A, Durr A, Martinez M, Gasser T, Bereznai B, Vaughan JR, Wood NW, Hardy J, Oostra BA, Breteler MM. The Ile93Met mutation in the ubiquitin carboxy-terminal-hydrolase-L1 gene is not observed in European cases with familial Parkinson's disease Neurosci Lett 1999; 270:1–4.
72. Den Hartog Jager WA, Bethlem J The distribution of Lewy bodies in the central and autonomic nervous system in idiopathic paralysis agitans. J Neurol Neurosurg Psychiatry 1960; 23:283–290.
73. Javoy-Agid F, Ruberg M, Taquet H, Bokobza B, Agid Y, Gaspar P, Berger B, N'Guyen-Legros J, Alvarez C, Gray F, Hauw JJ, Scatton B, Rouquier L. Biochemical neuropathology of Parkinson's disease. Adv Neurol 1984; 40:189–198.
74. Ohama E, Ikuta F. Parkinson's disease: distribution of Lewy bodies and monoamine neuron system. Acta Neuropathol (Berl) 1976; 34:311–319.
75. Jellinger K Overview of morphological changes in Parkinson's disease. Adv Neurol 1987; 45:1–18.
76. Buttlar-Brentano Von K. Das Parkinson-Syndrom in Lichte des lebensgeschichtlichen Veränderungen des Nucleus basalis. J Hirnforsch 1955; 2:56–76.
77. Forno LS, Alvord EC. The Pathology of parkinsonism. Some new observations and correlations (Part I). In McDowell R, Markham M, eds. Recent Advances in Parkinson's Disease. Philadelphia: F.A. Davis, 1971:47–63.
78. Candy JM, Perry RH, Perry EK, Irving D, Blessed G, Fairbairn AF, Tomlinson BE. (1983) Pathological changes in the nucleus of Meynert in Alzheimer's and Parkinson's diseases. J Neurol Sci 1983; 59:277–289.
79. Arendt T, Bigl V, Arendt A, Tennstedt A. Loss of neurons in the nucleus basalis of Meynert in Alzheimer's disease, paralysis agitans and Korsakoffs disease. Acta Neuropathol (Berl) 1983; 61:101–108.
80. Gaspar P, Gray F. Dementia in idiopathic Parkinsons disease—a neuropathological study of 32 cases. Acta Neuropathol (Berl) 1984; 64:43–52.
81. Tagliavini F, Pilleri G, Bouras C, Constantinidis J. The basal nucleus of meynert in idiopathic Parkinson's disease. Acta Neurol Scan 1984; 70:20–28.
82. Nakano I, Hirano A. Parkinson's disease—neuron loss in the nucleus basalis without concomitant Alzheimers' disease. Ann Neurol 1984; 15:415–418.
83. Langston JW, Forno LS. The hypothalamus in Parkinson disease. Ann Neurol 1978; 3:129–133.
84. Jellinger KA. Postmortem studies in Parkinson's disease—is it possible to detect brain areas for specific symptoms? J Neural Transm Suppl 1999; 56:1–29.
85. Hunter S. The rostral mesencephalon in Parkinson's disease and Alzheimer's disease. Acta Neuropathol (Berl) 1985; 68:53–58.
86. Fujimura H, Umbach I. Pathological correlations between dementia, Parkinson's disease and lesions of the reticular formation. Rev Neurol 1987; 143:108–114.
87. Oppenheimer DR. Neuropathology of progressive autonomic failure. In: Bannister R, ed. Autonomic Failure. Oxford: Oxford University Press, 1983:267–283.
88. Yoshimura M. Cortical changes in the parkinsonian brain: a contribution to the delineation of "diffuse Lewy body disease". J Neurol 1983; 229:17–32.
89. Gibb WR, Esiri MM, Lees AJ. Clinical and pathological features of diffuse cortical Lewy body disease

(Lewy body dementia). Brain 1987; 110(Pt 5):1131–1153.
90. Kosaka K, Yoshimura M, Ikeda K, Budka H. Diffuse type of Lewy body disease: progressive dementia with abundant cortical Lewy bodies and senile changes of varying degree—a new disease? Clin Neuropathol 1984; 3:185–192.
91. Lennox G, Lowe J, Landon M, Byrne EJ, Mayer RJ, Godwin-Austen RB. Diffuse Lewy body disease: correlative neuropathology using anti-ubiquitin immunocytochemistry. J Neurol Neurosurg Psychiatry 1989; 52:1236–1247.
92. Dickson DW, Ruan D, Crystal H, Mark MH, Davies P, Kress Y, Yen SH. Hippocampal degeneration differentiates diffuse Lewy body disease (DLBD) from Alzheimer's disease. Light- and electron-microscopic immunocytochemistry of CA2-3 neurites specific to DLBD. Neurology 1991; 41:1402–1409.
93. Dickson DW, Schmidt ML, Lee VM, Zhao ML, Yen SH, Trojanowski JQ. Immunoreactivity profile of hippocampal CA2/3 neurites in diffuse Lewy body disease. Acta Neuropathol (Berl) 1994; 87:269–276.
94. Braak H, Braak E, Yilmazer D, De Vos RA, Jansen EN, Bohl J, Jellinger K. Amygdala pathology in Parkinson's disease. Acta Neuropathol (Berl) 1994; 88:493–500.
95. Gai WP, Blessing WW, Blumbergs PC. Ubiquitin-positive degenerating neurites in the brainstem in Parkinson's disease. Brain 1995; 118(Pt 6):1447–1459.
96. Pellise A, Roig C, Barraquer-Bordas LI, Ferrer I. Abnormal, unbiquitinated cortical neurites in patients with diffuse Lewy body disease. Neurosci Lett 1996; 206:85–88.
97. Bugiani O, Perdelli F, Salvarani S, Leonardi A, Mancardi GL. Loss of striatal neurons in Parkinson's disease: a cytometric study. Eur Neurol 1980; 19:339–344.
98. Sabuncu N. Quantitative Untersuchungen am menschlichen Pallidum. Fälle ohne extrapyramidale Bewegungssterungen. Dtsch Z Nervenheilkd 1969; 195:57–63.
99. Sabuncu N. Untersuchungen am Pallidum beim Parkinsonsyndrom. Dtsch Z Nervenheilkd 1969; 196: 40–48.
100. Goetz CG, Olanow CW, Koller WC, Penn RD, Cahill D, Morantz R, Stebbins G, Tanner CM, Klawans HL, Shannon KM. (1989) Multicenter study of autologous adrenal medullary transplantation to the corpus striatum in patients with advanced Parkinson's disease [see comments]. N Engl J Med 1989; 320:337–341.
101. Defer GL, Geny C, Ricolfi F, Fenelon G, Monfort JC, Remy P, Villafane G, Jeny R, Samson Y, Keravel Y, Gaston A, Degos JD, Peschanski M, Cesaro P, Nguyen JP. Long-term outcome of unilaterally transplanted parkinsonian patients. 1. Clinical approach. Brain 1996; 119:41–50.
102. Kordower JH, Freeman TB, Snow BJ, Vingerhoets FJG, Mufson EJ, Sanberg PR, Hauser RA, Smith DA, Nauert GM, Perl DP, Warren Olanow C. Neuropathologic evidence of graft survival and striatal reinervation after the transplantation of fetal mesencephalic tissue in a patient with Parkinson's disease. N Engl J Med 1995; 332:1118–1124.
103. Conley SC, Kirchner JT. Medical and surgical treatment of Parkinson's disease. Strategies to slow symptom progression and improve quality of life. Postgrad Med 1999; 106:41–4, 49, 52.
104. Haberler C, Alesch F, Hainfeller JA, Mazal P, Pilz P, Jellinger K, Pinter M, Budka. H. Brain pathology after long-term-electrical neurostimulation in Parkinson's disease [abstrct]. Neuropathol Appl Neurobiol 1999; 25 (suppl 1):59.
105. Dejerine J, Thomas AA. L'atrophie olivo-ponto-cérébelleuse. Nouv Iconog Salpètrière 1900; 13:330–370.
106. Van Der Eeken H, Adams RD, Van Bogaert L. Striopallidal-nigral degeneration. An hitherto undescribed lesion in paralysis agitans. J Neuropathol Exp Neurol 1960; 19:159–161.
107. Adams RD, Van Bogaert L, Van Der Eeken H. Dégénérescences nigro-striées et cérébello-nigrigrostriées. Psychiatr Neurol 1961; 142:219–259.
108. Shy GM, Drager GA. A neurologic syndrome associated with orthostatic hypotension. Arch Neurol 1960; 2:511–527.
109. Graham JG, Oppenheimer DR. Orthostatic hypotension and nicotine sensitivity in a case of multiple system atrophy. J Neurol Neurosurg Psychiatry 1969; 32:28–34.
110. Gilman S, Low PA, Quinn N, Albanese A, Ben-Shlomo Y, Fowler CJ, Kaufmann H, Klockgether T, Lang AE, Lantos PL, Litvan I, Mathias CJ, Oliver E, Robertson D, Schatz I, Wenning GK. Consensus statement on the diagnosis of multiple system atrophy. J Auton Nerv Syst 1998; 74:189–192.
111. Bower JH, Maraganore DM, McDonnell K, Rocca WA. Incidence of progressive supranuclear palsy and multiple system atrophy in Olmsted County, Minnesota, 1976 to 1990. Neurology 1997; 49:1284–1288.
112. Wenning GK, Tison F, Benshlomo Y, Daniel SE, Quinn NP. Multiple system atrophy: a review of 203 pathologically proven cases. Mov Disord 1997; 12: 133–147.
113. Wenning GK, Ben Shlomo Y, Magalhaes M, Daniel SE, Quinn NP. Clinical features and natural history of multiple system atrophy. An analysis of 100 cases. Brain 1994; 117(Pt 4):835–845.
114. Nakamura S, Ohnishi K, Nishimura M, Suenaga T, Akiguchi I, Kimura J, Kimura T. Large neurons in the tuberomammillary nucleus in patients with Parkinson's disease and multiple system atrophy. Neurology 1996; 46:1693–1696.
115. Ozawa T, Oyanagi K, Tanaka H, Horikawa Y, Takahashi H, Morita T, Tsuji S. Suprachiasmatic nucleus in a patient with multiple system atrophy with abnormal circadian rhythm of arginine-vasopressin secretion into plasma. J Neurol Sci 1998; 154:116–121.
116. Gray F, Vincent D, Hauw JJ. Quantitative study of lateral horn cells in 15 cases of multiple system atrophy. Acta Neuropathol (Berl) 1988; 75:513–518.
117. Terao S, Sobue G, Hashizume Y, Mitsuma T, Takahashi A. Disease-specific patterns of neuronal loss in the spinal ventral horn in amyotrophic lateral sclerosis, multiple system atrophy and X-linked recessive bulbospinal neuronopathy, with special reference to the loss of small neurons in the intermediate zone. J Neurol 1994; 241:196–203.
118. Kanda T, Tsukagoshi H, Oda M, Miyamoto K, Tanabe H. Changes of unmyelinated nerve fibers in su-

ral nerve in amyotrophic lateral sclerosis, Parkinson's disease and multiple system atrophy. Acta Neuropathol (Berl) 1996; 91:145–154.
119. Probst-Cousin S, Rickert CH, Schmid KW, Gullotta F. Cell death mechanisms in multiple system atrophy. J Neuropathol Exp Neurol 1998; 57:814–821.
120. De La Monte SM, Sohn YK, Ganju N, Wands JR. P53-and CD95-associated apoptosis in neurodegenerative diseases. Lab Invest 1998; 78:401–411.
121. Papp MI, Kahn JE, Lantos PL. Glial cytoplasmic inclusions in the CNS of patients with multiple system atrophy (striatonigral degeneration, olivopontocerebellar atrophy and Shy-Drager syndrome). J Neurol Sci 1989; 94:79–100.
122. Papp MI Lantos PL. Accumulation of tubular structures in oligodendroglial and neuronal cells as the basic alteration in multiple system atrophy. J Neurol Sci 1992; 107:172–182.
123. Chin SSM, Goldman JE. Glial inclusions in CNS degenerative diseases. J Neuropathol Exp Neurol 1996; 55:499–508.
124. Feany MB, Dickson DW. Neurodegenerative disorders with extensive tau pathology: a comparative-study and review. Ann Neurol 1996; 40:139–148.
125. Takeda A, Mallory M, Sundsmo M, Honer W, Hansen L, Masliah E. Abnormal accumulation of NACP/alpha-synuclein in neurodegenerative disorders. Am J Pathol 1998; 152:367–372.
126. Lantos PL. The definition of multiple system atrophy: a review of recent developments. J Neuropathol Exp Neurol 1998; 57:1099–1111.
127. Golbe LI. The epidemiology of progressive supranuclear palsy. Adv Neurol 1996; 69:25–31.
128. Hynd GW, Pirozzolo FJ, Maletta GJ. Progressive supranuclear palsy. Int J Neurosci 1982; 16:87–98.
129. Kristensen MO. Progressive supranuclear palsy—20 years later. Acta Neurol Scan 1985; 71:177–189.
130. Golbe LI, Davis PH, Schoenberg BS, Duvoisin RC. Prevalence and natural history of progressive supranuclear palsy. Neurology 1988; 38:1031–1034.
131. Maher ER, Lees AJ. The clinical features and natural history of the Steele-Richardson-Olszewski syndrome (progressive supranuclear palsy). Neurology 1986; 36:1005–1008.
132. David NJ, Mackey EA, Smith JL. Further observations in progressive supranuclear palsy. Neurology 1968; 18:349–356.
133. Brown J, Lantos P, Stratton M, Roques P, Rossor M. Familial progressive supranuclear palsy. J Neurol Neurosurg Psychiatry 1993; 56:473–476.
134. Rojo A, Pernaute RS, Fontan A, Ruiz PG, Honnorat J, Lynch T, Chin S, Gonzalo I, Rabano A, Martinez A, Daniel S, Pramstaller P, Morris H, Wood N, Lees A, Tabernero C, Nyggard T, Jackson AC, Hanson A, de Yebenes JG. Clinical genetics of familial progressive supranuclear palsy. Brain 1999; 122:1233–1245.
135. Conrad C, Andreadis A, Trojanowski JQ, Dickson DW, Kang D, Chen XH, Wiederholt W, Hansen L, Masliah E, Thal LJ, Katzman R, Xia Y, Saitoh T. Genetic evidence for the involvement of tau in progressive supranuclear palsy. Ann Neurol 1997; 41:277–281.
136. Bennett P, Bonifati V, Bonuccelli U, Colosimo C, De Mari M, Fabbrini G, Marconi R, Meco G, Nicholl DJ, Stocchi F, Vanacore N, Vieregge P, Williams AC. Direct genetic evidence for involvement of tau in progressive supranuclear palsy. European Study Group on Atypical Parkinsonism Consortium. Neurology 1998; 51:982–985.
137. Morris HR, Janssen JC, Bandmann O, Daniel SE, Rossor MN, Lees AJ, Wood NW. The tau gene AO polymorphism in progressive supranuclear palsy and related neurodegenerative diseases. J Neurol Neurosurg Psychiatry, 1999; 66:665–667.
138. Steele JC, Richardson JC, Olszewski J Progressive supranuclear palsy. Arch Neurol 1964; 10:333–359.
139. Dubas F, Gray F, Escourolle R. Maladie de Steele-Richardson-Olszewski sans ophthalmoplegie. Six cas anatomo-clinique. Rev Neurol 1983; 139:407–416.
140. Davis PH, Bergeron C, Mclachlan DR. Atypical presentation of progressive supranuclear palsy. Ann Neurol 1985; 17:337–343.
141. Matsuo H, Takashima H, Kishikawa M, Kinoshita I, Mori M, Tsujihata M, Nagataki S. Pure akinesia—an atypical manifestation of progressive supranuclear palsy. J Neurol Neurosurg Psychiatry 1991; 54:397–400.
142. De Bruin VMS, Lees AJ. The clinical features of 67 patients with clinically definite Steele-Richardson-Olszewski syndrome. Behavi Neurol 1992; 5:229–232.
143. Daniel SE, De Bruin VMS, Lees AJ. The clinical and pathological spectrum of Steele-Richardson-Olszewski syndrome (progressive supranuclear palsy)—a reappraisal. Brain 1995; 118:759–770.
144. Litvan I, Campbell G, Mangone CA, Verny M, McKee A, Chaudhuri KR, Jellinger K, Pearce RK, D'Olhaberriague L. Which clinical features differentiate progressive supranuclear palsy (Steele-Richardson-Olszewski syndrome) from related disorders?—A clinicopathological study. Brain 1997; 120:65–74.
145. Litvan I, Agid Y, Calne D, Campbell G, Dubois B, Duvoisin RC, et al. Clinical research criteria for the diagnosis of progressive supranuclear palsy (Steele-Richardson-Olszewski syndrome): report of the NINDS-SPSP international workshop. Neurology 1996; 47:1–9.
146. Jellinger K, Bancher C. Neuropathology. In: Agid Y, Litvan I, eds. Progressive Supranuclear Palsy, Clinical and Research Approaches. New York: Oxford University Press, 1992:44–88.
147. Gearing M, Olson DA, Watts RL, Mirra SS. Progressive supranuclear palsy: neuropathologic and clinical heterogeneity. Neurology 1994; 44:1015–1024.
148. Daniel SE, Geddes JF, Revesz T. Glial cytoplasmic inclusions are not exclusive to multiple system atrophy. J Neurol Neurosurg Psychiatry 1995; 58:262–262.
149. Revesz T, Sangha H, Daniel SE. The nucleus raphe interpositus in the Steele-Richardson-Olszewski syndrome (progressive supranuclear palsy). Brain 1996; 119:1137–1143.
150. Hauw JJ, Verny M, Delaere P, Cervera P, He Y, Duyckaerts C. Constant neurofibrillary changes in the neocortex in progressive supranuclear palsy—basic differences with Alzheimer's disease and aging. Neurosci Lett 119:182–186.
151. Verny M, Duyckaerts C, Agid Y, Hauw JJ. The significance of cortical pathology in progressive supran-

uclear palsy—clinicopathological data in 10 cases. Brain 1996; 119:1123–1136.
152. Schmidt ML, Huang R, Martin JA, Henley J, Mawal-Dewan M, Hurtig HI, Lee VM, Trojanowski JQ. Neurofibrillary tangles in progressive supranuclear palsy contain the same tau epitopes identified in Alzheimer's disease PHFtau. J Neuropathol Exp Neurol 1996; 55:534–539.
153. Bancher C, Lassmann H, Budka H, Grudke-Iqbal I, Iqbal K, Wiche G, Seitelberger F, Wisniewski HM. Neurofibrillary tangles in Alzheimer's disease and progressive supranuclear palsy: antigenic similarities and differences. Microtubule-associated protein tau antigenicity is prominent in all types of tangles. Acta Neuropathol (Berl) 1987; 74:39–46.
154. Yamada T, McGeer PL, McGeer EG. Appearance of paired nucleated, tau-positive glia in patients with progressive supranuclear palsy brain tissue. Neurosci Lett 1992; 135:99–102.
155. Yamada T, Calne DB, Akiyama H, McGeer EG, McGeer PL. Further observations on tau-positive glia in the brains with progressive supranuclear palsy. Acta Neuropathol (Berl) 1993; 85:308–315.
156. Ikeda K, Akiyama H, Haga C, Kondo H, Arima K, Oda T. Argyrophilic thread-like structure in corticobasal degeneration and supranuclear palsy. Neurosci Lett 1994; 174:157–159.
157. Ikeda K, Akiyama H, Kondo H, Haga C, Tanno E, Tokuda T, Ikeda S. Thorn-shaped astrocytes—possibly secondarily induced tau-positive glial fibrillary tangles. Acta Neuropathol (Berl) 1995; 90:620–625.
158. Matsusaka H, Ikeda K, Akiyama H, Arai T, Inoue M, Yagishita S. Astrocytic pathology in progressive supranuclear palsy: significance for neuropathological diagnosis. Acta Neuropathol (Berl) 1998; 96:248–252.
159. Rebeiz JJ, Kolodny EH, Richardson EPJ. Corticodentatonigral degeneration with neuronal achromasia: a progressive disorder of late adult life. Trans Am Neurol Assoc 1967; 92:23–26.
160. Rebeiz JJ, Kolodny EH, Richardson EPJ. Corticodentiatonigral degeneration with neuronal achromasia. Arch Neurol 1968; 18:20–33.
161. Riley DE, Lang AE, Lewis A, Resch L, Ashby P, Hornykiewicz O, Black S. (1990) Cortical-basal ganglionic degeneration. Neurology, 40, 1203–1212.
162. Rinne JO, Lee MS, Thompson PD, Marsden CD. Corticobasal degeneration. A clinical study of 36 cases. Brain 1994 117:1183–1196.
163. Brown J, Lantos PL, Roques P, Fidani L, Rossor MN. Familial dementia with swollen achromatic neurons and corticobasal inclusion bodies: a clinical and pathological study. J Neurol Sci 1996; 135:21–30.
164. Lang AE, Riley DE, Bergeron C. Cortical-basal ganglionic degeneration. In: Calne DB, ed. Neurodegenerative Diseases. Philadelphia: W.B. Saunders, 1994:877–894.
165. Thompson PD, Day BL, Rothwell JC, Brown P, Britton TC, Marsden CD. The myoclonus in corticobasal degeneration. Evidence for two forms of cortical reflex myoclonus. Brain 1994; 117:1197–1207.
166. Thompson PD, Marsden CD. Corticobasal degeneration. In: Rossor MN, ed. Balliere's Clinical Neurology. Unusual Dementias, Vol. 1 (no. 3). London: Balliere Tindall, 1992:677–686.
167. Bergeron C, Pollanen MS, Weyer L, Black SE, Lang AE. Unusual clinical presentations of cortical basal ganglionic degeneration. Ann Neurol 1996; 40:893–900.
168. Bhatia KP, Lee MS, Rinne JO, Revesz T, Scaravilli F, Davies L, Marsden CD. Corticobasal degeneration look-alikes. Adv Neurol 2000; 82:169–82.
169. Revesz T, Daniel SF. Corticobasal degeneration. In: Markesbery WR, Neuropathology of Dementing Disorders. London: Arnold, 1998:257–267.
170. Gibb WR, Luther PJ, Marsden CD. Corticobasal degeneration. Brain 1989; 112(Pt 5):1171–1192.
171. Paulus W, Selim M. Corticonigral degeneration with neuronal achromasia and basal neurofibrillary tangles. Acta Neuropathol (Berl) 1990; 81:89–94.
172. Horoupian DS, Chu PL. Unusual case of corticobasal degeneration with tau/gallyas-positive neuronal and glial tangles. Acta Neuropathal (Berl) 1994; 88:592–598.
173. Wakabayshi K, Oyanagi K, Makifuchi T, Ikuta F, Homma A, Homma Y, et al. Corticobasal degeneration: etiopathological significance of the cytoskeletal alterations. Acta Neuropathol (Berl) 1994; 87:545–553.
174. Dickson DW, Yen SH, Suzuki KI, Davies P, Garcia JH, Hirano A. Ballooned neurons in select neurodegenerative diseases contain phosphorylated neurofilament epitomes. Acta Neuropathol (Berl) 1986; 71:216–223.
175. Lowe J, Errington DR, Lennox G, Pike I, Spendlove I, Landon M, Mayer RJ. Ballooned neurons in several neurodegenerative diseases and stroke contain alpha B crystallin. Neuropathol Appl Neurobiol 1992; 18:341–350.
176. Feany MB, Ksiezakreding H, Liu WK, Vincent I, Yen SHC, Dickson DW. Epitope expression and hyperphosphorylation of tau protein in corticobasal degeneration: differentiation from progressive supranuclear palsy. Acta Neuropathol (Berl) 1995; 90:37–43.
177. Smith TW, Lippa CF, De Girolami U. Immunocytochemical study of ballooned neurons in cortical degeneration with neuronal achromasia. Clin Neuropathol 1992; 11:28–35.
178. Halliday GM, Davies L, McRitchie DA, Cartwright H, Pamphlett R, Morris JGL. Ubiquitin-positive achromatic neurons in corticobasal degeneration. Acta Neuropathol (Berl) 1995; 90:68–75.
179. Feany MB, Dickson DW. Widespread cytoskeletal pathology characterizes corticobasal degeneration. Am J Pathol 1995; 146:1388–1396.
180. Arima K, Uesugi H, Fujita I, Sakurai Y, Oyanagi S, Andoh S, Izumiyama Y, Inose T. Corticonigral degeneration with neuronal achromasia presenting with primary progressive aphasia: ultrastructural and immunocytochemical studies. J Neurol Sci 1994; 127:186–197.
181. Feany MB, Mattiace LA, Dickson DW. Neuropathologic overlap of progressive supranuclear palsy, Pick's disease and corticobasal degeneration. J Neuropathol Exp Neurol 1996; 55:53–67.
182. Ksiezak-Reding H, Morgan K, Mattiace LA, Davies P, Liu WK, Yen SH, Weidenheim K, Dickson DW. Ultrastructure and biochemical composition of paired helical filaments in corticobasal degeneration. Am J Pathol 1994; 145:1496–1508.

183. Mori H, Nishimura M, Namba Y, Oda M. Corticobasal degeneration—a disease with widespread appearance of abnormal tau and neurofibrillary tangles, and its relation to progressive supranuclear palsy. Acta Neuropathol (Berl) 1994; 88:113–121.
184. Bancher C, Jellinger KA. Neurofibullary tangle predominant form of senile dementia of Alzheimer type: a rare subtype in very old subjects. Acta Neuropathol (Berl) 1994; 88:565–570.
185. Revesz T, Geddes JF, Daniel SE. Corticobasal degeneration. In: Ravid R, Cuzner ML, Neuropathological Diagnostic Criteria for Brain Banking. Cruz-Sanchez, Amsterdam: IOS Press, 1995; 99–104.
186. Bergeron C, Davis A, Lang AE. Corticobasal ganglionic degeneration and progressive supranuclear palsy presenting with cognitive decline. Brain Pathol 1998; 8:355–365.
187. Daniel SE, Geddes JF, Revesz T. Clinicopathological overlap between cases of Pick's disease and corticobasal degeneration [abstract]. Brain Pathol 1994; 4:516–516.
188. Jendroska K, Rossor MN, Mathias CJ, Daniel SE. Morphological overlap between corticobasal degeneration and Pick's disease—a clinicopathological report. Mov Disord, 1995; 10:111–114.
189. Cambier J, Masson M, Dairou R, Henin D. A parietal form of Pick's disease: clinical and pathological study [in French] Rev Neurol (Paris) 1981; 137:33–38.
190. Lang AE, Bergeron C, Pollanen MS, Ashby P. Parietal Picks disease mimicking cortical-basal ganglionic degeneration. Neurology 1994; 44:1436–1440.
191. Spillantini MG, Goedert M, Crowther RA, Murrell JR, Farlow MR, Ghetti B. Familial multiple system tauopathy with presenile dementia: a disease with abundant neuronal and glial tau filaments. Proc Natl Acad Sci USA 1997; 94:4113–4118.
192. Mirra SS, Murrell JR, Gearing M, Spillantini MG, Goedert M, Crowther RA, Levey AI, Jones R, Green J, Shoffner JM, Wainer BH, Schmidt ML, Trojanowski JQ, Ghetti B. Tau pathology in a family with dementia and a P301L mutation in tau. J Neuropathol Exp Neurol 1999; 58:335–345.
193. Goedert M, Spillantini MG, Davies SW. Filamentous nerve cell inclusions in neurodegenerative diseases. Curr Opin Neurobiol 1998; 8:619–632.
194. Hanger DP, Brion JP, Gallo JM, Cairns NJ, Luthert PJ, Anderton BH. Tau in Alzheimer's disease and Down's syndrome is insoluble and abnormally phosphorylated. Biochem J 1991; 275:99–104.
195. Goedert M. Tau protein and the neurofibrillary pathology of Alzheimer's disease. Trends Neurosci 1993; 16:460–465.
196. Flament S, Delacourte A, Verny M, Hauw JJ, Javoyagid F. Abnormal tau-proteins in progressive supranuclear palsy—similarities and differences with the neurofibrillary degeneration of the Alzheimer type. Acta Neuropathol (Berl), 1991; 81:591–596.
197. Revesz T, Gibb GM, Anderton BH, Daniel SE. Tau patterns in typical and atypical cases of the Steele-Richardson Olszewski syndrome (SROS). J Neuropathol Exp Neurol 1997; 56:80–80.
198. Sergeant N, Wattez A. Delacourte A. Neurofibrillary degeneration in progressive supranuclear palsy and corticobasal degeneration: tau pathologies with exclusively "exon 10" isoforms. J Neurochem 1999; 72: 1243–1249.
199. Delacourte A, Sergeant N, Wattez A, Gauvreau D, Robitaille Y. Vulnerable neuronal subsets in Alzheimer's and Pick's disease are distinguished by their tau isoform distribution and phosphorylation. Ann Neurol 1998; 43:193–204.
200. Okazaki H, Lipkin LS, Aronson SM. Diffuse intracytoplasmic ganglionic inclusions (Lewy type) associated with progressive dementia and quadriparesis in flexion. J Neuropathol Exp Neurol 1961; 20:237–244.
201. Ince PG, Perry EK, Morris CM. Dementia with Lewy bodies. A distinct non-Alzheimer dementia syndrome? Brain Pathol 1998; 8:299–324.
202. Lennox G, Lowe J. Morrell K, Landon M, Mayer RJ. Anti-ubiquitin immunocytochemistry is more sensitive than conventional techniques in the detection of diffuse Lewy body disease. J Neurol Neurosurg Psychiatry 1989; 52:67–71.
203. Perry RH, Irving D, Blessed G, Fairbairn A, Perry EK. Senile dementia of Lewy body type. A clinically and neuropathologically distinct form of Lewy body dementia in the elderly. J Neurol Sci 1990; 95:119–139.
204. McKeith I, Fairbairn A, Perry R, Thompson P, Perry E. Neuroleptic sensitivity in patients with senile dementia of Lewy body type [see comments]. BMJ 1992; 305:673–678.
205. Khachaturian ZS. Diagnosis of Alzheimers disease. Arch Neurol, 1985; 42:1097–1104.
206. Dickson DW, Davies P, Mayeux R, Crystal H, Horoupian DS, Thompson A, Goldman JE. Diffuse Lewy body disease. Neuropathological and biochemical studies of six patients. Acta Neuropathol (Berl) 1987; 75:8–15.
207. Wakabayashi K, Hansen LA, Masliah E. Cortical Lewy body–containing neurons are pyramidal cells: laser confocal imaging of double-immunolabeled sections with anti-ubiquitin and SMI32. Acta Neuropathol (Berl) 1995; 89:404–408.
208. Hansen LA, Masliah E, Terry RD, Mirra SS. A neuropathological subset of Alzheimer's disease with concomitant Lewy body disease and spongiform change. Acta Neuropathol (Berl), 1989; 78:194–201.
209. Lennox GG, Lowe JS. Dementia with Lewy bodies. In: Neuropathology of Dementing Disorders. Markesbery WR, ed. London: Arnold, 1998; 181–192.
210. Pollanen MS, Dickson DW, Bergeron C. Pathology and biology of the Lewy body. J Neuropathol Exp Neurol, 1993; 52:183–191.
211. Love S, Nicoll JA. Comparison of modified Bielschowsky silver impregnation and anti-ubiquitin immunostaining of cortical and nigral Lewy bodies. Neuropathol Appl Neurobiol 1992; 18:585–592.
212. Hansen LA, Masliah E, Terry RD, Mirra SS. A neuropathological subset of Alzheimer's disease with concomitant Lewy body disease and spongiform change. Acta Neuropathol (Berl) 1989; 78:194–201.
213. Hansen L, Salmon D, Galasko D, Masliah E, Katzman R, Deteresa R, Thal L, Pay MM, Hofstetter R, Klauber M, Rice V, Butters N, Alford M. The Lewy body variant of Alzheimer's disease: a clinical and pathologic entity [see comments]. Neurology 1990; 40:1–8.

214. Lantos PL, Ovenstone IM, Johnson J, Clelland CA, Roques P, Rossor MN. Lewy bodies in the brain of two members of a family with the 717 (Val to Ile) mutation of the amyloid precursor protein gene. Neurosci Lett 1994; 172:77–79.
215. Revesz T, McLaughlin JL, Rossor MN, Lantos PI. Pathology of familial Alzheimer's disease with Lewy bodies. J Neural Transm Suppl 1997; 51:121–135.
216. Lippa CF, Fujiwara H, Mann DMA, Giasson B, Baba M, Schmidt ML, Nee LE, O'Connell B, Pollen DA, St George-Hyslop P, Ghetti B, Nochlin D, Bird TD, Cairns NJ, Lee VM, Iwatsubo T, Trojanowski JQ. Lewy bodies contain altered alpha-synuclein in brains of many familiar Alzheimer's disease patients with mutations in presenilin and amyloid precursor protein genes. Am J Pathol 1998; 153:1365–1370.
217. Lippa CF, Schmidt ML, Lee VM, Trojanowski JQ. Antibodies to alpha-synuclein detect Lewy bodies in many Down's syndrome brains with Alzheimer's disease. Ann Neurol, 1999; 45:353–357.
218. Ueda K, Fukushima H, Masliah E, Xia Y, Iwai A, Yoshimoto M, et al. Otero DA, Kondo J, Ihara Y, Saitoh T. Molecular cloning of cDNA encoding an unrecognized component of amyloid in Alzheimer disease. Proc Natl Acad Sci USA 1993; 90:11282–11286.
219. McKeith IG, Galasko D, Kosaka K, Perry EK, Dickson DW, Hansen LA, Salmon DP, Lowe J, Mirra SS, Byrne EJ, Lennox G, Quinn NP, Edwardson JA, Ince PG, Bergeron C, Burns A, Miller BL, Lovestone S, Collerton D, Jansen EN, Ballard C, de Vos RA, Wilcock GK, Jellinger KA, Perry RH. Consensus guidelines for the clinical and pathologic diagnosis of dementia with Lewy bodies (DLB): report of the consortium on DLB international workshop. Neurology 1996; 47:1113–1124.
220. Knopman DS, Mastri AR, Frey WH, Sung JH, Rustan T. Dementia lacking distinctive histologic features: a common non-Alzheimer degenerative dementia. Neurology 1990; 40:251–256.
221. Giannakopoulos P, Hof PR, Bouras C. Dementia lacking distinctive histopathology: clinicopathological evaluation of 32 cases. Acta Neuropathol (Berl) 1995; 89:346–355.
222. Snowden JS, Neary D, Mann DMA, Fronto-Temporal Dementia, Progressive Aphasia, Sementic Dementia. Edinburgh: Churchill Livingstone, 1996.
223. Brun A. Frontal-lobe degeneration of non-Alzheimer type. 1. Neuropathology. Arch Gerontol Geriatr 1987; 6:193–208.
224. Brun A, Englund B, Gustafson L, Passant U, Mann DMA, Neary D, Snowden JS. Clinical and neuropathological criteria for frontotemporal dementia. J Neurol Neurosurg Psychiatry 1999; 57:416–418.
225. Neary D, Snowden JS, Gustafson L, Passant U, Stuss D, Black S, Freedman M, Kertesz A, Robert PH, Albert M, Boone K, Miller BL, Cummings J, Benson DF. Frontotemporal lobar degeneration—a consensus on clinical diagnostic criteria. Neurology 1998; 51:1546–1554.
226. Cooper PN, Jackson M, Lennox G, Lowe J, Mann DMA. Tau, ubiquitin, and alpha B-crystallin immunohistochemistry define the principal causes of degenerative frontotemporal dementia. Arch Neurol 1995; 52:1011–1015.
227. Jackson M, Lowe J. The new neuropathology of degenerative frontotemporal dementias. Acta Neuropathol (Berl) 1996; 91:127–134.
228. Mann DMA, South PW, Snowden JS, Neary D. Dementia of frontallobe type—neuropathology and immunohistochemistry. J Neurol Neurosurg Psychiatry 1993; 56:605–614.
229. Mann DMA. Dementia of frontal type and dementias with subcortical gliosis. Brain Pathol 1998; 8:325–338.
230. Foster NL, Wilhelmsen K, Sima AAF, Jones MZ, Damato CJ, Gilman S. Frontotemporal dementia and parkinsonism linked to chromosome 17: a consensus conference. Ann Neurol 1997; 41:706–715.
231. Spillantini MG, Bird TD, Ghetti B. Frontotemporal dementia and parkinsonism linked to chromosome 17: a new group of tauopathies. Brain Pathol 1998; 8:387–402.
232. Poorkaj P, Bird TD, Wijsman E, Nemens E, Garruto RM, Anderson L, Andreadis A, Wiederholt WC, Raskind M, Schellenberg GD. Tau is a candidate gene for chromosome 17 frontotemporal dementia. Ann Neurol 1998; 43:815–825.
233. Lynch T, Sano M, Marder KS, Bell KL, Foster NL, Defendini RF, Sima AAF, Keohane C, Nygaard TG, Fahn S, Mayeux R, Rowland LP, Wilhelmsen KC. Clinical characteristics of a family with chromosome 17–linked disinhibition-dementia-parkinsonism-amyotrophy complex [see comments]. Neurology 1994; 44:1878–1884.
234. Wszolek ZK, Pfeiffer RF, Bhatt MH, Schelper RL, Cordes M, Snow BJ, Rodnitzky RL, Wolters EC, Arwert F, Calne DB. Rapidly progressive autosomal dominant parkinsonism and dementia with pallido-ponto-nigral degeneration. Ann Neurol 1992; 32:312–320.
235. Knopman DS. Overview of dementia lacking distinctive histology: pathological designation of a progressive dementia. Dementia 1993; 4:132–136.
236. Lanska DJ, Currier RD, Cohen M, Gambetti P, Smith EE, Bebin J, Jackson JF, Whitehouse PJ, Markesbery WR. Familial progressive subcortical gliosis. Neurology 1994; 44:1633–1643.
237. Sima AA, Defendini R, Keohane C, D'amato C, Foster NL, Parchi P, Gambetti P, Lynch T, Wilhelmsen KC. The neuropathology of chromosome 17–linked dementia. Ann Neurol, 1996; 39:734–743.
238. Spillantini MG, Crowther RA, Kamphorst W, Heutink P, Van Swieten JC. Tau pathology in two Dutch families with mutations in the microtubule-binding region of tau. Am J Pathol 1998; 153:1359–1363.
239. Petersen RB, Tabaton M, Chen SG, Monari L, Richardson SL, Lynch T, Manetto V, Lanska DJ, Markesbery WR, Currier RD, Autiliogambetti L, Wilhelmsen KC, Gambetti P. Familial progressive subcortical gliosis: presence of prions and linkage to chromosome 17 [published erratum appears in Neurology 1995; 45(7):1430]. Neurology 1995; 45:1062–1067.
240. Sumi SM, Bird TD, Nochlin D, Raskind MA. Familial presenile dementia with psychosis associated with cortical neurofibrillary tangles and degeneration of the amygdala. Neurology 1992; 42:120–127.
241. Hutton M, Lendon CL, Rizzu P, Baker M, Froelich S, Houlden H, Pickering-Brown S, Chakraverty S, Isaacs A, Grover A, Hackett J, Adamson J, Lincoln S, Dickson D, Davies P, Petersen RC, Stevens M,

241. de Graaff E, Wauters E, van Baren J, Hillebrand M, Joosse M, Kwon JM, Nowotny P, Che LK, Norton J, Morris JC, Reed LA, Trojanowski J, Basun H, Lannfelt L, Neystat M, Fahn S, Dark F, Tannenberg T, Dodd PR, Hayward N, Kwok JBJ, Schofield PR, Andreadis A, Snowden J, Craufurd D, Neary D, Owen F, Oostra BA, Hardy J, Goate A, van Swieten J, Mann D, Lynch T, Heutink P. Association of missense and 5'-splice-site mutations in tau with the inherited dementia FTDP-17. Nature 1998; 393:702–705.
242. Clark LN, Poorkaj P, Wszolek Z, Geschwind DH, Nasreddine ZS, Miller B, Li D, Payami H, Awert F, Markopoulou K, Andreadis A, D'Souza I, Lee VM, Reed L, Trojanowski JQ, Zhukareva V, Bird T, Schellenberg G, Wilhelmsen KC. Pathogenic implications of mutations in the tau gene in pallido-pontonigral degeneration and related neurodegenerative disorders linked to chromosome 17. Proc Natl Acad Sci USA 1998; 95:13103–13107.
243. Spillantini MG, Murrell JR, Goedert M, Farlow MR, Klug A, Ghetti B. Mutation in the tau gene in familial multiple system tauopathy with presenile dementia. Proc Natl Acad Sci USA 1998; 95:7737–7741.
244. Spillantini MG, Goedert M. Tau protein pathology in neurodegenerative diseases. Trends Neurosci 1998; 21:428–433.
245. Rizzu P, Van Swieten JC, Joosse M, Hasegawa M, Stevens M, Tibben A, Niermeijer MF, Hillebrand M, Ravid R, Oostra BA, Goedert M, van Duijn CM, Heutink P. High prevalence of mutations in the microtubule-associated protein tau in a population study of frontotemporal dementia in The Netherlands. Am J Hum Genet 1999; 64:414–421.
246. Houlden H, Baker M, Adamson J, Grover A, Waring S, Dickson D, Lynch T, Boeve B, Petersen RC, Pickering-Brown S, Owen F, Neary D, Craufurd D, Snowden J, Mann D, Hutton M. Frequency of tau mutations in three series of non-Alzheimer's degenerative dementia. Ann Neurol 1999; 46:243–248.
247. Lopez OL, Becker JT, Dekosky ST Dementia accompanying motor neuron disease. Dementia 1994; 5:42–47.
248. Okamoto K, Hirai S, Yamazaki T, Sun XY, Nakazato Y. New ubiquitin-positive intraneuronal inclusions in the extra-motor cortices in patients with amyotrophic lateral sclerosis. Neurosci Lett 1991; 129:233–236.
249. Wightman G, Anderson VE, Martin J, Swash M, Anderton BH, Neary D, Mann D, Luthert P, Leigh PN. Hippocampal and neocortical ubiquitin-immunoreactive inclusions in amyotrophic lateral sclerosis with dementia. Neurosci Lett 1992; 139:269–274.
250. Kew J, Leigh PN. Unusual forms of dementia. In: Burns A, Levy R, eds. Dementia London: Chapman and Hall, 1994; 789–811.
251. Jackson M, Lennox G, Lowe J. Motor neurone disease–inclusion dementia. Neurodegeneration 1996; 5:339–350.
252. Holton JL, Revesz T, Crooks R, Scaravilli F. Motor neuron disease–inclusion dementia: evidence for pathological involvement of the spinal cord [abstract]. Neuropathol Appl Neurobiol 1999; 25:164.
253. Rossor MN, Revesz T, Lantos PL, Warrington E. Semantic dementia with tau negative ubiquitin positive inclusion bodies. Brain 2000; 123:267–276.
254. Hirano A, Kurland LT, Krooth RS, Lessell S. Parkinsonism–dementia complex, an endemic disease of the island of Guam. I. Clinical features. Brain 1961; 84:642–661.
255. Garruto RM, Yanagihara RT, Gajdusek DC. Disappearance of high-incidence amyotrophic lateral sclerosis and parkinsonism–dementia on Guam. Neurology 1985; 35:193–198.
256. Shiraki H, Yase Y. Amyotrophic lateral sclerosis in Japan. In: Vinken PJ, Bruyn GW, eds. Handbook of Clinical Neurology, Vol. 22. New York: Elsevier, 1975; 353–419.
257. Gajdusek DC, Salazar AM. Amyotrophic lateral sclerosis and parkinsonism syndromes in high incidence among the Auyu and Jakai people in West New Guinea. Neurology 1980; 32:107–126.
258. Hirano A, Malamud N, Kurland LT. Parkinsonism–dementia complex, an endemic disease of the island of Guam. II. Pathological features. Brain 1961; 84:662–679.
259. Hirano A, Arumugasamy N, Zimmerman HM. Amyotrophic lateral sclerosis: a comparison of Guam and classical cases. Arch Neurol 1967; 16:357–363.
260. Malamud N, Hirano A, Kurland LT. Pathoanatomic changes in amyotrophic lateral sclerosis on Guam. Neurology 1961; 5:401–414.
261. Hirano A, Dembitzer HM, Kurland LT. The fine structure of some intraganglionic alterations: neurofibrillary tangles, granulovacuolar bodies and "rod-like" structures as seen in Guam amyotrophic lateral sclerosis and parkinsonism–dementia complex. J Neuropathol Exp Neurol 1968; 27:167–182.
262. Garruto RM, Gajdusek DC, Chen KM. Amyotrophic lateral sclerosis and parkinsonism–dementia among Filipino migrants to Guam. Ann Neurol 1981; 10:341–350.
263. Yanagihara RT, Garruto RM, Gajdusek DC. Epidemiological surveillance of amyotrophic lateral sclerosis and parkinsonism–dementia in the Commonwealth of the Northern Mariana Islands. Ann Neurol 1983; 13:79–86.
264. Laspada AR, Wilson EM, Lubahn DB, Harding AE, Fischbeck KH. Androgen receptor gene mutations in X-linked spinal and bulbar muscular atrophy. Nature 1991; 352:77–79.
265. Ashizawa T, Dubel JR, Dunne PW, Dunne CJ, Fu YH, Pizzuti A, Caskey CT, Boerwinkle E, Perryman MB, Epstein HF, Hejtmancik JF. Anticipation in myotonic dystrophy. II. Complex relationships between clinical findings and structure of the GCT repeat. Neurology 1992; 42:1877–1883.
266. Koshy BT, Zoghbi HY. The CAG/polyglutamine tract diseases: gene products and molecular pathogenesis. Brain Pathol 1997; 7:927–942.
267. Berciano J. Olivopontocerebellar atrophy. A review of 117 cases. J Neurol Sci 1982; 53:253–272.
268. Harding AE. The clinical features and classification of the late onset autosomal dominant cerebellar ataxias. A study of 11 families, including descendants of the the Drew family of Walworth. Brain 1982; 105:1–28.
269. Subramony SH, Currier RD. The classification of familial ataxias. In: de Jong. JMBV, ed. Hereditary

270. Schut JW. Hereditary ataxia: clinical study through six generations. Arch Neurol Psychiatr 1950; 63:535–568.
271. Zoghbi HY, Pollack MS, Lyons LA, Ferrell RE, Daiger SP, Beaudet AI. Spinocerebellar ataxia—variable age of onset and linkage to human-leukocyte antigen in a large kindred. Ann Neurol 1988; 23:580–584.
272. Robitaille Y, Schut L, Kish SJ. Structural and immunocytochemical features of olivopontocerebellar atrophy caused by the spinocerebellar ataxia type-1 (SCA-1) mutation define a unique phenotype. Acta Neuropathol (Berl) 1995; 90:572–581.
273. Gilman S, Sima AA, Junck L, Kluin KJ, Koeppe RA, Lohman ME, Little R. Spinocerebellar ataxia type 1 with multiple system degeneration and glial cytoplasmic inclusions. Ann Neurol 1996; 39:241–255.
274. Robitaille Y, Lopescendes I, Becher M, Rouleau G, Clark AW. The neuropathology of CAG repeat diseases: review and update of genetic and molecular features. Brain Pathol 1997; 7:901–926.
275. Orr HT, Chung MY, Banfi S, Kwiatkowski TJ, Servadio A, Beaudet AL, McCall AE, Duvick LA, Ranum LP, Zaghbitty. Expansion of an unstable trinucleotide CAG repeat in spinocerebellar ataxia type-1. Nat Genet 1993; 4:221–226.
276. Ranum LPW, Lundgren JK, Schut LJ, Ahrens MJ, Perlman S, Aita J, Binol TD, Gomez C, Ozz HT. Spinocerebellar ataxia type-I and Machado-Joseph disease—incidence of CAG expansions among adult-onset ataxia patients from 311 families with dominant, recessive, or sporadic ataxia. Am J Hum Genet 1995; 57:603–608.
277. Servadio A, Koshy B, Armstrong D, Antalffy B, Orr HT, Zoghbi HY. Expression analysis of the ataxin-1 protein in tissues from normal and spinocerebellar ataxia type-1 individuals. Nat Genet 1995; 10:94–98.
278. Paulson HL, Das SS, Crino PB, Perez MK, Patel SC, Gotsdiner D, Fischbeck KH, Pittman RN. Machado-Joseph disease gene product is a cytoplasmic protein widely expressed in brain. Ann Neurol 1997; 41:453–462.
279. Paulson HL, Perez MK, Trottier Y, Trojanowski JQ, Subramony SH, Das SS, vif P, Mendel J-L, Fischbeck KH, Pittman RN. Intranuclear inclusions of expanded polyglutamine protein in spinocerebellar ataxia type 3. Neuron 1997; 19:333–344.
280. Orozco G, Estrada R, Perry TL, Arana J, Fernandez R, Gonzalez Quevedo A, Galariaga J, Hansen S. Dominantly inherited olivopontocerebellar atrophy from eastern Cuba—clinical, neuropathological, and biochemical findings. J Neurol Sci 1989; 93:37–50.
281. Ihara T, Sasaki H, Wakisaka A, Takada A, Yoshiki T, Matsuura T, Hamada T, Sujuki Y, Tashizok. Genetic heterogeneity of dominantly inherited olivopontocerebellar atrophy (OPCA) in the Japanese: linkage study of two pedigrees and evidence for the disease locus on chromosome 12q (SCA2). Jpn J Hum Genet 1994; 39:305–313.
282. Durr A, Smadja D, Cancel G, Lezin A, Stevanin G, Mikol J, Bellance R, Buisson GG, Bellance R, Chnaiweiss H, Agid V, Brice A. Autosomal dominant cerebellar ataxia type I in Martinique (French West Indies). Clinical and neuropathological analysis of 53 patients from three unrelated SCA2 families. Brain 1995; 118(Pt 6):1573–1581.
283. Lezin A, Cancel G, Stevanin G, Smadja D, Vernant JC, Durr A, Martial J, Buisson GG, Bellance R, Chnaiweiss H, Agid Y, Brice A. Autosomal dominant cerebellar ataxia type I in Martinique (French West Indies): genetic analysis of three unrelated SCA2 families. Hum Genet 1996; 97:671–676.
284. Cancel G, Durr A, Didierjean O, Imbert G, Burk K, Lezin A, Belal J, Benomar A, Abada Bendibm, Viale, Guimaraes, Chnaiweiss H, Stevanin G, Yvert G, Abbag N, Saudow F, Lobre AS, Yahyaui M, Hentauti F, Verubauty C, Klockfether T, Maudely C, Agiol Y, Brice A. Molecular and clinical correlations in spinocerebellar ataxia 2: a study of 32 families. Hum Mol Genet 1997; 6:709–715.
285. Pulst SM, Nechiporuk A, Nechiporuk T, Gispert S, Chen XN, Lopescendes I, Pearlman S, Starkman S, Orozco-Diaz G, Lunkes A, DeJony P, Rouleau GA, Auburger G, Korenberg JR, Figuersa C, Sohba S. Moderate expansion of a normally biallelic trinucleotide repeat in spinocerebellar ataxia type 2. Nat Genet 1996; 14:269–276.
286. Nechiporuk A, Lopescendes I, Nechiporuk T, Starkman S, Andermann E, Rouleau GA, Weissenback JS, Kort E, Pulst SM. Genetic mapping of the spinocerebellar ataxia type 2 gene on human chromosome 12. Neurology 1996; 46:1731–1735.
287. Trottier Y, Lutz Y, Stevanin G, Imbert G, Devys D, Cancel G, Saudon F, Weber C, David G, Fora L. et al. Polyglutamine expansion as a pathological epitope in Huntington's disease and four dominant cerebellar ataxias. Nature 1995; 378:403–406.
288. Coutinho P, Andrade C. Autosomal dominant system degeneration in Portuguese families of the Azores Islands. A new genetic disorder involving cerebellar, pyramidal, extrapyramidal and spinal cord motor functions. Neurology 1978; 28:703–709.
289. Lima L, Coutinho P. Clinical criteria for diagnosis of Machado-Joseph disease: report of a non-Azorean Portuguese family. Neurology 1980; 30:319–322.
290. Nakano KK, Dawson DM, Spence A. Machado disease. A hereditary ataxia in Portuguese emigrants to Massachusetts. Neurology 1972; 22:49–55.
291. Woods BT, Schaumburg HH. Nigro-spino-dentatal degeneration with nuclear ophthalmopleagia. A unique and partially treatable clinico-pathological entity. J Neurol Sci 1972; 17:149–166.
292. Coutinho P, Guimaraes A, Scaravilli F. The pathology of Machado-Joseph disease. Report of a possible homozygous case. Acta Neuropathol (Berl) 1982; 58:48–54.
293. ST George-Hyslop P, Rogaeva E, Huterer J, Tsuda T, Santos J, Haines JL, Schlumpf K, Rofaev E, Liangy, McLachlan DR. Machado-Joseph disease in pedigrees of Azorean descent is linked to chromosome 14. Am J Hum Genet 1994; 55:120–125.
294. Takiyama Y, Nishizawa M, Tanaka H, Kawashima S, Sakamoto H, Karube Y, Shimakazi H, Soutorne M, Eudo K, Onta S, et al. The gene for Machado-Joseph disease maps to human chromosome 14q. Nat Genet 1993; 4:300–304.
295. Durr A, Stevanin G, Cancel G, Duyckaerts C, Abbas N, Didierjean O, Chnaweiss H, Benomar A, Lyon-Cain O, Sulien J, Serdaru M, Penete, Afid Y, Brice A. Spinocerebellar ataxia 3 and Machado-Joseph dis-

295. ease: clinical, molecular, and neuropathological features. Ann Neurol 1996; 39:490–499.
296. Subramony SH, Fratkin JD, Manyam BV, Currier RD. Dominantly inherited cerebello-olivary atrophy is not due to a mutation at the spinocerebellar ataxia-I, Machado-Joseph disease, or dentato-rubro-pallido-luysian atrophy locus. Mov Disord, 1996; 11: 174–180.
297. Diriong S, Lory P, Williams ME, Ellis SB, Harpold MM, Taviaux S. Chromosomal localization of the human genes for alpha 1A, alpha 1B, and alpha 1E voltage-dependent Ca^{2+} channel subunits. Genomics 1995; 30:605–609.
298. Zhuchenko O, Bailey J, Bonnen P, Ashizawa T, Stockton DW, Amos C, Dobyns, Subramony SH, Zoghbi HY, Lee CC Autosomal dominant cerebellar ataxia (SCA6) associated with small polyglutamine expansions in the alpha 1A-voltage-dependent calcium channel. Nat Genet 1997; 15:62–69.
299. Benton CS, De Silva R, Rutledge SL, Bohlega S, Ashizawa T, Zoghbi HY. Molecular and clinical studies in SCA-7 define a broad clinical spectrum and the infantile phenotype. Neurology 1998; 51:1081–1086.
300. Holmberg M, Duyckaerts C, Durr A, Cancel G, Gourfinkel-An I, Damier P, Faucheux B, Trottier Y, Hizsch EC, Agiol Y, Brice A. Spinocerebellar ataxia type 7 (SCA7): a neurodegenerative disorder with neuronal intranuclear inclusions. Hum Mol Genet, 1998; 7:913–918.
301. David G, Giunti P, Abbas N, Coullin P, Stevanin G, Horta W, Gemmill R, Weissenbach J, Wood N, Cunhas S, Drabkin H, Harding AE, Agiol Y, Brice A. The gene for autosomal dominant cerebellar ataxia type II is located in a 5-cM region in 3p12-p13: genetic and physical mapping of the SCA7 locus. Am J Hum Genet 1996; 59:1328–1336.
302. Gouw LG, Digre KB, Harris CP, Haines JH, Ptacek LJ. Autosomal dominant cerebellar ataxia with retinal degeneration: clinical, neuropathologic, and genetic analysis of a large kindred. Neurology 1994; 44: 1441–1447.
303. Stevanin G, Giunti P, Belal S, Durr A, Ruberg M, Wood N, Brice A. De novo expansion of intermediate alleles in spinocerebellar ataxia 7. Hum Mol Genet 1998; 7:1809–1813.
304. Grewal RP, Tayag E, Figueroa KP, Zu L, Durazo A, Nunez C, Pulst SM. Clinical and genetic analysis of a distinct autosomal dominant spinocerebellar ataxia. Neurology 1998; 51:1423–1426.
305. Ranum LPW, Schut LJ, Lundgren JK, Orr HT, Livingston DM. Spinocerebellar ataxia type-5 in a family descended from the grandparents of President Lincoln maps to chromosome 11. Nat Genet 1994; 8:280–284.
306. Koeppen AH. The hereditary ataxias. J Neuropathol Exp Neurol 1998; 57:531–543.
307. Koskinen T, Santavuori P, Sainio K, Lappi M, Kallio AK, Pihko H Infantile onset spinocerebellar ataxia with sensory neuropathy: a new inherited disease. J Neurol Sci 1994; 121:50–56.
308. Nikali K, Isosomppi J, Lonnqvist T, Mao JI, Suomalainen A, Peltonen L. Toward cloning of a novel ataxia gene: refined assignment and physical map of the IOSCA locus (SCA8) on 10q24. Genomics 1997; 39:185–191.
309. Ross CA. Intranuclear neuronal inclusions: a common pathogenic mechanism for glutamine-repeat neurodegenerative diseaes? Neuron 1997; 19:1147–1150.
310. Difiglia M, Sapp E, Chase KO, Davies SW, Bates GP, Vonsattel JP, Azonin N. Aggregation of huntingtin in neuronal intranuclear inclusions and dystrophic neurites in brain. Science 1997; 277:1990–1993.
311. Becher MW, Kotzuk JA, Sharp AH, Davies SW, Bates GP, Price DL, Ross CA. Intranuclear neuronal inclusions in Huntington's disease and dentatorubral and pallidoluysian atrophy: correlation between the density of inclusions and IT15 CAG triplet repeat length. Neurobiol Dis 1998; 4:387–397.
312. Skinner PJ, Koshy BT, Cummings CJ, Klement IA, Helin K Servadio A, Zoghbi HV, Ozz HT. Ataxin-1 with an expanded glutamine tract alters nuclear matrix–associated structures [published erratum appears in Nature 1998; 391 (6664):307]. Nature 1997; 389:971–974.
313. Davies SW, Turmaine M, Cozens BA, Difiglia M, Sharp AH, Ross CA, Scherzinger E, Wanker EE, Mangiarini L., Bates GP. Formation of neuronal intranuclear inclusions underlies the neurological dysfunction in mice transgenic for the HD mutation. Cell 1997; 90:537–548.
314. Goldberg YP, Nicholson DW, Rasper DM, Kalchman MA, Koide HB, Graham RK, Bromm U, Kazemi-Esfarjarm P, Thornberry NA, Vaillancourt JP, Hayden MR. Cleavage of huntingtin by apopain, a proapoptotic cysteine protease, is modulated by the polyglutamine tract [see comments]. Nat Genet 1996; 13:442–449.
315. Sung JH, Ramirez-Lassepas M, Mastri AR, Larkin SM. An unusual degenerative disorder of neurons associated with a novel intranuclear hyaline inclusion (neuronal intranuclear hyaline inclusion disease). A clinicopathological study of a case. J Neuropathol Exp Neurol 1980; 39:107–130.
316. Haltia M, Somer H, Palo J, Johnson WG. Neuronal intranuclear inclusion disease in identical twins. Ann Neurol 1984; 15:316–321.
317. Kimber TE, Blumbergs PC, Rice JP, Hallpike JF, Edis R, Thompson PD, Suthers G. Familial neuronal intranuclear inclusion disease with ubiquitin positive inclusions. J Neurol Sci 1998; 160:33–40.
318. Schuffler MD, Bird TD, Sumi SM, Cook A. A familial neuronal disease presenting as intestinal pseudoobstruction. Gastroenterology 1978; 75:889–898.
319. Janota I. Widespread intranuclear neuronal corpuscles (Marinesco bodies) associated with a familial spinal degeneration with cranial and peripheral nerve involvement. Neuropathol Appl Neurobiol 1979; 5:311–317.
320. Munoz-Garcia D, Ludwin SK. Adult-onset neuronal intranuclear hyaline inclusion disease. Neurology 1986; 36:785–790.
321. Weidenheim KM, Dickson DW. Intranuclear inclusion-bodies in an elderly demented woman—a form of intranuclear inclusion-body disease. Clin Neuropathol 1995; 14:93–99.
322. Lieberman AP, Robitaille Y, Trojanowski JQ, Dickson DW, Fischbeck KH. Polyglutamine-containing aggregates in neuronal intranuclear inclusion disease. Lancet 1998; 351:884.

323. Jellinger K. Neuropathologic finds after neuroleptic long-term therapy. In: Shiraki H, Grcevic N, eds. Neurotoxicology. New York: Raven Press, 1977:25–42.
324. Rajput AH, Rozdilsky B, Hornykiewicz O, Shannak K, Lee T, Seeman P. Reversible drug-induced parkinsonism. Clinicopathologic study of two cases. Arch Neurol 1982; 39:644–646.
325. Langston JW, Ballard P, Tetrud JW, Irwin I. Chronic Parkinsonism in humans due to a product of meperidine-analog synthesis. Science 1983; 219:979–980.
326. Forno LS, Langston JW, Delanney LE, Irwin I, Ricaurte GA. Locus ceruleus lesions and eosinophilic inclusions in MPTP-treated monkeys. 1986; Ann Neurol 1986; 20:449–455.
327. Von Economo C. Encephalitis Lethargica. Its Sequelae and Treatment. Oxford: Oxford University Press, 1931.
328. Howard RS, Lees AJ. Encephalitis lethargica. A report of four recent cases. Brain, 1987; 110(Pt 1):19–33.
329. Elizan TS, Casals J, Swash M. No viral antigens detected in brain tissue from a case of acute encephalitis lethargica and another case of post-encephalitic parkinsonism [letter]. J Neurol Neurosurg Psychiatry 1989; 52:800–801.
330. Duvoisin RC, Yahr MD. Encephalitis and parkinsonism. Arch Neurol 1965; 12:227–239.
331. Litvan I, Jankovic J, Goetz CG, Wenning GK, Sastry N, Jellinger K, McKee A, Lai EC, Brandel JP, Verny M, Ray-Chaudhuri K, Pearce RK, Bartko JJ, Agid Y. Accuracy of the clinical diagnosis of postencephalitic parkinsonism: a clinicopathologic study. Eur J Neurol 1998; 5:451–457.
332. Torvik A, Meen D. Distribution of the brain stem lesions in postencephalitic parkinsonism. Acta Neurol Scand 1966; 42:415–425.
333. Ishii T, Nakamura Y. Distribution and ultrastructure of Alzheimer's neurofibrillary tangles in postencephalitic parkinsonism of Economo type. Acta Neuropathol (Berl) 1981; 55:59–62.
334. Martin JP. The globus pallidus in postencephalitic parkinsonism. J Neurol Sci 1965; 3:566–576.
335. Wisniewski H, Terry RD, Hirano A. Neurofibrillary pathology. J Neuropathol Exp Neurol 1970; 29:163–176.
336. Ikeda K, Akiyama H, Kondo H. Anti-tau-positive glial fibrillary tangles in the brain of postencephalitic parkinsonism of Economo type. Neurosci Lett 1993; 162:176–178.
337. Geddes JF, Hughes AJ, Daniel SE. Pathological overlap in cases of parkinsonism associated with neurofibrillary tangles. A study of recent cases of postencephalitic parkinsonism and comparison with progressive supranuclear palsy and guamanian parkinsonism–dementia complex. Brain 1993; 116:281–302.
338. Lennox G, Lowe J, Morrell K, Landon M, Mayer RJ. Ubiquitin is a component of neurofibrillary tangles in a variety of neurodegenerative diseases. Neurosci Lett, 94:211–217.
339. Bussiere T, Hof PR, Mailliot C, Brown CD, Caillet Boudin ML, Perl DP, Perl DP, Buee L, Delacourte A. Phosphorylated serine 22 on tau proteins is a pathological epitope found in several diseases with neurofibrillary degeneration. Acta Neuropathol (Berl) 1999; 97:221–230.
340. Buee-Scherrer V, Buee L, Leveugle B, Perl DP, Vermersch P, Hof PR, et al. Pathological tau proteins in postencephalitic parkinsonism: comparison with Alzheimer's disease and other neurodegenerative disorders. Ann Neurol 1997; 42:356–359.
341. Van Rossum A. Spastic pseudosclerosis (Creutzfeldt-Jakob disease). In: Vinken PJ, Bruyn GW, (eds, Handbook of Clinical Neurology, Vol. 6, Disease of the Basal Ganglia. Amsterdam: North Holland, 1968:726–760.
342. Revesz T, Daniel SE, Lees AJ, Will RG. A case of progressive subcortical gliosis associated with deposition of abnormal prion protein (PrP). J Neurol Neurosurg Psychiatry, 1995; 58:759–760.
343. Desoille H. Les troubles nerveux dus aux asphyxies aiguës (et plus particulierement a l'asphyxie oxycarbonée). Thése Medecine, University of Paris. Paris: le François, 1932.
344. Lapresle J, Fardeau M. The central nervous system and carbon monoxide poisoning. II. Anatomical study of brain lesions following intoxication with carbon monixide (22 cases). Prog Brain Res 1967; 24 31–74.
345. Edsall DL, Drinker CT. The Clinical Aspect of Chronic Manganese Poisioning. Contribution to Medical and Biological Research. Dedicated to Sir William Osler. New York: Paul B. Hoeber, 1919.
346. Stadler H. Zur Histopathologie des Gehirns bei Manganvergiftung. Z Ges Neurol Psychiatr 1935; 154:62–76.
347. Parnitzke KH, Pfeiffer J. Zur Klinik und pathologischen Anatomie der chronischen Braunsteinvergiftung. Arch Psychiatr Nervenheilkd 192: 1954; 192:405–429.
348. Canavan MM, Cobb S, Drinker CK. Chronic manganese poisoning. Report of a case with autopsy Arch Neurol Psychiatr (Chic) 1934; 32:501–512.
349. Pentschew A, Ebner FF, Kovatch RM. Experimental manganese encephalopathy in monkeys. J Jeuropathol Exp Neurol 1963; 22:488–499.
350. Souques A. Les syndromes parkinsoniens. Rev Neurol (Paris) 1921; 1:534–576.
351. Alvord EC Jr. An interpretation with special reference to other changes in the aging brain. In: McDowell, R, Markham M eds. The Pathology of Parkinsonism. Philadelphia: F.A. Davis, 1971:125–137.
352. Eadie MJ, Sutherland JM. Arteriosclerosis in parkinsonism. J Neurol Neurosurg Psychiatry 1964; 27:237–240.
353. Schwab RS, England AC. Parkinson syndromes due to various specific causes. In: Vinken PJ, Bruyn GW, eds. Handbook in Clinical Neurology. Vol. 6, Diseases of the Basal Ganglia. Amsterdam: North Holland, 1968:227–247.
354. Fenelon G, Houeto JL. Les syndromes parkinsoniens vasculaires: un concept controverse. Rev Neurol (Paris) 1998; 154:291–302.
355. Hunter R, Smith J, Thomson T, Dayan AD. Hemiparkinsonism with infarction of the ipsilateral substantia nigra. Neuropathol Appl Neurobiol 1978; 4:297–301.
356. Sciarra D, Sprofkin BE. Symptoms and signs referable to the basal ganglia in brain tumors. Arch Neurol Psychiatr 1953; 69:450–461.

357. Tolosa E, Vilato J, Fuemayor B. Parkinsonisme tumoral. Neurochirurgie, 12:555–559.
358. Blocq P, Marinesco G. Sur un cas de tremeblement parkinsonien hémiplégique symptomatique d'une tumeur du pédoncule cérébral. Rev Neurol (Paris) 1894; 2:265.
359. Gherardi R, Roualdes B, Fleury J, Prost C, Poirier J, Degos JD. Parkinsonian syndrome and central nervous system lymphoma involving the substantia nigra. A case report. Acta Neuropathol (Berl) 1985; 65:338–343.
360. Van Eck JH. Parkinsonism as a misleading brain tumor syndrome. Psychiatr Neurol Neurochir 1961; 64:109.
361. Krauss JK, Paduch T. Mundinger F, Seeger W. Parkinsonism and rest tremor secondary to supratentorial tumours sparing the basal ganglia. Acta Neurochir (Wien) 1995; 133:22–29.
362. Garcia DY, Gervas JJ Iglesias J, Mena MA, Martin DR, Somoza E. Biochemical findings in a case of parkinsonism secondary to brain tumor. Ann Neurol 1982; 11:313–316.
363. Lhermitte F, Agid Y, Serdaru M, Guimaraes J. Syndrome parkinsonien, tumeur frontale et L-dopa. Rev Neurol (Paris) 1984; 140:138–139.
364. Grant FC. The parkinsonian syndrome and brain tumor: a report of a case. Arch Neurol Psychiatr 1951; 65:784–785.
365. Coers C, Kleyntjens F, Brihaye J. Syndrome parkinsonien d'origine tumorale. Acta Neurol Belg 1952; 52:737–765.
366. Grimberg L. Paralysis agitans and trauma. J Nerv Ment Dis 1934; 79:14–42.
367. Lindenberg R. Die Schaedigungsmechanismen der Substantia nigra bei Hirntraumen und das Problem des posttraumatischen Parkinsonismus. Dtsch Z Nervenheilkd, 1964; 185:637–663.
368. Corsellis J, Bruton CJ, Freeman-Browne D. The aftermath of boxing. Psychol Medi, 1973; 3:270–303.
369. Roberts GW, Allsop D, Bruton C. The occult aftermath of boxing. J Neurol Neurosurg Psychiatry, 1990; 53:373–378.
370. Hof PR, Bouras C, Buee L, Delacourte A, Perl DP, Morrison JH. Differential distribution of neurofibrillary tangles in the cerebral cortex of dementia pugilistica and Alzheimer's disease cases. Acta Neuropathol (Berl) 1992; 85:23–30.
371. Geddes JF, Vowles GH, Nicoll JA, Revesz T. Neuronal cytoskeletal changes are an early consequence of repetitive head injury. Acta Neuropathol (Berl), 1999; 98:171–178.

10. The Scientific Basis of Parkinsonian Syndromes

ROBERT J. SCHWARTZMAN AND GUILLERMO M. ALEXANDER

This chapter will review the epidemiology, genetics, and newer concepts of the neuroanatomical pathways that form the basis of parkinsonian syndromes. These mechanisms will be reviewed in the context of the experimental 1-methyl-4-phenyl-1,2,3,6 tetrahydropyridine (MPTP) model of the disease and imaging techniques used in parkinsonian patients. The two major putative mechanisms of substantia nigra pars compacta cell death that underly many of the clinical manifestations will be discussed in light of current theory.

EPIDEMIOLOGY

Parkinson's disease (PD) is one of the most common neurodegenerative diseases encountered in the elderly, affects both sexes approximately equally, and occurs throughout the world in all ethnic groups.[1,2] The prevalence rates vary in different parts of the world, possibly because of exposure to different environmental substances, and increases exponentially with age.[3,4] At age 65–90 years, 0.3% of the general population is afflicted.[5] As the population ages, this prevalence will increase. At present, one million patients suffer from the disease in North America.[6] The mortality of those affected is two to five times greater than age matched controls and results in a reduction of life expectancy.[7,8] Age is the single most important risk factor, but several large case–control studies have suggested that rural living, herbicides, pesticides, well water, and industrial or chemical exposure, as possible environmental agents causative of the disease.[7] Smoking is associated with a reduced chance of getting Parkinson's.[9] A recent study has found that the reduction in risk in those who smoke is restricted to those with a relatively young age at onset.[10] A study to assess diet in PD found that vitamin E intake was lower in PD patients than in controls.[11]

GENETICS

Parkinson's disease in most patients is sporadic, although patients with familial disease are increasingly reported.[12] There are no accurate statistics for the prevalence of familial PD.[12] The advent of imaging studies using the uptake of 6^{18}F fluorodopa in position emission topography (PET; measures dopa decarboxylase activity in striatal terminals) increases the accuracy of diagnosis and has shown a concordance rate of 45% in monozygotic twins and 29% for dizygotic twins.[13] First-degree relatives of PD patients have twice the risk of developing the illness as that of controls.[14]

Autosomal Dominant Parkinson's Disease

Autosomal dominant Lewy body–positive familial PD comprises most of the familial cases, which may vary widely in their clinical expression.[15] The Contursi family of Southern Italy, in which 60 of 592 members are affected, provided the first evidence of a genetic mutation causing PD.[16,17] The mutation of the α-synuclein gene (*SNCA*) located on chromosome 4q 21–22 (mutation at bp 209), causes an alanine to threonine substitution at position 53 of the protein and is responsible for the disease in the Contursi kindred and possibly two distantly related Greek families. The other α-synuclein mutation found in PD that produces an Ala 30 Pro substitution was found in a German kindred.[18] These patients have a somewhat atypical course of illness with a younger age at onset (mean 46 years) and an aggressive, rapidly progressive course, with fewer tremors than in PD. The one family member who has been autopsied had Lewy bodies in the substantia nigra.[19] Secondary protein structure analysis suggests that Ala produces an α-helix structure and the substituted Thr^{53} results in a β-sheet structure that results in increased polymerization of the abnormal protein.

Several studies have failed to detect mutations in the *SNCA* gene in both familial and sporadic cases of Parkinson's disease.[20] Two recent studies have not supported the mutation in exon-4 of the α-synuclein gene, so this mutation may cause only one form of early-onset PD.[21] Recently, six families with more typical signs and symptoms of PD have been found to have linkage to chromosome 2p13.[22] There are many autosomal dominant Lewy body–positive familial parkinsonian families with atypical features.[23]

The Lewy body–negative autosomal dominant families have both young- and late-onset varieties. Autosomal dominant parkinsonism in which the presence or absence of Lewy body pathology has not been established frequently demonstrates anticipation or dystonia.[24]

Autosomal Recessive Parkinson's Disease

Autosomal recessive parkinsonism is much rarer than the dominant form. Recently, the gene for one family with autosomal recessive parkinsonism has been mapped to chromosome 6q 25.2–27 near the sod 2 (Mn SOD gene) locus.[25] This gene is novel and spans >500 kb with 12 exons that encode a 465 amino acid protein. Homozygous deletions between exons 3 and 7 are associated with the disease phenotype. The gene protein is named "Parkin." Rare maternal inheritance has been reported.[26]

Possible Genetic Predisposition in Sporadic Parkinson's Disease

The ability to detoxify or eliminate a toxin may be genetically determined and may be important in the susceptibility to PD. Liver enzymes that increase the metabolism of xenobiotic substances (the microsomal P450 system) may protect against the development of PD by destroying environmental toxins. The enzyme debrisiquine-4-hydroxylase is encoded by the *CYP2D6* gene and metabolizes a wide range of substances. It has been hypothesized that inadequate metabolism by debrisoquine may predispose patients to the toxic effects of a substance not adequately destroyed by this system. Some studies have shown that a higher risk of developing PD is associated with alleles that translate low enzyme activity.[27] More recent evidence does not support this association.[28] The inheritance of the *C4P2D6* allele of the P450 complex combined with a mutant allele of a second-phase detoxification enzyme, GST MI, may increase the risk of developing PD.[29] A further complicating issue of this hypothesis is the finding that the slow-acetylator gene type for *N*-acetyltransferase 2 is more often seen in familial PD (69% prevalence) than in control patients (37%), but the frequency of this gene type is intermediate in sporadic PD patients.[30] The possible association of *MAO B, COMT, CYPIAI* detoxification genes in the pathogenesis of PD is under investigation.[29,32] A genetic defect of complex I function of the mitochondrial respiratory chain has been demonstrated in some patients with PD (discussed in Pathogenesis of Oxidative Stress, below).

PARKINSONIAN SYNDROMES WITH KNOWN GENETIC LOCI

Segawa's disease (dopa-responsive dystonia) presents in childhood with limb dystonia, occurs with marked diurnal fluctuation, and is exquisitely responsive to L-dopa. These patients have mutations in the GTP cyclohydrolase gene (*GTPCH-I*). *GTPCH-I* is the rate-limiting step for biopterin production, a cofactor for tyrosine hydrolase that causes a defect in dopamine synthesis but does not kill dopaminergic neurons in the substantia nigra pars compacta (SNpc)[33]

Autosomal recessive early-onset parkinsonism with diurnal fluctuation (AR-EPDF) is a rare condition characterized by onset under the age of 40, akinesia, and rigidity; improvement by sleep is linked to chromosome 6 q 25.2-27, and AR-EPDF has been found in Japanese families. There is degeneration of dopaminergic cells of the SNpc, but Lewy bodies are absent.[25] Dominantly inherited early-onset parkinsonism has also been reported.

X-Linked Dystonia–Parkinson's Disease Complex

This disease was first described from the island of Panay in the Philippines. Patients present with parkinsonism, have intermittent truncal and mouth dystonia, and respond poorly to L-dopa. Linkage to xq12-13 has been established and the primary pathology is in the striatum rather than the ventrolateral tier of the SNpc.[34]

Disinhibition–Dementia–Parkinsonism–Amyotrophy Complex

Disinhibition–dementia–parkinsonism–amyotrophy complex (DDPAC) is an autosomal dominant disease that is linked to chromosome 17q 21–22. Patients present with personality and behavioral changes, rigidity, bradykinesia, loss of postural reflexes, and amyotrophy. The process is rapidly progressive with a mean survival of 13 years. Atrophy and spongiform degeneration are seen in the frontotemporal cortex. Neuronal loss and gliosis are most severe in the amygdala, SNpc, and anterior horn cells. There is no evidence of Lewy bodies, neurofibrillary tangles, or amyloid bodies, a finding similar to the pathology of temporal dementia with motor neuron degeneration.[35]

Familial Progressive Subcortical Gliosis

Familial progressive subcortical gliosis (FPSG) is an autosomal dominant disease and is also linked to chromosome 17q 21–22. It is characterized by dementia, personality changes, and extrapyramidal signs and symptoms. Neuronal accumulation of prion protein and degeneration of the frontotemporal lobes also occur. Some familial prion diseases are linked to chromosome 20pter-p12.[36]

Other syndromes with prominent parkinsonian features and known genetic loci are Machado-Joseph disease (spinocerebellar atrophy type 3) on chromosome 14q 24.3–32, Hallervorden-Spatz disease on chromosome 20p 12.3, Huntington disease on chromosome 4p 16.3, dentato-rubro-pallidoluysian atrophy (12p13.3), and Wilson's disease on 13q 14–21.[37–43]

The genetic etiology of many parkinsonian syndromes has been clearly identified, as noted above. That PD can be a single gene disorder is supported by the a-synuclein gene mutation in the Contursi kindred. The twin and family studies suggest a complex polygenic inheritance of PD. Further complicating the genetic picture is the possibility that functional polymorphic genes may determine susceptibility to the disease. Association studies suggest that specific polymorphism genes may determine dopamine metabolism and detoxification of possible external toxins. At the moment there is no clear picture of the influence of environmental or genetic factors in the initiation of sporadic Parkinson's disease.

NEUROANATOMICAL CONNECTIONS UNDERLYING THE PATHOPHYSIOLOGY OF PARKINSON'S DISEASE

The dopamine-deficient state that characterizes PD is thought to arise from excessive gamma aminobutyric acid (GABAergic) inhibition of the ventroanterior and ventrolateral motor nuclei of the thalamus.[1] These motor nuclei of the thalamus are excitatory (glutaminergic) to the premotor, supplementary motor (SMA), and motor cortex.[44] Thus, if these thalamic nuclei are inhibited, the motor initiation and executive cortex will not be stimulated and bradykinesia and akinesia will result.[44] The two major motor loops of this proposed anatomy are the direct and indirect, the former utilizing the D1 dopamine receptor and the latter the D2 receptor.[44] The action of dopamine is excitatory at the D1 receptor and inhibitory at the D2 receptor. The direct loop consists of (SNpc) neurons that project to and excite a subset of striatal GABAergic neurons that project and inhibit the major output neurons of the basal ganglia, the internal segment of the globus pallidus internus (GPi), and pars reticulata of the substantia nigra (SNpr). Thus normally, this direct loop inhibits the GABAergic output of the basal ganglia and decreases inhibition of the motor loop. The indirect loop consists of SNpc projections to the striatum, which inhibits D2 receptors and decreases the GABAergic descending projections to the external portion of the globus pallidus externus (GPe). This segment of the pallidum would be less inhibited and thus would depress the efferent activity of its major projection to the subthalamic nucleus (STN) by release of GABA. This nucleus (STN) is glutaminergic and directly stimulates the GPi and the SNpr (the major outflow of the basal ganglia), which would increase the GABAergic tone of the motor thalamus.[44-46] This concept has been used for many years to explain the most devastating features of idiopathic PD, namely akinesia and bradykinesia. This model is clinically strengthened by the recent demonstration that potent D1 and D2 agonists reverse the abnormal suppression of the SMA and premotor cortex in PD patients.[47] This finding supports the concept that dopamine reduces the increased firing rate of the GPi that has been demonstrated both in the MPTP model of PD and in parkinsonian patients.[48]

Recent anatomical work and the effects of both GPi and thalamic surgery suggest that this model is incomplete and must be revised.[49] Anatomical studies demonstrate that the functional separation of direct and indirect striatofugal pathways is inaccurate. The striatofugal axons are highly collateralized and project to GPe, GPi, and SNpr. This high degree of collateralization suggests that striatal neurons project efferent copies throughout the basal ganglia.[50,51] The current model of basal ganglia organization predicts that substance P (SP) neurons would project to GPi and the SNpr while enkephalin (ENK) neurons would project to GPe. Recent studies demonstrate SP and ENK terminals in equal numbers in the SNpr.[52] In the current model, GPe is the primary relay to the subthalamic nucleus but has recently been demonstrated to project to all components of the basal ganglia including the GPi, SNpr, and the striatum (STR).[46] It appears that the GPe is part of a disynaptic indirect pathway (STR-GPe-STN-GPi-SNpr) that would enhance its postulated role in modifying basal ganglia output.[46] The functional anatomy of the subthalamic nucleus (STN) is much more complicated than formerly thought. It receives afferents from the cerebral cortex, SNpc, the dorsal raphe nuclei, the pedunculopontine nucleus (PPN), and the centromedian parafascicular complex (CM/PF) and projects to almost all basal ganglia nuclei.[46,49] It is solely modified by the GPe, a fundamental concept of the indirect loop as presently conceived. The descending projections of the GPi, and SNpr to the deep layers of the superior colliculus and the pedunculopontine tegmental nuclei (PPN), which project back to the GPi, STN, and SNpc, may be important for initiation of gait, eye movements, and dystonia. Extrastriatal dopamine is liberated in the STN, GPi, and SNpr, which may be important in the modulation of basal ganglia output.[50]

Functional studies in both humans and MPTP parkinsonian monkeys show that (1) the GPe is not hypoactive in parkinsonian patients;[53,54] (2) GPe excitotoxic injections do not produce increased activity of STN and GPi/SNpr neurons;[52] and (3) excitotoxic lesions in GPe in MPTP monkeys increase L-dopa–induced dyskinesias rather than decrease them (STN would drive GPi and SPpr to inhibit the thalamus and thus the motor cortex) according to the present model.[55] The conclusions from these data must be that the hyperactivity demonstrated in STN in PD may not depend solely on the reciprocal GPe-STN connections. The important excitatory cerebral cortex projection to STN and the (CM/PF) complex are not accounted for in the present model, although they can excite nonstriatal basal ganglia nuclei.[56]

Stereotatic lesions of the ventral tier thalamic nuclei relieve rigidity and tremor. According to the present model, the lack of thalamic glutamatergic activation of the SMA and premotor cortex should make movement more difficult.[44,54,56] Lesions of GPi would be expected to increase L-dopa–induced dyskinesia by disinhibiting the motor thalamus. Paradoxically, the best result of this lesion is the reduction of dyskinesia caused by L-dopa therapy.[57] High-frequency stimulation of the STN relieves bradykinesia and induces dyskinesia in parkinsonian patients.[58] Stereotactic thalamotomy does not worsen hypokinesia or cause PD.[50] The expected neurotransmitter changes in specific nuclei have not been found in PD.[51]

PATHOGENESIS OF THE MPTP MODEL OF PARKINSONISM: CORROBORATOR OF ANATOMICAL CONNECTIONS AND PREDICTOR OF FUNCTIONAL STUDIES

Administration of the neurotoxin 1-methyl-4-phenyl-1,2,3,6 tetrahydro pyridine (MPTP) produces parkinsonism in nonhuman primates and humans.[59,60] The mode of administration of MPTP determines the neuropathological findings in this primate model of PD. Intravenous (IV) administration of MPTP causes a symmetric model of parkinsonism due to bilateral destruction of the SNpc and concomitant cell loss in the ventral tegmental area (VTA) and locus ceruleus.[59,61,62] A unilateral hemiparkinsonian model is produced by unilateral intracarotid injection of MPTP, which primarily destroys the SNpc on the ipsilateral injected side.[63] The unilateral model may not be as an accurate a reflection of the parkinsonian state as that produced by IV administration of MPTP because (1) there are bilateral projections of the SNpc; and (2) the VTA (A10) and the locus ceruleus (A5) are not affected. The latter nucleus may be important in the progression of PD.[64] The results of the systemic administration of MPTP will be discussed here, primarily because this model reflects the anatomical neuropathological and clinical features of human parkinsonism more accurately than any other. MPTP administration produces a parkinsonian syndrome characterized by hypophemia, akinesia, bradykinesia, rigidity, tremor, and flexed posture—features very similar to those seen within days to weeks in the idiopathic form of the disease in humans.[60]

The autoradiographic 2-deoxy (^{14}C) glucose (2-DG) method permits the quantitative measurement of local rates of glucose utilization throughout the brain and spinal cord.[65] Energy metabolism is closely coupled with glucose utilization, which is a measure of functional activity in central nervous system (CNS) structures.[66] Most glucose utilization occurs at synapses (90%) rather than in the neuronal cell body, so those nuclei that demonstrate increased glucose utilization reflect the afferent projections to that nucleus.[65] The sign of this activity (inhibitory or excitatory) is determined by electrophysiological means.

Measurement of glucose utilization prior to 21 days after the last IV dose of MPTP may reflect residual MPTP and 1-methyl-4-phenylpyridine (MPP$^+$), the toxic conversion product of MPTP in the circulation, that may affect regional brain glucose utilization.[6–69] Evaluation of the local cerebral metabolic rate for glucose (LCMRg) in MPTP-induced parkinsonism in monkeys after 21 days ("steady-state condition") and whose striatal dopamine was <3% of control values (severely depleted) showed increases of metabolism in the putamen, both internal and external segments of the globus pallidus, ventrolateral medial (VLM) nucleus of the thalamus, and the anterior dorsolateral segment of the substantia nigra pars compacta (SNpc). There was no change in LCMRg in the SNr or the STN. The LCMRg of the mesocortical limbic system did not differ from control values. The locus ceruleus demonstrated a significant increase in LCMRg, as did the motor cortex. The visual cortex was depressed metabolically.[69]

In acutely intoxicated animals, LCMRg measured 3 days following the last dose of MPTP caused metabolic depression of all cortical areas due to monoaminergic terminal destruction. The prolonged depression of visual cortex metabolism may be due to direct

MPTP damage of the dopaminergic retinal projection systems.[67] The increase in LCMRg of the motor cortex may be due to disinhibition of its afferent dopaminergic projections from the SNpc or through the basal ganglia, which may be inhibitory.[70,71] In both the acute and steady-state MPTP-intoxicated monkeys, the external and internal segments of the pallidum showed increased LCMRg.[72] The SNpc metabolism was increased at 3 days in the MPTP monkeys but returned to normal, except for the anterodorsolateral region, at 21 days.[69] MPTP-intoxicated monkeys evaluated at 3 months after their last dose of MPTP showed no increase in LCMRg in the motor cortex, locus ceruleus, and putamen. They still maintained increased metabolic activity in the GPe, but to a lesser extent than at 21 days.[72] In the acutely intoxicated animals, metabolic depression of the cortex and striatum is a reflection of monoaminergic terminal destruction. As the animal recovers, the effects of dopaminergic and noradrenergic system damage is more prominent and is reflected in the increased LCMRg of the motor cortex, midputamen, GPe, and GPi.

In clinically effective chronic L-dopa therapy of MPTP parkinsonian rhesus monkeys, widespread increases of glucose utilization have been noted throughout the brain, compared to that in normal animals receiving the same dose of L-dopa.[70] Significant increases in the LCMRg of the SNpc, STN, GPe, frontal eye fields, and medial dorsal nucleus of the thalamus have been found in untreated animals.[21] In normal monkeys, administration of L-dopa did not change LCMRg in any region of the brain other than the lateral hypothalamus.[70] L-dopa therapy in MPTP parkinsonian monkeys increased the LCMRg in the caudate, putamen, STN, prefrontal cortex, orbitofrontal cortex, frontal eye fields, motor, striate, entorrhinal cortex, mediodorsal thalamus, ventrolateral thalamic nucleus, and the lateral geniculate body. In many regions, the LCMRg rate was significantly greater than under normal conditions.[70] These widespread metabolic changes noted after L-dopa treatment suggest that circuits other than those mediating the clinical manifestations of PD may be involved in this model. The "overshoot of LCMRg" produced by L-dopa therapy may be produced by dopamine receptor hypersensitivity in these areas, increased receptor density, changes in dopamine release, or uptake mechanisms.[70]

Recent molecular studies that measure glutamate decarboxylase mRNA levels suggest that only the high-molecular-weight isoform (GAD67 rather than GAD65) is regulated by dopamine projections from the SNpc.[71] GABAergic neuronal projections from the striatum to GP/SNr and GPe are pivotal elements underlying the behavioral manifestations of PD.[44] In MPTP parkinsonism, there is an increase of mRNA GAD 67 levels in neurons of the striatum and pallidum.[72] The increase is noted in the dorsolateral zone of the anterior putamen throughout the striatum at postcommisural caudal levels and in the GPe and GPi, which reflect increased GABAergic activity.[72] The area of highest increase in GAD 67 labeling, the dorsolateral putamen, receives the major sensorimotor cortical projection to the striatum, which regulates *GAD 67* gene expression.[73,74] The dorsolateral putamen in MPTP parkinsonian monkeys demonstrates increased preproenkephalin mRNA, which suggests that these neurons project to pallidal neurons that express GABA and ENK.[75] GAD 67 mRNA levels are increased in GPe in the MPTP monkey and in the rat after 6-hydroxydopamine lesions of ascending dopaminergic systems, which supports the role of the SNpc dopaminergic afferents in the regulation of gene expression in this nucleus.[76] The correlation of increased GAD 67 labeling in striatal neurons, which have a major projection to this nucleus, is further evidence for striatal control of GABAergic neurons of the GPe.

GAD 67 mRNA levels are increased in GPi of both the squirrel and *Macaca fascicularis* monkey after treatment with MPTP; this finding support, the role of dopamine in GAD 67 regulation of neurons in the GPi.[77] GAD 67 mRNA labeling in the GPi is not correlated with striatal neurons that project to GPe. These complex changes in gene regulation of GAD 67 in MPTP monkeys support the metabolic 2DG studies reviewed above. Positron emission tomographic (PET) metabolic studies and 6^{18}F-fluoro-L-dopa (FDOPA) tracer techniques have demonstrated decreased striatal dopa decarboxylase activity in patients with PD.[78,79] FDOPA uptake is proportional to remaining striatal dopaminergic nerve terminals, transporters, and SNpc neurons.[80] Patients with less severe PD, Hoehn and Yahr (HY) stage I–II, had reduced caudate and putaminal FDOPA metabolism, which decreased further with advancing clinical disease (stages HY III–IV).[81] In general PD patients with HY I–II disease show increased ^{11}C raclopride (RACLO) uptake (a measure of binding to D_2 receptors) in the putamen, with returns to normal as the disease progresses. The caudate nucleus RACLO index is normal in HY I–II disease but declines with disease progression.[81] Putaminal glucose metabolism is increased in all stages of disease.[79]

Position emission tomographic measurements of presynaptic nigrostriatal dopaminergic function correlate closely with bradykinesia and rigidity but not with tremor.[78] Focal vascular lesions of the substantia nigra that spare the rubroolivocerebellar and cerebellothalamic pathways cause rigidity and bradykinesia without tremor.[82] Recent PET studies have shown that the metabolic anatomy of tremor in PD involves the motor association cortices, thalamus, and pons.[83] These findings are consistent with magnetoencephalographic (MEG) data of thalamocortical oscillation that involve sequential discharges of the thalamus and premotor and motor cortices.[84] Electrophysiological studies have shown that ventral thalamic discharges synchronized with tremor that is improved or abolished by thalamotomy, and these studies support the thalamus as being the generator of PD tremor.[85,86]

Patients with PD demonstrate bradykinesia of free movement, which is associated with metabolic underactivity of the supplementary motor area, dorsal prefrontal cortex, and frontal association areas that receive afferents from the basal ganglia. There is increased metabolic activity of the lateral premotor and parietal cortex, whose primary role is facilitating motor responses to visual and auditory cues.[87] Dopaminergic medication, GPi pallidotomy, high-frequency stimulation of STN, and mesencephalic fetal tissue transplantation tend to restore normal activation patterns of the SMA and dorsal prefrontal cortex.[87] Recent imaging studies US (1231) beta computed tomography (CT) and single-photon emission computed tomography (SPECT) suggest decreased striatal uptake in relatives of patients with PD who may be at high risk for developing PD.[88]

Through the recent use of precise anatomical mapping methods, the basic connections of the functional loops involved in parkinsonian syndromes have been outlined; however, the complexity of these methods must also be addressed, as suggested recently by Parent.[50] The 2-DG analysis of the MPTP model has suggested the major nuclear groups and their connections that are important in parkinsonism. The effects of dopamine depletion on gene expression of GAD 67, the isomer of this enzyme under dopaminergic control, have shown the sensitivity of these studies, which in turn have aided researchers to combining anatomical and functional views of the underlying physiology in PD. Position emission tomography and fluorodeoxyglucose and receptor imaging have allowed the application of these basic science methods to patients suffering from this disease.

The pathogenesis of PD is at present unknown. Genetic, environmental, and toxic etiologies have all been implicated. Recent experimental studies suggest both mitochondrial defects and oxidative stress as possible fundamental mechanisms.

Pathogenesis of Oxidative Stress

Free radicals are entities that contain unpaired electrons.[89] The predominant free radicals are oxygen based and along with peroxides are the normal products of cellular aerobic metabolism, such as energy generation from mitochondria. These compounds are referred to as "reactive oxygen species" (ROS), the most important being the superoxide ($O_2^{\cdot}$) and hydroxyl ($OH^{\cdot}$) free radicals, hydrogen peroxide (H_2O_2) and peroxynitrite ($ONOO^-$).[90,91] In addition, iron is a pro-oxidant and can donate an electron to enhance redox reactions.[92] Hydrogen peroxide in the presence of iron can, via the Fenton reaction, lead to the formation of the much more reactive hydroxyl free radical.[93]

There are a number of cellular protective mechanisms whose function is the prevention and repair of damage from ROS. The cellular antioxidant defense mechanisms include enzymatic and non-enzymatic antioxidants consisting of superoxide dismutase (SOD), catalase, glutathione peroxidase (GSH-Px), glutathione reductase (GSH-red) and quinone reductase (QR), the vitamins C and E, and uric acid. In addition, reduced nicotinamide adenine dinucleotide (NADH), reduced nicotinamide adenine dinucleotide phosphate (NADPH), and reduced glutathione (GSH) provide reducing equivalents for many of the antioxidant enzymes. Also, entities that prevent the accumulation of iron can be protective against oxidative stress. Transferrin binds iron and reduces its participation in lipid peroxidation and ceruloplasmin oxidizes iron without the release of ROS.[94] These compounds can be considered part of the antioxidant defenses that protect against oxidative stress.

Oxidative stress is an imbalance between the production of ROS and the ability of antioxidant defenses to reduce their concentrations. The hypothesis that oxidative stress plays a role in the pathogenesis of PD is well supported.[95] The dopaminergic neurons of the SNpc are extremely vulnerable to ROS.[96] Dopamine contains an unstable catechol moiety that can undergo enzymatic oxidation as well as non-enzymatic auto-oxidation leading to the formation of hydrogen peroxide, superoxide, and reactive quinones and semiquinones.[96] These oxidation products can cause alterations in lipids, proteins, and DNA.[97,98]

There is evidence for increased lipid peroxidation and decreased levels of reduced glutathione in the substantia nigra of patients with PD.[99–101] Oxidative stress can cause protein damage and generate protein carbonyl groups.[102,103] Increased protein oxidation and a generalized increase in protein carbonyls have been demonstrated in the brain of patients with PD.[104,105]

A number of investigators have shown that iron is elevated in PD.[106,107] The accumulation of iron in the SNpc can promote oxidative stress and has been shown to facilitate lipid peroxidation. The increase in iron content in the SNpc of PD patients,[106] along with the hydrogen peroxide produced during dopamine metabolism,[108] can lead to highly reactive hydroxyl radicals by the Haber-Weiss or Fenton reactions.[94] In addition, patients with PD show a systemic decrease in ferritin and transferrin as well as a decrease in the mean density of transferrin-binding sites in SNpc.[108,109] The increase in SNpc iron along with altered iron metabolism may accelerate free-radical formation, leading to neuronal cell death.

Damage by ROS includes DNA strand breaks.[110–112] Mitochondrial DNA (mtDNA) is particularly susceptible to oxidative damage because of its limited repair capabilities and proximity to the electron transport chain.[91,113] Patients with PD show decreased activity and immunostaining of NADH-ubiquinone oxidoreductase, complex I of the mitochondrial respiratory chain, in SNpc.[114,115] Reductions in complex I activity have also been reported in platelet and skeletal muscle mitochondria of patients with PD.[116,117] That decreased complex I activity is important in the pathophysiology of PD is clearly demonstrated by a decrease in its activity caused by the neurotoxin MPTP.

The neurotoxicity of MPTP requires passage across the blood–brain barrier, its oxidation to MPP$^+$, a reaction catalyzed by monoamine oxidase B (MAO-B), and the uptake of MPP$^+$ by the monoamine transport system.[118,119] Inhibition of mitochondrial complex I by MPP$^+$ is felt to be the critical event in the lethal cell injury resulting from exposure to MPTP.[120–122] The fact that MPP$^+$ is a mitochondrial toxin suggests the possibility of mitochondrial dysfunction as the basis for idiopathic PD.

Oxidative stress has also been implicated in excitotoxicity, which is the lethal effect of high concentrations of excitatory amino acids on neuronal populations. Glutamate is the major excitatory amino acid transmitter in the CNS. Reactive oxygen species have been shown to increase glutamate release and inhibit its reuptake.[123,124] Peroxynitrite (ONOO$^-$) is formed spontaneously by the combination of superoxide with nitric oxide (NO). Nitric oxide is generated by nitric oxide synthase (NOS), which is activated by CA^{2+}/calmodulin following glutamate stimulation of NMDA receptors.[125] The oxidative stress caused by peroxynitrite has been shown to inhibit all brain glutamate transporters.[126] Inhibition of glutamate reuptake results in an increase in its extracellular concentration, with a concomitant increase in NMDA receptor stimulation. By these mechanisms, a lethal cycle of increased production of ROS is initiated that leads to increased extracellular levels of glutamate, which activates NMDA receptors and causes a further increase in ROS. The age-related onset and progressive nature of PD may be due to a cyclic process including impaired energy metabolism, excitotoxicity, and oxidative stress caused by inadequate antioxidant defenses.

Great advances in our understanding of the scientific basis of parkinsonian syndromes have been made over the past 30 years. The recent re-introduction of stereotactic neurosurgical techniques and the use of functional magnetic resource imaging (MRI), metabolic and receptor imaging, and possible gene therapy make the possibility of enhanced patient care in the near future very real.

REFERENCES

1. Zhang ZX, Roman GC. Worldwide occurrence of Parkinson's disease: an updated review. Neuroepidemology 1993; 12:195–208.
2. Rajput AH, Rozdilsky B, Rajput A. Accuracy of clinical diagnosis in parkinsonism—a prospective study. Can J Neurol Sci 1991; 18:275–278.
3. Sutcliffe RLG, Meara. Parkinson's disease epidemiology in the Northampton district, England. Acta Neurol Scand 1992; 92:443–450.
4. Seidler A, Hellenbrand W, Robra BP, Vieregge P, Nischan P, Joerg J. Oertel WH, Ulm G, Schneider E. Possible environmental, occupational and other etiologic factors for Parkinson disease: a case control study in Germany. Neurology 1996; 46:1275–84.
5. Moghal S, Rajput AH, D'Arcy C, Rajput R. Prevalence of movement disorders in elderly community residents. Neuroepidemology 1994; 13:175–178.
6. Lang AE, Lozano AM. Parkinson's disease. N Engl J Med 1999; 339:1045–1053.
7. Morens DM, Davis JW, Grandinetti A, Ross GW, Popper JS, White LR. (1996). Epidemiologic observations on Parkinson's disease: incidence and mortality in a prospective study of middle aged men. Neurology 1996; 46:1044–1050.
8. Louis ED, Marder K, Conti L, Tang M, Mayeux R. Mortality from Parkinson's disease. Arch Neurol 1997; 54:260–264.
9. Gradinetti A, Morens DM, Reed D, MacEachern D. Prospective study of cigarette smoking and the risk of developing idiopathic Parkinson's disease. Am J Epidemiol 1994; 139:1129–1138.
10. Tzourio C, Rocca WA, Breteler MM, Baldereschi M, Dartigues JF, Lopez-Pousa S, Manubens-Bertran JM, Alperovitch A. Smoking and Parkinson's disease: an age dependent risk effect? Neurology 1997; 49:1267–1272.
11. deRijk MC, Breteler MM, denBreeijen JH, Lavner LJ, Grobbee DE, van der Meche FG, Hofman A. Dietary antioxidants and Parkinson's disease. The Rotterdam Study. Arch Neurol 1997; 54:762–765.
12. Mizuno Y, Hattori N, Matsumine H. Neurochemical and neurogenetic correlates of Parkinson's disease. J Neurochem 1998; 71:893–902.
13. Tanner CM, Ottman R, Ellenberg JH, Goldman SM, Mayeux R, Piu Chan J, Langston W. Parkinson's disease (PD) concordance in elderly male monozygotic (MZ) and dizygotic (DZ) twins. [abstract]. Neurology 1997; 48:(Suppl A333)
14. Marder K, Tang M-X, Mejia H. Risk of Parkinson's disease among first degree relatives: a community based study. Neurology 1996; 47:155–160.
15. Lazzarini AM, Myers RH, Zimmerman TR Jr. A clinical genetic study of Parkinson's disease: evidence for dominant transmission. Neurology 1994; 44:499–506.
16. Polymeropoulos MH, Higgins JJ, Golbe LI, Johnson WG, Ide SE, DiIorio G, Sanges G, Stenroos ES, Pho LT, Schaffer AA, Lazzarini AM, Nussbaum R., Duvoisisin RC. Mapping of a gene for Parkinson's disease to chromosome 4q21–q23. Science 1996; 274: 1197–1199.
17. Golbe LI, DiLorio G, Sanges G, Lazzarini AM, LaSala S. Clinical genetic analysis of Parkinson's disease in the Contursi kindred. Ann Neuro 1996; 40: 767–775.
18. Kruger R, Kuhn W, Muller T, Woitalla D, Graeber M, Kosel S, Przuntek H, Epplen JT, Schols L Riess O. Ala30Pro mutation in the gene encoding α-synuclein in Parkinson's disease. Nat Genet 1998; 18: 106–108.
19. Degl'Innocenti F, Maurello MT, Marini P. A parkinsonian kindred. Ital J Neurol Sci 1989; 10:307–310.
20. Scott WK, Staijich JM, Yamaoka LH. Genetic complexity and Parkinson's disease. Science 1997; 277: 388–389.
21. Munoz E, Oliva R., Orbach V, Marti MJ, Pastor P, Ballesta F, Tolosa E. Identification of a Spanish familial Parkinson's disease and screening for the Ala 53 Thr mutation of the α synuclein gene in early onset patients. Neurosci Lett 1997; 235:57–60.
22. Gasser T, Müller-Myhsok B, Wszolek ZK. A susceptibility locus for Parkinson's disease maps to chromosome 2 p13. Nat Genet, 1998;18:262–265.
23. Yoshikuni M, Hattori N, Matsume H. Neurochemical and neurogenetic correlates of Parkinson's disease. J Neurochem 1998; 71:893–902.
24. Dobyns WB, Ozelius LJ, Kramer PL, Brashear A, Farlow MR, Perry TR, Walsh LE, Kasarskis EJ, Butler IJ Breakefield XO. Rapid onset dystonia-parkinsonism. Neurology 1993; 43:2596–2602.
25. Matsumine H, Saito M, Shimoda-Matsutayashi S, Tanaka H, Ishikawa A, Nakagawa-Hattori Y, Yokochi M, Kobayashi T, Igarashi S, Takano H, Sanpei K, Koike R, Mori H, Kondo T, Mizurtaini Y, Schaffer AA, Yamamura Y, Nakamura S, Kuzuhara S, Tsuji S, Mizuno Y. Localization of a gene for an autosomal recessive form of juvenile parkinsonism to chromosome 6 q25.2–27. Am J Hum Genet 1997; 60:588–596.
26. Wooten GF, Currie LJ, Bennett JP. Maternal inheritance in Parkinson's disease. Ann Neurol 1997; 41: 265–268.
27. Steiger MJ, Lleda P, Quinn NP. Debrisoquine hydroxylation in Parkinson's disease. Acta Neurol Scand 1992; 86:159–164.
28. Riedl AG, Watts PM, Jenner P. P 450 enzymes and Parkinson's disease: the story so far. Mov Disord 1998; 13:212–220.
29. Marsden CD, Olanow CW. The causes of Parkinson's disease are being unraveled and rational neuroprotective therapy is close to reality. Ann Neurol 1998; 44(Suppl 1):S189–S196.
30. Bandmann O, Vaughan J, Holmans P, Marsden CD,

Wood NW, (1997). Association of slow acetylator gene type for N-acetyltransferase 2 with familial Parkinson's disease. Lancet 1997; 350:1136–1139.
31. Marsden CD, Obeso JA. The functions of the basal ganglia and the paradox of stereotatic surgery in Parkinson's disease. Brain 1994; 117:877–897.
32. Nanko S, Veki A, Hattori M. No association between Parkinson's disease and monoamine oxidase A and B gene polymorphisms. Neurosci Lett 1996;204:125–127.
33. Ichinose H, Ohye T, Takahashi E, Seki N, Hori T, Segawa M, Nomura Y, Endo K, Tanaka H Tsuji S, Fujita K, Nagatsu T. Hereditary progressive dystonia with marked diurnal fluctuation caused by mutations in the GTP cyclohydrolase I gene. Nat Genet 1994; 8:236–242.
34. Wilhelmsen KC, Weeks DE, Nygaard TG, Moskowitz CB, Rosales RL, dela Paz DC, Sobrevega EE, Fahn S, Gilliam TC. Genetic mapping of "Lubag" (x-linked dystonia-parkinsonism) in a Filipino kindred to the pericentromeric region of the x-chromosome. Ann Neurol 1991; 29:124–131.
35. Wilhelmsen KC, Lynch T, Pavlow E. Localization of disinhibition dementia-parkinsonism–amyotrophy complex to 17q 21–22. Am J Hum Genet 1994; 55: 1159–1165.
36. Hsiao K, Baker HF, Crow TJ, Poulter M, Owen F, Terwilliger JD, Westaway D, Ott J, Prusiner SB. Linkage of a prion protein missense variant to Gerstmann-Straussler syndrome. Nature 1989; 338: 342–345.
37. Kawaguchi Y, Okamoto T, Taniwaki M, Aizawa M, InouE M, Katayama S, Kawakami H, Nakamura S, Nishimura M, Akiguchi I, Kimura J, Narumiya S, Kakizuka A. CAG expansion in a novel gene for Machado-Joseph disease at chromosome 14 q32.1. Nat Genet 1994; 8:221–228.
38. Taylor TD, Litt M, Kramer P, Pandolfo M, Angelini L, Nardocci N, Davis S, Pineda M, Hattori H, Flett PJ, Cilio MR, Bertini E, Hayflick SJ. Homozygosity mapping of Hallervorden-Spatz syndrome to chromosome 20p 12.3–p 13. Nat Genet 1996; 14:479–481.
39. Tanzi RE, Petrukhin K, Chernov I, Pellequer JL, Wasco W, Ross B, Romano DM, Parano E, Pavone L, Brzustowicz LM, Devotor M, Peppercorn J, Bush AI, Sternlieb I, Pirastu M, Gusella JF, Evgrafov O, Penchaszadeh GK, Honig B, Edelman IS, Soares MB, Scheinberg IH, Gilliam TC. The Wilson disease gene is a copper transporting ATPase with homology to the Menkes disease gene. Nat Genet 1993; 5:344–350.
40. Takano T, Yamanouchi Y, Nagafuchi S, Yamada M. Assignment of the dentatorubral and pallidoluysian atrophy (DRPLA) gene to 12 p13.31 by fluorescence in situ hybridization. Genomics 1996; 32:171–172.
41. The Huntington's Disease Collaborative Research Group. A novel gene containing a trinucleotide repeat that is expanded and unstable on Huntington's disease chromosomes. Cell 1993; 72:971–983.
42. Filion M, Tremblay L. Abnormal spontaneous activity of globus pallicus neurons in monkeys with MPTP induced parkonsonism. Brain Res 1991; 547:142–151.
43. Jenkins IH, Fernandez W, Playford ED, Lees AJ, Frackowiak RS, Passingham RE, Brooks DJ. Impaired activation of the supplementary motor area in Parkinson's disease is reversed when akinesia is treated with apomorphine. Ann Neurol 1992; 32:749–757.
44. Albin RL, Young AB, Penney JB. The functional anatomy of basal ganglia disorders. Trends Neurosci 1989; 12:366–375.
45. DeLong MR. Primate models of movement disorders of basal ganglia origin. Trends Neurosci 1990; 13:281–285.
46. Parent A, Hazrati LN. Functional anatomy of the basal ganglia II. The place of subthalamic nucleus and external pallidum in basal ganglia circuitry. Brain Res Rev 1995; 20:128–154.
47. Jenkins IH Fernandez W, Playford ED, Lees AJ, Frackowiak RS, Passingham RE, Brooks DJ. Impaired activation of the supplementary motor area in Parkinson's disease is reversed when akinesia is treated with apomorphine. Ann Neurol 1992; 32:749–757.
48. Hutchinson WD, Lozono AM, Davis KD. Differential neuronal activity in segments of globus pallidus in Parkinson's disease patients. Neuroreport 1997; 42: 767–775.
49. Parent A, Cicchetti F. The current model of basal ganglia organization under scrutiny. Mov Disord 1998; 13:199–202.
50. Wichmann T, DeLong MR. Functional and pathophysiological models of the basal ganglia. Curr Opin Neurobiol 1996; 6:751–758.
51. Kawaguchi Y, Wilson CJ, Emson PC. Projection subtypes of rat neostriatal matrix cells revealed by intracellular injection of biocytin. J Neurosci 1990; 10: 3421–3438.
52. Parent A, Cote PY, Lavoie B. Chemical anatomy of primate basal ganlia. Prog Neurobiol 1996; 46:131–197.
53. Vila M, Levy R, Herrero MT, Ruberg M, Faucheux B, Obeso JA, Agid Y, Hirsch EC. Consequences of nigrostriatal denervation on the function of the basal ganglia in human and nonhuman primates: in situ hybridization study of cytodrome oxidase subunit I mRNA. J Neurosci 1997; 17:765–773.
54. Chesselet MF, Delfs JM. Basal ganglia and movement disorders: an update. Trends Neurosci 1996; 19:417–422.
55. Blanchet PJ, Boucher R, B'edard PJ. Excitotoxic lateral pallidotomy does not relieve L-dopa induced dyskinesia in MPTP parkinsonian monkeys. Brain Res 1994; 650:32–39.
56. Feger J. Updating the functional model of the basal ganglia [letter]. Trends Neurosci 1997; 20:152–153.
57. Baron MS, Vitek JL, Bakay RA, Green J, Kaneoke Y. Treatment of advanced Parkinson's disease by GPi pallidotomy: 1 year pilot study results. Ann Neurol 1996; 40:355–366.
58. Siegfried J, Lippitz B. Bilateral chronic electrostimulation of ventroposterolateral pallidum: a new therapeutic approach for alleviating all parkinsonian symptoms. Neurosurgery 1994; 35:1126–1130.
59. Burns ST, Chiueh CC, Markey SP, Ebert MH, Jacobowitz DM, Kopin IJ. A primate model of parkinsonism: A selective destruction of dopaminergic neurons in the pars compacta of the substantia nigra by N-methyl-4-phenyl-1,2,3,6-tetrahydropyridine. Proc Natl Acad Sci USA 1983; 80:4546–4550.
60. Burns SR, Markey SP, Phillips JM, Chiueh CC. The

neurotoxicity of 1-methyl-4-phenyl-1,2,3,6-tetrahydropyridine in the monkey and man. Can J Neurol Sci 1184; 11:166–168, 1984.
61. Mitchell IJ, Cross AJ, Sambrook MA, Crossman AR. Sites of the neurotoxic action of 1-mthyl-4-phenyl-1,2,3,6-tetrahydropyridine in the macaque monkey include the ventral tegmental area of the locus coeruleus. Neurosci Lett 1985; 61:195–200.
62. Forno LS, Langston JW, DeLanney LE, Irwin I, Ricaurte GA. Locus ceruleus lesions and eosinophilic inclusions in MPTP-treated monkeys. Ann Neurol 1986; 20:449–455.
63. Bankiewicz KS, Oldfield EH, Chiueh CC. Doppman JL, Jacobowitz DM, Kopin IJ. Hemiparkinsonism in monkeys after unilateral internal carotid artery infusion of 1-methyl-4-phenyl-1,2,3,6-tetrahydropyridine (MPTP). LifSci 1986; 39:7–16.
64. Mitchell IJ, Clarke CE, Boyce S, Robertson RG, Peggs D, Sambrook MA, Crossmann AR. Neural mechanisms underlying parkinsonian symptoms based upon regional uptak of 2-deoxyglucose in monkeys exposed to 1-methyl-4-phenyl-1,2,3,6-tetrahydropyridine. Neuiroscience 1989; 32:213–226.
65. Sokoloff L, Reivich M, Kennedy C, DesRosiers MH, Patlak CS, Pettigrew KD, Sakurada O, Shinohara M. The (14C) doxyglucose method for the measurement of local cerebral utilization: theory, procedure and normal values in the conscious and anesthetized albino rat. J Neurosci 1977; 28:897–916.
66. Sokoloff L. Localization of functional activity in the central nervous system by measurement of glucose utlization with radioactive deoxyglucose. J Cereb Blood Flow Metab 1981; 1:7–36.
67. Schwartzman RJ, Alexander GM. Changes in local cerebral metabolic rate for glucose in the MPTP primate model of Parkinson's disease. Brain Res 1985; 358:137–143.
68. Schwartzman RJ, Alexander GM, Memlo M. Changes in regional glucose metabolism in the mesocortical dopaminergic system of a primate model of Parkinson's disease. Neurology 1985; 35:116.
69. Schwartzman RJ, Alexander GM, Ferraro TN, Grothusen JR, Stahl SM. Cerebral metabolism of parkinsonian primates 21 days after MPTP. Exp Neurol 1988; 102:307–313.
70. Porrino LJ, Burns RS, Crane AM, Palombo E, Kopin IJ, Sokoloff L. Local cerebral metabolic effects of L-dopa therapy in 1-mthyl-4-phenyl-1,2,3,6-tetrahydropyridine–induced parkinsonian monkeys. Proc Natl Acad Sci USA 1987; 84:5995–5999.
71. Soghomonion JJ, Chesselet MF. Effects of dopamine nigrostratal lesions on the levels of messenger RNAs encoding two isoforms of glutamate decarboxylase in the globus pallidus and entopedicular nucleus of the rat. Synapse 1992; 11:124–133.
72. Soghomonion JJ, Pedneault S., Audet G, et al. Increased glutamate decarboxylase mRNA levels in the striatum and pallidum of MPTP treated primates. J Neurosci 1994; 14:6256–6265.
73. Parent A. Extrinsic connections of the basal ganglia. Trends Neurosci 1990; 13:254–258.
74. Salin P, Chesselet MF. Expression of GAD (M,67,000) and its messenger RNA in basal ganglia and cerebral cortex after ischemic corticallesions in rats. Exp Neurol 1993; 119:291–301.
75. Soghomonion JJ, Cote PY, Parent A. Preproenkephalin mRNA levels in the neurostriatum of normal and parkinsonian monkeys. Soc Neurosci Abstr 1993; 19:782.
76. Kincaid AE, Albin RE, Newman SW, Penney JB, Young AB. 6-hydroxydopamine lesions of the nigrostriatal pathway alter the expression of glutamate decarboylase messenger RNA in rat globus pallidus projection neurons. Neuroscience 1992; 51:705–718.
77. Herrero M-T, Ruberg M, Hirsch EC, Guridi Jm Linquin M-T, Ruberg M, Agid EC, Agid Y, Obeso JA. Changes in GAD mRNA expression in neurons of the internal pallidum in parkinsonian monkeys after L-dopa therapy. Soc Neurosci Abstr 1993; 19:132.
78. Leenders KL, Palmer AJ, Quinn N, Clark JC, Firnau G, Garnett ES, Nahmias C, Jones T, Marsden CD. Brain dopamine metabolism in patients with Parkinson's disease measured with positron emission tomography. J Neurol Neurosurg Psychiatry 1986; 49:853–860.
79. Eidelberg D, Moeller JR, Dhawan V, Sidtis JJ, Ginos JZ, Strother SC, Cedarbaum J, Greene P, Fahn S, Rottenberg DA. The metabolic anatomy of Parkinson's disease: complementary (18F) flurodeoxyglucose and (18F) fluorodopa positron emission tomography studies. Mov Disord 1990; 5:203–213.
80. Snow BJ, Tooyama I, McGreer EG, Yamada T, Calne DB, Takahashi H, Kimura H. Human positron emission tomographic (18F) fluorodopa studies correlate with dopamine cell counts and levels. An Neurol 1993; 34:324–330.
81. Antonni A, Vontobel P, Psylla M, Gunther I, Maguire PR, Missimer J, Leenders KL. Complementary positron emission tomographic studies of the striatal dopaminergic system in Parkinson's disease. Arch Neurol 1995; 52:1183–1190.
82. Boecker H, Weindl A, Leenders K, Antonini A, Kuwert T, Kruggel F, Grafin von Einsiedel H, Conrad B. Secondary parkinsonism due to focal substantia nigra lesions: regional cerebral glucose utilization and dopa-decarboxylase studied using PET. Acta Neurol Scand 1996; 93:387–392.
83. Antonini, A, Moeller JR, Nakamura T, Spetsicris P, Dhawan V, Eidelberg D. The metabolic anatomy of tremor in Parkinson's disease. Neurology 1998; 57:803–810.
84. Volkmann J, Joliot M, Mogilner A, Ioannides AA, Lado F, Fazzini E, Ribary U, Llinas R. General motor look oscillations in parkinsonian resting tremor revealed by magnetoencephalography. Neurol 1996; 46:1359–1370.
85. Lenz FA, Tasker RR, Schnider S, Kwong R, Murayama Y, Dostrovsky JO, Murphy JT. Single-unit analysis of the human ventral thalamic nuclear group: correlation of thalamic "tremor cells" with the 3–6 Hz component of parkinsonian tremor. J Neurosci 1988; 8:754–764.
86. Burchiel KJ. Thalamotomy for movement disorders. Funct Neurosurg 1995; 6:55–71.
87. Brooks DJ. Functional imaging of Parkinson's disease: is it possible to detect brain areas for specific symptoms? J Neurol Transm Suppl 1999; 56:139–153.
88. Maraganore DM, O'Conner MK, Bower JH, Kuntz KM, McDonnell SK, Schaid DJ, Rocca WA. Detection of preclinical Parkinson's disease in at-risk family members with use of (123I) beta-CT and SPECT: an exploratory study. Mayo Clin Proc 1999; 74:681–685.

89. Halliwell B. Oxidants and human disease: some new concepts. FASEB J 1987; 1:358–364
90. Simonian NA, Coyle JT. Oxidative stress in neurodegenerative diseases. Annu Rev Pharmacol Toxicol 1996; 36:83–106.
91. Bowling AC, Beal MF. Bioenergetic and oxidative stress in neurodegenerative diseases. Life Sci 1995; 56:1151–1171.
92. Jenner P, Olanow CW. Understanding cell death in Parkinson's disease. Ann Neurol 1998; 44(1):S72–S84.
93. McCord JM. Oxygen-derived free radicals in postischemic tissue injury. N Engl J Med 1985; 312:159–163.
94. Simonian NA, Coyle JT. Oxidative stress in neurodegenerative diseases. Annu Rev Pharmacol Toxicol 1996; 36:83–106.
95. Olanow CW, Arendash GW. Metals and free radicals in neurodegeneration. Curr Opin Neurol 1994; 7:548–558.
96. Marsden CD, Olanow CW. The cause of Parkinson's disease are being unraveled and rational neuroprotective therapy is close to reality. Ann Neurol 1998; 44(1):S189–S196.
97. Adams JD Jr, Odunze IN. Oxygen free radicals and Parkinson's disease. Free Radic Biol Med 1991; 10:161–169.
98. Freeman BA, Crapo JD. Biology of disease: free radicals and tissue injury. Lab Invest 1982; 47:412–426.
99. Dexter DT, Carter CJ, Wells FR, Javoy-Agid F, Agid Y, Lees A, Jenner P, Marsden CD. Basal lipid peroxidation in substantia nigra is increased in Parkinson's disease. J Neurochem 1989; 52:381–389.
100. Jenner P, Dexter DT, Sian J, Schapira AH, Marsden CD. Oxidative stress as a cause of nigral cell death in Parkinson's disease and incidental Lewy body disease. The Royal Kings and Queens Parkinson's Disease Research Group. Ann Neurol. 1992; 32(Supp 1):S82–S87.
101. Sian J, Dexter DT, Lees AJ, Daniel S, Agid Y, Javoy-Agid F, Jenner P, Marsden CD. Alterations in glutathione levels in Parkinson's disease and other neurodegenerative disorders affecting basal ganglia. Ann Neurol 1994; 36:348–355.
102. Oliver CN, Ahn BW, Moerman EJ, Goldstein S, Stadtman ER. Age-related changes in oxidized proteins. J Biol Chem 1987; 262:5488–5491.
103. Smith CD, Carney JM, Starke-Reed PE, Oliver CN, Stadtman ER, Floyd RA, Markesbery WR. Excess brian protein oxidation and enzyme dysfunction in normal aging and in Alzheimer disease. Proc Natl Acad Sci USA 1991; 88:10540–10543.
104 Alam ZI, Daniel SE, Lees AJ, Marsden DC, Jenner P, Halliwell B. A generalised increase in protein carbonyls in the brain in Parkinson's but not incidental Lewy body disease. J Neurochem 1997; 69:1326–1329.
105. Floor E, Wetzel MG. Increased protein oxidation in human substantia nigra pars compacta in comparison with basal ganglia and prefrontal cortex measured with an improved dinitrophenylhydrazine assay. J Neurochem 1998; 70:268–275.
106. Sofic E, Riederer P, Heinsen H, Beckmann H, Reynolds GP, Hebenstreit G, Youdim MB. Increased iron (III) and total iron content in post mortem substantia nigra of parkinsonian brain. J Neural Transm 1988; 74:199–205.
107. Hirsch EC, Faucheux BA. Iron metabolism and Parkinson's disease. Mov Disord 1998; 13(1):39–45.
108. Ben-Shachar D, Riederer P, Youdim MB. Iron-melanin interaction and lipid peroxidation: implications for Parkinson's disease. J Neurochem 1991; 57:1609–1614.
109. Logroscino G, Marder K, Graziano J, Freyer G, Slavkovich V, LoIacono, N, Cote L, Mayeux R. Altered systemic iron metabolism in Parkinson's disease. Neurology 1997; 49:714–717.
110. Faucheux BA, Hauw JJ, Agid Y, Hirsch EC. The density of [125I]-transferrin binding sites on perikarya of melanized neurons of the substantia nigra is decreased in Parkinson's disease. Brain Res. 1997; 749:170–174.
111. Devasagayam TP, Steenken S, Obendorf MS, Schulz WA, Sies H. Formation of 8-hydroxy (deoxy) guanosine and generation of strand breaks at guanine residues in DNA by singlet oxygen. Biochem 1991; 30:6283–6289.
112. Brawn K, Fridovich I. DNA strand scission by enzymically generated oxygen radicals. Arch Biochem Biophys 1981; 206:414–419.
113. Wallace DC. Mitochondrial genetics: a paradigm for aging and degenerative diseases? Science 1992; 256:628–632.
114. Mizuno Y, Hattori N, Matsumine H. Neurochemical and neurogenetic correlates of Parkinson's disease. J Neurochem 1998; 71:893–902.
115. Schapira AH., Cooper JM, Dexter D, Clark JB, Jenner P, Marsden CD. Mitochondrial complex I deficiency in Parkinson's disease. J Neurochem. 1990; 54:823–827.
116. Parker WD Jr, Boyson SJ, Parks JK. Abnormalities of the electron transport chain in idiopathic Parkinson's disease. Ann Neurol 1989; 26:719–723.
117. Schoffner JM, Watts RL, Juncos JL, Torroni A, Wallace DC. Mitochondrial oxidative phosphorilation defects in Parkinson's disease. Ann Neurol 1991; 30:332–339.
118. Langston JW, Irwin I, Lanston EB, Forno LS. Methyl-4-phenylpyridinium ion (MPP+): identification of a metabolite of MPTP, a toxin selective to the substantia nigra. Neurosci Lett 1984; 48:87–92.
119. Namura I, Douillet P, Sun CJ, Pert A, Cohen RM, Chiueh CC. MPP+ (1-methyl-4-phenylpyridine) is a neurotoxin to dopamine, norepineprine- and serotonin-containg neurons. Eur J Pharmacol 1987; 136:31–37.
120. Nicklas WJ, Vyas I and Heikkila RE. Inhibition of NADH-linked oxidation in brain mitochondria by N-methyl-4-phenylpyridine, a metabolite of the neurotoxin N-methyl-4-phenyl l-1,2,5,6-tetrahydropyridine. Life Sci 1985; 36:2503–2508.
121. Langston JW, Irwin I, Lanston EB, Forno LS. Pargyline prevents MPTP-induced parkinsonism in primates. Science 1984; 225:1480–1482.
122. Ramsay RR, Salach JI, Dadgar J, Singer TP. Inhibition of mitochondrial NADH dehydrogenase by pyridine derivatives and its possible relation to experimental idiopathic parkinsonism. Biochem Biophys Res Commun 1986; 135:269–275.
123. Volterra A. Inhibition of high-affinity glutamate transport in neuronal and glial cells by arachidonic

124. Volterra A, Trotti D, Racagni G. Glutamate uptake is inhibited by arachidonic acid and oxygen radicals via two distinct and additive mechanisms. J Pharmacol Exp Ther 1994; 46:986–992.

125. Garthwaite J, Boulton CL. Nitric oxide signaling in the central nervous system. Annu Rev Physiol 1995; 57:683–706.

126. Trotti D, Rossi D, Gjesdal O, Levy LM, Racagni G, Danbolt NC, Volterra A. Peroxynitrite inhibits glutamate transporter subtypes. J Biol Chem 1996; 271: 5976–5979.

(continued from previous) acid and oxygen-free radicals. Molecular mechanisms and neuropathological relevance. Renal Physiol Biochem 1994; 17:165–167.

11. Degenerative Diseases of the Cerebellum

UMBERTO DE GIROLAMI AND MEL FEANY

For the past 200 years, the cerebellum has been recognized to be of fundamental importance in the modulation, planning, and control of movement. For historical overviews of cerebellar functional anatomy, the reader is referred to the selected studies cited in the References section.[1–8] Landmark studies on the microscopic anatomy of the cerebellum include those performed at the turn of the century by Golgi[9] and Ramón y Cajal[10] (Fig. 11–1A; see also reviews by Jansen and Brodal.[11,12]). The magnificently illustrated textbook by Palay and Chan-Palay gives a comprehensive account of the ultrastructural anatomy of the cerebellar cortex and remains current 25 years after publication.[13] It has long been recognized that there is a group of slowly progressive, often hereditary, "degenerative" diseases of the nervous system that involve principally the cerebellum and its afferent and efferent connections. The seminal publication by Greenfield in 1954 forms the basis for morphologic classification of the spinocerebellar degenerations[14] (Fig. 11–1B). Koeppen[15] has recently reviewed the neuropathology and genetics of the hereditary ataxias. Comprehensive accounts of the epidemiologic and clinical aspects of this group of diseases are available in several texts.[16–19] In this chapter we first provide a general review of the functional neuroanatomy of the cerebellum, then briefly discuss the clinical aspects of cerebellar disease, with particular emphasis on the hereditary ataxias. Lastly, we discuss in depth the neuropathologic and genetic aspects of the hereditary cerebellar ataxias, particularly of those illnesses that begin or extend well into adulthood.

ANATOMIC CONSIDERATIONS

Macroscopic Anatomy and General Organization

The human cerebellum, together with the cerebrum and brain stem, is one of the three major subdivisions of the brain, accounting for about 10% of its total volume and 50% of the total neuronal population, and taking up about 80% of the content of the posterior fossa. It is a bihemispheral structure overlying the fourth ventricle, joined at the midline by the vermis and connected to the brain stem via the superior, middle, and inferior cerebellar peduncles. The cerebellum is organized anatomically into an outer region of gray matter (the cerebellar cortex), a deeper subcortical portion (the corpus medullare—the subcortical white matter containing the afferent and efferent fiber systems), and the cerebellar peduncles and a paraventricular region (containing the paired cerebellar or roof nuclei—dentate, emboliform, globose, fastigial; in lower vertebrates the emboliform and globose nuclei are fused into the nucleus interpositus). Topographic regions of the cerebellum can also be separated on the basis phylogenetic age and functional domains into three regions:[20] (1) the relatively newer *neocerebellum*, or *cerebrocerebellum*, (most of the hemispheres and midportion of vermis), which is responsible for coordination of motor function and other poorly understood functions, discussed below; (2) the older *paleocerebellum*, or *spinocerebellum*, (portions of the anterior lobe, vermis, and paraflocular regions), which is concerned with the regulation of muscle tone; and (3) the oldest region, the *archicerebellum*, or vestibulocerebellum, (paired flocculi and nodulus), which is closely related to the vestibular system.

Functional Neuroanatomic Connections

The afferent and efferent cerebellar connections are summarized briefly below. *Afferent* projections to the cerebellum include olivocerebellar fibers, spinocerebellar tracts, corticopontocerebellar systems, vestibulocerebellar tracts, and reticulocerebellar tracts. There are two categories of afferent fibers to the cerebellar cortex: *climbing fibers* and *mossy fibers*. These two populations of afferents are present within all three divisions of the cerebellum. The axons of neurons of the inferior olivary nuclei and accessory olivary nuclei (olivocerebellar) are distributed as climbing fibers to the contralateral Purkinje cells throughout the cortex of cerebellar hemispheres and vermis and also to cerebellar nuclei. Olivocerebellar fibers form the largest component of the inferior cerebellar peduncle (restiform body). The other afferent fiber system, the mossy fibers, arise from spinal (spinocerebellar), brain stem (reticulocerebellar, vestibulocerebellar), and pontine (pontocerebellar) neurons and terminate as "rosettes" on the claw-like dendrites of several granule cells in complex synapses (glomeruli). The spinocerebellar system conveys impulses concerning proprioception from the legs and trunk, which enter the cord via posterior roots. These posterior root fibers send axon terminals to synapse with the neurons of Clarke's column in the thoracolumbar cord, among other synaptic targets. These neurons, in turn, give rise to the dorsal spinocerebellar tract (uncrossed), which continues into the inferior cerebellar peduncle to terminate in the granule layer of the cerebellum. Spinal border cells located in the anterior horn of the lumbosacral segments send crossed fibers into the ventral spinocerebellar tract, which enters the cerebellum with the superior cerebellar peduncle. The corresponding fiber system to the dorsal spinocerebellar tract from the arms and neck makes synaptic connections with neurons of the external cuneate nucleus in the low medulla (cuneocerebellar) and continues to the cerebellum in the inferior cerebellar peduncle. Reticulocerebellar fibers originating from several of the brain stem reticular nuclei enter the cerebellum via the superior, inferior, and middle cerebellar peduncles and are distributed principally to the flocculonodular lobe, vermis/paravermian areas, and to the roof nuclei. Primary vestibulocerebellar fibers originating from the semicircular canals, utricle, and saccule project ipsilaterally to the flocculonodular lobe. Fibers originating from the inferior and, to some extent, medial, vestibular nuclei (secondary) enter the juxtarestiform body and terminate bilaterally in portions of the cerebellar hemispheres, vermis, and fastigial nuclei. Virtually all regions of the cerebral cortex send corticopontine axons to the griseum pontis—these axons are the major input of that structure. The griseum pontis (pontine nuclei) in turn sends pontocerebellar axons across the midline, which form the middle cerebellar peduncle and end in virtually all regions of the cerebellar cortex (except the nodulus). All major lobes of the cerebral cortex also send a much smaller contingent of axons to the ipsilateral inferior olivary complex, which receives additional inputs from the red nucleus, the spinal cord, and other structures. The tectum also sends information to the cerebellum by way of axon pathways that make synaptic connections in the griseum pontis and enter the cerebellum via the middle cerebellar peduncle.

Cerebellar efferents arise either from the cerebellar cortex or from the cerebellar nuclei and are distinct for the different cerebellar units. The Purkinje cell axon in the cerebellar cortex is the foremost efferent fiber, making ipsilateral connections from the hemispheres to the dentate nucleus or exiting the cerebellum directly from the paleo- and archicerebellar cortex (e.g., cerebellovestibular projections). Ipsilateral connections between the Purkinje cells of the vermis/flocculonodular regions of the cortex and the globose and emboliform nuclei also exist. The most massive emerging fiber system arises from the dentate through the ipsilateral superior cerebellar pe-

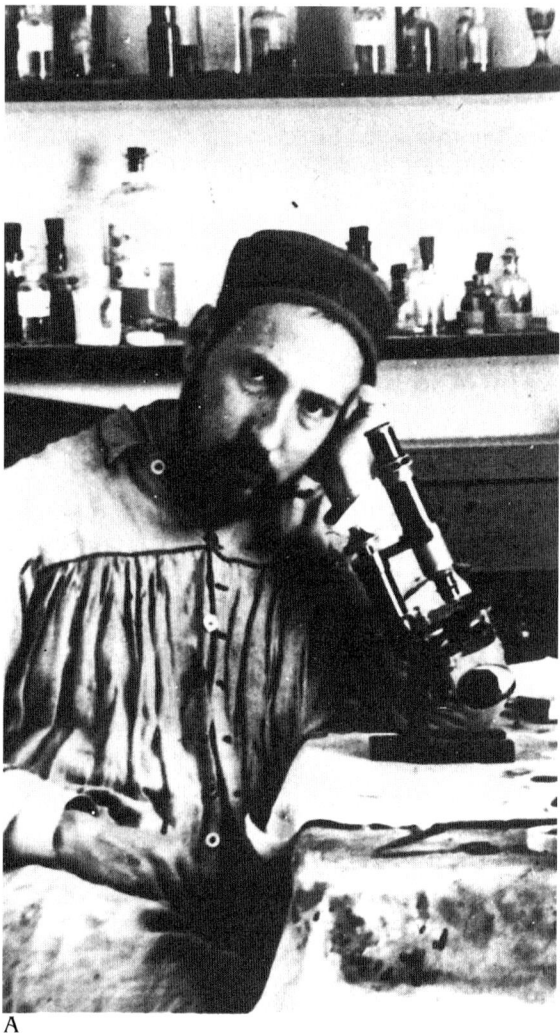

Figure 11-1. Historic figures. A. Santiago Ramon y Cajal, pioneer neurohistologist, described the detailed microscopic anatomy of the cerebellum. B. J. Goodwin Greenfield introduced a comprehensive neuropathologic classification of the spinocerebellar degenerations.

duncle, crosses the midline anterior to the inferior colliculi, and continues rostrally through and around the red nucleus to the thalamus (dentatorubrothalamic projection). Some of these fibers connect with the anterior portions of the red nuclei, tectal nuclei, and oculomotor nuclei, but most of them proceed forward to make synaptic connections with the ventrolateral (VL) nucleus of the thalamus. Still others connect with ventral posterolateral (VPL; pars oralis) and other (intralaminar, mediodorsal) nuclei of the thalamus. From the thalamus the efferent fibers project mainly to the motor parts of the cerebrum. Thus a circuit is completed whereby the cerebrum is connected with the cerebellum via the corticopontocerebellar system and receives information from it via the dentatorubrothalamic system.

Other axons from dentate nucleus neurons traveling the superior cerebellar peduncle ascend uncrossed and a third contingent turns sharply, descending to the pons and medulla to terminate in the lateral vestibular nucleus (Deiter's), the paramedian reticular nuclei, reticulotegmental nuclei, and inferior olivary nuclei. Fibers exiting the cerebellum in the superior cerebellar peduncle and emerging from the emboliform and globose nuclei project to the contralateral caudal red nucleus and to different regions of the same nuclei of

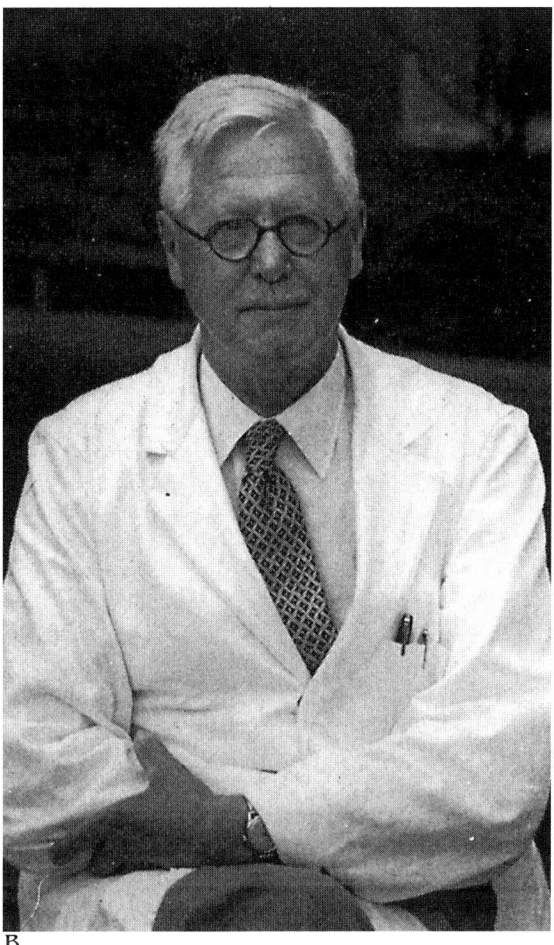
B

the thalamus as fibers from the dentate nucleus. Fastigial nucleus axons exit the cerebellum largely in the contralateral uncinate fasciculus (of Russell), which curves over the superior cerebellar peduncle, but some also emerge ipsilaterally in the juxtarestiform body. These fastigial projections terminate in multiple nuclei of the brain stem: fastigiovestibular, fastigioreticular projections are bilateral projections that go to the lateral and inferior vestibular nuclei; other projections go to pontine nuclei; and ascending projections go to the superior colliculus and the thalamus. The fastigial projections also terminate in the anterior horns of the cervical spinal cord (fastigiospinal).

Some Purkinje cell axons exit the cerebellum without making synaptic contact with the cerebellar nuclei. The cell bodies of these cerebellovestibullar fibers, located in the paleo- and archicerebellum, emerge ipsilaterally to reach the lateral and inferior vestibular nuclei (vermis), superior and medial vestibular nuclei (flocculus) superior, and the medial and inferior vestibular nuclei (nodulus and uvula). For further details, the reader is referred to standard texts.[8,21]

Microscopic Anatomy

Most of the cerebellar cortex is thrown into folds, called "folia." Histologically, the folia are quite uniform, regardless of their anatomic position, and are composed of a regular array of cells organized into three strata: *molecular, Purkinje cell,* and *granular cell layers*. There are five major types of neurons in the cerebellar cortex: Purkinje, granule, Golgi type II, basket, and stellate cells. The *Purkinje cell* (Fig. 11–2), located in the single-cell Purkinje cell layer of the cerebellar cortex, is a remarkable cell with an enormous arborization of dendrites that are flattened in the sagittal plane and arrayed vertically through the molecular layer like a climbing plant on a trellis. The Purkinje cell neuron has a flask-shaped cell body with a single stout axon that descends on one of the neurons of the nuclei of the cerebellum. Some of these Purkinje cell axons also send off a collateral branch to make synaptic contact with Golgi neurons, while others exit the cerebellum without making contact with the roof nuclei. The granule cells, situated in the granular cell layer of the cerebellar cortex, are among the smallest neurons in the nervous system, and their packing density is remarkable. Granule cells and their claw-like dendrites form small aggregates (glomeruli) around mossy afferent fiber branches (mossy fiber rosettes). Their very thin axons course upward, and when they reach the molecular layer, they branch at right angles and run in transversely oriented, closely packed bundles (parallel fibers) to make synaptic contacts with Purkinje cells. In the molecular layer granule cell axons also make synaptic contacts with stellate and basket cells and Golgi neurons. The cell bodies of Golgi neurons are located throughout the granular and Purkinje cell layers; their dendrites extend to the molecular layer and their axons make synaptic contacts with cerebellar glomeruli. The molecular layer is composed largely of the dendritic arborization of the Purkinje cells and their synaptic connections with granule cell axons. In addition, the outer portions contain the cell bodies and dendrites of stellate cells and, in the deeper layers, those of the basket cells. Stellate cells are small neurons that make synaptic contacts with Purkinje cell dendrites. Basket cell neurons are located near the Purkinje cell body and have long axons running deep and at right angles to the parallel fibers with collaterals that enmesh and make synaptic contacts with as many as 150 Purkinje cell bodies. These "baskets" enveloping the Purkinje cell soma may contain the axon terminals of as many as 30 basket cells. Glial cells (astrocytes, oligodendrocytes, ependyma, and microglia) populate the cerebellar gray and white matter, as they do other parts of the brain. Protoplasmic astrocytes in the cerebellar cortex have been subdivided on the basis of their morphology and anatomic position: lamellar astrocytes reside in the granular cell layer; and Bergmann astrocytes (Golgi "epithelial" cells) and the feathery cells of Fañanas reside in the Purkinje cell layer (some researchers believe that Bergmann and Fañanas astrocytes are identical). Bergmann astrocytes are believed to be developmentally related to radial glia, whose function is to guide the migration of Purkinje cells and granule cells from their origin in the paraventricular region and the outer cortex, respectively, to their final position.

Cerebellar Cortical Circuitry

Figure 11–3 is a schematic drawing of the cerebellar cortical circuitry, described here briefly (see also original work by Llinás[22] and recent reviews[23]). Afferent climbing fiber cerebellar projections (olivocerebellar) make multiple synaptic contacts with the smooth, proximal portions of Purkinje cell dendrites and are excitatory inputs; afferent mossy (pontocerebellar, vestibulocerebellar, reticulocerebellar, spinocerebellar) fibers terminating on granule cells have an excitatory input. Granule cell neurons have unmyelinated axons that extend upward into the molecular layer, where they bifurcate (parallel fibers) and course transversely to Purkinje dendrites upon whose terminal spines they make synaptic contacts; they thus impart excitatory inputs to rows of Purkinje cells, as well as to interneurons. Basket cells, situated deep in the molecular layer, and stellate cells in the superficial parts of the cortex are also stimulated by granule cells. The axons of basket cells, which run in the sagittal plane and envelop rows of Purkinje cells so that their influence is widely distributed, are believed to inhibit the Purkinje cells. Golgi cell axon terminals invade the mossy fiber–granule cell dendrite glomeruli exerting inhibitory influence. This geometric arrangement of cell processes allows a given series of Purkinje cells to be stimulated while the adjacent ones

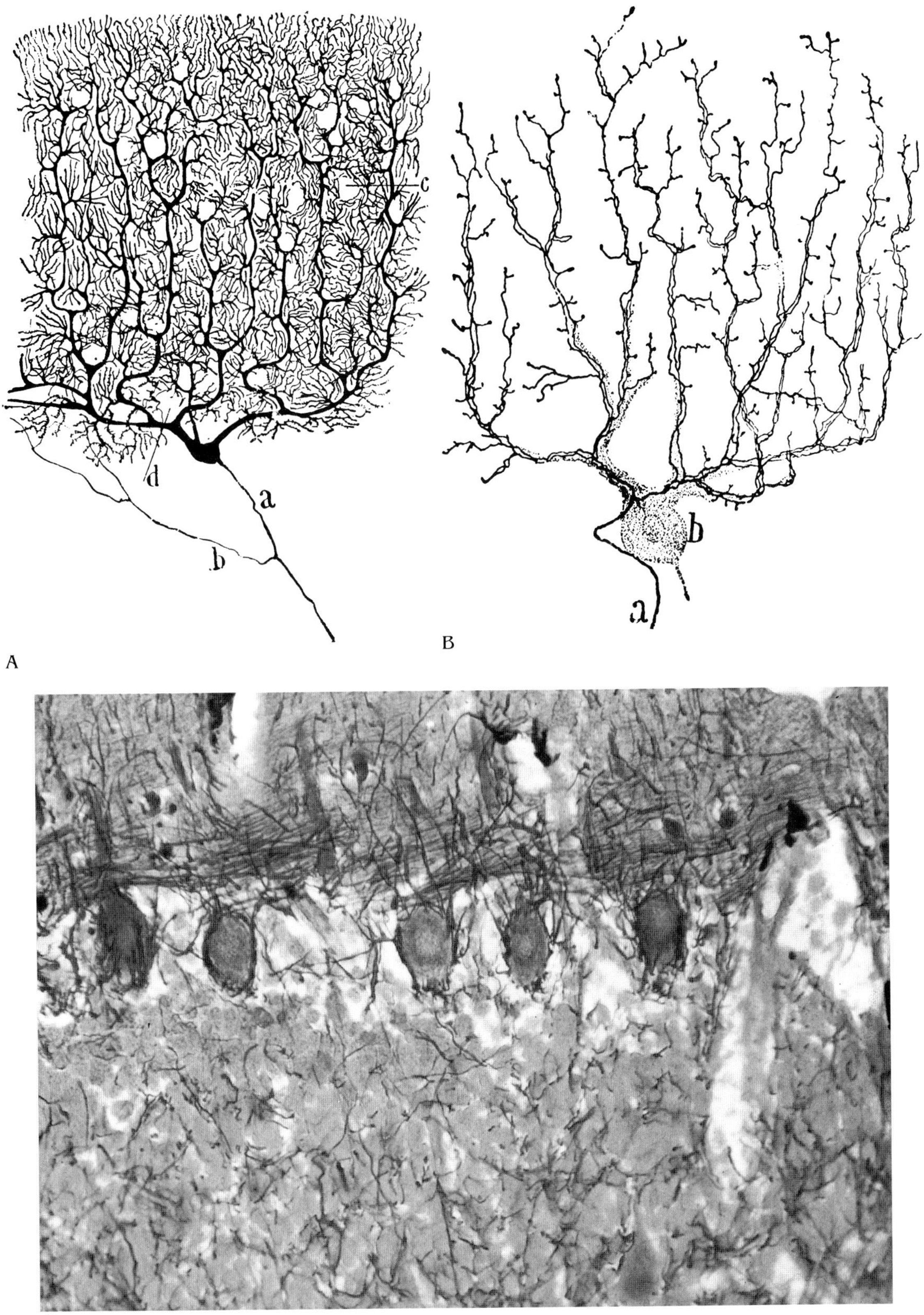

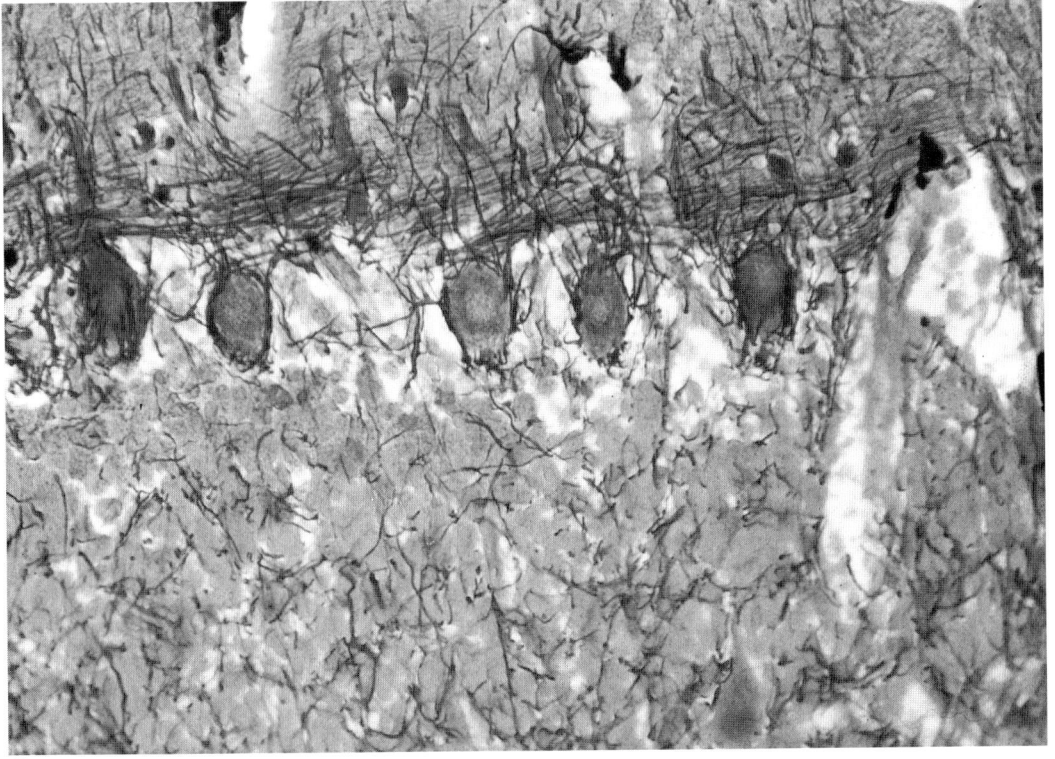

Figure 11–2. Cells of the cerebellum. A. Drawing of Purkinje cell stained with Golgi method showing dendritic arborization: (a) axon, (b) collateral branch (c) and (d) spaces within the arborization for stellate cells B. Drawing of Purkinje cell body (b) with dendritic arborization intertwined by climbing fiber branches (a) [From Ramón y Cajal,[10] with permission.] C. Cerebellar cortex showing Purkinje cells within baskets. Bielschowsky, ×400.

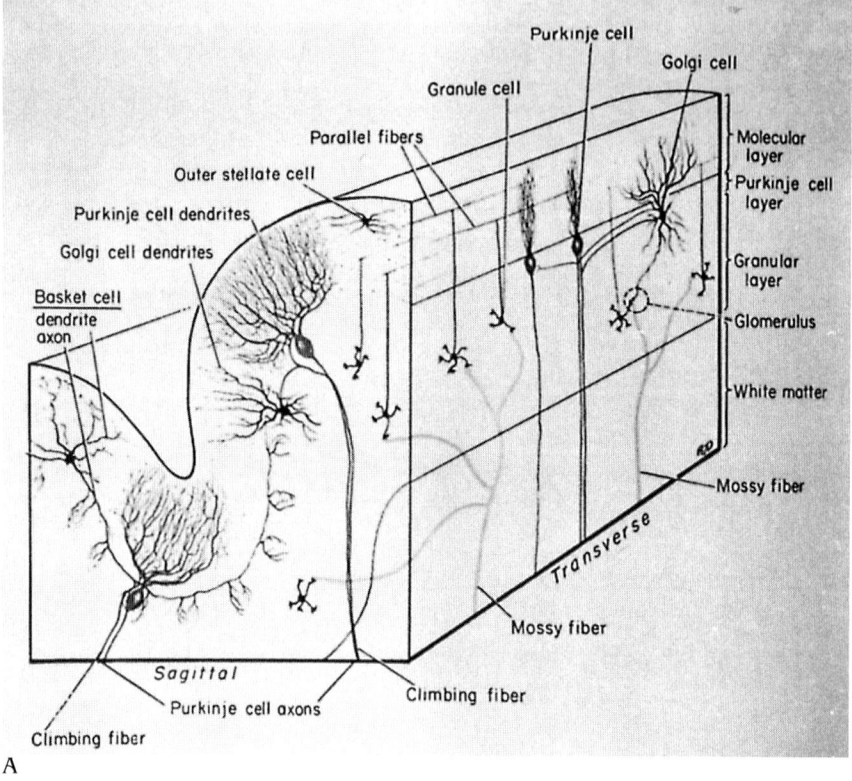

Figure 11–3. Drawings of functional organization of cerebellar connections. A. Cerebellar cortex in sagittal and transverse planes showing cell and fiber organization. B. Cellular and fiber elements of the cerebellar cortex in the longitudinal axis of a folium. [A, B from Parent,[8] with permission.]

on either side are inhibited. To summarize, granule cells are excitatory while all other cells in the cerebellum are inhibitory and therefore when excited, the stellate and basket cells inhibit Purkinje neurons with which they make contact. The net effect of a localized mossy fiber input is brief firing of a sharply defined population of Purkinje cells.

Chemical Neuronatomy

Definitive data concerning types of cerebellar neurotransmitters are just beginning to be collected.[24,25] Of the five intrinsic neurons of the cerebellar cortex, three (Purkinje, Golgi, basket) have γ-aminobutyric acid (GABA) as their inhibitory neurotransmitter. Glycine is co-localized in Golgi neurons and nitric oxide synthase (NOS) in basket cells. The inhibitory neurotransmitter of stellate cells is uncertain, but taurine is a likely candidate. The excitatory neurotransmitter that modulates the climbing and mossy fibers and is released by granule cells is glutamate. Purkinje cells also express various polypeptides. The neurons of the cerebellar nuclei are thought to be excitatory and glutamate and asparate are their primary neurotransmitters; a population of inhibitory GABAergic neurons is also recognized. Aminergic, afferent fiber systems from the brain stem to the cerebellum are also known to exist, including (1) serotonergic projections from the raphe nuclei to the cerebellar cortex and nuclei; (2) noradrenergic fibers from the locus ceruleus to vermis and fastigial nucleus via the middle and superior cerebellar peduncle; and (3) dopaminergic input to the cerebellar nuclei and cortex from the substantia nigra.

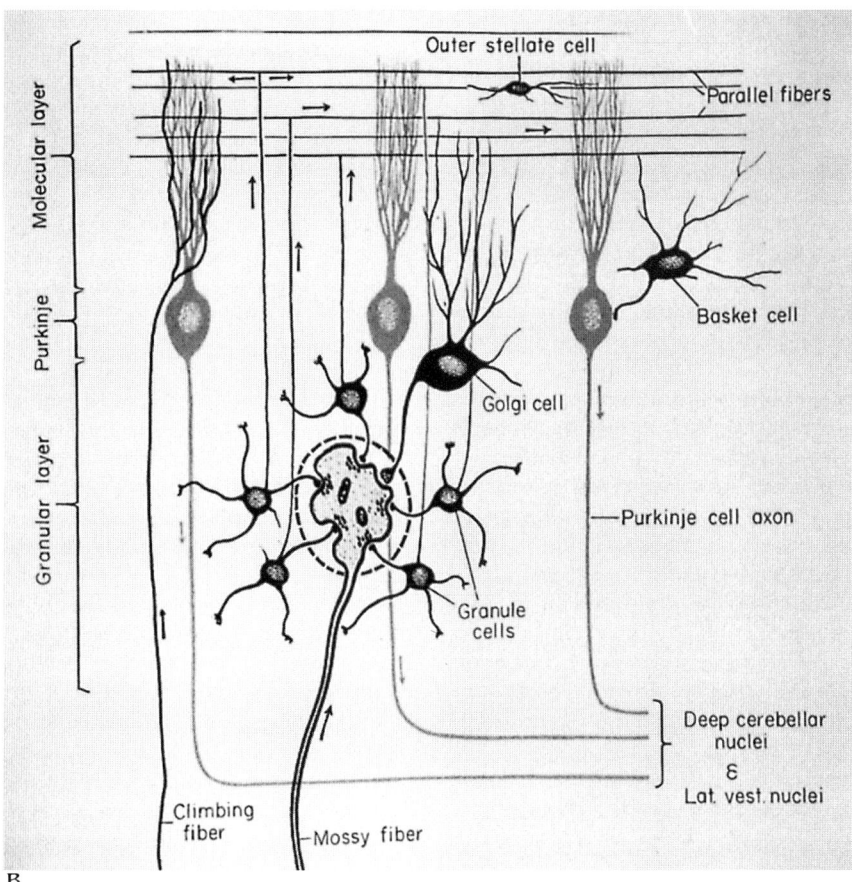

B

CLINICAL MANIFESTATIONS OF DEGENERATIVE DISEASES OF THE CEREBELLUM

Clinical Manifestations of Cerebellar Dysfunction

Disturbances in movement and posture that result from lesions of the cerebellum in human beings were first clearly documented in the clinical studies of Babinski[26,27] and Holmes,[28,29] whose observations were based on the motor status of patients with gunshot wounds sustained during World War I. From these clinical studies they concluded that the main function of the human cerebellum is to modulate and coordinate muscles in planned voluntary movements of the limbs. Without cerebellar control there is slowness in initiating movement or in arresting the movement on target. The agonist–antagonist–agonist sequence is disturbed, resulting in hypermetria (overshoot) or hypometria (undershoot or failure to reach the target) in a single, swift movement. Important signs and symptoms of cerebellar disease include hypotonia, incoordination of limbs (dysmetria), speech (dysarthria) and eye movements (nystagmus), tremor, and disorders of equilibrium and gait (see discussion by Adams et al.[18]). Controversy exists as to whether nystagmus should be considered a symptom of "cerebellar pathway" dysfunction rather than a manifestation of a purely cerebellar lesion.

Hypotonia is usually a clinical manifestation of an acute cerebellar lesion; the phenomenon is inconsistently displayed in chronic cerebellar diseases and it is presumably based on a reduction in activity of muscle spindle fibers. The most characteristic manifestation of cerebellar dysfunction is abnormalities of volitional movement, or cerebellar incoordination (ataxia). This is manifest clinically as dyssynergia, dysmetria, and disdiadokokinesia. Myoclonic movements may be combined with cerebellar ataxia. In cerebellar dysarthria the speech is slow, effortful, and at times of uneven volume. Often the enunciation of consonants is "staccato" or poorly articulated (scanning speech). Simple tongue movements are strong enough but rapid repetitive movements are markedly slowed. The variety of clinically observed ocular movement abnormalities recorded in patients with suspected cerebellar diseases range from loss of smooth pursuit movements, dysmetria of lateral and vertical eye movements, gaze-paretic and rebound (alternating) nystagmus on attempted lateral and vertical fixation, to ocular flutter, opsoclonus, and rhythmic clonus. Patients with intention tremor have a rhythmic oscillation of an arm or leg during the performance of a projected movement, i.e., as it approaches a target. Inability to stand and walk with proper balance are widely recognized signs of cerebellar disease and they may be present even though the movements of the limbs are well coordinated. The patient may stand with feet wide apart and take steps that are uneven, with improper placement of the feet and lurching to the side, forward, or backward. The gait disorder may or may not be accompanied by a truncal and head tremor (titubation). Patients with cerebellar lesions may complain of nonrotational dizziness, made worse at times by movement, but this has not been associated with lesions of a specific part of the cerebellum.

Neuroanatomists have subdivided cerebellar syndromes into three groups on the basis of ablation studies of archicerebellar, paleocerebellar, and neocerebellar structures. In animals, the midline zone of the cerebellum, including the fastigial nuclei, participates in the control of eye movements by regulating the vestibulo-ocular reflex (interactions between floculonodular lobe and vestibular nuclei) and the maintenance of body equilibrium. The intermediate zone, if damaged, results in tremor of the trunk and legs and ataxia of these parts, with stiffening of legs and a wide stance, probably the result of voluntary correction. The syndrome of the neocerebellum causes ataxia of the limbs, dysarthria, nystagmus, and other ocular disorders.

Neuropathologists have encountered difficulty in attempting to match clinical syndromes in humans to the three anatomic divisions of the cerebellum. Part of the problem may be due to the fact that the connections of these functional zones in human beings are more widely organized. Thus the midline zone receives information from the cerebrum as well as the vestibular nuclei. The midline zone sends projections rostrally as well as to the spinal cord and the lateral zone connects with the spinal cord as well as the forebrain.

While "classic" types of degenerative diseases of the cerebellum exist, many patients with these illnesses show aberrant and transitional forms on both clinical examination and neuropathologic study. Furthermore, the function of a large part of the human neocerebellum is very poorly understood and is not easily testable by clinical examination. However, researchers have learned that portions of the so-called silent cerebellar cortex that are concerned with unconscious motor learning and memory of motor events may also have a role in emotion, sensory acquisition, and cognition.[30–34] Thus, a damaged cerebellar hemisphere may be discovered at postmortem examination in an individual who had no symptoms of cerebellar deficit during life. Also, cerebellar symptoms from acute cortical lesions that spare the cerebellar nuclei have a way of disappearing, a phenomenon attributed to compensation by other parts of the nervous system. Finally, it is well known that lesions of the brain stem, spinal cord, and parietal lobe may cause a cerebellar type of ataxia with no visible abnormality being noted in the cerebellum itself. This is possible because of the manifold links among the cerebellum and the cerebrum, brain stem, and spinal cord, as discussed above.

Epidemiology of Degenerative Diseases of the Cerebellum

The hereditary ataxias are uncommon. Prevalence estimates in major geographic areas range from 1 to 23 cases per 100,000 (see review[35]). Detailed epidemiologic studies in western Norway have documented the prevalence of Friedreich's ataxia (1/100,000), autosomal dominant cerebellar ataxia (ADCA) (6.4/100,000), and non-Friedreich's recessive ataxias (3/100,000[36]). In Great Britain, Friedreich's ataxia is the most common hereditary ataxia, with a prevalence of approximately 2 per 100,000.[37] The hereditary ataxias are about as common as Huntington's disease (prevalence 5–10/100,000 in the United States[38]), and are approximately 10-fold less prevalent than Parkinson's disease.[39] Specific hereditary ataxias may be substantially more common in particular geographic areas. Spinocerebellar ataxia type 3 (SCA3; Machado-Joseph disease) has a prevalence of 1 per 3600 in the Portuguese islands of the Azores, while the prevalence in mainland Portugal is 1 per 100,000.[40] One in 140 individuals is affected in the Azorean island of Flores. Similarly, the prevalence of SCA2 is as high as 133 per 100,000 in certain towns in eastern Cuba.[41] These geographic clusters of increased prevalence likely represent genetic founder effects.

CLINICAL ASPECTS, NEUROPATHOLOGY, AND GENETICS OF HEREDITARY ATAXIC DISEASES OF THE CEREBELLUM AND RELATED DISORDERS

Greenfield reviewed the many early clinical and pathologic reports of heredofamilial spinocerebellar diseases[14] and the comprehensive chapter by Ule reviews the neuropathologic studies up to 1957.[42] Over the past 20 years there has been enormous expansion in the understanding of these diseases, principally as a result of the progress in the field of molecular genetics. The discussion that follows reviews the clinical aspects and neuropathology of this group of illnesses, and what is now known of their etiology. The classification presented here is an attempt to merge traditional clinicopathologic understanding of hereditary degenerative diseases of the cerebellum with recent advances in molecular genetics. Currently, there are genetically distinct kindreds with little or neuropathologic data, as well as established clinicopathologic entities for which the molecular genetic basis is unknown. Furthermore, considerable clinical overlap exists between what are now recognized as genetically distinct hereditary ataxias. Lastly, for an important subset of these diseases, recent advances in molecular and cellular biology suggest some common underlying pathogenetic mechanisms.

Many hereditary ataxias, including Friedreich's, ataxia-telangiectasia, and other rarer, recessive ataxias, affect primarily children and young adults (see Table 11–1): only Friedreich's ataxia is discussed here in detail. The genetic defects underlying many adult hereditary ataxias have been defined (Table 11–1). Genetic data have prompted a practical reclassification of many of these disorders. For example, ADCAs classified as type I by Harding[37] now include SCAs 1, 2, and 3. The relatively pure cerebellar syndromes correspond to ADCA III of Harding, and Greenfield's Holmes type, and are represented by the SCA6 locus. Harding's ADCA II, or cerebellar ataxia with retinal degeneration, corresponds to SCA7. However, the current genetic classification remains incomplete. In 20% to 40% of families, linkage to the known hereditary ataxia loci, including SCA1–7, dentatorubral pallidoluysian atrophy (DRPLA), and Friedreich's ataxia, have been excluded.[43-45] In addition, a number of traditionally described heredofamilial spinocerebellar disorders exist. These include the non-Friedreich ataxia of Sanger Brown and others, and Ramsay-Hunt dentatorubral degeneration (reviewed by Greenfield[14]). Such classically delineated clinical and pathological entities have not yet been defined in terms of their genetic locus.

Both the ADAs and Friedreich's ataxia are caused by a specific type of genetic alteration: the expansion of a trinucleotide repeat sequence. Mutations arise when a naturally occurring, relatively short stretch of trinucleotides expands in the germline. The resulting expanded allele is transmitted to the offspring. If the expansion is long enough, clinical disease develops and the age of onset of the disease decreases as the repeat length increases. Successive generations often show genetic anticipation by expressing symptoms earlier in life, which has been associated with subsequent expansion of the repeat. Expansion of triplet repeats has been implicated in a number of neurologic disorders in addition to the hereditary ataxias, including Huntington's disease, myotonic dystrophy, spinobulbar mus-

Table 11–1. Molecular Genetics of Hereditary Ataxias

Disease	Inheritance	Chromosomal Location	Protein	Mutation
Disorders affecting older adults				
SCA1	AD	6p23	ataxin 1	CAG repeat
SCA2	AD	12q24	ataxin 2	CAG repeat
SCA3 (Machado-Joseph disease)	AD	14q32.1	ataxin 3	CAG repeat
SCA4	AD	16q22.1		
SCA5	AD	11q13.1-q13.3		
SCA6	AD	19q13	alpha-1A calcium channel	CAG repeat
SCA7	AD	3p12-13	ataxin 7	CAG repeat
Dentatorubral pallidoluysian atrophy	AD	12p13	DRPLA	CAG repeat
Episodic ataxia 1 (EA1)	AD	12p13	delayed rectifier potassium channel	P
Episodic ataxia 2 (EA2)	AD	19q13	alpha-1A calcium channel	P
Disorders typically affecting children and young adults				
Friedreich's ataxia	AR	9q13	frataxin	GAA repeat
Familial vitamin E deficiency	AR	8q13	alpha-tocopherol transfer protein	P,T
Ataxia-telangiectasia	AR	11q22	phosphatidyl-inositol 3-kinase-like	P,T,D

Ch, chromosome; P, point mutation; T, truncation; D, deletion.

cular atrophy, and the fragile X syndrome (see review by Gusella and MacDonald[46]). In Huntington's disease and the SCAs, the triplet sequence expanded is (CAG). Friedreich's ataxia patients show GAA expansions, while individuals with myotonic dystrophy have CTG repeats, and patients with fragile X have expansions of the CGG trinucleotide. Some distinct clinical features, such as genetic anticipation, are common to almost all the trinucleotide repeat disorders. However, diseases such as the ADCAs that are caused by expansion of CAG repeat sequences are clinically and pathologically distinct. A growing body of experimental evidence indicates that the observed differences reflect fundamentally different pathogenetic mechanisms. Disorders caused by CAG expansions usually show a dominant mode of inheritance, relatively late onset, and specific intranuclear inclusions. In contrast, diseases arising from expansions of the other repeat sequences are typically recessive, often affect younger individuals, and usually do not have inclusion bodies. In correlation with these clinical and neuropathological distinctions are clear molecular mechanistic differences (diagrammed in Fig. 11–4) between the two types of repeats.

In contrast to all non-CAG repeats described to date, CAG expansions are located in coding portions of the gene. The CAG trinucleotides are translated into polyglutamine stretches in the resulting protein. Although the details of the mechanism are still unclear, the polyglutamine tract apparently endows the enlarged protein with a novel, toxic activity that ultimately results in neuronal death. Much experimental work has contributed to the suggested pathogenetic hypothesis. The most important evidence is the ability to model the disorders in mice with pathologic polyglutamine expansions,[47,48] but not gene knockouts.[49] Also key is the lack of human mutations predicted to produce simple loss of

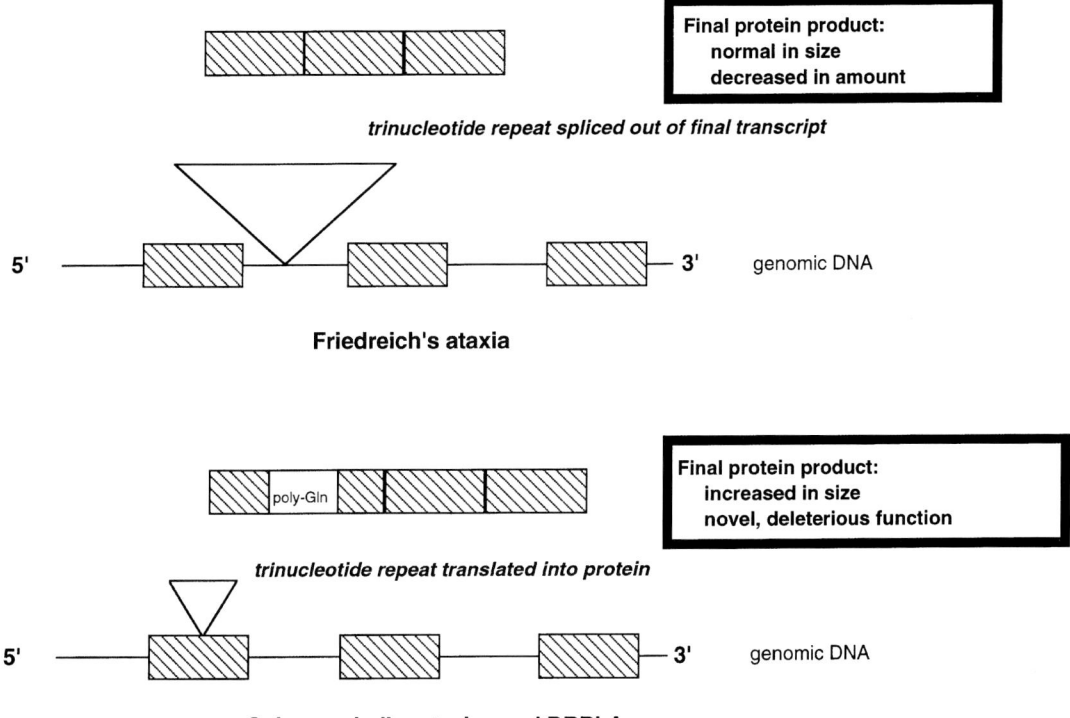

Figure 11–4. Diagram of mechanism of representative trinucleotide mutations.

gene function, such as the point mutants, truncations, and deletions observed in other types of trinucleotide disorders (see Table 11–1). The postulated toxic gain of function mechanism correlates well with the observed dominant pattern of inheritance of the SCAs and DRPLA.

Molecular insights have yet to address a number of important clinical and pathologic features of the CAG repeat disorders. As discussed in detail below for the SCAs and DRPLA, individual disorders display clear clinical and anatomic specificities. However, normal and mutant proteins are usually widely expressed throughout the nervous system. With limited exceptions, neither the normal expression pattern nor the accumulation of polyglutamine-enriched gene products reflects the neuropathologic pattern of neuronal loss and gliosis. Anatomic specificity may reflect the presence of a cofactor that does show appropriately restricted expression; such cofactors have not yet been identified. The mechanism of neuronal injury also awaits clarification. Again, interacting factors appear to be plausible mediators of cellular damage. A number of proteins that specifically interact with mutant huntingtin have been identified, but their role in the disease process remains unclear.[50]

In contrast to the polyglutamine-encoding CAG repeats, other repeat sequence expansions are located within noncoding portions of the gene. In Friedreich's ataxia the expanded GAA sequences are found within the first intron. The presence of extra sequences within the intron presumably interferes with efficient processing or translation of the mRNA transcript, resulting in markedly reduced frataxin (the gene product).[51] Most patients with Friedreich's ataxia are homozygous for an expanded GAA allele. Approximately 5% of patients carry instead an expanded allele on one chromosome and a point mutation on the opposite chromosome. The presence of point mutations in at least some patients supports a loss of function mechanism. If the disease state is produced by inadequate production of frataxin, then experimental animals carrying a targeted disruption of the frataxin gene might be ataxic. Although characterization of frataxin-negative animals has not been reported, a similar experiment was performed with the murine homolog of the fragile X gene product. Mice lacking the FMR1 product of the fragile X locus showed macroorchidism and learning defects, both features of the human disorder.[52] These results support a loss-of-function mechanism for non-coding trinucleotide expansions.

As might be expected for mutations altering protein-coding sequences, CAG repeat expansions are usually rather modest. Although there is some variability from disorder to disorder, normal CAG repeat lengths are usually between 5 to 40, whereas pathologically expanded alleles are usually between 40 and 90 repeats in length. In contrast, non-CAG, non-coding repeat expansions are often quite long. Clinically unaffected individuals typically have between 6 and 42 copies of the GAA repeat in the first intron of the frataxin gene. Friedreich's ataxia patients have between 200 and 1700 repeats.[53]

Advances in molecular genetics have not only had important implications for the classification and mechanistic understanding of the hereditary ataxias but also added to the neuropathologic understanding of these disorders. Histologic comparisons can now be made with certainty between genetically distinct disorders. In addition, development of immunologic reagents has allowed subcellular localization of the abnormal proteins. As was first demonstrated in Huntington disease,[54] nuclear inclusions are a prominent feature of CAG repeat disorders. To date, inclusions have been demonstrated in SCA1,[55,56] SCA3 (Machado-Joseph disease),[57] SCA7,[58] and DRPLA.[59] On electron microscopic examination the inclusions are a heterogeneous mixture of granular and filamentous structures. Inclusions are specifically immunolabeled with antibodies against the normal protein as well as those recognizing the abnormal repeat sequence. Many inclusions also show ubiquitin immunoreactivity. As with inclusions in many other neurodegenerative disorders, the pathogenetic significance of the nuclear inclusions remains to be demonstrated. Elegant recent experiments in a mouse model of SCA1,[60] and in cell culture,[61] suggest that although nuclear localization of the polyglutamine-containing proteins is necessary for toxicity, inclusion formation is not required for neuronal death. Further studies promise to shed additional light on the relationship of inclusion formation to disease progression in the CAG repeat disorder and perhaps in other neurodegenerative conditions.

Immunologic reagents that recognize expanded polyglutamine epitopes have not only allowed localization of the mutant proteins but also facilitated molecular and cellular analysis of previously uncharacterized ADCAs. The pathologic proteins in SCA2, SCA3, and SCA7 were all initially detected using an antibody recognizing polyglutamine-encoded epitopes.[62] Methods have also been developed to clone novel polyglutamine-encoding DNA sequences. Specific techniques for isolating abnormal CAG repeat sequences and the polyglutamine-containing proteins they encode may speed characterization of additional cerebellar ataxia loci.[63]

SPECIFIC HEREDITARY ATAXIAS

Spinocerebellar Ataxia Type 1

CLINICAL MANIFESTATIONS

The clinical and pathologic manifestations of SCA1 and those of one form of "classic," dominantly inherited disease olivopontocerebellar atrophy (OPCA), have been described.[14,64,65] However, it is now recognized that there are also other forms of OPCA that are entirely different from the SCAs and are part of the spectrum of multiple systems atrophy (MSA); these other forms do not have trinucleotide repeats and have a complex multisystem degenerative disease characterized microscopically by the presence of oligodendroglial inclusions containing α-synuclein (these are discussed in Chapter 9). The clinical syndrome of SCA1 is characterized by development of progressive cerebellar ataxia in adulthood or late mid-life. The movement disorder involves the upper and lower extremities, and in the trunk there is slowness of voluntary movements, impairment of equilibrium and gait, scanning speech, nystagmus, and tremor of the head and trunk. Pyramidal signs, amyotrophy, and sensory disturbances (posterior column function) are also seen. Dementia develops in a minority of patients; sphyncteric disturbances are commonly observed. Dysarthria, dysphagia, and involvement of cranial motor nerves (oculomotor, facial) are also observed in some patients.

MOLECULAR GENETICS AND NEUROPATHOLOGY

The wild-type SCA1 gene encodes ataxin-1, an 816 amino acid protein with no homology to previously identified molecules.[66] Ataxin-1 expression is widespread in neuronal and non-neuronal tissues.[67] A high degree of conservation is noted among species. SCA1 provided the first successful animal model of polyglutamine-mediated neurotoxicity.[47] Expression of an SCA1 transgene carrying an expanded CAG repeat produces ataxia and Purkinje cell degeneration. In contrast, mice lacking ataxin-1 are viable and fertile and do not show any evidence of ataxia or neurodegeneration.[68] The cerebellar leucine-rich acidic nuclear protein (LANP) interacts with ataxin-1 in vitro.[69] Interaction with a protein enriched in the cerebellum suggests a mechanism for some of the cellular specificity observed in SCA1; however, ataxin-1 interaction with LANP has not been demonstrated in vivo.

The neuropathology of SCA1 appears to be distinctive. In genetically confirmed cases, a relatively consistent pattern of degeneration has been observed.[70–72] On gross examination of the brain stem and cerebellum there is atrophy of the ventral pons, middle cerebellar peduncles, entire cerebellum, and inferior olives. On sectioning, basal ganglia usually appear normal, as do the substantia nigra and locus ceruleus. The dentate nucleus is markedly atrophic. The spinal cord is thin and flat. Microscopic examination (Fig. 11–5) reveals variable neuronal loss and reactive gliosis in the brain stem and spinal cord. The cerebral cortex is normal. The most constant and severe changes are seen in the cerebellar cortex, dentate nucleus, pontine nuclei, and inferior olives. In the cerebellum, Purkinje cell loss is extensive and is accompanied by Bergmann gliosis. The granule cell layer is less affected. The pathological changes are most marked in the upper vermis. Neuronal loss and gliosis may also be severe in the red nucleus, third and twelfth cranial nerve nuclei, and gracile and cuneate nuclei, but are less constant. The striatum, globus pallidus, thalamus, subthalamic nucleus, and substantia nigra are generally relatively spared (although involvement of the external pallidum is reported in patients from Japan). In the spinal cord, the posterior columns and Clarke's column are invariably atrophic and gliotic. Anterior and posterior spinocerebellar tracts show moderate myelin pallor. There is extensive anterior horn cell loss at all levels accompanied by moderate atrophy of the pyramidal tracts. The intermediolateral column is spared. Immunohistochemical studies demonstrate widespread intranuclear neuronal inclusions. Inclusions are somewhat more prominent in severely affected areas such as the pons, but are also found in unaffected areas, including the cortex.[56]

Ubiquitinated inclusions of the MSA type are not a feature of SCA1 or any of the other ADCAs examined thus far, with rare possible exceptions.[73]

Spinocerebellar ataxia type 1 is distinguished from SCA2 by involvement of the substantia nigra and relative sparing of the dentate nucleus in SCA2. In SCA3 there is variable involvement of the globus pallidus, and the subthalamic nucleus and substantia nigra, degenerate. Cerebellar Purkinje cells are mostly spared in SCA3, whereas the intermediolateral column is often involved. In DRPLA there is generally much more extensive involvement of the globus pallidus and subthalamic nucleus whereas Purkinje cells are spared.

Spinocerebellar Ataxia Type 2

CLINICAL MANIFESTATIONS

A second clinical phenotype of ADCA was described initially for Cuban pedigrees and subsequently for patients from other geographic regions.[41,75,75] Considerable clinical variability has been reported among patients with age of onset being in childhood or adulthood. Also, there is much clinical overlap with SCA1, except that some patients show less marked py-

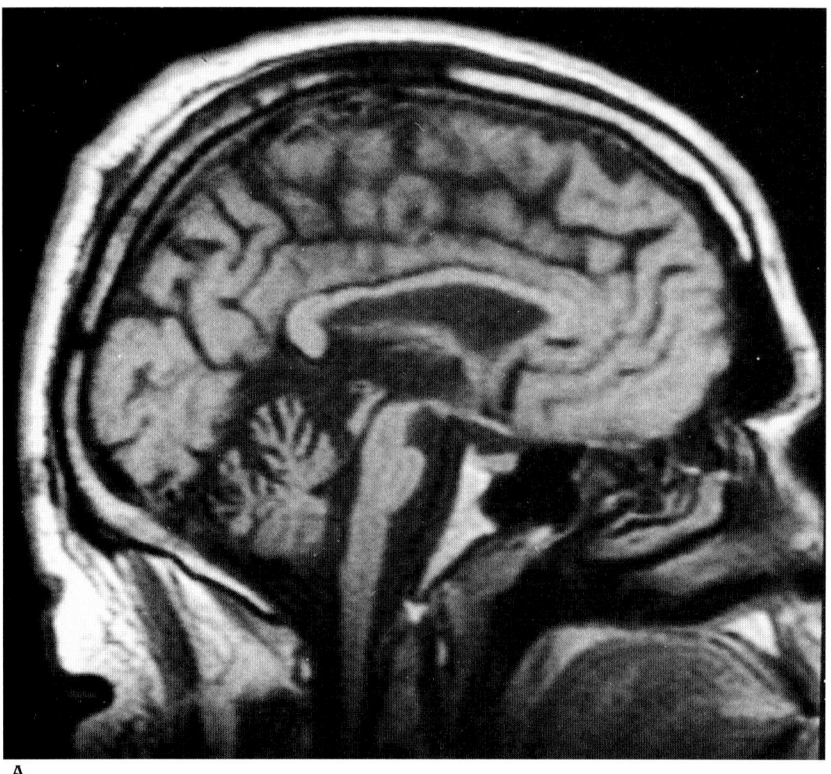

A

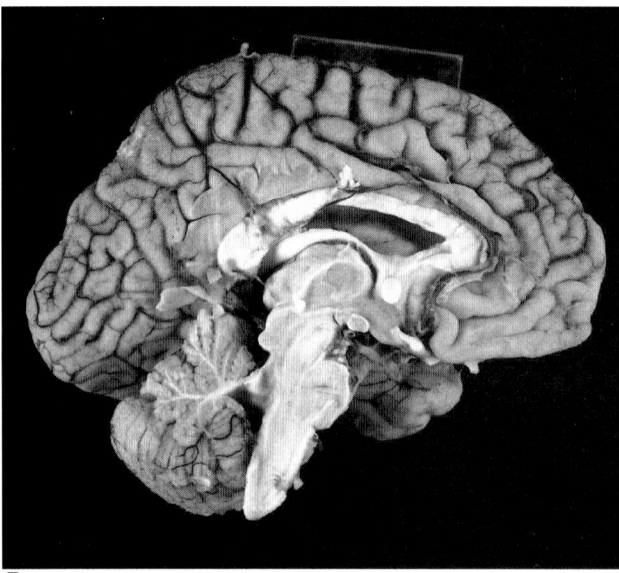

B

Figure 11–5. Spinocerebellar ataxia type 1. *A.* MRI sagittal view of brain of patient with olivopontocerebellar Atrophy OPCA; (genetics unknown) showing atrophy of vermis. [Courtesy of Dr. L. Hsu, Department of Radiology, Brigham and Women's Hospital, Boston, MA.] *B.* Sagittal view of brain. Note atrophy of vermis and some dilatation of the fourth ventricle. *C, D.* Sections of cerebellar cortex at low and high magnification showing patchy loss of Purkinje cells and gliosis. Cresyl violet stains; C: ×40, ×100. *E.* Dentate nucleus showing neuronal loss and gliosis. Cresyl violet stain, ×100. *F.* Inferior olivary nucleus showing neuronal loss and gliosis. Cresyl violet stain, ×100 [Figures B–F are courtesy of Dr. A. Koeppen, Department of Neurology, Stratton Station V.A. Medical Center, Albany, NY.] *(continued)*

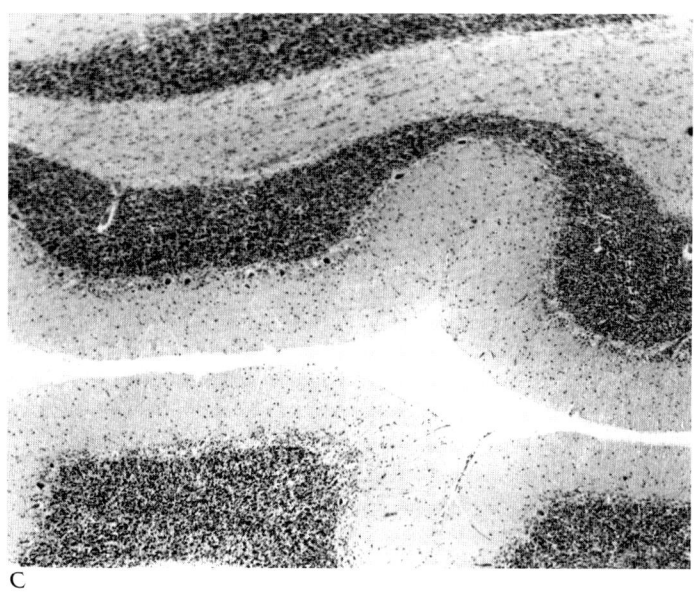

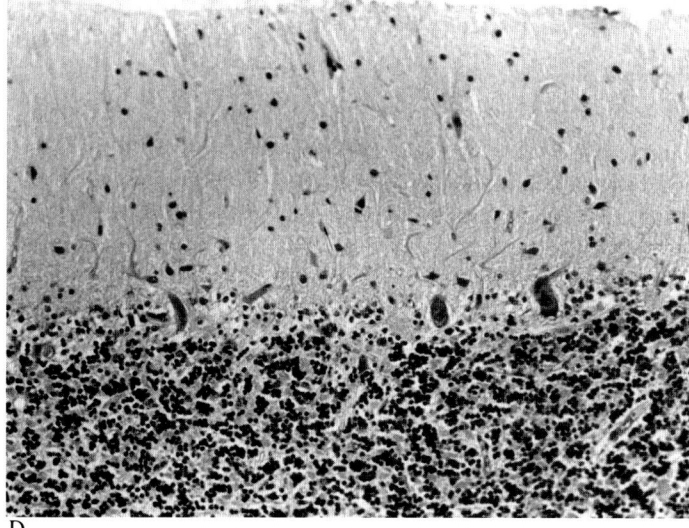

Figure 11–5. (continued)

ramidal and extrapyramidal findings. Intellectual deterioration seems to be more commonly observed in SCA2 than in SCA1.

MOLECULAR GENETICS AND NEUROPATHOLOGY

Like ataxin-1, ataxin-2 is an ubiquitously expressed protein of unknown function.[63,76,77] Repeat lengths in normal and pathologic alleles tend to be somewhat shorter in SCA2 than in most other CAG repeat genes. In addition, an unusually steep inverse relations between repeat number and age of onset suggests that the SCA2 locus is particularly sensitive to polyglutamine expansion.[75,76]

Spinocerebellar ataxia type 2 resembles SCA1 in the marked degeneration of the cerebellar cortex (Fig. 11–6A–D) pontine nuclei, and inferior olive but is distinguished by moderate to severe involvement of the substantia nigra.[41,74,78] In addition, compared to SCA1,

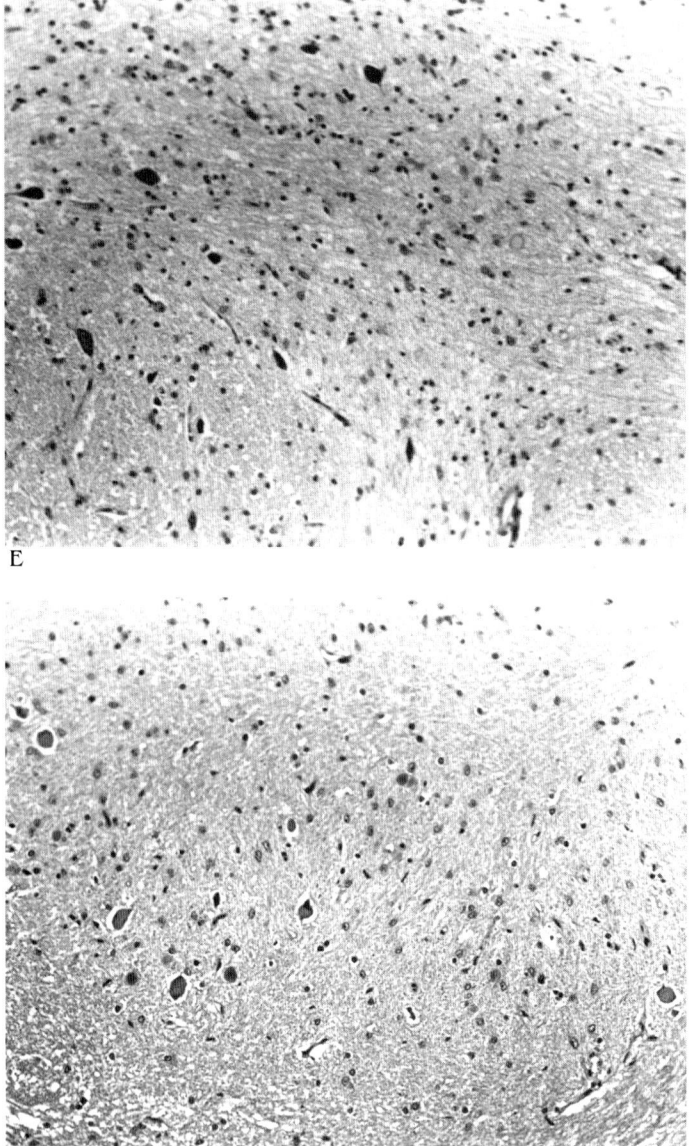

Figure 11–5.

the dentate nucleus is relatively spared in SCA2 (Fig. 11–6E), as is the red nucleus. Synaptic degeneration, as assessed by immunohistochemical testing with antibodies directed against the presynaptic protein SNAP-25, was found to be particularly severe in the cerebellar cortex and brain stem.[79] The cerebral cortex, basal ganglia, thalamus, subthalamic nucleus, and oculomotor nuclei are generally spared in SCA2, although in some cases there has been neuronal loss in the cerebral cortex. In the spinal cord, there is degeneration of the dorsal columns, Clarke's column, and the spinocerebellar tracts. The pyramidal tracts are spared.

Spinocerebellar Ataxia Type 3 (Machado Joseph Disease)

CLINICAL MANIFESTATIONS

This is a hereditary ataxia originally described in patients of Portuguese-Azorean origin, but

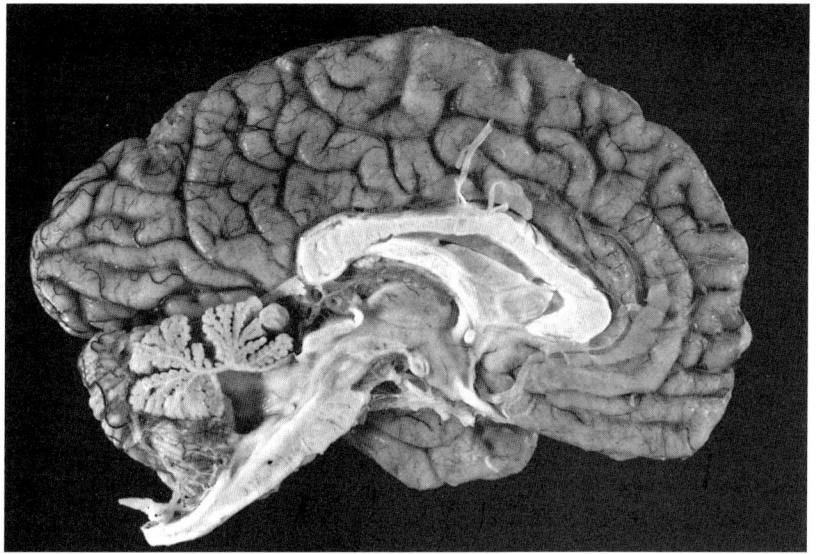

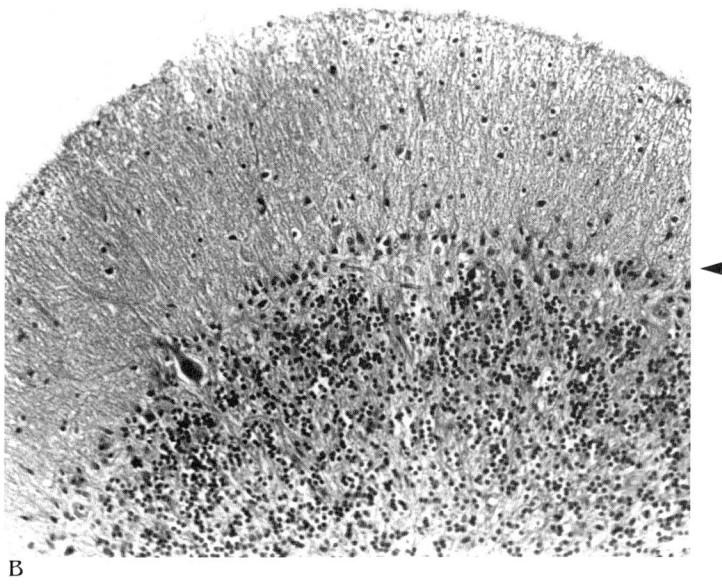

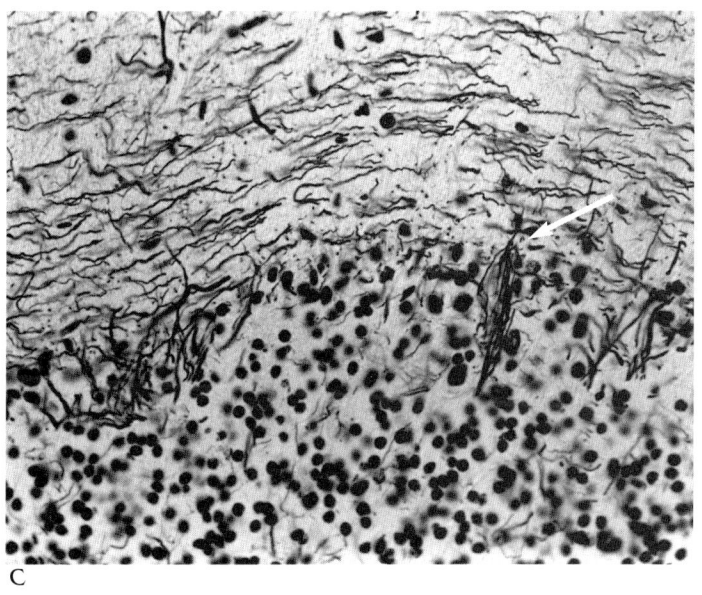

Figure 11–6. Spinocerebellar ataxia type 2. *A.* Sagittal view of brain. Note severe atrophy of vermis, small cerebellar hemisphere, and some dilatation of the fourth ventricle. *B.* Section of cerebellar cortex showing extensive loss of Purkinje cells. H&E, ×160. *C.* Section of cerebellar cortex showing loss of Purkinje cells (empty baskets). Bodian, ×400. *D.* Section of cerebellar cortex showing abnormally shaped proximal Purkinje cell axons ("torpedoes"). Immunocytochemical reaction with antibody against phosphorylated neurofilament protein (SMI-31), ×160. *(continued)*

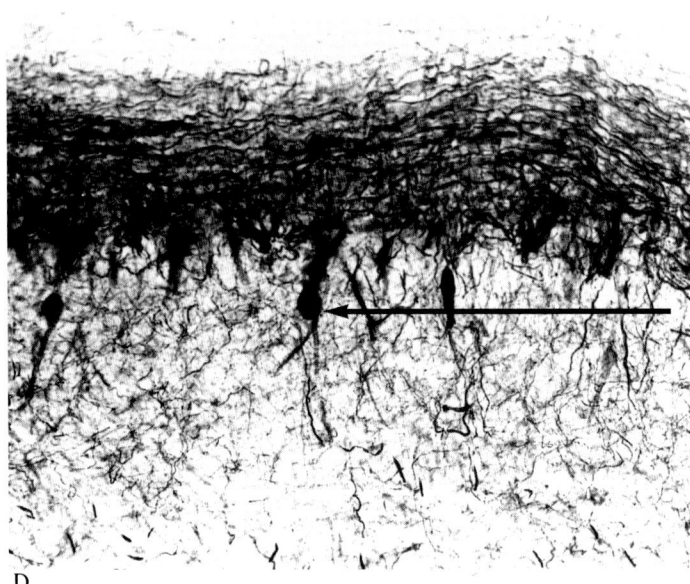

Figure 11–6.

D

it has also been recognized in individuals of other ancestry.[80–83] Several clinical phenotypes have been described, with some overlap between the subtypes.[84] This autosomal dominant disease is characterized by ataxia of gait, generally manifest first between the ages of 20 and 40, progressing to incoordination of limbs, extrapyramidal rigidity, and dysarthria. Other important clinical signs and symptoms are hyperreflexia, bulbar signs, sensory disturbances (loss of position and vibration sense), and abnormalities of eye movements (ophthalmoplegia).

MOLECULAR GENETICS AND NEUROPATHOLOGY

The SCA3 gene is alternatively spliced and encodes several isoforms of a novel, ubiquitously expressed protein.[85–87] Expression of mutant ataxin-3 causes neuronal degeneration not only in mice,[88] but also in *Drosophila*,[89] which suggests that polyglutamine proteins activate a highly conserved program of cellular injury.

The neuropathological features of SCA3 have been reported in both Azorean and non-Azorean kindreds.[71,80–82,90,91] Gross atrophy of the pontine base, cerebellum, and spinal cord may be seen (Fig. 11–7). The globus pallidus, subthalamic nucleus, and substantia nigra are often shrunken and discolored. Microscopically, neuronal loss and gliosis are most marked in the internal segment of the globus pallidus, subthalamic nucleus, dentate nucleus ("grumose degeneration"), oculomotor nuclei, spinocerebellar tracts, and Clark column. Variable involvement of the substantia nigra, hypoglossal nucleus, trigeminal nucleus, the intermediolateral column, the anterior horn of the spinal cord, and the anterior spinal roots is seen. The cerebral cortex, thalamus, striatum, inferior olivary nucleus and cerebellar Purkinje cells, and pyramidal tracts are relatively spared. Preservation of the olive and cerebellar cortex facilitates the distinction between SCA1 and SCA2.[92] In addition, the intermediolateral column is spared in SCA1.[72]

Aggregates of abnormal ataxin-3 accumulate in the nucleus and can be detected with antibodies against ataxin-3, polyglutamine epitopes, and ubiquitin. Unlike the widespread nuclear inclusions observed in SCA1, nuclear inclusions in SCA3 are apparently only detectable in affected regions of the nervous system.[87]

Spinocerebellar Ataxia Types 4 and 5

CLINICAL MANIFESTATIONS

In addition to cerebellar ataxia, clinical manifestations in these autosomal dominantly inherited ataxias have included pyramidal tract signs, a prominent peripheral sensory axonal

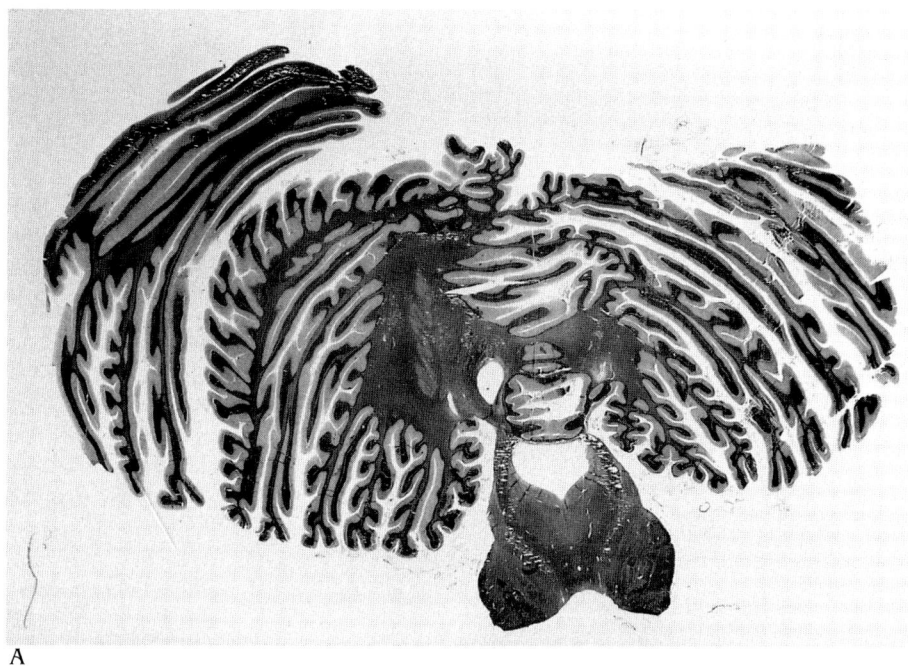

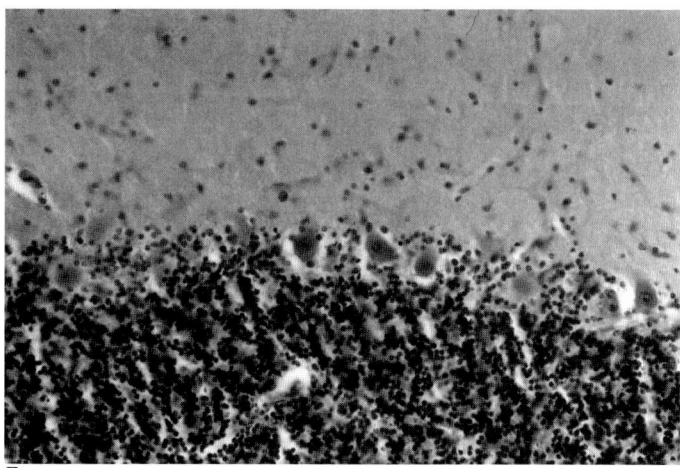

Figure 11–7. Spinocerebellar ataxia type 3, Machado-Joseph disease. *A.* Horizontal section through anterior portion of cerebellum and pons showing pallor of myelin staining around dentate nucleus (only one dentate shown in section), thinning of superior cerebellar peduncles, and dilatation of the fourth ventricle. Heidenhain-Woelke stain for myelin. *B.* Section of cerebellar cortex showing relatively good preservation of nuerons. H&E ×100. *C.* Section of dentate nucleus showing severe depopulation of neurons and gliosis. H&E, ×100. *D.* Section through XII nerve nucleus showing neuronal loss and gliosis. H&E, ×100. *E.* Horizontal section of thoracic spinal cord showing loss of neurons in the nucleus dorsalis of Clark Luxol fast blue-PAS, ×40. *(continued)*

neuropathy.[93] The family studied by Nachmanoff et al.[94] was clinically indentical to Biemond's posterior column ataxia.[95]

MOLECULAR GENETICS AND NEUROPATHOLOGY

SCA4 has been linked to chromosome 16q22, but molecular cloning has not yet been reported. Postmortem analysis of one patient with the clinical syndrome of ataxia with sensory neuronopathy revealed Purkinje cell loss, gliosis of the cerebellar molecular layer, degeneration of the dentate nucleus, and marked myelin pallor of the posterior columns accompanied by loss of dorsal root ganglion cells. (Fig. 11–8)[94] Other systems appeared relatively well preserved. The SCA5 locus has

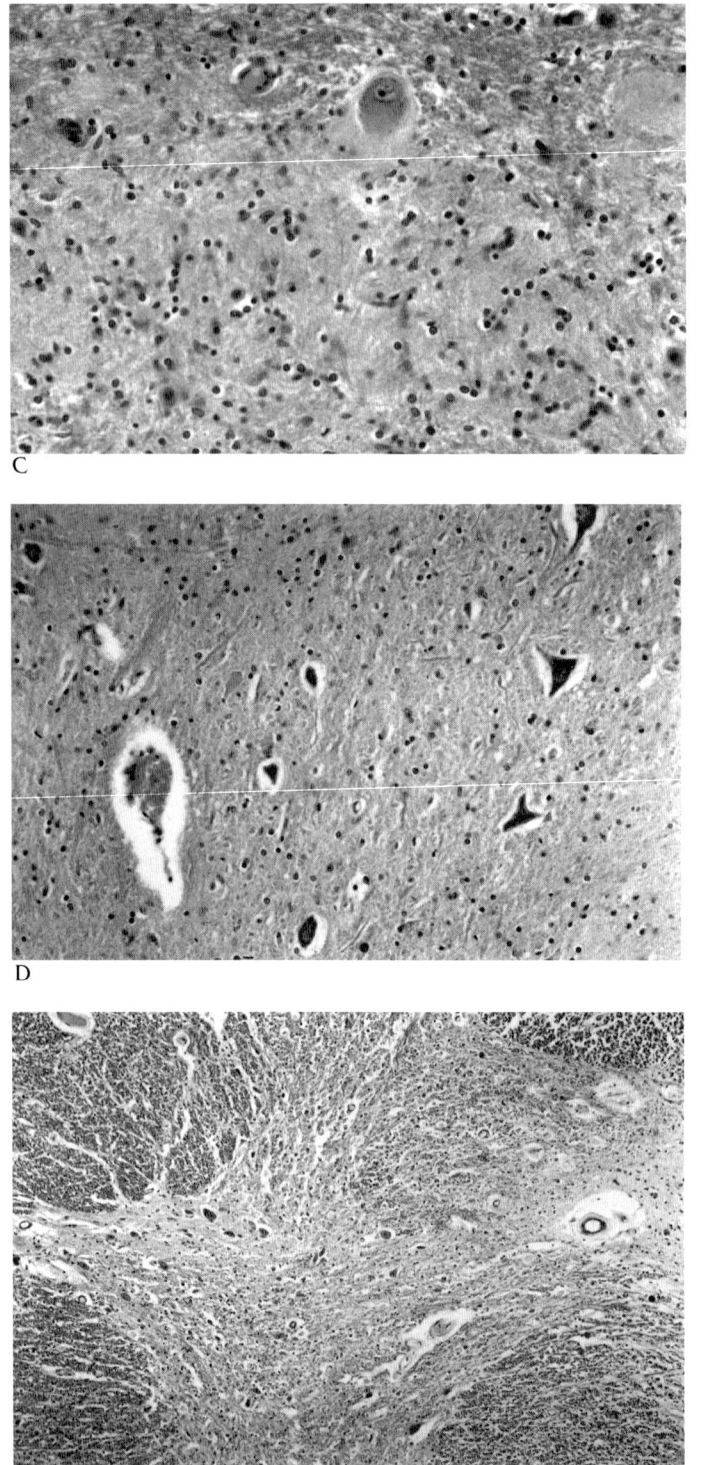

Figure 11–7.

been defined genetically, but molecular cloning or neuropathologic analysis has not been reported.

Spinocerebellar Ataxia Type 6 and Episodic Ataxia Type 2

MOLECULAR GENETICS AND NEUROPATHOLOGY

Spinocerebellar ataxia type 6 is the only ADCA whose gene product has a known function. Trinucleotide expansions in the carboxy-terminal cytoplasmic tail of the alpha$_{1A}$-voltage-dependent calcium channel (CACNL1A4) result in the clinical and neuropathologic syndrome of SCA6.[96] Missense and frameshift mutations are found in the CACNL1A4 gene in two other autosomal dominant disorders: episodic ataxia type 2 (EA2) and familial hemiplegic migraine.[97] Thus, three traditionally distinct neurologic diseases are caused by different types of mutations in the same gene. However, some patients with SCA6 may show an episodic course, particularly early in the disease process.[98] Conversely, EA2 may sometimes be progressive. These observations suggest that mutations causing SCA6, unlike other CAG trinucleotide expansions, may act by interfering with the normal function of CACNL1A4. Several other lines of evidence also support at least a partial loss of function component. CACNL1A4 is expressed throughout the nervous system but is markedly enriched in Purkinje and cerebellar granular cells.[97,99] Loss-of-function mutations in the mouse calcium channel homolog cause ataxia and seizures.[99]

Pathologic expansions in SCA6 are unusually small. Expansions of just 21 to 27 repeats can result in clinical symptoms, compared to 4 to 16 repeats in normal individuals.[96] CACNL1A4 may be particularly sensitive to small genetic alterations, with resulting dominant ataxic syndromes. Genetic anticipation is a less prominent feature in SCA6 families, compared to other ADCAs families.

The neuropathology of only a few cases of genetically confirmed SCA6 has been reported.[15,100–103] In these cases a good correlation was found with the relatively pure cere-

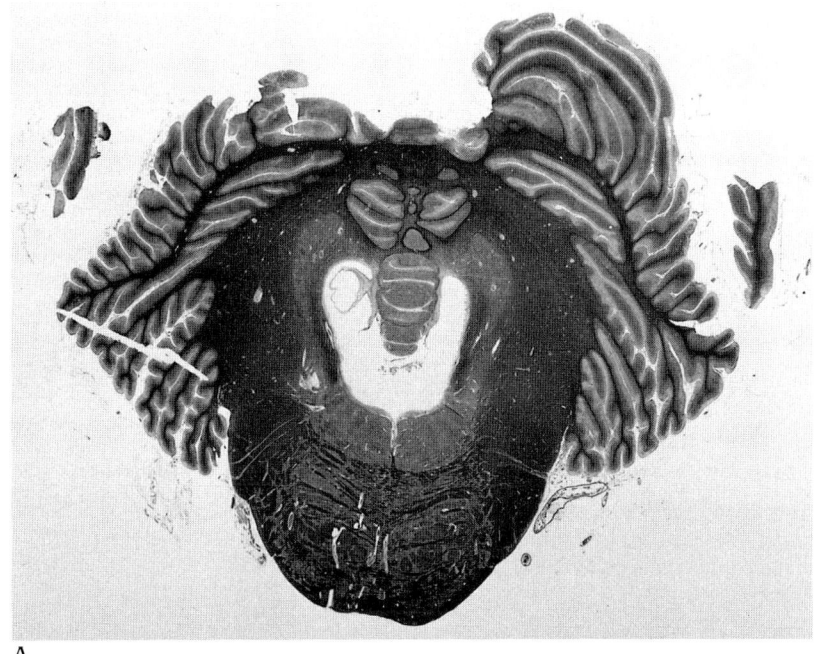

Figure 11–8.

A

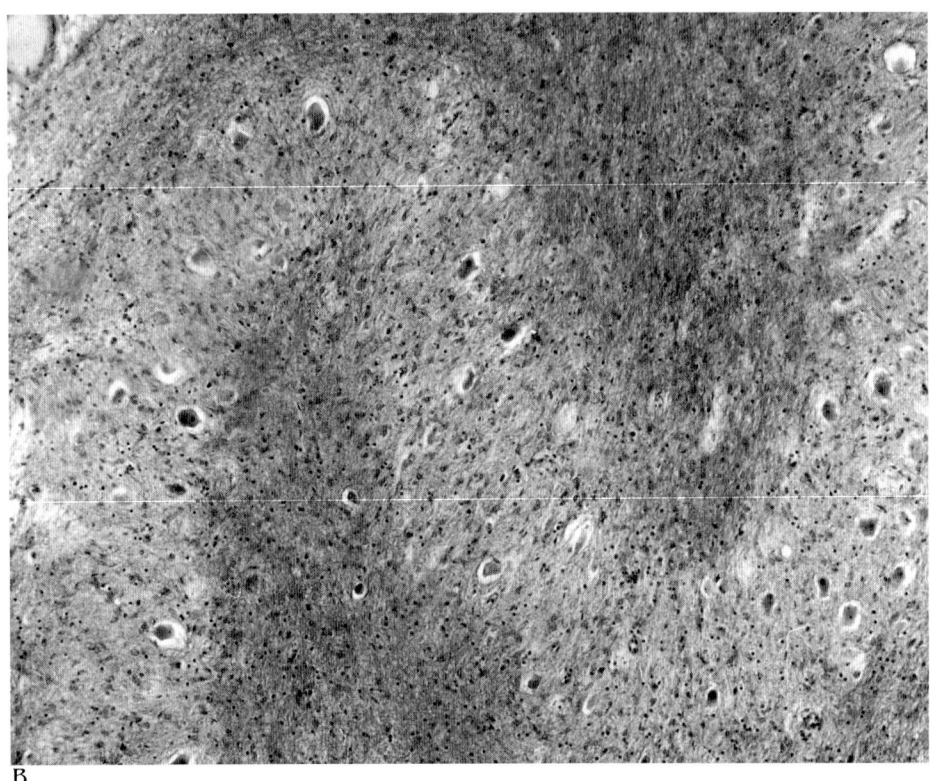

B

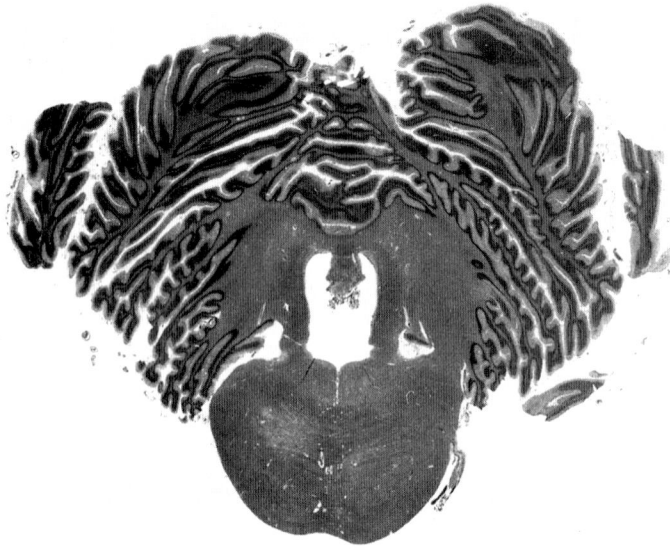

C

Figure 11–8. Spinocerebellar ataxia type 4. *A.* Horizontal section through mid-portion of cerebellum and pons showing pallor of myelin staining around dentate nucleus and dilatation of the fourth ventricle. Heidenhain-Woelke stain for myelin. *B.* Section of dentate nucleus showing neuronal loss and gliosis. Luxol fast blue-PAS, ×100. *C.* Horizontal section through anterior portion of cerebellum and pons showing thinning of superior cerebellar peduncle and dilatation of fourth ventricle. *D.* Section of cerebellar cortex showing loss of Purkinje cells (empty baskets). Bielschowsky, ×400. *E, F.* Horizontal sections of spinal cord at the cervical (E) and lumbar (F) enlargements showing pallor of posterior columns. Heidenhain-Woelke stain for myelin. *G.* Section of dorsal root ganglion showing extensive loss of sensory ganglion cells and nodules of Nageotte. Cresyl violet, ×100. *(continued)*

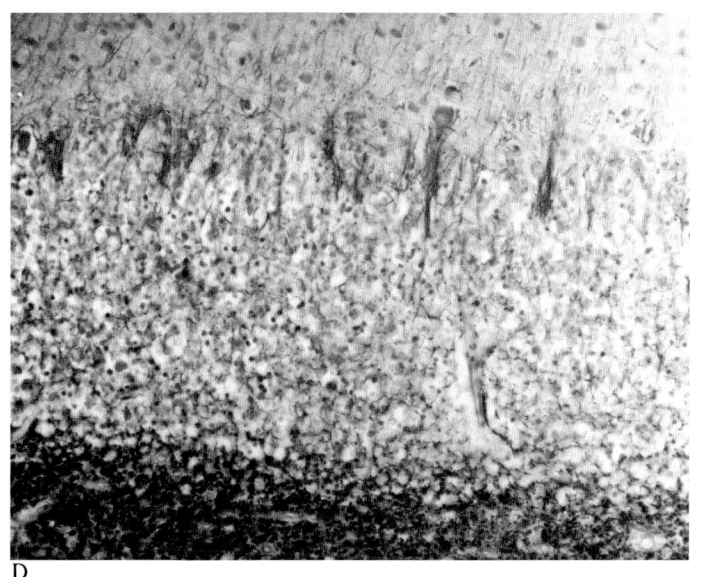

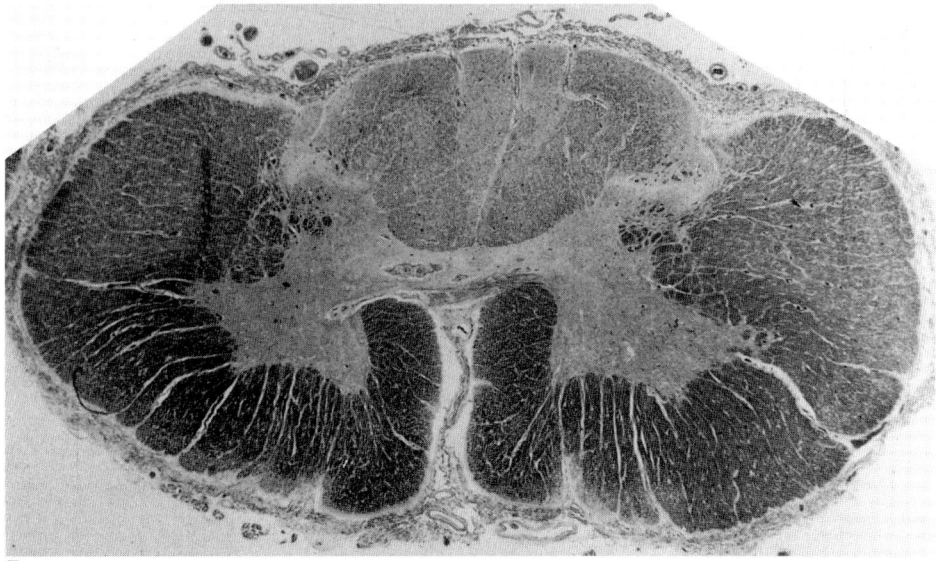

Figure 11–8. *(continued)*

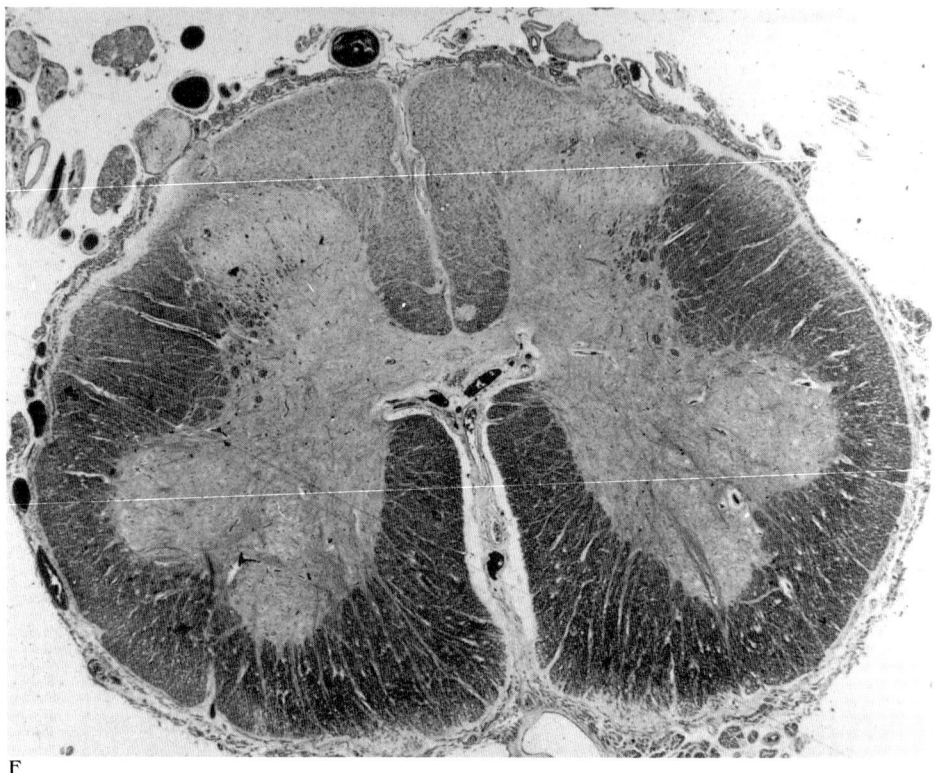

F

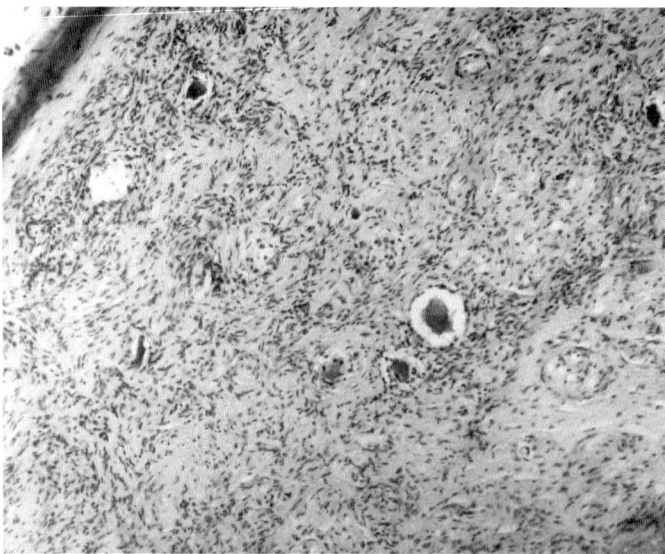

G

Figure 11-8.

bellar syndrome observed clinically. In the patient reported by Sasaki et al.,[102] pathology was restricted to the cerebellum. Vermal atrophy was noted grossly with relative preservation of the hemispheres. The cerebellar white matter and dentate nuclei were well preserved. On histological examination, the number of Purkinje cells was decreased to approximately one-third to one-fourth of age-matched controls; some of the surviving Purkinje cells showed proximal axonal expansions ("torpedoes") but most appeared entirely normal. The number of granule cells was mildly decreased. The cerebral cortex, white matter, basal ganglia, brain stem, including the inferior olive, and spinal cord were normal. Neuropathologic analysis of two individuals from another family[100] who carried the SCA6 mutation,[96] showed that they had very similar pathology in the cerebellum. In addition, there was neuronal loss in the inferior olive in these patients. The patients of Gomez et al.[101] showed similar cerebellar pathology and displayed mild to severe neuronal loss and gliosis in the inferior olivary nucleus. Neuropathologic analysis of EA2 patients has not been reported.

Spinocerebellar Ataxia Type 7

CLINICAL MANIFESTATIONS

This is a dominantly inherited spinocerebellar atrophy associated with retinal degeneration.

MOLECULAR GENETICS AND NEUROPATHOLOGY

The SCA7 gene encodes a ubiquitously expressed protein of unknown function.[104] CAG repeat sequences are particularly variable and unstable in SCA7. Mutated alleles range from 38 to 130 repeats and include the longest CAG repeat documented thus far in the ADCAs. Normal alleles range from 7 to 17 repeats in length. Intergenerational instability is higher in SCA7 than in any of the other diseases caused by CAG repeat enlargement and is greatest during paternal transmission. An expansion of 85 repeats has been documented in one generation. As expected, age of onset decreases with increasing repeat length. These observations correlate very well with the observations by Harding[37] that ADCA II (cerebellar ataxia with retinal degeneration) includes many more young adults and children than does ADCA I or III.

Neuropathologic analyses of genetically confirmed cases of SCA7 are now beginning to be available,[58] (unpublished observations; see Fig. 11–9); furthermore, the pathology of a number of cases of ADCA associated with retinal degeneration and marked genetic anticipation has been reported.[37,105,106] These cases seem likely candidates for SCA7 mutations. Correlating with the multisystem clinical findings, many areas of the nervous system are affected pathologically. As expected, retinal degeneration is seen, with loss of photoreceptors, bipolar cells, and ganglion cells. The retinal pigment epithelium is degenerated and the choroid is atrophic. The optic nerves and tracks are atrophic and the lateral geniculate nucleus shows neuronal loss and gliosis. The cerebral cortex is spared. The cerebellum is grossly atrophic. There is marked loss of Purkinje and granule cells, and myelin pallor and gliosis of the cerebellar white matter. The dentate nucleus and inferior olive show neuronal loss and gliosis. The subthalamic nucleus is atrophic, with lesser involvement of the globus pallidus and substantia nigra. Motor neurons of the brain stem are depleted. In the spinal cord, atrophy of the dorsal and ventral spinocerebellar tracts is present. The dorsal columns and pyramidal tracts are variably involved.

Dentatorubral Pallidoluysian Atrophy

CLINICAL MANIFESTATIONS

This rare disease was originally described by Titica and van Bogaert[107] in Europe and subsequently by Smith and collaborators[108] in the United States. The disease is characterized by symptoms of cerebellar ataxia associated with dystonia and choreoathetosis (thereby resembling the presentation of Huntington's chorea) and sometimes includes myoclonus, epilepsy, and dementia. Patients begin to show symptoms and signs between the second and fifth decade, these progress relentlessly over a course of 10 years or more.

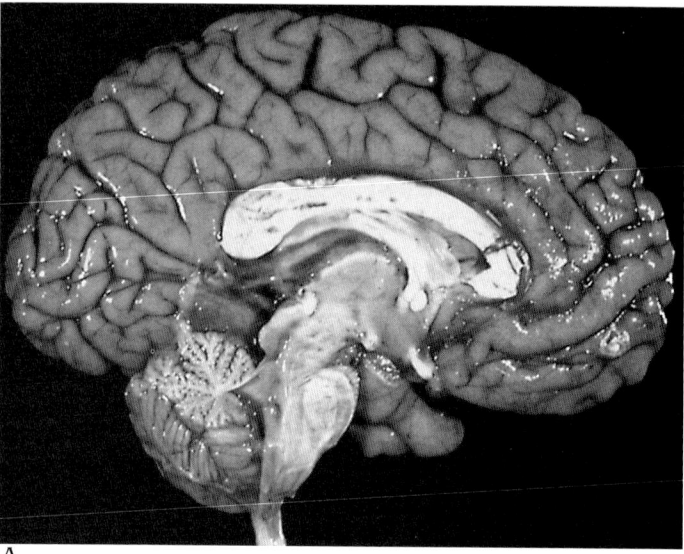

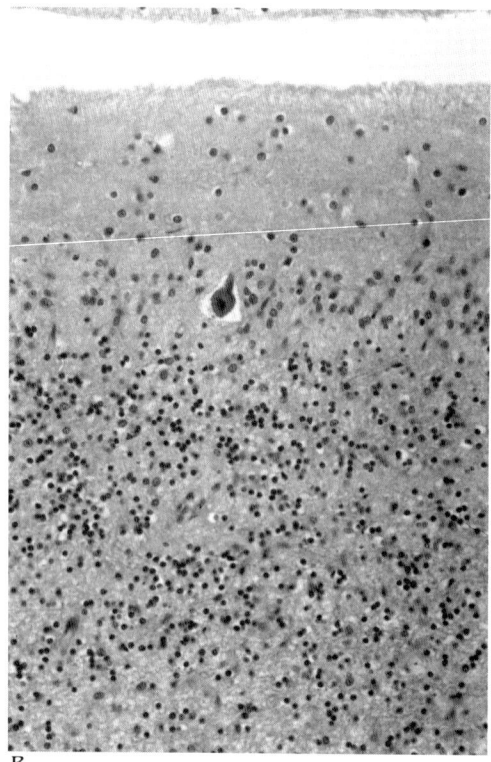
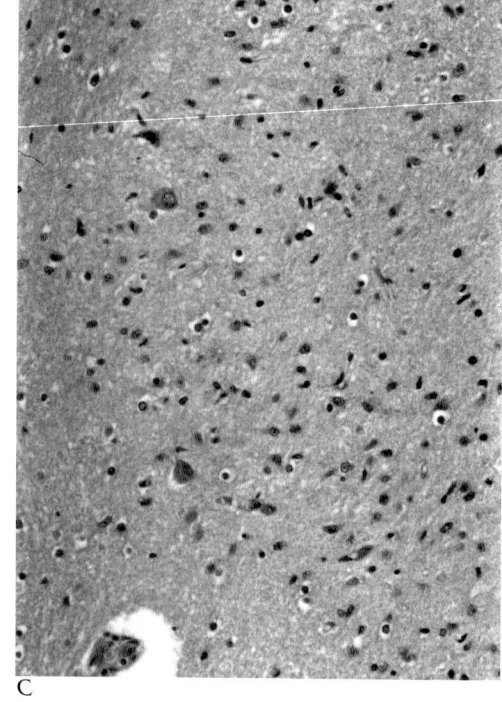

Figure 11-9.

MOLECULAR GENETICS AND NEUROPATHOLOGY

The normal DRPLA gene encodes a widely expressed protein of 190 KDa and unknown function.[109,110] Cases of combined dentatorubral and pallidoluysian atrophy show substantial neuropathologic heterogeneity, but common to most is severe involvement of the dentate nucleus, atrophy of the superior cer-

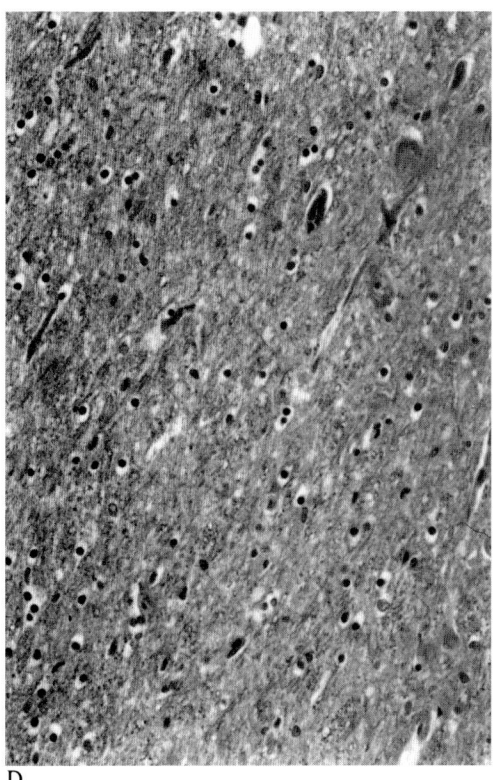

Figure 11–9. Spinocerebellar ataxia type 7 A. Sagittal view of brain. Note atrophy of vermis and some dilatation of the fourth ventricle. B. Section of cerebellar cortex showing severe loss of Purkinje cells and some loss of granule cells. H&E, ×100. C. Section of inferior olivary nucleus showing loss of cells and gliosis. H&E, ×100. D. Section of substantia nigra showing neuronal loss and gliosis. H&E, ×100. This case was contributed through the courtesy of Dr. M. Frosch from the archives of the Department of Pathology (Neuropathology), Massachusetts General Hospital, Boston, MA.

ebellar peduncle, and some injury to the red nuclei. Genetic cloning of the DRPLA locus has been important in clarifying the relationships of these disorders. The features common to genetically confirmed cases of DRPLA include marked neuronal loss and gliosis of the dentate nucleus and degeneration of the cerebellar white matter.[111] Although considered typical of DRPLA, neuronal loss is not always observed in the outer segment of the globus pallidus, subthalamic nucleus, or red nucleus. Varying degrees of degeneration may be seen in the thalamus, inferior olivary nucleus, gracile nucleus, and posterior columns of the spinal cord. The cerebral cortex, substantia nigra, Purkinje cells, and motor neurons are relatively spared in many cases. These findings are similar to those reported as DRPLA in some Japanese kindreds.[112,114] However, disorders previously considered distinct from DRPLA on clinical and neuropathologic grounds are now known to be caused by CAG expansions in the DRPLA gene.[114,115] Neuropathologic findings in the Haw River syndrome include extensive demyelination of the subcortical white matter and parenchymal mineralization of the globus pallidus, features thought to be atypical for DRPLA.[116] Typical neuronal loss and astrocytosis of the globus pallidus and subthalamic nucleus are not observed. Nonetheless, pathologic expansions of the DRPLA gene do underlie the Haw River syndrome.[114] Repeat expansions in the Haw River syndrome are similar in size to those seen in the Japanese population, implicating other factors in the clinical and neuropathological differences.

Typical neuronal intranuclear inclusions can be identified in DRPLA using antibodies against either ubiquitin[117] or the DRPLA protein.[59] Inclusions are widespread and do not concentrate in affected areas. In DRPLA, unlike other polyglutamine disorders, inclusions are found in glial as well neuronal nuclei.[117]

Friedreich's Ataxia

CLINICAL MANIFESTATIONS

This is the prototype of all forms of hereditary ataxia and accounts for about 50% of all cases of hereditary ataxia. Because of its importance it is included here, even though it is characteristically not a disease of the aged. The disease was well described by Friedreich of Heidelberg, Germany in 1861 and 1863,[118,119] who emphasized its hereditary aspects in contradistinction to other forms of locomotor ataxia (e.g., tabes dorsalis). Later, after considerable debate (see historical reviews[14,120]), Duchenne in France and others in Britain and the United States, confirmed its nosologic identity and in 1882, Brousse[121], attached Friedreich's name to the new entity. The disease characteristically starts during puberty with slowly progressive unsteadiness of gait (ataxia and weakness);[122] the characteristic findings on initial clinical examination include cerebellar signs, extensor plantar reflexes (Babinski), deep sensory loss, and depressed deep tendon reflexes. Both sexes are equally affected. Subsequently, important clinical manifestations include involvement of the upper extremities, speech disturbances (dysarthria), nystagmus and other eye movement abnormalities, extensor plantar responses, kyphoscoliosis, foot deformities, and peripheral neuropathy (sensorimotor with decrease tendon reflexes). Other signs and symptoms are deafness, optic atrophy with pigmentary degeneration of the retina, and tremor. Cardiac disturbances (EKG abnormalities, myocardial insufficiency) are an important manifestation of the disease and tend to occur in mid-course; a minority of patients have developed diabetes mellitus. Mentation is preserved in most patients. Most patients die within 20 years from onset of the disease. Clinically atypical forms of Friedreichs's ataxia having the same mutations on the frataxin gene as classic Friedreich's ataxia have been described: late-onset Friedreich's ataxia (LOFA)[44,123,124] and Friedreich's ataxia with retained reflexes (FARR).[44,125] These patients manifest clinical symptoms after the age of 20, sometimes in their late 20s and 30s. The neurologic manifestations are similar to those of classic Friedreich's ataxia, except that the rate of progression of the disease is slower. Eventually severe neurologic impairment ensues, muscle wasting, foot deformities, and diabetes have been found to be absent.[126] Oddly enough, the clinical course in some pedigrees appears to be markedly different despite the sibs' genetic similarity with regard to the length of the repeat expansions in the frataxin gene.[127]

MOLECULAR GENETICS AND NEUROPATHOLOGY

The disease is transmitted as an autosomal recessive disorder. The gene locus is on chromosome 9. The gene product of the Friedreich's ataxia locus encodes a 210 amino acid protein, frataxin, which shows some similarities to a yeast protein important in mitochondrial respiration[53] (see reviews[128,129]). Frataxin is localized to mitochondria and seems to be important in the activity of the mitochondrial respiratory chain.[51] Yeast organisms deficient in the frataxin homologue accumulate iron in mitochondria and show increased sensitivity to oxidative stress; a parallel mechanism is believed to occur in cultured fibroblasts from patients with Friedreich's ataxia.[130] The mutation in most cases of Friedreich's ataxia is an expanded trinucleotide (GAA) repeat in an intron of both alleles of the frataxin gene. The expansion has been found to be between 120 and 1700 repeats and there is a tendency toward an inverse correlation between the number of repeats and age of onset of the disease.

Pathologic changes in Friedreich's ataxia are concentrated in the spinal cord, dorsal root ganglia, and dorsal roots; all three are atrophic on macroscopic examination.[14] The principal neuropathologic changes include loss of the large neurons in dorsal root ganglia, thinning of dorsal roots, and ascending degeneration of the fasciculus gracilis and cuneatus.[14,131–133] There is also loss of dorsal root fibers destined for the nucleus of Clark and ascending degeneration of the dorsal spinocerebellar tract; the ventral spinocerebellar tract may be involved as well, though to a lesser extent. The corticospinal fibers are affected and transverse sections of the cord show pallor of myelin staining (Fig. 11–10E) and gliosis of both the crossed and uncrossed fibers, which is most severe in the most distal portions of the fibers. Biopsy studies of sensory nerves show severe axonal loss and the few autopsy studies that have carefully looked at multiple peripheral nerves have shown loss of fibers and connective tissue ingrowth. Study of the cerebellum in a number of autopsy cases, has shown loss of neurons and gliosis in the dentate nucleus (as well as the other cerebellar nuclei) and loss of fibers in the superior cerebellar peduncle, (Fig. 11–10C). Although the cerebellar cortex has usually not shown dramatic changes (Fig. 11–

10A, B) several studies suggest there may be a loss of Purkinje cells in the superior vermis in advanced cases. In the brain stem, the inferior olivary nucleus has generally been normal (Fig. 11–10D), while the gracile and cuneate nuclei and the accessory cuneate nucleus have been found to be moderately depleted; there have also been isolated reports describing neuronal loss in several other sensory and autonomic brain stem nuclei. In some cases there is neuronal loss in all vestibular and cochlear nuclei. There have been no constant abnormalities described in the cerebrum; some have seen loss of Betz cells, neuronal loss and gliosis in the subthalamic nucleus, or depletion of neurons in the globus pallidus. The cardiac abnormality is a hypertrophic cardiomyopathy with extensive replacement fibrosis of the myocardium and iron deposition (Fig. 11–10F, G).

Sporadic Ataxias

Approximately two-thirds of degenerative ataxias with adult onset are apparently sporadic. Although about 10% of these cases represent one of the ADCAs or atypical Friedreich's ataxia,[44] the majority fall into the category of multisystem atrophy (MSA) (see Chapter eight). The presence of characteristic ubiquitinated glial and neuronal inclusions can confirm the diagnosis of MSA. Sporadic, adult-onset ataxias also include historically de-

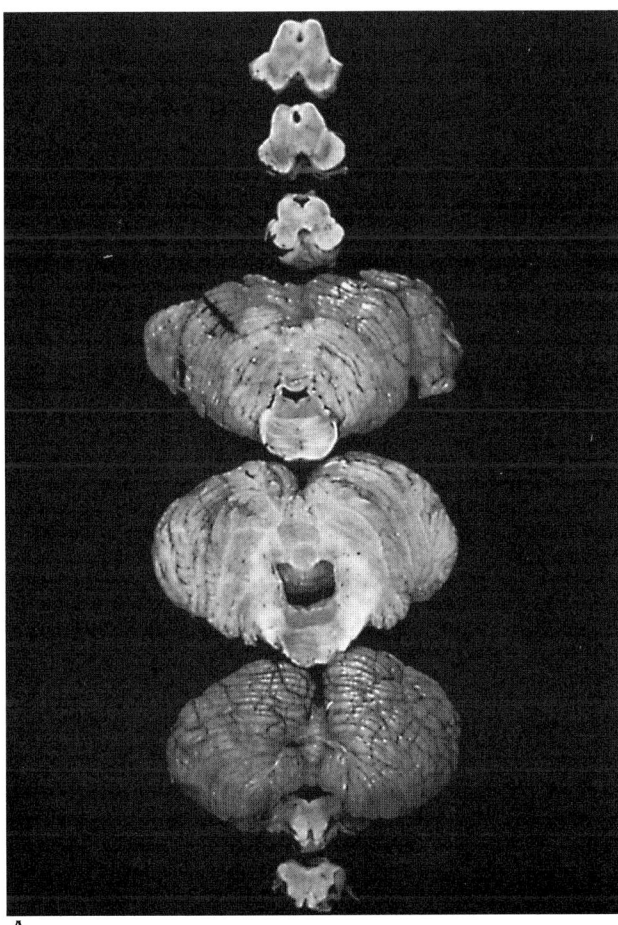

Figure 11–10. Friedreich's ataxia. A. Serial views of the posterior fossa structures showing relatively good preservation of the cerebellum and brain stem. The substantia nigra is somewhat depigmented and the fourth ventricle is moderately dilated. B. Horizontal section through midportion of cerebellum and pons showing normal myelin staining around dentate nucleus and dilation of the fourth ventricle. The cerebellar cortex is normal. Klüver-Barrera stain for myelin. C. Horizontal section through anterior portion of cerebellum and pons showing thinning of superior cerebellar peduncle and dilation of fourth ventricle. Klüver-Barrera stain for myelin. D. Section through midportion of medulla showing normal inferior olivary nucleus and normal pyramidal tracts. Heidenhain-Woelke stain for myelin. E. Transverse section of cervical spinal cord showing pallor of myelin staining in the posterior columns, corticospinal tracts (lateral and anterior), and spinocerebellar tracts (dorsal, especially). Heidanhain-Woelke stain for myelin. F. Cross section of ventricles through mid-portion of heart showing some right ventricular dilation. Masson trichrome. G. Section of left ventricle showing extensive interstitial fibrosis (pale areas). Masson trichrome, ×40. This case and some of its illustrations were contributed through the courtesy of Dr. M. Frosch from the archives of the Department of Pathology (Neuropathology), Brigham and Women's Hospital, Boston, MA. *(continued)*

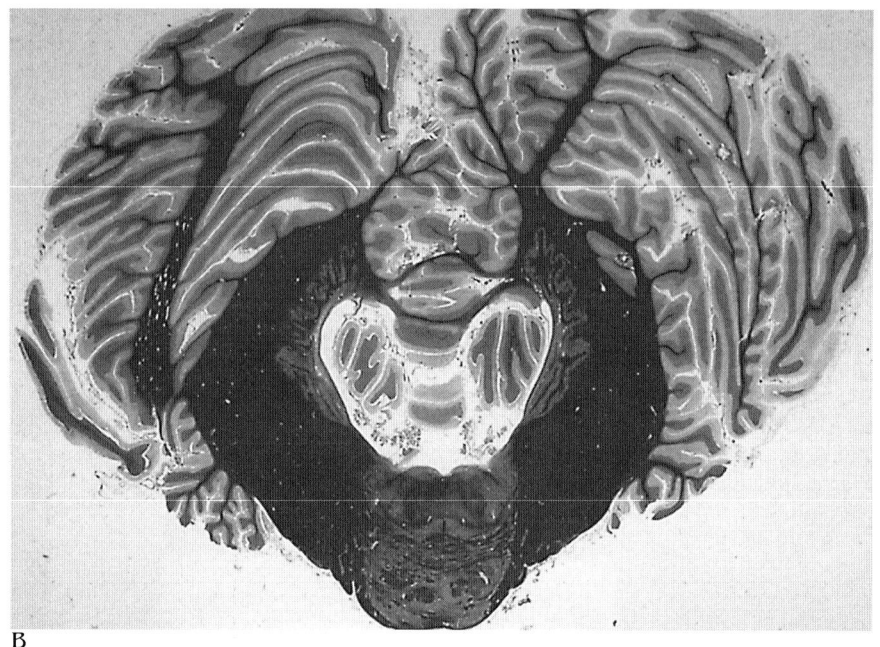

B

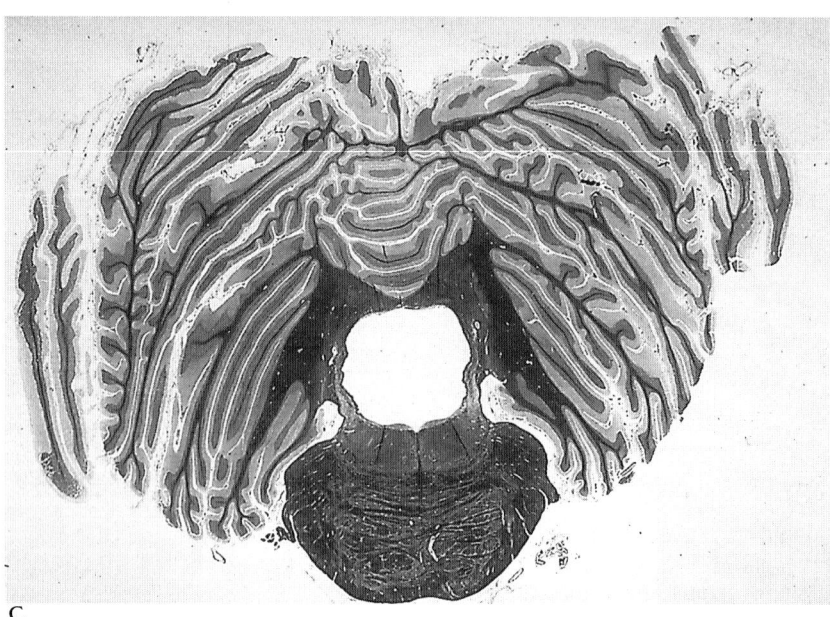

C

Figure 11–10. *(continued)*

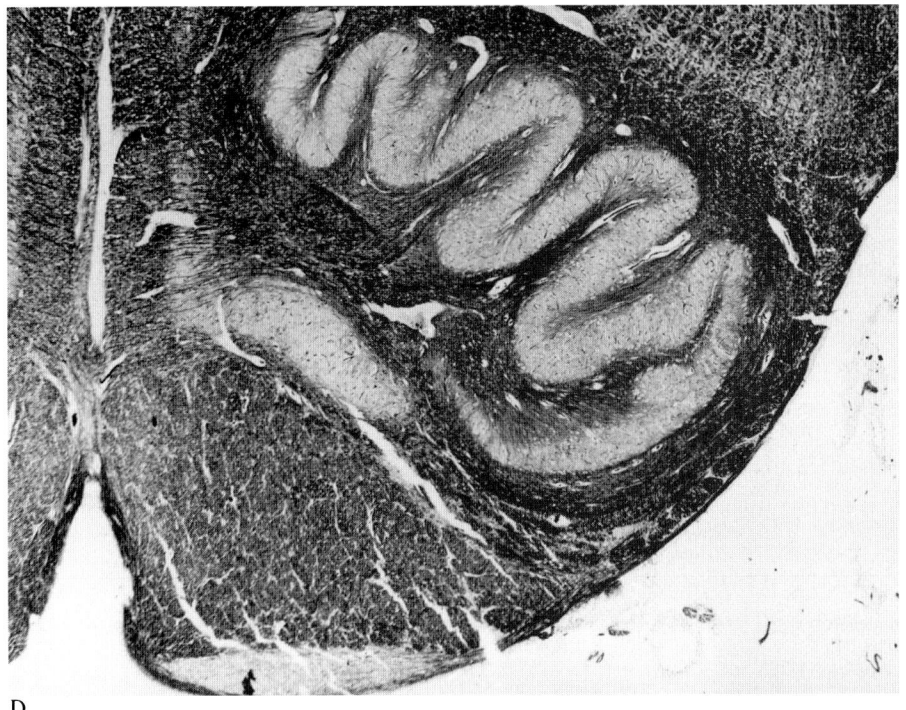

D

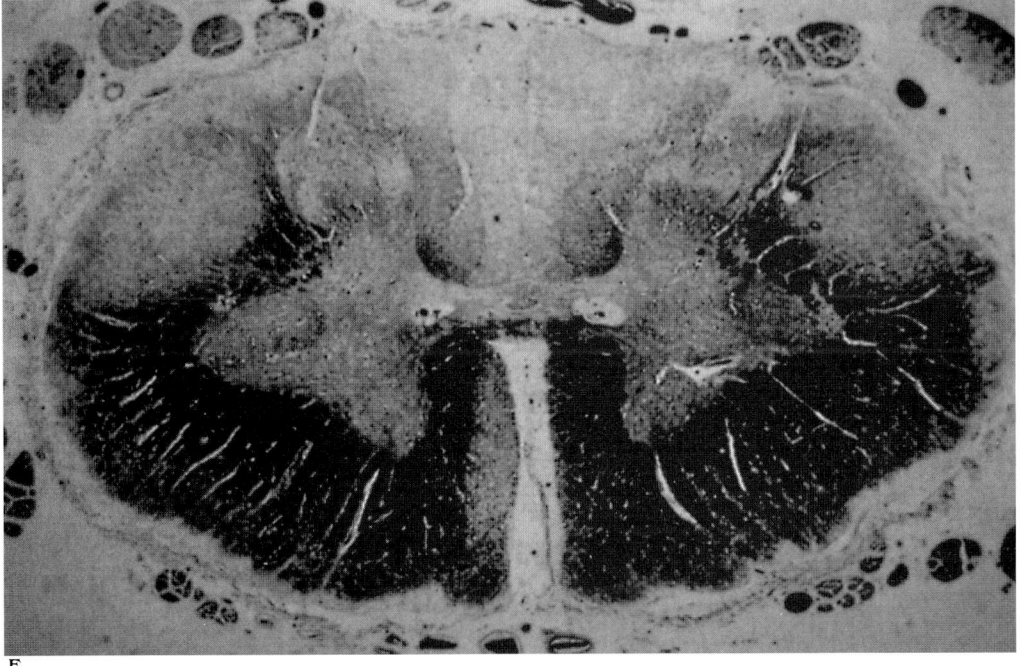

E

Figure 11–10. *(continued)*

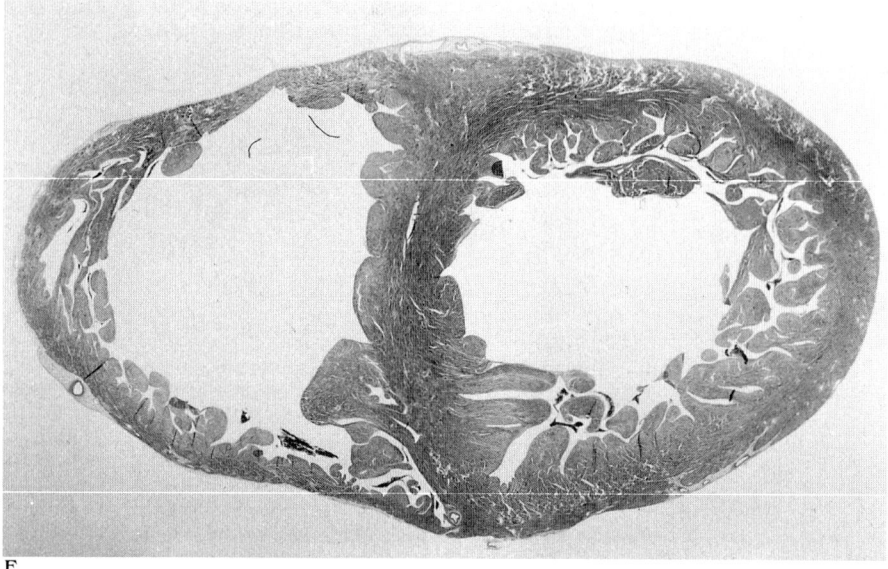

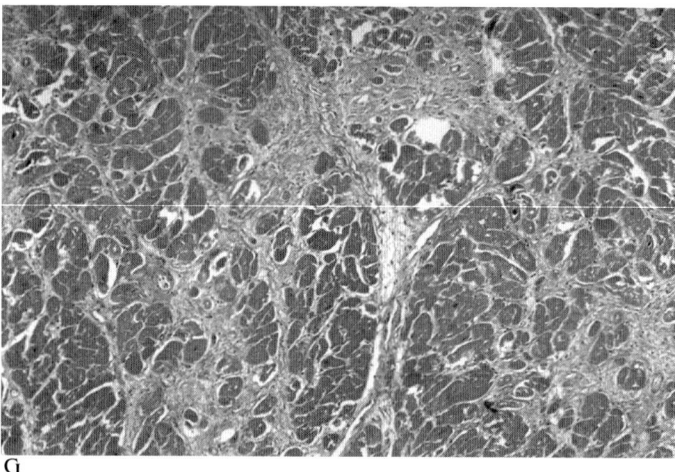

Figure 11–10.

scribed entities such as the *heredoataxie cerebelleuse* of Marie-Foix-Alajouanine, more recently categorized as late-onset sporadic ataxia.[37] The etiology of the non-MSA sporadic disorders remains unknown.

Dentatorubral degeneration was originally described in 1921 by Ramsay Hunt (*dyssynergia cerebellaris myoclonica*)[134] as a sporadic ataxia with onset in childhood and associated with prominent myoclonus. The precise nosologic status of this entity is now uncertain; it may well be a syndrome with multiple causes and heterogeneous neuropathologic findings.

The authors thank Drs. C. Duyckaerts, M. P. Frosch, A. Koeppen, J. D. Schmahmann, and M. K. Wolf for kindly reviewing portions of the text; we especially thank Dr. Koeppen and the National Ataxia Foundation for contributing illustrative material.

REFERENCES

1. Luciani L. Il Cervelletto. Nuovi Studi di Fisiologia Normale e Patologica. Florence: Le Monnier, 1891.
2. Probst M. Zur Anatomie und Physiologie des Kleinhirns. Arch Psychiatrie Nervenkrankheiten 1902; 35: 692–777.

3. Bolk L. Das Cerebellum der Saugetiere: Eine Vergleichende Anatomische Untersuchung. Haarlem: Fischer, 1906.
4. Dow RS, Moruzzi G. The Physiology and Pathology of the Cerebellum. Minneapolis: University Minnesota Press, 1958.
5. Fox CA, Snider RS, (eds). The cerebellum Prog Brain Res 1967; 25:1–135.
6. Fields WS, Willis WD. The Cerebellum in Health and Disease. Saint Louis: W.H. Green, 1970.
7. Brodal A. The cerebellum. In: Brodal As eds. Neurological Anatomy in Relation to Clinical Medicine. New York: Oxford University Press, 1981:294–393.
8. Parent A. Cerebellum. In Parent AS eds. Carpenter's Neuroanatomy. Baltimore: Williams and Wilkins, 1996:583–629.
9. Golgi C. Sulla Fine Anatomia del Cervelletto Umano. Milan: Hoepli, 1903 (1874):99–111.
10. Ramón y Cajal S. Histologie du Système Nerveux de l'Homme et des Vertébrés. Madrid: Consejo Superior de Investigaciones Científicas. Instituto Ramón y Cajal, (1904) 1952.
11. Jansen J. On the morphogenesis and morphology of the mammalian cerebellum. In: Jansen J, Brodal AS, eds. Aspects of Cerebellar Anatomy. Oslo: Tanun, 1954:13–81.
12. Jansen J, Brodal A. Das Kleinhirn. In: von Mollendorff W, Gragmann WS, eds. Handbuch der Mikroskopischen Anatomie des Menschen, Volume IV/8. Berlin: Springer Verlag, 1958:1–323.
13. Palay SL, Chan-Palay V. Cerebellar Cortex. Cytology and Organization: Berlin: Springer-Verlag, 1974.
14. Greenfield JG. The Spino-cerebellar Degenerations. Springfield, IL: Charles C. Thomas, 1954.
15. Koeppen AH. The hereditary ataxias. J Neuropathol Exp Neurol 1998; 57:531–543.
16. Gilman S, Bloedel JR, Lechtenberg R. Disorders of the Cerebellum. Philadelphia: F.A. Davis, 1981.
17. Harding AE. The clinical features and classification of the late onset autosomal dominant cerebellar ataxias. A study of 11 families, including descendants of "the Drew family of Walworth." Brain 1982; 105:1–28.
18. Adams RD, Victor M, Ropper AH. Principles of Neurology. New York: McGraw-Hill, 1997.
19. Iwabuchi K, Tsuchiya K, Uchihara T, Yagishita S. Autosomal dominant spinocerebellar degenerations. Clinical, pathological, and genetic correlations. Rev Neurol 1999; 55:255–270.
20. Altman J, Bayer SA. The Development of the Cerebellar System in Relation to its Evolution, Structure, and Systems. New York: CRC Press, 1997.
21. Nieuwenhuys R, Donkelaar HJ, Nicholson C. (ed). The Central Nervous System of Vertebrates, Vol 1. Berlin: Springer-Verlag, 1998:
22. Llinás RR. The cortex of the cerebellum. Sci Amer 1975; 232:56–71.
23. Voogd J, Glickstein M. The anatomy of the cerebellum. Trends Neurosci 1998; 21:370–375.
24. Voogd J, Jaarsma D, Mariani E. The cerebellum: chemoarchitecture and anatomy. In: Björklund A, Hökfelt TS, eds. Handbook of Chemical Neuroanatomy, Vol 12. Amsterdam: Elsevier, 1996:1–370.
25. De Zeew CI, Strata P, Voogd J (eds). The Cerebellum: from Structure to Control, Vol. 114. Amsterdam: Elsevier 1997.
26. Babinski J. De l'asynergie cérébelleuse Rev Neurol 1899; 7:806–816.
27. Dejerine J, Thomas A. Maladies de la Moelle Epinère. Paris: Baillière, 1909.
28. Holmes G. The Croonian Lectures of the clinical symptoms of cerebellar disease and their interpretation. Lancet 1922; 1, 2:1177–1182; 59–65.
29. Holmes GM. The cerebellum of man. Hughlings Jackson Lecture. Brain 1939; 62:1–30.
30. Schmahmann JD. An emerging concept. The cerebellar contribution to higher function. Arch Neurol 1991; 48:1178–1187.
31. Gao J-H, Parsons L, Bower JM, Xiong J, Li J, Fox PT. Cerebellum implicated in sensory acquisition and discrimination rather than motor control. Science 1996; 272:545–547.
32. Allen G, Buxton RB, Wong EC, Courchesne E. Attentional activation of the cerebellum independent of motor movement. Science 1997; 275:1940–1943.
33. Schmahmann JD, Pandya DN. The cerebrocerebellar system. In: Schmahmann JDS (eds). Int Rev Neurobiol 1997; 41:31–60.
34. Schmahmann JD. The cerebellar cognitive affective syndrome. Brain 1998; 121:561–579.
35. Schoenberg BS. Epidemiology of the inherited ataxias. Adv Neurol 1979; 21:15–32.
36. Skre H. Epidemiology of spinocerebellar degenerations in western Norway: hereditary ataxias. In: Soubue IS ed. Spinocerebellar Degenerations. Baltimore: University Park Press, 1978:103–120.
37. Harding A. The Hereditary Ataxias and Related Disorders. Edinburgh: Churchill Livingstone, 1984.
38. Koroshetz WJ, Myers RH, Martin JB. The neurology of Huntington's disease. In: Joseph AB, Young RH, eds. Movement Disorders in Neurology and Neuropsychiatry. Boston: Blackwell, 1992:167–177.
39. Cummings JL. Parkinson's disease and parkinsonism. In: Joseph AB, Young RH, eds. Movement Disorders in Neurology and Neuropsychiatry. Boston: Blackwell, 1992:195–203.
40. Sequeiros J, Coutinho P. Epidemiology and clinical aspects of Machado-Joseph disease. 1993:61:139–153.
41. Orozco G, Estrada R, Perry TL, Arana J, Fernandez R, Gonzales-Quevedo A, Galarraga J, Hansen J. Dominantly inherited olivopontocerebellar atrophy from eastern Cuba. Clinical, neuropathological, and biochemical findings. J Neurol Sci 1989; 93:37–50.
42. Ule G. Die systematischen Atrophien des Kleinhirns. In: Lubarsch O, Henke F, Rössle R, eds. Handbuch der Speziellen Pathologischen Anatomie und Histologie, Volume XIII/1/A. Berlin: Springer-Verlag, 1957: 934–998.
43. Grewal RP, Tayag E, Figueroa KP, Zu L, Durazo A, Nunez C, Pulst SM. Clinical and genetic analysis of a distinct autosomal dominant spinocerebellar ataxia. Neurology 1998; 51:1423–1426.
44. Moseley ML, Benzow KA, Schut LJ, Bird TD, Gomez CM, Barkhous PE, Blindauer KA, Labuda M, Pandolfo M, Koob MD, and others. Incidence of dominant spinocerebellar and Friedreich triplet repeats among 361 ataxia families. Neurology 1998; 51:1666–1671.
45. Silveira I, Coutinho P, Maciel P, Gaspar C, Hayes S, Dias A, Guimaraes J, Loureiro L, Sequeiros J, Rouleau GA. Analysis of SCA1, DRPLA, MJD, SCA2, and

SCA6 CAG repeats in 48 Portuguese ataxia families. Am J Med Genet 1998; 28:134–138.
46. Gusella JF, MacDonald ME. Trinucleotide instability: a repeating theme in human inherited disorders. Annu Rev Med 1996; 47:201–209.
47. Burright EN, Clark HB, Servadio A, Matilla, Feddersen RM, Yunis WS, Duvick LA, Zoghbi HY, Orr HT. SCA1 transgenic mice: a model for neurodegeneration caused by an expanded CAG trinucleotide repeat. Cell 1995; 82:937–948.
48. Mangiarini L, Sathasivam K, Seller M, Cozens B, Harper A, Hetherington C, Lawton M, Trottier Y, Lehrach H, Davies SW, and others. Exon 1 of the HD gene with an expanded CAG repeat is sufficient to cause a progressive neurologic phenotype in transgenic mice. Cell 1996; 87:493–506.
49. Duyao MP, Auerbach AB, Ryan A, Persichetti F, Barnes GT, McNeil SM, Ge P, Vonsattel J-P, Gusella JF, Joyner AL, and others. Inactivation of the mouse Huntington's disease gene homolog Hdh. Nature 1995; 269:407–409.
50. Wellington CL, Hayden MR. Of molecular interactions, mice and mechanisms: new insights into Huntington's disease. Neurology 1997; 10:291–298.
51. Campuzano V, Montermini L, Lutz Y, Cova L, Hindelang C, Jiralerspong S, Trottier, Y, Kish SJ, Faucheux B, Trouillas P, and others. Frataxin is reduced in Friedreich ataxia patients and is associated with mitochondrial membranes. Hum Mol Genet 1997; 6: 1771–1780.
52. The Dutch-Belgian Fragile X Consortium. Fmr1 knockout mice: a model to study fragile X mental retardation. Cell 1994; 78:23–33.
53. Campuzano V, Montermini L, Molto MD, Pianese L, Cossée M, Cavalcanti F, Monros E, Rodius F, Duclos F, Monticelli A, and others. Friedreich's ataxia: autosomal recessive disease caused by an intronic GAA triplet repeat expansion. Science 1996; 271:1423–1427.
54. DiFiglia M, Sapp E, Chase KO, Davies SW, Bates GP, Vonsattel JP, Aronin N. Aggregation of huntingtin in neuronal intranuclear inclusions and dystrophic neurites in brain. Science 1997; 277:1990–1993.
55. Skinner PJ, Koshy BT, Cummings CJ, Klement IA, Helin K, Servadio A, Zoghbi HY, Orr HT. Ataxin-1 with an expanded glutamine tract alters nuclear matrix–associated structures. Nature 1997; 389:971–978.
56. Duyckaerts C, Dürr A, Cancel G, Brice A. Nuclear inclusions in spinocerebellar ataxia type 1. Acta Neuropathol 1999; 97:201–207.
57. Paulson HL, Perez MK, Trottier Y, Trojanowski JQ, Subramony SH, Das SS, Vig P, Mandel J-L, Fischbeck KH, Pittman RN. Intranuclear inclusions of expanded polyglutamine protein in spinocerebellar ataxia type 3. Neuron 1997; 19:333–344.
58. Holmberg M, Duyckaerts C, Dürr A, Cancel G, Gourfinkel-An I, Damier P, Faucheux B, Trittier Y, Hirsch EC, Agid Y, and others. Spinocerebellar ataxia type 7 (SCA7): a neurodegenerative disorder with neuronal intranuclear inclusions. Hum Mol Genet 1998; 7:913–918.
59. Igarashi S, Koide R, Shimohata T, Yamada M, Hayashi Y, Takano H, Date H, Oyake M, Sato T, Sato A, and others. Suppression of aggregate formation and apoptosis by transglutaminase inhibitors in cells expressing truncated DRPLA protein with an expanded polyglutamine stretch. Nat Genet 1998; 18:111–117.
60. Klement IA, Skinner PJ, Kaytor MD, Yi H, Hersh SM, Clark HB, Zoghbi HY, Orr HT. Ataxin-1 nuclear localization and aggregation: role in polyglutamine-induced disease in SCA1 transgenic mice. Cell 1998; 95:41–53.
61. Saudou F, Finkbeiner S, Devys D, Greenberg ME. Huntingtin acts in the nucleus to induce apoptosis but death does not correlate with the formation of intranuclear inclusions. Cell 1998; 95:55–66.
62. Trottier Y, Lutz Y, Stevanin G, Imbert G, Devys D, Cancel G, Saudou F, Weber C, David G, Tora L, and others. Polyglutamine expansion as a pathologic epitope in Huntington's disease and four dominant cerebellar ataxias. Nature 1995; 378:403–406.
63. Sanpei K, Takano H, Igarashi S, Sato T, Oyake M, Sasaki H, Wakisaka A, Tashiro K, Ishida Y, Ikeuchi T, and others. Identification of the spinocerebellar ataxia type 2 gene using a direct identification of repeat expansion and cloning technique, DIRECT. Nat Genet 1996; 4:277–284.
64. Dejerine J, Thomas A. L'atrophie olivo-ponto-cérébelleuse. Nouv Iconogr Salpêtrière 1900; 13:330–370.
65. Critchley M, Greenfield JG. Olivo-ponto-cerebellar atrophy. Brain 1948; 71:343–364.
66. Banfi S, Servadio A, Chung M-Y, Kwiatkowski TJ, McCall AE, Duvick LA, Shen Y, Roth EJ, Orr HT, Zoghbi HY. Identification and characterization of the gene causing type 1 spinocerebellar ataxia. Nat Genet 1994; 7:513–519.
67. Servadio A, Koshy B, Armstrong D, Antalffy B, Orr HT, Zoghbi HY. Expression analysis of the ataxin-1 protein in tissues from normal and spinocerebellar ataxia type 1 individuals. Nat Genet 1995; 10:94–98.
68. Matilla A, Roberson ED, Banfi S, Morales J, Armstrong D, Burright EN, Orr HT, Sweatt JD, Zoghbi HY, Matzuk MM. Mice lacking ataxin-1 display learning deficits and decreased hippocampal paired-pulse facilitation. J. Neurosci 1998; 18:5508–5516.
69. Matilla A, Koshy B, Cummings CJ, Isobe T, Orr HT, Zoghbi HY. The cerebellar leucine-rich acidic nuclear protein interacts with ataxin-1. Nature 1997; 389:974–978.
70. Genis D, Matilla T, Volpini V, Rosell J, Davalos A, Ferrer I, Molins A, Estivill X. Clinical neuropathologic and genetic studies of a large spinocerebellar ataxia type 1 (SCA1) kindred: (CAG)n expansion and early premonitory signs and symptoms. Neurology 1995; 45:24–30.
71. Robitaille Y, Schut L, Kish SJ. Structural and immunocytochemical features of olivopontocerebellar atrophy caused by the spinocerebellar ataxia type 1 (SCA-1) mutation define a unique phenotype. Acta Neuropathol 1995; 90:572–581.
72. Yagishita S, Inoue M. Clinicopathology of spinocerebellar degeneration: its correlation to the unstable CAG repeat of the affected gene. Pathol Int 1997; 47: 1–15.
73. Gilman S, Sima AAF, Junck L, Kliun KJ, Koeppe RA, Lohman ME, Little R. Spinocerebellar ataxia type 1 with multiple system degeneration and glial cytoplasmic inclusions. Ann Neurol 1996; 39:241–255.

74. Dürr A, Smadja D, Cancel G, Lezin A, Stevanin G, Mikol J, Bellance R, Buisson G-G, Chneiweiss H, Dellanave J, and others. Autosomal dominant cerebellar ataxia type I in Martinique (French West Indies): clinical and neuropathological analysis of 53 patients from three unrelated SCA2 families. Brain 1995; 18:1573–1581.

75. Sasaki H, Wakisaka A, Sampei K, Takano H, Igarashi S, Ikeuchi T, Iwabuchi K, Fukazawa T, Hamada T, Yuasa T, and others. Phenotype variation correlates with CAG repeat length in SCA2—a study of 28 Japanese patients. J Neurol Sci 1998; 59:202–208.

76. Imbert G, Saudou F, Yvert G, Devys D, Trottier Y, Garneir J-M, Weber C, Mandel J-L, Cancel G, Abbas N, and others. Cloning of the gene for spinocerebellar ataxia 2 reveals a locus with high sensitivity to expanded CAG/glutamine repeats. Nat Genet 1996; 14: 285–291.

77. Pulst S-M, Nechiporuk A, Nechiporuk T, Gispert S, Chen X-N, Lopes-Cendes I, Pearlman S, Starkman S, Orozco-Diaz G, Lunkes A, and others. Moderate expansion of a normally biallelic trinucleotide repeat in spinocerebellar ataxia type 2. Nat Genet 1996; 4:269–276.

78. Estrada R, Galarraga J, Orozco G, Nodarse A, Auburger G. Spinocerebellar ataxia 2 (SCA2): morphometric analyses in 11 autopsies. Acta Neuropathol 1999; 97:306–310.

79. Koeppen AH, Dickson AC, Lamarche JB, Robitaille Y. Synapses in hereditary ataxias. J Neuropathol Exp Neurol 1999; 58:748–764.

80. Nakano KK, Dawson DM, Spence A. Machado disease. A hereditary ataxia in Portuguese emigrants to Massachusetts. Neurology 1972; 22:49–55.

81. Woods BT, Schaumburg HH. Nigro-spino-dentatal degeneration with nuclear ophthalmoplegia. A unique and partially treatable clinico-pathological entity. J Neurol Sci 1972; 17:149–166.

82. Romanul FCA, Fowler HL, Radvany J, Feldman RG, Feingold M. Azorean disease of the nervous system. N Engl J Med 1977; 296:1505–1508.

83. Rosenberg RN, Nyhan WL, Coutinho P, Bay C. Joseph's disease: an autosomal dominant neurological disease in the Portuguese of the United States and the Azores Islands. Adv Neurol 1978; 21:33–57.

84. Matilla T, McCall A, Subramony SH, Zoghbi HY. Molecular and clinical correlations in spinocerebellar ataxia type 3 and Machado-Joseph disease. Ann Neurol 1995; 38:68–72.

85. Kawaguchi Y, Okamoto T, Taniwaki M, Aizawa M, Inoue M, Katayama S, Kawakami H, Nakamura S, Nishimura M, Akiguchi I, and others. CAG expansions in a novel gene for Machado-Joseph disease at chromosome 14q32.1. Nat Genet 1994; 8:221–227.

86. Paulson HL, Das SS, Crino PB, Perez MK, Patel SC, Gotsdiner D, HFK, Pittman RN. Machado-Joseph disease gene product is a cytoplasmic protein widely expressed in brain. Ann Neurol 1997; 41:453–462.

87. Schmidt T, Landwehrmeyer GB, Schmitt I, Trottier Y, Auburger G, Laccone F, Klockgether T, Völpel M, Epplen JT, Schöls L, and others. An isoform of ataxin-3 accumulates in the nucleus of neuronal cells in affected brain regions of SCA3 patients. Brain Pathol 1998; 8:669–679.

88. Ikeda H, Yamaguchi M, Sugai S, Aze Y, Narumiya S, Kakizuka A. Expanded polyglutamine in the Machado-Joseph disease protein induces cell death in vitro and in vivo. Nat Genet 1996; 13:196–201.

89. Warrick JM, Paulson HL, Gray-Board L, Bui QT, Fischbeck KN, Pittman RN, Bonini NM. Expanded polyglutamine protein forms nuclear inclusions and causes neural degeneration in Drosophila. Cell 1998; 93:939–949.

90. Coutinho P, Guimarães A, Scaravilli F. The pathology of Machado-Joseph disease. Report of a possible homozygous case. Acta Neuropathol 1982; 58:48–54.

91. Sachdev HS, Forno LS, Kane CA. Joseph disease: a multisystem degenerative disorder of the nervous system. Neurology 1982; 32:192–195.

92. Takiyama Y, Oyanagi S, Kawashima S, Sakamoto H, Saito K, Yoshida M, Tsuji S, Mizuno Y, Nishizawa M. A clinical and pathologic study of a large Japanese family with Machado-Joseph disease tightly linked to the DNA markers on chromosome 14q. Neurology 1994; 44:1302–1308.

93. Bennett RH, Ludvigson P, DeLeon G, Berry G. Large fiber sensory neuronopathy in autosomal dominant spinocerebellar degeneration. Arch Neurol 1984; 41:175–178.

94. Nachmanoff DB, Segal RA, Dawson DM, Brown RB, De Girolami U. Hereditary ataxia with sensory neuronopathy: Biemond's ataxia. Neurology 1997; 48:273–275.

95. Biemond A. La forme radiculo-cordonnale postérieure des dégénerescences spino-cérébelleuses. Rev Neurol 1954; 91:3–21.

96. Zhuchenko O, Bailey J, Bonnen P, Ashizawa T, Stockton DW, Amos C, Dobyns WB, Subramony SH, Zoghbi HY, Lee CC. Autosomal dominant cerebellar ataxia (SCA6) associated with small polyglutamine expansions in the alpha1A-voltage-dependent calcium channel. Nat Genet 1997; 15:62–69.

97. Ophoff RA, Terwindt GM, Vergouwe MN, van Eijk R, Oefner PJ, Hoffmen SMG, Lamerdin JE, Mohrenweiser HW, Bulman DE, Ferrari M, and others. Familial hemiplegic migraine and episodic ataxia type-2 are caused by mutations in the Ca^{2+} channel gene CACNL1A4. Cell 1996; 87:543–552.

98. Geshwind DH, Perlman S, Figueroa KP, Karrim J, Baloh RW, Pulst SM. Spinocerebellar ataxia type 6. Frequency of the mutation and genotype-phenotype correlations. Neurology 1997; 649:1247–1251.

99. Fletcher CF, Lutz CM, O'Sullivan TN, Shaughnessy JD, Hawkes R, Frankel WN, Copeland NG, Jenkins NA. Absence epilepsy in tottering mutant mice is associated with calcium channel defects. Cell 1996; 87:607–617.

100. Subramony SH, Fratkin JD, Manyam BV, Currier RD. Dominantly inherited cerebello-olivary atrophy is not due to a mutation at the spinocerebellar ataxia-1 Machado-Joseph disease, or dentato-rubro-pallido-luysian atrophy locus. Mov Disord 1996; 11: 174–180.

101. Gomez CM, Thompson RM, Gammack JT, Perlman SL, Dobyns WB, Truwit CL, Zee DS, Clark HB, Anderson JH. Spinocerebellar ataxia type 6: gaze-evoked and vertical nystagmus, Purkinje cell degeneration, and variable age of onset. Neurology 1997; 42:933–950.

102. Sasaki H, Kojima H, Yabe I, Tashiro K, Hamada T, Sawa H, Hiraga H, Nagashima K. Neuropathological and molecular studies of spinocerebellar ataxia type 6 (SCA6). Acta Neuropathol 1998; 95:199–204.

103. Tsuchiya K, Ishikawa K, Watabiki S, Tone O, Taki K, Haga C, Takashima M, Ito U, Okeda R, Mizusawa H, and others. A clinical, genetic, neuropathological study in a Japanese family with SCA 6 and a review of Japanese autopsy cases of autosomal dominant cortical cerebellar atrophy. J Neurol Sci 1998; 160:54–59.

104. David G, Abbas N, Stevaini G, Dürr A, Yvert G, Cancel G, Weber C, Imert G, Saudou F, Antoniou E, and others. Cloning of the SCA7 gene reveals a highly unstable CAG repeat expansion. Nat Genet 1997; 17:65–69.

105. Gouw LG, Digre KB, Harris CP, Haines JH, Ptacek LJ. Autosomal dominant cerebellar ataxia with retinal degeneration: clinical, neuropathologic, and genetic analysis of a large kindred. Neurology 1994; 44:1441–1447.

106. Martin JJ, Van Regemorter N, Krols L, Brucher JM, de Barsy T, Szliwowski H, Evrard P, Ceuterick C, Tassignon MJ, Smet-Dieleman H, and others. On an autosomal dominant form of retinal-cerebellar degeneration: an autopsy study of five patients in one family. Acta Neuropathol 1994; 88:277–286.

107. Titica J, van Bogaert L. Heredo-degenerative hemiballismus. A contribution to the question of primary atrophy of the corpus Luysii. Brain 1946; 69:251–263.

108. Smith JK, Gonda VE, Malamud N. Unusual form of cerebellar ataxia. Combined dentato-rubral and pallido-Luysian degeneration. Neurology 1958; 8:205–209.

109. Nagafuchi S, Yanagisawa H, Sato K, Shirayama T, Ohsaki E, Bundo M, Takeda T, Tadokoro K, Kondo I, Murayama N, and others. Dentatorubral and pallidoluysian atrophy expansion of an unstable CAD trinucleotide on chromosome 12p. Nat Genet 1994; 6:14–18.

110. Yazawa I, Nukina N, Hashida H, Goto J, Yamada M, Kanazawa I. Abnormal gene product identified in hereditary dentatorubralpallidoluysian atrophy (DRPLA) brain. Nat Genet 1995; 10:99–103.

111. Becher MW, Rubinsztein DC, Leggo J, Wagster MV, Stine OC, Ranen NG, Franz ML, Abbott MH, Sherr M, MacMillan JC, and others. Dentatorubral and pallidoluysian atrophy (DRPLA). Clinical and neuropathological findings in genetically confirmed North Ameican and European pedigrees. Mov Disord 1997; 12:519–530.

112. Takahashi H, Ohama E, Naito H, Takeda S, Nakashima S, Makifuchi T, Ikuta F. Hereditary dentatorubral-pallidoluysian atrophy: clinical and pathologic variants in a family. Neurology 1988; 38:1065–1070.

113. Tsuchiya K, Oyanagi S, Arima K, Ikeda K, Akashi T, Ando S, Kurosawa T, Ikeuchi T, Tsuji S. Dentatorubropallidoluysian atrophy: clinicopathological study of dementia and involvement of the nucleus basalis of Meynert in seven autopsy cases. Acta Neuropathol 1998; 96:502–508.

114. Burke JR, Wingfield MS, Lewis KE, Roses AD, Lee JE, Hulette C, Pericak-Vance MA, Vance JM. The Haw River syndrome: dentatorubropallidoluysian atrophy (DRPLA) in an African-American family. Nat Genet 1994; 7:521–524.

115. Warner TT, Williams L, Harding AE. DRPLA in Europe. Nat Genet 1994; 6:225.

116. Farmer TW, Wingfield MS, Lynch SA, Vogel FS, Hulette C, Katchinoff B, Jacobson PL. Ataxia, chorea, seizures and dementia. Pathologic features of a newly defined familial disorder. Arch Neurol 1989; 46:774–779.

117. Hayashi Y, Kakita Z, Yamada M, Koide R, Igarashi S, Takano H, Ikeuchi T, Wakabayashi K, Egawa S, Tsuji S, and others. Hereditary dentatorubralpallidoluysian atrophy: detection of widespread ubiquitinated neuronal and glial intranuclear inclusions in the brain. Acta Neuropathol 1998; 96:547–552.

118. Friedreich N. Ueber degenerative Atrophie der spinalen. Hinterstränge Beilage zum Tagblatt der 36. Versammlung deutscher Naturforscher und Aerzte, Speyer 1861(18 Sept); 21;29;30.

119. Friedreich N. Ueber degenerative Atrophie der spinalen Hinterstränge. Virchows Arch 1863; 26:391–419; 433–459; 27–26.

120. Ladame P. Friedreich's disease. Brain 1890;13:467–537.

121. Brousse A. De l'Ataxie Héréditaire (Maladie de Friedreich). Paris: Doin, 1882.

122. Harding AE. Friedreich's ataxia: a clinical and genetic study of 90 families with an analysis of early diagnostic criteria and interfamilial clustering of clinical features. Brain 1981; 104:589–620.

123. De Michele G, Filla A, Barbieri F, Perretti A, Santoro L, Trombetta L, Santorelli F, Campanella G. Late onset recessive ataxia with Friedreich's disease phenotype. J Neurol Neurosurg Psychiatry 1989; 52:1398–1401.

124. De Michele G, Filla A, Barbieri F, Di Maio L, Pianese L, Castaldo I, Calabrese O, Monticelli A, Varrone S, Campanella G, and others. Late onset Friedreich's disease: clinical features and mapping of mutation to FRDA locus. J Neurol Neurosurg Psychiatry 1994; 52:977–979.

125. Dürr A, Cossee M, Agid Y, Campuzano V, Mignard C, Penet C, Mandel JL, Brice A, Koenig M. Clinical and genetic abnormalities in patients with Friedreich's ataxia. N Engl J Med 1996; 335:1169–1175.

126. Klockgether T, Chamberlain S, Wüllner U, Fetter M, Dittman H, Petersen D, Dichgans J. Late-onset Friedreich's ataxia. Molecular genetics, clinical neurophysiology, and magnetic resonance imaging. Arch Neurol 1993; 50:803–806.

127. Klopstock T, Charhrokh-Zadeh S, Holinski-Feder, E Meindl A, Gasser T, Pongrantz D, Müller-Feder W. Markedly different course of Friedreich's ataxia in sib pairs with similar GAA repeat expansions in the frataxin gene. Acta Neuropathol 1999; 97:139–142.

128. Klockgether T, Evert B. Genes involved in hereditary ataxias. Trends Neurosci 1998; 21:413–418.

129. Pandolfo M. Molecular pathogenesis of Friedreich ataxia. Arch Neurol 1999; 56:1201–1208.

130. Delatycki MB, Camakaris J, Brooks H, Evans-Whipp T, Thorburn DR, Williamson R, Forrest SM. Direct evidence that mitochondrial iron accumulation oc-

curs in Friedreich ataxia. Ann Neurol 1999; 45:673–675.
131. Rennie GE. A case of Friedreich's hereditary ataxia with necropsy. BMJ 1899; 2:129–131.
132. Philippe C, Oberthür J. Deux autopsies de maladie de Friedreich. Rev Neurol 1901; 9:971–980.
133. Oppenheimer DR. Brain lesions in Friedreich's ataxia. Can J Neurol Sci 1979; 6:173–176.
134. Hunt JR. Dyssynergia cerebellaris myoclonica—primary atrophy of the dentate system: a contribution to the pathology and symptomatology of the cerebellum. Brain 1921; 44:490–538.

12. Immunocytochemistry and Molecular Genetics of Amyotrophic Lateral Sclerosis

NICHOLAS K. GONATAS

Amyotrophic lateral sclerosis (ALS) is a fatal disease characterized by the progressive degeneration of motor neurons in the spinal cord, brain stem, and motor cortex and by gliosis, which has been assumed to be secondary to neuronal loss. The dramatic neurogenic atrophy of skeletal muscles is caused by the progressive degeneration of motor neurons. The disease has been named after Charcot, who wrote its first comprehensive description, or Lou Gehrig, the legendary American baseball player who died from ALS at the age of 36.[1,2] Amyotrophic lateral sclerosis is often discussed together with a variety of motor neuronopathies (MND) that comprise a heterogeneous group of disorders. This review focuses on classical ALS, with emphasis on recent advances accomplished with molecular genetic and immunocytochemical methods.

The neuropathological diagnosis of ALS depends on the topographical distribution of neuronal loss in the spinal cord, brain stem, and motor cortex; the atrophy of peripheral nerves and skeletal muscles; and on the detection of a variety of characteristic cellular lesions seen in the cytoplasm of neurons and astrocytes. In this regard, ALS is similar to two other neurodegenerative diseases, Parkinson's disease and Alzheimer's disease, although the cellular lesions in ALS are considerably different from the Lewy bodies of the former and the senile plaques and neurofibrillary tangles of the latter.[2]

Immunocytochemical analysis has been a useful tool in the diagnosis of ALS. Recent studies, summarized by Hirano,[3] have identified a variety of inclusions and lesions of the motor neuron, such as the accumulation of phosphorylated neurofilaments, the skein-like or granular ubiquitin-positive inclusions, the Lewy body–like hyaline inclusions (LBHIs), the Bunina bodies, the astrocytic hyaline inclusions (Ast-HIs), and the fragmentation of the Golgi apparatus. The recognition of these cytoplasmic lesions and inclusions contributes to the diagnosis of ALS and introduces insights into the pathogenesis of the disease.[3,4]

The cause of sporadic ALS, which accounts for over 90% of cases, is unknown. A small percentage of cases of ALS is familial (FALS). Fifteen percent of FALS cases are autosomal dominant with mutations of the gene encoding the enzyme Cu,Zn superoxide dismutase (SOD-1), located in chromosome 21, while a smaller number of autosomal FALS cases are recessive because of a defect of an unknown gene located in chromosome 2q23.[5,6] A few cases of FALS have been associated with changes of genes encoding neurofilament proteins.[7,8]

In addition to cases of FALS with a typical clinical symptomatology, evolution, and pathology, which involve predominantly the upper and lower motor neurons, certain cases of FALS have been described with involvement of the posterior and Clark's columns, the spinocerebellar tracts, the Onuf's nucleus, the brain stem reticular formation, and other nuclei.[9–19] These disorders are characterized by a variety of neuronal inclusion bodies, such as the Bunina body, LBHIs, hyaline inclusions (Ast-HIs), and conglomerate neurofilamentous inclusion bodies (CIs), several of which, however, may also be found in typical sporadic ALS, although less frequently. The molecular genetic basis of FALS with a variety of neuronal cytoplasmic inclusion bodies and involvement of several neuronal systems has not yet been elucidated.

Motor neuronopathies or axonopathies that are virtually identical or resemble ALS have been described in transgenic mice expressing mutant forms of the SOD-1 protein and the wild-type human neurofilament heavy gene (NF-H), and in mice expressing three to four times the normal levels of the wild-type murine light-chain neurofilament gene (NF-L).[20–23] These animal models offer unique opportunities to study the pathogenesis of ALS and to test therapies.

LITERATURE REVIEW AND DISCUSSION

Classical Neuropathology of Amyotrophic Lateral Sclerosis

Amyotrophic lateral sclerosis is rarely associated with systemic cancer and the occurence of both disorders is considered coincidental.[24] Nevertheless, a routine autopsy on a patient suspected of suffering either from typical ALS or from another MND should include a detailed examination of the brain, spinal cord, spinal roots, peripheral nerves, and skeletal muscle as well as of all organs. Samples of brain, spinal cord, and blood should be routinely obtained and kept at −80°C for biochemical and molecular genetic studies, which may be used for diagnosis and future research.

The gross examination of the spinal cord often reveals a selective atrophy of the anterior roots, which is highly suggestive of the diagnosis of ALS. Typically, a myelin stain of sec-

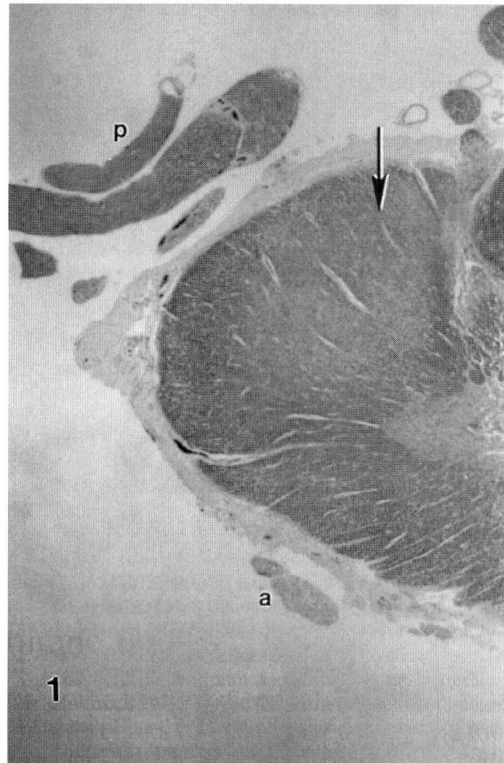

Figure 12–1. Hemisection of the cervical segment of the spinal cord from a patient with sporadic amyotrophic lateral sclerosis, stained for myelin with the method of Weil. There is atrophic and pale staining of the anterior root, (a), and larger and better myelination of the posterior root (b). The corticospinal tract in the lateral column is pale (arrow) because of Wallerian degeneration of axons secondary to the loss of upper motor neurons in the cerebral cortex, brain stem, and medulla.

tions of the spinal cord reveals palor and atrophy of the anterior roots and often palor of the lateral columns due to Wallerian degeneration of axons of the corticospinal tract, especially in cases with severe involvement of the upper motor neuron (Fig. 12–1). The pathology is concentrated in the anterior horn area where loss of the large α-motor neurons, gliosis, and deposits of masses of neurofilaments in enlarged dystrophic axons are invariably noted (Figs. 12–2, and 12–3).

Neurofilaments

Accumulations of neurofilaments in the perikarya of motor neurons are rare in most cases

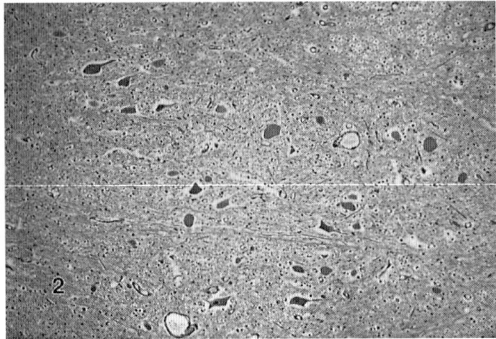

Figure 12–2. Section of cervical segment of spinal cord from a patient with sporadic amyotrophic lateral sclerosis, stained using the Bodian's silver impregnation method. Note numerous processes stained with silver corresponding to dystrophic axons containing masses of neurofilaments.

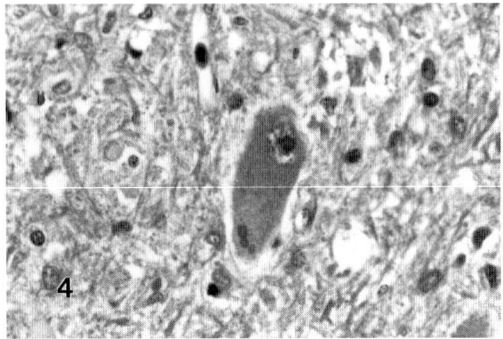

Figure 12–4. Spinal cord motor neuron from a patient with sporadic amyotrophic lateral sclerosis, stained with hematoxylin and eosin, contains an eosinophilic bilobed Bunina body.

of sporadic ALS, although occasionally they can be found in cases with a short clinical course.[25,26] It should be emphasized, however, that accumulations of neurofilaments in neuronal perikarya have been encountered in certain cases of familial ALS[15,17]. Therefore, silver impregnation stains, such as with the Bodian or Bielchowski methods, and immunostaining of spinal cord sections with antibodies against neurofilament phosphorylated and nonphosphorylated epitopes should be included in a routine neuropathological study of a case of ALS.

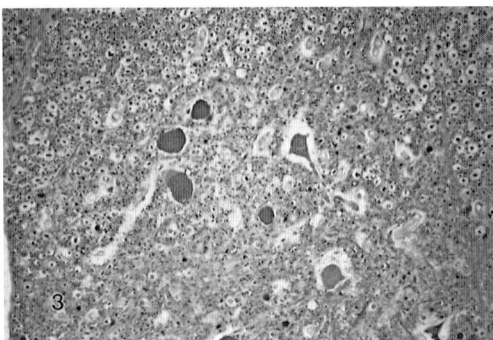

Figure 12–3. Spinal cord section from a patient with sporadic amyotrophic lateral sclerosis, immunostained with the anti-neurofilament antibody SMI 32, reacting with a nonphosphorylated epitope of the heavy neurofilament chain [from Sternberger Monoclonals, Baltimore, MD]. Note prominent staining of several dystrophic axons.

The Bunina Body

Bunina bodies are small cytoplasmic eosinophilic inclusions found in spinal cord motor neurons in familial, sporadic, and Guam ALS (Fig. 12–4).[27] Bunina bodies have been immunostained with an antiserum against cystatin C, a 13 kDa inhibitor of lysosomal cysteine proteinases, thought to be involved in the regulation of cysteinase activity.[28] Bunina bodies contain electron-dense amorphous material and vesicular and tubular structures.[29] The role of Bunina bodies in the pathogenesis of ALS is unknown; however, ALS cases with numerous Bunina bodies had the highest percentage of spinal cord motor neurons with fragmented Golgi apparatus.[30] A similar correlation exists between spinal cord motor neurons containing fragmented Golgi apparatus and ubiquitin-positive inclusions.[31]

Fragmentation of the Golgi Apparatus of Motor Neurons

This unusual lesion of the Golgi apparatus of motor neurons was detected with organelle-specific antibodies and was subsequently confirmed in several studies of spinal cords from patients with sporadic and Guam ALS.[32,33,34] The recent finding of fragmented Golgi apparatus of Betz cells in the motor cortex strongly suggests that the fragmentation of the organelle of spinal cord motor neurons is not secondary to deafferentation.[35] Motor neurons

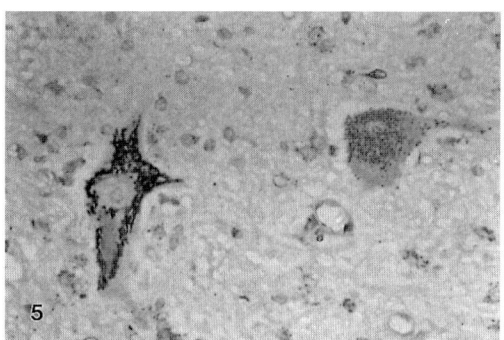

Figure 12–5. Fragmentation of the Golgi apparatus of a spinal cord motor neuron from a patient with sporadic amyotrophic lateral sclerosis. The section was immunostained with an antibody against MG160, a medial Golgi sialoglycoprotein.[34] Compare the normal Golgi network of the neuron on the left with the fragmented Golgi apparatus of the neuron on the right. From Gonatas et al., Histochemistry and Cell Biology 1998; 109: 592,[56] with permission.

with fragmented Golgi apparatus contain isolated small, immunostained elements of the organelle instead of the usual network of interconnected cisternae of the normal Golgi apparatus (Fig. 12–5). Earlier experimental studies had shown that fragmentation of the Golgi apparatus, such as that seen in ALS, was not produced by chromatolysis following axonotomy, neuronal deafferentation, or in a proximal axonopathy induced by β,β'-iminodipropionitrile.[31,36]

The significance of fragmented Golgi apparatus in the pathogenesis of sporadic ALS was unknown until an identical lesion was detected in both asymptomatic and paralyzed transgenic mice expressing the G93A mutation of the human gene encoding the enzyme Cu,Zn superoxide dismutase ($SOD1^{G93A}$).[20,37] The presence of fragmented Golgi apparatus of spinal cord motor neurons in asymptomatic transgenic mice expressing $SOD1^{G93A}$) months before the onset of paralysis suggests that it is an early lesion in the cascade of events leading to the degeneration and death of the motor neuron. A lesion of the Golgi apparatus should have deleterious consequences on axons and presynaptic terminals since most proteins destined for the fast axoplasmic transport are processed by the organelle.[38] Lastly, the recognition of fragmented neuronal Golgi apparatus in both sporadic ALS and in transgenic mice expressing $SOD1^{G93A}$ strongly suggests that common pathogenetic mechanisms operate in both the nonfamilial form of the disease and in FALS associated with mutations of the $SOD1$ gene.

Ubiquitin Inclusions

As the term indicates, the protein ubiquitin is present in virtually all cells and tissues where it plays a central role in intracellular but extralysosomal proteolysis. Two recently published books on ubiquitin have summarized its importance in intracellular protein degradation and in pathology.[39,40] The application of anti-ubiquitin antibodies to ALS and other neurodegenerative diseases has introduced new insights into their nosology and pathogenesis.[41] At least four types of ubiquitin positive inclusions have been observed in motor neurons in most cases of sporadic and familial ALS. These inclusions, summarized by Lowe, are in the form of skein-like (Fig. 12–6), sperical, or granular hyaline bodies, or LBHIs.[4]

Most mammalian proteins conjugated to ubiquitin are destined for degradation by the 26-S proteasome, an ATP-dependent protease composed of about 30 different proteins.[42,43] The molecular composition of the protein substrate(s) conjugated with ubiquitin in the various ubiquitin positive inclusions

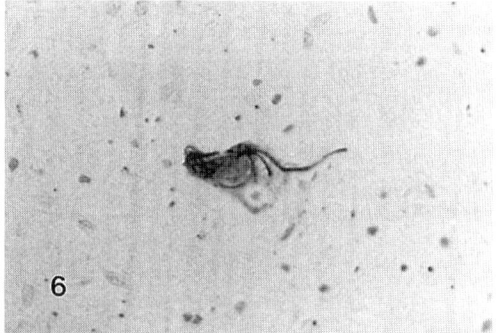

Figure 12–6. Spinal cord motor neuron from a patient with sporadic amyotrophic lateral sclerosis contains a "skein-like" ubiquitin-positive inclusion.[31] The section was immunostained with an anti-ubiquitin antibody obtained from Dako (Carpinteria, CA). [From Mourelatos et al., America Journal Pathology 1994; 144: 1294,[31] with permission.]

found in ALS is unknown. The characterization of these proteins is a major challenge for the future; their accumulation in the form of ubiquitin-positive inclusions may signify that a fundamental molecular lesion in ALS results from the failure of degradation of aggregates of abnormal neuronal proteins. Furthermore, the study of ALS tissues with antibodies against ubiquitin have led to the recognition of the involvement of several non-motor systems, in addition to the primary involvement of the motor neuron.[4] The discussion of these ALS-related syndromes is beyond the scope of this review.

Intraneuronal Lewy Body–Like Hyaline Inclusions

Unusual hyaline or Lewy body–like hyaline inclusions were seen in the cytoplasm of motor neurons and axons and in astrocytes from several cases of familial disease, which were "clinically indistinguishable from ALS" (Fig. 12–7).[11] Furthermore, in addition to the typical involvement of lower and upper motor neurons, these cases showed loss of neurons in the column of Clark and demyelination of the mid-root zones of the spinocerebellar tracts and the posterior colums. On hematoxylin and eosin stains, the hyaline inclusions consisted of a poorly stained homogeneous peripheral zone around a deeply stained central round or oval core resembling a Lewy body (Fig. 12–7). Future studies are needed

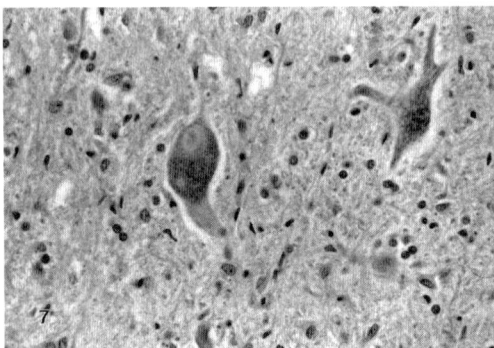

Figure 12–7. Spinal cord motor neuron from a case of familial amyotrophic lateral sclerosis containing a Lewy body–like hyaline inclusion. [From Hirano et al., Archives of Neurology 1967; 16: 232–243,[11] with permission.]

to establish the molecular genetic basis of the inheritance of these unusual cases of FALS.

Familial Amyotrophic Lateral Sclerosis Caused by Mutations of the Gene Encoding Cu,Zn Superoxide Dismutase

Two research groups have recently reported the association of mutations of the *SOD1* gene with FALS.[44,45] Subsequently, a transgenic mouse generated to express $SOD1^{G93A}$ "recapitulated" virtually all clinical and histopathological manifestations of sporadic ALS, including the fragmentation of the Golgi apparatus of motor neurons.[20,37] These molecular genetic studies and the generation of a transgenic mouse model of the disease represent important landmarks in ALS research. The availability of transgenic mice that are faithful models of the human disease is now enabling investigators to examine systematically the pathogenesis of the disease and to test therapies that may be applicable to human ALS.

The mechanism of neurotoxicity exerted by the mutant SOD1 protein has been the subject of numerous but still inconclusive studies. A recent report, however, showed that neurotoxicity in SOD1 transgenic mice correlated with aggregation of the mutant protein in the form of neuronal inclusions; furthermore, elevation of the wild-type SOD1 in these mice did not affect the clinical course of SOD1 mutant–mediated disease.[46] These results suggest that the use of SOD1 mimetics as therapeutic agents may not be effective and have raised the question of whether superoxide-mediated cellular stress is an important component of the neurotoxic action.[46]

Studies with transgenic mice expressing mutations of the *SOD1* gene are directly applicable to the small number of FALS cases caused by similar mutations. However, the identification of SOD1 immunoreactivity in Lewy body–like inclusions in 10 of 20 patients with sporadic ALS raises the interesting question of whether a significant percentage of sporadic ALS is also associated with undegraded SOD1.[47,48]

Role of Astrocytes in the Pathogenesis of Familial Amyotrophic Lateral Sclerosis

In several cases of FALS, some of which are associated with mutations of the *SOD1* gene, neuronal Lewy body–like and astrocytic hyalin inclusions were noted.[49] The astrocytic inclusions were immunostained with antibodies against SOD1, ubiquitin, and several other proteins including α and β tubulin, tau, S-100, and heat shock protein 27 (HSp-27). Similar inclusions were seen in astrocytes in transgenic mice expressing the $SOD1^{G85R}$ mutant.([49] In these mice there was a 50% reduction of the level of the glutamate transporter 1 (GLT-1), normally found predominantly in glia. Furthermore, the astrocytic inclusions increased as the disease progressed and were paralleled by a decrease in GLT-1. These findings suggest that an important component of neurotoxicity might have been caused by an excess of glutamate due to the presumed failure of the glutamate transporter of astrocytes to remove from the extracellular space this potentially toxic amino acid.[49] These studies suggest that astrocytes may not play their assumed "reactive" role in producing scar tissue but instead may be active participants in the disease process.

SUMMARY AND PERSPECTIVE

Amyotrophic lateral sclerosis has a worldwide incidence with strikingly uniform mortality rates. The mortality rates in Harris County, Texas differ little from mortality data from Europe. In Texas, deaths from ALS peak in the 65- to 74-year age-group, amounting to almost 7 per 100,000 per year, with lower mortality rates under the age of 45 and declining rates after the age of 75.[52] Considering the multiethnic character of the population studied, the data from Texas are probably representative of worldwide ALS. The only exception to a uniformly low worldwide mortality rate of ALS had been noted in the island of Guam in the Western Pacific, where the disease commonly appears in combination with parkinsonism and dementia.[53] However, the recent striking decrease in the incidence of the disease in Guam suggests that demographic and other factors may play a role in its pathogenesis.[51]

The occurrence of ALS in combination with Parkinson's and Alzheimer's diseases in Guam suggests that the three disorders may share similar pathogenetic mechanisms, although their initial causative factors are obviously different. This suggestion is supported by the frequent finding of a variety of ubiquitin-positive neuronal and glial inclusions in ALS, in neurites in Alzheimer's disease, in dementia with Lewy bodies, and in Huntington disease.[54] These observations suggest that during the course of ALS and of other neurodegenerative diseases with ubiquitin-positive inclusions, there is extralysosomal degradation of mostly unknown protein substrates, presumably by the ubiquitin–proteasome system.[41–42] A deficiency in the neuronal and glial ubiquitin–proteasome system for degrading pathological protein aggregates may be central to the pathogenesis of ALS and other neurodegenerative diseases.

In view of the increasing value of immunocytochemical analysis in the identification of a variety of neuronal and glial inclusions that appear in both sporadic and more prominently, familial ALS, the neuropathologist should routinely use a variety of immunostains, which might include at least antibodies against various epitopes of neurofilament proteins, ubiquitin, SOD1, and markers of the Golgi apparatus.

The recent discovery of mutations of the gene encoding the SOD1 enzyme in certain cases of FALS[44,45] and the subsequent development of the first transgenic animal model expressing mutant SOD1 of FALS represent major landmarks in ALS research.[20] Thus a better appreciation of the contribution of genetic factors in the pathogenesis of ALS is likely to develop in the near future.

The detection of near-normal levels of SOD1 activity in transgenic mice expressing mutant human *SOD1* has led to formulation of the gain-of-function-hypothesis which proposes that the degeneration of motor neurons is caused by a new, dominant toxic function in *SOD1* mutations, and not by a deficiency in SOD1 enzymatic activities. The nature of the toxic function of mutant forms of the SOD1 protein needs to be clarified before a rational treatment of the MND is attempted in this transgenic animal model of familial ALS.

A few cases of ALS may be associated with abnormal genes encoding neurofilament proteins[7,8]. Neurofilaments, however, need not always play pathological roles; to the contrary, neurofilaments may have salutary effects, as in the case of the protective role of overexpressed neurofilaments in a motor neuron disease induced by mutant *SOD1*.[53,54] Similarly, two mouse models of a neurodegenerative disease, dystonia musculorum and an SOD1-mediated form of a human ALS-like disease, progressed with no change in clinical course in a transgenic mouse background in which axons did not contain neurofilaments[4]. These results indicate that the role of neurofilaments in the pathogenesis of sporadic and familial ALS must be reassessed. Also, it should be re-emphasized that in most cases of sporadic ALS, in contrast to the frequent accumulation of neurofilaments in dystrophic or swollen axons, significant focal accumulations of neurofilaments in neuronal cell bodies are either rare, requiring extensive sampling and sectioning, or do not occur at all.

The relevance of conclusions reached from studies of transgenic mice expressing mutations of the *SOD1* gene of FALS to sporadic ALS remains to be proven. The identical nature of certain neuronal lesions, such as the ubiquitin-positive inclusions and fragmentation of the Golgi apparatus, found in both transgenic SOD1 mice and in sporadic ALS suggests that common "downstream" pathogenetic pathways exist despite obvious differences in the initiating causes.[32,38] In this regard, the recent question posed by Bredesen et al. is of great interest and their hypothesis deserves further testing.[55] Specifically they proposed that age-associated post-translational modifications of SOD1 (namely glycations, carbonyl modifications of amino acid residues, and disulfide formation) may produce structural and functional effects on SOD1 similar to those produced by the over 50 described single amino acid substitutions in FALS. If this is proven to be correct, therapies tried in transgenic mice expressing mutations of *SOD1* may be applicable not only to FALS with *SOD1* mutations but also to sporadic ALS.

This work was supported by NS 36732-01 from the National Institutes of Health of the U.S. Public Health Service. We wish to thank Anna Stieber for the immunocytochemical stains of the Golgi protein MG160, neurofilaments, and ubiquitin; Jackie Gonatas for the polyclonal antibody against MG160, Eileen Heatherby for the neurohistological stains; and Asao Hirano of the Neuropathology Division, Montefiore Hospital and Medical Center, Bronx, NY, for Figure 12–7.

REFERENCES

1. Charcot JM, Joffroy A. Deux cas d'atrophie musculaire progressive avec lésions de la substance grise et des faisceaux antérolatéraux de la moelle épinière. Arch Physiol Normal Pathol Par 1869; 2:354, 629, 744.
2. Hirano A. Cytopathology of amyotrophic lateral sclerosis. Adv Neurol 1989; 56:91–101.
3. Hirano A. Neuropathology of ALS: an overview. Neurology 1996; 47 (Suppl 2): S63–S66.
4. Lowe J. New pathological findings in amyotrophic lateral sclerosi. J Neurol Sci 1994; 124:38–51.
5. Siddique T, Nijhawan D, Hentati A. Familial amyotrophic lateral sclerosis. JR Neural Transm Suppl 1997; 49:219–233.
6. Siddique T, Deng H-X. Genetics of amyotrophic lateral sclerosis. Hum Mol Genet 1996; 5:1465–1470.
7. Figlewicz DA, Krizus A, Martinoli MG, Meininger, V, Dib, M, Rouleau GA, Julien, J-P. Variants of the heavy neurofilament subunit are associated with the development of amyotrophic lateral sclerosis. Hum Mol Genet 1994; 3:1757–1761.
8. Julien J-P, Mushynski ME. Neurofilaments in health and disease. Prog Nucl Acid Res Mol Biol 1998; 61: 1–23.
9. Horton WA, Eldridge R, Brody JA. Familial motor neuron disease. Evidence for at least three different types. Neurology 1976; 26:460–465.
10. Engel WK, Kurland LT, Klatzo I. An inherited disease similar to amyotrophic lateral sclerosis with a pattern of posterior column involvement. An intermediate form? Brain 1959; 82:203–220.
11. Hirano A, Kurland LT, Sayer GP. Familial amyotrophic lateral sclerosis: a subgroup characterized by posterior and spinocerebellar tract involvement and hyaline inclusions in the anterior cells. Arch Neurol, 1967; 16:232–243.
12. Kihira T, Yoshida S, Uebashi Y, Yase Y, Yoshimesu F. Involvement of Onuf's nucleus in ALS. Demonstration of intraneuronal conglomerate inclusions and Bunina bodies. J Neurol Sci 1991; 104:119–128.
13. Takayashi K, Nakamura H, Okada E. Hereditary amyotrophic lateral sclerosis. Histochemical and electron microscopic study of hyaline inclusions in motor neurons. Arch Neurol 1972; 27:292–299.
14. Mizusawa H, Hirano A, Yen SH. Anterior horn cell inclusions in familial amyotrophic lateral sclerosis contain ubiquitin and phosphorylated neurofilament epitopes. Neuropathology 1991; 11–20.
15. Hirano A, Nakano, I, Kurland LT, Mulder, DW, Holley, PW, Sacco Manno G. Fine structural study of neurofibrillary changes in a family with amyotrophic lateral sclerosis. J Neuropathol Exp Neurol 1984; 43: 471–480.

16. Schochet SS, Hardmann JM Ladewig PP, Earle, KM Intraneural conglomerates in sporadic motor neuron disease. Arch Neurol 1969; 20:548–553.
17. Mizusawa H, Matsumoto S, Yen SH, Hirano A, Corona-Rojas, RR, Donneyfeld H. Focal accumulation phosphorylated neurofilaments within anterior horn cell in familial amyotrophic lateral sclerosis. Acta Neuropathol 1989; 79:37–43.
18. Takahashi K, Nakamura H, Okada E. Hereditary amyotrophic lateral sclerosis. Histochemical and electron microscopic study of hyaline inclusions in motor neurons. Arch Neurol 1972; 27:292–299.
19. Kato S, Hayashi H, Nakashima K, Nanba E, Kato M, Hirano A, Nakano I, Asayama K, Ohama E. Pathological characterization of astrocytic hyaline inclusions in familial amyotrophic lateral sclerosis. Am J Pathol 1997; 151:611–620.
20. Gurney ME, Pu H, Chiu AY, Motor neuron degeneration in mice that express a human Cu, Zn superoxide dismutase mutation. Science, 1994; 264:1772–1775. Dal Canto MC, Polchow CY, Alexander DD, Caliendo J, Hentati A, Kwon YW, Deng HX, Chen W, Zhai P, Sufit RL, Siddique T.
21. Coté F, Collard JF, Julien JP. Progressive neuronopathy in transgenic mice expressing the human neurofilament heavy gene. Cell 1993; 73:35–46.
22. Xu Z-S, Cork LC, Griffin JW, Cleveland PW. Increased expression of neurofilament subunit NF-L produces morphological alterations that resemble the pathology of human motor neuron disease. Cell 1993; 73:23–33.
23. Price DL, Sidodia SS, Borchelt DR. Genetic neurodegenerative diseases: the human illness and transgenic models. Science 1998; 282:1079–1083.
24. Forsyth PA, Dalmau J, Graus F, Cwik V, Rosenblum MK, Posner JB. Motor neuron syndromes in cancer patients. Ann Neurol 1997; 41:722–730.
25. Gambetti P, Shecket G, Ghetti Hirano A, Dahl D. Neurofibrillary changes in human brain. An immunocytochemical study with neurofilament antiserum. J Neuropathol Exp Neurol 1983; 42:69–79.
26. Hirano A, Inoue K. Early pathological changes of amyotrophic lateral sclerosis. Electron microscopy study of chromatolysis, spheroids and Bunina bodies. Neurol Med (Tokyo) 1980; 13:148–160.
27. Okamoto K. Bunina bodies in amyotrophic lateral sclerosis. Neuropathology (Tokyo) 1993; 13:193–199.
28. Okamoto K, Hirai S, Amari M, Watanabe M, Sakurai A. Bunina bodies in amyotrophic lateral sclerosis immunostained with rabbit anti-cystatin C antiserum. Neurosci Lett 1993; 162:125–128.
29. Okamoto K, Hirai S, Shoji M, Harigaya Y Fokuda T. Widely distributed Bunina bodies and spheroids in a case of atypical sporadic amyotrophic lateral sclerosis. Acta Neuropathol 1991; 81:349–352.
30. Stieber A, Chen YJ, Wei S, Mourelatos Z, Gonatas J, Okamoto K, Gonatas NK. The fragmented neuronal Golgi apparatus in amyotrophic lateral sclerosis includes the trans-Golgi network: functional implications. Acta Neuropathol 1998, 95:245–253.
31. Mourelatos, Z, Hirano A, Rosenquist AC, Gonatas NK. Fragmentation of the Golgi apparatus of motor neurons in Amyotrophic Lateral Sclerosis (ALS). Clinical studies in ALS of Guam and experimental studies in deafferented neurons and in β,β'-Iminodipropionitrile axonopathy. Am. J Pathol 1994; 144:1288–1300.
32. Mourelatos Z, Adler H, Hirano A Donnenfeld H, Gonatas J, Gonatas NK, A. Fragmentation of the Golgi apparatus of motor neurons in amyotrophic lateral sclerosis revealed by organelle-specific antibodies. Proc Natl Acad Sci, USA 1990; 87:4393–4395.
33. Mourelatos Z, Yachnis A, Rorke LI, Mikol J, Gonatas NK. The Golgi apparatus of motor neurons in amyotrophic lateral sclerosis. Ann Neurol 1993; 33:608–615.
34. Gonatas NK. Contributions to the physiology and pathology of the Golgi apparatus. Am J Pathol 1994; 140:731–737.
35. Fujita Y, Okamoto K, Sakurai A, Amari A, Nakazato Y, Gonatas NK. Fragmentation of the Golgi apparatus of Betz cells in patients with amyotrophic lateral sclerosis. J Neurol Sci 1999; 163:81–85.
36. Croul SE, Mezitis SGE, Gonatas NK. An anti-organelle antibody in pathology. The chromatolytic reaction studied with a monoclonal antibody against the Golgi apparatus. Am J Pathol 1988; 133:355–362.
37. Mourelatos Z, Gonatas NK, Stieber A, Gurney ME, Dal Canto MC. The Golgi apparatus of spinal cord motor neurons in transgenic mice expressing mutant Cu,Zn superoxide dismutase becomes fragmented in early, preclinical stages of the disease. Proc Natl Acad Sci USA 1996; 93:5472–5277.
38. Hammerschlag, R, Stone GC, Bolen E, Lindsey JD, Ellisman MH. Evidense that all newly synthesized proteins destined for fast axonal transport pass through the Golgi apparatus. J Cell Biol 1982; 93: 568–575.
39. Rechsteiner M, ed. Ubiquitin. New York: Plenum Press, 1998.
40. Peters J-M, Robin Harris J, Finley D, eds. Ubiquitin and the Biology of Cell. New York: Plenum Press, 1998.
41. Mayer JR, Lowe J. Ubiquitin and the molecular pathology of human disease. In: Peters J-M, Harris JR, Finley D, eds. Ubiquitin and the Biology of the Cell. New York: Plenum Press, 1998:429–462.
42. Hershko A. Lessons from the discovery of the ubiquitin system. Trends 1996; 21:445–449.
43. Rechsteiner M. The 26 S proteasome. In Peters J-M, Harris JR, Finley D, eds. Ubiquitin and the Biology of the Cell. 1998:147–189.
44. Rosen DR, Siddique T, Patterson D, Figlewicz DA, Sapp P, Hentati A, Donaldson D, Goto J, O'Regan JP, Deng HX, Rahmani Z, Krizus A, McKenna-Yasek D, Cayabyab A, Gaston SM, Berger R, Tanzi RE, Halperin JJ, Herzfeldt B, Van den Bergh R, Hung HY, Brid T, Deng G, Mulder DW, Smyth C, Laing NG, Soriano E, Pericak-Vance MA, Haines J, Rouleau GA, Gusella JS, Horvitz HR, Brown RH Jr. Mutations in Cu/Zn superoxide dismutase gene are associated with familial amyotrophic lateral sclerosis. Nature 1993; 362:59–62.
45. Deng HX, Hentati A, Tainer JA, Iqbal Z, Cayabyab A, Hung WY, Getzoff ED, Hu P, Herzfeldt B, Roos RP, Warner C, Deng G, Soriano E, Smyth C, Parge HE, Ahmed A, Roses AD, Hallewell RA, Pericak-Vance MA, Siddique T. Amyotrophic lateral sclerosis and structural defects in Cu,Zn superoxide dismutase. Science 1993; 261:1047–1051.
46. Bruijn LI, Houseweart MK, Kato S, Anderson KL,

Anderson, SD, Ohama, E, Reaume AG, Scott RW, Cleveland, DW. Aggregation and motor neuron toxicity of an ALS-linked SOD1 mutant independent from wild-type SOD1. Science 1998; 281:1851–1854.

47. Shibata N, Hirano A, Kobayashi M, Sasaki S, Kato T, Matsumoto, S, Shiozawa Z, Komori T, Ikemoto A, Umaharas T, Asayama K. Cu/Zn superoxide dismutase-like immunoreactivity in Lewy body-like inclusions of sporadic amyotrophic lateral sclerosis. Neurosci Lett 1994; 179:149–152.

48. Kato S, Shimoda M, Watanabe Y, Nakashima K, Takahashi K, Ohama E. Familial amyotrophic lateral sclerosis with a two base pair deletion in superoxide dismutase 1 gene: multisystem degeneration with intracytoplasmic hyaline inclusions in astrocytes. J Neuropathol Exp Neurol 1996; 55:1089–1101.

49. Bruijn LI, Becher MW, Lee MK, Anderson KL, Jenkins NA, Copeland NG, Sisodia SS, Rothstein JD, Borchelt DR, Price DL, Cleveland DN. ALS-linked SOD1 mutant G85R mediates damage to astrocytes and promotes rapidly progressive disease with SOD1-containing inclusions. Neuron 1997; 18:327–338.

50. Annegers JF, Appel SH, Perkins P, Lee J. Amyotrophic lateral sclerosis mortality rates in Harris County, Texas. Adv Neurol 1991; 56:239–243.

51. Lavine L, Steele JC, Wolfe N, Calne DB, O'Brien PC, Williams DB, Kurland LT, Schoenberg BS. Amyotrophic lateral sclerosis/parkinsonism-dementia complex in southern Guam: is it disappearing? Adv Neurol 1991; 56:271–285.

52. Mayer RJ, Landon M, Lowe J. Ubiquitin and the molecular pathology of human disease. In: Peters J-M, Robin Harris J, Finley D, eds. Ubiquitin and the Biology of Cell. New York: Plenum Press, 1998:429–462.

53. Couillard-Despress S, Zhu Q, Wong PC, Price DL, Cleveland DW, Julien J-P. Protective effect of neurofilament heavy gene overexpression in motor neuron disease induced by mutant superoxide dismutase. Proc Natl Acad Sci USA 1998; 95:9626–9630.

54. Eyer J, Cleveland DW, Wong PC, Peterson AC. Pathogenesis of two axonopathies does not require neurofilaments. Nature 1998; 391:584–587.

55. Bredesen DE, Ellerby LM, Hart PJ, Wiedau-Pazos M, Valentine, JS. Do post-translational modifications of CuZnSOD lead to sporadic amyotrophic lateral sclerosis? Ann Neurol 1997; 42:135–137.

13. Huntington Disease with Emphasis on Late Onset and Aging

JEAN PAUL G. VONSATTEL, E. TESSA HEDLEY-WHYTE, AND MARIAN DIFIGLIA

In memory of Dr. Edward Peirson Richardson, Jr.

Huntington disease (HD) is an autosomal dominant illness with mid-life onset and psychiatric, cognitive, and motor symptoms. Death occurs 12–15 years from the time of symptomatic onset.[1]

The HD mutation consists of an unstable expansion of CAG (trinucleotide) repeats within the coding region of the gene *IT15* (for "interesting transcript" referred to as "HD-IT15 CAG repeats"). This gene, on chromosome 4 (4p63), encodes the protein huntingtin.[2] The mutation in huntingtin produces expanded glutamine residues. The function of normal huntingtin and the mechanism of pathogenicity of the polyglutamine expansion in mutant huntingtin are unknown. The abnormal huntingtin still retains some functions of the normal huntingtin since individuals homozygous for the HD gene produce only mutant huntingtin and yet appear to have the same clinical features as heterozygous HD patients. The abnormal huntingtin is present in all organs, yet the pathology of HD is apparently restricted to the brain, where degeneration occurs initially in the striatum and cortex and eventually may appear throughout the brain as a constellation of the toxic effect of the mutation and the ensuing secondary changes. Among the theories for the selective cellular damage in HD, the most compelling involve impaired energy metabolism and excitotoxicity.

Recent reports demonstrating the aggregation of mutant huntingtin in HD brain, the interaction of mutant huntingtin with novel and known proteins, and the development of HD-transgenic mice have provided opportunities for identifying the cause of neuronal loss in HD.

CLINICAL AND GENETIC FEATURES OF HUNTINGTON DISEASE

The diagnostic criteria for HD include (1) a family history of Huntington chorea; (2) progressive motor disability with chorea or rigidity of no other cause, and (3) psychiatric disturbance with gradual dementia of no other cause. The disease is universal. The prevalence of patients with HD in North America and Europe is 5–10/100,000. It is highest in populations of western European origin and lowest in African or Asian populations. Apparently, new mutations rarely occur.[3]

Most persons with the HD mutation develop and function normally into early adulthood. Involuntary movements may begin any time after infancy. Chorea is the most com-

We recently published a review on Huntington disease from which this report is derived.

Table 13-1. Number of CAG Repeats in *IT15* Gene on Chromosome 4 (4p63) with or without Huntington Disease

Individuals	(HD-IT15 CAG)$_n$ Trinucleotide Repeats on Chromosome 4
General population (both alleles); nonaffected allele of HD carriers	6–34
Possible HD carriers; some HD patients (commonly one allele, the other allele as above)	Diagnostically uncertain range: 35–39 (rare, apparently normal elderly individuals[18])
HD nonagenarians	Likely to be in the lower range (38–40); however, may be longer than 40[15]
Most HD patients (usually only one allele affected)	40–55
HD patients with juvenile onset (6% of all HD patients;[5] usually only one allele affected)	Commonly 70 or more—up to 259—usually paternal transmission; expansion exceeding 100 is rare

HD, Huntington disease.

mon involuntary movement in adult patients with HD. Rigidity is seen in patients with juvenile onset. Deficits in attention and memory are often present at the time of onset of motor dysfunction and gradually worsen. Comprehensive reviews of dementia in HD are provided by Hayden,[4] Folstein,[5] and Harper.[6]

The mean age of patients at onset of movement disorders is 40 years. In 9% of patients symptoms are present before the age of 20. Twenty-five percent of subjects remain asymptomatic until age 50 or later.[7] Young et al. reported that 94% of patients were adult onset, and 6% were juvenile onset in the Venezuelan cohort.[8] In 90% of patients with age of onset under 10 years, the gene is paternally transmitted.[6]

In normal subjects or in affected ones, the HD-IT15 CAG segment of the *huntingtin* gene is inherited in a mendelian fashion, is polymorphic and unstable, and undergoes changes during meiosis, including increases or decreases of 1–5 CAG repeat units.[9–11] Larger increases may occur, particularly in paternal transmissions. Table 13-1 summarizes the HD-IT15 CAG length repeats observed in the general and HD populations. Individuals with 34 or fewer HD-IT15 CAG repeats on the longest allele will not develop HD, those with 35 to 39 may or may not develop HD, and those with 40 or more will develop the disease. Most HD patients with adult onset of symptoms have expansions ranging from 40 to 55 HD-IT15 CAG units.[9,12–14] The HD-IT15 CAG repeats in HD nonagenarians are likely to be in the lower range (38–40), thus carriers of the HD mutation with repeats in this range may develop HD if they live long enough.[15] Expansions of 70 or more repeats usually occur in patients with juvenile onset of symptoms. Rarely, patients have expansions exceeding 100 repeats. The number of repeats correlates inversely with age of onset or with age at death.[16] More than 99% of patients with the clinical and pathological hallmarks of HD have an expanded huntingtin allele.[10,13,17] A few individuals with the phenotype of HD have been reported to have HD-IT15 CAG repeat lengths in the normal range.[2,17] Furthermore, apparently normal elderly individuals were found to have 36–39 repeats.[18] Nevertheless, evaluation of the HD-IT15 CAG repeat length is the most powerful diagnostic test now available to clinicians.[13] Such a test, however, should be offered only if a set of recommended provisions is followed.[19]

ORGANIZATION OF THE BASAL GANGLIA SYSTEM

Nomenclature

The *basal ganglia* consist of the corpus striatum and the amygdaloid nucleus. Because of their connections, the subthalamic nucleus and substantia nigra are often included among the basal ganglia. The *corpus striatum* includes the neostriatum (caudate nucleus and putamen) and paleostriatum (globus pallidus). The *globus pallidus* (GP), or *paleostriatum*, is divided into *external* (GPe) and *internal* (GPi) segments. The *neostriatum* is commonly referred to as the "striatum." The *substantia nigra* (SN) has two main zones: the *pars reticulata* (SNr) and the *pars compacta* (SNc).

Pathways

The striatum collects inputs from the entire neocortex. It processes the signals and then sends them through other parts of the basal ganglia to areas of frontal cortex that have been implicated in motor planning and execution.[20] A useful model of the functional anatomy of disorders of the basal ganglia was proposed by Albin et al.[21] The model is a practical conception of basal ganglia pathophysiology with emphasis on chorea, parkinsonism, and hemiballism. According to this model, the basal ganglia concerned with motor functions have two compartments—one for input and one for output. The *input compartment* consists of the caudate nucleus (CN) and putamen, which receive inputs from the entire cerebral cortex and the SN. The *output compartment* includes the subthalamic nucleus, SNr, and GPi. The target nuclei of the output compartment are in the thalamus, which has an excitatory action upon the cortex.

Two major pathways (a direct and an indirect) integrate the input compartment with the output compartment. The direct (monosynaptic) striatal pathway projects to the GPi. The indirect pathway passes first to the GPe, subthalamic nucleus, and SNr, and then to the GPi, which sends projections to the thalamus. These two efferent systems of the striatum have apparently opposing effects upon the output nuclei and thalamic target nuclei.[22] The disruption of these striatal efferent pathways in HD leads to the development of motor dysfunction. A selective loss of striatal neurons that give rise to the indirect pathway reduces the inhibitory action of the GPe upon the subthalamic nucleus. The subthalamic nucleus then becomes hypofunctional and causes reduction of the inhibitory action of the GPi upon the thalamus. This subsequent disinhibition of the thalamus leads to chorea. Albin et al. hypothesized that chorea might result from preferential loss of striatal neurons projecting to the GPe, and that rigid–akinetic HD might be due to the additional loss of striatal neurons projecting to the GPi.[23] Recent data suggest that dyskinesia results not only from an imbalance of activity between the two pallidal segments (GPe, hyperactivity; GPi, hypoactivity) but also from imbalance within each pallidal segment.[24]

The Striosome–Matrix Compartments

The primate neostriatum is heterogeneously organized based on levels of acetylcholinesterase (ACh) activity. The intensity of histochemical staining for ACh is weak in the 300- to 600-μm–wide striosomes and dense in the surrounding matrix.[25,26] Many other molecular markers, including huntingtin, exhibit an uneven distribution corresponding to the striosome–matrix compartments. Afferent and efferent connections of the striatum contribute to the striosome–matrix configuration. Afferents to the striosomes originate in the SNc, prefrontal cortex, and limbic system. Efferents from the striosomes terminate in the SNc. Afferents to the matrix originate in the motor and somatosensory cortices and in the parietal, occipital, and frontal cortices. Efferents from the matrix terminate in the GPe, SNr, and GPi.[27,28] The striosome–matrix organization detected by ACh activity is relatively preserved in the HD neostriatum.[29] Neuronal loss and gliosis occur in both compartments and appear first in the striosomes, indicating that the neurons in striosomes may be more vulnerable at an early stage of HD than those in the matrix.[30] Matrix neurons projecting to the GPe appear to degenerate before matrix neurons projecting to the GPi.

Classification of Neostriatal Neurons

Two groups of neostriatal neurons can be distinguished with Cresyl violet staining. One group consists of small or medium-sized neurons, and a second consists of large neurons (40 μm in diameter and larger). The ratio of small–medium to large neurons averages 175:1 (range 130:1–258:1). Golgi and ultrastructural studies identify at least six categories of neurons.[31,32] The two main categories consist of neurons with spiny dendrites (spiny neurons) and those with smooth dendrites (aspiny neurons).[31] Both the spiny and aspiny neurons are represented by small to medium-sized and large neurons.[33] Spiny neurons account for at least 80% of neostriatal neurons and all contain γ-aminobutyric acid (GABA). They are the principal input and output neurons of the neostriatum. Subsets of spiny neurons contain enkephalin, dynorphin, substance P (SP), or calbindin. Enkephalin is a reliable marker for the indirect pathway and SP is a reliable marker for the direct pathway. Aspiny neurons are interneurons with local connections. Medium-sized aspiny neurons colocalize nicotinamide adenine dinucleotide phosphate diaphorase (NADPH-d), somatostatin (SS), neuropeptide Y (NPY), and nitric oxide synthase (NOS). Other medium-sized aspiny neurons contain cholecystokinin (CCK) or the calcium-binding protein parvalbumin. The large aspiny neurons utilize ACh.

Glutamate and Dopamine Neurotransmission in the Striatum

Corticostriatal projections use glutamate as a neurotransmitter, which is the principal excitatory neurotransmitter in the brain. Glutamate activates ionotropic glutamate receptors (iGluR), which control ion channels, and metabotropic glutamate receptors (mGluR), which control the activity of membrane enzymes via G proteins.[34] The iGluR activated by glutamate are N-methyl-D-aspartate (NMDA), α-amin-3-hydroxy-5-methyl-4-isoxazole-propionic acid (AMPA), and kainate receptors. So far, five subtypes of NMDA receptors (NMDAR) can be distinguished. The neostriatal spiny neurons, which are the most vulnerable in HD, contain predominantly NMDAR-1 and NMDAR-2B. Aspiny neurons, which are relatively preserved in HD, contain mainly NMDAR-2D. Among the three known subtypes of AMPA receptors, GluR1 predominates in the striosomes and in aspiny interneurons.

The mGluR family includes three groups of G protein–coupled receptors, which modulate excitatory synaptic transmission. Individual mGluR subtypes mediate distinct, facilitatory (group I subtype), or inhibitory (group II and group III subtypes) actions on neuronal degenerative processes. Their activation might lead to either neurotoxicity or neuroprotection. Neostriatal spiny neurons express mainly mGlu5 (group I) and mGlu3 (group II) receptors.

Excitotoxic mechanisms are thought to play a major role in the pathophysiology of HD. Overstimulation of iGluR (notably NMDAR) increases the neuronal cytoplasmic concentration of Ca^{2+}, causing cell death. Overstimulation of group I mGluR opens voltage-operated Ca^{2+} channels and facilitates glutamate release, resulting in neurotoxicity. Dopaminergic innervation of neostriatal neurons originates in the SNc. The five subtypes of dopamine (DA) receptors (D1 to D5) identified in the neostriatum can be subdivided into D1-like (D1 and D5) and D2-like (D2, D3, and D4) receptors as per pharmacological criteria. D1 receptors are localized in striatal spiny neurons that give rise to the direct pathway, and D2 receptors are present in spiny neurons of the indirect pathway. There is a marked loss of D1 and D2 receptors in asymptomatic mutation carriers of HD.[35] This suggests that altered DA receptors contribute to the pathophysiology of HD.

NEUROPATHOLOGY

Historical View

Anton initially observed an association between bilateral atrophy of the putamen and choreic movements in the presence of an apparently normal cerebral cortex and spinal cord.[36] Jelgersma later correlated the atrophy of the caudate nucleus with chorea in HD.[37] Alzheimer attributed the chorea of HD mainly to atrophy of the striatum.[38] There was disagreement in early reports about the extent of involvement of the claustrum,[39–42] hypothalamus,[43] hypothalamic lateral tuberal nucleus,[44] amygdala,[45,46] hippocampal formation,[41,47] thalamus,[39,42,48] subthalamic nucleus,[42,49] red nucleus,[50] substantia nigra, especially pars reticulata,[42,48,49,51–53] locus coeruleus,[54] superior olivary nucleus,[41,49,55,56] pons and medulla oblongata,[39,57] cerebellum,[42,58,59] and spinal cord.[41,48,49,58,60] The discrepancies between early reports on the pathology of HD are due in part to the wide spectrum of pathological features that can exist across HD brains and the lack of a large series of HD brains available for study by the same group of investigator(s). In our HD research center, the opportunity to systematically evaluate more than 1000 HD brains during the past 19 years has enhanced our knowledge of HD pathology.

Current understanding of HD pathology is based on information gathered from the use of conventional and morphometric approaches and histochemical, immunohistochemical, and in situ hybridization techniques. Distinct topographic and cellular alterations, notably in the striatum and cerebral cortex, are characteristic of HD pathology. A grading system that stages the extent of striatal pathology has been developed and is widely used as a research tool.

General Features

On external examination, 80% of HD brains show atrophy of the frontal lobes and 20% are apparently normal. The mean brain weight at postmortem examination ($n = 163$) was 1067 g (normal is about 1350 g) with a sample modal weight of 1140 g.[61] Examination of coronal sections reveals bilateral, symmetric atrophy of the striatum in 95% of HD brains. This striatal atrophy is prominent in 80%, mild in 15%, and subtle, if at all, in 5% of the brains[1] (Fig. 13–1 and Fig. 13–2). Nonstriatal regions show atrophy of variable severity or have a normal appearance (Fig. 13–3). As a rule, the brain is diffusely smaller than normal in the late stage of disease. Increased atrophy may occur in nonstriatal regions of HD brain with superimposed morbidity. For example, enhanced atrophy of the limbic system (cingulate gyrus, amygdala, hippocampal formation) with severe widening of the temporal horn of the lateral ventricle may occur when HD coexists with Alzheimer's disease (Fig. 13–4). Morphometric analyses using five standardized coronal sections each from 30 graded HD brains revealed a 21%–29% cross-sectional area loss in the cerebral cortex, a 28% loss in the thalamus, a 57% loss in the CN, and a 64% loss in the putamen.[62] The white matter also showed a 29%–34% loss in area; this finding supports

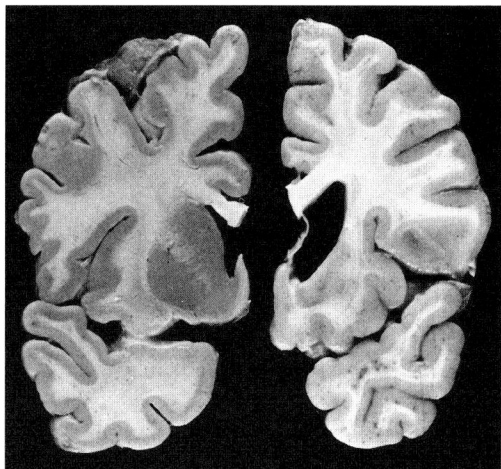

Figure 13–1. Coronal sections passing through the nucleus accumbens of a 94-year-old woman (*left*) (HD-IT15 CAG, long allele 40; grade 1) and of a 12-year-old boy (*right*) (HD-IT15 CAG, long allele 80, grade 4), both with Huntington disease. The anterior neostriatum of the 94-year-old woman (left) is apparently normal, while that of the 12-year-old boy (right) is severely atrophic with a concave, ventricular margin of the head of the caudate nucleus. Note the volumetric difference of the centrum semi-ovale in grade 1 (left) and grade 4 (right). However, the corpus callosum of the nonagenarian (left) is thinner than that of the boy. There is no significant difference in thickness of the cerebral cortex between the two specimens.

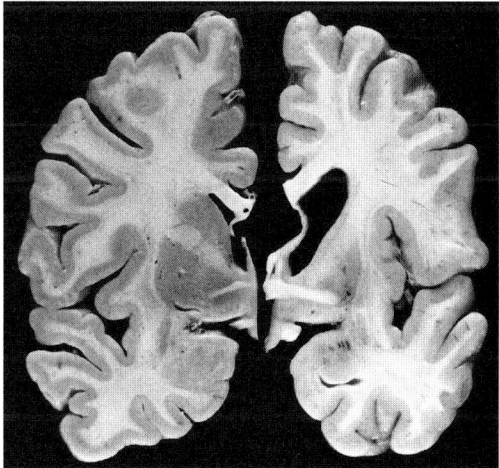

Figure 13–2. Coronal sections passing through the anterior commissure of the same patients as in Figure 13–1. The striatum and centrum semi-ovale of the 94-year-old woman (*left*; grade 1) are apparently normal, while those of the 12-year-old are severely atrophic (*right*). Note the difference in thickness of the anterior white commissures.

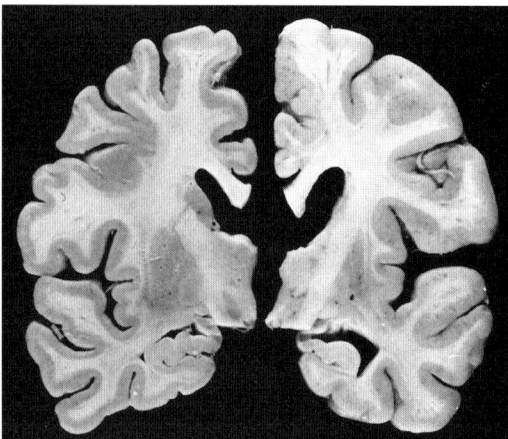

Figure 13–3. Coronal sections passing through the subthalamic nucleus of the same patients as in Figure 13–1. The tail of the caudate nucleus of both patients is indistinguishable. The atrophy of the body of the caudate nucleus and lenticular nucleus is notable only in the section of the 12-year-old boy (*right*; grade 4) in contrast to that of the 94-year-old woman (*left*; grade 1). The thalamus is more atrophic in grade 4 (right) than in grade 1 (left) despite a difference of 82 years between the two patients.

early observations by Kiesselbach in 1914[63] and by Dunlap in 1927.[64] With volumetric analyses from six HD brains, Lange et al. found a 20% loss of the "hemisphere and cortex," 58% loss of the "striatum," 57% loss of the GPe, 50% loss of the GPi, and a 24% loss of the subthalamic nucleus.[65]

In HD, the striatum is the only site where neuronal loss is associated with "active" reactive, fibrillary astrocytosis (Fig. 13–5). An increased density of oligodendrocytes, up to twice that of controls, is observed, notably in the anterior neostriatum.[39,41,48,66] Usually, by conventional methods of evaluation, there is no visible reactive gliosis in the nonstriatal parts of the HD brain, even when there is atrophy. There is no lymphoplasmatic infiltration. However, scattered, reactive microgliocytes are present and can be detected with appropriate antibodies within the striatum, neocortex (Fig. 13–6) and white matter.[67]

Grading of Striatal Neuropathology

The pathological hallmark of HD is the gradual atrophy of the neostriatum. Neostriatal de-

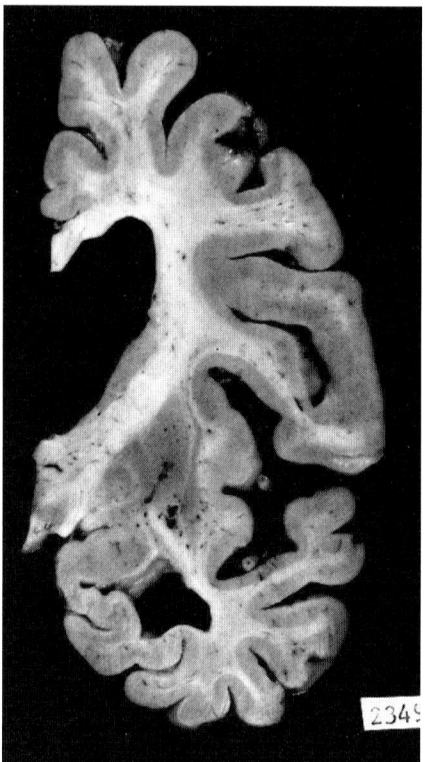

Figure 13–4. Coronal section passing through the amygdaloid nucleus of an 88-year-old woman with Huntington disease (HD-IT15 CAG 17/39, grade 2) and concomitant Alzheimer disease (case 4, Table 13–3). There is marked atrophy of the striatum, centrum semi-ovale, amygdaloid nucleus, and neocortex.

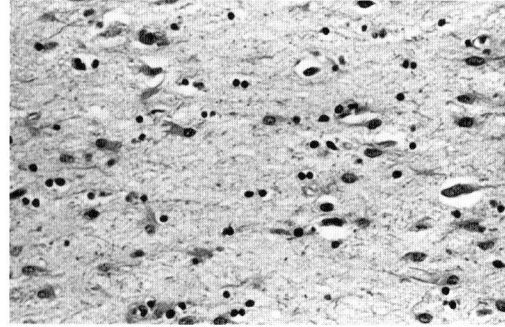

Figure 13–5. Microphotograph of the head of the caudate nucleus, dorsal, at midpoint between the ependyma and medial border of the internal capsule. Neuronal loss and fibrillary astrocytosis are severe (grade 3), in contrast to the relative preservation of the nucleus accumbens (see Figure 13–8, same case, same histological section). Luxol fast blue, counterstained with hematoxylin and eosin; original magnification, ×312.

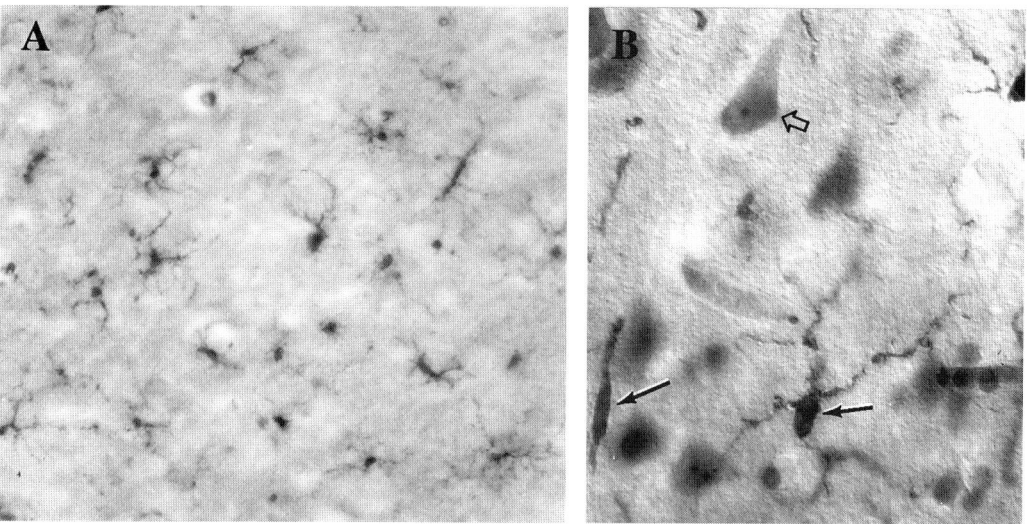

Figure 13–6. Reactive microglia in neocortex of patient with Huntington disease, grade 3. *A.* Reactive microglia labeled with antibody to thymosin β4. *B.* Reactive microglia (arrows) are rod shaped and have short, stout, or radiating processes. Section was counterstained with Cresyl violet to show pyramidal neurons (open arrow).

generation has an ordered and topographic distribution.[39,41,42,48,52,58,61,63,64,68–70] The tail of the caudate nucleus (TCN) shows more degeneration than the body (BCN), which in turn is more involved than the head (HCN) (Fig. 13–7). Similarly, the caudal portion of the putamen is more degenerated than the rostral portion. Along the coronal axis of the neostriatum, the dorsal neostriatal regions (Fig. 13–5) are more involved than the ventral ones (Fig. 13–8). With progression of the disease, neostriatal degeneration appears to simultaneously move in a caudorostral direction and in a dorsoventral/mediolateral direction. Fibrillary astrogliosis parallels the loss of neurons along caudorostral and dorsoventral gradients of decreasing severity. Most remaining neostriatal neurons in the postmortem brains have normal morphology but contain more lipofuscin and may be smaller than normally expected. In addition, scattered atrophic neurons stain darker with Luxol fast blue counterstained with hematoxylin and eosin (LHE) than the apparently healthy neurons.

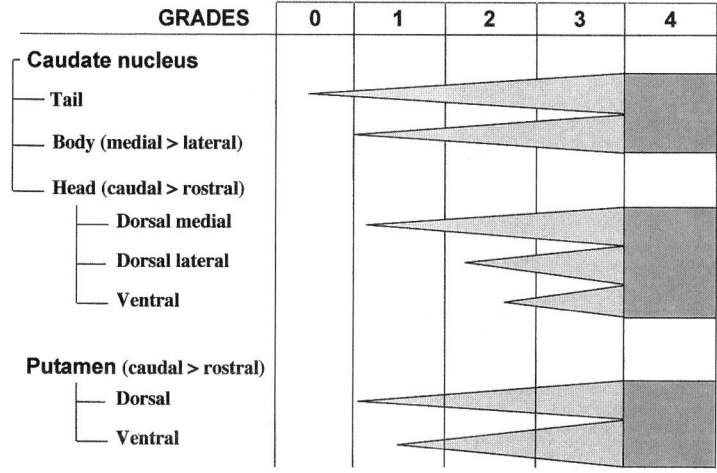

Figure 13–7. Diagram depicting the grades and variation of striatal neuronal loss and gliosis observed in Huntington disease. There is a decreasing gradient of neuronal loss and gliosis along the caudorostral, mediolateral, and dorsoventral axes of the striatum. In grade 4, these gradients are blurred because of the extent of the degeneration.

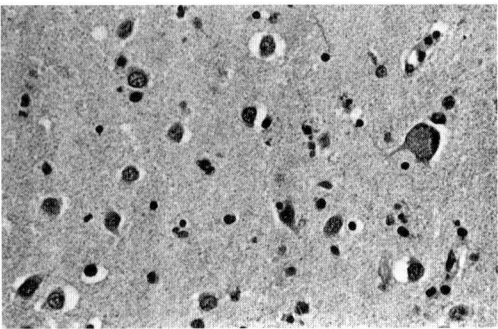

Figure 13–8. Microphotograph of the nucleus accumbens (grade 3) at midpoint between the ependyma and lateral border of putamen. Both neuronal loss and gliosis are mild in contrast to that in the dorsal portion of the neostriatum (see Figure 13–5, same case and same histologic section). Luxol fast blue, counterstained with hematoxylin and eosin; original magnification, ×312.

Thus, they are referred to as "neostriatal dark neurons" (NDN). These neurons have a scalloped cellular membrane, a granular dark cytoplasm, and a nucleus with condensed chromatin (Fig. 13–9). They are scarce in both the atrophic and in the relatively preserved zones; however, their density increases in the intermediary zone, which lies between the two other zones. About 20% of NDN are labeled with TdT-mediated dUTP-biotin nick end labeling (TUNEL) methods, suggesting that they may be undergoing apoptosis, a hypothesis supported by observations made using a cellular model of HD.[71]

Less than 5% of HD brains show unusual microscopical changes in the anterior neostriatum. They consist of one to five (rarely more) discrete round islets of relatively intact parenchyma. The cross sections of the islets measure about 0.5–1.0 mm and thus are larger than striosomes. The density of neurons in islets is the same as or slightly lower than that in the normal neostriatum, but the density of astrocytes is increased.[72] Islets are found more frequently in patients with juvenile than adult onset of clinical symptoms. The reason for this is unclear.

The distinctive pattern of degeneration in the HD striatum was the framework for the grading system developed by Vonsattel et al.[61] The assignment of a grade of neuropathological severity is based on gross and microscopic findings of the striatum obtained from three standardized coronal sections that include the striatum. This system has five grades (0–4) of severity of striatal involvement. Grade 0 comprises <1% of all HD brains. Gross examination shows features indistinguishable from normal brains. Cell counts indicate a 30%–40% loss of neurons in the HCN and no visible reactive gliosis. Grade 1 comprises 3% to 4% of all HD brains. The TCN is much smaller than normal and atrophy of the BCN may also be present (Fig. 13–3, left). Neuronal loss and astrogliosis are evident in the TCN and less so in the BCN and dorsal portion of both the head and nearby dorsal putamen. Cell counts show 50% or greater loss of neurons in the HCN. A careful examination of the entire length of the TCN is necessary for assignment of grade 1 since the body and head of the CN and putamen may appear normal on gross examination. The TCN of neurologically normal subjects may show variations including periodic constriction or segmentation (Fig.13–10). In contrast to HD, the normal variations are focal and therefore likely to be apparent in only one or two coronal sections.

Brains assigned grade 2 comprise 16%, those assigned grade 3 comprise 52%, and those assigned grade 4 comprise 28% of all HD brains. Gross striatal atrophy is mild to moderate in grade 2 and severe in grade 3. The microscopical changes in grades 2 and 3 are more severe than in grade 1 and less than

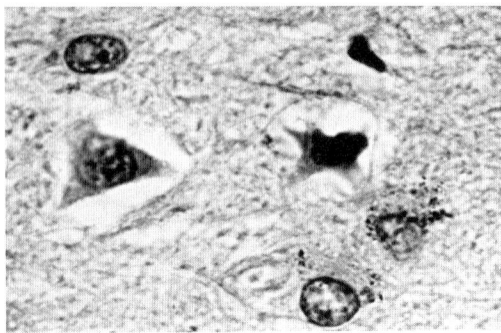

Figure 13–9. Neostriatal dark neurons. Scant neostriatal neurons are atrophic and have a scalloped cellular membrane with a granular dark cytoplasm and a nucleus with condensed chromatin. They are more readily found in the transition zone between the severely involved and the relatively preserved parts of the neostriatum. Luxol fast blue, counterstained with hematoxylin and eosin; original magnification ×500.

TAIL OF THE CAUDATE NUCLEUS IN NORMAL AND IN HUNTINGTON DISEASE

Sagittal representation

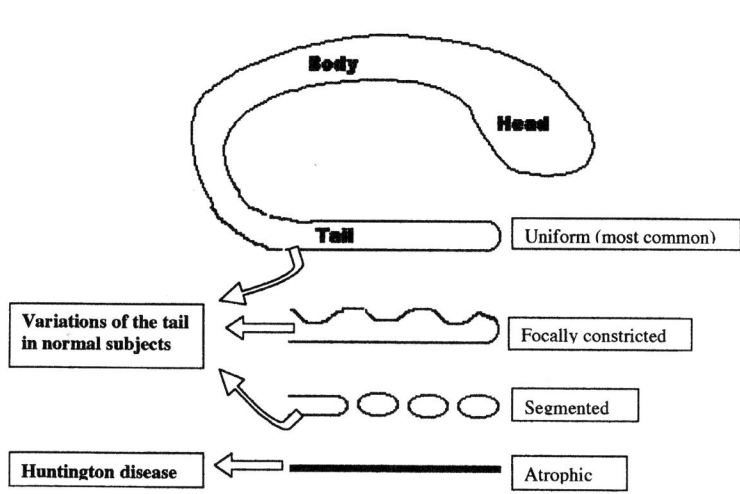

Figure 13–10. Sagittal representation of the caudate nucleus. Variations of the tail of the caudate nucleus are occasionally seen in subjects without neurological disorder. The variations include segmental constrictions or segmental absence of the tail that mimics Huntington disease findings in grades 1 and 2 and especially in older patients with HD-IT15 CAG repeat expansion between 37 and 40. A careful examination of the entire length of the tail of the caudate nucleus is necessary for assignment of grade 1 or 2. Notably in grade 1, the anterior striatum is apparently normal on gross examination while the tail of the caudate nucleus may be severely atrophic (see Figs. 13–1, 13–2, and 13–3).

in grade 4 brains. In grade 4, the striatum is severely atrophic and the neostriatum depleted of 95% or more of neurons. In at least 50% of grade 4 brains the underlying nucleus accumbens remains remarkably preserved.

Relationship of Neostriatal Pathology to Changes in Other Brain Regions

In general, there is a good correlation between the grade of striatal disease and the atrophy of brain regions other than the striatum in HD. In grades 1 and 2, nonstriatal structures of the brain are unremarkable or show only mild atrophy (Fig. 13–3, left) unless there is age-related volumetric loss or a superimposed disease (Fig. 13–4). However, in grades 3 and 4, non-neostriatal structures of HD brains including globus pallidus or paleostriatum, neocortex, thalamus, subthalamic nucleus, SN, white matter, and cerebellum are slightly to markedly smaller than normally expected (Fig. 13–3, right). As further detailed below, these gray matter structures may show minimal or marked neuronal loss, usually without reactive astrocytosis. Similarly, the white matter atrophy may be severe, yet without any microscopical abnormality recognized by conventional methods.

GLOBUS PALLIDUS

The GP shows atrophy in grades 3 and 4, with the external segment much more involved than the internal segment. In grade 4, there is a 50% volume reduction of the GP (Fig. 13–3, right). Microscopically, the GP is less abnormal than would be expected from the degree of macroscopic atrophy. The neurons of the GP are more densely packed than normal in grade 3, and even more so in grade 4, which suggests that although tissue bulk decreases, neurons are relatively preserved. Lange et al. found that in HD the absolute number of pallidal neurons decreases up to 40%, but the neuronal density is up to 42% higher than normal in the GPe and 27% higher in the GPi.[65] Thus, in the GP the atrophy is apparently chiefly due to loss of neuropil and hence of striatal fiber connections and fiber passage, and to a lesser extent to loss of neurons.[39,52,53,61,68] Reactive gliosis is usually confined to the external segment and is visible in grade 4 and to a lesser extent in grade 3. The ansa lenticularis is thinner than normal in grades 3 and 4.

CEREBRAL CORTEX

Atrophy of the cerebral cortex may or may not be pronounced in grades 3 and 4. Even when atrophy is marked, neuronal loss in the HD cerebral cortex is hard to appreciate on general survey of histological sections, resulting in contradictory statements in the literature. On the one hand, Dunlap found the HD cortex ($n = 30$) to be "slightly thinner than in the controls but the difference was very little," and he found no cell loss.[64] On the other hand, Terplan claimed that neocortical neuronal loss is severe in HD. Terplan compared the normal cortex from a 20-year-old executed convict with that of the severely atrophic cortex from a 38-year-old woman with HD who died after a 10-year history of chorea and was found to have lung gangrene at autopsy.[58] Forno and Jose stated that changes in the cerebral cortex were often subtle and difficult to evaluate on histologic examination, so that to the naked eye, the thinning of the cortical ribbon was the more reliable finding.[41] Lange found that the volume loss of the cerebral cortex in HD was more severe in the occipital lobe than in the other lobes.[50] Zalneraitis et al. observed little or no neuronal loss, normal astrocytes, and a relatively normal content of glial fibrillary acidic protein in the cortex of 14 HD brains.[73]

Braak and Braak detected "a layer-specific" loss of neurons without an increase in astrocytes in the entorhinal cortex and subiculum of seven HD patients with grades 3 or 4 striatal atrophy.[47] Sotrel et al. performed morphometric studies of 81 HD prefrontal cortices and showed a loss of large pyramidal neurons in layers III, V, and VI in grades 2–4, with the greatest loss being in grade 4. There was no astrogliosis, however, and cortical oligodendrocytic density was increased.[74] Cudkowicz and Kowall found a loss of cortical long projecting neurons but a normal number of local circuit neurons in graded HD brains.[75] Contrary to Sotrel et al., they did not find a correlation between the grades and the severity of cortical neuronal loss. Selemon et al. measured the cortical thickness of Brodmann area (BA) 9 from nine grade 3 or grade 4 HD brains.[76] They noticed an overall 28% reduction in the cortical thickness with a range from normal thickness to severe thinning (up to 46%) and they observed that cortical neuronal density was increased in three of them.[76] In a later study, using eight of the nine HD brains, Selemon et al. recorded a 35% increase in neuronal density, a 61% increased glial density, and 30% cortical thinning in BA46.[77] Furthermore, Rajkowska et al. evaluated BA9 and BA17 of seven HD brains from the same series as that used by Selemon et al. and reported a 50% to 80% reduction in density of "extra large neurons" in layers I, III, V, and VI. In addition, Rajkowska et al. observed in layer VI a 23% decrease in the density of large neurons associated with a 150% increase in the density of small neurons.[78] Hedreen et al. found a 57% neuronal loss in layer VI and a 71% loss in layer V in BA10 of five HD brains with grade 4 striatal atrophy.[79]

THALAMUS, SUBSTANTIA NIGRA, AND SUBTHALAMIC NUCLEUS

In the thalamus, astrocytosis and neuronal loss in the centrum medianum is regularly observed in grade 4 and to a lesser extent in grade 3 brains; otherwise, the thalamus is apparently normal in lower grades. There is a loss of neurons in the SNr.[42,48,49,51–53] The SNc is thinner than normal, yet its number of neurons is apparently normal in all grades, giving the impression of an increased density of pigmented neurons.[51,53] In the subthalamic nucleus, there is a discrepancy between the marked atrophy present in grades 3 and 4 (up to 25% volumetric loss[65]) and the scarcity of reactive astrocytes.

CEREBELLUM

There is no consensus on cerebellar findings in HD. Dunlap's comprehensive report on 29 patients with chronic chorea (17 with proven family history) found only 1 patient with HD who had cerebellar atrophy. He identified the fraction of the weight of cerebrum to cerebellum to be 1/5.8 in HD compared to 1/7.2 in controls.[64] McCaughey found "possible patchy loss of Purkinje's cells" in 6 HD brains and loss of neurons in the dentate nucleus in 9 of his series of 21 HD brains.[39] In a series of "about 300" HD brains, Rodda found only three with "severe atrophy of the cerebellum" at postmortem examination.[80] Two of those three patients had adult-onset symptoms and no unequivocal family history of HD. The third patient had epilepsy and a family history of HD, had epilepsy, and died at the age of 6 years. Jeste et al. conducted a quantitative study of the cerebellar cortex of 17 HD patients, 2 of whom had epilepsy.[81] There was no cerebellar atrophy noticed on gross examination. They found a decrease (up to 50%) in the density of Purkinje cells but normal thickness of granular and molecular layers. The Purkinje cell loss was variable in its extent in different patients.

Cerebellar atrophy is often reported in patients with juvenile onset. The four HD patients with juvenile onset and severe cerebellar atrophy reported by Jervis all had epilepsy.[82] The 9-year-old HD patient reported by Markham and Knox had epilepsy and severe cerebellar atrophy but "no focal atrophy in Sommer's sector."[83] Byers et al. reported four juvenile HD patients, all with severe cerebellar atrophy.[84] The hippocampal formation was available in three of the four patients; of these three hippocampi, two showed neuronal loss and reactive gliosis, suggesting that to some extent the cerebellar atrophy may have been secondary to remote hypoxic-ischemic events. Juvenile HD patients are prone to seizures, which may account for some cerebellar or hippocampal neuronal loss, two sites notably vulnerable to hypoxic-ischemic events.

In our extensive collection of HD brains, we found that the cerebellum is smaller than normally expected in grades 3 and 4 but relatively less atrophic than the cerebral cortex and GP. Despite the clear presence of atrophy, neuronal density in the cerebellar cortex frequently appears within normal limits. Segmental loss of Purkinje cells with or without Bergmann gliosis may occur; however, these changes are inconsistent and seem not to be specific for HD. Extensive loss of neurons in the cerebellar cortex occurs rarely in our cases and most of the time it is associated with agonal or remote hypoxic-ischemic events. Indeed, concomitant neuronal changes indistinguishable from those caused by ischemia were often found in the Sommer sector or in neocortical watershed territories in our series of HD brains with marked cerebellar neuronal loss. The cerebellum of all of our nine patients with juvenile onset was smaller than normal, and the Purkinje cell density was either apparently normal or slightly decreased, except in one case where it was marked. The advent of antiepileptic drugs prevents hypoxic episodes and may explain why cerebellar changes in juvenile HD patients are less striking now than before, despite the possible toxicity of phenytoin on Purkinje cells. Quantitative studies are needed to determine whether the cerebellum is a site of primary degeneration in HD.

RELATIVE VULNERABILITY OF NEOSTRIATAL NEURONS

Medium-sized spiny projection neurons bear the brunt of the degenerative process in HD. As visualized by Golgi impregnation, dendritic changes (recurving of dendrites, decrease or increase in the density of spines, and altered shape and size of spines) were observed in spiny neurons in contrast to aspiny neurons, indicating that there is selective neuronal degeneration in the spiny neuron population in HD.[85] Variable rates of degeneration among different types of spiny neurons occur. Enkephalin-containing spiny neurons projecting to the GPe are more affected than SP-containing neurons projecting to the Gpi.[86–88]

The NADPH-d aspiny interneurons are relatively resistant to degeneration in HD, perhaps because of the types of glutamate receptors they express.[89] Interestingly, infusion of the endogenous NMDAR agonist quinolinic acid in rat striatum causes loss of spiny neurons with sparing of NADPH-d aspiny neurons. This experimental selective neuronal vulnerability resembles the one that occurs in HD. Furthermore, the intrastriatal infusion of the non-NMDA receptor agonist, kainate or quisqualate, causes loss of both spiny and NADPH-d aspiny neurons, yet local injection of s-4-carboxy-3-hydroxyphenylglycine, which is both an agonist of group II and an antagonist of group I mGluR, protects striatal neurons against quinolinic acid.[34,90,91] Thus, NADPH-d–enriched neurons may lack NMDAR and instead have a preponderance of kainate receptors. Likewise, subtypes of mGluR may have protective effects. These observations indicate that the selective neuronal vulnerability and variable rates of neuronal degeneration may be a function of specific glutamate receptors—either iGluR or mGluR or both. In short, striatal projection neurons degenerate in a specific temporal sequence: striato-SNc are followed by striato-GPe and striato-SNr, then followed by striato-GPi.[92] The extreme striatal atrophy and the loss of neurons in grade 4 indicates that both spiny and aspiny neurons are vulnerable at the end stage of the disease. That both medium-sized and large neostriatal neurons eventually degenerate in HD is repeatedly mentioned in the literature.[38,42,48,50,52,58]

Impaired energy metabolism may also play a role in the selective vulnerability of medium-sized spiny neurons. Indeed, regional and selective neostriatal neuronal loss (projection neurons > interneurons) can be induced by subacute systemic injection of 3-nitropropionic acid, which causes irreversible inhibition of succinate dehydrogenase–complex II of the mitochondrial respiratory chain.[93] The toxic effect of 3-nitropropionic acid can be blocked by NMDA antagonists. Gu et al. reported increased cerebral lactic acid levels in patients with HD and decreased succinate dehydrogenase activity in postmortem HD striata, which further supports the hypothesis of impairment of energy metabolism in HD.[94] Impaired energy metabolism results in decreases in high-energy phosphate stores and a deteriorating membrane potential. Under these conditions, the voltage-sensitive Mg^{2+} block of NMDA receptors is relieved, allowing the receptors to be activated by glutamate, which may lead to neuronal death by a slow excitotoxic mechanism.[95]

THE GRADING SYSTEM IN HUNTINGTON DISEASE RESEARCH

Since 1985, most investigations using HD postmortem tissue include correlation with the grade of neuropathologic severity. The use of the grading system has helped to identify the earliest histopathological and biochemical changes in HD. The analysis of low-grade HD striatum showed that immunoreactive enkephalin-containing neurons projecting to the GPe were more affected than the SP-containing neurons projecting to the Gpi.[86,87] Histochemical studies of NADPH-d–labeled aspiny neurons showed that these cells were relatively spared in low and high grades of striatal pathology.[89]

Some alterations in the HD cortex are not synchronized with those involving the gradient of striatal neurodegeneration.[96] For example, there was no relationship found between elevated peptide levels in the HD cortex and the grade.

There is a correlation between the HD-IT15 CAG lengths and grades of neuropathological severity.[97,98] Correlation of HD-IT15 CAG repeat lengths and grades using 310 brains from clinically diagnosed HD patients showed that repeat stretches of 37–40 units occurred in all grades but that the largest alleles (>50 units) occurred only in grades 3 and 4.[97] Furtado et al. found that greater numbers of trinucleotide repeats were associated with higher grades or greater neuronal loss in both the caudate nucleus and putamen.[97] Gutekunst et al. observed that aggregates of huntingtin increase in size in higher grades.[99] Sapp et al. reported a grade-dependent increase in reactive microglia in both neocortex and striatum.[67]

CHARACTERISTICS OF WILD-TYPE AND MUTANT HUNTINGTIN

Huntingtin is a protein of about 350 kDa and is expressed in neurons throughout the brain.[100,101] In the normal striatum, huntingtin immunoreactivity is weak in the striosomes and conspicuous in the matrix with variability in staining intensity among medium-sized neurons.[102] It is found in the cytoplasm of cell bodies, dendrites, and axon terminals.[99,103] Huntingtin associates with vesicle membranes and microtubules and therefore may function in vesicle transport.[104] An important role for huntingtin in embryogenesis is suggested by the finding that deletion of both huntingtin alleles in mice is lethal in utero.[105,106]

Mutant huntingtin with its elongated NH2-terminal polyglutamine stretch can be distinguished from the wild type by its slower migration in SDS-PAGE and detection on Western blot with anti-huntingtin antisera.[99,103] Mutant huntingtin co-distributes with wild

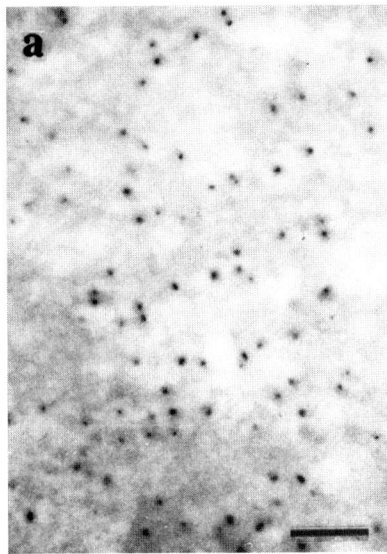
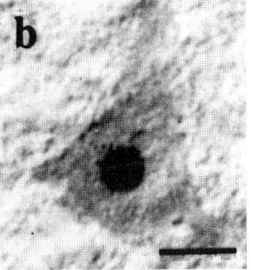

Figure 13–11. Nuclear inclusions in Huntington disease neocortex. A. Immunoperoxidase method and antibody to N-terminus of huntingtin shown with the Nomarski optics reveal many nuclear inclusions. Scale bar = 1 μm. B. A pyramidal neuron with a large nuclear inclusion. The adjacent nucleolus is not labeled. Scale bar = 10 μm.

type in all regions and in both gray and white matter. Mutant huntingtin is also detected with the wild type in cortical synaptosomes of HD heterozygotes' brain tissue, indicating that the abnormal protein is expressed and transported with the normal one to nerve endings.[107]

In the HD brain, huntingtin immunoreactivity is increased in neurons, compared to that in control brains. Labeling appears diffusely elevated in the nucleus and cytoplasm and in multivesicular organelles of affected neurons.[108] The N-terminal region of mutant huntingtin accumulates in the nucleus and cytoplasm of cortical, allocortical, hippocampal, and neostriatal neurons.[99,103,109] Cortical neurons with nuclear (Fig. 13–11) or cytoplasmic inclusions or both are more prevalent in the brains of patients with juvenile onset of symptoms than patients with adult onset of symptoms.[103] Cytoplasmic accumulation of N-terminal mutant huntingtin also appears in degenerating corticostriatal axons in brains with low-grade Huntington pathology.[110] This observation suggests that cortical projections to the striatum may be among the earliest affected by the mutant protein.

Mice transgenic for exon 1 of the HD gene encoding a highly expanded polyglutamine tract develop nuclear inclusions before the onset of motor deficits. The results in mice suggest that nuclear inclusions may be involved in HD pathogenesis. However, the HD brains of patients with adult onset of symptoms and low-grade pathology (grades 1 or 2) show only scant nuclear inclusions.[110] Studies in cultured cells suggest that cell death is caused by the presence of mutant protein in the nucleus, but not by the formation of nuclear inclusions.[71,111] Other studies in cultured cells and in transgenic mice suggest that the cytoplasmic accumulation of mutant huntingtin may be sufficient to cause neurotoxicity.[111–113]

PUTATIVE PATHOGENIC MECHANISMS INVOLVING MUTANT HUNTINGTIN

A toxic gain of function by mutant huntingtin may lead to neurodegeneration in HD. Inhibition of normal huntingtin function does not appear to be involved in HD pathogenesis, based on the observation that heterozygous knock out mice with only one wild-type huntingtin allele develop a normal phenotype.

The elongation of the polyglutamine track in huntingtin may alter the configuration of the protein and hence modify its solubility or its interactions with other cellular proteins. Burke et al. found that huntingtin interacts through its polyglutamines with the enzyme glyceraldehyde-3-phosphate dehydrogenase

(GAPDH), and they postulate that inhibition of GAPDH results in a loss-of-energy metabolism.[114] This enzymatic inhibition supports the hypothesis of impairment of energy metabolism as a possible mechanism of the selective neurodegeneration in HD. Li et al. identified a protein (huntingtin-associated protein, or HAP-1) of unknown function, which binds to huntingtin. This binding is enhanced by an expanded polyglutamine stretch, which may induce a change of function.[115] Saudrou et al., using an in vitro model of HD that exhibits features of neurodegeneration of HD in vivo, reported cytopathological features of apoptosis in degenerating striatal neurons transfected by mutant huntingtin.[71] Furthermore, they demonstrated that striatal but not hippocampal neurons were susceptible to the effects of mutant huntingtin. Wheeler et al. hypothesized that the effect of the glutamine tract of mutant huntingtin may act by altering interaction with a critical cellular constituent or by depleting a form of huntingtin essential to medium-sized spiny neurons.[116]

Many theories have been proposed to explain the formation of insoluble aggregates by mutant huntingtin.[117,118] The co-distribution of ubiquitin with mutant huntingtin in the aggregates suggests that ubiquitin-dependent proteolysis of mutant huntingtin is incomplete. Whether the presence of the aggregates contributes to the altered cell function is not known.[119] These aggregates may alter the regulation of gene transcription, protein interactions, and protein transport within the nucleus and cytoplasm, and vice versa.[116,118,120] Vesicle transport may also be affected since mutant and wild-type huntingtins associate with vesicle membranes and co-distribute in axon endings.[104] Recent observations suggest that caspase-1 may play an important role in the pathogenesis of HD. Indeed, in a transgenic mouse model of HD, expression of a dominant-negative caspase-1 mutant extends survival and delays both symptomatic onset and appearance of neuronal inclusions. Furthermore, in this model, mice receiving intraventricular caspase inhibitors have later onset of symptoms, less symptoms, and longer life expectancy than those without administration of caspase inhibitors.[121] Cell-specific factors may be crucial in determining the selective neuronal and regional toxicity of mutant huntingtin in the striatum and cortex. Given the clinical and pathological spectra of HD, however, additional genetic factors are also likely to influence disease phenotype.

OCCURRENCE OF FEATURES ATTRIBUTED TO USUAL AGING IN HUNTINGTON DISEASE BRAINS

With increasing age, the human brain undergoes changes that are commonly ascribed to usual aging if the individual was without neurological symptoms. The changes are qualitatively similar in Alzheimer's disease (AD) except that they are more prominent, widespread, and symptomatic. These changes include cerebral atrophy, enlargement of the ventricular system, neuronal loss, amyloid deposition, cerebral amyloid angiopathy, and formation of neuritic, immature, and diffuse plaques; formation of neurofibrillary tangles of Alzheimer's; granulovacuolar degeneration; and accumulation of Marinesco, Hirano, or Lewy bodies. These features span a continuum between physiological aging and neurodegeneration and require a certain threshold of severity or frequency for individuals to become symptomatic, provided they live long enough.

The evaluation of changes ascribed to usual aging or to AD are challenging in the HD population for the following reasons. First, HD brains from older patients are rare since the life expectancy of the HD population is shorter than the non-HD population; this suggests that AD would be unusual in the HD population.[41,122–124]

Second, the symptoms due to the HD mutation are likely to predominate and mask those of Alzheimer's disease, thus the diagnosis of coexistent AD depends on neuropathological evaluation. Third, it is not known whether the HD mutation influences the occurrence, extent, and phenotype of changes assigned to old age or to AD. Fourth, the striatal susceptibility to degeneration caused by the HD mutation may be less severe in individuals with both HD and AD than in individuals with HD alone, since the cortical Alzheimer's pathology is likely to reduce the corticostriate glutamate afferents. This reduction would putatively lessen the cytotoxic effect of glutamate on neostriatal neurons in patients with both HD and AD compared to patients with HD alone.

As mentioned above, during usual aging, plaques or tangles or both may be present in brains of cognitively normal, elderly individuals, notably in the limbic system.[125–127] The consensus is that Hirano bodies in the Sommer sector result from an age-related alteration of microfilaments.[128] The number of Marinesco bodies increases with age.[129] Although Lewy bodies are characteristically found in idiopathic Parkinson's disease and in Lewy body dementia, they may be present in neurologically normal, older individuals.[130] Therefore, one could assume that patients with late-onset HD who are older than 50 years of age are more likely to develop cerebral changes associated with usual aging than those with adult onset who are less than 50 years of age, unless the HD mutation prevents or increases it.

To determine the frequency of changes related to usual aging in HD brains, we recorded the presence or absence of neuritic plaques; neurofibrillary tangles of Alzheimer's; Hirano bodies in CA2, CA1, and subiculum of hippocampal formation; Marinesco bodies in the pars compacta of the substantia nigra and nucleus coeruleus; Lewy bodies in the substantia innominata, hypothalamus, and pigmented nuclei of the brain stem; and cerebral amyloid angiopathy (CAA). Those brains containing plaques or tangles or both in a quantity that was not sufficient to meet the criteria for the diagnosis of AD were designated "Alzheimer changes." We assigned the additional diagnosis of AD (see below) only to those HD brains with Alzheimer's-related cortical lesions corresponding to stages V or VI, or isocortical stages according to Braak and Braak.[131]

The occurrence of selected, cerebral changes associated with usual aging that were recorded in HD brains, is summarized in Table 13–2. We identified Alzheimer's changes insufficient to meet the neuropathological criteria of AD in 13% of HD brains from patients of all ages. The morphologic and topographic

Table 13–2. Occurrence of Features Attributed to Usual Aging and of Lewy Bodies in Huntington Disease

		AGE AT DEATH (YEARS)		
	N (%)	Mean (SD)	Range	M/F*
Alzheimer changes (tangles or neuritic plaques or both) in 565 HD brains				
With	72 (12.7)	72 (10.5)	37–97	33/39
Without	493	57 (15)	9–89	238/211 (44)
Hirano bodies in 431 HD brains				
With	55 (12.8)	72 (11)	45–96	201/174
Without	376	57 (14)	14–97	22/33
Marinesco bodies in 427 HD brains				
With	77 (18)	69 (12)	40–97	37/38
Without	350	57 (15)	14–90	183/166 (1)
Lewy bodies in 433 HD brains				
With	9 (2.1)	76 (14)	50–97	5/4
Without	424	59 (15)	14–90	220/203 (1)
Cerebral amyloid angiopathy in 539 HD brains				
With	34 (6.3)	73 (11.2)	50–97	17/17
Mild[a]	24	72 (12.6)	50–97	
Moderate[a]	8	72 6.2)	70–89	
Severe[a]	2	75 (2.8)	73–77	
Without	505	59 (14.4)	14–96	255/246

HD, Huntington disease; N, total number; SD, standard deviation; *unknown.

features of Alzheimer's changes in the HD brains were identical to those observed in non-HD individuals. Those HD patients with Alzheimer's changes were older (mean 72 years) than those without (mean 57 years). The occurrence of Hirano bodies, Marinesco bodies, Lewy bodies, and CAA had a similar correlation with age (Table 13–2). Thus, selected cerebral features attributed to usual aging do occur in HD and as well as in the non-HD population.

COEXISTENCE OF HUNTINGTON DISEASE AND ALZHEIMER'S DISEASE

To ascertain the frequency of AD in the HD population we determined the frequencies of diagnoses of interest assigned to brains collected between 1978 and 1996 by the Harvard Brain Tissue Resource Center and the Alzheimer Disease Resource Center. Among 4050 brains, we found 18 with coexisting HD and AD (Table 13–3), 866 (including 361 from patients who were 65 years or older at death) with HD, and 1201 with AD or AD–Lewy body variant. As mentioned before, we assigned the additional diagnosis of AD only to those HD brains with Alzheimer's-related cortical lesions corresponding to stages V or VI, or isocortical stages according to Braak and Braak.[131]

The group with coexisting HD and AD consisted of 13 women and 5 men (mean age 75.7, ±SD 8.8 years). There was only one person who carried the two diagnoses intra vitam. Indeed, the coexistence of HD with AD

Table 13–3. Clinical, Genotype, and Neuropathological Characteristics of Patients with Huntington Disease Coexisting with Alzheimer's Disease

Case	Age/Sex	Duration[a] (years)	CAG	NEUROPATHOLOGICAL DIAGNOSES	
				HD Grade[b]	AD Stage[c]
1	90/F	50	24/38	2	V
2	75/M	13	17/39	2	V
3	83/F	18	18/39	2	V
4	88/F	18	17/39	2	VI
5	77/F	17	21/40	3	VI
6	85/F	14	23/40	2	V
7	82/M	18	19/40	3	VI
8	66/F	NA	17/41	3	V
9	59/F	15	23/42	3	V
10	74/F	16	17/42	4	V
11	85/F	NA	17/42	3	V
12	73/F	23	21/42	3	V
13	65/F	NA	20/43	2	V
14	68/M	32	23/43	4	V
15	68/F	21	23/44	4	V
16	71/F	15	21/44	2	V
17	82/M	7	NA	2	V
18	72/F	18	NA	1	V

AD, Alzheimer's disease; CAG: cytosine, adenine, guanine; HD, Huntington disease; NA, not available.
[a] Duration from onset of symptoms to death.
[b] HD grade of neuropathological severity (4-point scale) according to Vonsattel et al. (1985).[61]
[c] AD staging (6-point scale) according to Braak and Braak (1993).[131]

is almost never identified intra vitam.[61,122,124,132] However, dementia was documented in the rest of the patients and was thought to have been secondary to HD. Details on dementia were lacking in the clinical notes for enabling distinction between cortical versus subcortical dementia. The mean expanded HD-IT15 CAG allele of this group was 41.1 ± 1.89 repeats (shortest 38, longest 44 repeats).

In our series, the pathology of HD coexisted with that of AD in 2% of HD patients irrespective of their age at death, or in 5% of those who were 65 years or older at death. Therefore, the frequency of AD in the HD population resembles that of the general population since an estimated 3% to 11% of people older than 65 years are thought to have AD.[133-135]

We sought to determine whether the HD-IT15 CAG expansion influences the phenotype of Alzheimer pathology when AD coexists with HD. Both HD and AD cause atrophy of the brain and characteristic changes in the stratum striatum. In HD, the striatum bears the brunt of the deleterious effect of the mutation, which occurs in an ordered and topographic distribution (Fig. 13–7). In AD, the striatum shows neuritic plaques and amyloid, with mild to moderate neuronal loss and gliosis in the caudate nucleus, putamen, and internal segment of the GP.[136-138] Neurofibrillary tangles often involve the large, cholinergic, caudate and putaminal interneurons.[139-141] In addition, the AD brain shows neuronal loss involving amygdala, hippocampus, entorhinal cortex, and the neocortex, as well as Aβ-amyloid deposits with neuritic plaques and neurofibrillary tangles.[136,142] In our series, the HD or AD pathology, when combined, appeared to develop independently of one another. In general, patients with combined HD-AD were older and their expanded HD-IT15 CAG size was smaller than in those patients with HD alone. We found no evidence that the striatal HD pathology was less extensive in the presence of AD pathology than in its absence. On the basis of these observations, our impression is that the degenerative process of HD is independent of AD pathology. If a loss of corticostriatal input occurs because of the cortical Alzheimer pathology, this loss is not reflected in a detectable reduction in HD pathology when HD is associated with AD.

NONAGENARIANS WITH HUNTINGTON DISEASE

The symptoms of HD in older individuals (old-old [75 to 85 years], and oldest-old [85 years or older][143]) may be enigmatic even to clinicians familiar with the disease. Coexisting cerebral pathologies are frequent in nonagenarians, which may mask the clinical and neuropathological features of HD. Furthermore, the cerebral HD pathology may be subtle since patients of this group may have an HD-IT15 CAG repeat expansion that is in the diagnostically uncertain range of 35–39 (Table 13–1). Thus, the evaluation of the neostriatal sites involved early in the course of the disease may be crucial to determine whether the changes are caused by the HD mutation. For example, in grade 1 HD, the tail of the caudate nucleus (Fig. 13–7) is more atrophic than both the body and the head (Fig. 13–3).

We have identified six HD nonagenarians (Table 13–4). Their HD-IT15 CAG long allele ranged between 38 and 40. Three of them had minimal or no cognitive impairment. Preservation of cognition even 10 to 30 years following the onset of chorea may occur in late-onset HD, which exemplifies the variation occurring in this disease.[144] One of the three demented HD nonagenarians had coexistent AD, one had coexistent Pick disease (with Pick bodies and Pick cells), and one had hippocampal sclerosis.

This series of HD nonagenarians conveys three messages. First, there is a risk of attributing a case of HD to a new mutation in an individual whose carrier parent had mild symptoms with pathologic changes ascribed to aging or who died before symptom onset. Second, individuals with an HD-IT15 CAG expansion of up to 40 or even 41 repeats may have far longer life expectancies than patients with higher repeat sequences. The variability of symptoms and striatal atrophy seen in this group of patients support the hypothesis that extra genes influence the pathophysiology of HD, a hypothesis suggested as early as 1935.[145] Third, the severity of striatal atrophy in HD nonagenarians may range from mild to severe. When subtle, the HD pathology is visible only in sites involved early in the course of the disease and may be obscured by concomitant changes such as neuritic plaques,

Table 13–4. Nonagenarians with Huntington Disease

Age (year) / Sex	CAG	HD Grade[a]	Additional Diagnosis	Comment
91/F	19/38	3	Infarcts; hippocampal sclerosis	See Sax and Vonsattel[123]
96/M	17/40	3	Lewy body; Alzheimer changes, mild	
90/F	24/38	2	AD	
90/F	21/40	3	Pick disease, type A	See Tissot et al.[146]
97/F	NA	3	Alzheimer changes, mild; Lewy body; CAA	
94/F	40	1	Possible AD[b]	See Mirra et al.;[147] no dementia

AD, Alzheimer disease; CAA, cerebral amyloid angiopathy; CAG, cytosine, adenine, guanine; HD, Huntington disease; NA, not available.
[a] HD grade of neuropathological severity according to Vonsattel et al. (1985).[61]
[b] By Consortium to Establish a Register for Alzheimer's Disease (CERAD) criteria.[147]

neurofibrillary tangles of Alzheimer, or gliosis.[15] The condition of elderly subjects with long-standing, slowly worsening, hereditary chorea and mild striatal atrophy is at times referred to as "status subchoreaticus" or "subchorea."[65,145] Striatal lesions due to vasculopathies are frequently observed in older individuals and may be superimposed upon the HD pathology, thus masking it. The presence of ubiquitin-labeled nuclear inclusions in scattered cortical and neostriatal neurons supports the diagnosis of HD.

We thank E.D. Bird, M.D. for his immense support. The HD-IT15 CAG repeat lengths were kindly performed in the laboratories of J.F. Gusella, Ph.D., and M.E. MacDonald, Ph.D. We are truly grateful to W. Hobbs for her help and support. We gratefully acknowledge L. Cherkas for his photography and advice. We also express our appreciation to the numerous pathologists who referred case material to the Harvard Brain Tissue Resource Center. We are especially grateful to the families of the patients for providing brain tissue for research. This work was supported in part by NIH grants NINCDS 31862 (Harvard Brain Tissue Resource Center), NS 16367 (Huntington's Disease Center Without Walls), and NIA 2P50-AG0 5134 (J.P.V, E.T.H.-W.), and by grants from the Vaughn Foundation and Hereditary Disease Foundation.

REFERENCES

1. Vonsattel J-PG, DiFiglia M. Huntington disease. J Neuropathol Exp Neurol 1998; 57:369–384.
2. The Huntington's Disease Collaborative Research Group:, MacDonald ME, Ambrose CM, Duyao MP, Myers RH, Lin C, Srinidhi L, Barnes G, Taylor SA, James M, Groot N, MacFarlane H, Jenkins B, Anderson MA, Wexler NS, Gusella JF. A novel gene containing a trinucleotide repeat that is expanded and unstable on Huntington's disease chromosomes. Cell 1993; 72:971–983.
3. Myers RH, MacDonald ME, Koroshetz WJ, Duyao MP, Ambrose CA, Taylor SAM, Barnes G, Srinidhi J, Lin CS, Whaley WL, Lazzarini AM, Schwarz M, Wolff G, Bird ED, Vonsattel J-P, Gusella JF. De novo expansion of a (CAG)n repeat in sporadic Huntington's disease. Nat Gen 1993; 5:168–173.
4. Hayden MR. Huntington's Chorea. New York: Springer-Verlag, 1981.
5. Folstein SE. Huntington's disease. A Disorder of Families. London: The Johns Hopkins University Press, 1990.
6. Harper PS. Huntington's disease. In: Major Problems in Neurology (31), 2nd ed. London: W.B. Saunders Company, 1996:xx–xx.
7. Myers RH, Sax DS, Schoenfeld M, Bird ED, Wolf PA, Vonsattel JP, White RF, Martin JB. Late onset of Huntington's disease. J Neurol Neurosurg Psychiatry 1985; 48:530–534.
8. Young AB, Shoulson I, Penney JB, Starosta-Rubinstein S, Gomez F, Travers H, Ramos-Arroyo MA, Snodgrass SR, Bonilla E, Moreno H, Wexler NS. Huntington's disease in Venezuela: neurologic features and functional decline. Neurology 1986; 36:244–249.
9. Duyao M, Ambrose C, Myers R, Novelletto A, Persichetti F, Frontali M, Folstein S, Ross C, Franz M, Abbott M, Gray J, Conneally P, Young A, Penney J, Hollingsworth Z, Shoulson I, Lazzarini A, Falek A, Koroshetz W, Sax D, Bird E, Vonsattel J, Bonilla E, Alvir J, Bickham Conde J, Cha J-H, Dure L, Gomez F, Ramos M, Sanchez-Ramos J, Snodgrass S, de

Young M, Wexler N, Moscowitz C, Penchaszadeh G, MacFarlane H, Anderson M, Jenkins B, Srinidhi J, Barnes G, Gusella J, MacDonald M. Trinucleotide repeat length instability and age of onset in Huntington's disease. Nat Gen 1993; 4:387–392.

11. Telenius H, Almqvist E, Kremer B, Spence N, Squitieri F, Nichol K, Grandell U, Starr E, Benjamin C, Castaldo I, Calabrese O, Anvret M, Goldberg YP, Hayden MR. Somatic mosaicism in sperm is associated with intergenerational $(CAG)_{11}$ changes in Huntington disease. Hum Mol Genet 1995; 4:189–195.

12. MacMillan JC, Snell RG, Tyler A, Houlihan GD, Fenton I, Cheadle JP, Lazarou LP, Shaw DJ, Harper PS. Molecular analysis and clinical correlations of the Huntington's disease mutation. Lancet 1993; 342:954–958.

13. Kremer B, Goldberg P, Andrew SE, Theilmann J, Telenius H, Zeisler J, Squitieri F, Lin B, Bassett A, Almqvist E, Bird TD, Hayden MR. A worldwide study of the Huntington's disease mutation. The sensitivity and specificity of measuring CAG repeats. N Engl J Med 1994; 330:1401–1406.

14. Albin RL, Tagle DA. Genetics and molecular biology of Huntington's disease. Trends Neurosci 1995; 18:11–14.

15. Karluk D, Myers RH, DiFiglia M, Gusella JF, MacDonald ME, Penney JB, Jr., Young AB, Hobbs W, Lenzi S, Srinidhi S, Hedley-Whyte ET, Vonsattel J-P. Nonagenarians with Huntington disease (HD) have low CAG repeats [abstract] J Neuropathol Exp Neurol 1999; 58:549.

16. Persichetti F, Ambrose CM, Ge P, McNeil SM, Srinidhi J, Anderson MA, Jenkins B, Barnes GT, Duyao MP, Kanaley L, Wexler NS, Myers RH, Bird ED, Vonsattel JP, MacDonald ME, Gusella JF. Normal and expanded Huntington's disease gene alleles produce distinguishable proteins due to translation across the CAG repeat. Mol Med 1995; 1:374–383.

17. Persichetti F, Srinidhi J, Kanaley L, Ge P, Myers RH, D' Arrigo K, Barnes GT, MacDonald ME, Vonsattel J-P, Gusella JF, Bird ED. Huntington's disease CAG trinucleotide repeats in pathologically confirmed post-mortem brains. Neurobiol Dis 1994; 1:159–166.

18. Rubinsztein DC, Leggo J, Coles R, Almqvist E, Biancalana V, Cassiman J-J, Chotai K, Connarty M, Craufurd D, Curtis A, Curtis D, Davidson MJ, Differ A-M, Dode C, Dodge A, Frontali M, Ranen NG, Stine OC, Sherr M, Abbott MH, Franz ML, Graham CA, Harper PS, Hedreen JC, Jackson A, Kaplan J-C, Losekoot M, MacMillan JC, Morrison P, Trottier Y, Novelletto A, Simpson S, Theilmann J, Whittaker JL, Folstein SE, Ross CA, Hayden Phenotypic characterization of individuals with 30–40 CAG repeats in the Huntington disease (HD) gene reveals HD cases with 36 repeats and apparently normal elderly individuals with 36–39 repeats. Am J Hum Genet 1996; 59:16–22.

19. Guidelines for the molecular genetics predictive test in Huntington's disease. Neurology 1994; 44:1533–1536.

20. Graybiel AM, Aosaki T, Flaherty AW, Kimura M. The basal ganglia and adaptive motor control. Science 1994; 265:1826–1831.

21. Albin RL, Young AB, Penney JB. The functional anatomy of basal ganglia disorders. Trends Neurosci 1989; 12:366–375.

22. Alexander GE, Crutcher MD. Functional architecture of basal ganglia circuits: neural substrates of parallel processing. Trends Neurosci 1990; 13:266–271.

23. Albin RL, Reiner A, Anderson KD, Penney JB, Young AB. Striatal and nigral neuron subpopulations in rigid Huntington's disease: implications for the functional anatomy of chorea and rigidity-akinesia. Ann Neurol 1990; 27:357–365.

24. Matsumura M, Tremblay L, Richard H, Filion M. Activity of pallidal neurons in the monkey during dyskinesia induced by injection of bicuculline in the external pallidum. Neuroscience 1995; 65:59–70.

25. Goldman-Rakic PS. Cytoarchitectonic heterogeneity of the primate neostriatum: subdivision into *island* and *matrix* cellular compartments. J Comp Neurol 1982; 205:398–413.

26. Holt DJ, Graybiel AM, Saper CB. Neurochemical architecture of the human striatum. J Comp Neurol 1997; 384:1–25.

27. Gerfen CR, Herkenham M, Thibault J. The neostriatal mosaic: II. Patch- and matrix-directed mesostriatal dopaminergic and non-dopaminergic systems. J Neurosci 1987; 7:3915–3934.

28. Graybiel AM. Neurotransmitters and neuromodulators in the basal ganglia. Trends Neurosci 1990; 13:244–254.

29. Ferrante RJ, Kowall NW, Richardson EP Jr. Cellular composition of striatal patch and matrix compartments in Huntington's disease [abstract]. Soc Neurosci 1989; 15:935.

30. Hedreen JC, Folstein SE. Early loss of neostriatal striosome neurons in Huntington's disease. J Neuropathol Exp Neurol 1995; 54:105–120.

31. DiFiglia M, Pasik P, Pasik T. A Golgi study of neuronal types in the neostriatum of monkeys. Brain Res 1976; 114:245–256.

32. Braak H, Braak E. Neuronal types in the striatum of man. Cell Tissue Res 1982; 227:319–342.

33. Graveland GA, Williams RS, DiFiglia M. A Golgi study of the human neostriatum: neurons and afferent fibers. J Comp Neurol 1985; 234:317–333.

34. Nicoletti F, Bruno V, Copani A, Casabona G, Knöpfel T. Metabotropic glutamate receptors: a new target for the therapy of neurodegenerative disorders? Trends Neurosci 1996; 19:267–271.

35. Weeks RA, Harding AE, Brooks DJ. Striatal D1 and D2 dopamine receptor loss in asymptomatic mutation carriers of Huntington's disease. Ann Neurol 1996; 40:49–54.

36. Anton G. Über die Beteiligung der grossen basalen Gehirnganglien bei Bewegungstörungen und insbesondere bei Chorea. Jahrbücher Psychiatr Neurol (Lpz) 1896; 14:141–181.

37. Jelgersma G. Neue anatomische Befunde bei Paralysis agitans und bei chronischer Chorea. Neurol Centralblatt 1908; 27:995–996.

38. Alzheimer A. Über die anatomische Grundlage der Huntingtonschen Chorea und der choreatischen Bewegungen überhaupt. Neurol Centralblatt 1911; 30:891–892.

39. McCaughey WTE. The pathologic spectrum of Huntington's chorea. J Nerv Ment Dis 1961; 133:91–103.

40. Bruyn GW. Huntington's chorea; historical, clinical

41. Forno LS, Jose C. Huntington's chorea: a pathological study. In: Barbeau A, Chase TN, Paulson GW, eds. Advances in Neurology, Vol. 1, Huntington's Chorea. New York: Raven, 1973:453–470.
42. Lewy FH. Die Histopathologie der choreatischen Erkrankungen. Zeitschr Ges Neurol Psychiatr (Berl) 1923; 85:622–658.
43. Bruyn GW. Neuropathological changes in Huntington's chorea. In: Barbeau A, Chase TN, Paulson GW, eds. Huntington's chorea 1872–1972. Advances in Neurology, Vol. 1. New York: Raven, 1973: 399–403.
44. Kremer HPH, Roos RAC, Dingjan GM, Bots GTAM, Bruyn GW, Hofman MA. The hypothalamic lateral tuberal nucleus and the characteristics of neuronal loss in Huntington's disease. Neurosci Lett 1991; 132: 101–104.
45. Davison C, Goodhart SP, Shlionsky H. Chronic progressive chorea. The pathogenesis and mechanism; a histopathologic study. Arch Neurol Psychiatry (Chicago) 1932; 27:906–928.
46. Bruyn GW, Bots GTAM, Dom R. Huntington's chorea: current neuropathological status. In: Chase TN, Wexler NS, Barbeau A, eds. Advances in Neurology, Vol. 23, Huntington's Disease. New York: Raven, 1979:83–93.
47. Braak H, Braak E. Allocortical involvement in Huntington's disease. Neuropathol Appl Neurobiol 1992; 18:539–547.
48. Hallervorden J. Huntingtonsche Chorea (Chorea chronica progressiva hereditaria). In: Lubarsch O, Henke F, Rössle R, Scholz W, eds. Handbuch der Speziellen Pathologischen Anatomie und Histologie (XIII/1 Bandteil A). Heidelberg: Springer-Verlag, 1957:793–822.
49. Spielmeyer W. Die anatomische Krankheitsforschung am Beispiel einer Huntingtonschen Chorea mit Wilsonschem Symptombild. Zeitschr Ges Neurol Psychiatr (Berl) 1926; 101:701–728.
50. Lange HW. Quantitative changes of telencephalon, diencephalon, and mesencephalon in Huntington's chorea, postencephalitic, and idiopathic parkinsonism. Verh Anat Ges 1981; 75:923–925.
51. Richardson EP Jr. Huntington's disease: some recent neuropathological studies. Neuropathol Appl Neurobiol 1990; 16:451–460.
52. Schroeder K. Zur Klinik und Pathologie der Huntingtonschen Krankheit. J Psychol Neurol 1931; 43:183–201.
53. Campbell AMG, Corner B, Norman RM, Urich H. The rigid form of Huntington's disease. J Neurol Neurosurg Psychiatry 1961; 24:71–77.
54. Zweig RM, Ross CA, Hedreen JC, Peyser C, Cardillo JE, Folstein SE, Price DL. Locus coeruleus involvement in Huntington's disease. Arch Neurol 1992; 49: 152–156.
55. Weisschedel E. Über eine systematische Atrophie der Oberen Olive. Arch Psychiatrie 1938; 108:219–227.
56. Weisschedel E. Über histopathologische Befunde an der oberen Olive und deren Beziehung zur Hörfunktion. Zeitschr Ges Neurol Psychiatr (Berl) 1939; 165: 248–256.
57. Zweig RM, Koven SJ, Hedreen JC, Maestri NE, Kazazian HH Jr, Folstein SE. Linkage to the Huntington's disease locus in a family with unusual clinical and pathological features. Ann Neurol 1989; 26:78–84.
58. Terplan K. Zur pathologischen Anatomie der chronischen progressiven Chorea. Virchow's Arch Pathol Anat (Berl) 1924; 252:146–176.
59. Tokay, L. (1930). "Studien über die Chorea chronica und die Beziehung des Striatum zu dieser." Arbeiten aus dem Institut für Anatomie und Physiologie des Centralnervensystems an der Wiener Universität 32: 209–230.
60. Jéquier M. Remarques sur la chorée de Huntington: le rôle des lésions médullaires. Schweiz Arch Neurol Psychiatr 1947; 60:405–407.
61. Vonsattel J-P, Myers RH, Stevens TJ, Ferrante RJ, Bird ED, Richardson EP Jr. Neuropathological classification of Huntington's disease. J Neuropathol Exp Neurol 1985; 44:559–577.
62. de la Monte SM, Vonsattel JP, Richardson EP Jr. Morphometric demonstration of atrophic changes in the cerebral cortex, white matter, and neostriatum in Huntington's disease. J Neuropathol Exp Neurol 1988; 47:516–525.
63. Kiesselbach G. Anatomischer Befund eines Falles von Huntingtonscher Chorea. Monatsschr Psychiatr Neurol 1914; 35:525–543.
64. Dunlap CB. Pathologic changes in Huntington's chorea. Arch Neurol Psychiatry (Chicago) 1927; 18:867–943.
65. Lange H, Thörner G, Hopf A, Schröder KF. Morphometric studies of the neuropathological changes in choreatic diseases. J Neurol Sci 1976; 28:401–425.
66. Myers RH, Vonsattel JP, Paskevich PA, Kiely DK, Stevens TJ, Cupples LA, Richardson EP Jr., Bird ED. Decreased neuronal and increased oligodendroglial densities in Huntington's disease caudate nucleus. J Neuropathol Exp Neurol 1991; 50:729–742.
67. Sapp E, Kegel KB, Aronin N, Hashikawa T, Uchiyama Y, Tohyama K, Bhide PG, Vonsattel JP, DiFiglia M. Early and progressive accumulation of reactive microglia in the Huntington disease brain. J Neuropathol Exp Neurol 2001; 60 (in press).
68. Neustaedter M. Concerning the striatal localization in chronic progressive chorea. With a report of three cases, two of the Huntington type in siblings and one senile arteriosclerotic, with necropsies. Nerv Ment Dis 1933; 78:470–491.
69. Birnbaum G. Chronisch-progressive Chorea mit Kleinhirnatrophie. Arch Psychiatrie 1941; 114:160–182.
70. Roos RAC, Pruyt JFM, de Vries J, Bots GTAM. Neuronal distribution in the putamen in Huntington's disease. J Neurol Neurosurg Psychiatry 1985; 48:422–425.
71. Saudou F, Finkbeiner S, Devys D, Greenberg ME. Huntingtin acts in the nucleus to induce apoptosis but death does not correlate with the formation of intranuclear inclusions. Cell 1998; 95:55–66.
72. Vonsattel J-P, Myers RH, Bird ED, Ge P, Richardson EP Jr. Maladie de Huntington: sept cas avec îlots néostriataux relativement préservés. Rev Neurol 1992; 148:107–116.
73. Zalneraitis EL, Landis DMD, Richardson EP Jr, Selkoe DJ. A comparison of astrocytic structure in cerebral cortex and striatum in Huntington's disease. Neurology 1981; 31:151.

74. Sotrel A, Paskevich PA, Kiely DK, Bird ED, Williams RS, Myers RH. Morphometric analysis of the prefrontal cortex in Huntington's disease. Neurology 1991; 41:1117–1123.
75. Cudkowicz M, Kowall NW. Degeneration of pyramidal projection neurons in Huntington's disease cortex. Ann Neurol 1990; 27:200–204.
76. Selemon LD, Rajkowska G, Goldman-Rakic PS. Abnormally high neuronal density in the schizophrenic cortex. Arch Gen Psychiatry 1995; 52:805–818.
77. Selemon LD, Rajkowska G, Goldman-Rakic PS. Elevated neuronal density in prefrontal area 46 in brains from schizophrenic patients: application of a three-dimensional, stereologic counting method. J Comp Neurol 1998; 392:402–412.
78. Rajkowska G, Selemon LD, Goldman-Rakic PS. Neuronal and glial somal size in the prefrontal cortex. A postmortem morphometric study of schizophrenia and Huntington disease. Arch Gen Psychiatry 1998; 55:215–224.
79. Hedreen JC, Peyser CE, Folstein SE, Ross CA. Neuronal loss in layers V and VI of cerebral cortex in Huntington's disease. Neurosci Lett 1991; 133:257–261.
80. Rodda RA. Cerebellar atrophy in Huntington's disease. J Neurol Sci 1981; 50:147–157.
81. Jeste DV, Barban L, Parisi J. Reduced Purkinje cell density in Huntington's disease. Exp Neurol 1984; 85:78–86.
82. Jervis GA. Huntington's chorea in childhood. Arch Neurol 1963; 9:244–257.
83. Markham CH, Knox JW. Observations on Huntington's chorea in childhood. J Pediatr 1965; 67:46–57.
84. Byers RK, Gilles FH, Fung C. Huntington's disease in children. Neurology 1973; 23:561–569.
85. Graveland GA, Williams RS, DiFiglia M. Evidence for degenerative and regenerative changes in neostriatal spiny neurons in Huntington's disease. Science 1985; 227:770–773.
86. Reiner A, Albin RL, Anderson KD, D'Amato CJ, Penney JB, Young AB. Differential loss of striatal projection neurons in Huntington disease. Proc Natl Acad Sci USA 1988; 85:5733–5737.
87. Sapp E, Ge P, Aizawa H, Bird E, Penney J, Young AB, Vonsattel J-P, DiFiglia M. Evidence for a preferential loss of enkephalin immunoreactivity in the external globus pallidus in low grade Huntington's disease using high resolution image analysis. Neuroscience 1995; 64:397–404.
88. Richfield EK, Maguire-Zeiss KA, Cox C, Gilmore J, Voorn P. Reduced expression of preproenkephalin in striatal neurons from Huntington's disease patients. Ann Neurol 1995; 37:335–343.
89. Ferrante RJ, Kowall NW, Beal MF, Martin JB, Bird ED, Richardson EP. Morphologic and histochemical characteristics of a spared subset of striatal neurons in Huntington's disease. J Neuropathol Exp Neurol 1987; 46:12–27.
90. Beal MF, Kowall NW, Ellison DW, Mazurek MF, Swartz KJ, Martin JB. Replication of the neurochemical characteristics of Huntington's disease by quinolinic acid. Nature 1986; 321:168–171.
91. Koh J-Y, Peters S, Choi DW. Neurons containing NADPH-diaphorase are selectively resistant to quinolinate toxicity. Science 1986; 234:73–76.
92. Albin RL. Selective neurodegeneration in Huntington's disease. Ann Neurol 1995; 38:835–836.
93. Beal MF, Brouillet E, Jenkins BG, Ferrante RJ, Kowall NW, Miller JM, Storey E, Srivastava R, Rosen BR, Hyman BT. Neurochemical and histologic characterization of striatal excitotoxic lesions produced by the mitochondrial toxin 3-nitropropionic acid. J Neurosci 1993; 13:4181–4192.
94. Gu M, Gash MT, Mann VM, Javoy-Agid F, Cooper JM, Schapira AHV. Mitochondrial defect in Huntington's disease caudate nucleus. Ann Neurol 1996; 39:385–389.
95. Beal MF, Hyman BT, Koroshetz W. Do defects in mitochondrial energy metabolism underlie the pathology of neurodegenerative diseases? Trends Neurosci 1993; 16:125–131.
96. Mazurek MF, Garside S, Beal MF. Cortical peptide changes in Huntington's disease may be independent of striatal degeneration. Ann Neurol 1997; 41:540–547.
97. Furtado S, Suchowersky O, Rewcastle B, Graham L, Klimek ML, Garber A. Relationship between trinucleotide repeats and neuropathological changes in Huntington's disease. Ann Neurol 1996; 39:132–136.
98. Penney JB, Vonsattel J-P, MacDonald ME, Gusella JF, Myers RH. CAG repeat number governs development rate of pathology in Huntington's disease. Ann Neurol 1997; 41:689–692.
99. Gutekunst C-A, Li S-H, Mulroy JS, Kuemmerle S, Jones R, Rye D, Ferrante RJ, Hesh SM, Li X-J. Nuclear and neuropil aggregates in Huntington's disease: Relationship to neuropathology. J Neurosci 1999; 19:2522–2534.
100. Landwehrmeyer GB, McNeil SM, Dure LS, IV, Ge P, Aizawa H, Huang Q, Ambrose CM, Duyao MP, Bird ED, Bonilla E, de Young M, Avila-Gonzales AJ, Wexler NS, DiFiglia M, Gusella JF, MacDonald ME, Penney JB, Young AB, Vonsattel JP. Huntington's disease gene: regional and cellular expression in brain of normal and affected individuals. Ann Neurol 1995; 37:218–230.
101. Gutekunst C-A, Levey AI, Heilman GJ, Whaley WL, Yi H, Nash NR, Rees HD, Madden JJ, Hersch SM. Identification and localization of huntingtin in brain and human lymphoblastoid cell lines with anti-fusion protein antibodies. Proc Natl Acad Sci USA 1995; 92:8710–8714.
102. Ferrante RJ, Gutekunst C-A, Persichetti F, McNeil SM, Kowall NW, Gusella JF, MacDonald ME, Beal MF, Hersch SM. Heterogeneous topographic and cellular distribution of huntingtin expression in the normal human neostriatum. J Neurosci 1997; 17:3052–3063.
103. DiFiglia M, Sapp E, Chase KO, Davies SW, Bates GP, Vonsattel JP, Aronin N. Aggregation of huntingtin in neuronal intranuclear inclusions and dystrophic neurites in brain. Science 1997; 277:1990–1993.
104. DiFiglia M, Sapp E, Chase K, Schwarz C, Meloni A, Young C, Martin E, Vonsattel J-P, Carraway R, Reeves SA, Boye FM, Aronin N. Huntingtin is a cytoplasmic protein associated with vesicles in human and rat brain neurons. Neuron 1995; 14:1075–1081.
105. Duyao MP, Auerbach AB, Ryan A, Persichetti F, Barnes GT, McNeil SM, Ge P, Vonsattel JP, Gusella JF, Joyner AL, MacDonald ME. Inactivation of the

mouse Huntington's disease gene homolog (*Hdh*). Science 1995; 269:407–410.
106. White JK, Auerbach W, Duyao MP, Vonsattel J-P, Gusella JF, Joyner AL, MacDonald ME. Huntingtin is required for neurogenesis and is not impaired by the Huntington's disease CAG expansion. Nat Genet 1997; 17:404–410.
107. Aronin N, Chase K, Young C, Sapp E, Schwarz C, Matta N, Komreich R, Landwehrmeyer B, Bird E, Beal MF, Vonsattel JP, Smith T, Carraway R, Boyce FM, Young AB, Penney JB, DiFiglia M. CAG expansion affects the expression of mutant huntingtin in the Huntington's disease brain. Neuron 1995; 15:1193–1201.
108. Sapp E, Schwarz C, Chase K, Bhide PG, Young AB, Penney J, Vonsattel JP, Aronin N, DiFiglia M. Huntingtin localization in brains of normal and Huntington's disease patients. Ann Neurol 1997; 42:604–612.
109. Maat-Schieman MLC, Dorsman JC, Smoor MA, Siesling S, van Duinen SG, Verschuuren JGM, den Dunnen JT, van Ommen G-JB, Roos AC. Distribution of inclusions in neuronal nuclei and dystrophic neurites in Huntington disease brain. J Neuropathol Exp Neurol 1999; 58:129–137.
110. Sapp E, Penney J, Young AB, Aronin N, Vonsattel J-P, DiFiglia M. Axonal transport of N-terminal huntingtin suggests early pathology of corticostriatal projections in Huntington disease. J Neuropathol Exp Neurol 1999; 58:165–173.
111. Kim M, Lee H-S, LaForet G, McIntyre C, Martin EJ, Chang P, Kim TW, Williams M, Reddy PH, Tagle D, Boyce FM, Won L, Heller A, Aronin N, DiFiglia M. Mutant huntingtin expression in clonal striatal cells: dissociation of inclusion formation and neuronal survival by caspase inhibition. J Neurosci 1999; 19:964–973.
112. Hodgson JG, Agopyan N, Gutekunst C-A, Leavitt BR, LePiane F, Singaraja R, Smith DJ, Bissada N, McCutcheon K, Nasir J, Jamot L, Li X-J, Stevens ME, Rosemond E, Roder JC, Phillips AG, Rubin EM, Hersch SM, Hayden MR. A YAC mouse model for Huntington's disease with full-length mutant huntingtin, cytoplasmic toxicity, and selective striatal neurodegeneration. Neuron 1999; 23:182–192.
113. Reddy PH, Williams M, Charles V, Garrett L, Pike-Buchanan L, Whetsell WO, Jr., Miller G, Tagle DA. Behavioural abnormalities and selective neuronal loss in HD transgenic mice expressing mutated full-length HD cDNA. Nat Genet 1998; 20 20:198–202.
114. Burke JR, Enghild JJ, Martin ME, Jou Y-S, Myers RM, Roses AD, Vance JM, Strittmatter WJ. Huntingtin and DRPLA proteins selectively interact with the enzyme GAPDH. Nature Med 1996; 2:347–350.
115. Li X-J, Li S-H, Sharp AH, Nucifora FC, Jr., Schilling G, Lanahan A, Worley P, Snyder SH, Ross CA. A huntingtin-associated protein enriched in brain with implications for pathology. Nature 1995; 378:398–402.
116. Wheeler VC, White JK, Gutekunst C-A, Vrbanac V, Weaver M, Li X-J, Li S-H, Yi H, Vonsattel J-P, Gusella JF, Hersch S, Auerbach W, Joyner AL, MacDonald ME. Long glutamine tracts cause nuclear localization of a novel form of huntingtin in medium spiny striatal neurons in Hdh^{Q92} and Hdh^{Q111} knock-in mice. Hum Mol Genet 2000; 9:503–513.

117. Perutz MF, Johnson T, Suzuki M, Finch T. Glutamine repeats as polar zippers: Their possible role in inherited neurodegenerative diseases. Proc Natl Acad Sci USA 1994; 91:5355–5358.
118. Persichetti F, Trettel F, Huang CC, Fraefel C, Timmers HTM, Gusella JF, MacDonald ME. Mutant huntingtin forms in vivo complexes with distinct context-dependent conformations of the polyglutamine segment. Neurobiol Dis 1999; 6:364–375.
119. Kuemmerle S, Gutekunst C-A, Klein AM, Li X-J, Li S-H, Beal MF, Hersch SM, Ferrante RJ. Huntingtin aggregates may not predict neuronal death in Huntington's disease. Ann Neurol 1999; 46:842–849.
120. Huang CC, Faber PW, Persichetti F, Mittal V, Vonsattel J-P, MacDonald ME, Gusella JF. Amyloid formation by mutant huntingtin: Threshold, progressivity and recruitment of normal polyglutamine proteins. Somat Cell Mol Genet 1998; 24:217–233.
121. Ona VO, Li M, Vonsattel JPG, Andrews LJ, Khan SQ, Chung WM, Frey AS, Menon AS, Li X-J, Stieg PE, Yuan J, Penney JB, Young AB, Cha J-HJ, Friedlander RM. Inhibition of caspase-1 slows disease progression in a mouse model of Huntington's disease. Nature 1999; 399:263–267.
122. McIntosh GC, Jameson HD, Markesbery WR. Huntington disease associated with Alzheimer disease. Ann Neurol 1978; 3:545–548.
123. Sax DS, Vonsattel J-P. Case Records of the Massachusetts General Hospital. Case 2-1992. Chorea and progressive dementia in an 88-year-old woman. N Engl J Med 1992; 326:117–125.
124. Reyes MG, Gibbons S. Dementia of the Alzheimer's type and Huntington's disease. Neurology 1985; 35:273–277.
125. Morris JC, Storandt M, McKeel DW, Jr., Rubin EH, Price JL, Grant EA, Berg L. Cerebral amyloid deposition and diffuse plaques in "normal" aging: evidence for presymptomatic and very mild Alzheimer's disease. Neurology 1996; 46:707–719.
126. Mizutani T, Shimada H. Neuropathological background of twenty-seven centenarian brains. J Neurol Sci 1992; 108:168–177.
127. Gómez-Isla T, Price JL, McKeel DW Jr, Morris JC, Growdon JH, Hyman BT. Profound loss of layer II entorhinal cortex neurons occurs in very mild Alzheimer's disease. J Neurosci 1996; 16:4491–4500.
128. Hirano A. Hirano bodies and related neuronal inclusions. Neuropathol Appl Neurobiol 1994; 20:3–11.
129. Yuen P, Baxter DW. The morphology of Marinesco bodies (paranucleolar corpuscles) in the melanin-pigmented nuclei of the brain-stem. J Neurol Neurosurg Psychiatry 1963; 26:178–183.
130. Forno LS. Concentric hyalin intraneuronal inclusions of Lewy type in the brains of elderly persons (50 incidental cases): relationship to parkinsonism. J Am Geriatr Soc 1969; 17:557–575.
131. Braak H, Braak E, Bohl J. Staging of Alzheimer related cortical destruction. Eur Neurol 1993; 33:403–408.
132. Moss RJ, Mastri AR, Schut LJ. The coexistence and differentiation of late onset Huntington's disease and Alzheimer's disease. A case report and review of the literature. J Am Geriatr Soc 1988; 36:237–241.
133. Corey-Bloom J, Thal LJ, Galasko D, Folstein M, Drachman D, Raskind M, Lanska DJ. Diagnosis and

evaluation of dementia. Neurology 1995; 45:211–218.
134. Van Broeckhoven CL. Molecular genetics of Alzheimer disease: identification of genes and gene mutations. Eur Neurol 1995; 35:8–19.
135. Tucker GJ, Popkin M, Caine ED, et al. Delirium, Dementia, and Amnestic and Other Cognitive Disorders Work Group. In: Diagnostic and Statistical Manual of Mental Disorders. DSM-IV, 4th ed. Washington, DC. American Psychiatric Association, 1994:123–163.
136. Alzheimer A. Über eigenartige Krankheitsfälle des späteren Alters. Zeitschr Ges Neurol Psychiatr (Berl) 1911; 4:356–385.
137. Rudelli RD, Ambler MW, Wisniewski HM. Morphology and distribution of Azheimer neuritic (senile) and amyloid plaques in striatum and diencephalon. Acta Neuropathol 1984; 64:273–281.
138. Suenaga T, Hirano A, Llena JF, Yen S-H, Dickson DW. Modified Bielschowsky stain and immunohistochemical studies on striatal plaques in Alzheimer's disease. Acta Neuropathol 1990; 80:280–286.
139. Herz E, Fünfgeld E. Zur Klinik und Pathologie der Alzheimerschen Krankheit. Arch Psychiatrie 1928; 84:633–664.
140. Lehéricy S, Hirsch EC, Cervera P, Hersh LB, Hauw J-J, Ruberg M, Agid Y. Selective loss of cholinergic neurons in the ventral striatum of patients with Alzheimer disease. Proc Natl Acad Sci USA 1989; 86:8580–8584.
141. Selden N, Mesulam M-M, Geula C. Human striatum: the distribution of neurofibrillary tangles in Alzheimer's disease. Brain Res 1994; 658:327–331.
142. Braak H, Braak E. Pathology of Alzheimer's disease. In: Calne DB, ed. Neurodegenerative Diseases. Philadelphia: W.B. Saunders, 1994:585–613.
143. Katzman R. The aging brain. Limitations in our knowledge and future approaches. Arch Neurol 1997; 54:1201–1205.
144. Britton JW, Uitti RJ, Ahlskog JE, Robinson RG, Kremer B, Hayden MR. Hereditary late-onset chorea without significant dementia: genetic evidence for substantial phenotypic variation in Huntington's disease. Neurology 1995; 45:443–447.
145. Patzig B. Vererbung von Bewegungsstörungen. Zeitschrift für Induktive Abstammungs- und Vererbungslehre 1935; 70:476–484.
146. Tissot R, Constantinidis J, Richard J. La Maladie de Pick. Paris: Masson, 1975.
147. Mirra SS, Heyman A, McKeel D, Sumi SM, Crain BJ, Brownlee LM, Vogel FS, Hughes JP, van Belle G, Berg L. The Consortium to Establish a Registry for Alzheimer's Disease (CERAD). Part II. Standardization of the neuropathologic assessment of Alzheimer's disease. Neurology 1991; 41:479–486.

14. Effects of Malnutrition and Alcoholism on the Aging Nervous System

CLIVE HARPER AND SERGE DUCKETT

The term *"malnutrition"* is a general expression that includes not only its main manifestation, undernutrition, but also overnutrition and unbalanced nutrition. Undernutrition is the most common cause of ill health and death in humans, maiming or killing 10 million humans per year, striking particularly those at the most vulnerable stages of life—children and the elderly. Yet, undernutrition is preventable and treatable if dealt with in a timely fashion. Malnutrition is caused primarily by war, incarceration, poverty, dietary ignorance, moral inertia, or tardiness in assistance to others facing natural or human-made catastrophes (e.g, Ethiopia, Sudan, Rwanda, Yugoslavia). The media have been successful in informing the public, sometimes dramatically, of the horrors of malnutrition. The clinical and pathologic consequences of undernutrition were described in great detail by physicians studying the victims of famine during the French Commune[1] and World War I,[2] in post-World War II Germany,[3] during the Spanish Civil War,[4] and in the concentration camps of Nazi Germany.[5,6]

Undernutrition, sometimes referred to as "protein-energy or protein-calorie malnutrition," may be an absence of any nutrition, as in concentration camps on areas of famine or as the result of self-imposed abstinence or disinterest in food. Undernutrition may be specific, caused by the absence of one and/or other normal dietary components such as proteins, carbohydrates, fats, vitamins, and trace element. Malnutrition may be caused by a lack of appetite, resulting from psychological problem, such as depression, bereavement, loneliness, disinterest, or disease.[7–11]

Malnutrition causes 12% of global mortality; almost one billion humans do not have their basic daily nutritional requirements and over two billion, one-third of the world population, present with micronutrient deficiencies. The tragedy of malnutrition will be even more striking if the percentage of death and incapacitation from malnutrition is projected in light of future population numbers. The world population is currently 6 billion and will rise to 9 to 12 billion by 2049.[12,13] There were 35.3 million individuals over the age of 65 in the United States in 1996 and it is projected that there will be 70 million in 50 years.[14] There were 40,000 centenarians in 2000 in the United States and there will be 60,000 in 2050. Asia had a population of 150 million individuals over the age of 65 in 1990, currently this age-group numbers 200 million, and there will be 500 million in 2050.[15] Malnutrition causes, or plays a role in, the pathogenesis of most cases of neurological and psychiatric diseases. In the United States over the past two decades half the patients over age 65 have been incapacitated by neurological disease and 90% of these individuals were severely incapacitated.[16–18] These figures provide a view of the potential human and financial problems caused by malnutrition that will result from a growing elderly population if preventive steps are not taken, be they education, prevention, treatment, or making sure that every citizen is correctly fed.

Our concern in this chapter is the effect of malnutrition and alcoholism on the human nervous system after the age of 65. Total caloric food intake is determined by energy needs, which decrease significantly with age and are the result of a decline in muscular mass. Thus a 30% reduction in energy needs will be translated into a 30% decrease in food intake. Compared to younger individuals, humans over the age of 70 consume a third less calories, yet the requirements for virtually every other nutrient except carbohydrates do not decline significantly with age.

The clinical and mental manifestations of malnutrition in the elderly may be difficult to recognize because of the patient's confusion, mutism, or disinterest, memory problems, associated diseases, physical weakness, or lack of family and friends, and sometimes because of the extended period between the cause of the problem and its clinical manifestations. Dehydration and ionic anomalies, a frequent problem in the elderly, are also deficiency syndromes and their clinical manifestations are difficult to interpret.

DISEASES ASSOCIATED WITH MALNUTRITION

The most frequent types of encephalopathies are those related to either hypoglycemia or vitamin-deficiency states—particularly the Wernicke-Korsakoff's syndrome (WKS; vitamin B1 deficiency). Peripheral neuropathy is also common and patients with WKS may develop central pontine myelinolysis or Marchiafava-Bignami disease. Other B vitamin deficiencies that can affect the nervous system include nicotinic acid, riboflavin, pyridoxine (B6) and B12 and folic acid. These are all water-soluble vitamins. The most important fat-soluble vitamin-deficiency state affecting the nervous system is vitamin E and abetaliproteinemia. Although all of these disorders can be seen in populations suffering from general malnutrition, there are certain groups of people who are particularly susceptible. For example, thiamin deficiency is frequently seen in alcoholics. This is not only the result of poor diet but the alcohol can interfere with the absorption, storage, and metabolism of thiamin.

Hypoglycemic Encephalopathy

The normal brain uses 100 to 150 g of glucose daily and this is its only source of energy. It has a reserve of only 2 g glucose. When glycemia is 2.2 mmol/liter, the brain diminishes its energy needs and uses amino acids and lipids. Thus in the undernourished and gastrectomized individual who abuses alcohol there is the danger of an hypoglycemic encephalopathy, particularly if complicated by an unknown and/or untreated diabetes. The result can be a progressive mental deterioration and signs of psychosis. Additionally, the patient presents with epilepsy and pyramidal and extrapyramidal signs.

The neuropathological changes caused by hypoglycemia resemble those observed in anoxia, in that they both cause selective neuronal necrosis. However, there are differences that may relate to the biochemical changes in the brain. For example, in hypoglycemia there is reduced lactate and pyruvate production, resulting in alkalosis of the tissues, whereas in ischemia there is increased lactate production and acidosis of tissues. The length of survival and the extent of the glucose deficiency determine the severity of the brain damage. Neurons in the cerebral cortex, hippocampus, and caudate nucleus are particularly susceptible. Ultimately, in long-term survivors, atrophy of the cerebral cortex with consequent dilatation of the ventricles can develop. In short, hypoglycemia causes a polioencephalopathy with possible diffuse secondary Wallerian degeneration of the white matter.

Wernicke-Korsakoff Syndrome

Thiamin deficiency is associated with beri-beri (see below and Chapter 20) and WKS. Beri-beri is a disease of the peripheral nerves (dry beri-beri) or of the heart (wet beri-beri). The peripheral neuropathy is characterized by a sensation of "pins and needles" in the feet and hands. The daily requirement of thiamin is

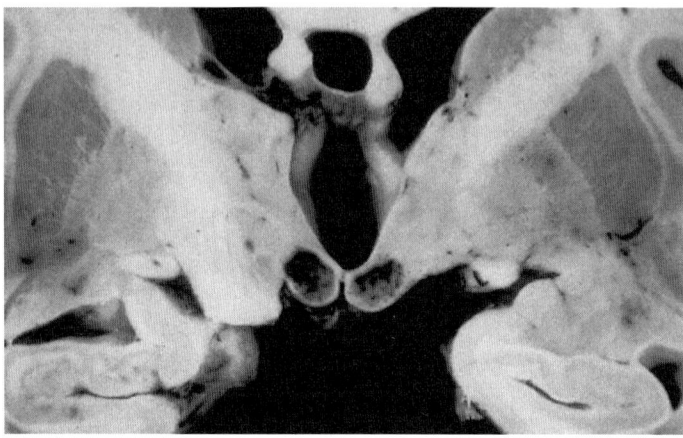

Figure 14–1. Coronal section of cerebral hemispheres at the level of the mamillary bodies (arrow) shows small hemorrhages in areas typically damaged in acute Wernicke's encephalopathy—the mamillary bodies and the walls of the third ventricle.

1.0–1.5 mg/day and body stores can be depleted within 3 weeks. The role of thiamin is that of a coenzyme in the form of thiamin pyrophosphate. There are two clinical entities within the WKS spectrum: Wernicke's encephalopathy (WE) and Korsakoff's psychosis (KP). These are separate clinical syndromes yet associated so often as to be referred to as the WKS. This disorder is seen most commonly in the alcoholic population but there are a number of other at-risk groups; patients on starvation diets, those who have undergone gastric stapling or prolonged intravenous feeding, and those suffering from other causes of severe malnourishment. Patients with WE present with eye symptoms (ophthalmoplegia and/or nystagmus), ataxia, and mental symptoms such as confusion, drowsiness, or even coma.[19] It is important to note that many patients will not have all of these clinical signs and often will only exhibit a change in their conscious state.[20] Patients with KP have loss of anterograde episodic but not semantic memory, with few deficits in nondeclarative memory. Korsakoff's psychosis is most likely the end result of repeated episodes of WE. It has been suggested that some episodes of WE may be subclinical.[21] Korsakoff's psychosis may also occur as the result of other diencephalic lesions such as tumors and trauma. Interestingly, calorie-deprived prisoners of war developed WE but this did not progress to KP, perhaps because of the absence of alcohol as a cofactor. The anomaly of these two apparently distinctive clinical syndromes is that the neuropathological changes have been said to be identical in the chronic stages of the diseases (Fig. 14–1). The most characteristic lesions are seen in the mamillary bodies and in the periventricular regions of the third and fourth ventricles and aqueduct. The macroscopic and microscopic features depend upon the stage and severity of the disease—that is, acute, subacute, or chronic. Repeated episodes are common so that acute on chronic changes are seen frequently. In one study, 17% were acute, 66% were chronic, and 17% acute on chronic.[22] Hemorrhages are only seen in about 5% of cases, and it is possible to miss the diagnosis unless sections are taken for microscopic examination. The most consistent abnormality in chronic WE is shrinkage (30% of normal volume) and brown discoloration of the mamillary bodies (Fig. 14–2). The mamillary bodies may also be shrunken in Alzheimer's disease (AD), posterior cerebral artery territory infarction, and hippocampal sclerosis.[23] Microscopic changes give an indication of the duration of the disease. In the acute phase there is edema and extravasation of red blood cells into the perivascular spaces. These may extend outward into the parenchyma to cause visible petechia. Within 1 or 2 days the endothelial cells become hypertrophic and neovascularization commences. These changes are maximal at about 7–10 days. Frank tissue necrosis is seen occasionally. In most areas neurons show relatively little change and do not appear to be the main target of the disease process. However, thalamic and olivary neurons appear to be an exception and may show "red cell change."[24] An astrocytic reaction is

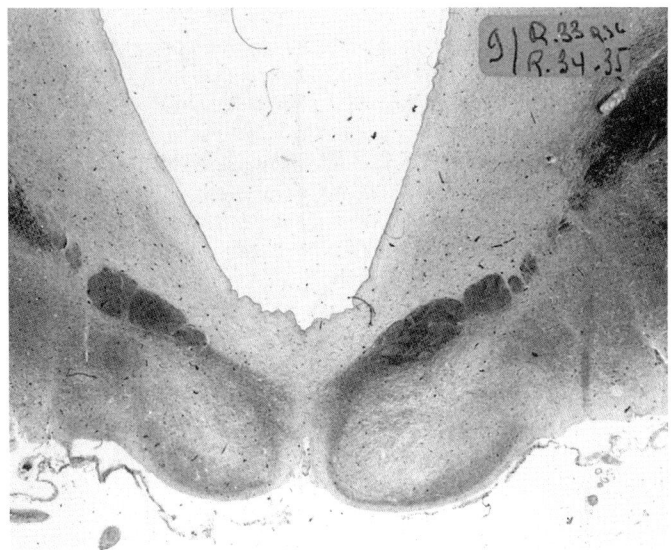

Figure 14–2. Coronal section of cerebral hemispheres at the level of the mamillary bodies shows that they are shrunken and discolored (brown) and typical of chronic Wernicke's encephalopathy. In addition, there is some dilatation of the third ventricle due to brain shrinkage.

noted by the third or fourth day and myelin and axons may be destroyed. There is almost no cellular reaction in the damaged areas. In chronic lesions there is tissue loss and spongiosis with an increase in the density of thin-walled capillaries. Chronic changes in other vulnerable regions are similar but less severe and can be quite difficult to identify. A number of other less characteristic changes have been described recently in cerebral cortex, white matter, and subcortical and brain stem regions. There is a reduction in white matter volume of between 10% and 15%.[25] We have shown a 22% reduction in the number of neurons in the superior frontal cortex (Brodmann's area 8) but no significant change in the primary motor (area 4), frontal cingulate (area 32), or inferior temporal (areas 20 and 36)[26] (discussed further in Alcohol and Aging, below). Studies of subcortical structures are summarized in Table 14–1. Noradrenergic neurons in the locus coeruleus do not appear to be vulnerable to damage in WKS but serotonergic neurons in the raphe nuclei are particularly susceptible. The neuronal loss, however, does not correlate with specific clinical symptoms such as the severe amnesia of KP.[27] Basal forebrain nuclear changes in alcoholics with WKS do appear to correlate with impairments in attention and information processing.[28] The most interesting recent data relate to changes in the thalamic nuclei. The dorsomedial thalamic nuclei are severely damaged in the chronic WE, however, the anterior principal thalamic nuclei are much more severely damaged in those alcoholics with KP. These findings suggest that this is the anatomical site of the lesion that correlates with the characteristic amnestic state.[27]

Table 14–1. Distribution and Severity of Pathological Lesions in Wernicke-Korsakoff Syndrome

	Chronic WE	KP
Cerebral cortex (frontal)	+	+
White matter	++	++
Hippocampus	−	−
Mamillary bodies	++	++
Thalamus (dorsomedial)	++	++
Thalamus (anterior principal)	+	+++[a]
Basal forebrain	++	++
Locus ceruleus	−	−
Raphe nuclei	++	++
Cerebellum	++	++

Chronic WE, non-amnestic Wernicke-Korsakoff syndrome; KP, amnestic Wernicke-Korsakoff syndrome.

[a] The anterior principal nucleus of the thalamus appears to be the discriminant region causing the amnesia of KP.

Most patients with WE respond rapidly to treatment with parenteral thiamin. Resolution of clinical signs usually occurs within 24–48 hrs. The likelihood of progression from WE to KP is difficult to predict, with figures varying from 56% to 84% of cases.[19,29] Once patients have developed KP, the response is much less favorable and the amnestic state is said to persist in about half of the cases. Mandatory enrichment of bread flour with thiamin was introduced in Australia in 1991 because of the high prevalence rates of WKS in two autopsy studies. In a subsequent study in 1996–97, the prevalence rate had dropped from 4.7% in 1983 to 1.1%.[30] Thus, thiamin enrichment programs seem to be useful public health measures and are already in place in many other countries of the world including the United States, Canada, and the United Kingdom.[23]

Central Pontine Myelinolysis

This relatively uncommon disorder usually occurs in alcoholics with WKS. Other nonalcoholic groups can be affected, the most common being patients with severe liver disease (especially post orthotropic liver transplant), severe burns, malnutrition, anorexia, and severe electrolyte disorders. Too-rapid correction of a profound hyponatremia seems to be an important contributing factor, but alternative hypotheses have been proposed, such as hypophosphatemia.[31] The disease usually evolves rapidly in very sick patients and they may be confused or demented, with focal signs such as flaccid or spastic quadriparesis, supranuclear opththalmoplegia, and difficulties in swallowing and eating. Central pontine myelinolysis (CPM) was thought to have a very high mortality, but magnetic resonance imaging (MRI) scans have enabled the identification of early cases that have progressed to complete recovery.[31,32] Most cases of CPM have a similar topography, with lesions in the center of the basis pontis and sparing of the tegmentum. The area of demyelination is often triangular or butterfly shaped and symmetrical in transverse sections (Fig. 14–3) The diagnosis can be missed on macroscopic examination but is easily seen on myelin-stained sections as a sharply demarcated area of pallor within the basis pontis and a relative preservation of axons (seen with silver stains only). Extra-pontine myelinolytic lesions have also been reported in about 10% of cases. With regard to the management of the hyponatremia, most workers believe that it is the absolute change in serum sodium rather than the rate of change which is critical.

Marchiafava-Bignami Disease

This extremely rare condition is seen in middle-aged and elderly men and women and is caused by the continued excessive con-

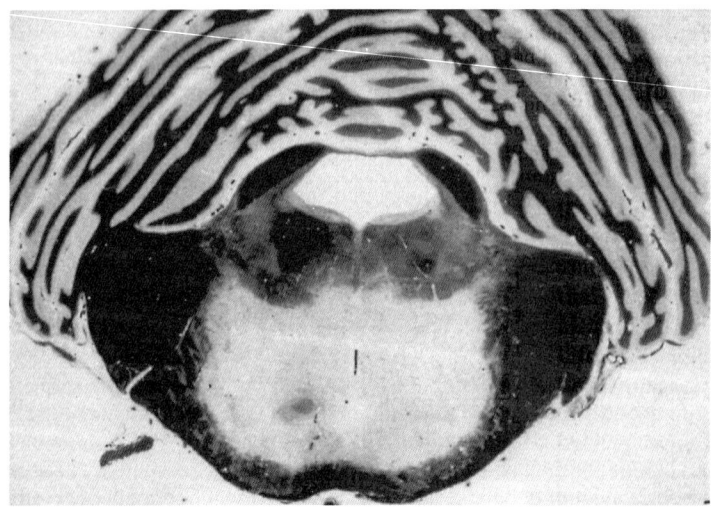

Figure 14–3. Horizontal section of the pons shows pallor of the central zone of the basis pontis, which was shown on histology to be demyelination. This is typical of central pontine myelinolysis.

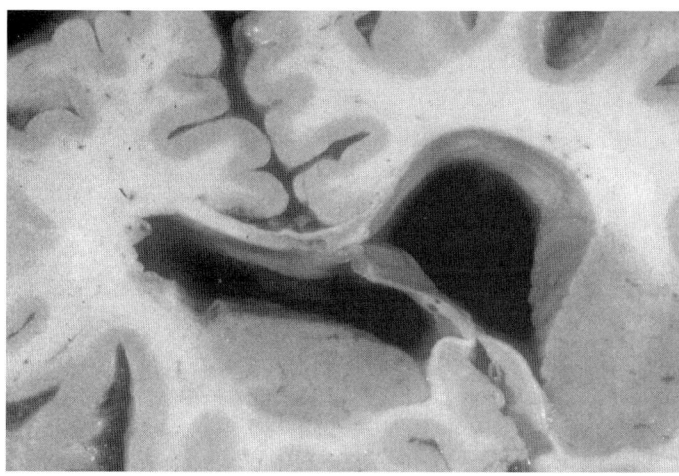

Figure 14–4. Coronal section of cerebral hemispheres shows assymetrical thinning and pallor of the corpus callosum, which, on histological examination was found to be demyelination. This is characteristic of Marchiafava-Bignami disease.

sumption of alcohol, be it red or white wine, gin, or other beverages. It is occasionally seen in poorly nourished non-drinkers. Marchiafava-Bignami disease (MBD) has been found in association with WE and CPM. Although there is no typical clinical presentation, some patients can present acutely with seizures and disorders of consciousness progressing to death. Alternatively, some present with a more chronic form with progressive dementia or interhemispheric disconnection syndromes lasting several years. The diagnosis was often not made until autopsy, but more recently cases have been diagnosed with CT and MRI, and by sequential imaging, patients surviving MBD have been identified.[33] Pathologically, MBD is characterized by necrotizing demyelinating lesions of the corpus callosum, which can extend into the adjacent white matter (Fig. 14–4). Occasionally there is an associated cortical laminar sclerosis.[34] The pathogenesis of MBD disease is still unknown.

Other Vitamin Deficiencies

NIACIN DEFICIENCY

Niacin (nicotinic acid) deficiency causes pellagra. It is much less common today than during the epidemic prevalence of the early part of the twentieth century. Niacin has been added to foods such as flour and bread for many years, which has reduced the prevalence of pellagra. It is seen in the alcoholic population and in patients with tuberculosis who are being treated with isoniazid. Pellagra is more likely to occur in patients who are vegetarians or vegans. The characteristic clinical triad in endemic pellagra is dermatitis, diarrhea, and dementia. Many patients with non-endemic pellagra do not exhibit dermatitis and diarrhea and the diagnosis can be very difficult to make.[35] Neurological signs and symptoms include insomnia, anxiety, depression, and confusion or more specific signs such as gait disturbances, extrapyramidal signs, and spastic paraplegia. Many patients also develop a peripheral neuropathy.

The brain appears macroscopically normal but microscopically neurons may be chromatolytic. Chromatolysis is most common in the pontine nuclei and dentate nuclei of the cerebellum.[36] Cranial nerve nuclei (mainly the third, sixth, seventh, and eighth), the reticular nuclei, arcuate nuclei and posterior horn cells may also be affected.

COBALAMINE (B12) DEFICIENCY

Vitamin B-12 is absorbed from the ileum by binding to intrinsic factor and deficiency is still most common in patients with Addisonian pernicious anemia who fail to produce intrinsic factor. This is an autoimmune disease that affects women, particularly those over the age of 60. Gastric surgery and a variety of small intestinal disorders may also be causative factors. Vitamin B12 deficiency of dietary origin is rare but can occur in vegetarians. Haemopoietic tissues, epithelial surfaces, and the nervous system are all affected. Subacute degeneration of the spinal cord is the principle disorder and is characterised by symmetrical sensory disturbances in the feet, with loss of sensation along with a feeling of "pins and needles". The symmetrical sensory polyneuropathy that is seen in B12 deficiency may or may not be associated with the myelopathy. The fully developed case may have ataxia, spasticity, and loss of reflexes; mental changes have been observed. Neuropsychiatric problems were reported in 28% of cases in one study.[37] Pathologically, some studies indicate a demyelinating neuropathy[39] whereas others describe predominantly axonal degeneration.[38] The brain appears macroscopically normal but the spinal cord may be shrunken and, when cut in the transverse plane, the posterior and lateral columns appear gray-white in color and have an almost translucent appearance. Microscopically, there are multifocal vacuolated and demyelinated lesions in the white matter of the spinal cord, particularly affecting the posterior and lateral columns, but with occasional involvement of the anterior columns (Fig. 14–5). The mid-thoracic segments are most severely affected, but more rostral cervical segments and even the medulla can be involved.

VITAMIN E AND ABETALIPROTEINEMIA

Vitamin E plays an important role in the nervous system, acting as a scavenger of free radicals and preserving the structural integrity of the tissues.[39] A deficiency state rarely occurs on a dietary basis but all forms of malabsorption can lead to a secondary deficiency. Neurological signs and symptoms are similar to those of Friedrich's ataxia. There is a progressive cerebellar ataxia with muscle weakness, areflexia in the lower limbs, sensory loss, and ophthalmoplegia. Neuropathological studies show degeneration of axons in the posterior columns. Swollen dystrophic axons (spheroids) are present in the gracile and cuneate nuclei. Lipofuscin accumulates in neurons and endothelial cells. It has been suggested that this disorder may be related to oxidative stress as proposed for other progressive degenerative neurologic disorders such as Parkinson's disease.[40] Biopsies of peripheral sensory nerves

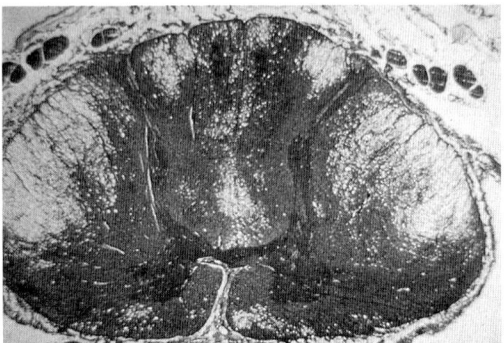

Figure 14–5. Transverse section of the thoracic spinal cord stained with a myelin technique shows spongy vacuolation of the white matter, particularly in the lateral and posterior columns, typical of subacute combined degeneration of the spinal cord.

have shown that there may be an associated loss of the larger myelinated nerves and that the disorder is a central–peripheral distal axonopathy.[41]

Cerebellar Cortical Degeneration

Atrophy of the cerebellum is commonly associated with alcoholism and/or malnutrition. It can develop abruptly or over a period of weeks and is usually associated with a neuropathy. Clinically, patients present with progressive unsteadiness and difficulty in walking. The feet become more widely based and the gait is hesitant. This is associated with ataxia of the legs and trunk. The incidence in a general hospital population is about 5% and in an alcoholic population, about 25%.[42] The atrophy is readily identified on CT and MRI.[43] (Fig. 14–6). Macroscopically, there is shrinkage of the folia, particularly the anterior superior vermis (Fig. 14–7). There is a reduction in the volume of white matter, which accounts for a proportion of the shrinkage. Microscopically, there is a loss of Purkinje cells with proliferation of Bergmann glia. There is a significant reduction in the number and size of Purkinje cells, which is most marked in the smaller rostral and caudal lobes of the vermis (lobes I–IV, IX, and X).[44] The Purkinje cell loss and shrinkage are most marked in those alcoholics with WKS. Studies

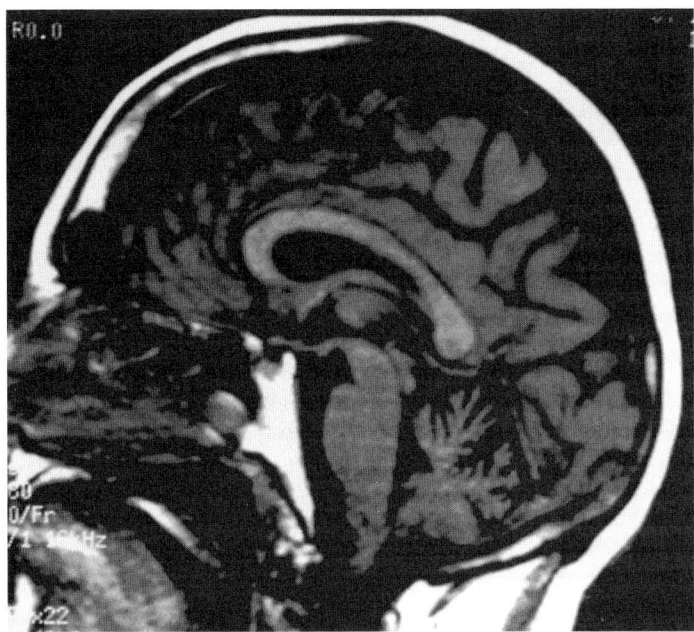

Figure 14–6. Magnetic resonance imaging scan of the brain of a 46-year-old man with a history of alcoholism. The sagittal image shows severe atrophy of anterior superior vermal segments.

have shown that the Purkinje cells have a reduced dendritic arbor.[45] Debate continues as to whether alcohol or thiamin deficiency causes the cerebellar degeneration. Adams[46] described a disease identical to alcoholic cerebellar degeneration in malnourished individuals without alcoholism. Additional evidence pointing toward the importance of thiamin deficiency as the principal pathogenetic factor in alcoholic cerebellar degeneration is the fact that the clinical features of the disorder have been shown to be reversed by the administration of thiamin, even in the presence of continued alcohol consumption. The most recent neuropathological study of "alcoholic" cerebellar degeneration suggests that thiamin deficiency is the principle etiological factor.[42]

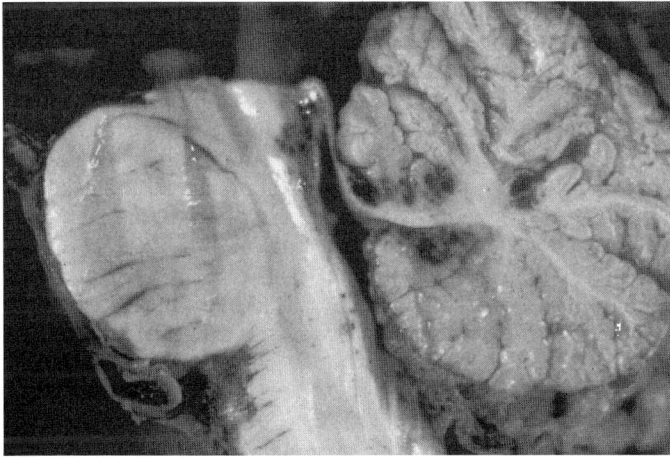

Figure 14–7. Sagittal section of the cerebellar hemispheres and brain-stem of a 56 year old woman with a history of drinking 10 standard drinks a day for 30 years. Note the severe atrophy of the anterior superior segment of the vermis, typical of cerebellar cortical degeneration.

Peripheral Neuropathies

The elderly are particularly prone to neuropathies caused by vitamin deficiencies, particularly those of thiamin (B1), pyridoxine (B6) and niacin or nicotinic acid (pellagra). They have also been described in vitamin B12 deficiency and in vitamin E deficiency. These disorders are discussed briefly in the sections above and in some detail in Chapter 20.

ALCOHOL AND AGING

It is difficult to estimate the number of elderly people who consume alcohol at hazardous or harmful levels, but a recent national survey from Australia showed that 8.5% of men aged 65–74 consumed 40–60 g/day (hazardous level) and 5.7% consumed >60 g/day (harmful level).[47] In a group of veterans of a similar age, 19% drank at the hazardous level and 21% at the harmful level.[48] Data from the United States are limited but in a recent review, Zucker claimed that between 2% and 4% of the elderly population meet criteria for alcohol abuse or dependence and up to 10% are heavy or problem drinkers.[49] An important additional consideration is that there is generally a dramatic increase in total body fat with aging and a concomitant reduction in body water. This results in higher and more dangerous blood alcohol levels in older people for the same dose of alcohol.[50] To determine the relationship (if any) between alcohol and aging, pathological changes that are truly age-related and alcohol-related must be identified. Harper and colleagues have compared their quantitative data for aging and alcohol-related brain damage to address this issue.[51] The parameters discussed include brain weight and volume, pericerebral space volume (see below for definition), cerebral hemisphere and cerebellar volumes, cerebral cortical gray and white matter volumes, and basal ganglia volumes. Cortical neuronal counts and densities, and measurements of neuronal dendritic arborization are also addressed.

Alcohol-related neuropathological changes can occur as a result of other medical complications such as thiamin (vitamin B-1) deficiency and cirrhosis of the liver, but these cases were excluded in the Caine report, using the recently described operational criteria.[52] All cases were screened to eliminate neurological abnormalities such as strokes, AD, and severe head injuries. Cases used in their studies included controls who drank <20 g alcohol per day (most cases had nil intake), moderate drinkers who consumed 30–80 g/day, and uncomplicated alcoholics who consumed >80 g/day. Most of the latter group drank >120 g/day and had a 20- to 30-year drinking history. They had no other medical complications such as cirrhosis or WKS. The mean age of the drinking groups was in the sixth decade and their drinking histories were in excess of 25 years. The mean age of the control group was also in the sixth decade.

Brain Weight and Volume

One of the changes that is common to both aging and the long-term effects of alcohol is brain shrinkage. The MRI data are particularly interesting in that the age-related loss of brain volume in the alcoholic group is over and above that expected in normal aging.[53] The changes are particularly evident in the temporal cortex and the white matter. Mean reductions in brain weight in our alcoholic cases are shown in Table 14–2. However, a Scandinavian group showed no difference in brain weight between controls and alcoholics after 70 years of age.[54]

Brain weights and volumes exhibit a wide range of variation, even in the normal population and a more reliable parameter for detecting brain shrinkage is measurement of the pericerebral space (PICS), which is illustrated in Figure 14–8. This measure effectively excludes individual variation based on physical parameters such as height and weight and

Table 14–2. Fresh Brain Weight in Controls, Moderate Drinkers, and Alcoholics

Group	n	Weight (g)	Sem
Control	56	1433	17
Moderate	16	1415	34
Alcoholic	38	1352°	27

SEM, standard error of the mean.
°$P < .01$.

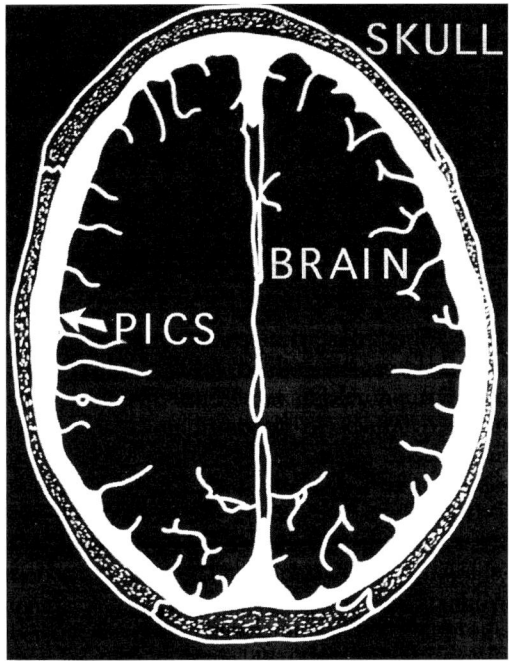

Figure 14–8. The pericerebral space (PICS) lies between the skull and the brain and is filled with cerebrospinal fluid. This volume will increase if there is brain shrinkage. The calculation of the PICS is discussed below.

gender differences. Any reduction in brain volume will cause an increase in the PICS value which can be calculated from the following equation:

$$\text{PICS} = \frac{\text{intracranial volume} - \text{brain volume}}{\text{intracranial volume}} \times \frac{100\%}{1}$$

A simple technique for measuring intracranial volume is based on the production of a permanent polyurethane cast of the intracranial cavity.[55] Table 14–3 gives the mean PICS val-

Table 14–3. Pericerebral Space Values in Controls and Alcoholics

Group	n	PICS (%)	Sem
Control	51	7.8	0.5
Moderate	13	8.8	1.2
Alcoholic	32	11.3*	1.0

PICS, pericerebral space; SEM, standard error of the mean.
*$P < 0.001$.

ues and standard errors for the controls, moderate drinkers, and uncomplicated alcoholics. As shown in previous studies,[56,57] there is a statistically significant difference between controls and uncomplicated alcoholics and even in the moderate drinkers there is a trend suggesting that an intake of <80 g alcohol per day may cause loss of brain tissue.

Regression analyses show that there is a strong correlation between brain shrinkage and age in both the control and alcoholic groups (Fig. 14–9). Moreover, the older alcoholic patients have much higher PICS values than controls. This finding suggests that there may be a cumulative effect of age and alcohol.

Volume Changes Within the Cerebral Hemispheres

Macroscopic examination of the cerebral hemispheres of both aging and alcoholic patients has provided generally little information on volume change. In alcoholics, Courville[58] and others have commented that the frontal lobes seem to be more severely atrophic. Imaging studies of alcoholics have also shown that the frontal lobes are more shrunken than other brain regions.[59] Frontal atrophy has also been noted in aging and AD. Quantitative studies have shown that there is a different pattern of atrophy in aging and AD, the frontal cortex being more severely affected in AD whereas the frontal white matter tends to bear the brunt of the atrophy in aging.[60] The latter is similar to the documented white matter loss in alcoholics (see Reversibility of White Matter Loss, below). Regression analyses of cortical gray matter volume for both groups show surprisingly little change with respect to age (Table 14–4).

Cerebral cortical gray matter can be assessed during life by means of MRI and by pathological studies after death. Animal studies of aging highlight the relative lack of change in the cerebral cortex of aging primates (Rhesus monkeys).[61] The most recent human pathological studies support the contention that cortical gray matter is relatively intact in "normal" old people.[60] Although brain atrophy is a common finding in aged humans, it is not an inevitable consequence. Moreover, the selection of noncognitively impaired aged subjects for these types of studies may not be

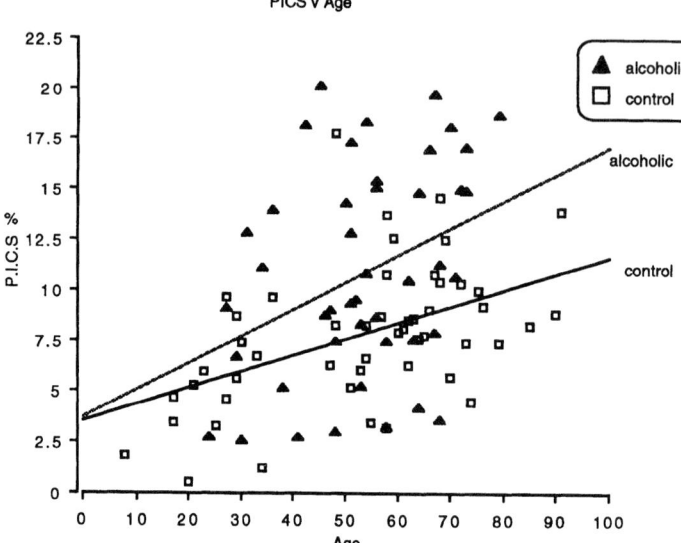

Figure 14–9. Relationship between brain shrinkage and age for the control (aging) and alcoholic groups. For the alcoholic group, pericerebral space (PICS) = 3.715 + 0.134 × age; R^2 = 0.127. For the control group, PICS = 3.529 + 0.081 × age; R^2 = 0.242

representative of the whole population—that is, we may be selecting a successfully aging population. Many of the older quantitative neuropathological studies showed a progressive decrease in neuronal density with age. However, the techniques applied in these studies are now considered inaccurate and inappropriate. There is, however, neuronal loss in some regions of the brain with age: the basal forebrain,[62] and locus coeruleus,[63] for example, but neurons in the cerebral cortex appear to be preserved.[64] Although studies of alcoholic patients do not show significant changes in cortical gray matter volume,[56,65] there are selected regions where neuronal loss

Table 14–4. Percentage of Gray and White Matter in Cerebral Hemispheres

		GRAY MATTER		WHITE MATTER	
	n	Volume (%)	Sem	Volume (%)	Sem
Control	26	53.8	0.6	40.5	0.5
Moderate	13	55.3	0.7	39.4	0.7
Alcoholic	34	54.3	0.5	39.1°	0.4

SEM, standard error of the mean.
°$P < .01$

is significant. The superior frontal association cortex has reduced neuronal density[26] and reduced total neuronal counts.[65] Neuronal loss in alcoholics has also been documented in subcortical regions.[66] The findings in these studies are listed in Table 14–5, which shows a comparison of patterns of neuronal loss in aging and alcoholism. An important point to note is that neuronal loss in the thalamus, basal forebrain, and raphe nuclei is only seen in those alcoholics with thiamin deficiency (WKS).[27,67] Our most recent study showed that there is no consistent change in the number of neurons or in volume for any of the cerebellar regions in chronic alcoholics without clinical signs of WE.[42] Not all authors agree that alcohol causes cortical neuronal loss. Jensen and Pakkenberg[68] found no neuronal loss in their study of alcohol toxicity; they used an unbiased stereological technique. However, as Kril and colleagues have shown, there is a substantial variation in the number of neurons from case to case within cortical regions and the large variations in neuronal number could mask the small selective loss observed (in frontal association cortex) when regions are averaged.[65] It is interesting to note that the correlation between neuronal loss and alcohol consumption is dose related in the supraoptic and paraventricular nuclei of the hypothalamus.[69]

A number of other findings have been made

Table 14–5. Regional Neuronal Loss in Aging and Alcoholism

Brain Region	Aging	Alcohol
Cerebral cortex	−	+
Basal ganglia	−	−
Thalamus	−	+[a]
Substantia nigra	−	−
Basal forebrain	+	+[a]
Hippocampus	−	−
Locus coeruleus	+	−
Raphe nuclei	−	+[a]
Cerebellum	−	+[a]

[a] Neuronal loss only seen in cases with Wernicke-Korsakoff syndrome.

in experimental models that suggest links between aging and alcohol toxicity. Lipofuscin is generally considered to be a marker of aging in central nervous system (CNS) neurons and several groups have found an increase in intracellular lipofuscin deposition in the hippocampal and cerebellar neurons of rats given alcohol chronically.[70,71]

Given that neuritic plaques and neurofibrillary tangles are a common finding in the brains of aging subjects and that they are two of the pathological hallmarks of AD, it is reasonable to propose that, if alcohol induces premature aging, the brains of alcoholics should have greater numbers of these pathological markers than comparable controls. We have found no significant difference in these markers between controls and alcoholics of the same age (unpublished data). However, Cullen and co-workers have shown that the magnocellular neurons of the basal nucleus of Meynert are particularly susceptible to neurofibrillary tangle formation in alcoholics who also have WKS, but this was not seen in uncomplicated alcoholics.[67]

Dendritic arborization of layer III pyramidal neurons from the frontal and motor cortices has been studied in controls and alcoholics. A significant relationship was found between age and total dendritic length, number of branches, and maximal width of dendritic field in both control and alcoholic groups.[25] The dendritic arborization was more severely affected in the alcoholics than in controls.

Although authors have long noted a reduction in the volume of the white matter with aging,[72] this finding has been largely overlooked. This is partly because both macroscopic and microscopic changes in the white matter of normal aged patients are minimal, or at least very subtle. It has become evident from recent neuropathological studies however, that white matter loss is a feature of aging and appears to account for most of the cerebral tissue loss.[60] This finding is supported by MRI studies. A similar reduction in white matter volume has been noted in studies of alcohol-related brain damage.[56,65] The loss is most severe in those alcoholics who have additional complications such as WKS and cirrhosis of the liver. The white matter of the cerebellar vermis is also reduced in volume in alcoholics when compared to controls.[42] Regression analyses of white matter volumes for the control (aging) and alcoholic groups are shown in Fig. 14–10.

There were relatively few alcoholics in the older age-groups which may account for the apparent convergence of the regression lines in the latter decades. In a previous study,[73] both controls and alcoholics showed significant decreases in volume of white matter with age (controls: slope = 0.08, P = 0.005; alcoholics: slope = 0.11, P = 0.04). It should be noted however, that the alcoholic group included patients with no complications and those with cirrhosis and WKS. In one study it has been shown that the loss of white matter correlates negatively with life-long alcohol consumption.[65]

Microscopic studies show pale staining of the white matter (myelin stains) in older patients but not in young patients.[74] Diffuse pallor of white matter has also been reported in alcoholics, particularly those with WKS. Alling and Bostrom found significantly lower concentrations of phospholipids, cholesterol, and cerebroside, implying a loss of myelin in alcoholic cases.[75] Studies of aging in Rhesus monkeys have show a significant loss of white matter with age and a concomitant increase in the size of the ventricles. Using 1 µm plastic embedded sections, these workers noted degeneration of myelinated axons, which was most obvious in the deeper layers of the cortex and in the subcortical white matter. On electron microscopy there were frequent profiles of large nerve fibers in which the myelin sheaths

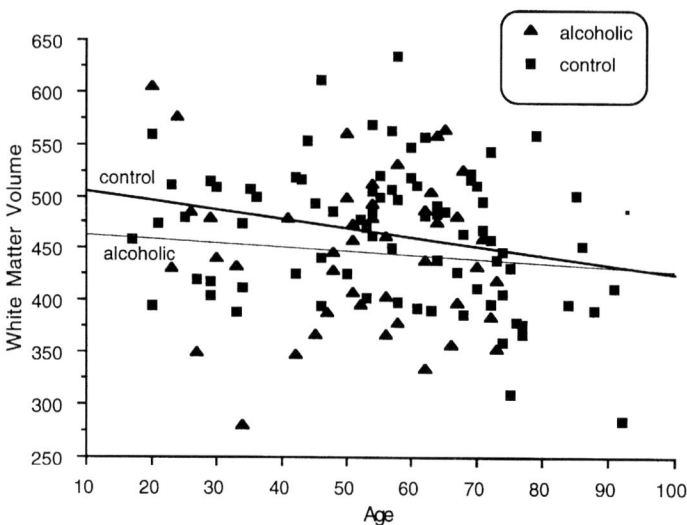

Figure 14–10. Relationship between cerebral white cerebral white matter volume and age for the control (aging) and alcoholic groups. For the alcoholic group, white matter volume = 467.169 − 0.402 × age; $R^2 = 7.031E - 3$. For the control group, the white matter volume = 513.708 − 0.87 × age; $R^2 = 0.062$.

appeared to be empty or to contain debris. Splitting of the myelin was a common finding and many of the medium-sized nerve fibers had dark, presumably degenerating axons. It was shown that there was a good correlation between the extent of myelin degeneration and performance deficits of the monkeys.[61] In an animal model of alcohol toxicity combined with thiamin deficiency, Langlais and Zhang have also shown degeneration in the white matter.[76]

Ultrastructural studies of the effects of alcohol on the structure of developing optic nerve in a rat model show that alcohol causes a reduction in the relative thickness of myelin sheaths.[77] The subtle nature of the white matter changes are borne out by physical and chemical studies of the white matter of aging and alcoholic subjects.[78,79]

Reversibility of White Matter Loss

An important difference in the white matter changes in aging and alcoholism is the fact that, at least in some cases, the loss of white matter in alcoholics appears to be reversible. Using sequential MRIs, Shear and co-workers showed that after 3 months of abstinence, there was an increase in the volume of white matter.[53] Young patients with the shortest drinking histories seem to have the greatest chance for reversibility,[80] which suggests that there is probably both a reversible and an irreversible component of white matter damage in alcoholics. It is conceivable that the irreversible component is similar to the change in aging and is likely to relate to neuronal loss and Wallerian degeneration of myelinated axons.

The most common clinical change in aging patients is a generalized slowing of cognitive processes.[81,82] This slowing may be the result of decreased nerve conduction through the central white matter, but this is difficult to evaluate until the pathological substrate for the change is identified. A recent MRI study showed a correlation between the magnitude of white matter loss and cognitive decline.[83] Similar radiological and cognitive changes have been reported in alcoholics.[84]

In summary, the question, does alcohol affect the aging process of the brain, has been addressed by comparing the neuropathological changes that have been identified in both aging and alcohol-related brain damage studies. One of the disappointing features of this review is the fact that some of the regression analyses failed to reveal statistical significance, even though the slopes of the lines were fairly consistent among different parameters (e.g., brain weight, volume, cerebral hemisphere volume). The reason for this may be the great variability in individual biological measures—alternatively, to identify age-related changes, a number of time points might have to be employed. The same almost certainly applies to studies of the changes caused by a neurotoxin that appears to act slowly over a long period of time—i.e., alcohol. Moreover, it may well be that both factors act in a non-linear fashion, thus more specialized statistically analyses should be applied to the problem. Nevertheless, a number of conclusions can be drawn from these data. There is loss of brain tissue with aging and alcoholism and the loss is greater in alcoholics (PICS data). The loss is mainly from the cerebral hemispheres and is predominantly white matter. The loss of white matter is greater in alcoholics and correlates with life-long alcohol intake. There is also a correlation between loss of white matter and cognitive dysfunction in both aging and alcoholism.

Alcoholic Myopathy

Alcohol abuse can result in an acute or a chronic myopathy. The acute form is a dramatic disorder that begins abruptly with muscle weakness, pain, edema, and swelling of limbs, and myoglobinuria, and it can progress to renal failure. Muscle biopsy shows acute rhabdomylysis (see Chapter 22). Alcohol-induced chronic myopathy is a painless disorder with proximal muscle weakness and atrophy involving primarily the pelvic girdle and thighs and sometimes the shoulder girdle. There is often an associated cardiomyopathy and neuropathy. The history, clinical examination, and examination of the muscle biopsy (see Chapter 22) suggest a diagnosis that is confirmed by the relative success of the treatment: alcohol withdrawal.

REFERENCES

1. Parrot J. Clinique des Nouveaux-nés. L'Athrepsie, Paris: G. Masson 877:291–354.
2. Nobécourt P. Des hypotrophies et des cachexies des nourrissons. Arch Med Enf 1916; 19:113.
3. Jackson CM. The Effects of Inanation and Malnutrition upon Growth and Structure. Philadelphia: Blakiston, 1925:173–190.
4. Grande F, Peraita M. Avitaminosis y Systema Nervoso. Madrid, 1941.
5. Spillane JD. Nutritional Disorders of the Nervous System. Edinburgh: E. & S. Livingstone, 1947.
6. Helweg-Larson P, Hoffmeyer H, Kilder J, et al. Famine disease in German concentration camps: complications and sequels. Acta Med Scand 1952; 144:3–460, 244:1.
7. Sone Y. Age-associated problems in nutrition. Appl Hum Sci 1995; 14:201–210.
8. Casper RC. Nutrition and its relationship to aging. Exp Gerentol 1995; 30:299–314.
9. Nickols-Richardson SM, Johnson MA, Poon LW, Martin P. Mental health and number of illnesses are predictors of nutritional risk in elderly persons. Exp Aging Res 1996; 22:141–54.
10. Aihie Sayer A, Cooper C. Undernutrition and aging. Gerentology 1997; 43:203–205.
11. Lesourd BM, Mazari L, Ferry M. The role of nutrition in immunity in the aged. Nutr Rev 1998; 56:S113–S125.
12. United Nations. United Nations Human Development Report. New York: Oxford University Press, 1998.
13. United Nations. The 1996 Revision. World Population Prospects. New York: United Nations Publications 1998:6–18.
14. Katzman R. The aging brain. Limitations in our knowledge and future approaches [editorial]. Arch Neurol 1997; 54:1201–1205.
15. Rowland DT. Population Policies and Ageing in Asia: a Cohort Perspective. New York: United Nations Publications, 1994.
16. Riggs JE. Changing demographics and neurologic disease in the elderly. Neurol Clin 1996; 14:477–486.
17. Riggs JE. The aging population. Neurol Clin 1998; 16:555–560.
18. Odenheimer GL. Geriatric neurology. Neurol Clin 1998; 16:561–567.
19. Victor M, Adams RD, Collins GH. The Wernicke-Korsakoff Syndrome, 2nd ed. Philadelphia: Davis, 1989.
20. Harper CG, Giles M, Finlay-Jones R. Clinical signs in the Wernicke-Korsakoff complex—a retrospective analysis of 131 cases diagnosed at autopsy. J Neurol Neurosurg Psychiatry 1986; 49:341–345.
21. Lishman WA, Jacobson RR, Acker C. Brain damage in alcoholism: current concepts. Acta Med Scand [Suppl] 1987; 717:5–17.
22. Harper CG. The incidence of Wernicke's encephalopathy in Australia—a neuropathological study of 131 cases. J Neurol Neurosurg Psychiatry 1983; 46:593–598.
23. Harper C, Fornes P, Duyckaerts C, Lecomte D, Hauw J-J. An international perspective on the prevalence of the Wernicke-Korsakoff syndrome. Metab Brain Dis 1995; 10:17–24.
24. Byrne C, Halliday G, Ellis J, Harper C. Thalamic vacuolation in acute Wernicke's encephalopathy. Metab Brain Dis 1993; 8:107–113.
25. Harper CG, Kril JJ. Neuropathology of alcoholism. Alcohol Alcoholism 1990; 25:207–216.

26. Harper C, Kril J, Daly J. Are we drinking our neurones away? Br Med J 1987; 294:534–536.
27. Halliday GM, Cullen K, Harding A. Neuropathological correlates of memory dysfunction in the Wernicke-Korsakoff syndrome. Alcohol Alcohol Suppl 1994; 2:245–251.
28. Cullen KM, Halliday GM, Caine D, Kril JJ. The nucleus basalis (Ch4) in the alcoholic Wernicke-Korsakoff syndrome: reduced cell number in both amnesic and non-amnesic patients. J Neurol Neurosurg Psychiatry 1997; 63:315–320.
29. Wood B, Currie J, Breen K. Wernicke's encephalopathy in a metropolitan hospital. Med J Aust 1986; 144: 12–15.
30. Harper CG, Sheedy DL, Lara AI, Garrick TM, Hilton JM, Raisanen J. Prevalence of Wernicke-Korsakoff syndrome in Australia: has thiamin fortification made a difference? Med J Aust 1998; 168:542–545.
31. Peeters A, Van de Wyngaert F, Van Lierde M, Sindic CJ, Laterre EC. Wernicke's encephalopathy and central pontine myelinolysis induced by hyperemesis gravidarum. Acta Neurol Belg 1993; 93:276–282.
32. Wakui H, Nishimura S, Watahiki Y, Endo Y, Nakamoto Y, Miura AB. Dramatic recovery from neurological deficits in a patient with central pontine myelinolysis following severe hyponatremia. Jpn J Med 1991; 30:281–284.
33. Yamashita K, Kobayashi S, Yamaguchi S, Koide H, Nishi K. Reversible corpus callosum lesions in a patient with Marchiafava-Bignami disease: serial changes on MRI. Eur Neurol 1997; 37:192–193.
34. Logak M, Feve A, Samson Y, Guillard A, Rancurel G. Contribution of position emission tomography in a case of Marchiafava Bignami disease: Morel's laminar sclerosis? Rev Neurol (Paris) 1996; 152:47–50.
35. Serdaru M, Hausser-Hauw C, Laplane D, Buge A, Castaigne P, Goulon M, Lhermitte F, Hauw J. The clinical spectrum of alcoholic pellagra encephalopathy. Brain 1988; 111:829–842.
36. Hauw J-J, De Baecque C, Hausser-Hauw C, Serdaru M. Chromatolysis in alcoholic encephalopathies. 1988; Brain 111:843–857.
37. Lindenbaum J, Healton EB, Savage DG, Brust JC, Garrett TJ, Podell ER, Marcell PD, Stabler SP, Allen, RH. Neuropsychiatric disorders caused by cobalamin deficiency in the absence of anaemia or macrocytosis. N Engl J Med 1988; 318:1720–1728.
38. McCombe PA, McLeod JG The peripheral neuropathy of vitamin B12 deficiency. J Neurol Sci 1984; 66: 117–126.
39. Sokol RJ. Vitamin E and neurologic function in man. Free Radic Biol Med 1989; 6:189–207.
40. Dexter DT, Brooks DJ, Harding AE, Burn DJ, Muller DP, Gross-Sampson MA, Jenner PG, Marsden CD. Nigrostriatal function in vitamin E deficiency: clinical, experimental and positron emission tomographic studies. Ann Neurol 1994; 35:298–303.
41. Wichman A, Buchthal F, Pezeshkpour GH, Gregg RE. Peripheral neuropathies in abetalipoproteinemia. Neurology 1985; 35:1279–1289.
42. Baker KG, Harding AJ, Halliday GM, Kril JJ, Harper CG. Neuronal loss in functional zones of the cerebellum of chronic alcoholics with and without Wernicke's encephalopathy. Neuroscience 1999; 91(2)429–438 (In press).
43. Pfefferbaum A, Rosenbloom M. In vivo imaging of morphological brain alterations associated with alcoholism. In: Hunt WA, Nixon SJ, eds. Alcohol-Induced Brain Damage. Research Monograph No. 22. Rockville, MD: U.S. Department of Health and Human Services, 1993:71–87.
44. Phillips SC, Harper CG, Kril J. A quantitative histological study of the cerebellar vermis in alcoholic patients. Brain 1987; 110:301–314.
45. Ferrer I, Fabreques I, Pineda M, Gracia, I, Ribalta T. A Golgi study of cerebellar atrophy in human chronic alcoholism. Neuropathol Appl Neurobiol 1984; 10:245–253.
46. Adams RD, Nutritional Cerebellar Degeneration. Amsterdam: Elsevier, 1976.
47. Castles I. National Health Survey: Summary of Results. Canberra: Australian Bureau of Statistics, 1991.
48. Dent OF, Sulway MR, Broe GA, Creasey H, Kos SC, Jorm AF, Tennant C, Fairley MJ. Alcohol consumption and cognitive performance in a random sample of Australian soldiers who served in the second world war. BMJ 1997; 314:1655–1657.
49. Zucker RA. Developmental aspects of aging, alcohol involvement, and their interrelationship. In: Gomberg ESL, Hegedus AM, Zucker RA, eds. Alcohol Problems and Aging, eds. Vol. 33. Bethesda, MD: NIH Publications, 1998:3–23.
50. Dufour MC, Archer L, Gordis E. Alcohol and the elderly. Clin Geriatr Med 1992; 8:127–141.
51. Harper C, Sheedy D, Halliday G, Double K, Dodd P, Lewohl J, Kril J. Neuropathological studies: the relationship between alcohol and aging. In: Gomberg ESL, Hegedus AM, Zucker RA, eds. Alcohol Problems and Aging, Vol. 33. Bethesda, MD: NIH Publications, 1998:117–134.
52. Caine D, Halliday GM, Kril JJ, Harper CG. Operational criteria for the classification of chronic alcoholics: identification of Wernicke's encephalopathy. J Neurol Neurosurg Psychiatry 1997; 62:51–60.
53. Shear PK, Jernigan TL, Butters N. Volumetric magnetic resonance imaging quantification of longitudinal brain changes in abstinent alcoholics. Alcohol Clin Exp Res 1994; 18:172–176.
54. Lindboe CF, Loberg EM. The frequency of brain lesions in alcoholics. J Neurol Sci 1988; 88:107–113.
55. Harper C, Kril J, Raven D, Jones N. Intracranial cavity volumes: a new method and its potential applications. Neuropathol Appl Neurobiol 1984; 10:25–32.
56. Harper CG, Kril JJ, Holloway RL. Brain shrinkage in chronic alcoholics—a pathological study. BMJ 1985; 290:501–504.
57. Harper C, Kril J, Daly J. Does a "moderate" alcohol intake damage the brain? J Neurol Neurosurg Psychiatry 1988; 51:909–913.
58. Courville CB. Effects of Alcohol on the Nervous System of Man. San Lucas Press: Los Angeles, 1966.
59. Jernigan TL, Butters N, DiTraiglia G, Schafer K, Smith T, Irwin M, Grant I, Schuckit M, Cermak LS. Reduced cerebral grey matter observed in alcoholics using magnetic resonance imaging. Alcohol Clin. Exp Res 1991; 15:418–427.
60. Double KL, Halliday GM, Kril JJ, Harasty J, Cullen K, Brooks WS, Creasey H, Broe GA. Topography of brain atrophy during normal aging and Alzheimer's disease. Neurobiol Aging 1996; 17:513–521.
61. Peters A, Rosene DL, Moss MB, Kemper TL, Abraham CR, Tigges J, Albert MS. Neurobiological bases

62. Halliday GM, Cullen K, Cairns MJ. Quantitation and three-dimensional reconstruction of Ch4 nucleus in the human basal forebrain. Synapse 1993; 15:1–16.
63. Halliday G, Baker K. Noradrenergic locus coeruleus neurons [letter]. Alcohol Clin Exp Res 1996; 20:191–192.
64. Wickelgren I. For the cortex, neuron loss may be less than thought. Science 1996; 273:48–50.
65. Kril JJ, Halliday GM, Svoboda MD, Cartwright H. The cerebral cortex is damaged in chronic alcoholics. Neuroscience 1997; 79:983–998.
66. Harper C, Butterworth R. Nutritional and metabolic disorders. In: Graham DI, Lantos PL, eds. Greenfield's Neuropathology. Vol. 1, London: Arnold, 1997: 601–642.
67. Cullen KM, Halliday GM. Neurofibrillary tangles in chronic alcoholics. Neuropathol Appl Neurobiol 1995; 21:312–318.
68. Jensen GB, Pakkenberg B. Do alcoholics drink their neurons away? Lancet 1993; 342:1201–1204.
69. Harding AJ, Halliday GM, Ng JLF, Harper CG, Kril JJ. Loss of vasopressin-immunoreactive neurons in alcoholics. Neuroscience 1996; 73:699–708.
70. Tavares MA, Paula-Barbosa MM. Lipofuscin granules in Purkinje cells after long-term alcohol consumption in rats. Alcohol Clin Exp Res 1983; 7:302–306.
71. Borges MM, Paula-Barbosa MM, Volk B. Chronic alcohol consumption induces lipofuscin deposition in the rat hippocampus. Neurobiol Aging 1986; 7:347–355.
72. Haug H, Eggers R. Morphometry of the human cortex cerebri and corpus striatum during aging. Neurobiol Aging 1991; 12:336–338.
73. Harper C, Kril J. Brain atrophy in chronic alcoholic patients: a quantitative pathological study. J Neurol Neurosurg Psychiatry 1985; 48:211–217.
74. Kemper TL. Neuroanatomical and Neuropathological Changes During Aging and Dementia. New York: Oxford University Press, 1994.
75. Alling C, Bostrom K. Demyelination of the mammillary bodies in alcoholism. A combined morphological and biochemical study. Acta Neuropathol 1980; 50:77–80.
76. Langlais PJ, Zhang S. Cortical and subcortical white matter damage without Wernicke's encephalopathy after recovery from thiamine deficiency in the rat. Alcohol Clin Exp Res 1997; 21:434–443.
77. Phillips DE, Krueger SK, Rydquist JE. Short-and long-term effects of combined pre-and postnatal ethanol exposure (three trimester equivalent) on the development of myelin and axons in rat optic nerve. Int J Dev Neurosci 1991; 9:631–647.
78. Harper CG, Kril JJ, Daly JM. Brain shrinkage in alcoholics is not caused by changes in hydration: a pathological study. J Neurol Neurosurg Psychiatry 1988; 51:124–127.
79. Wiggins RC, Gorman A, Rolsten C, Samorajski T, Ballinger WEJ, Freund G. Effects of aging and alcohol on the biochemical composition of histologically normal human brain. Metab Brain Dis 1988; 3:67–80.
80. Jacobson R. The contributions of sex and drinking history to the CT brain scan changes in alcoholics. Psychol Med 1986; 16:547–559.
81. Boone KB, Miller BL, Ledder IM, Mehringer C, Hill-Gutierrez E, Goldberg MA, Berman NG. Neuropsychological correlates of white-matter lesions in healthy elderly subjects. Arch Neurol 1992; 49:549–554.
82. Ylikoski R, Ylikoski A, Erkinjuntti T, Sulkava R, Raininko R, Tilvis R. White matter changes in healthy elderly persons correlate with attention and speed of mental processing. Arch Neurol 1993; 50:818–824.
83. Leuchter AF, Dunkin JJ, Lufkin RB, Anzai Y, Cook IA, Newton TF. Effect of white matter disease on functional connections in the aging brain. J Neurol Neurosurg Psychiatry 1994; 57:1347–1354.
84. Pfefferbaum A, Lim KO, Zipursky RB, Mathalon DH, Rosenbloom MJ, Lane B, Ha CN, Sullivan EV. Brain gray and white matter volume loss accelerates with aging in chronic alcoholics: a quantitative MRI study. Alcohol Clin Exp Res 1992; 16:1078–1089.

15. Brain Tumors in the Elderly

GEOFFREY J. PILKINGTON

The subject area of neoplasia in the elderly is of considerable significance. Although the death rate from heart disease in the elderly is steadily falling, the same cannot be said for cancer, as a steady increase in death from malignant neoplasms has been documented over the past couple of decades. Indeed, age is the greatest risk factor for the development of cancer and human cancer incidence increases exponentially with increasing age.[1,2] Moreover, in excess of 50% of all cases of cancer diagnosed exist in the over-65-year-old-age-group, and this age-group currently represents approximately 10%–15% of the population. With increasing life expectancy, the significance of these figures becomes more marked.[3] In the case of brain tumors, much attention is focused upon pediatric cases, where tumors of the Central Nervous System (CNS) account for 23% of all cancers (as compared to 31% for the leukemias) presenting during the period of birth to 15 years of age. The overall incidence of CNS tumors during this early period of life is, however, considerably lower than that in later life and, as with other cancers, brain tumors may in many respects be considered to be a disease associated with increasing age.

Tumors within or on the brain may be broadly divided into the categories of *intrinsic* (arising from the neuroectoderm) or *extrinsic* (arising either from the meninges or nerve sheaths or as secondary, or metastatic deposits from other somatic cancers). The terms "malignant" and "benign" may also be used, although these refer to the generally accepted histological criteria for malignancy and should be qualified by the location of the neoplasm within the brain. Indeed, any tumor arising in the regions of the brain that control vital functions, such as respiration and heart rate, in the brain stem must be considered biologically malignant or life threatening, irrespective of histological grade of malignancy. Indeed, the effect of any space-occupying lesion within the brain, together with peritumoural edema and the local neoplastic cell invasion that accompany many intrinsic, glial neoplasms, is raised intracranial pressure and associated neurological sequelae. From the sixth decade of life onward the most common tumors affecting the brain are secondary malignancies, glioblastoma multiforme (the most malignant form of glial neoplasm in adulthood), Schwannomas (accoustic neuromas) and meningiomas. There has been a reported incidence of some 35% to 45% in incidence of and mortality from brain tumors in developed countries over the past three decades. While putative risk factors such as mobile telephones and pesticides, and various food additives such as artificial sweeteners, may contribute to this increase, as may better diagnostic imaging approaches (e.g., MRI scans), as with other cancers, brain tumors are predominantly, although by no means exclusively, associated with aging.

In general, the clinical presentation, pathology, and biology of intrinsic brain tumors in the elderly mirror the situation in earlier adult life. There may be occasions when a clinical diagnosis is hampered by the possibility of stroke, and coexisting medical conditions in older people may complicate both diagnosis and treatment. Moreover, symptoms in the elderly tend to be reported as somewhat lower in intensity than in the general population of cancer patients; the reason for this is not clear.

Table 15–1. Incidence Rates (per 100,000 Person-Years) of Major Types of Brain Tumor Afflicting the Elderly

	AGE AT PRESENTATION (YEARS)							
	0–19	20–34	35–44	45–54	55–64	65–74	75–84	85+
Meningioma	0.08	0.59	1.83	4.26	6.65	11.05	13.72	13.32
Glioblastoma multiforme	0.15	0.42	1.12	3.87	8.47	12.22	10.83	4.95
Anaplastic astrocytoma	0.11	0.43	0.56	0.72	1.02	1.37	1.03	0.41
Astrocytoma (not otherwise specified)	0.51	0.73	0.87	1.02	1.58	2.50	2.72	1.09
Pituitary adenoma	0.13	0.86	1.21	1.31	1.96	2.24	2.24	0.77
Lymphoma	0.02	0.37	0.63	0.46	0.97	1.46	1.57	0.68†
Tumors of cranial and spinal nerves: nerve sheath, benign and malignant	0.06	0.45	0.96	1.75	1.91	1.86	1.19	0.68

Data are taken from the Central Brain Tumor Registry of the United States Annual Report 1997 for the period 1990–1994.[4]

It is also documented that the elderly are relatively under-treated compared to other age-groups; the poor prognosis and tolerance of the aged patient to invasive or toxic therapeutic regimens must, of course, be taken into consideration. Recent knowledge of the molecular genetics of CNS tumors may, in the foreseeable future, enable researchers to distinguish evolutionary trends in brain tumor diagnosis linked to age at onset or clinical appearance and may provide prognostic indicators and a reliable means with which to assess the efficacy of various treatment regimens.

INCIDENCE AND ETIOLOGY

Incidence

According to the Central Brain Tumor Registry of the United States (CBTRUS) figures for the period 1990–1994, the mean age at diagnosis for both glioblastoma multiforme and meningioma was 62 years. The mean age at diagnosis for anaplastic astrocytoma was 50 years; for nerve sheath tumors 51 years; and for lymphoma, 54 years[4] (see Table 15–1). The most frequently reported histological types of tumor in this recent large study from the United States were meningiomas (24.0%) and glioblastoma multiforme (22.6%), and the overall annual incidence rate for all primary brain and CNS tumors was 11.5 per 100,000 person-years.

A specific study of the incidence of primary intracranial tumors in a well-defined population of 271 brain tumor patients from a cohort of 216,000 people over the age of 70 years in the Kumamoto prefecture in Japan between 1989 and 1995 showed an average annual incidence rate of 18.1 cases per 100,000 population per year.[5] In this study, in which there was a higher incidence in women (20.3/100,000 population) than in men (15.2/100,000 population), the age-specific incidence was 23.2, 18.1, 15.1, and 7.6 per 100,000 population for those 70–74 years old, 75–79 years old, 80–84 years old, and those over 85 years respectively. Again, meningiomas (50.6%) and malignant gliomas (13.3%) were the most commonly encountered neoplasms.

Etiology

The suggestion of an increased incidence of brain tumors has prompted the search for risk factors. A variety of environmental agents have been considered as potential neurocarcinogens. Among these are organic solvents, ionizing radiation/electromagnetic fields, viruses, pesticides, and crop fertilizers, and dietary additives.

Nitrosocompounds are a group of potentially carcinogenic agents consisting of the nitrosamines, which are present in food such as cured meats to which nitrite preservatives have been added, and the nitrosamides which, although absent from foodstuffs, can be manufactured in the body from nitrites and amine precursors. Such nitrites are taken into the body both as food preservatives and with green vegetables, which contain relatively large amounts of these substances because of the use of nitrogenous crop fertilizers and pesticides. Common species of fungi can also reduce nitrates to nitrites and decompose proteins, thereby increasing the amount of amines in moldy foods and facilitating the formation of nitrosamines. In the Henan Province of China, for example, a region with a high incidence of esophageal cancer, more than half the samples of bread grains tested contained dietary nitrosamines. Nitrosocompounds therefore constitute a possible risk factor as environmental and dietary neurocarcinogens. Druckrey and colleagues[6] established that a single injection of ethylnitrosourea (ENU) into a pregnant rat could induce CNS tumors in the offspring. Pilkington and Lantos went on to suggest that some, if not all, brain tumors may arise as a result of fetal exposure to carcinogens in utero and proposed a hypothesis for the cellular pathogenesis of brain tumors[7,8] based on a sequential ultrastructural study of the subependymal plate of neonatal and adult rats that had been exposed transplacentally to ENU. The tumors that arose were pleomorphic, reflecting a diverse range of cellular origins. On the basis of these studies, the authors proposed that gliomas frequently arise as a result of early insult to the undifferentiated, mitotically active progenitor cells of the subependymal plate, which provide a highly susceptible target for carcinogenic stimuli. Although this initiating event may take place in early life, overt neural neoplasia may not be evidenced until a later age, possibly following various "promoter" events. The multi-step process of malignant transformation begins with enzyme-independent hydrolization of the proximate carcinogens to the electrophilic alkylating agents that covalently bind to nucleophilic centers in DNA and RNA. While the 06-position of guanine appears to be the critical target for methylnitrosourea (MNU), other 06-alkylated bases are similarly important for ENU. The net result is point mutations. In most tissues, 06-alkylguanine is rapidly removed by the DNA repair enzyme 06-alkylguanine DNA transferase (AT), a 22 kDa enzyme that removes the alkyl group from the 06-position of guanine to one of its own cysteine residues. Since the cysteine acceptor site is not regenerated, there is a stoichiometric relationship between the amount of enzyme present and the number of alkylated guanine residues that can be repaired.[9] During a limited susceptible period, the brain is deficient in this enzyme. The deficiency in the brain of this enzyme is believed to be responsible for the persistence of alkylated DNA bases and hence for the selective induction of tumors in the CNS by ENU and MNU. Epidemiological evidence has linked dietary sources of nitrosocompounds with the development of gliomas in adults,[10] however, more substantial reports of a link between maternal exposure to nitrosocompounds and incidence of primary brain tumors[11,12] have concentrated on pediatric and young patient cohorts. In addition, attention has focused on aspartame, an artificial sweetener, which has been consumed worldwide since its commercial introduction in 1981; the market for this product was worth £607 million ($1,000 million) in 1995. Relatively large amounts of this chemical product are used to artificially sweeten soft drinks (approximately 480 mg/liter), yoghurt (41 mg/100 g) and confectionary (100 mg/100 g). Aspartame has been implicated in brain tumorigenesis[13] because of (a) the temporal correlation between its introduction to the food market in 1981 and increased incidence of brain tumors since that time, (b) the suggestion that it can induce aggressive glial tumors in laboratory rats and (c) the change in predominant type of brain tumors seen in humans from astrocytomas to glioblastomas during the period that aspartame was introduced commercially.

Shephard and co-workers[14] demonstrated that nitrosation of aspartame for 10 to 30 min with 40 mM nitrite elicits considerable mutagenic potential in *Salmonellla typhimurium* TA100. These in vitro studies suggest that aspartame, or its diketopiperazine breakdown product, could be nitrosated in vivo in the human gastrointestinal tract to form a potentially carcinogenic nitrosocompound such as a nitrosourea-like agent. This could be of major significance since nitrosoureas, including ENU, are the most potent agents known to induce malignant brain tumors in experimental animals as outlined above.

Although a number of oncogenic viruses have been shown experimentally to be able to induce tumors of the nervous system in laboratory animals, the identification of virus or virus-like particles in brain tumors has not been shown to have a causal relationship and may be reflective of incidental or co-pathogenic findings. Recently, however, cases for the etiological role of SV40 in pleural mesothelioma[15] and brain tumors,[16] respectively, have been made. Although SV40 can transform human cells in vitro, it is not normally infective in humans. The current interest in this agent has come following the accidental inoculation of SV40 as a contaminant of polio vaccines given in the late 1950s and early 1960s and the perceived increase in incidence of both mesothelioma and glioblastoma multiforme in the ensuing years.

The oncogenicity and transforming ability of SV40 depends upon expression of the early region of the viral genome that encodes the Tag, or Large T antigen, a 96 kDa nuclear phosphoprotein with multiple biological properties. Large T has ATPase and helicase activities and binds to viral and cellular DNA, inducing their replication. Large T inactivates a variety of growth-regulatory nuclear proteins through complex formation. Targets include p53 protein, p105, RB-1, topoisomerase I, and a p107 host cell protein. It remains to be shown if association with these proteins is responsible for tumor induction by Large T.

In one study[16] polymerase chain reaction (PCR) amplification and Southern blot hybridization were used to study human brain tumors and cell lines. SV40 early region sequences were detected in 47% of astrocytomas, 33% of glioblastomas, and 14% of meningiomas, while 33% of astrocytoma cell lines and 50% of glioblastoma cell lines also expressed the same viral sequence. However, although no expression was seen in "normal" brain tissue, the virus was detected in peripheral blood cells and sperm fluids from apparently healthy individuals. The association between SV40 and brain tumors remains, therefore, a matter of conjecture.

Radiation has long been suspected as being connected with regional increased cancer incidence, although, apart from reported cases of therapeutic radiation-induced neoplasia following radiotherapy of the head, little hard evidence exists for a link between the development of brain tumors and exposure to radiation. A recent study of occupational exposure to magnetic fields and the likelihood of developing glioma and meningioma in which 100 tumor cases were compared with 155 controls concluded that results based on magnetic field measurements give some support to the hypothesis that magnetic field exposure may contribute to the development of brain tumors.[17] In addition, in recent years, cellular mobile telephones have been cited in law suits as playing causative roles in neural neoplastic cell transformation. A recent case-control study of the use of cellular telephones in Sweden by brain tumor patients between 20 and 80 years showed a nonsignificant increased risk of tumor in the temporal or occipital lobe on the same side that a cellular telephone had been used. However, increased risk was only found with the older analogue NMT system, whereas the newer digital GSM system remains to be accurately assessed.[18]

The role of pesticide residues in the evolution of cancer may be of significance. For example, levels of the chlorinated chemicals dichlororodiphenyl-dichloroethylene (DDE; a breakdown product of the pesticide dichlorodiphenyl-trichloroethane [DDT], which is currently used in certain regions of the world and especially in orange and grapefruit production as a by-product of the pesticide Kelthane) and polychlorinated biphenyls (PCBs; from fluorescent light fixtures and coolants in power transformers on telephone poles) have been assessed in individuals suffering from cancer and from other diseases (Tables 15–2, 15–3, and 15–4). Cancer patients were seen to have around twice the levels of these chemicals in their bodies. This phenomenon appears to be cumulative with age.

Elevated DDE and PCB levels found in cancer patients may contribute to the disease either by damage to the structure of genes controlling cell proliferation and differentiation or by interference with immune function. Although they may not directly cause the neoplasm, they may accelerate its onset or

Table 15–2. Dichlorodiphenyl-dichloroethylene and Polychlorinated Biphenyl Levels Detected in Adipose Tissue of Cancer and Non-cancer Patients at Postmortem with Respect to Age

Age (years)	DDE in Males with Cancer (ppm)	DDE in Males with No Cancer (ppm)	DDE in Females with Cancer (ppm)	DDE in Females with No Cancer (ppm)	PCB in Males with Cancer (ppm)	PCB in Males with No Cancer (ppm)	PCB in Females with Cancer (ppm)	PCB in Females with No Cancer (ppm)
0–24	—	0.74	0.817	0.933	—	3.718	4.418	2.866
25–49	4.078	3.088	1.872	1.522	11.092	9.260	3.537	3.684
50–74	4.084	3.637	5.904	2.584	7.987	5.685	8.935	4.801
>75	12.809	2.562	6.689	2.788	6.276	6.217	13.115	6.183
All	5.668	2.840	5.026	2.138	8.805	5.912	8.686	4.515

DDE, dichlorodiphenyl-dichloroethylene; PCB, polychlorinated biphenyl.
Source: Adapted from Unger and Olsen.[19]

Table 15–3. Dichlorodiphenyl-dichloroethylene Levels Detected in Patients with Various Forms of Malignant Disease

Neoplasm	DDE Level Base level found in non-cancer patients = 2.5 ppm (ppm)
Rectum cancer	11.2
Lymphosarcoma	9.3
Glioblastoma multiforme	6.4
Colon cancer	5.6
Breast cancer	5.4
Malignant lymphoma	4.3
Adenocarcinoma	3.4
Lung cancer	3.4

DDE, dichlorodiphenyl-dichloroethylene.
Source: Adapted from Unger and Olsen.[19]

growth. Indeed, both DDE and PCB levels may be of specific importance in glioblastoma multiforme, the levels of DDE and PCB being 2.5 ppm and 5.2 ppm, respectively in non-cancer patients, whereas in glioblastoma patients they are 6.4 ppm and 12.7 ppm, respectively.[19] From a group of eight tumor types studied, these levels for glioblastoma ranked third only to rectal cancer (11.2 ppm) and lymphosarcoma (9.3 ppm) (DDE) and fourth only to lymphosarcoma (24.1 ppm), adenocarcinoma (15.9 ppm), and malignant lymphoma (15.7 ppm) (PCB).

During the past decade, both the mortality from,[20] and incidence of,[21] brain tumors in elderly people have substantially increased. Indeed, annual average increases of 7.0%, 20.4%, and 23.4% in the incidence of brain tumors in the age-groups 75–79, 80–84 and 80+ years, respectively, have been reported[21] between the years 1973 and 1985. The combined increase for all age-groups was only 0.9% during this time period.

This increase may, however, be artifactual, as a result of an increased elderly population or more intensive and improved investigation, diagnosis, and treatment of older people. For example, in one study the use of computed tomography scan was relatively stable for patients between 65 and 74 years of age whereas it increased among those patients over 85 years of age.[22] The number of patients in this cohort is, of course, low, and the case for the increased exposure to environmental risk factors as outlined above is equally important.

A further explanation for the occurrence of neoplasms in elderly patients relates to the relative ineffectiveness, with increasing age, of biological mechanisms protecting against cancer. For example, it has been proposed that high levels of soluble tumor necrosis factor alpha receptors (TNF-α-R) in the serum of elderly patients may counteract the protective effects of TNF by interference with receptor binding, thereby contributing to susceptibility of the elderly to neoplastic disease.[23]

Table 15–4. Polychlorinated Biphenyl Levels Detected in Patients with Various Forms of Malignant Disease

Neoplasm	PCB Level Base level found in non-cancer patients = 5.2 ppm (ppm)
Lymphosarcoma	24.1
Adenocarcinoma	15.9
Malignant lymphoma	15.7
Glioblastoma multiforme	12.7
Colon cancer	12.6
Breast cancer	10.9
Rectum cancer	9.8
Lung cancer	8.7

PCB, polychlorinated biphenyl.
Source: Adapted from Unger and Olsen.[19]

IMAGING STRATEGIES

Computed tomography (CT) and magnetic resonance imaging (MRI) are the most common and useful technical approaches to imaging brain tumors. The rapid development and accessibility of MRI over the past couple of decades threatened to totally overshadow CT; however, with the advent of subsecond and spiral CT scanning, modern MRI and CT may be considered complementary[24] and the detection rate for tumors above the tentorium

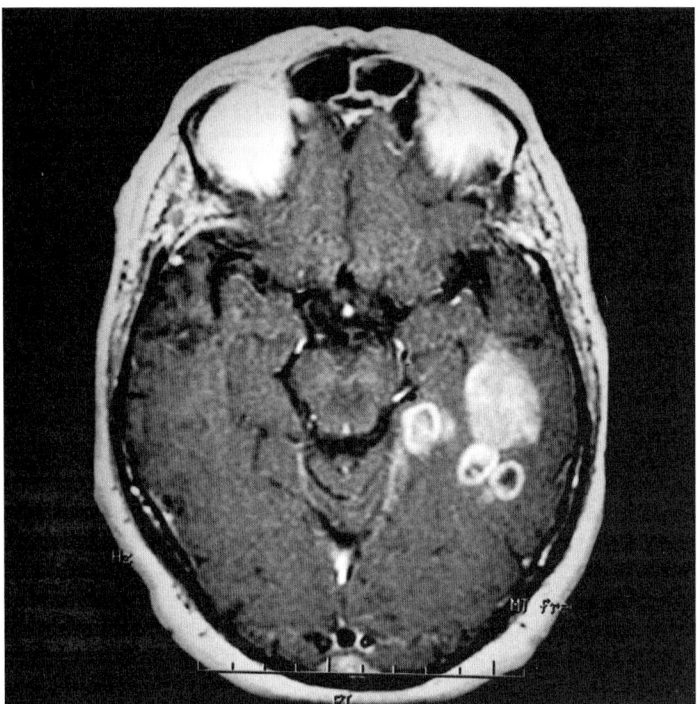

Figure 15–1. Multiple ring-enhancing lesions characteristic of cerebral metastases on MRI scan.

is approximately the same.[25] Moreover, CT can offer three advantages over MRI: (*1*) better detection of small amounts of calcium[26] such as may be seen in oligodendroglioma, (*2*) identification of early acute hemorrhage and (*3*) easier execution in very ill or elderly patients. The advantages of MRI over CT include the detection of smaller lesions, more accurate localization, prolonged evidence of hemorrhage (due to hemosiderin in macrophages), and the greater sensitivity of MRI contrast-enhancing agents to areas of blood–brain barrier disruption (this may be of some value in planning stereotactic biopsy of a low-grade tumor).

The ultimate value of imaging is to provide the neurosurgeon with information that will aid in determining whether there is a space-occupying lesion present, the location of the mass, the nature of the lesion, the best surgical approach, and, perhaps significantly in the case of elderly patients, whether surgery is implicated. Requirements for initial or primary diagnosis and for follow-up scanning are different. At primary diagnosis the function is to ascertain not only whether a neoplasm may be present but also whether this is solitary or multiple in nature. In considering a diagnosis the two most important considerations are location of the lesion and age of the patient. In many cases the age of the patient and the location are intrinsically liked. For example, cerebellar lesions are frequently astrocytamas in childhood and metastases in adulthood (Fig. 15–1). In other instances, the location tends to determine the diagnosis irrespective of age. Such is the case with acoustic neuromas, which are the most common tumor type in the cerebellopontine angle in all age-groups (Fig. 15–2). Sampling of tissue by biopsy may be considerably assisted by imaging and, while it is accepted that for primary brain tumors, neoplastic cells exist some considerable distance from the enhancing margin of the tumor (the enhancing region identifies the main tumor bulk while the non-enhancing region surrounding abnormal tissue represents vasogenic edema and reactive gliosis), some tissue should always be taken from the area of enhancement. The neurosurgical problem of how to approach the tumor is also critically dependent upon the quality and interpretation

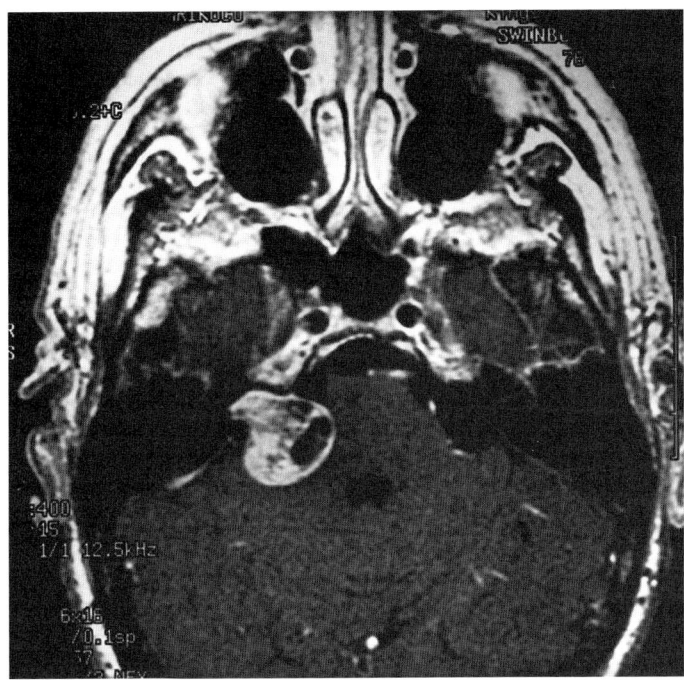

Figure 15–2. Cerebellopontine acoustic neuroma (Schwannoma) with cystic change on MRI scan.

of imaging. Through a CT- or MRI-based stereotactic surgical approach, accurate positioning within a couple of millimeters can be achieved.

Follow-up scans usually serve to assess local recurrence, distant metastases, and complications of treatment but are less commonly used in the elderly where prognosis may be expected to be much poorer than in younger patients. The time of follow-up scan after surgery is a matter of controversy, but it should be noted that biological changes affecting the CT or MRI images occur during both early and late postoperative periods. For example, enhancement seen soon after surgical debulking is probably a reflection of residual tumor since the neovascularity necessary for tissue healing does not occur for around 1 week postoperatively. Conversely, subsequent patterns of enhancement may provide evidence of reaction rather than neoplasia, but around 3 months after surgery, enhancement probably reflects residual or recurrent tumor rather than simple postoperative biological changes within normal tissue. Diffuse meningeal enhancement is seen frequently, however, on MRI following surgery and may persist for several months without providing evidence for or against tumor dissemination.[27]

CELLULAR AND MOLECULAR PATHOBIOLOGY: DIAGNOSIS AND PROGNOSTIC SIGNIFICANCE

Secondary (Metastatic) Brain Tumors

Secondary neoplasia in the brain is thought to be a non-random event, that involves host–tumor cell interaction. Of all cancers 24% are said to metastasize to the brain,[28,29] the main tissues of origin being lung, breast, skin, kidney, and gastrointestinal tract, respectively, in order of frequency. While metastatic tumors in the brain are generally well-circumscribed lesions (Fig. 15–3), intrinsic, or primary, brain tumors—most frequently derived from the glial cell (astrocyte, oligodendrocyte, and ependymal cell) population—show a marked difference at the brain–tumor interface. Here, motile, so-called guerilla cells from the pri-

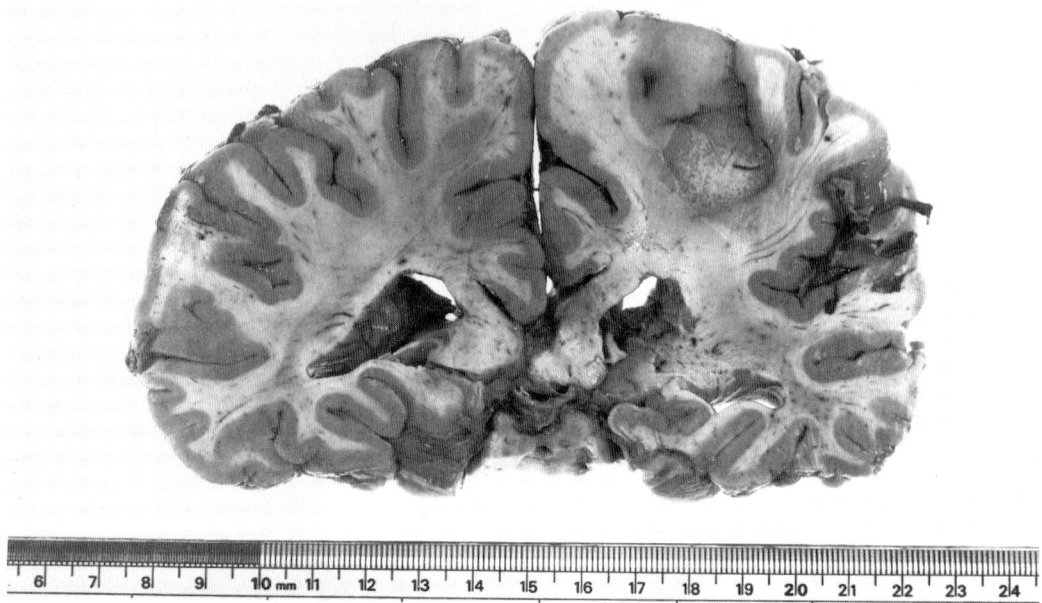

Figure 15–3. Macroscopic view of a coronal brain slice showing a large, well-circumscribed space-occupying lesion indicative of a secondary carcinoma.

mary glial neoplasm may migrate several millimeters or even centimeters away from the tumor mass, resulting in poor definition of the tumor edge. The existence and behavior of these migratory neoplastic glial cells probably explain the recurrence of tumors arising adjacent to the original site of presentation despite surgical resection and adjuvant radio- and chemotherapy.[30] Even neuroepithelial tumors of low-grade, malignancy are poorly demarcated and are never properly encapsulated. Somewhat paradoxically, intrinsic brain tumors seldom metastasize to distant organs.[31] Theories for the absence of metastases from glial neoplasms include immune surveillance, fatality from the primary tumor before manifestation of secondaries, the so-called seed-and-soil hypothesis (whereby cells from the original tumor fail to grow in a different organ microenvironment), and the presence of the blood–brain barrier.[32] Although these have been generally dismissed, two further explanations have been substantiated by experimental evidence. First, correlative in vitro/in vivo studies have shown that neither rat nor human brain tumor cells are able to intravasate through vital basal laminae.[33] The absence of an effective blood–brain barrier in primary brain tumors and surgical intervention could still, allow neoplastic cells into the vascular lumen. The second postulated mechanism for metastatic failure is based on the absence of the cell adhesion molecule CD15 from the cell surface of neoplastic glia.[34] CD15 expression has been shown to correlate with metastatic behavior of cancer cells, and transfection of cells with the CD15 gene confers enhanced metastatic potential upon cells. This molecule facilitates heterophilic and homophilic binding of tumor cells with vascular endothelium. Accordingly, even if CD15-negative neoplastic glia did breach the brain vascular basal laminae, their entry into new host "target" tissues would be barred by an inability to adhere to the non-brain endothelium.

Primary (Intrinsic) Brain Tumors

In addition to their diffuse invasive behavior and metastatic failure, intrinsic brain tumors exhibit a number of characteristic biological features that distinguish them from cancers of other organs. In particular, the expansive growth of brain tumors within the unyielding bony cranium gives rise to the life-threatening consequences of raised intracranial pressure. In addition, the location of the tumor within the brain determines to a considerable extent the clinical picture and prognosis. Cellular heterogeneity of gliomas[35] is also a prominent feature since the divergent processes of differentiation and anaplasia give rise to a mixture of morphological appearances as well as antigenic differences and differential resistance to drug and radiation therapies. This phenomenon may, not infrequently, give rise to differing degrees of malignancy becoming manifest in different regions of the same tumor. In addition, truly mixed tumors exist, reflecting derivation from different cell lineages. A new, dynamic approach to the diagnosis of intrinsic brain tumors in which novel cellular and molecular biological tools are used to supplement the conventional histological approach has provided a welcome insight into the cellular origins and mechanisms of malignant progression of this debilitating and distressing group of tumors.[36]

During the last century a variety of different systems were used for the diagnosis and classification of CNS tumors as well as for allocating degrees of malignancy. These relied to a considerable extent upon the diagnostic technologies available at the time, from classical histology to electron microscopy, immunohistochemistry, and molecular biology.[37] The current World Health Organization (WHO) system of classification for CNS tumors[38] and the malignancy grading systems of Kernohan[39] and Daumas-Duport[40] form the basis of neuropathological diagnosis in most laboratories. In this chapter the major macroscopic, histological, and biological features, that may be used for diagnostic and prognostic purposes are described for the types of tumor that most commonly affect an elderly population of patients. These tumors include astrocytoma, glioblastoma multiforme, meningioma, Schwannoma, secondary tumors, and primary malignant lymphoma of the brain.

ASTROCYTOMA

Astrocytic neoplasms account for some 20% of all neuroepithelial tumors, constituting the single largest group thought to be derived from glial elements or their progenitors. Although they can occur at any age, they occur most frequently from the sixth decade of life on (Table 15–5) and show a 3:2 male to female prevalence. They can develop anywhere along the neuroaxis but in adulthood are most commonly found in the cerebral white matter. The astrocytic nature of these tumors is usually confirmed by immunohistochemical analysis with antibodies against glial fibrillary acidic protein (GFAP), a 47 kDa protein comprising the 10 nm intermediate filaments, that characterize terminally differentiated astrocytes.[41] This specificity was extended to the study of astrocytic tumors,[42,43] where it has proved invaluable in the context of both diagnosis and research. The major cytoskeletal protein of immature astrocytes is vimentin,[44] which has a molecular weight of 57 kDa and can coexist in both reactive and neoplastic astrocytes, showing a predominance over GFAP in less well–differentiated cells. Since anaplasia is a frequent feature of these tumors other markers, such as the cytosol enzyme glutamine synthetase, may also be employed;[45] however, some reactivity has been reported in oligodendrogliomas, meningiomas, and metastases,[46] so caution should be taken in interpretation. Fibrillary, protoplasmic, and gemistocytic variants of astrocytoma can be distinguished histologically; while fibrillary forms are most commonly encountered, these are less frequently seen in later life. More malignant (anaplastic) forms of astrocytoma are seen in the aged population. The Ki-67 labeling index for proliferating cells in astrocytic tumors shows direct correlation with histological degree of malignancy of the tumor.[47] Indeed, percentages of Ki-67 positive cells have been reported to range from 1% in benign pilocytic astrocytomas to 40%–50% in glioblastoma multi-

Table 15–5. Five-year Survival Rates Following Diagnosis of Primary Malignant Brain Tumor in Relation to Age

	AGE IN YEARS			
	0–20	21–44	45–64	65+
Surviving at 5 years (%)	59.6	48.1	12.9	4.5

Source: Data taken from Ries et al.[95]

fome.[48] Hoshino and colleagues[49] concluded from a series of 174 astrocytic brain tumors that probability of survival is function of both age and bromodeoxyuridine (BudR) labeling index.

Certain monoclonal antibodies such as M2 are expressed less in juvenile astrocytomas than in malignant astrocytomas of adulthood[50] and may be indicative of oncogene products associated with increased malignancy. Anaplastic astrocytomas show generalized or focal features of malignancy, including cellular and nuclear pleomorphism, increased cellularity and mitotic activity, and reduced GFAP expression. In addition to the invariable recurrence of low-grade astrocytic tumors in adults due to their infiltrative nature, these tumors frequently undergo malignant transition to anaplastic astrocytoma and glioblastoma multiforme (see below). In particular, the gemistocytic form of astrocytoma appears particularly prone to follow this progressive course.

GLIOBLASTOMA MULTIFORME

Glioblastoma multiforme (GBM) is generally thought to arise from cells of astrocytic lineage; however, oligodendroglial or progenitor cell derivation may also be possible (see below). These are highly malignant neoplasms that are characterized by their high mitotic rate, cellular pleomorphism, nuclear atypia, necrosis, and microvascular proliferation (endothelial hyperplasia) (Fig. 15–4). The component neoplastic cells may vary considerably in both size and shape, ranging from small, undifferentiated cells with hyperchromatic nuclei to pleomorphic astrocytes and even multinucleate giant cells.

Mitotically active endothelial cells frequently aggregate to form characteristic glomeruloid structures. Vascular endothelial growth factor (VEGF),[51,52] derived from neoplastic cells, has been demonstrated at high levels in glioblastoma tissue and may serve to drive this phenomenon. Hypoxia as a result of the blood supply failing to match the growth rate of the tumor may result in areas of frank necrosis surrounded by pseudopalisades of neoplastic cells. The cells comprising these pseudopalisades may serve to secrete the VEGF in order to attempt further angiogenesis within the tumor.

Glioblastoma multiforme frequently arises in the deep white matter of the cerebral hemispheres and may spread by diffuse cellular invasion via the corpus callosum into the contralateral hemisphere, giving rise to a characteristic butterfly pattern. The large size at clinical presentation, high growth rate, frequently resulting in midline shift, and diffuse invasion of contiguous brain tissues (Fig. 15–5) render these tumors difficult to treat and almost invariably fatal.

Biologically, two forms of GBM are thought to exist: those that arise through different stages of malignant progression from a lower grade of astrocytic tumor and those that appear de novo, in older patients. Indeed, there is now considerable information of the molecular genetic events that underlie these diverse pathways of pathogenesis (Fig. 15–6).

The expression and role of previously undetected progenitor cells in adult brain have recently attracted considerable attention from neuropathologists. The NG2 transmembrane chondroitin sulphate proteoglycan is known to be expressed by oligodendroglial progenitors in the developing and adult mammalian CNS and by oligodendrocyte/type 2 astrocyte (O-2A) progenitors in vitro. In addition, O-2A cells are characterized by expression of gangliosides recognized by the monoclonal antibodies A2B5 and GD3, as well as by platelet-derived growth factor alpha receptor (PDGF-R) and O4 antibodies. Very recently, NG2 has been reported to be expressed in cells from multiple sclerosis brains[53] and in human brain tumors.[54] Increased expression was seen in tumors with a higher grade of malignancy whereas NG2-positive and-negative subpopu-

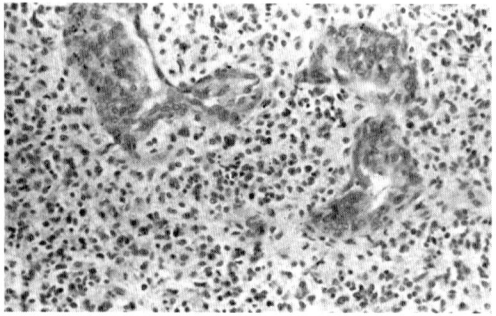

Figure 15–4. Hematoxylin and eosin–stained section of glioblastoma multiforme (GBM). Microvascular proliferation (endothelial hyperplasia) is a major histological criterion in the diagnosis of GBM.

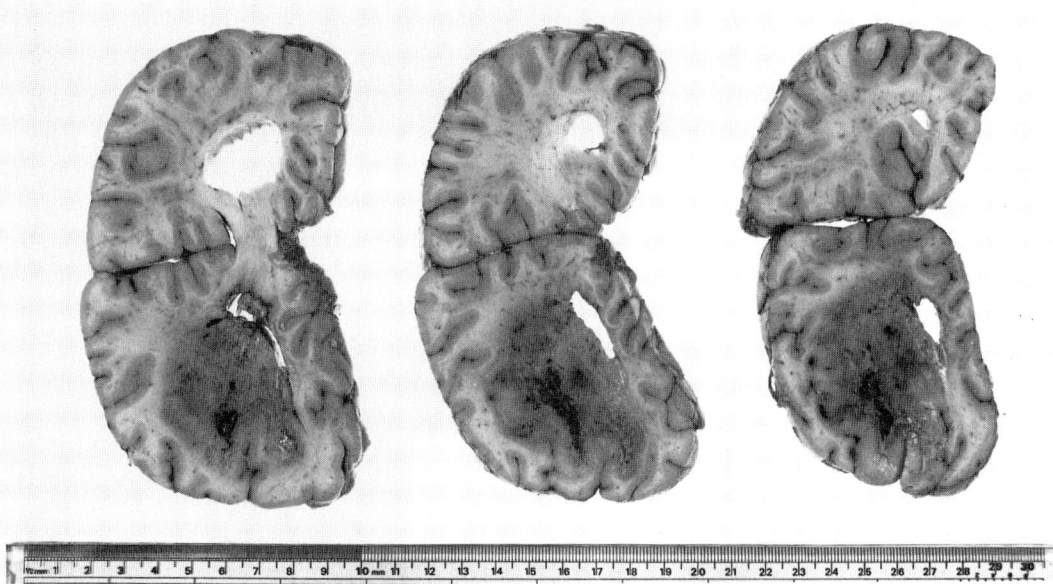

Figure 15–5. Macroscopic view of glioblastoma multiforme showing serial coronal slices of a large neoplasm of the left frontal lobe compressing the lateral ventricle, causing midline shift and invading contiguous normal brain tissue.

lations were morphologically distinct; NG2-positive cells showed higher migratory potential and NG2-positive cells showed greater proliferative potential. Subsequent work has shown that there are NG2-positive/GD3-negative and NG2-negative/GD3-positive subpopulations, the former being indicative of invasion while the latter is representative of the proliferative pool.[54] Moreover, blocking of PDGF-R sites results in ablation of NG2 expression and subsequent retirement from proliferative activity and induction of migration. This is in keeping with the "migration or proliferation" characteristics of neoplastic glia as described by Pilkington.[30] Indeed, NG2 expression occurs predominantly within the main tumor mass of growing neoplastic cells while GD3 is evidenced strongly at the brain–tumor interface,[54] where diffuse infiltration of the normal contiguous brain by migratory tumor cells occurs. The expression of such neoplastic glial progenitor cell populations in adult brain tumors may, therefore, indicate not only a stem cell origin (whereby microenvironment dictates to some extent the histological appearance of the tumor) but also the biological activity of the neoplasm. Molecular interference with this "switch-on/switch-off" mechanism for invasion/proliferation in neoplastic glia may offer some hope in the future for biological therapeutic intervention for these tumors.

Primary or de novo GBM appears clinically in older patients who have not previously presented with astrocytic brain tumors of lower grade. The most common genetic alterations in this form of GBM are epidermal growth factor receptor (EGFR) amplification and overexpression, CDKN2A deletion, and mutation in the PTEN gene, so-called since it codes for a peptide of the tyrosine phosphatase family which has extensive sequence homology to the cytoskeletal protein tensin. Moreover, murine double minute 2 (MDM2) overexpression with or without gene amplification is a genetic hallmark of de novo GBM, while TP53 mutations are typically lacking.[55]

Both amplification (40% of cases) and overexpression (60% of cases) of the EGFR are characteristic in this form of GBM. Increased EGFR has been reported to correlate with malignancy in gliomas[56,57] and patients with EGFR amplification show shorter survival times, although this appears to be irrespective of sex, treatment, histological features, and, perhaps most significantly, age.[58] Similarly, the MDM2 gene[59] is also seen to be amplified (up to 10% of cases) and more frequently over-

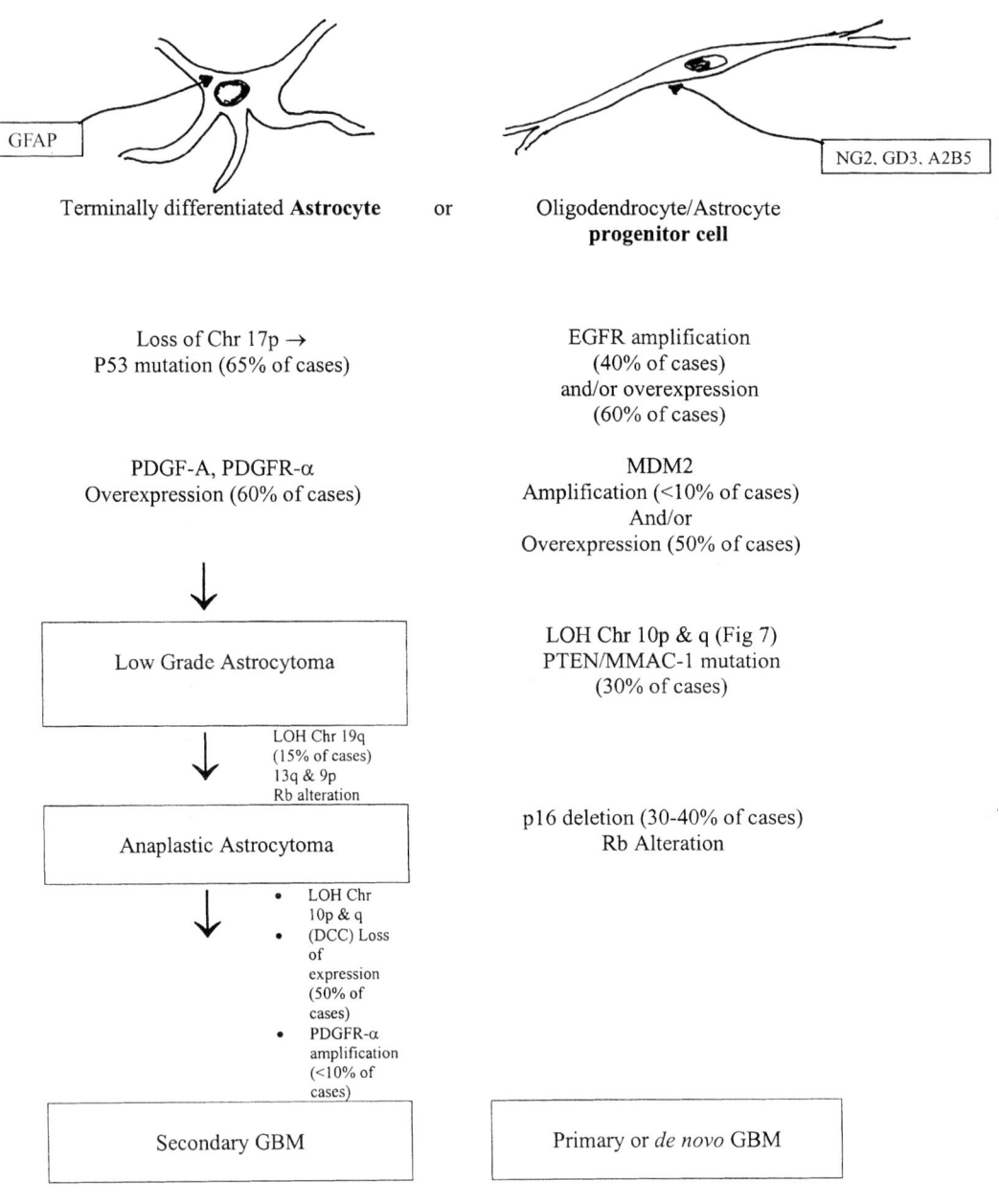

Figure 15–6. Schematic representation of possible genetic evolution of primary (de novo) and secondary glioblastoma multiforme.

expressed (50% of cases), and this probably contributes to some extent to the resistance of GBM in the elderly to chemotherapeutic approaches. The PTEN (phosphatase and tensin h0omologue)[60] or MMAC-1 (multiple mutated in advanced cancers 1)[61] tumor suppressor gene has been found by various groups to be mutated in around 30% of glioblastomas,[62,63] such mutations occurring almost exclusively (32% of cases) in de novo GBM and only rarely (4% of cases) in secondary GBM.[64] Moreover, TP53, which is seen in secondary but not primary GBM, and PTEN mutations appear to be mutually exclusive.[64]

Relatively recently, oligodendrocytic differentiation (both in overt oligodendrogliomas and within GBMs) has been shown to be linked to a favorable response to chemotherapy. This is based on allelic loss or loss of heterozygosity of chromosome 1p and combined loss involving chromosomes 1p and 19q in certain of these tumors.[65] The increased survival times following chemotherapy in patients with such genetic losses suggests that molecular genetic analysis of brain tumors may have considerable diagnostic and prognostic value in neuropathology in the future. The molecular investigation of oligodendroglial differentiation in GBM may shed light on the origins of these tumors and their response to various therapeutic regimens. Putative tumor suppressor gene loci have been identified, by cytogenetic and molecular genetic analyses, on various chromosomes, including 10, 19q, and 17p in astrocytic tumors.

MENINGIOMA

This group of tumors shows a predilection for the mid–late decades of life and there is a considerable female preponderance. They are common, generally benign, neoplasms accounting for 14% of all primary intracranial tumors. Although they are most frequently found over the convexity of the brain related to the sagittal sinus (parasagittal meningiomas) (Figs. 15–7 and 15–8), they may be seen in the Sylvian fissures, at the base of the sphenioidal ridges, olfactory grooves, and pituitary fossa, as well as within the ventricular system. Eleven subtypes are described in the WHO classification system,[38] the most common being meningothelial (or syncytial), fibrous (or fibroblastic), transitional (Fig. 15–9), and psammomatous; more than one type often occurs within the same tumor. A fifth, papillary subtype is more cellular and can be aggressive, carrying a worse prognosis. Additionally, atypical and anaplastic (malignant) meningiomas are noted. Epithelial membrane antigen (EMA) immunostaining may help to distinguish between meningiomas and Schwannomas.[66] There is little information on the contribution of molecular genetics to the evolution and pathogenesis of meningiomas. The neurofibromatosis type 2 (NF2) gene does, however, play an important role in the development of transitional, fibroblastic, and malig-

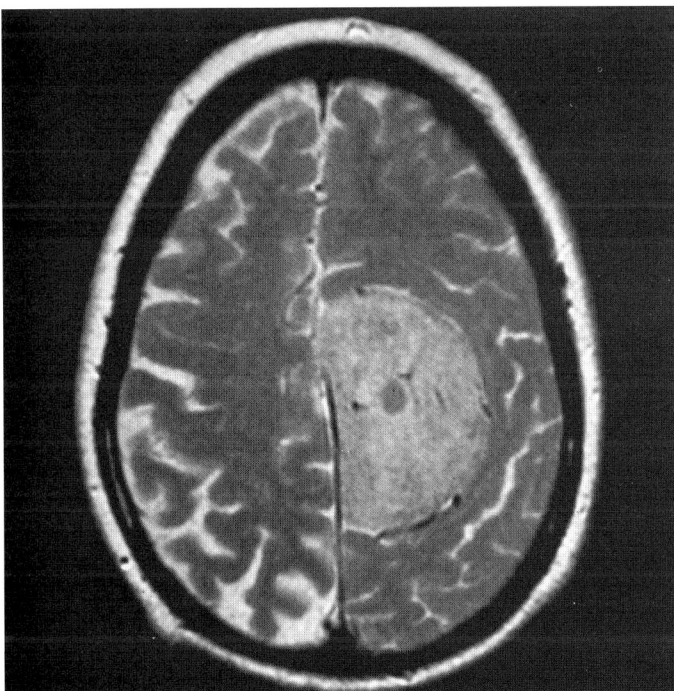

Figure 15–7. Neuroimaging of parasaggital meningioma with evidence of cystic change (center) and clear demarcation of tumor from surrounding brain tissue.

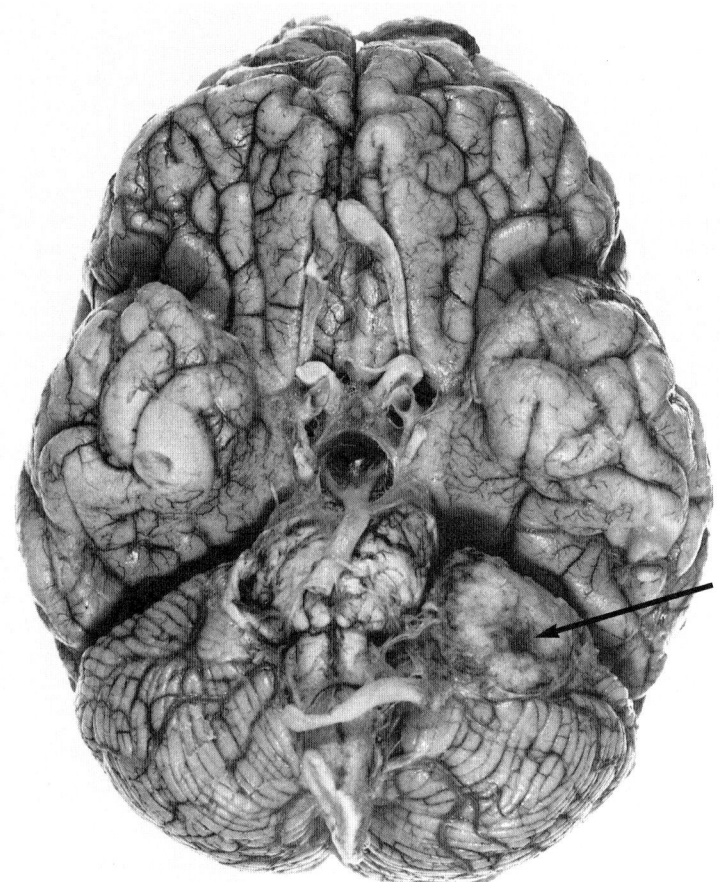

Figure 15–8. Macroscopic view of ventral area of a meningioma (arrow) in the cerebellopontine angle.

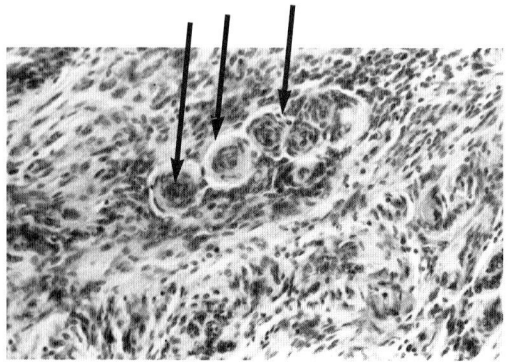

Figure 15–9. Transitional meningioma with characteristic "onion bulb" whorl formations (arrows). Hematoxylin and eosin–stained section.

nant variants of meningioma.[67] Allelic losses on chromosomes 1p, 10q, 14q, and 22 have been reported to contribute to the malignant progression of these neoplasms (Fig.15–10).[68–71] Moreover, PTEN/MMAC1 mutations, while absent from low-grade meningiomas, may contribute to malignant progression in a fraction of anaplastic meningiomas.[72]

SECONDARY CARCINOMA/ MELANOMA

Carcinomas are the most common source of secondary tumors in the brain, with bronchial

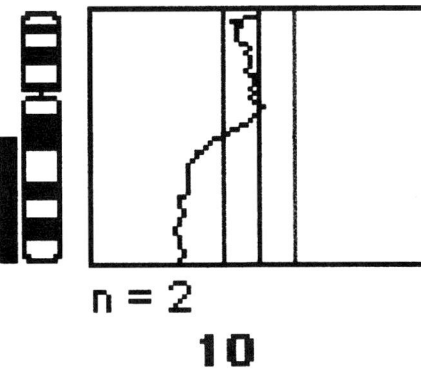

Figure 15–10. Loss of chromosome 10q demonstrated by comparative genomic hybridization (CGH).

and breast carcinomas being the most frequent primary lesions in men and women, respectively. Such secondaries are generally well circumscribed and multiple, while secondary lymphomas and leukemias are generally more diffuse and frequently involve the meninges. Carcinomas may be immuohistochemically identified by the use of cytokeratin-recognizing antibodies[73] and EMA.[74] Melanomas are negative for both cytokeratin and EMA but express vimentin, neutronspecific enolase (NSE), and S-100 protein.[75] The precise origin and nature of metastatic carcinomas may be determined by the use of chromagranin[76] and carcinoembryonic antigen (CEA).[77]

Although these tumors do not show the high degree of diffuse invasive behavior characteristic of gliomas, they are invariably multiple rather than solitary lesions, a fact that together with the likely dissemination of the disease throughout other somatic tissues, renders then particularly difficult to treat, particularly in elderly patients.

SCHWANNOMA

Schwannomas, which may occur in the cranial nerves (Fig. 15–11), spinal nerve roots, and peripheral nerves, constitute some 8% of intracranial tumors.[78] Although they generally present in the middle decades of life and show a female preponderance, they may continue a slow growth pattern or recur following surgery or radiotherapy in later life. The vestibular cranial nerves are most commonly affected whereas the trigeminal, vagus, and glossopharyngeal nerves are rarely involved. Although multiple tumors are associated with von Recklinghausen's disease, Schwannomas tend to be solitary lesions that are firm, encapsulated, and well circumscribed. They are generally benign and slow growing, carrying a good prognosis following surgical removal. Malignant change is exceptionally rare.[79] A biphasic histological pattern of so-called Antoni A and Antoni B type tissues is apparent (Fig. 15–12). The former reflects interwoven bundles of fusiform Schwann cells with elongated nuclei while the latter consists of randomly distributed pleomorphic cells within an eosinophilic matrix; microcystic and xanthomatous appearances may also be apparent. On electron microscopy the component neoplastic cells are surrounded by basal laminae and, accordingly, reticulin staining is marked at the light microscopical level. Immunohistochemical staining for Leu-7[80] and S-100 protein[81] differentiates Schwannomas from other nerve sheath neoplasms.

PRIMARY MALIGNANT LYMPHOMA

Although these neoplasms have shown a considerable rise in incidence in young, immunosupressed, HIV-infected patients[82] in recent years, their presentation in the absence of these conditions is more frequent in the fifth

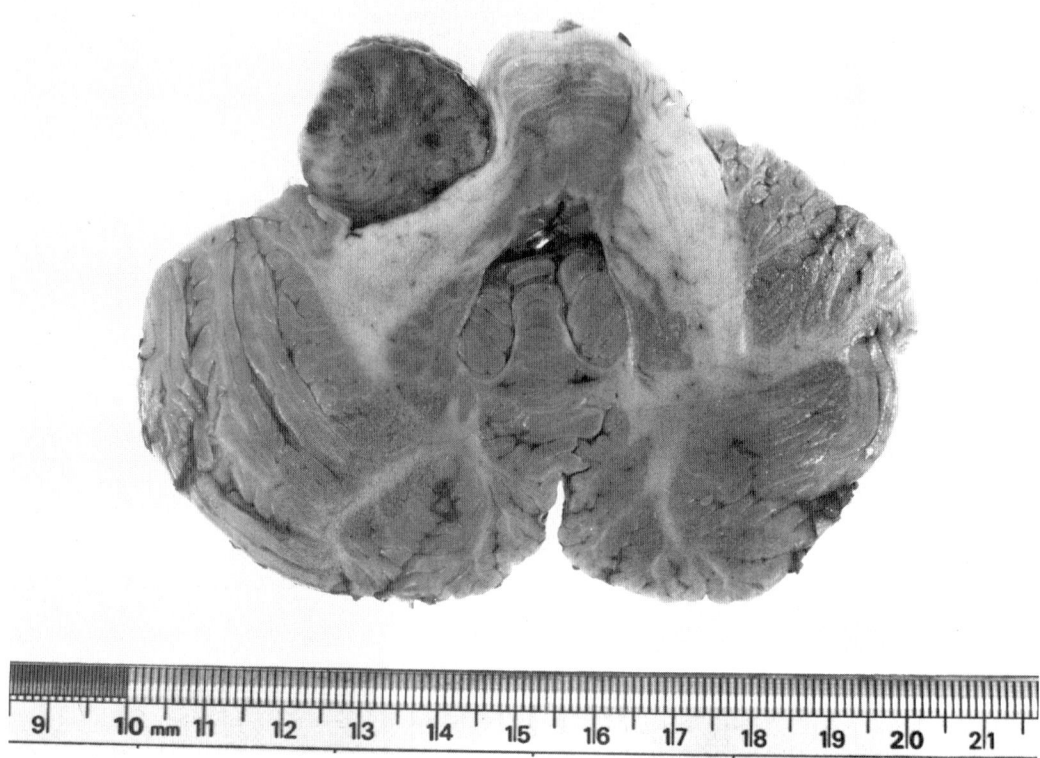

Figure 15–11. Macroscopic view of a Schwannoma of the cerebellopontine angle.

and sixth decades of life. Primary lymphomas are cellular, pleomorphic lesions that surround blood vessels and may be single, multiple, or diffuse. Initially, both perivacular space (Fig. 15–13) and vascular walls are infiltrated by neoplastic cells, with subsequent diffuse invasion of the brain substance. Perivascular neoplastic lymphocytes are surrounded by a rich reticulin (basal laminar) network, probably reflecting an abortive attempt by the pericytes and reactive astrocytes to limit spread of the tumor cells. In previous nomenclature systems these tumors were referred to as "microglioma," their reclassification resulting largely from immu-

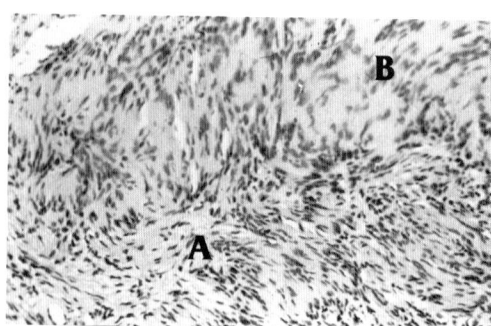

Figure 15–12. Hematoxylin and eosin–stained section of a Schwannoma demonstrating characteristic Antoni A (A) and hypocellular Antoni B (B) regions.

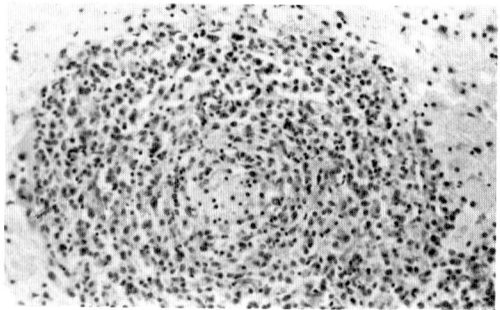

Figure 15–13. Hematoxylin and eosin–stained section of a primary malignant CNS lymphoma showing characteristic perivascular pattern of neoplastic B cells.

nohistochemical staining for B- and T-cell differentiation. Indeed, most lymphomas are B-cell derived[83] with a characteristic, reactive T-cell component in the perivascular region.[84] T-cell derived lymphomas do, however, exist and commonly present within the leptomeninges.[85]

MANAGEMENT, THERAPY, AND PALLIATIVE CARE

As far as intrinsic glial neoplasms are concerned, age is undeniably the single most important prognostic factor and younger patients live significantly longer than older patients (Table 15–5). Indeed, the input of other prognostic factors can be influenced by age to such an extent that these additional factors are invalidated.[87] The 18-month survival rate for patients under 40 years of age who suffer from malignant glioma has been cited as 64% while that for patients over the age of 60 years is only 8%.[88]

Brain tumor surgery in the elderly has a relatively poor outcome and a high rate of complication; however, careful patient selection can result in substantial benefit to patients from aggressive intervention along with customized treatment.[89] Whittle,[90] however, argues that tissue confirmation of a neuroradiological diagnosis of malignant glioma in the elderly may not be appropriate when there is a history of progressive neurological or cognitive deficits and disability. This pragmatic approach is based on the poor prognosis in elderly patients with poor functional status.[91]

While radiation has been accepted since the late 1970s as being of value in the treatment of malignant glioma, age and performance status are the two most critical factors in assessment of benefit.[92] The value of such an approach is therefore less apparent in older patients. Interstitial radiotherapy with implanted iodine[125] seeds may be indicated in elderly patients with meningioma.[93] In addition, clinical depression and anxiety may be experienced in these patients[94] and may contribute to the morbidity in the elderly suffering from advanced neural neoplasia.

I am indebted to Dr. Joe Jarosz for CT and MRI scans, Dr. Tracy Warr for the comparative genomic hybridization (CGH) preparation, and Dr. Andrew King for provision of clinical material. Mr. Alan Brady prepared the photographs. I also gratefully acknowledge the contribution of Dr. Teresa Beynon, Mr. Richard Gullan, Dr. Ron Beaney, and Dr. Philip Barnes for helpful discussions with particular reference to their own areas of expertise (palliative medicine, neurosurgery, radiotherapy, and clinical neurology, respectively).

REFERENCES

1. Miller DG. On the nature of susceptibility to cancer. The presidential address. Cancer 1980; 15:1307–1318.
2. Newell GR, Spitz MR, Sider JG. Cancer and age. Semin Oncol 1989; 16:3–9.
3. Redmond K, Aapro MS, eds. Cancer in the Elderly: A Nursing and Medical Perspective. European School of Oncology, Scientific Updates 2. New York: Elsevier 1997.
4. Surawicz TS, McCarthy BJ, Kupelian V, Jukich PJ, Bruner JM, Davis FG. Descriptive epidemiology of primary brain and CNS tumors: results from the Central Brain Tumor Registry of the United States, 1990–1994. Neuro-Oncology 1999; 1:14–25.
5. Kuratso J, Ushio Y. Epidemiological study of primary intracranial tumors in elderly people. J Neurol Neurosurg Psychiatry 1997; 63:116–118.
6. Druckrey H, Ivankovic S, Preussmann R. Teratogenic and carcinogenic effects in the offspring after single injection of ethylnitrosourea to pregnant rats. Nature 1966; 210:1378–1379.
7. Lantos PL, Pilkington GJ. The development of experimental brain tumors: a sequential light and electron microscope study of the subependymal plate. I. Early lesions (abnormal cell clusters). Acta Neuropathol (Berl) 1979; 45:167–175.
8. Pilkington GJ, Lantos PL. The development of experimental brain tumors: a sequential study of the subependymal plate. II. Microtumours. Acta Neuropathol (Berl) 1979; 45:177–185.
9. Pegg AE. Properties of the O6-alkylguanine-DNA repair system of mammalian cells. In: O'Neill IK, Von Borstel RC, Miller CT, Long J, Bartsch, eds. N-Nitroso Compounds: Occurrence, Biological Effects and Relevance to Human Cancer. IARC Sci Publ 1984; 57:575–580.
10. Blowers L, Preston-Martin S, Mack WJ. Dietary and other lifestyle factors of women with brain gliomas in Los Angeles County (California USA). Cancer Causes Control 1997; 8:5–12.
11. Preston-Martin S, Henderson BE. N-Nitroso compounds and human intracranial tumors. IARC Sci Publ 1984; 57:887–894.
12. Bunin GR, Kuitjen RR, Boesel CP, Buckley JD, Meadows AT. Maternal diet and risk of astrocytic glioma in children: a report from the Children's Cancer Group (United States and Canada). Cancer Causes Control 1994; 5:177–187.
13. Olney JW, Farber NB, Spitznagel E, Robins LN. Increasing brain tumor rates: is there a link to aspartame? J Neuropathol Exp Neurol 1996; 55:1115–1123.
14. Shephard SE, Wakabayashi K, Nagao M. Mutagenic

activity of peptides and the artificial sweetener aspartame after nitrosation. Food Chem Toxicol 1993; 31: 323–329.
15. Pepper C, Jasani B, Navabi H, Wynford-Thomas D, Gibbs AR. Simian virus 40 large T antigen (SV40LTAg) primer specific DNA amplification in human pleural mesothelioma tissue. Thorax 1996; 51: 1074–1076.
16. Martini F, Iaccheri L, Lazzarin L, Carinci P, Corallini A, Gerosa M, Iuzzolino P, Barbanti-Brodano G, Tognon M. SV40 early region and large T antigen in human brain tumors, peripheral blood cells, and sperm fluids from healthy individuals. Cancer Res 1996; 56: 4820–4825.
17. Rodvall Y, Ahlbom A, Stenlund C, Preston-Martin S, Lindh T, Spannare B. Occupational exposure to magnetic fields and brain tumors in central Sweden. Eur J Epidemoil 1998; 14:563–569.
18. Hardell L, Nasma A, Pahlson A, Hallquist A, Hansson MK. Use of cellular telephones and the risk for brain tumors: a case–control study. Int J Oncol 1999; 15: 113–116.
19. Unger M, Olsen J. Organochloride compounds in the adipose tissue of deceased people with and without cancer. Environ Res 1980; 23:257–263.
20. Davis DL, Ahlbom A, Hoel D, Percy C. Is brain cancer mortality increasing in industrial countries? Am J Ind Med 1990; 19:412–431.
21. Greig NH, Ries LG, Yancik R, Rapoport SI. Increasing annual incidence of primary malignant brain tumors in the elderly. J Natl Cancer Inst 1990; 82:1621–1624.
22. Legler JM, Gloeckler Reis LA, Smith MA, Warren JL, Heineman EF, Kaplan RS, Linet MS. Brain and other central nervous system cancers: recent trends in incidence and mortality. J Natl Cancer Inst 1999; 91: 1382–1390.
23. Hasegawa Y, Sawada M, Ozaki N, Inagaki T, Suzumura A. Increased soluble tumor necrosis factor receptors in the serum of elderly people. Gerontology 2000; 46(4):185–188.
24. Kingsley D. Imaging strategies for brain tumors. Neuropathol Appl Neurobiol 1996; 22:418–421.
25. Moseley IF. Imaging the adult brain. J Neurol Neuropathol Psychiatry 1995; 58:7–21.
26. Oot RF, New PJF, Pile-Spellman J, Rose BR, Shoukumas GM, Davies KR. The detection of intracranial calcification by MR. Am J Neuroradiol 1986; 7:801–809.
27. Osbourne AG. Diagnostic Neuroradiology. St Louis: Mosby, 1994:520.
28. Posner JB, Chernik NL. Intracranial metastases from systemic cancer. Adv Neurol 1978; 19:575–587.
29. Steck PA, Nicholson GL. Metastases to the central nervous system. In: Levine AJ, Schmidek HH, eds. Molecular Genetics of Nervous System Tumors. New York: Wiley-Liss, 1993:371–379.
30. Pilkington GJ. Tumor cell migration in the central nervous system. Brain Pathol 1994; 4:157–166.
31. Pilkington GJ. The paradox of neoplastic glial cell invasion of the brain and apparent metastatic failure. Anticancer Res 1997; 17:4103–4106.
32. Pilkington GJ. The biology, pathogenesis and spread of malignant glioma. Strahlenther Onkol 1989; 165: 235–238.
33. Bernstein JJ, Woodard CA. Glioblastoma cells do not intravasate into blood vessels. Neurosurgery 1995; 36: 124–132.
34. Martin K, Akinwunmi J, Rooprai HK, Kennedy AJ, Linke A, Ognjenovic N, Pilkington GJ. Non-expression of CD15 and selectins by neoplastic glia: a barrier to metastasis? Anticancer Res 1995; 15: 1159–1165.
35. Pilkington GJ. Glioma heterogeneity in vitro: the significance of growth factors and gangliosides. Neuropathol Appl Neurobiol 1992; 18:434–442.
36. Merzak A, Pilkington GJ. The molecular and cellular pathology of intrinsic brain tumors. Cancer Metastasis Rev 1997; 16:155–177.
37. Lantos PL, Pilkington GJ. Biological markers for tumors of the brain. In: Simon L, Calliau L, Cohadon F, Lobo J, Loew F, Nornes H, Pásztor E, Pickard JD, Strong AJ, Yasargil MG, eds. Advances and Technical Standards in Neurosurgery, Vol. 21. New York: Springer-Verlag, 1994:3–41.
38. Kleihues P, Burger PC, Scheithauer BW. The new WHO classification of brain tumors. Brain Pathol 1993; 3:255–268.
39. Kernohan JW, Habon RF, Svien HJ, Adson AW. A simplified classification of gliomas. Proc Mayo Clin 1949; 24:71–75.
40. Daumas-Duport C, Scheithauer B, O'Fallon J, Kelly P. Grading of astrocytomas. A simple and reproducible method. Cancer 1988; 62:2152–2165.
41. Eng LF, Vanderhaeghen JJ, Bignami A, Gerstl B. An acidic protein isolated from fibrous astrocytes. Brain Res 1971; 28:351–354.
42. Duffy PE, Graf L, Rapport MM. Identification of glial fibrillary acidic protein by the immunoperoxidase method in human brain tumors. J Neuropathol Exp Neurol 1977; 36:645–652.
43. Deck JHN, Eng LF, Bigbee J, Woodcock SM. The role of glial fibrillary acidic protein in the diagnosis of central nervous system tumors. Acta Neuropathol (Berl) 1978; 42:183–190.
44. Dahl D, Rueger DC, Bignami A, Weber K, Osborn M. Vimentin, the 57,000 MW protein of fibroblast filaments, is the major cytoskeletal component in immature glia. Eur J Cell Biol 1981; 24:191–196.
45. Pilkington GJ, Lantos PL. The role of glutamine synthetase in the diagnosis of cerebral tumors. Neuropathol Appl Neurobiol 1982; 8:227–236.
46. McCormick D, McQuaid S, McClusker C, Allen IV. A study of glutamine synthetase in normal brain and intracranial tumors. Neuropathol Appl Neurobiol 1990; 16:205–211.
47. Schiffer D, Cavalla P, Pilkington GJ. Proliferative properties of malignant brain tumors. In: Mikkelsen T, Bjerkvig R, Laerum O-D, Rosenblum ML, eds. Brain Tumour Invasion: Biological, Clinical and Therapeutic Considerations. New York: John Wiley & Sons, 1998:161–184.
48. Giangaspero F, Doglioni C, Rivano MT, Pileri S, Gerdes J, Stein H. Growth fraction in human brain tumors defined by the monoclonal antibody Ki-67. Acta Neuropathol (Berl) 1987; 74:179–182.
49. Hoshino T, Ahn D, Prados MD, Lamborn K, Wilson CB. Prognostic significance of the proliferative potential of intracranial gliomas measured by bromodeoxyuridine labelling. Int J Cancer 1993; 53:550–555.
50. Sarawar SR, Bonshek RE, Marsden HB, Yates PO, Kumar S. A monoclonal antibody which discriminates

between sub-types of astrocytoma. Anticancer Res 1991; 11:1429–1432.
51. Plate KH, Breier G, Weich HA, Risau W. Vascular endothelial growth factor is a potential tumour angiogenesis factor in human gliomas in vivo. Nature 1992; 359:845–848.
52. Plate KH, Breier G, Weich HA, Mennel HD, Risau W. Vascular endothelial growth factor and glioma angiogenesis: coordinate induction of VEGF receptors, distribution of VEGF protein and possible in vivo regulatory mechanisms. Int J Cancer 1994; 59:520–529.
53. Scolding N, Franklin R, Stevens S, Heldin CH, Compston A, Newcombe J. Oligodendrocyte progenitors are present in the normal adult human CNS and in lesions of multiple sclerosis. Brain 1998; 121:2221–2228.
54. Chekenya M, Rooprai HK, Davies D, Butt AM, Pilkington GJ. NG2, a proteoglycan marker for O-2A adult progenitor phenotype: expression and role in human gliomas. Int J Dev Neurosci 1999; 17:421–435.
55. Kleihues P, Ohgaki H. Primary and secondary glioblastomas: from concept to clinical diagnosis. Neuro-Oncology 1999; 1:44–51.
56. Schmidek HH. The molecular genetics of nervous system tumors. J Neurosurg 1987; 67:1–16.
57. Torp SH, Helseth E, Dalen A, Unsgaard G. Epidermal growth factor receptor expression in human gliomas. Cancer Immunol Immunother 1991; 33:61–64.
58. Hurtt MR, Moossy J, Donovn-Peluso M, Locker J. Amplification of epidermal growth factor receptor gene in gliomas: histopathology and prognosis. J Neuropathol Exp Neurol 1992; 51:84–90.
59. Reifenberger G, Reifenberger J, Ichimura K, Meltzer PS, Collins VP. Amplification of multiple genes from chromosomal region 12q13–14 in human malignant gliomas: preliminary mapping of the amplicons shows preferential involvement of CDK4, SAS and MDM2. Cancer Res 1994; 54:4299–4303.
60. Li J, Yen C, Liaw D, Podsypanina K, Bose S, Wang SI, Puc J, Miliaresis C, Rodgers L, McCombie R, Bigner SH, Giovanella BC, Ittmann M, Tycko B, Hibshoosh H, Wigler MH, Parsons R. PTEN, a putative protein tyrosine phosphatase gene mutated in human brain, breast and prostate cancer. Science 1997; 275:1943–1947.
61. Steck PA, Jesser SA, Yung WK, Lin H, Ligon AH, Langford LA, Baumgard ML, Hattier T, Davis T, Frye C, Hu R, Swedlund B, Teng DHF, Tavtigian SV. Identification of a candidate tumour suppressor gene, MMAC1, at chromosome 10q23.3 that is mutated in multiple advanced cancers. Nat Genet 1997; 15:356–362.
62. Bostrom J, Cobbers JMJL, Wolter M, Tabatabai G, Weber RG, Lichter, P, Collins VP, Reifenberger G. Mutation of the PTEN (MMAC1) tumor suppressor gene in a subset of glioblastomas but not in meningiomas with loss of chromosome arm 10q[1]. Cancer Res 1998; 58:29–33.
63. Duerr E-M, Rollbrocker B, Hayashi Y, Peters N, Meyer-Puttlitz B, Louis DN, Schramm J, Wiestler OD, Parson R, Eng C, von Deimling A. PTEN mutations in gliomas and glioneuronal tumors. Oncogene 1998; 16:2259–2264.
64. Tohma Y, Gratas C, Biernat W, Peraud A, Fukuda M, Yonekawa Y, Kleihues P, Ohgaki H. PTEN (MMAC1) mutations are frequent in primary glioblastomas (de novo) but not in secondary glioblastomas. J Neuropathol Exp Neurol 1998; 57:684–689.
65. Cairncross JG, Ueki K, Zlatescu MC, Lisle DK, Finkelstein DM, Hammond RR, Silver JS, Stark PC, MacDonald DR, Ino Y, Ramsay DA, Louis DN. Specific genetic predictors of chemotherapeutic response and survival in patients with anaplastic oligodendrogliomas. J Natl Cancer Inst 1998; 90:1473–1479.
66. Perentes E, Rubinstein LJ. Recent application of immunoperoxidase histochemistry in human neuro-oncology. Acta Pathol Lab Med 1987; 111:796–812.
67. Wellenreuther R, Kraus J, Lenartz D, Menon AG, Schramm J, Louis DN, Ramesh V, Gusella JF, Wiestler OD, von Deimling A. Analysis of the neurofibromatosis 2 gene reveals molecular variants of meningioma. Am J Pathol 1995; 146:827–832.
68. Lindblom A, Ruttledge M, Collins VP, Nordensjoeld M, Dumanski JP. Chromosomal deletions in anaplastic meningiomas suggest multiple regions outside chromosome 22 as important in tumour progression. Int J Cancer 1994; 56:354–357.
69. Menon AG, Rutter JL, von Sattel JP, et al. Frequent loss of chromosome 14 in atypical and malignant meningioma: identification of a putative tumour progression locus. Oncogene 1997; 14:611–616.
70. Rempel SA, Schwechheimer K, Davis RL, Cavenee WK, Rosenblum ML. Loss of heterozygosity for loci on chromosome 10 is associated with morphologically malignant meningioma progression. Cancer Res 1993; 53:2386–2392.
71. Simon M, von Deimling A, Larson JJ, Wellenreuther, Kaskel P, Waha A, Warmick RE, Tow JM Jr, Menon AG. Allelic losses on chromosomes 14, 10 and 22 in atypical and malignant meningiomas: a genetic model of meningioma progression. Cancer Res 1995; 55:4696–4701.
72. Peters N, Wellenreuther R, Rollbrocker B, Hayashi Y, Meyer-Puttlitz B, Duerr E-M, Lenartz D, Marsh DJ, Schramm J, Weistler OD, Parsons R, Eng C, von Deimling A. Analysis of the PTEN gene in human meningiomas. Neuropathol Appl Neurobiol 1998; 24:3–8.
73. Ramaekers FCS, Puts JJG, Moesker O, Kant A, Huysmans A, Haag D, Jap PHK, Herman CJ, Vooijs GP. Antibodies to intermediate filament proteins in the immunohistochemical identification of human tumors: an overview. Histochem J 1983; 15:691–713.
74. Pinkus G, Etheridge CL, O'Connor EM. Are keratin proteins a better tumor marker than epithelial membrane antigen? A comparative immunohistochemical study of various paraffin-embedded neoplasms using monoclonal and polyclonal antibodies. Am J Clin Pathol 1986; 85:269–277.
75. Loffel SC, Gillespie Y, Mirmiran SA, Miller EW, Golden P, Askin FP, Siegel GP. Cellular immunolocalization of S-100 protein within fixed tissue sections by monoclonal antibodies. Arch Pathol Med 1985; 109:117–122.
76. Heitz PU. Neuroendocrine tumor markers. In: Seifert G, ed. Morphological Tumor Markers. Curr Top Pathol 1987; 77:279–306.
77. Wachter R, Wittekind C, Von Kleist S. Localization of CEA, β-HCG, SP1 and keratin in the tissue of lung

carcinomas. An immunohistochemical study. Virchows Arch 1984; 402:415–420.
78. Casadei GP, Komori T, Scheithauer BW, Miller GM, Parisi JE, Kelly PJ. Intracranial parenchymal schwannoma. A clinicopathological an neuroimaging study of nine cases. J Neurosurg 1993; 79:217–222.
79. Woodruff JM, Selig AM, Crowley K, Allen PW. Schwannoma (neurilemoma) with malignant transformation. A rare, distinctive peripheral nerve tumor Am J Surg Pathol 1994; 18:882–895.
80. Perentes E, Rubinstein LJ. Immunohistochemical recognition of human nerve sheath tumors by anti-Leu 7 (HNK-1) monoclonal antibody. Acta Neuropathol (Berl) 1985; 68:319–324.
81. Johnson HD, Glick AD, Davis BW. Immunohistochemical evaluation of Leu-7, myelin basic protein, S100 protein, glial fibrillary acidic protein and LN3 immunoreactivity in nerve sheath tumors and sarcomas. Arch Pathol Lab Med 1988; 112:155–160.
82. Morgello S, Petito CK, Mouradian JA. Central nervous system lymphoma in the acquired immunodeficiency syndrome. Clin Neuropathol 1990; 9:205–215.
83. Kumanishi T, Washiyama K, Saito T, Nishiyama A, Abe S, Tanaka T. Primary malignant lymphoma of the brain: an immunohistochemical study of eight cases using a panel of monoclonal and heterologous antibodies. Acta Neuropathol (Berl) 1986; 71:190–196.
84. Murphy JK, O'Brien CJ, Ironside JW. Morphologic and immunophenotypic characterization of primary brain lymphomas using paraffin-embedded tissue. Histopathology 1989; 15:449–460.
85. Grove A, Vyberg M. Primary leptomeningeal T-cell lymphoma: a case and a review of primary T-cell lymphoma of the central nervous system. Clin Neuropathol 1993; 12:7–12.
86. Salcman M. Epidemiology and factors affecting survival. In: Apuzzo MLJ, ed. Malignant Cerebral Glioma. Neurosurgical Topics. Park Ridge: American Association of Neurological Surgeons, 1990:95–109.
87. Walker MD, Green SB, Byar DP, et al Randomized comparisons of radiotherapy and nitrosoureas for the treatment of malignant glioma after surgery. N Engl J Med 1980; 303:1323–1329.
88. Chang CH, Horton J, Schoenfeld D, et al. Comparison of postoperative radiotherapy and combined postoperative radiotherapy and chemotherapy in the multidisciplinary management of malignant gliomas. A Joint Radiation Therapy Oncology and Eastern Cooperative Oncology Group study. Cancer 1983; 52: 997–1007.
89. Bernstein M. Brain tumor surgery in the elderly: a brief reappraisal. Can J Surg 1996; 39:147–150.
90. Whittle IR. Management of primary malignant brain tumors. J Neurol Neurosurg Psychiatry 1996; 60:2–5.
91. Fine HA. The basis for current treatment recommendations for malignant gliomas. J Neurooncol 1994; 20: 111–120.
92. Rampling R. Modern aspects of radiation therapy for glial tumors of the brain. Forum Reports (Genova) 1998; 8:289–301.
93. Vuorinen V, Heikkonen J, Brander A, Setala K, Sane T, Randell T, Paetau A, Pohjola J, Mantyla M, Jaaskelainen J. Interstitial radiotherapy of 25 parasellar/clival meningiomas and 19 meningiomas in the elderly. Analysis of short-term tolerance and responses. Acta Neurochir (Wien) 1996; 138:495–508.
94. Kaplan CP, Miner ME. Anxiety and depression in elderly patients receiving treatment for cerebral tumors. Brain Injury 1997; 11:129–135.
95. Ries LAG, Kosary CL, Hankey BF, Miller BA, Edwards BK. SEER Cancer Statistics Review, 1973–1995. Bethesda, MD: National Cancer Institute, 1998.

16. Neurometabolic Disorders and the Aging Human Nervous System

HANS H. GOEBEL

Neurometabolic disorders belong to the category of neurodegenerative disorders, but their biochemistry, especially that caused by enzymatic defects, has been only partially elucidated. They share with neurodegenerative diseases the features of progression and often fatal outcome. They differ from certain neurodegenerative diseases, however, in their systemic nature, i.e., involvement of noncerebral tissues and organs besides the brain, and in age of onset. When hereditary, neurometabolic disorders represent inborn errors of metabolism, with the temporal peak occurring during childhood, often even in infancy. When acquired, they usually show involvement of the brain, but an extracerebral origin of the disease may lie at the root of the process, e.g., in uremic and hepatic encephalopathies, endocrinopathies, and paraneoplastic syndromes. While certain neurodegenerative diseases of the brain occur during childhood, others may be seen only in adulthood or during aging. The groups of neurodegenerative diseases developing in these two different periods of life belong to entirely different categories, as there is no Alzheimer disease of infancy and no recorded senile neuroaxonal dystrophy. Moreover, at this stage in our knowledge of neurodegenerative diseases, the diseases of advanced adulthood and old age are purely cerebral conditions, whereas childhood neurodegenerative diseases, e.g., neuroaxonal dystrophies, Lafora disease, and giant axonal neuropathy, show both intracerebral and extracerebral morphological manifestations.

Several neurometabolic disorders in children are biochemically and morphologically characterized as disorders of single organelles or multi-organs, such as those involving abnormalities in the lysosomes, peroxisomes, and mitochondria in the respective familial neurometabolic disorders—the lysosomal disorders, peroxisomal diseases, and mitochondriopathies. The terminal axon in infantile neuroaxonal dystrophy, aggregation of intermediate filaments in giant axonal neuropathy, and fibrillar cytoplasmic glycogen in polyglucosan disorders, the latter being genetically and biochemically still incompletely understood, mark these neurodegenerative diseases of children.

Hereditary and neurometabolic disorders of adulthood and aging fall into two separate categories: those commencing early and running a very protracted course in adulthood and those displaying a late clinical onset. We have yet to learn the extent to which these adult forms of inborn errors of metabolism show genetic peculiarities and characteristics that distinguish them from genetic abnormalities in childhood types. With increasing longevity of the population, the number of patients affected by neurometabolic disorders of long duration and late clinical onset is expected to increase. Although recognition of the disease and correct diagnosis may be achieved in individuals before old age sets in, the complete disease pathology, especially that of the central nervous system (CNS), may only become known during the end stage of the patient's neurometabolic disease through postmortem studies, after the patient has died from the respective neurometabolic disease or from causes independent of it.

HEREDITARY DISORDERS

Metabolic Leukodystrophies

Leukodystrophies generally fall into two categories: those affecting the lipid components of the myelin sheath and those affecting proteins of the myelin sheath. Some are genetically and thus nosologically well defined including the lysosomal metachromatic and globoid cell leukodystrophies and peroxisomal adrenoleukodystrophy/adrenomyeloneuropathy, and the forms of proteolipid protein (PLP) deficiencies.[1] The hereditary protein deficiencies occur in childhood, and the lysosomal and peroxisomal lipid–related leukodystrophies occur in both children and adults, the latter also affecting the myelin of the peripheral nervous system.

Metachromatic leukodystrophy

This progressive demyelinating disorder is caused by mutations in the gene coding for arylsulphatase A. Demyelination, which spares the subcortical or U fibers during early phases of the disease, is of a diffuse type and mainly affects the centrum ovale. Active demyelination at the border between demyelinated and normally myelinated areas is marked by rather large macrophages that can contain lysosomal metachromatic material, i.e., sulphatides, the noncatabolized substrate of the deficient arylsulphatase A. Metachromasia, which means "change in color," is imparted to these macrophages when the acid crystal-violet stain is used on fixed but unembedded frozen tissues, resulting in a change in color from violet to a brownish hue. Electron microscopically, the sulphatide-replete lysosomes form in oligodendrocytes and, after their destruction and associated breakdown of myelin sheaths, they accrue in the respective macrophages. Ultrastructurally, the intralysosomal accrued sulfatides show a similar pattern in early- and late-onset metachromatic leukodystrophy (MLD), with prismatic, tuff-stone, and herring-bone formations (Fig. 16–1). Myelinated regions outside of the centrum ovale are also affected, but to a lesser extent. However, lysosomal storage is more prominent when demyelination is incomplete.

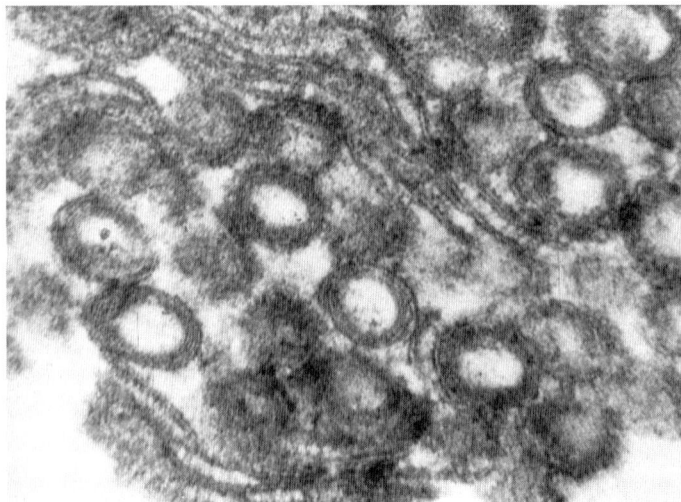

Figure 16–1. Metachromatic leukodystrophy, with tuff-stone profiles of sulphatides. ×307,400.

Arylsulphatase A is the enzyme deficient in metachromatic leukodystrophy. The milder form of adult MLD is associated with residual activity of arylsulphatase A and a small immunohistochemical amount of the respective enzyme protein. Its gene, which is located on the long arm of chromosome 22, appears in a number of variations, including those responsible for the infantile type, ARA[1]. One ARA gene showing a point mutation Pro to Leu, found in patients with adult MLD, is called "ARA[A] gene," which is homozygously mutated in adult patients.

Of the few patients afflicted with late-onset adult MLD,[2,3] one was identified as having compound heterozygous point mutations and its C2381T allelic component has been found to be present in some 50% of adult MLD alleles.[4] This same compound heterzygosity had been determined retrospectively[5] in archival material reported earlier.[6,7] Genotype–phenotype correlations in MLD, including an explanation for late-onset adult forms, are incompletely defined.[4]

Globoid Cell Leukodystrophy

Although this lysosomal disorder, marked by a deficiency of galactosyl ceramidase, is a classical childhood demyelinating disorder of infantile or late-infantile onset, called Krabbe disease, older adult–onset forms have recently been described.[8,9] The gene for galactosyl-ceramidase has been mapped to human chromosome 14. The globoid cell is a macrophage harboring the unmetabolized substrate of galactosyl ceramidase, galactoceramide, in its lysosomal compartment. This arrangement gives oligodendrocytes and Schwann cells of the peripheral nervous system a needle-like appearance at the ultrastructural level; a slightly different ultrastructure may appear in late-onset forms.[10] While secretory eccrine sweat gland epithelial cells show needle-like lysosomal inclusions similar to those seen in Schwann cells in childhood forms of globoid cell leukodystrophy, it is not known whether such diagnostic features are also present within secretory eccrine sweat gland epithelial cells in late-onset forms.

Adrenoleukodystrophy (Adrenomyeloneuropathy)

Adrenoleukodystrophy (ALD),[11,12] also called the "adrenotesticulo-leuko-myeloneuropathic complex" and "adrenomyeloneuropathy" (AMN), is the longest known member of the growing group of rare diseases, the peroxisomal disorders.[13] This disease shows a mutated gene for an ATP-binding transporter protein (ALDP), which is a transporter protein for very long–chain fatty acids and in vivo is located in mature oligodendrocytes of the corpus callosum, internal capsule, and commissura anterior, in endothelial cells, and in microglia.[14] It contains 745 amino acids and has been localized to the peroxisomal membrane. It is coded by a 20 kb Xq28-located gene of 10 exons. Mutations in this gene are now considered the cause of ALD and AMN. Immunohistochemically, the ALDP is absent in some 70% of studied tissues.[15] Long duration of ALD as a marker of nosological severity is not related to presence or absence of ALDP.

Adrenoleukodystrophy occurs more often in children and only rarely in adults; occurrence in adults has been termed "adult cerebral ALD."[13] Adrenomyeloneuropathy shows diffuse demyelination of the centrum ovale (Fig. 16–2). The adult variant has the same distributional patterns as childhood ALD, with a rather long duration into senescence,[16] and may appear as either a purely neuropathic, an AMN-pure, or mixed (AMN-cerebral) demyelinating disorder of the central and peripheral nervous systems.[13] While cerebral white matter has been found to be little affected in AMN, the cerebellar white matter has shown more profound pathology.[13] Although some 20% of females are heterozygous for ALD and may develop clinical symptoms, though of a milder form, usually the AMN form, they may live to an older age than that of ALD- or AMN-affected male patients. As in the lysosomal leukodystrophies, the breakdown products of demyelination are stored in large macrophages that cluster around white matter vessels (Fig. 16–3) but are nonmetachromatic. The inclusions contain needle-like structures (Fig. 16–4) that resemble those of glo-

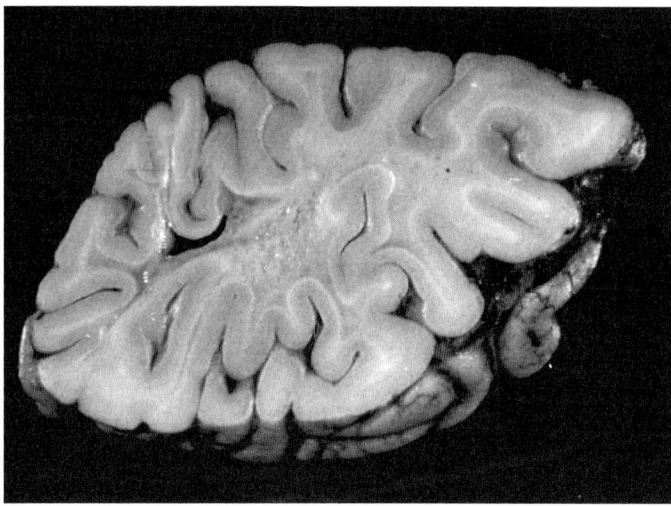

Figure 16–2. Demyelination of the centrum semi-ovale in adrenomyeloneuropathy [courtesy of Dr. J. Bohl, Johannes Gutenberg University Medical Center, Mainz, Germany.]

boid cell leukodystrophy. They occur in oligodendrocytes, Schwann cells, and macrophages, as well as in adrenoepithelial and testicular cells. A peculiar feature not seen in other metabolic leukodystrophies is the sometimes considerable infiltration and perivascular cuffing of the white matter by inflammatory lymphocytes, (T cells); this is considered an immunological reaction to the demyelinating process. This perivascular lymphocytic inflammation has been thought to occur subsequent to an earlier dysmyelinated process in both ALD and AMN. Thus, the myelin pathology in these two related conditions appears in a two-stage process.[13]

Sphingolipidoses

Just as many other lysosomal diseases are defined as hereditary lysosomal enzyme deficiencies with intralysosomal accumulation of respective lysosomal enzyme-related substrates, adult forms are often marked by residual activity of the respectively deficient lysosomal enzyme. This deficiency causes the cell to accumulate intracellular lysosomal residual bodies for a longer period than seen in earlier forms with often completely deficient activity of the respective lysosomal enzyme. As more mutations in genes coding for proteins of lysosomal enzymes become known, it remains

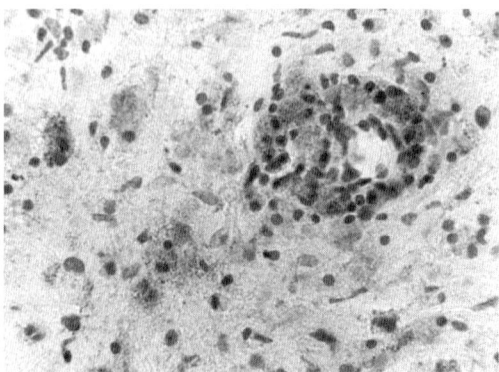

Figure 16–3. Adrenomyeloneuropathy marked by perivascular assembly of lipid-laden macrophages and round lymphocytes. Sudan red, ×740.

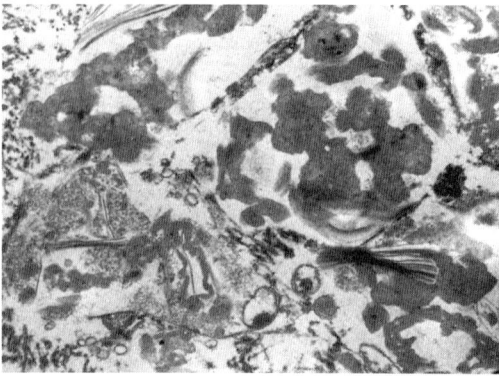

Figure 16–4. Adrenoleukodystrophy in which a macrophage contains numerous needle-like inclusions. ×36,400.

to be seen to what extent certain mutations may be responsible for residual enzyme activities in respective lysosomal disorders of long duration or late onset. The overall scarcity of adult forms among lysosomal disorders may delay such genotype–phenotype correlations. Aside from the lysosomal leukodystrophies mentioned above, other types of adult lysosomal diseases are certain sphingolipidoses, such as the gangliosidoses and Fabry disease, some mucopolysaccharidoses and oligosaccharidoses, Niemann Pick disease type C and aspartylglucosaminuria, and the adult form of neuronal ceroid lipofuscinosis, or Kufs' disease.

Among the GM1 gangliosidoses, a chronic, adult form (type III), in addition to the infantile (type I) and juvenile (type II) forms, has been reported,[17] especially in Japan.[18] This adult form is due to β-galactosidase deficiency and marked by intralysosomal accumulation of GM1 ganglioside in neuronal cells, which on electron microscopy appears as membraneous cytoplasmic bodies (Fig. 16–5) and similar lamellar inclusions. Neuronal storage, which includes the formation of meganeurites, appears prominent subcortically, especially in the basal ganglia. β-galactosidase activity is severely decreased but residual activity is present, apparently owing to a point mutation I-51-T in the β-galactosidase gene.[19,20] The missense or point mutations seen in type III GM1 gangliosidosis have not been found in patients or families afflicted with GM1 gangliosidosis of earlier onset.

The late-onset, chronic forms of GM2 gangliosidosis fall into the categories of hexosaminidase A deficiency (Tay-Sachs type) or hexosaminidases A and B deficiencies (Sandhoff type), this can only be distinguished by respective biochemical studies. Subcortical involvement manifests itself when spinocerebellar or motor neuron dysfunctions show intraneuronal storage of GM2 gangliosides as membraneous cytoplasmic bodies both in the perikaryon and the proximal meganeurite. In patients with the chronic, adult forms of GM2 gangliosidosis[21–25] of either the Tay-Sachs and Sandhoff types, certain mutations have been observed that differ from those seen in earlier forms.[26]

Fabry disease, which is due to α-galactosidase A deficiency, is mainly a vascular dis-

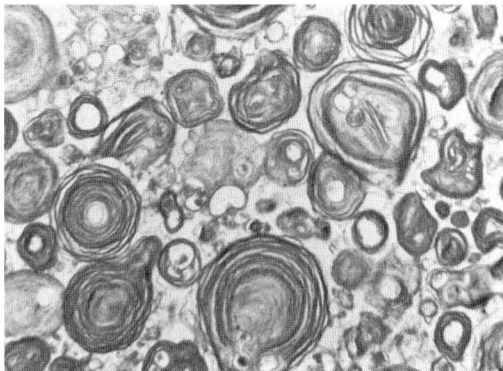

Figure 16–5. GM1 gangliosidosis, showing numerous membranous cytoplasmic bodies are within a neuronal perikaryon. ×40,000.

ease with conspicuous accumulation of lysosomal lamellar bodies in mural small vessel cells throughout the body, including in the visceral and neural organs, resulting in telangiectatic vessels and considerable narrowing of the vascular lumen. Because Fabry disease is an X-linked disorder of not only hemizygous males but also heterozygous females, regardless of whether they are clinically manifesting carriers or not, it may show the same pathology and ultrastructure of the intralysosomally accreted glycosphingolipids. In addition to mural vascular cells, neurons of both the central and peripheral nervous systems may accumulate large lamellar lysosomes.[27] Patients with a mild form and thus a long duration, and those with late onset of the disorder or who remain asymptomatic show largely cardiac rather than neurological involvement. Unlike severely affected hemizygous male patients, those with milder symptoms also have residual lysosomal activity of α-galactosidase and their mutations of the α-galactosidase gene are different from those in patients who have the severe form. Mild involvement may mean absense of clinical symptoms, thus discovery of the disease may occur only postmortem.[28,29]

Neuronal Ceroid-Lipofuscinosis

Recent genetic data have confirmed earlier conclusions based on morphological features of lysosomal lipopigment formation that the

Table 16–1. Nosology of Neuronal Ceroid Lipofuscinoses

Gene Type	Gene Locus	Gene Product
CLN1 (Childhood)	1p32	Lysosomal palmitoyl protein thioesterase
CLN2 (Late infantile)	11p15	Lysosomal pepstatin-insensitive peptidase/tripeptidyl peptidase I
CLN3 (Juvenile)	16p12	Lysosomal transmembrane CLN3 protein
CLN4 (Adult)	Not known	Not known
CLN5 (Late infantile variant)	13q31-32	Transmembrane CLN5 protein
CLN6 (Early juvenile variant)	15q21–23	Not known
CLN7 (Early juvenile variant)	Not known	Not known
CLN8 (Northern epilepsy)	8p23	Transmembrane CLN8 protein

neuronal ceroid-lipofuscinoses (NCL) are true lysosomal disorders.[30] The NCL are a large group of genetically diverse conditions that prevail nosologically during childhood but that also show a separate late-onset, adult type called "Kufs' disease." For the individual clinical types of NCL, genes have been located on at least six different chromosomes (Table 16–1). The gene mutated in infantile NCL codes for a lysosomal enzyme, palmitoyl protein thioesterase (PPT), and the gene mutated in late-infantile NCL, CLN2, codes for lysosomal pepstatin-resistant peptidase. The genes mutated in juvenile NCL, CLN3, and the Finnish late-infantile variant, CLN5, are thought to code for transmembraneous proteins of lysosomal membranes, proteins previously undescribed and of unknown functions.

Within the catalogue of gene-related forms of NCL, adult NCL is currently numbered CLN4; a lack of familial disease has prevented the gene from being assigned to any human chromosome. Autosomal dominant and autosomal recessive as well as a large number of sporadic cases of adult NCL suggest nosological heterogeneity rather than a single nosological entity. Nonetheless, only CLN4, a preliminary genetic form among the various types of CLN 1–8, can currently be considered for adult NCL.

Certain neurodegenerative diseases that appear in late adulthood and in the elderly have been considered model diseases of aging, among them Alzheimer's disease, (AD), Parkinson's disease (PD), amyotrophic lateral sclerosis (ALS), and NCL.[31] The first three disorders which may not represent single entities but a group of nosologically and genetically diverse conditions, are marked by features that generally encompass loss of nerve cells, although the distribution of nerve cell loss varies among the three neurodegenerative diseases, and the formation of intracellular inclusions, i.e., neurofibrillary tangles in AD, Lewy bodies in PD (and generalized Lewy body disease), and intraneuronal inclusions in ALS. In addition, AD and aging are marked by the formation of extracellular amyloid-containing plaques. Unlike these three disorders, the NCL are biochemically defined as lysosomal disorders, even if adult NCL has not been shown to express abnormal lysosomal biochemistry. In this respect, adult NCL still conforms to the earlier categorization as a lysosomal disease, based on the formation of lysosomal lipopigments. Thus, like aging and the three neurodegenerative disorders adult NCL, as well as the other forms of NCL, is characterized by a loss of nerve cells and the additional accumulation of intracellular material—

in adult NCL, of lysosomal lipopigments. Therefore, adult NCL may also be considered a model disease of aging, as lipofuscin is the typical pigment in aging neurons.

Clinical and possible nosological heterogeneity of adult NCL is corroborated by the wide spectrum of onset of clinical symptoms during adulthood. Recently, even a pre-senile type of adult NCL has been described.[32]

Adult NCL[33] is a progressive disorder that is morphologically marked by the accumulation of lipopigments within cerebral and extracerebral neurons as well as non-neuronal cells. In this respect, this accumulation parallels the widespread distribution of lipopigments in other non-adult forms of NCL. Lipopigments accruing within the lysosomal compartment are autofluorescent, PAS positive, stain with Luxol fast blue, and stain like neutral lipids. Their ultrastructure shows fingerprint profiles (Fig. 16–6), curvilinear profiles, and granular material in varying association. Precise topographic and ultrastructural descriptions of the lipopigments inside and outside of the brain in adult NCL have not yet been reported, and the biochemical analysis of lipopigments in adult NCL, non-adult NCL, and other disorders of aging that involve lipopigment accrual remains incomplete. Immunohistochemical studies (Fig. 16–7) in which antibodies were used against subunit C of mitochondrial ATP synthase (SCMAS) and, to a lesser degree, sphingolipid activator proteins (SAPs) have shown the presence of these proteins among lipopigments of adult NCL.

As in other neuronal lysosomal disorders,

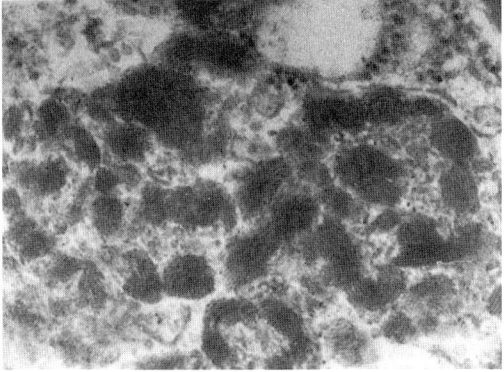

Figure 16–6. Adult neuronal ceroid lipofuscinosis showing fingerprint profiles within a cerebral neuron. ×187,880.

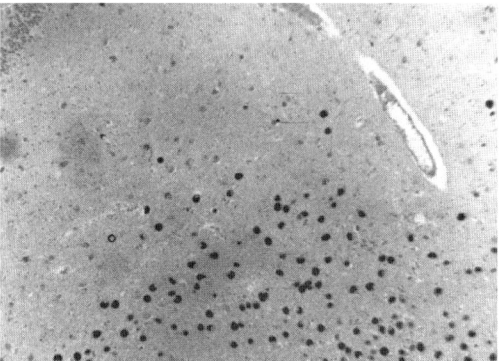

Figure 16–7. Adult neuronal ceroid lipofuscinosis. Hippocampal neurons are loaded with subunit C of mitochondrial ATP synthase. ×104.

the lipopigments accrue most in the neuronal perikaryon, which may become ballooned over time. In addition, proximal axonal segments may be incorporated into the formative process of lipopigments, resulting in conspicuous axon spindles or meganeurites. This ballooning and formation of axon spindles may serve as differential diagnostic criteria for distinguishing between true adult NCL and disorders marked by nonspecific accumulation of lipofuscin, as adult NCL may be both over- and under-diagnosed[34] morphologically and clinically.

In adult NCL and other forms of NCL, lipopigments also accrue in non-neuronal cells, extracerebrally in viscera, in the striated muscle fibers, and in dermal eccrine sweat glands and vessel walls. Thus, adult NCL may be diagnosed through biopsy, the results of which can confirm clinical and radiological data; skin and skeletal muscle are most suitable for biopsy. Contrary to findings in non-adult NCL, circulating lymphocytes have not yet been shown to contain disease-specific lipopigments in adult NCL.

The second hallmark of the NCL, loss of nerve cells, is less obvious in adult NCL, although it certainly occurs. Cortical atrophy and reduction in brain weight may be inconspicuous (Fig. 16–8). On pigmentoarchitectonic analysis,[35] it appears that the loss of nerve cells in the cerebral cortex is more subtle than in childhood forms of NCL but it follows the same pattern in that small pigmented nerve cells of layer II disappear early, as do pyramidal cells of layer V. On 100 μm–thick

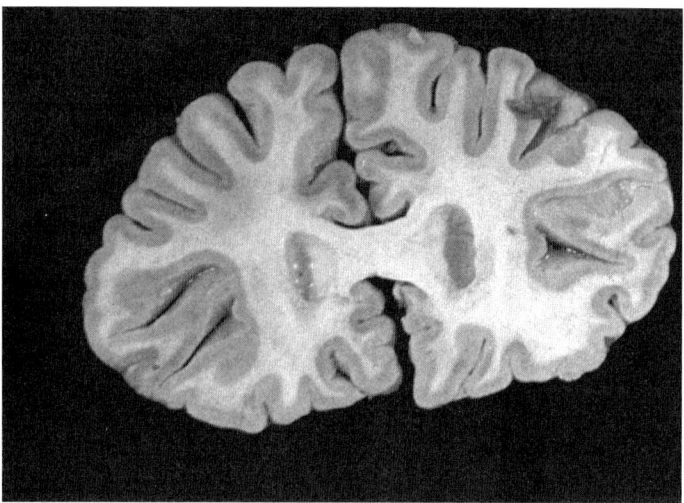

Figure 16–8. Adult neuronal ceroid lipofuscinosis in a brain weighing 1256 g, with no conspicuous cerebral atrophy.

sections used in the pigmentoarchitectonic technique of Braak, distribution of this neuronal loss is not uniform across the cerebral mantle but rather spares the occipital lobes. The loss of subcortical neurons is less well known because it is less well studied.[36] In adult NCL, activation of microglia is a sensitive feature that accompanies damage to nerve parenchyma. This activation of microglia, demonstrated immunohistochemically[37] can be observed in adult NCL both cortically and subcortically, indicating subtle damage to or even loss of nerve cells and their processes.

The non-adult forms of NCL are marked by severe atrophy of the retina due to neuronal cell loss commencing at the level of photoreceptors and resulting in glial scarring of the entire atrophic retina at the end stage of the disorder. One nosological criterion of adult NCL is that the retina does not undergo progressive neurodegeneration, but the retina is not exempted from the formation of intraneuronal lipopigments.[38,39] These lipopigments in the retina may be of granular[39] or fingerprint[38] types.

The formation of lipopigments and preservation of retinal neurons in adult NCL raise the question of whether formation of lipopigments are responsible for loss of nerve cells or whether loss of nerve cells show, in an early phase of neuronal degeneration, pathological accumulation of lipopigments. Likewise, the relationship between the accumulation of SCMAS, and, to a lesser degree, of SAPs, and the underlying biochemical and genetic defects in NCL is still unknown, as there are no biochemical and genetic data available, particularly for adult NCL. Only correct recognition and awareness of adult NCL may aid in supplementing the knowledge already accumulated of non-adult forms of NCL.

A pigment variant of NCL has also been observed in adults[40] that is marked by the accumulation of lipopigments, even extracellularly, in subcortical gray matter, and the formation of axonal spheroids that resemble the neuropathology of neuroaxonal dystrophies.

Mucopolysaccharidoses

As with many other lysosomal disorders, the mucopolysaccharidoses (MPS) occur primarily in childhood and adolescence; adult and late-onset, usually mild, forms have been observed only occasionally. Since the MPS represent dysfunction and metabolic abnormalities of mesenchymal cells, neurological symptoms in such patients may be rare, mild, or absent. However, lysosomal storage in mesenchymal cells may also be present within the nervous system where meningeal coverings and the vasculature (Fig. 16–9) are composed of mesenchymal cells. The respective lesions within the nervous system as well as around it occasionally result in secondary lesions, mostly of the nervous system parenchyma, by compression. Moreover, there is also primary lysoso-

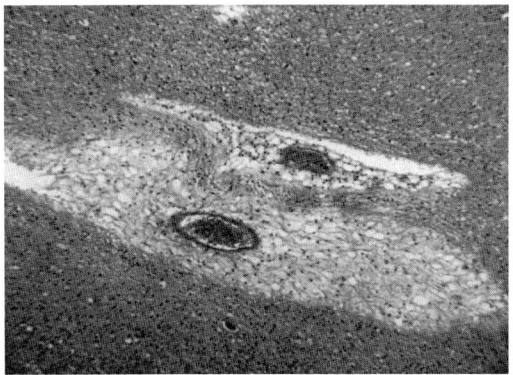

Figure 16–9. Mucopolysaccharidosis with enlarged Virchow-Robin space composed of vacuolated mesenchymal cells. Hematoxylineosin, ×145.

mal storage within nerve cells in MPS, which results in severe clinical deficits in early-onset forms. The extent to which this intraneuronal lysosomal storage occurs in late-onset or mild adult forms of MPS is largely unknown because biopsy and postmortem studies of the nervous system in such patients and electron microscopic data to verify subtle intraneuronal lysosomal storage are not available.

Ten lysosomal enzymes have been found to be deficient in the group of MPS (Table 16–2), with more than one of the lysosomal enzymes assigned to MPS being of the same MPS category. Mild variants marked by long duration of disease into adulthood, even into senescence,[41] but not necessarily marked by neurological symptoms are MPS I-S, Scheie syndrome; MPS II, mild Hunter disease;[41,42] MPS III-B, Sanfilippo syndrome;[43,44] MPS VI, Maroteaux-Lamy disease; and MPS VII, Sly syndrome.[45] MPS IVB, late-onset Morquio disease, is caused by β-galactosidase deficiency, which is not only present in an early form of clinically greater severity but may also be responsible for GM1 gangliosidosis.

Niemann-Pick Disease

Niemann-Pick disease (NPD) appears biochemically and genetically as a group of lysosomal entities. The childhood forms, NPD A and B, are marked by deficiencies of sphingomyelinase, with NPD B being a milder, non-neuronopathic form that can last into adulthood. Type NPD C, which is a cholesterol lipidosis, has its own clinical spectrum that includes patients with late onset. Niemann-Pick disease type C and its allelic variant, type D, of Nova Scotia, are now considered a lysosomal cholesterol storage disorder. One gene of this type, NPC-1, has been mapped to chromosome 18q11 and coded for a transmembraneous 1278 amino acid protein of still unknown function.[46] Morphologically, the NPD A to C types are marked by neuronal

Table 16–2. Nosology of Mucopolysaccharidoses

	Type	Gene Product	Gene Locus
MPS I-H	Hurler	α-iduronidase	4p16.3
MPS I-S	Scheie	α-iduronidase	4p16.3
MPS I-H/S	Variants	α-iduronidase	4p16.3
MPS II	Hunter	Iduronate-2-sulphatase	Xq28
MPS III-A	Sanfilippo A	Sulphamidase	17q25.3
MPS III-B	Sanfilippo B	α-N-acetylglucosaminidase	17q21
MPS III-C	Sanfilippo C	Acetyl-CoA:α-glucosaminide-N-acetyltransferase	?
MPS III-D	Sanfilippo D	N-acetylglucosamine-6-sulphatase	12q14
MPS IV-A	Morquio A	Galactosamine 6-sulphatase	16q24
MPS IV-B	Morquio B	β-galactosidase	3p14-p21
MPS VI	Maroteaux-Lamy	N-acetylgalactosamine-4-sulphatase	5q13
MPS VII	Sly	β-glucuronidase	7q21-q22

Source: Courtesy of Dr. Michael Beck, Department of Pediatrics, Mainz University Medical Center, Mainz, Germany.

lysosomal storage and lysosomal storage in cells of the reticuloendothelial system and epithelial cells, primarily hepatocytes. Within the CNS, lysosomal storage affects neurons along the entire neuraxis that are ultrastructurally characterized by lamellar inclusions, some of them resembling Zebra bodies; by membraneous cytoplasmic bodies; and by others appearing amorphic. In non-neuronal cells, lysosomal storage may display a characteristic combination of an electron-lucent component and electron-dense lamellar profiles.[47–50] Neurofibrillary tangles have been observed intraneuronally in patients with long-standing disease.[51–52] On immunohistochemical and immunoblot analysis, these neurofibrillary tangles are identical to those seen intraneuronally in AD, as they consist of paired helical filaments.[53] Axons may show dystrophic enlargement.[54]

Sialic Acid– and Neuraminic Acid–related Disorders

These lysosomal disorders of sialic acid metabolism include sialidoses I and II, which are marked by deficient sialidase, and galactosialidosis, which is marked by combined sialidase and β-galactosidase deficiencies resulting from a defective lysosomal "protective" protein coded by a gene on chromosome 20q13.1. This group of disorders also includes those in which lysosomal accumulation of sialic acid occurs due to a carrier defect, infantile sialic acid storage disease and Salla disease. Although sialidosis I is milder than sialidosis II, commencing in adolescence or even adulthood, only Salla disease has a long duration and an occasional unimpaired life span.[55] Salla disease is largely one of the inborn errors of metabolism in patients of Finnish descent, although a few non-Finnish patients have also been described. Neuropathologically, it is marked by severe impairment of myelination, vacuolar lysosomal storage, and considerable formation of intraneuronal lipopigments.[56] Only recently has the gene been localized to chromosome 6q,[57] but the allelic gene product has not been identified.

An adult form of galactosialidosis appears quite frequently in patients approaching old age. Lysosomal storage in cerebral and extracerebral cell types involves lysosomal vacuoles and some vacuolar lysosomal residual bodies frequently associated with accumulation of intraneuronal lipopigments.[58] This vacuolar and nonvacuolar lysosomal storage mimics the pattern of other lysosomal disorders, e.g., MPS, GM1 gangliosidosis, and certain oligosaccharidoses.

Other Oligosaccharidoses

Mild forms of β-mannosidosis[59] fucosidosis,[60] and aspartylglucosaminuria, another error of metabolism occurring predominantly in patients of Finnish descent marked by lysosomal vacuoles in a variety of cell types may occur in patients reaching adulthood and old age.

Glycogenoses

Of the ten different groups of glycogenosis, adult type II glycogenosis, which is marked by a deficiency in lysosomal acid maltase or α-1, 4-glucosidase, may show morphological accumulation of lysosomal glycogen in a variety of CNS cell types, based on the ubiquity of the lysosomal storage of glycogen. Clinical symptoms may not accompany the morphological cerebral changes and may only be detected on electron microscopy, which shows the lysosomal storage of glycogen within cellular compartments.

Other disorders marked by fibrillar accumulation of glycogen are glycogenosis type IV and polyglucosan body disease. Although glycogenosis type IV is primarily a disorder of childhood and adolescence, an adult form deficient in glycogen-branching enzyme activity has been noted.[61] The adult form may affect the skeletal muscle more than any other organ. Polyglucosan body disease, however, is a disorder of the nervous system and includes CN simulating dementia[62–63] and amyotrophic lateral sclerosis.[64] The glycogen that is not membrane bound and therefore not of lysosomal type accumulates as round, strongly PAS-postive bodies within neurons and neuronal processes (Fig. 16–10)[65] as well as in white matter, apparently within astrocytic processes.[66] Appearing in white matter and subpial regions, these polyglucosan bodies in astrocytic processes are actually corpora

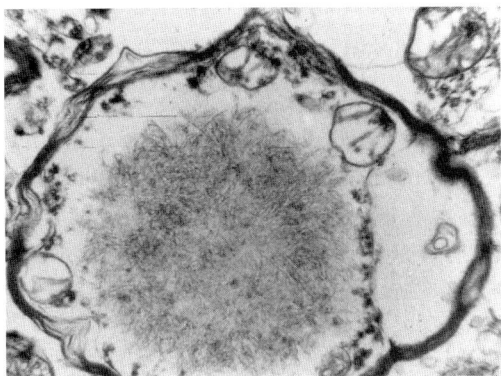

Figure 16–10. An intra-axonal polyglucosan body consisting of fibrillar glycogen. ×52,000.

amylacea. A nosological similarity between type IV glycogenosis and polyglucosan body pathology, even of the late-onset or adult type, has recently been recognized. Mutations in the glycogen-branching enzyme were discovered in elderly Ashkenazi Jewish patients with adult polyglucosan body disease.[61] Thus it appears that, depending on the molecular biological and biochemical techniques, polyglucosan diseases (Table 16–3), including those of late adulthood, may be considered metabolic disorders marked by metabolic defects within an expanded spectrum of glycogenosis IV because of the mutational and biochemical abnormalities of the glycogen-branching enzyme.

Mitochondrial Disorders

The concept of mitochondrial diseases evolved from the identification of ultrastructurally abnormal mitochondria, the light microscopic equivalent in skeletal muscle fibers being ragged red fibers, and the biochemical recognition of usually multiple, sometimes mildly, sometimes severely, diminished mitochondrial enzyme activity. At the molecular level, diverse mutations in the mitochondrial and nuclear genomes affecting mitochondrial functions were also noted. The ubiquitous presence of mitochondria in all cell types except circulating erythrocytes, and in organs may result in a diverse clinical, morphological, biochemical, and molecular genetic spectrum of mitochondrial entities. The principle of mitochondrial heteroplasmy and the observation that mitochondria may undergo genomic changes during life, especially with increasing age, underscore this diversity.

Biochemically defects in mitochondria comprise oxidative phosphorylation involving respiratory chain complexes I–V, some defects in transportation across mitochondrial membranes, and defects in substrate utilization and in the tricarbonic cycle.

Mutations in the nuclear genome, the mitochondrial genome, and both genomes, so-called bi-genomic defects, involve single deletions, multiple deletions, duplications, and point mutations, i.e., the entire spectrum of mutations. Such a wealth of mutational abnormalities has rendered genotype–phenotype correlations extremely difficult. The concept of mitochondrial disorders is further complicated by the fact that a single mutation may cause different clinical entities, and a single clinical entity may be caused by different mutations.

From a morphological standpoint, among the mitochondriopathies, mitochondrial my-

Table 16–3. Nosology of Polyglucosan Disorders

Forms	Enzyme Defect	Gene Locus
Type IV glycogenosis	Brancher enzyme:	⎫
Infantile form	Complete	⎪
Juvenile form	Partial (muscle, heart, liver)	⎬ 3p12
Adult form	Partial (muscle)	⎪
Polyglucosan body disease/ encephalopathy	Partial	⎭
Lafora disease		6q24

opathies were first identified as a group, followed by mitochondrial encephalomyopathies, when lesions of the central and peripheral nervous systems were found. Mitochondrial encephalopathies without skeletal muscle involvement may also occur, i.e., hereditary optic neuroretinopathy and ataxia–retinitis pigmentosa–dementia.[67] The involvement of other organs renders the mitochondrial cytopathies a group of truly single-organelle (mitochondria), multi-organ diseases.

Mitochondrial encephalomyopathies affect the CNS during childhood, adolescence, and adulthood. The three classical forms are Kearns-Sayre syndrome, mitochondrial encephalopathy with lactic acidosis and stroke-like episodes (MELAS), and myoclonic epilepsy with ragged red fibers (MERRF). Ragged red fibers in muscle biopsy specimens are the common morphological hallmark in these three disorders. MERRF and MELAS are caused by point mutations in the mitochondrial DNA (mtDNA), whereas large single lesions, one of which is common, of mtDNA are responsible for the Kearns-Sayre syndrome.[68] The nervous system is affected centrally and peripherally;[69] encephalopathy and neuropathy may occur separately or in combination.

Morphologically, the encephalopathic lesions are characterized by sponginess, necrosis, and mineralization; neuronal loss, demyelination, capillary proliferation, and gliosis affect gray and white matter to different degrees in different conditions. The leukoencephalopathy is often described radiologically, but this feature often lacks a morphological equivalent, reflecting a wealth of nonmorphological data but a paucity of morphological data—i.e., postmortem findings, on mitochondrial encephalomyopathies.

Because there are only a few relevant autopsy reports, the data are scant on the neuropathology in the CNS of the full spectrum of mitochondrial encephalomyopathies and encephalopathies. However, leaving the paucity of postmortem data aside, certain patterns have been noted concerning the three classical forms of mitochondrial encephalomyopathies. Kearns-Sayre syndrome is marked by spongiform encephalopathy, neuronal loss, and demyelination, followed by cellular and fibrillar astrocytosis. Using antibodies against mtDNA-encoded subunits of respiratory chain proteins, a decrease in neurons of the dentate nucleus, accompanied by sponginess of the cerebellar white matter and loss of Purkinje neurons, has been documented.[70] Neuronal loss and degeneration of myelinated tracts characterize MERRF, which are followed by cellular and fibrillar astrocytosis. The hallmarks of MELAS, however, are multifocal necrosis (Fig. 16–11), spongy degeneration (Fig. 16–12), mineral deposits, and neuronal loss with ensuing astrocytosis. Occasionally, the neuropathological pattern of Leigh syndrome, i.e., proliferation of capillaries, astrocytosis, and demyelination in gray matter but preser-

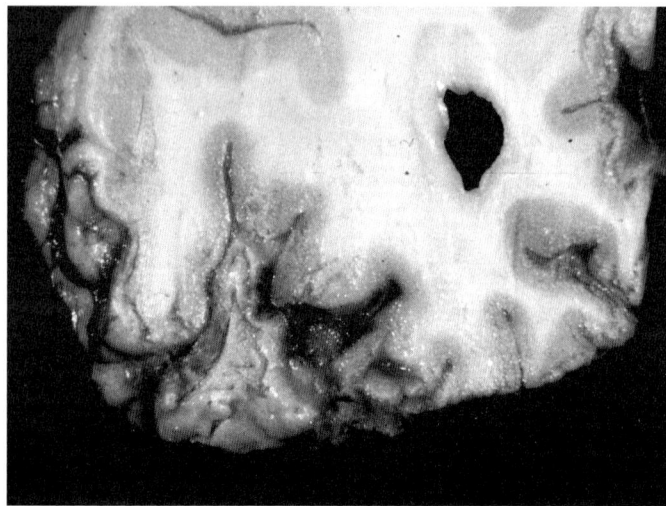

Figure 16–11. Cerebrocortical necrosis in mitochondrial encephalopathy with lactic acidosis and stroke-like episodes (MELAS). [Courtesy of Dr. A. Bornemann, Johannes Gutenberg University Medical Center, Mainz.]

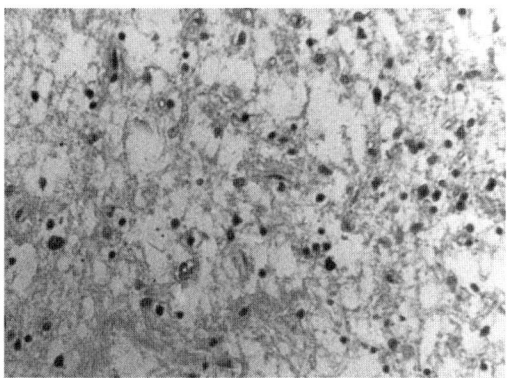

Figure 16–12. Spongy degeneration of the cerebral cortex, in MELAS, ×504. [Courtesy of Dr. A. Bornemann, Johannes Gutenberg University Medical Center, Mainz, Germany.]

vation of neuronal cell bodies in a spongy neuropil, may fall into this category, as has recently been shown by retrospective molecular genetic studies of archival paraffin-embedded tissues.[71] Necrosis resembling small infarcts occurs predominantly in the cortex, particularly in the occipital lobe, and may be caused by vascular obstruction on account of accumulation of abnormal mitochondria in mural smooth muscle and endothelial cells.

A leukoencephalopathy that is part of the rare mitochondrial neurogastrointestinal encephalomyopathy (MNGIE) syndrome is apparent on radiographic findings but has no morphological white matter lesions.[72] It is also marked by accumulation of mitochondria and smooth muscle cells and has been recently identified in biopsied intestine;[67] it may also be present in mural cells of the cerebral white matter vessels.

The mitochondrial genome is prone to undergo mutations during aging[73] that also affect the brain.[74] Thus, it is not surprising to learn that certain model diseases of aging, particularly Alzheimer's disease, may also show an increased number of mitochondrial deletions in CNS regions[74] or reduced function of mitochondria, especially of the respiratory chain complexes.[75] It is conceivable, therefore, that certain neurodegenerative diseases, e.g., Alzheimer's and Parkinson's diseases, may some day be considered neurometabolic rather than neurodegenerative diseases, given more extensive knowledge of abnormal mitochondrial metabolism in respective CNS regions and cell types. Thus individuals of families affected by inherited mitochondrial mutations may additionally suffer from age-related mitochondrial mutations. This combination may explain the occurrence of mitochondrial encephalomyopathies such as MERRF, even in senescence.[73]

ACQUIRED CONDITIONS

Central Pontine and Extrapontine Myelinolysis

Central pontine myelinolysis (CPM) is a purely demyelinating lesion (Fig. 16–13) that is often small and coincidental at autopsy but occasionally of sufficient size to cause clinical symptoms. Through the use of MRI, awareness of this disorder has been enhanced and the dynamics of some of these lesions which may subside during the course of the disease, have become better understood. Survival of CPM and extrapontine myelinolytic lesions may be recognized by fibrillar gliosis. In the differential diagnosis of CPM and extrapontine myelinolytic lesions, the lesions have to be distinguished from infarcts[76] and multiple sclerosis plaques. Central pontine myelinolysis is secondary to a number of different unrelated conditions, such as liver disease from liver transplantation, chronic alcoholism, malnutrition, and human immunodeficiency virus (HIV) infection.[77,78] Currently it is thought to be an iatrogenic disorder—i.e., characterized by too rapid correction of hyponatremia. Extrapontine lesions, which occasionally occur

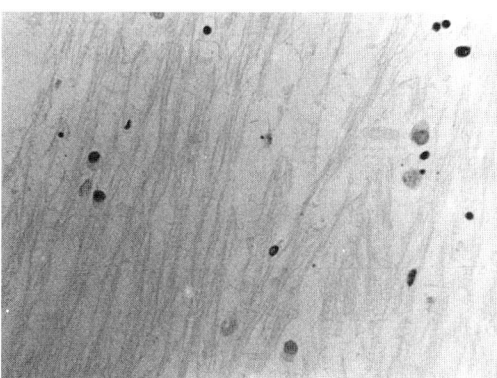

Figure 16–13. Central pontine myelinolysis. A few oligodendrocytes have remained among myelin-denuded separated nerve fibers. Hematoxylin-eosin, ×700.

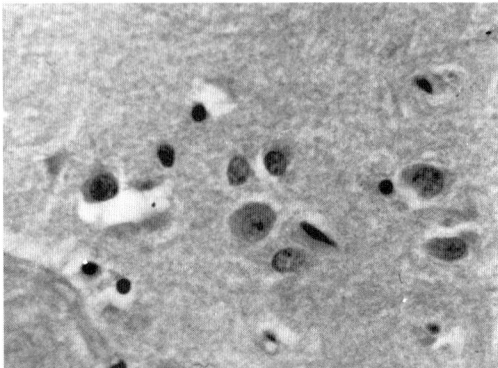

Figure 16–14. Hepatic encephalopathy with large astroglial nuclei and Alzheimer type II glia in putamen. Hematoxylin-eosin, ×800.

without pontine lesions,[79] have the same etiopathogenesis as CPM.[80] They affect myelin in the basal ganglia and thalamus,[81] producing chorea and parkinsonian symptoms.[82]

Hepatic and Uremic Encephalopathies

Encephalopathies, which are marked predominantly by obtundation and neuropsychiatric abnormalities, develop when failure of the liver and kidney occur during hepatic and uremic encephalopathies. The former is caused by increased circulation of ammonium, the latter by that of uremic toxins. Astrocytes of particularly the subcortical gray matter swell, and this can be recognized in large and round, watery nuclei (Fig. 16–14) of type II Alzheimer glia. These astrocytes do not stain for the glial fibrillary acidic protein when liver failure is acute. Generalized swelling of the brain from cytotoxic edema may also occur.

Type II Alzheimer's astroglial cells are also encountered in autosomal recessive hepatocerebral degeneration, or Wilson's disease, a condition of disturbed copper metabolism. Large, sometimes multinucleated astrocytes called "Alzheimer type I glia" (Fig. 16–15), and other large round cells with distinct nuclei called "Opalski cells," whose cytological origin is still unknown, may be encountered.

Financial support from the the European Union, Brussels, Belgium (ECA-NCL: BIOMED 2 programme BMH 4-CT 95-0563) as well as photography by Walter Meffert and editorial assistance from Astrid Wöber are gratefully acknowledged.

REFERENCES

1. Hodes ME, Zimmerman AW, Aydanian A, Naidu S, Miller NR, Garcia-Oller JL, Barker B, Aleck KH, Hurley TD, Dlouhy SR. Different mutations in the same codon of the proteolipid protein gene, *PLP*, may help in correlating genotype with phenotype in Pelizaeus-Merzbacher disease/X-linked spastic paraplegia (PMD/SPG2). Am J Med Genet 1999; 82:132–139.
2. Bosch EP, Hart MN. Late adult-onset metachromatic leukodystrophy: dementia and polyneuropathy in a 63-year-old man. Arch Neurol 1978; 35:475–477.
3. Duyff RF, Weinstein HC. Late-presenting metachromatic leukodystrophy. Lancet 1996; 348:1382–1383.
4. Perusi C, Lira MG, Duyff RF, Weinstein HC, Pignatti PF, Rizzuto N, Salviati A. Mutations associated with very late–onset metachromatic leukodystrophy [letter to the editor]. Clin Genet 1999; 55:130.
5. Berger J, Löschl B, Bernheimer H, Lugowska A, Tylki-Szymanska A, Gieselmann V, Molzer B. Occurrence, distribution, and phenotype relations of arylsulphatase A in patients with metachromatic leukodystrophy. Am J Med Genet 1997; 69:335–340.
6. Pilz H, Duensing I, Heipertz R, Seidel D, Lowitzsch K, Hopf HC, Goebel HH. Adult metachromatic leukodystrophy. Eur Neurol 1977; 15:301–307.
7. Goebel HH, Argyrakis A, Shimokawa K, Seidel D, Heipertz R. Adult metachromatic leukodystrophy. IV Ultrastructural studies on the central and peripheral nervous system. Eur Neurol 1980; 19:294–307.
8. Hedley-Whyte ET, Boustany RM, Riskind P, Raghavan S, Zuniga G, Kolodny EH. Peripheral neuropathy due to galactosylceramide-β-galactosidase deficiency (Krabbe's disease) in a 73-year-old woman. [Brit Neuropathol Soc Proc]. Neuropathol Appl Neurobiol 1988; 14:515–516.

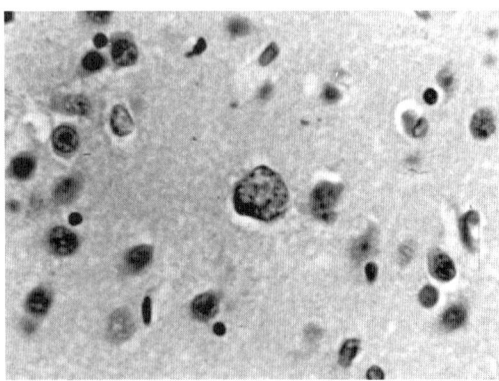

Figure 16–15. Large Alzheimer type I glial nucleus in Wilson's disease, with striate body. Hematoxylin-eosin, ×1100.

9. Choi KG, Sung JH, Clark HB, Krivit W. Pathology of adult-onset globoid cell leukodystrophy (GLD) [abstract # 142]. J Neuropathol Exp Neurol 1991; 50: 336.
10. Goebel HH, Harzer K, Ernst JP, Bohl J, Klein H. Late-onset globoid cell leukodystrophy: unusual ultrastructural pathology and subtotal β-galactosidase deficiency. J Child Neurol 1990; 5:299–307.
11. Moser HW, Moser AB, Naidu S, Bergin A. Clinical aspects of adrenoleukodystrophy and adrenomyeloneuropathy. Dev Neurosci 1991; 13:254–261.
12. Moser HW, Smith KD, Moser AB. X-linked adrenoleukodystrophy. In: Scriver CR, Beaudet AL, Sly WS, Valle D, eds. The Metabolic and Molecular Bases of Inherited Disease, Vol. 2. New York: McGraw-Hill, 1995; 2325–2347.
13. Powers JM, Moser HW. Peroxisomal disorders: genotype, phenotype, major neuropathologic lesions, and pathogenesis. Brain Pathol 1998; 8:101–120.
14. Fouquet F, Zhou JM, Ralston E, Murray K, Tralen F, Magal E, Robain O, Dubois-Dalcq M, Aubourg P. Expression of the adrenoleukodystrophy protein in the human and mouse central nervous system. Neurobiol Dis 1997; 3:271–285.
15. Watkins PA, Gould SJ, Smith MA, Braiterman LT, Wei HM, Kok F, Moser AB, Moser HW, Smith KD. Altered expression of ALDP in X-linked adrenoleukodystrophy. Am J Hum Genet 1995; 57:292–301.
16. Moser HW. Adrenoleukodystrophy: phenotype, genetics, pathogenesis and therapy. Brain 1997; 120: 1485–1508.
17. Goldman JE, Katz D, Rapin I, Purpura DP, Suzuki K. Chronic G_{M1}-gangliosidosis presenting as dystonia: I. Clinical and pathological features. Ann Neurol 1981; 9:465–475.
18. Suzuki Y, Nakamura N, Fukuoka K, Shimada Y, Uono M. β-galactosidase deficiency in juvenile and adult patients. Report of six Japanese cases and review of literature. Hum Genet 1977; 36:219–229.
19. Yoshida K, Oshima A, Shimmoto M, Fukuhara Y, Sakuraba H, Yanagisawa N, Suzuki Y. Human β-galactosidase gene mutations in G_{M1}-gangliosidosis: a common mutation among Japanese adult/chronic cases. Am J Hum Genet 1991; 49:435–442.
20. Yoshida K, Oshima A, Sakuraba H, Nakano T, Yanagisawa N, Inui K, Okada S, Uyama E, Namba R, Kondo K, Iwasaki S, Takamiya K, Suzuki Y. G_{M1}-gangliosidosis in adults: clinical and molecular analysis of 16 Japanese patients. Ann Neurol 1992; 31:328–332.
21. Oonk JGW, van der Helm HJ, Martin JJ. Spinocerebellar degeneration: hexosaminidase A and B deficiency in two adult sisters. Neurology 1979; 29:380–384.
22. Yaffe MG, Kaback M, Goldberg M, Miles J, Itabashi H, McIntyre H, Mohandas T. An amyotrophic lateral sclerosis-like syndrome with hexosaminidase-A deficiency: a new type of G_{M2} gangliosidosis [abstract #13]. Neurology 1979; 29:611.
23. Barbeau A, Plasse L, Cloutier T, Paris S, Roy M. Lysosomal enzymes in ataxia: discovery of two new cases of late onset hexosaminidase A and B deficiency (adult Sandhoff disease) in French Canadians. Can J Neurol Sci 1984; 11:601–606.
24. Navon R, Argov Z, Frisch A. Hexosaminidase A deficiency in adults. Am J Med Genet 1986; 24:179–196.
25. Karni A, Navon R, Sadeh M. Hexosaminidase A deficiency manifesting as spinal muscular atrophy of late onset. Ann Neurol 1988; 24:451–453.
26. Gravel RA, Clarke JTR, Kaback MM, Mahuran D, Sandhoff K, Suzuki K. The G_{M2}-gangliosidoses. (chap. 92). In: Scriver CR, Beaudet AL, Sly WS, Valle, D, eds. The Metabolic and Molecular Bases of Inherited Disease, Vol. 2. New York: McGraw-Hill, 1996:2839–2877.
27. deVeber GA, Schwarting GA, Kolodny EH, Kowall, NW. Fabry disease: Immunochemical characterization of neuronal involvement. Ann Neurol 1992; 31: 409–415.
28. Elleder M, Bradová V, Smid F, Budesinksy M, Harzer K, Kustermann-Kuhn B, Ledinova J, Belohlavek J, Kral V, Dorazilova V. Cardiocyte storage and hypertrophy as a sole manifestation of Farby's disease. Virchows Arch A 1990; 417:449–455.
29. Ogawa K, Sugamata K, Funamota N, Abe T, Sato T, Nagashima K, Ohkawa S. Restricted accumulation of globotriaosylceramide in the hearts of atypical cases of Fabry's disease. Hum Pathol 1990; 21:1067–1073.
30. Mole SE, Gardiner RM, Goebel HH. Workshop on the genetic and molecular basis of the neuronal ceroid-lipofuscinoses. London, U.K., Nov. 13–16, 1997. Eur J Pediatr Neurol 1998; 2:2(A1–18).
31. Zeman W. The neuronal ceroid-lipofuscinoses—Batten-Vogt syndrome: a model for human aging? Adv Gerontol Res 1971; 3:147–170.
32. Constantinidis J, Wisniewski KE, Wisniewski TM. The adult and a new late adult forms of neuronal ceroid lipofuscinosis. Acta Neuropathol (Berl) 1992; 83: 461–468.
33. Martin J-J, Gottlob I, Goebel HH, Mole SE. CLN4: adult NCL. In: Goebel HH, Mole SE, Lake BD, eds. The Neuronal Ceroid Lipofuscinoses (Batten Disease). Amsterdam: IOS Press, 1999; 77–90.
34. Martin J-J, Ceuterick C. Adult neuronal ceroid-lipofuscinosis—personal observation. Acta Neurol Belg 1997; 97:85–92.
35. Braak H, Braak E. Pathoarchitectonic pattern of iso- and allocortical lesions in juvenile and adult neuronal ceroid-lipofuscinosis. J Inherited Metab Dis 1993; 16: 259–262.
36. Braak H, Braak E. Projection neurons of basolateral amygdaloid nuclei develop meganeurites in juvenile and adult human neuronal ceroid lipofuscinosis. Clin. Neuropathol 1987; 6:116–119.
37. Goebel HH, Schochet SS, Jaynes M, Brück W, Kohlschütter A, Hentati F. Progress in neuropathology of the neuronal ceroid lipofuscinoses. Mol Genet Metab 1999; 66:367–372.
38. Martin J-J, Libert J, Ceuterick C. Ultrastructure of brain and retina in Kufs' disease (adult type-ceroid-lipofuscinosis). Clin Neuropathol 1987; 6:231–235.
39. Goebel HH, Schochet SS, Jaynes M, Gutmann L. Ultrastructure of the retina in adult neuronal ceroid lipofuscinosis. Acta Anat 1998; 162:127–132.
40. Jakob H, Kolkmann F-W. Zur Pigmentvariante der adulten Form der amaurotischen Idiotie (Kufs). Acta Neuropathol (Berl) 1973; 26:225–236.
41. Hobolth N, Pedersen C. Six cases of a mild form of the Hunter syndrome in five generations. Three affected males with progeny [abstract]. Clin. Genet 1978; 13:121.
42. Young ID, Harper PS. Mild form of Hunter's syn-

43. Van Schrojenstein-De Valk HMJ, van de Kamp HP. Follow-up on seven adult patients with mild Sanfilippo B disease. Am J Med Genet 1987; 28:125–129.
44. Di Natale P. Sanfilippo B disease: a re-examination of a particular sibship after 12 years. J Inherited Metab Dis 1991; 14:23–28.
45. de Kremer RD, Givogri I, Argaraña E, Hliba E, Conci R, Boldini CD, Capra AP. Mucopolysaccharidosis type VII (β-glucuronidase deficiency): a chronic variant with an oligosymptomatic severe skeletal dysplasia. Am J Med Genet 1992; 44:145–152, 1992.
46. Vanier MT, Suzuki K. Recent advances in elucidating Niemann-Pick C disease. Brain Pathol 1998; 8:163–174.
47. Longstreth WT Jr, Daven JR, Farrell DF, Bolen JW, Bird TD. Adult dystonic lipidosis: clinical, histologic and biochemical findings of a neurovisceral storage disease. Neurology 1982; 32:1295–1299.
48. Elleder M, Jirásek A, Vlk J. Adult neurovisceral lipidosis compatible with Niemann-Pick disease type C. Virchows Arch [A] 1983; 401:35–43.
49. Wherrett JR, Rewcastle NB. Adult neurovisceral lipidosis [abstract]. Clin Res 1969; 17:665.
50. Hulette CM, Earl NL, Anthony DC, Crain BJ. Adult onset Niemann-Pick disease type C presenting with dementia and absent organomegaly. Clin Neuropathol 1992; 11:293–297.
51. Love S, Bridges LR, Case CP. Neurofibrillary tangles in Niemann-Pick disease type C. Brain 1995; 118:119–129.
52. Suzuki K, Parker CC, Pentchev PG, Katz D, Ghetti B, D'Agostino AN, Carstea ED. Neurofibrillary tangles in Niemann-Pick disease type C. Acta Neuropathol (Berl) 1995; 89:227–238.
53. Auer IA, Schmidt ML, Lee VM-Y, Curry B, Suzuki K, Shin RW, Pentchev PG, Carstea ED, Trojanowski JQ. Paired helical filament tau (PHFtau) in Niemann-Pick type C disease is similar to PHFtau in Alzheimer's disease. Acta Neuropathol (Berl) 1995; 90:547–551.
54. Elleder M, Jirásek A, Smid F, Ledinova J, Besley GT. Niemann-Pick disease type C: study on the nature of cerebral storage process. Acta Neuropathol (Berl) 1985; 66:325–336.
55. Gahl W, Schneider JA, Aula PP. Lysosomal transport disorder: cystinosis and sialic acid storage disorders. In: Scriver CR, Beaudet AL, Sly WS, Valle D, eds. The Metabolic and Molecular Bases of Inherited Disease, Vol. 2. New York: McGraw-Hill, 1995:3763–3795.
56. Autio-Harmainen H, Oldfors A, Sourander P, Renlund M, Dammert K. Simila S. Neuropathology of Salla disease. Acta Neuropathol. (Berl) 1988; 75:481–490.
57. Haataja L, Schleutker J, Laine A-P, Renlund M, Savontaus ML, Dib C, Weissenbach J, Peltonen L, Aula P. The genetic locus for free sialic acid storage disease maps to the long arm of chromosome 6. Am J Hum Genet 1994; 54:1042–1049.
58. Amano N, Yokoi S, Akagi M, Sakai M, Yagishita S, Nakata K. Neuropathological findings of an autopsy case of adult β-galactosidase and neuraminidase deficiency. Acta Neuropathol (Berl) 1983; 61:283–290.
59. Cooper A, Sardhawalla IB, Roberts MM. Human β-mannosidase deficiency [letter]. N Engl J Med 1986; 315:1231.
60. Willems PJ, Gatti R, Darby JK, Romeo G, Durand P, Dumon JE, O'Brien JS. Fucosidosis revisited: a review of 77 patients. Am J Med Genet 1991; 38:111–113.
61. Lossos A, Meiner Z, Barash V, Soffer D, Schlesinger I, Abramsky O, Argov Z, Shpitzen S, Meiner V. Adult polyglucosan body disease in Ashkenazi Jewish patients carrying the Tyr[329]Ser mutation in the glycogen-branching enzyme gene. Ann Neurol 1998; 44:867–872.
62. Boulon-Predseil P, Vital A, Brochet B, Darriet D, Henry P, Vital C. Dementia of frontal lobe type due to adult polyglucosan body disease. J Neurol 1995; 242:512–516.
63. Bigio EH, Weiner MF, Bonte FJ, White CL 3rd. Familial dementia due to adult polyglucosan body disease. Clin Neuropathol 1997; 16:227–234.
64. McDonald TD, Faust PL, Bruno C, DiMauro S, Goldman JE. Polyglucosan body disease simulating amyotrophic lateral sclerosis. Neurology 1993; 43:785–790.
65. Gray F, Gherardi R, Marshall A, Janota I, Poirier J. Adult polyglucosan body disease (APBD). J Neuropathol Exp Neurol 1988; 47:459–474.
66. Chou SM, McMahon JT. Adult polyglucosan body disease (APBD): a white matter disease with intractable seizures? [abstract #143]. J Neuropathol Exp Neurol 1991; 50:336.
67. Perez-Atayde AR, Fox V, Teitelbaum JE, Anthony DA, Fadic R, Kalsner L, Rivkin M, Johns DR, Cox GF. Mitochondrial neurogastrointestinal encephalomyopathy. Am J Surg Pathol 1998; 22:1141–1147, 1998.
68. Zeviani M, Antozzi C. Defects of mitochondrial DNA. Brain Pathol 1992; 2:121–132.
69. Rose MR. Mitochondrial myopathies. Arch Neurol 1998; 55:17–24.
70. Tanji K, Vu TH, Schon EA, DiMauro S, Bonilla E. Kearns-Sayre syndrome: unusual pattern of expression of subunits of the respiratory chain in the cerebellar system. Ann Neurol 1999; 45:377–383.
71. Santorelli FM, Tanji K, Shanske S, Krishna S, Schmidt RE, Greenwood RS, DiMauro S, De Vivo DC. The mitochondrial DNA A8344G mutation in Leigh syndrome revealed by analysis in the paraffin-embedded sections: revisiting the past. Ann Neurol 1998; 44:962–964.
72. Bardosi A, Creutzfeldt W, DiMauro S, Felgenhauer K, Friede RL, Goebel HH, Kohlschütter A, Mayer G, Rahlf G, Servidei S, Van Lessen G, Wetterling T. Myo-neurogastrointestinal encephalopathy (MNGIE syndrome) due to partial deficiency of cytochrome c oxidase: a new mitochondrial multi-system disorder. Acta Neuropathol (Berl) 1987; 74:248–258.
73. Wallace DC. Mitochondrial DNA variation in human evolution, degenerative disease, and aging. Am J Hum Genet 1995; 57:201–223.
74. Corral-Debrinski M, Horton T, Lott MT, Shoffner JM, Beal MF, Wallace DC. Mitochondrial DNA deletions in human brain: regional variability and increase with advanced age. Nat Genet 1992; 2:324–329.
75. Bonilla E, Tanji K, Hirano M, Vu TH, DiMauro S, Schon EA. Mitochondrial involvement in Alzheimer's

disease. Biochim Biophys Acta Bioenergetics 1999; 1410:171–182.
76. Kleinschmidt-DeMasters BK, Anderson CA, Rubinstein D. Asymptomatic pontine lesions found by magnetic resonance imaging: are they central pontine myelinolysis? J Neurol Sci 1997; 149:27–35.
77. Miller RF, Harrison MJ, Hall-Craggs MA, Scaravilli F. Central pontine myelinolysis in AIDS. Acta Neuropathol (Berl) 1998; 96:537–540.
78. Mossakowski MJ, Zelman IB. Neuropathological syndromes in the course of full blown acquired immune deficiency syndrome (AIDS) in adults in Poland (1987–1995). Folia Neuropathol (Warsz) 1997; 35:133–193.
79. Waragai M, Satoh T. Serial MRI of extrapontine myelinolysis of the basal ganglia: a case report. J Neurol Sci 1998; 161:173–175.
80. Choe WJ, Cho BK, Kim IO, Shin HY, Wang KC. Extrapontine myelinolysis caused by electrolyte imbalance during the management of suprasellar germ cell tumors. Childs Nerv Syst 1998; 14:155–158.
81. Salvesen R. Extrapontine myelinolysis after surgical removal of a pituitary tumour. Acta Neurol Scand 1998; 98:213–215.
82. Ezpeleta D, de Andres C, Gimenez-Roldan S. Movimientos abnormales en un caso de mielinolisis extrapontina. Revision de literatura. Rev Neurol Esp 1998; 26:215–220.

17. Immunologic Diseases of the Aging Nervous System

ROBERT L. KNOBLER

Changes in the nervous system with age may be due to many different processes, and many disorders become more common with aging. The mnemonic VITAMIN D can be used, as a way of conducting a differential diagnosis; each letter represents a category of conditions. These include *vascular* lesions due to atherosclerotic disease or vasculitis; *infections*, such as reactivation of *Varicella zoster* in shingles (herpes zoster); *traumatic* lesions due to falls; *autoimmune* disorders, which include immune-mediated disorders reflecting divergent pathological processes such as vasculitis, atypical antibodies, paraneoplastic disorders, and as yet unknown immunological mechanisms; *metabolic* derangements, such as diabetes and renal failure; *iatrogenic* etiologies, such as chemotherapy-related axonopathies; *neoplasms*, such as carcinomas, lymphomas, and myeloma; and *degenerative* diseases affecting the brain, spinal cord, and nerve roots, which may reflect mechanical or genetic processes.

In this chapter the focus is on those changes that are mediated through the function of the immune system. To understand this process, it is essential to have some background information on the organization of the immune system.

IMMUNE ORGANIZATION

The immune system is appreciated as having a pivotal role in immune surveillance and host defense. These roles allow for the immune system to recognize malignant cells and infectious agents as potential threats, and to orchestrate their elimination. This is mediated through either humoral (antibodies) or cellular (T cells, natural killer cells, and macrophages) effector arms of the immune system to impart specificity. Another level of the effector arm is carried out through mediator molecules such as cytokines, lymphokines, and other mediator molecules.

In some cases, the immune inflammatory process involves the destruction of normal-appearing tissue. This has been described as "bystander" damage—that is, the tissue is destroyed by locally released mediators.[1] While this may happen as a consequence of tissue invasion by malignant cells and infectious agents, there is also the potential for direct attack as part of autoimmune disease. In this chapter, the immunological diseases that affect muscle, the neuromuscular junction (NMJ), peripheral nervous system (PNS), and central nervous system (CNS) tissues are explored (Table 17–1). These may be part of organ-specific diseases or may be secondary to a more systemic process.

Organ-specific tissues have a number of different molecules that serve as targets of immune-mediated destruction, in what are antigen-driven autoimmune diseases (e.g., myasthenia gravis, Lambert-Eaton syndrome). In other instances, the autoimmune disease remains without identification of a specific target antigen (e.g., multiple sclerosis, systemic lupus erythematosus).

A brief review of some of the components

Table 17-1. Immunologic Diseases of the Aging Nervous System

Muscle
Dermatomyositis (DM)
Polymyositis (PM)
Polymyalgia rheumatica (PR)

The Neuromuscular Junction (NMJ)
Myasthenia gravis (MG)
Lambert Eaton syndrome (LES)

Peripheral Nervous System (PNS)
Plasma cell dyscrasias (PCD)
Paraneoplastic
Guillain Barré syndrome (GBS)
Chronic inflammatory demyelinating neuropathy (CIDP)

Central Nervous System (CNS)
Multiple sclerosis (MS)
Systemic lupus erythematosus (SLE)

---

of the immune system helps to provide a conceptual framework for better understanding the pathogenesis of the autoimmune diseases. Further elaboration of these details can be obtained through any current standard textbook of immunology. The immune system consists of an afferent limb, which is the antigen-processing arm, and an efferent limb, which is the attack arm that functions to destroy the target antigen.[2,3] The mechanism for antigen processing involves the breakdown of target antigens into a series of small parts called an "epitope," a complex presentation of that epitope to the immune system, and then generation and execution of a specific attack directed against the epitope by the "activated" immune system.

There is a double signal for arming or activation of the effector arm[4] that of the trimolecular complex (antigen epitope, receptor, and HLA class II) and that of the costimulatory signal (B7). The T cells are subdivided into those which are $CD4^+$ first simply classified as helpers, and those which are CDb^+, first classified as cytotoxic/suppressor T cells. In reality, the picture is even far more complex, since there are precursors of the $CD8^+$ cells, that mature into separate cytotoxic T cell and "suppressor" T cell populations, and B cells that mature into antibody-producing cells that are dependent upon a subsets of cells of the $CD4^+$ population.

The $CD4^+$ cells have been further characterized as Th1 and Th2 subpopulations depending on their predominant cytokine profiles. Th1 cells produce γ-interferon (IFN-γ), tumor necrosis factor (TNF), and interleukin-2 (IL-2), which expands and amplifies the cellular humoral response, including the activation of macrophages. In contrast, the TH2 cells have a different profile, yielding interleukins-4, 5, 6 and-10, which elaborate humoral immunity. More perplexing still is the observation that cells of the $CD4^+$ subset may actually play a cytotoxic or suppressor role in specific circumstances. This level of complexity leaves the full picture of the role of the immune system in the various disorders under discussion here unclear at the present time.

Under normal circumstances, antigens that the immune system has been exposed to since early development have also generated an immune response. However, because of its exposure to these antigens during development, the immune system does not normally respond to these molecules with immune attack. This is because of immunoregulatory mechanisms in place which lead to immunological tolerance of these antigens, allowing the immune system to distinguish between "self" and "not-self." However, autoimmune diseases may occur when these protective mechanisms are bypassed, by such phenomena as occur during infections, exposure to certain drugs (e.g., low-dose cyclophosphamide), and radiation (Table 17–2).

Polyclonal activation represents the nonspecific activation of cells of the immune system to produce their specific products. In some

Table 17-2. Potential Immune Bypass Mechanisms

Polyclonal activation
Superantigens
Altered antigens
Molecular mimicry
Antigen spreading
Events of aging

cases this will be antibody that was not ordinarily being produced because of regulation through mechanisms of immune tolerance that has been "broken" through exposure to a polyclonal activation stimulus, such as infection with Epstein-Barr virus. A related phenomenon is the action of a toxic product of an infectious organism (e.g., staphylococcal enterotoxin B) as a "superantigen," which activates a cascade of immune activation of a whole subpopulation of immune cells that do not have specificity for this particular antigen.

Altered antigens can occur when an infectious agent, such as a virus, incorporates a portion of the infected cell into its structure, or when an altered form of cellular protein is generated because of mutation. When the immune system then recognizes this component of the infectious agent, it also generates a response against that portion of the cell.

Molecular mimicry is a specific situation in which the epitope under attack has either a configurational or sequence homology with a portion of an existing tissue molecule, resulting in an immune attack not only on the original epitope, but also on the resident molecule with which it shares homology. An example of molecular mimicry is found in Grave's disease, in which there is a long-acting thyroid stimulating (LATS) hormone produced, due to an immune response to the thyroid stimulating hormone (TSH) receptor. Ironically, rather than destroying the receptor, this antibody binds to and stimulates this receptor, leading to the overproduction of thyroid hormone, and a thyrotoxic state.

Antigen spreading is a situation that follows attack against an original epitope, with a subsequent release of previously sequestered antigens in the process. These released antigens themselves then come under attack. During aging there is more opportunity for multiple exposure to such processes, including viral infections and natural senescence, which could lead to immune dysregulation and unmasking of autoimmune reactivity.

All of these processes can lead to either altered immune regulation, immune-mediated structural and functionally impairing changes, or even functionally stimulatory changes, such as those observed in Grave's disease. In discussing those changes specifically as they relate to the muscle, the NMJ, peripheral nerves, and CNS, a good place to begin is with the identification of some of the target antigens of these different tissues.

IMMUNE TARGETS OF THE NERVOUS SYSTEM

There are many potential antigens that can be targets of the immune response. It is currently not clear whether these are basic to the mechanism of disease, as results from experimental animal models employing these antigens would suggest, or whether they are secondary to immune responses to them following their release during inflammatory lesions identified in these tissues. Table 17–3 lists those structures that have been identified as targets of immune destruction in the muscle, the NMJ, PNS, and CNS. These lesions include the accumulation of per-ivascular infiltrating cells, along with phagocytosis and subsequent resolution.

Table 17–3. Target Antigens of Immunological Diseases of Muscle, the Neuromuscular Junction, Peripheral Nervous System, and Central Nervous System

Vascular and connectective tissue diseases affecting muscle and nerves
Periarteritis nodosa (PN)
Systemic lupus erythematosus (SLE)
Polymyositis/dermatomyositis (PM/DM)
Temporal arteritis (TA) and polymyalgia rheumatica (PR)

Peripheral Nerve
Chronic inflammatory demyelinating neuropathy (CIDP)
Guillain Barré syndrome (GBS)
Myasthenia gravis (MG) and the neuromuscular junction

Neoplastic
Cerebellar degeneration (CD)
Lambert Eaton syndrome (LES)
Paraneoplastic neurologic disorders (PND)
Peripheral neuropathy (PN)
Plasma cell dyscrasia (PCD)

Multiple sclerosis

Table 17–4. Reasons for the Late Appearance of Symptoms and Signs

Lesion size overcomes redundancy within system
Time course of lesion onset is slowly progressive
Late onset of pathological process

In discussing the immune-mediated diseases of the aging nervous system, we will need to focus on those pathological processes that increase the specific involvement of the muscle, NMJ nerves, and CNS white matter with age. When we identify pathological changes we usually are visualizing the end result or transition into the final pathological presentation, rather than the initial precipitating event. Therefore, it is not surprising that there is typically a discrepancy between the onset of pathology and the onset of symptoms (Table 17–4).

The first concept to address when discussing immunological diseases of the aging nervous system is related to the reserve "safety factor" built into the organization of each neural pathway. This reserve is due in part, to redundancy in the number of fibers and connections. The degree of redundancy is variable for different pathways and in different individuals. However, because there are more functioning fibers than the minimum required to mediate the principal neural activity of the given pathway, a percentage of the pathway can be rendered nonfunctional before recognizable neurological symptoms or signs become apparent. There may also be functional fluctuations in the remaining elements of a given pathway, depending on their state of myelination (for example, thinly remyelinated fibers may decompensate in function with increasing body temperature, as after physical activity, in febrile states, or high ambient temperatures), or metabolic conditions (hypoglycemia, hyponatremia, or hypoxia).

The second concept is related to the time course of symptom development. A rapidly expanding mass, hemorrhage, or even the edema associated with an inflammatory infiltrate may produce devastating functional deficits very rapidly because of the way in which these processes may disrupt the normal cytoarchitecture. Steroid hormone therapies have proven to be clinically effective in such cases. Slower processes can progress unnoticed for some time before becoming clinically apparent. In this sense, clinical symptoms are just the tip of the pathological iceberg.

The third concept is related to the later onset of a pathological process because of a later developmental expression of a gene product. With this background in the workings of the immune system, we will explore features of selected neuroimmunologic diseases.

NEUROIMMUNOLOGIC DISEASES

Neuroimmunologic diseases are of clinical importance in the aging population because they become more prevalent with increasing age and because they have the potential to be quite disabling. The more common of these disorders are discussed from the periphery inward, beginning with muscle.

Muscle

Immunological disorders within muscle may be the consequence of infections with various agents, or may follow a reaction to an intramuscular immunization. Because muscle is readily accessible for biopsy, it is possible to gain greater insight into the disorders affecting muscle that have an immunological basis. Laboratory models can be developed with cultured myoblasts and myotubes and expansion of lymphocyte populations harvested from the biopsy.[5] There are three clinical disorders of note to discuss in this section: dermatomyositis (DM), polymyositis (PM), and polymyalgia rheumatica (PR). The latter also includes temporal arteritis. The first two are the most common inflammatory myopathies.[6]

Dermatomyositis is named for its involvement of the muscle and skin. It occurs in two populations, childhood and older adults, and is more common in females, as are many autoimmune disorders. The latter form has features not found in the childhood form, so it may represent a different etiology with shared pathologic expression. The adult form is more common in blacks than whites. Both DM and PM begin with slowly progressive weakness of the proximal muscles, affecting the neck, shoulders, and limb girdle. The progression may vary from weeks to years, and may be asymmetric or even localized to a particular limb. Pain may accompany weakness in about one-third of patients.

Skin manifestations in DM include the characteristic heliotrope discoloration and swelling of the eyelids, and a raised scaly erythematous rash on the face, shoulders, and upper trunk, as well as on the extensor surfaces of the limbs, particularly the fingers, wrists, elbows, and knees.

The muscle involvement in both DM and PM is evident in raised levels of circulating muscle enzymes, particularly creatine kinase (CK), abnormal electromyographic responses (a myopathic presentation of low-amplitude motor units mixed with fibrillation potentials and positive waves) and on muscle biopsy (necrosis and regeneration of muscle fibers, with foci of inflammatory cells). The erythrocyte sedimentation rate is elevated in about half of affected individuals.

In DM there is perifascicular atrophy, which spares the central portions of the muscle fascicle.[7] Expression of MHC class I antigens is quite intense within the atrophic fibers, but may also be seen in the absence of inflammation.[8] There is also ischemia, with endothelial cell hyperplasia of the intramuscular blood vessels. Focal depletion of capillaries is an early feature of DM, and deposition of complement membrane attack complex (MAC) has been identified in these vessels.[9] In DM there are more B cells and CD4+ cells than in PM, which, along with the observation of the complement MAC, suggests an antibody-mediated pathogenesis in DM.

These disorders may be triggered by an infectious agent, such as a virus, as exemplified by human immunodeficiency virus (HIV)–associated polymyositis.[10] There is epidemiological evidence for a role of coxsackie virus in other forms of DM and PM.[11] The adult forms of both DM and PM are associated with collagen vascular disorders such as rheumatoid arthritis, scleroderma, and systemic lupus erythematosus. There is an increased association of malignant diseases with DM.

In PM, but not DM, infiltrating CD8pl lymphocytes, expressing α β receptors and macrophages are present, and target expression of MHC class I antigen occurs, as in DM.[12] Another form of PM showed expression of γ δ T cells and expression of a known target of this receptor class, the 65 kDa heat shock protein.[13] A similar association of this receptor class with heat shock protein expression has been reported in multiple sclerosis.[14]

Temporal (giant cell) arteritis occurs most often in patients over age 60. These patients suffer visual loss as a result of ischemia to the optic nerve or retina. There are also symptoms of muscle aches (myalgia) that may be associated with fever, and often tender, pulseless arteries on the scalp. The erythrocyte sedimentation rate is significantly elevated; this along with a suggestion of visual loss and myalgias should prompt rapid initiation of steroids in the patient because of the increased risk of permanent visual loss and stroke. Skip lesions in temporal artery biopsies may result in a negative result. Polymyalgia rheumatica may also be present or may occur independently of the temporal arteritis.

The Neuromuscular Junction

The neuromuscular junction (NMJ) is affected by two significant disorders. These are myasthenia gravis, characterized by motor weakness that worsens with effort (fatigue), and Lambert Eaton syndrome, characterized by weakness that improves with effort.

MYASTHENIA GRAVIS

Myasthenia gravis (MG) is mediated by autoantibody-directed damage of the postsynaptic acetylcholine receptor portion of the NMJ.[15] This condition is frequently associated with thymoma in the older population, and removal of the tumor may contribute to improvement. Thymic hyperplasia is observed in younger individuals. It is more common in younger women and older men, with HLA-A1,-B8, and -DR3 being more common in younger patients, and HLA-A3,-B7, and -DR2 being more common in those older. Men outnumber women 3:2. Weakness of the eye muscles occurs in about 90% of patients.

The diagnosis of MG is corroborated with three tests beyond the history and physical examination. These include the edrophonium (Tensilon®) test, in which up to 10 mg of this short-acting anticholinesterase agent is injected intravenously, and reversal of muscle weakness is assessed. The second test is repetitive stimulation of a nerve, and recording a decremental response in the compound muscle action potential (CMAP) of 10%. The third test is the search for antibodies to the acetylcholine receptor. Neonatal myasthenia is a transient form of the disease that occurs when antibodies are inadvertently transferred across the placenta. Myasthenia gravis is often associated with other autoimmune diseases such as Hashimoto's thyroiditis, systemic lupus, and erythematosus and rheumatoid arthritis.

Because of the damage to the NMJ in MG, there is increased sensitivity to a number of drugs and chemicals that alter conduction across the remaining acetylcholine receptors. This group includes a variety of antibiotics, anticonvulsants, anti-arrhythmics, anti-rheumatics, anti-psychotics, tranquilizers, opioids, hypnotics, laxatives, and hormones. The use of corticosteroids may worsen myasthenic symptoms before there is stabilization of the MG.

LAMBERT EATON SYNDROME

Lambert Eaton syndrome (LES) may precede the diagnosis of an underlying malignant tumor by as long as 4 years. In about 50% of the patients it is associated with the presence of a tumor, most commonly, small cell lung cancer. Under these circumstances an immunoglobulin G (IgG) binds to and destroys the presynaptic voltage-gated calcium channels.[16] Consequently, reduced acetylcholine is released with resulting weakness and fatigue. Autonomic features include dry mouth, difficulties with sphincter control, and impotence. The diagnosis is usually corroborated with nerve conduction studies demonstrating a smaller than normal CMAP, while repetitive stimulation provides more than a 100% increase in amplitude. Patients may respond to plasmapheresis. In the non-cancer form of the disease, there is an association with other autoimmune disorders.

Peripheral Nervous System

Immunologic disorders of the PNS may have a variety of mechanisms. However, unlike muscle, which depends on a rich supply of blood to fulfill its metabolic requirements to perform work, the nerves have different needs and are shielded through a blood–nerve barrier provided by endoneurial endothelium and perineurial interaction. As a result, there is a higher level of endoneurial pressure which also supports the concept of a barrier mechanism.[17] The barrier is naturally leakiest at the ends of the line, surrounding the dorsal root ganglion and the peripheral nerve terminals. As with the blood–brain barrier, activated lymphocytes cross the blood–nerve barrier.[18] MHC class II molecules are not ordinarily expressed within the nerve, although the endothelial cells and perivascular macrophages are exceptions under unique circumstances.

Lesions are generally occur in two basic forms. They may lead to axonal destruction, or axonopathy, with secondary demyelination due to Wallerian degeneration of the nerve fiber. In contrast, there may be primary demyelination, due to direct involvement of the Schwann cell.

Damage may be mediated through specific mechanisms in which humoral immunity plays a role, such as in plasma cell dyscrasias and paraneoplastic syndromes. Cellular mechanisms are believed to be important in both the acute (Guillain Barré syndrome) and chronic (chronic inflammatory demyelinating polyneuropathy) forms of demyelinating polyneuropathy.[19] Nonspecific damage may occur in the context of vasculitic, infectious, and inflammatory disorders, as a variation of bystander damage following interruption of the blood–nerve barrier.

Lesion localization to sites of compression, with interruption of the blood–nerve barrier, is often found in forms of demyelinating neuropathy, while in other conditions there is localization to naturally more permeable sites, such as surrounding the dorsal root ganglia and at peripheral nerve terminals. Permeability is also influenced by the release of vasoactive amines from tissue mast cells that are also more prevalent at these very same locations.

In vasculitic lesions, immune complexes are deposited within the epineurial blood vessels, which secondarily bind inflammatory cells to their location. The disorder gives rise to a symmetrical sensorimotor distal axonal polyneuropathy. As a result, relative ischemia of the endoneurium occurs, as well as a patchy depletion of affected fascicles, primarily affecting the center of the fascicle. This leads to axonal degeneration with secondary demyelination. This pattern is observed in both periarteritis nodosa (PN) and systemic lupus erythematosus (SLE), in which systemic involvement may also include the joints, kidneys, and skin, in addition to multiple peripheral nerves (mononeuritis multiplex).

The concept of bystander demyelination has proven quite useful in explaining the sensitivity of the component structures of the nerve to damage.[1] However, on closer examination, axonal degeneration has proved to be the primary manifestation in an experimental model in which an antigen has been injected within the sciatic nerve of an animal previously sensitized to this antigen.[20] This result suggests the need for humoral or cellular elements for the development of more robust primary demyelination. Table 17–5 lists the differential diagnosis of these neuropathies.

PLASMA CELL DYSCRASIA

Plasma cell dyscrasia (PCD), in contrast, results in a gradually progressive motor and sensory, or purely sensory demyelinating polyneuropathy. The frequency of PCD increases with age, and may have invasion of bone and tissue in about half of those affected. In PCD a monoclonal gammopathy is produced, with an identifiable M protein. The M protein may be of the IgM, IgG, or IgA subtypes. The disorder is identified as Waldenstrom's macroglobulinemia when the M protein is IgM, and identified as multiple myeloma if it is IgG or IgA.

Peripheral neuropathy is found in about 10% of those with multiple myeloma, and in around 25% of those with Waldenstrom's macroglobulinemia. Pathological changes may reflect the deposition of the antibodies within the nerves or direct invasion by plasma cells.

Typically, a demyelinating neuropathy occurs in the context of a monoclonal IgM paraproteinemia, with axonal conduction maximally slowed distally. Nerve biopsy characteristically shows widely spaced myelin lamellae in the affected nerve, with deposited IgM identified as the IgM light chain of the IgM paraproteinemia. These patients often have a distal sensory loss that can evolve into a chronic demyelinating sensorimortor neuropathy. The IgM often is directed toward

Table 17–5. Common Neuropathies by Presentation

Motor Neuropathies
Motor neuron disease
Guillain Barré syndrome
Chronic inflammatory demyelinating neuropathy
Lead intoxication
Acute porphyria
Multifocal motor neuroathy
Hereditary motor sensory neuropathy (Charcot Marie Tooth disease)

Asymmetric Weakness
Motor neuron disease
Radiculopathy, cervical/lumbosacral
    Disk, osteoarthritis, shingles, meningeal carcinomatosis
Plexopathy, brachial/lumbosacral
    Immune, neoplastic infiltration, diabetic
Mononeuritis multiplex
    Vasculitis, Lyme disease, sarcoid, leprosy, HIV, hereditary pressure palsy
    Multifocal motor neuropathy
Compressive/entrapment
    Median, ulnar, radial
    Peroneal, posterior tibial

Painful Neuropathies
Diabetes
Vasculitis
Guillain Barré syndrome
Amyloidosis
Toxic (arsenic, thallium)
HIV
Fabry's disease
Idiopathic sensorimotor neuropathy

Sensory Neuropathies
Cancer
Cisplatin and related chemotherapeutic agents
Sjogren's syndrome
Vitamin B-6 toxicity
HIV-related sensory neuronopathy
Idiopathic sensory neuronopathy

Autonomic Neuropathies
Diabetes mellitus
Amyloid
Porphyria

myelin-associated glycoprotein (MAG) and/or myelin glycolipids, which produces some variability in the clinical picture from patient to patients.[21]

The reason for this antigenic specificity remains unknown, but this represents only about half of those affected. There is a subgroup termed the "GALOP syndrome," with *g*ait *a*taxia, *a*utoantibody, *l*ate-age *o*nset, and a sensory-motor *p*olyneuropathy. These patients have high titers of antibody to a CNS myelin antigen (CMA) preparation. The gait ataxia, which is wide-based and unsteady, causes falling, with only mild distal weakness. Sensory loss is mild to moderate and involves both large– and small-diameter nerve fibers. Demyelination was evident on nerve conduction studies in 80% of patients, who responded to treatment with immunomodulatory therapy.[22] Yet another subset has been identified with sensory loss and pain localized in the hands and feet, with distal weakness in the legs; reflexes may be lost at the ankles. Nerve conduction studies have demonstrated axonal loss in those with polyclonal anti-sulfatide antibodies, but demyelination when M proteins directed against sulfatide were present.[23]

In other paraproteinemias, IgG or A predominates, with unknown target antigens. In a rare disorder known by the acronym POEMS, there is monoclonal IgG or IgA with multisystem involvement of *p*olyneuropathy, *o*rganomegaly, *e*ndocrinopathy, *M* protein, and *s*kin changes. It has been suggested that the manifestations are mediated by proinflammatory cytokines.[24] In contrast, in some cases antibodies are directed against complex molecules such as chondroitin sulfate, gangliosides, or other glycolipids, and these more often result in axonal neuropathy, neuroparthy, [25] leading to implications for a role in some forms of motor neuron disease. However, it is an IgM that binds to a common portion of the gangliosides GM1 and GD1b.

PARANEOPLASTIC NEUROLOGIC DISORDERS

Paraneoplastic neurologic disorders (PND), such as a sensory neuropathy, can be found in the context of small cell lung cancer, although this pairing is not their full extent. These disorders may be the first sign of an occult malignant disease, predating the discovery of the cancer by upwards of 6 months. Ironically, the PND may symptomatically be more disabling than the cancer, and occur in 5% of unselected cancer patients. Awareness of PND occurrence clinically is important because PND may mimic other neurologic disorders, leading to the loss of time in the diagnosis and treatment of the underlying malignancy.

Sensory neuronopathy is characterized by inflammation of the dorsal root ganglion cell, with subsequent degeneration. An antibody, described as anti-Hu (from the first two letters of the first patient from whom it was identified, and also known as ANNA-1 for antineuronal nuclear antibody), has been noted to cross-react with an antigen common to both the affected neurons and the small cell lung cancer cells.[26] While the dorsal root ganglion neurons are most commonly affected, other neuron systems have also been damaged.

Sensory neuronopahty is characterized by pain and paresthesias, sometimes followed by severe asymmetric proprioceptive loss that results in ataxia. The onset can be abrupt or subacute, affecting large-diameter nerve fibers. Symptoms may begin affecting any part of the body and are usually progressive, following a subacute course. Motor conduction velocities are normal, while sensory conduction study results are decreased if they can be detected at all. Central nervous system features are also found in most patients, with elevated spinal fluid protein, increased intrathecal IgG synthesis, spinal fluid pleocytosis, and anti-Hu antibodies in the serum. Differential diagnosis includes idiopathic acute sensory neuropathy, sensory neuropathy of Sjogren's syndrome,[27] toxic neuropathies, and neuropathy associated with monoclonal gammopathy of undetermined significance (MGUS).

Motor neuronopathy is a progressive, usually symmetrical muscle weakness, which may stabilize or improve.[28] Motor neuronopathy typically occurs after the diagnosis of lymphoma (primarily Hodgkin's disease), even after clinical remission or radiotherapy. Kidney and lung tumors are also associated. Differential diagnosis includes amyotrophic lateral sclerosis (without upper motor neuron symptoms) and lower motor neuron disease (as anti-Hu paraneoplastic encephalomyelitis, with elevated IgG, oligoclonal bands, and cell counts).

Although the vast majority of patients have

small cell lung cancer, a variety of other tumors have also been associated, including non-small cell lung cancer, breast, seminoma, sarcoma, prostate, neuroblastoma, and colon cancer.[29,30] There is evidence that antibodies alone are insufficient to damage neuronal cells, and that antigen-specific cytotoxic (CD8$^+$) T cells are involved. While small cell lung cancer is more common in men, the paraneoplastic disorder is more common in women, as with other autoimmune diseases.

Other paraneoplastic syndromes have also been identified. An acute to subacute cerebellar syndrome with dysarthria and upbeat nystagmus has been associated with anti-Yo antibodies (also known as PCA-1) and ovarian, breast and uterine cancer. An opsoclonus–myoclonus syndrome has been associated with anti-Ri antibodies (also known as ANNA-2) and breast and small cell lung cancer. Although neuropathy is not a significant feature of the anti-Yo and anti-Ri syndromes, it may occur as part of the clinical picture. These antibodies and the molecules they recognize need more unifying classification.[31] Unfortunately, unlike paraneoplastic disorders affecting the NMJ (MG and LES), the response to therapy has not significantly reversed the deficits.[32]

Finally, there are other conditions that may occur. These include acute or subacute autonomic neuropathy, which can include isolated orthostatic hypotension; urinary retention; constipation; dry mouth and pupillary abnormalities in small cell carcinoma; and Hodgkin's disease.[33] Damage to the myenteric plexus occurs with chronic pseudo-obstruction, resulting in progressive loss of appetite, early filling, vomiting, and constipation with or without associated peripheral nerve symptoms. Subacute or chronic sensorimotor neuronopathy is estimated to be four times more common than sensory neuronopathy.[34] A glove-and-stocking sensory loss with paresthesias and distal foot muscle weakness are also symptoms.

GUILLAIN BARRÉ SYNDROME AND CHRONIC INFLAMMATORY DEMYELINATING POLYRADICULONEUROPATHY

Guillain Barré syndrome (GBS) and chronic inflammatory demyelinating polyradiculoneuropathy (CIDP) are two ends of a spectrum of acquired demyelinating polyneuropathies. There are also acute motor and acute motor and sensory axonal neuropathy variants that resemble GBS, in which the primary attack is focused on the axon rather than the myelin. While GBS peaks at 4 weeks,[35,36] CIDP usually takes twice as long to get fully underway.[37,38] Heavy inflammatory infiltration occurs at the dorsal root ganglion region; this condition closely resembles the acute and chronic forms of experimental allergic neuritis (EAN), which is precipitated by immunization with myelin antigens.[39] Magnetic resonance imaging (MRI) with gadolinium may show enhancement of the spinal nerve roots, which is consistent with breakdown of the blood–nerve barrier.

Relevant myelin antigens in GBS and CIDP include the myelin basic protein, P2 protein, the P0 glycoprotein, and galactocerebroside.[40] Axonal degeneration, rather than primary demyelination, is more frequent in those patients with antibodies to gangliosides such as GM1 and GD1b, which occurs in 20%, but there is an association of prior infection with certain strains of *Campylobacter jejuni*, especially in northern China.[41] This should be investigated further as an indication of poor prognosis, since it has been observed that patients with such antibodies tend to recover incompletely.

In GBS there is a fairly symmetrical, ascending paralysis, with loss of reflexes. The cerebrospinal fluid is characterized by elevated protein, yet typically less than five lymphocytes, the classical albuminocytologic dissociation. The nerve conductions are affected, with reduced conduction velocities, prolonged distal latencies, and temporal dispersion of the evoked potential responses. Lymphocytic infiltrates with macrophage-mediated demyelination are also present.

Miller Fisher syndrome (MFS) a variant of GBS, is characterized by ophthalmoplegia, ataxia, and areflexia, and other cranial nerve involvement affecting speech and swallowing.[42] This variant has some clinical resemblance to botulism, and the toxin is known to bind to the ganglioside GQ1b. Antibodies to GQ1b have been detected in the MFS variant.

In CIDP there is a progressive or relapsing course, with weakness in two or more limbs and decreased or absent deep tendon reflexes.

Electrophysiological findings of demyelination have been reported, as in GBS, but with a different clinical course, and a similar albuminocytologic dissociation. Absence of monoclonal IgM antibodies and antibodies to myelin-associated glycoprotein (MAG) is also needed to rule out a paraproteinemia.

Plasma exchange is useful in the treatment of GBS but is of less benefit in CIDP, where its impact is short-lived. Large doses of intravenous immunoglobulin have been demonstrated to be effective in reversing symptoms for longer periods in both GBS and CIDP. In contrast, steroids have no significant impact on GBS, although they are effective in CIDP. The reasons for these clinical discrepancies in response to treatment are not apparent at the present time.

Central Nervous System

Central nervous system immune-mediated involvement can occur in the context of primary disease, such as with multiple sclerosis, or may be secondary to other conditions, such as systemic lupus erythematosus.

MULTIPLE SCLEROSIS

Multiple sclerosis (MS) is a CNS disease in which the predominant feature is immune-mediated demyelination.[43] The inflammatory lesion not only leads to demyelination but may also produce axonal damage with more long-lasting neurologic sequelae. This consideration underscores why remyelination alone may be insufficient to ensure recovery.

In the lesions, there are perivascular cuffs of mononuclear cells that infiltrate into the white matter areas of the brain and spinal cord, as well as the optic nerves, which are also a part of the CNS.[44] This specificity of attack supports the notion that this immune-mediated attack is directed toward a CNS myelin-specific antigen, the identity of which remains unknown.

Myelin basic protein (MBP) has long been suspected as a candidate target antigen because of its pivotal role in the laboratory model of MS, experimental allergic encephalomyelitis (EAE). However, virtually any of the myelin antigens have been shown experimentally to be capable of inducing an EAE response. Epitope spreading could occur following the initial attack in this paradigm. Furthermore, it is possible that a principal MBP-specific clone initiates subsequent attacks, but that through epitope spreading, a variety of clones are also represented within the lesion. The mechanism by which, and when the first attack occurs in MS remains unknown.

Whether a single clone or a variety of clones contributes to initiating each subsequent lesion has important implications in the treatment approach to MS. Stem cell transplants are being investigated with the hope of deleting the clones that trigger MS. Understanding whether there is a single clone or multiple clones, and the basis of their entry into the CNS compartment are critical to the success of preventing recurrence of disease following stem cell reconstitution.

Viruses or other infectious agents, as yet unidentified have long been suspected as being the target of the immune attack in MS on the basis of three key findings in MS. First, the perivascular cuffs suggest an immune response to an infectious agent. Second, there are increased quantities of antibodies to a variety of common childhood infectious agents expressed within the CNS tissue and the spinal fluid. There are also a variety of clones expressed as oligoclonal bands, with evidence for expression of separate clones in separate lesions. Third, a massive increase in the presence of inflammatory cells occurs within the spinal fluid compartment. To date, a long list of potential candidate agents has been excluded. The exploration of human herpes virus-6 (HHV-6) and Chlamydia pneumonia as having a causative role in the development of MS is currently under investigation.

Multiple sclerosis is initially clinically characterized by relapses and remissions, which reflect lesions located in clinically expressive regions of the CNS. In fact, however, studies with magnetic resonance imaging (MRI) of the brain reveal lesion formation at a rate up to 10-fold more frequently than is apparent from the rate of onset of new clinical symptoms. Thus the clinical picture alone in MS is merely the tip of the iceberg, and there can be many more lesions evident (the lesion burden), which would not have necessarily been suspected from review of the number and severity of the clinical attacks alone. The relapsing–remitting pattern of MS may progress into a secondary progressive course as the individual grows older.

SUMMARY AND CONCLUSIONS

Age causes changes that are irreversible. Although we may gain wisdom and experience with age, there is a price to pay. As a clinician, it is obvious that when we reach age 40, we become aware of parts of our bodies that we never thought about before. When we reach age 50, they begin to hurt, and so on. From a review of the immune disorders affecting the nervous system associated with the aging process, we come to realize just how fortunate we are if we get away with a few aches and pains. However, one thing about pain is that it proves we are alive!

REFERENCES

1. Wisniewski HM, Bloom BR. Primary demyelination as a non-specific consequence of circulating immunocytes in Guillain-Barré syndrome. A cell-mediated immune reaction. J Exp Med 1975; 141: 346–359.
2. Pober JS. Cytokine-mediated activation of vascular endothelium. Am J Pathol 1988; 133: 426–433.
3. Springer TA. Adhesion receptors of the immune system. Nature 1990; 346: 425–434.
4. Weaver CT, Unanue ER. The costimulatory function of antigen presenting cells. Immunol Today 1990; 11: 49–55.
5. Hohlfeld R, Engel AG. Coculture with autologous myotubes of cytotoxic T cells isolated from muscle in inflammatory myopathies. Ann Neurol 1991; 29: 498–507.
6. Dalakas M. Polymyositis, dermatomyositis and inclusion body myositis. N Engl J Med 1991; 325: 1487–1498.
7. Whitaker JN. Inflammatory myopathy: a review of etiologic and pathologic factors. 1982; Muscle Nerve 5: 573–592.
8. Griggs RC, Karpati G. The pathogenesis of dermatomyositis. Arch Neurol 1991; 48: 21–22.
9. Emslie-Smith AM, Engel AG. Microvascular changes in early and advanced dermatomyositis: a quantitative study. Ann Neurol 1990; 27:343–356.
10. Illa I, Nath A, Dalakas M. Immunocytochemical and virological characteristics of HIV-associated inflammatory myopathies: similarities with seronegative polymyositis. Ann Neurol 1991; 29: 474–481.
11. Bowles NE, Dubowitz V, Sewry CA, Archard LC. Dermatomyositis, polymyositis and Coxsackie-B-virus infection. Lancet 1987; 1: 1004–1007.
12. Karpati G, Pouliot Y, Carpenter S. Expression of immunoreactive major histocompatibility complex products in human skeletal muscles. Ann Neurol 1988; 23: 64–72.
13. Hohlfeld R, Engel AG, Ii K, Harper MC. Polymyositis mediated by T lymphocytes that express the gamma-delta receptor. N Engl J Med 1991; 324: 877–881.
14. Selmaj K, Brosnan CF, Raine CS. Colocalization of lymphocytes bearing the γδ T-cell receptor and heat shock protein hsp 65$^+$ oligodendrocytes in multiple sclerosis. Proc Natl Acad Sci USA 1991; 88: 6452–6456.
15. Drachman DB. Myasthenia gravis. N Engl J Med 1994; 330: 1797–1810.
16. Lennon VA, Kryzer TJ, Greismann GE, Padraig MS, O'Suilleabhain E, Windebank AJ, Woppmann A, Miljanich GP, Lambert EH. Calcium-channel antibodies in the Lambert-Eaton syndrome and other paraneoplastic syndromes. N Engl J Med 1995; 332: 1467–1474.
17. Powell HC, Meyers RR, Costello MI, Lampert PW. Endoneurial fluid pressure in Wallerian degeneration. Ann Neurol 1979; 5: 550–573.
18. Wekerle H, Linington C, Lassmann H, Meyermann R. Cellular immune reactivity within the CNS. Trends Neurolog Sci 1986; 9: 271–277.
19. Thomas PK. The Guillain-Barré syndrome: no longer a simple concept. J Neurol 1992; 239: 361–362.
20. Powell HC, Braheny SL, Hughes RAC, Lampert PW. Antigen-specific demyelination and significance of the bystander effect in peripheral nerves. Am J Pathol 1984; 114: 43–453.
21. Latov N. Pathogenesis and therapy of neuropathies associated with monoclonal gammopathies. Ann Neurol 1995; 37 (SI): S32–S42.
22. Pestronk A, Choksi R, Bieser K, Goldstein JM, Adler CH, Caselli RJ, George EB. Treatable gait disorder and polyneuropathy associated with high titer serum IgM binding to antigens that copurify with myelin-associated glycoprotein. Muscle Nerve 1994; 17: 1293–1300.
23. Pestronk A, Li F, Griffin J, Feldman EL, Cornblath D, Trotter J, Zhu S, Yee WC, Phillips D, Peeples DM, Winslow B. Polyneuropathy syndromes associated with serum antibodies to sulfatide and myelin-associated glycoprotein. Neurology 1991; 41: 357–362.
24. Gherardi RK, Chouaib S, Malapert D, Belec L, Intrator L, Degos JD. Early weight loss and high serum tumor necrosis factor-alpha levels in polyneuropathy, organomegaly, endocrinopathy, M protein, skin changes syndrome. Ann Neurol 1994; 35: 501–505.
25. Brindel I, Preud'Homme J, Vallat J, Vincent D, Vasquez J, Jauberteau M. Monoclonal IgM reactive with several gangliosides in a chronic relapsing polyneuropathy. Neurosci Lett 1994; 181: 103–106.
26. Dalmau J, Furneaux HM, Rosenblum MK, Graus F, Posner JB. Detection of the anti-Hu antibody in specific regions of the nervous system and tumor from patients with paraneoplastic encephalomyelitis/sensory neuronopathy. Neurology 1991; 41: 1757–1764.
27. Gainsborough N, Hall SM, Hughes RAC, Leibowitz S. Sarcoid neuropathy. J Neurol 1991 Jun; 238(3): 177–180.
28. Nobile-Orazio E, Carpo M, Legname G, Meucci N, Sonnino S, Scarlato G. Anti-G_{M1} IgM antibodies in motor neuron disease and neuropathy. Neurology 1990; 40: 1747–1750.

29. Lennon VA. Paraneoplastic autoantibodies: The case for a descriptive generic nomenclature. Neurology 1994; 44: 2236–2240.
30. Moll JW, Vecht CJ. Immune diagnosis of paraneoplastic neurological disease. Clin Neurol Neurosurg 1995; 97: 71–81.
31. Dalmau J, Posner JB. Neurologic paraneoplastic antibodies (anti-Yo; anti-Hu; anti-Ri): the case for a nomenclature based on antibody and antigen specificity. Neurology 1994; 44: 2241–2246.
32. Stübgen J-P. Neuromuscular disorders in systemic malignancy and its treatment. Muscle Nerve 1995; 18: 636–648.
33. Hughes RAC, Britton T, Richards M. Effects of lymphoma on the peripheral nervous system. J R Soc Med 1994; 87: 526–530.
34. Peterson K, Forsyth PA, Posner JB. Paraneoplastic sensorimotor neuropathy associated with breast cancer. J Neurooncol 1994; 21: 159–170.
35. Prineas JW. Pathology of the Guillain-Barré syndrome. 1981; Ann Neurol 9 (Suppl.):6–19.
36. Hughes RAC. The concept and classification of Guillain-Barré syndrome and related disorders. Rev Neurol (Paris) 1995; 151: 291–294.
37. Ad Hoc Committee of the American Academy of Neurology HIV Task Force. Research criteria for the diagnosis of chronic inflammatory demyelinating polyradiculoneuropathy (CIDP). Neurology 1991; 41: 617–618.
38. Glass JD, Cornblath DR. Chronic inflammatory demyelinating polyneuropathy and paraproteinemic neuropathies. Curr Opin Neurol 1994; 7: 393–397.
39. Waksman BH, Adams RD. Allergic neuritis: Experimental disease of rabbits induced by injection of peripheral nervous tissue and adjuvants. J Exp Med 1955; 102: 213–225.
40. Khalili-Shirazi A, Atkinson P, Gregson N, Hughes RAC. 1993 Antibody responses to P_0 and P_2 myelin proteins in Guillain-Barré syndrome and chronic idiopathic demyelinating polyneuropathy. J Neuroimmunol 1993; 46: 245–252.
41. Griffin JW, Ho TWH. The Guillain-Barré syndrome at 75: The *Campylobacter* connection. Ann Neurol 1993; 34: 125–127.
42. Fross RD, Daube JR. Neuropathy in the Miller-Fisher syndrome: clinical and electrophysiologic findings. Neurology 1987; 37: 1493–1498.
43. McFarlin DE, McFarland HF. Multiple sclerosis. N Engl J Med 1982; 307: 1183–1188, 1246–1251.
44. Hickey WF, Hsu BL, Kimura H. T lymphocyte entry into the central nervous system. J Neurosci Res 1991; 28: 254–260.

18. Brain Trauma in the Elderly

J. C. DE LA TORRE

Traumatic injuries to the central nervous system (CNS) of elderly individuals are generally more damaging and present greater complications than similar injuries in younger subjects. The significance of this statistic has major neuropathologic and socioeconomic implications. Injury to the aged CNS takes a more alarming aspect when it is learned that the number of people 65 and over in the world makes up about 11% of the general population. In the United States, where such statistics are of growing concern, 12 million individuals are over age 75 and this figure is expected to increase exponentially during the twenty-first century.

Certain generalizations about the aging process may help explain the relative vulnerability of the CNS to traumatic injury. First, performance on reaction-timed tasks and speed of processing incoming information peak at age 20 and thereafter steadily decline during a life span.[1] Second, evidence shows reduced perception of sensory stimuli affecting visual and auditory systems. Since motor and sensory abilities decline during aging, body balance and postural maintenance involving gait disturbances can be compromised, a condition that exposes the elderly subject to more frequent accidents. Third, elderly individuals tend to take more medicines for a variety of ailments, appropriately called, "polypharmacy." If trauma is introduced, these medicines can pose a problem for surgical repair, pair alleviation, and drug interactions.[2] Fourth, problems can arise in assessing traumatic injury in confused or noncommunicative patients or patients with multiple medical conditions.[3] This chapter reviews data that may be useful to the neuropathologist in assessing CNS traumatic damage.

NEURONAL LOSS DURING AGING

Conventional wisdom since the 1950s[4-6] has held that significant neuronal loss occurs during aging. This notion has been reinforced by the fact that significant neuronal loss could account for waning memory recall in the elderly as well as some loss in language, abstraction, reasoning, and judgment associated with progressive aging. Findings in the last two decades, however, have challenged the premise that aging involves loss of large numbers of neurons, particularly if neurodegeneration can be ruled out at postmortem. Brains of normal elderly subjects examined postmortem show little if any neuronal loss. The question as to why the authors of more recent articles disagree with the older literature that neuronal loss during aging is not a normal phenomenon has to do with the term "normal." When "normal" health status in aging subjects was confirmed through rigorous examination at autopsy, histological analysis of brain tissue showed that pyknotic cortical neurons could occur in healthy aged subjects in the absence of degeneration of these neurons.[7-13] This together with the advent of more accurate stereological techniques for counting brain cells[14,15] has indicated no significant loss of neurons in elderly humans when entorhinal cortex and CA1, two hippocampal regions most responsible for memory function, are examined.[16,17]

Other confounding factors that need to be considered in neuron counts of the aged are tissue processing, sampling design, and individual anatomical variability that exists in the human brain. Individual anatomic variability in neuron counting of aged human brain can be appreciated through the comparison of two recent studies. In the first study,[16] neuron loss in normal aged subjects was observed in the hilus and subiculum, two subdivisions of the hippocampus related to memory and learning. A second study[18] demonstrated loss of neurons in CA1 and subiculum, in Alzheimer patients but not normal aged subjects. The discrepancy reported for normal aged brain in these two studies may be due to small quantification variability in the brain regions studied. Another explanation when finding neuronal loss in an otherwise healthy aged individual is the possibility of pre-existing damaged brain tissue.

The brain is not the only region where neuronal loss has been described. Progressive loss of motor neurons in the spinal cord has been reported to coincide with increased aging up to age 70 in individuals free of neurologic disease.[19] This loss of motor neurons was accompanied by a progressive increase in astrocytes in the anterior horn of the oldest cases examined.[19]

TRAUMA AND NEURODEGENERATION

Severe traumatic brain injury involving loss of consciousness has been reported to be a high risk factor leading to neurodegeneration. The leading example of this phenomenon is dementia pugilistica, when a professional boxer who has received repeated blows to the brain or has been frequently knocked unconscious develops a neurodegenerative condition that eventually leads to cognitive failure and dementia. It has been documented that neurodegeneration following brain trauma is associated with Alzheimer's disease.[20]

Since both conditions are generally more prevalent in the elderly population, it is assumed that brain injury sustained prior to reaching an advanced age may cause chronic or permanent damage to regions of the brain regulating cognitive ability, including primary and secondary memory.[21] A curious relationship in the development of neurodegeneration following trauma to the brain has been reported by many authors, i.e., that head injury is a strong risk factor for the development of Alzheimer's disease. However, several studies have indicated that head trauma is also a risk factor for vascular dementia, a condition that is characterized by infarcts of large or small brain vessels.[22,23] If these findings are correct, cerebral blood flow could be an important determinant of whether neurodegeneration results from acute brain injury in the elderly, since both Alzheimer's disease and vascular dementia are more prevalent in this age-group. Cerebral blood flow impairment could explain, at least in part, the increased vulnerability of neurons in the elderly subject who sustains a brain injury, since the more we age, the less blood flow reaches the brain. Nerve cells that receive less blood flow are more susceptible to developing metabolic energy dysfunction, a condition that may accelerate apoptotic necrotic cell-death pathways. The levels of cerebral blood flow during the acute period following head injury in the older subject may determine the neurologic and physiologic outcome in these individuals who have an additional age-related burden of a lowered cerebral perfusion prior to their injury.[24]

Clinical studies have suggested that age is an important predictor of pathologic sequelae following head injury. For example, increased cerebral blood flow or hyperemia is commonly found in children and young adults after traumatic brain injury but much less so in adults over the age of 40. Experiments in rodents have confirmed the above clinical observation. Rats exposed to a concussive brain injury reacted to increased cerebral blood flow when they were young, but aged rats showed a marked decreased in cerebral perfusion in the area of impact.[25] In similar experiments in rats exposed to brain trauma a progressive loss of cortical tissue associated with enlargement of the ventricles occurred during a 12-month observation period.[26] These rodents showed progressive atrophy of cortical and hippocampal neurons leading to neurodegenerative changes after a year's time.[26] These findings suggest that trauma can induce progressive neuronal damage that does not appear to stabilize soon after the injury and that a window of treatment opportunity even days after traumatic brain injury may arrest further extension of neuronal damage and eventual neurodegeneration.

Another factor that may lead to neurodegeneration after head injury is the accumulation of the excitatory neurotransmitters glutamate and aspartate.[27] The traumatized elderly brain shows an enhanced vulnerability to excitotoxic damage from these neurotransmitters, possibly because of reduced blood flow and metabolic compromise that leads to increased neuronal atrophy and death.[28] Interestingly, the N-methyl-D-aspartate (NMDA) receptor, which modulates glutamate entry into brain cells after brain trauma, appears to be more sensitive in early life, whereas non-NMDA receptors may be more active during aging and may play a greater role in the development of neurodegeneration in the elderly.[28]

CEREBRAL HEMODYNAMICS AFTER BRAIN TRAUMA

The subject of cerebrovascular resistance (CVR) brought on by progressive fibrosis and loss of vessel elasticity has been studied in the elderly.[29] In older subjects, CVR appears greatest in the distribution of the middle cerebral artery and least in vessels located in the cerebellar–brain stem region.[29] It also affects those blood vessels that show a tendency toward arteriosclerosis, such as the middle cerebral artery and the terminal extension of the carotid artery in the brain. The most susceptible vessels to CVR in the elderly are the small cerebral arteries and arterioles ranging from 50 to 500 μm in diameter, in contrast to the larger diameter vessels, which normally do not play a role in CVR.

A physiologic link between age-related increases in arterial vessel stiffness and blood pressure can result in increases in CVR.[30] Moreover, elevation of CVR in association with arterial stiffness appears to be inversely related to blood volume, stroke volume, and cardiac output in the elderly.[31] Pulse pressure also increases with aging.[32] These factors will maximize traumatic brain injury in older patients and generally involve reductions in the cerebral metabolic rate of oxygen, cerebral blood flow levels, glucose metabolic rate, and cerebral arteriovenous oxygen differences.[33] Consequently, severe hemodynamic disturbances in the brain of injured, older subjects is certain to create a more serious outcome than in similarly injured younger persons. This conclusion is reinforced by statistics gathered in the Trauma Coma Data Bank, which indicate that motor-sensory recovery in younger subjects is substantially greater than that in the older age-group.[34–41] On examination of categories ranging from good recovery to vegetative state or death for all age-groups following severe head trauma, the worst outcomes in terms of survival or neurologic deficits were observed in the 55–65 age-group and the best outcome was observed among the 16 to 25-year-olds (Fig. 18–1).[35–41]

Improvements of cerebral perfusion and autoregulation following severe head trauma have been shown to correlate positively with preservation of cognitive capacity.[42] For this reason, age-related cognitive impairment will

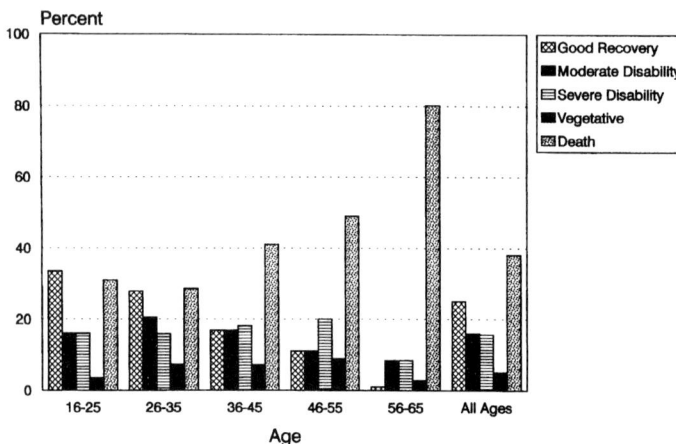

Figure 18–1. Glasgow Coma Scale as a function of increasing age. Bars show increase in death risk and vegetative state following traumatic brain injury in subjects ranging in age from 45 to 65 as compared to ages 16–45. From this scale, it can be seen that 80% of patients 56 years or older died from their trauma within 6 months post-injury in contrast to 40% at age 45 or less. Statistics from the Traumatic Coma Data Bank. [Modified from Jane JA, Francel PE. Age and outcome of head injury. In: Narayan RK, Willberger J, Povlishock JT, eds. Neurotrauma. McGraw-Hill, 1995: 793–804.]

be more severe in elderly individuals who may already show 15%–20% reduced blood flow to the brain due to their advanced age. Cerebral metabolic rates have been mapped out for glucose (CMRGlu) and oxygen ($CMRO_2$) in conscious elderly subjects using positron emission tomography (PET). Specific brain regions can be studied with PET using markers such as ^{15}O for $CMRO_2$ and ^{18}F-fluoro-2deoxy-D-glucose for CMRGlu activities.[43–45]

Since glucose is normally the sole substrate for cerebral energy metabolism and oxygen is required for oxidative phosphorylation and the formation of ATP, their metabolism in brain can reflect functional neuronal activity in relation to aging. By carefully screening healthy and asymptomatic elderly subjects to measure $CMRO_2$ and CMRGlu in brain activity, comparisons with these levels in age-matched individuals with a variety of organic brain disorders can be made. The range of $CMRO_2$ and CMRGlu levels for healthy elderly subjects can also be compared with those in other population groups for differences according to age, sex, race, nutrition, and demographics.

Most studies in which $CMRO_2$ in normal aging has been examined have concluded that oxygen utilization is reduced in most brain regions of the cerebral cortex.[46–50] One study has reported no changes in oxygen metabolism in healthy elderly individuals.[51] The $CMRO_2$ reduction in healthy aged subjects may be related to the decreased gray and white matter cerebral perfusion that generally occurs in the regions of low oxygen utilization.[50] Consequently, the age-related decline in cerebral blood flow observed in the elderly would presumably affect cerebral oxygen transport and eventual neural tissue utilization, a finding that has been amply confirmed using PET, and these changes are severely pronounced in the demented patient.[52,53] The $CMRO_2$ appears to positively correlate with cerebral blood flow and negatively correlate with blood viscosity. A study of elderly subjects with various types of polycythemia (increased red cell production and low $CMRO_2$) accompanied by reduced cerebral blood flow revealed that following phlebotomy, blood viscosity gradually decreased. The reduction in blood viscosity was sufficient to increase regional cerebral blood flow and $CMRO_2$ in these patients.[54]

There is no general agreement as to whether CMRGlu is affected in healthy, asymptomatic aged persons. Studies have shown either a decrease in regional CMRGlu activity in normal elderly brains[45,52,55] or no changes.[56–58] Since the metabolism of glucose involves countless anaerobic and aerobic pathways with the production of a variety of substrates, its rate of utilization may vary widely among different neuronal populations that have different energy requirements. Another factor that may explain the different findings for CMRGlu in normal aged brain, in contrast to those for $CMRO_2$ is the fact that glucose delivery to neurons requires a transporter at the blood–brain barrier level (Glut 1) and another transporter to deliver glucose to neurons (Glut 3), whereas oxygen transport is facilitated by diffusion through the blood–brain barrier.[59,60]

Alavi et al.[61] found a 26% reduction of glucose metabolism in psychometrically normal elderly subjects aged 72 years, compared to a control group 22 years of age. Overall, it has been shown that there is a reduction in CMRGlu of approximately 25% that which may occur with normal cerebral aging.[62,63] During hypoxia/ischemia of the brain, the elderly patient almost always suffers more extreme and prolonged changes in $CMRO_2$ and CMRGlu than the younger adult, and this effect results in a worse neurologic outlook with respect to morbidity and mortality.[64] These vascular insults can result in occlusive infarcts, encephalic hemorrhage, and dementia. All three conditions can severely affect the older subject in terms of cerebral blood flow, brain energy metabolism, and neuronoglial homeostasis.[65]

Other hemorhelogical changes that occur in the elderly individual can have an important impact on the evolution and outcome of severe head injury. Besides the normal reduction in cerebral blood flow seen during aging, studies show that normal elderly individuals also develop a rise in blood viscosity, fibrinogen, plasma viscosity, red cell rigidity, brain degradation products, and activation of the coagulating system. These factors all contribute to further reduce and impede blood flow circulation.[66] Increased blood and plasma viscosity is known to reduce cerebral perfusion whereas a high fibrinogen level is the most important marker for impending myocardial infarction. Red cell rigidity will reduce microcirculation and impede normal oxygen dissociation from hemoglobin, thus reducing oxygen availability to neurons. Hypercoagulability is also associated with reduced brain perfusion. Such hemorheologic events, as well as increased prevalence of diabetes mellitus and hypertension present in older people, will create a vulnerable and grim outlook in the presence of even mild brain trauma. Since cerebral blood flow and neuronal metabolism are tightly coupled, a reduction in flow will likely increase neuronal demand for essential nutrients whereas a lowering of metabolic activity will result in a stepped-up flow delivery as supply tries to meet demand.[67]

The neuropathology of brain trauma for all adults can be classified as primary or secondary, depending on the relationship between the time of injury and the development of pathologic events.[68] *Primary impact injury* includes epidural hematoma, skull fracture, brain confusion, and laceration, and intracerebral hemorrhage including subdural hematoma, diffuse axonal injury and diffuse vascular injury. *Secondary injury* entails hypoxia-ischemia, increased intracranial presuure, cerebral edema, and infectious agents.

DIFFUSE AXONAL INJURY

A considerable amount of research using animal and human postmortem brain tissues has demonstrated that diffuse axonal injury (DAI) can occur very quickly after brain trauma. This type of injury is characterized by axons injured in continuity, generally by shearing forces during acceleration–deceleration and rotational forces of the head. The morphologic and reactive changes of DAI in humans has been largely defined from controlled studies using animal models.[69–73] It has long been known that following brain trauma, DAI is more pronounced and has more severe consequences in the older population than in other age-groups.[74] The elderly are consequently doubly cursed by their increased risk of falling and their higher risk of sustaining brain injury after a fall.[71]

Diffuse axonal injury is characterized histologically by axonal swellings termed "axonal retraction balls," which can be seen microscopically using silver staining (Fig. 18–2). Other useful markers in the diagnosis of DAI

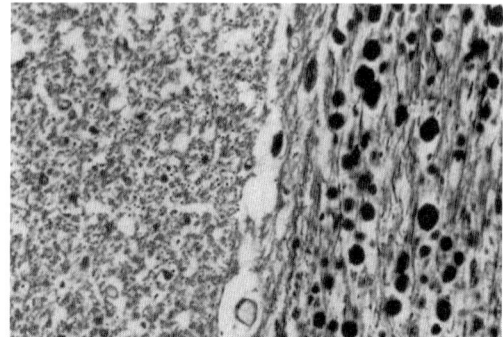

Figure 18–2. Brain stem axonal bulbs seen on the right are characteristic of diffuse axonal injury. These lesions are commonly found in brain stem structures involving medial lemnisci, central tegemental and corticospinal tracts, and in parasagittal white matter, corpus callosum, internal capsule, and deep gray matter. See also Figure 18–3. Palmgren, ×360. [From Graham DI. Neuropathology of head injury. In: Narayan RK, Willberger J, Povlishock JT, eds Neurotrauma. McGraw Hill, 1995: 47, with permission.]

include immunocytochemical staining for Aβ protein (most commonly found in Alzheimer's disease).[75,76] This protein may even be present before axonal retraction ball formation, which generally require 24 hr after trauma to be detected.[77,78] Ubiquitin and synaptophysin immunostaining are additional diagnostic markers for DAI, which can reveal increased numbers of axonal swellings over that seen with traditional silver or hematoxylin-eosin staining.[76,77] Microglial and astrocytic immunomarkers such as CD68 for the former and glial fibrillary acidic protein (GFAP) for the latter can also aid in the diagnosis of DAI.[79,80]

The brain regions most affected by DAI are the corpus callosum and the dorsolateral quadrant of the upper brain stem.[81] For neuropathologic grading purposes, DAI grade 1 involves the white matter of the cerebral hemispheres, corpus callosum, brain stem, and sometimes the cerebellum; in grade 2, there is additionally a focal lesion of the corpus callosum; grade 3 involves the dorsolateral quadrant(s) of the rostral brain stem (Fig. 18–3). When white matter is severely reduced from DAI, ventricular enlargement can develop and continue for a long period in the vegetative patient.[82]

Neuroradiologically, DAI can be diagnosed

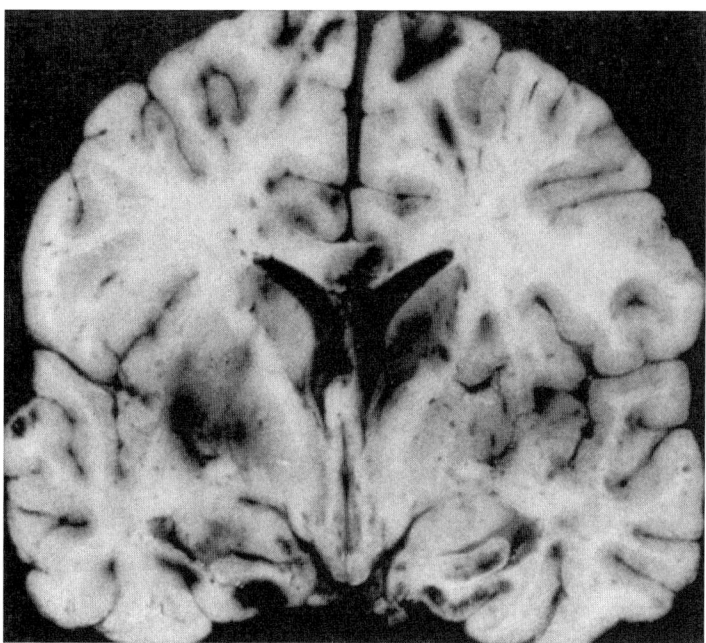

Figure 18–3. Diffuse axonal injury. Note the hemorrhagic lesion in the corpus callosum and the bilateral "gliding" contusions in the parasagittal areas. Small hematomas are seen in the right caudate nucleus and left lentiform nucleus with small hemorrhages scattered throughout the anteromedial regions of each medial lobe. [From Graham DI. Neuropathology of head injury. In: Narayan RK, Willberger J, Povlishock JT, eds. Neurotrauma. McGraw-Hill, 1995:46, with permission.]

acutely using computed tomography (CT) scans, which reveal characteristic punctate hemorrhages measuring <10 mm at gray–white junctions, and in upper brain stem, corpus callosum, and basal ganglia regions (Fig. 18–3).[83] Magnetic resonance (MR) imaging can detect both hemorrhagic and nonhemorrhagic (gliotic scars) involving DAI as well as blood-breakdown products such as hemosidesin.[70] Because of its technical versatility, MR imaging can be used to diagnose recent and chronic brain lesions much more effectively than with CT scans.[70]

Biochemical in vivo assessment of DAI can be done using MR spectroscopy. Analysis of animal data using MR spectroscopy shows that DAI has profound effects on intracellular metabolism of the white matter soon after experimental head injury. Severe metabolic disturbance is indicated by the presence of increased brain tissue levels of N-acetylaspartate (NAA), a marker of neuronal death, and by reduction in the high-energy metabolite phosphocreatine.[26,54,85]

The most likely cause of the initial loss of consciousness and development of coma following severe injury to the brain is DAI. There is also evidence that DAI may be responsible for the severe disability associated with the vegetative state following head injury.[72]

It is not clear why DAI is more devastating for elderly patients who sustain brain trauma than for younger subjects with similar injury. Since the DAI injury involves a shearing force that induces small blood vessel damage and hemorrhage in the brain, along with tearing and stretching of nerve fibers, it would be expected, at least from a neuropathologic (rather than clinical) point of view, that both young and old patients would have a similar neurologic and anatomic outcome. However, the elderly have a less compliant cerebrovascular distensibility than younger subjects because of an increase in the collagen/elastin ratio of blood vessels (COX). When the collagen/elastin ratio is increased, arterial walls tend to stiffen.[86–89] In addition, elderly patients with hypertension, cerebrovascular insufficiency, or increased vascular resistance resulting from vessel noncompliance may have dysfunctional endothelial cell elastin and smooth muscle, which are the distensible components of the arterial wall.[86–89] This phenomenon could explain the increased vulnerability to DAI and coma in older subjects.

EXCITOTOXICITY AFTER BRAIN TRAUMA

Glutamate is an excitatory neurotransmitter that appears to be most involved in neuronal secondary damage after brain injury. When large concentrations of this amino acid are released as a result of brain trauma, neurons may be chronically or permanently damaged.[90] High extracellular glutamate buildup is the key to excitotoxicity and cell death.[91] Excessive opening of the glutamate NMDA-operated ion channels and voltage-sensitive Ca^{2+} channels is believed to be responsible for excessive intracellular Ca^{2+} accumulation, which can trigger immediate cell death or progressive degeneration lasting hours or days.[92–94] This process has been aptly described as "delayed neuronal death."

Excitotoxic injury after brain trauma is characterized by axon-sparing dendritic damage that targets neuronal populations that are more vulnerable than others to glutamate-induced cytolysis.[28,95,96] Experimental animal data have shown that increased glutamate release occurs after induction of a subdural hematoma, resulting in reduced cerebral blood flow.[97,98] Since the development of acute subdural hematoma worsens the prognosis of head injury in older patients, this correlation between glutamate activity and brain blood flow becomes more clinically meaningful in the geriatric population sustaining a head injury. It should be pointed out that authors of biomechanical studies of rapid deceleration of parasagittal bridging veins, which often cause subdural hematomas as well as the "lucid period" many patients show after such subdural hematoma injury, argue in favor of an intracerebral mass lesion and not diffuse axonal injury as the cause of this pattern injury.[72,97]

Evidence that glutamate could be partly responsible for the secondary injury involved after brain trauma in older adults has stimulated a great deal of research in the search for NMDA receptor antagonists and blockers of glutamate and Ca^{2+}. However, the therapeutic window for NMDA receptor antagonists in animals is <60 min and it is likely that a similar time-related limit is also operable in humans. So far, no human therapy has been approved in the United States for glutamate antagonists.

Elderly patients who develop regional or global cerebral ischemia have a worse outcome than those subjects with normal cerebral perfusion. When cerebral blood flow reaches a critical threshold, defined as 18 ml/100 g/min or less flow, neuronal damage of ischemic-sensitive neurons may follow.[98] It has been shown that massive glutamate release is associated with sustained cerebral blood flow decline below the threshold required for neuronal damage in head injured humans.[99] This correlate would be most prevalent in the geriatric patient.

CLOSED HEAD INJURIES

Closed head injuries are usually associated with blunt trauma to the head. In the elderly they originate mainly from falls, vehicular accidents, and assault; the skull is not fractured. Blunt trauma can lead to epidural or subdural hematoma (Fig. 18–4). Epidural hematomas classically arise in the temporal fossa from laceration of the middle meningeal artery or dural sinus and are associated generally with skull fracture, but not always. Subdural hematomas occur from tearing of a bridging vein from the cortex to the sinus, although sometimes cortical arteries may be the source of bleeding.[100] When these mass-occupying lesions measure >5 cm on the radiograph, displacement of intracranial structures across the midline and compression or effacement of the

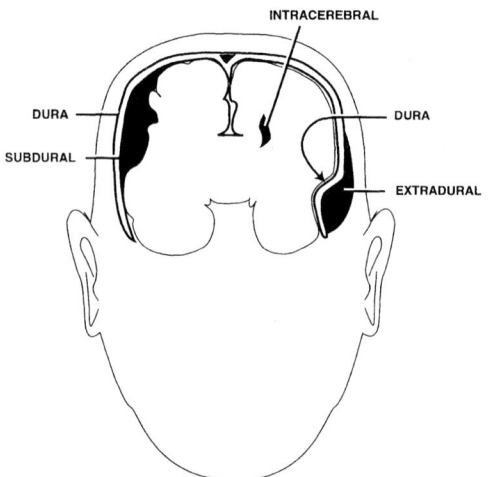

Figure 18–4. Various locations of traumatic intracranial hematomas. The clinical significance of such injuries in the elderly are discussed in the text.

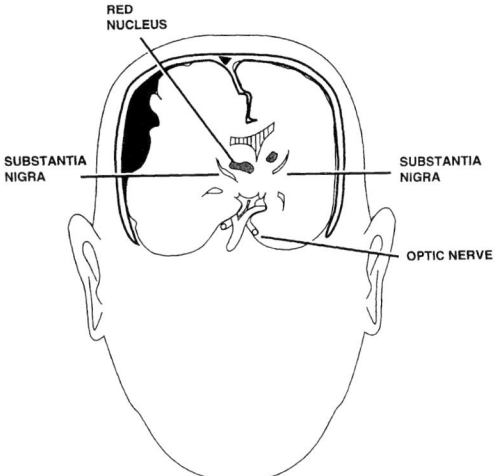

Figure 18–5. Schematic representation of an expanding intracranial hematoma. Note that displacement of midbrain (substantia nigra, red nucleus, third ventricle) can result in decerebrate rigidity. Direct compression of the cortex can result in contralateral motor and reflex changes. Displacement of midline structures and uncus of temporal lobe can lead to loss of consciousness. Stretching of the oculomotor nerve (beneath posterior cerebral artery) produces oculomotor palsy with dilation of pupil. Sketch illustrates a subdural clot. The physiological outcome is essentially similar, regardless of whether the clot lies in the epidural space or occupies the the space intracranially.

basal cisterns can occur (Fig. 18–5).[101] This condition constitutes a surgical emergency requiring immediate evacuation to relieve intracranial pressure (ICP) and brain swelling.[102] Contusions (bruises) of the brain are generally associated with small petechial hemorrhages in the area of the contusion.[103] This creates a mixture of blood and parenchyma, giving a "salt and pepper" appearance on CT scans.[103] Depending on the extensiveness and depth of the contusion, the blood-brain barrier may be focally disrupted, leading to infarction and further bleeding. This condition can be mistaken for an intracerebral hematoma.

OPEN HEAD INJURIES

Open or "penetrating" brain injuries can result from practically any trauma involving fracture of the skull, including gunshot wounds, which in some areas of the world have become more common than falls or automobile accidents.[104] Adult and elderly patients with penetrating skull injuries are at risk for seizures, infections, hematomas, and abscess formation as well as extensive injury of cerebral vessels and intracranial contents.[105]

Fractures of the skull may be linear (80% of cases), comminuted, or depressed (Fig. 18–6). Linear fractures occur when there is elastic deformation of the skull and generally result from falls or vehicular accidents. Depressed fractures occur when a sufficient force collapses the bone at the site of impact, for example, from a bullet or high-velocity traveling object. Comminuted fractures of the skull can occur from a slow-moving object with high kinetic energy. This type of impact can result in comminuted radial fractures extending outward from the lesion site.

The severity of closed and open head injuries can be classified in a number of ways, but the most widely used method is the Glasgow Coma Scale (GCS) (Table 18–1). This scaling system provides a rapid, simple, and generally reproducible assessment of the level of consciousness of the head-injured patient.[68] Injury severity can be categorized into three levels with the GCS numbering system that ranges from 15 (normal) to 3 (vegetative state): mild head injury, 13–15; moderate head injury, 12–9; and severe head injury, 8–3. These categories can provide useful prognostic information about the patient and can assess the relative success of a given therapy following brain trauma.[106,107] However, the GCS cannot measure crucial age-related variables of head trauma including cerebral perfusion pressure, cerebral flood flow, ICP, heart rate, and arterial oxygen saturation. Aged patients should have the above parameters monitored when even mild head trauma is present because of their increased vulnerability to head trauma and the presence of possible aggravating factors such as use of medication that may increase bleeding or thrombosis. Other conditions such as cardiac, pulmonary, renal, and liver disease can worsen the outcome of head injury in the elderly.

It has been estimated that 70% of the deaths due to falls occur in the older age population.[108] A mortality rate of 85% has been recorded for patients age 65 and over who sustain a head injury classified as a GCS 9 or less[109] in contrast to a rate of 50% for age-groups of 45–55.[20] Many older patients with fall-related injuries tend to develop acute subdural hematomas more commonly than

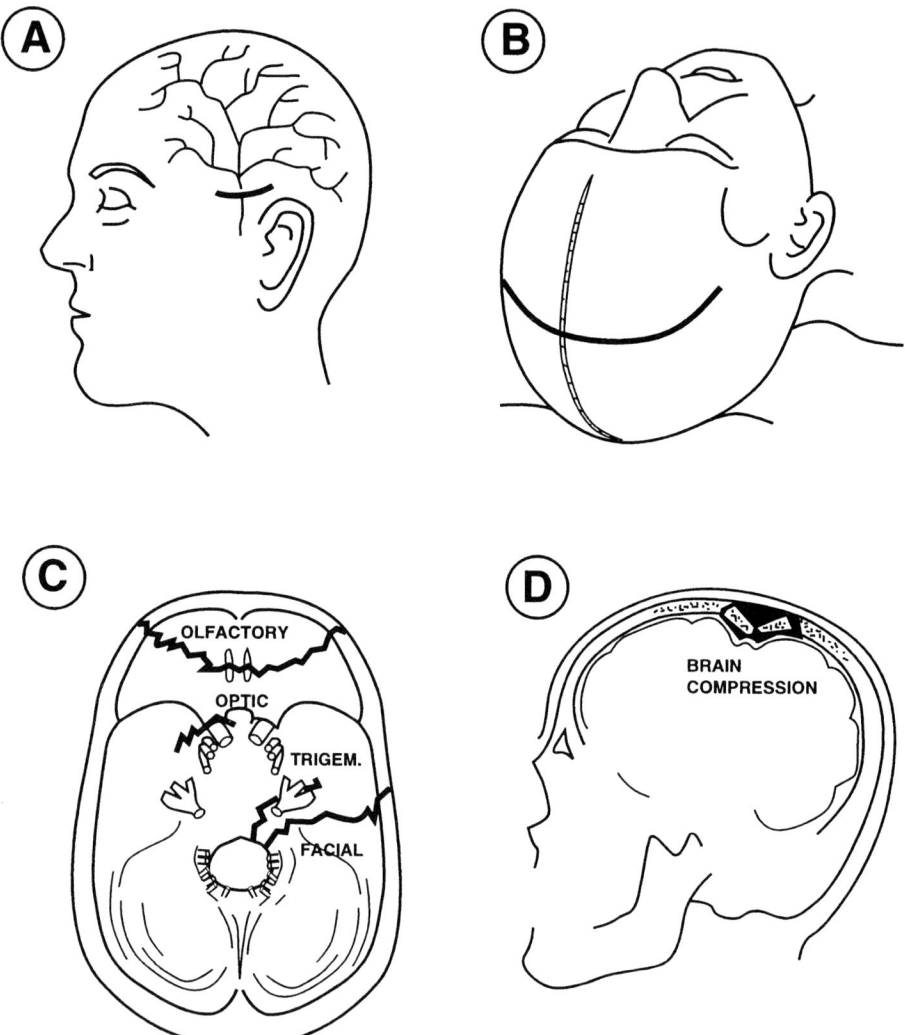

Figure 18–6. Fractures whose outcome may result in neural damage. *A.* Fracture line crosses middle meningeal artery (bold line), which can lead to extradural hematoma. *B.* Fracture crossing superior longitudinal (sagittal) sinus, which can cause tear leading to subdural hematoma (or more rarely, to extradural hematoma). *C.* Basilar fractures involving one or more cranial nerves. Four common fracture locations are shown. *D.* Depressed fracture showing inward displacement of bone with direct cerebral compression. Such fractures tend to extensively disrupt inner table of the skull more than the outer table.

extradural hematomas.[110] The reason is that the dura is often found adhering to the skull with advanced age and the brain can shrink leaving a potential space for blood to collect following concussive head trauma.[111] Since subdural hematomas have a worse prognosis than extradural hematomas, the mortality rate is bound to be greater in the older than the younger age-group.[111,112] Hypertension or hypotension in the brain-injured elderly subject can significantly reduce cerebral perfusion, while age-related cognitive difficulties often complicate and delay proper diagnosis.[42,113,114]

A recent study concluded that traumatic brain injury reduces significantly the time of onset in the development of Alzheimer's disease in those persons at risk.[115] These studies are of interest for three reasons:

1. The elderly may be more prone to hippocampal damage secondary to head in-

Table 18–1. Glasgow Coma Scale

Eye Opening
4 = Spontaneously
3 = To voice
2 = To pain
1 = None

Verbal Response
5 = Oriented
4 = Confused
3 = Inappropriate words
2 = Incomprehensible sounds
1 = None

Motor Response
6 = Follows commands
5 = Localizes to pain
4 = Withdrawal to pain
3 = Abnormal flexion
2 = Abnormal extension
1 = None

The Glasgow Coma Scale is used in assessing initial severity of traumatic brain injury and the subsequent course of the injury. The scale can be used to obtain a rough estimate of prognosis. Coma grades 3–5 are considered potentially fatal, particularly when accompanied by absence of oculovestibular responses and fixed pupils. Grades 3–8 are considered severe and are accompanied by loss of consciousness. Grades 9–15 correlate with increasing chances of good recovery. See text for details.

jury due to lower age-related cerebral perfusion.
2. The hippocampal CA1 region is linked in part to cognitive failure in Alzheimer's disease.
3. Head injury is a major risk factor for development of Alzheimer's disease.[116–120]

The collective findings above indicate that levels of cerebral blood flow in humans can be a positive or negative factor in the outcome of brain trauma and in the possible development of cognitive impairment or even Alzheimer's dementia. It is well known that head injury usually involves a reduction in regional or global cerebral blood flow. Aging also has a tendency to retard cerebrospinal fluid outflow, a condition that can result in hydrocephalus during brain swelling secondary to trauma.[121] Since normal elderly subjects develop cerebral perfusion decline associated with increased aging, monitoring of cerebral blood flow may be one of the best ways to assess, manage, and treat patients who sustain head trauma. For this purpose, Tc-99m single-photon emission computed tomography (SPECT) of the traumatized brain is a good choice because of its simplicity, sensitivity, and ability to record regional blood low changes.[122]

Studies have shown that when the (ICP) rises from non-missile head injury, hippocampal neuron damage, an area of the brain modulating memory and learning can undergo severe pathological changes even when the injury is not subjacent to the hippocampus.[82,96] Hippocampal neuron loss after traumatic brain injury may be due to the selective vulnerability of these nerve cells to hypoxia and ischemia.[88,123,124] In a study of 112 fatal head injuries, damage to the CA1 hippocampus was noted in 84% of the cases, 70% of these showing bilateral damage to the CA1 subfield.[109]

INTRACEREBRAL HEMATOMAS

Intracerebral hematomas arise from a torn vessel within the brain as a consequence of cerebral laceration or coalescence of petechrial hemorrhages following severe brain contusion. This space-occupying lesion can develop slowly over a period of days or weeks and can worsen the prognosis of the original traumatic insult. The symptoms and signs may be quite similar to those caused by a subdural hematoma, with progressive motor, sensory, reflex, speech, and visual changes and loss of consciousness, depending on the location of the hematoma. Indications for surgical evacuation depend on the size and location of the hematoma.[100] Lesions >5 cm in the frontal, occipital, or right temporal lobe are surgically accessible, however, there may be little benefit from evacuating deep hematomas, especially those subserving motor activity and speech. Many deep hematomas may become absorbed in time or may leave a harmless cystic cavity in communication with the ventricle. Delayed intracranial hematomas in the elderly are important because, in many cases, early treatment can limit secondary brain injury. The diagnosis can be made using CT scans or a newer technique, near-infrared spectroscopy, which in some cases can detect this lesion before a change in neurological status, a change in the CT scan, or an increase in ICP occurs.[125] Near-infrared spectroscopy is a noninvasive, direct, and continuous method of monitoring cerebral oxygenation (oxyhemoglobin/deoxyhemoglobin ratio) and cerebral blood volume that can be used to reliably detect changes in cerebral hemodynamics, particularly those seen after traumatic brain injury.[126]

TREATMENT

Elderly patients with head injury need effective and rapid treatment to prevent secondary neuronal damage and permanent neurologic impairment. Despite a considerable amount of research on potential pharmacotherapy for head injury, no effective compound has been found that is truly effective in limiting or reversing neuronal damage after brain trauma.

Standard treatments include use of osmotic diuretic agents, such as glycerol, urea, and mannitol[127] for the control of ICP. Osmotic agents also lower blood viscosity, which may be higher than normal in older patients. Mannitol is commonly administered to lower ICP but unfortunately repeated doses can induce hyperosmolar states that render it ineffective and potentially dangerous in inducing acute renal failure.[128] Additionally, high doses of mannitol can result in a rebound effect where ICP becomes higher than before treatment. Steroids have been used widely in the past to treat head injury, but many studies have shown it to be ineffective in reducing ICP or improving outcome.[129–134] Use of tirilazad, a non-glucocorticoid-21-amino steroid, showed great promise during animal experiments as a strong anti-oxidant and inhibitor of lipid peroxidation-induced free radicals. However, tirilazad was not demonstrated to be effective in human head injury trials.[135] Another highly touted anti-oxidant, polyethylene-glycol–conjugated superoxide dismutase (PEG-SOD), was reported to be ineffective in a multicenter trial[136] for severe head injury. Treatment with PEG-SOD has previously shown promise in limited clinical studies.[137]

Barbiturate therapy was originally suggested as a possible treatment for reducing ICP,[138,139] but subsequent prospective studies reported no improvement in outcome and a dangerous tendency of this agent to produce hypotension. This is a strict control indication in the elderly population,[140,141] who are more apt to develop severe hypotension, given their normally lower age-related decline in cerebral blood flow rate. Barbiturates could also worsen cardiovascular compromise by inducing hypotensive episodes, a condition also more likely to be found in the geriatric patient.[142] Other pharmacological agents that have been proposed as possible treatment for head injury include calcium channel blockers, prostaglandin metabolites, and anti-inflammatory compounds. However, none have shown consistent clinical efficacy.

Several promising agents have been tested clinically after extensive animal data indicated their potential in head injury treatment. CP-0127 (Bradycor) has been reported to prevent secondary brain swelling in 10 of 11 patients treated subsequent to mild brain trauma[29] (GCS 12). This agent acts predominantly on the bradykinin-2 receptor, which may prevent tissue inflammatory reaction, and the production of excessive free radicals,[143] which can further damage compromised neurons.

Another compound that has been tested for severe closed head injury is dimethyl sulfoxide. Dimethyl sulfoxide has three properties that may be useful in managing the elderly brain trauma patient: (1) it increases cerebral blood flow without altering blood pressure;[144–146] (2) it reduces intracranial pressure quickly without a rebound effect;[147–149] and (3) it is a potent diuretic that does not affect cardiac rate or output.[144,146] Twenty patients with a GCS of 8 or less (in coma) were treated intravenously with dimethyl sulfoxide and all showed a quick reduction in ICP after treatment.[149,150] The ICPs ranging from 40 to 130 mm Hg were reduced to normal within 6 days of treatment with dimethyl sulfoxide and the GCS returned to normal (15) or near normal (13) in all but three patients.[149,150] These results indicate that restoration of cerebral perfusion pressure without affecting blood pressure or cardiac function may be a key element in the successful management of the older patient with trauma to the brain.

In summary, traumatic brain injury in the elder subject involves a cascade of cellular and molecular events that can lead to apoptotic or necrotic neuronal death pathways.[151] Although many factors can influence the neurologic outcome and mortality, advanced age is generally a negative influence on recovery. Head injury therapy, aimed specifically at the somatic vulnerabilities of the aged, needs to be developed with some urgency in view of the changing demographics and extended life span of this population group in the next two decades.

REFERENCES

1. Stuss DT, Stethem LL, Picton TW, Leech EE, Pelchat G. Traumatic brain injury, aging and reaction time. Can J Neurol Sci 1989; 16:161–.
2. Nusbaum NJ. How do geriatric patients recover from surgery? South Med J 1996; 89:950–.
3. Zwimpfer TJ, Moulton RJ. Neurologic trauma concerns. Crit Care Clin 1993; 9:727–.
4. Dayan AD. Quantitative histological studies on the aged human brain. I. Senile plaques and neurofibrillary tangles in "normal" patients. Acta Neuropathol 1970; 16:85–.
5. Coleman PD, Flood DG. Neuron numbers and dendritic extent in normal aging and Alzheimer's disease. Neurobiol Aging 1987; 8:521–.
6. Colon EJ. Quantitative cytoarchitectonics of the human cerebral cortex. Psychiatr Neurol Neurochir 1971; 74:291–.
7. Haug H. Nervous tissue. In: Weibel ER, ed. Stereological Methods, Vol. 1: Practical Methods for Biological Morphometry. London: Academic Press, 1979: 311–322.
8. Haug H. The evaluation of cell densities and of nerve-cell size distribution by stereological procedures in a layered tissue (cortex cerebri). Microsc Acta 1979; 82: 147–.
9. Meier-Ruge WR. Morphometric methods and their potential value for gerontological brain research. Top Gerontolo 1988; 25:90–.
10. Haug H, Barmwater U, Eggers R, Fischer D, Kuhl S, Sass NL. Anatomical changes in aging brain: morphometric analysis of the human prosencephalon. In: Cervos-Navarro J, Sarkander HI, eds. Brain Aging: Neuropathology and Neuropharmacology. New York: Raven Press, 1983:1–12.
11. Haug H. Macroscopic and microscopic morphometry of the human cortex. A survey in the light of new results. Brain Pathol 1984; 1:123–.
12. Morrison JH, Huf PR. Life and death of neurons in the aging brain. Science 1997; 278:412–419.
13. Stadtman ER. Protein oxidation and aging. Science 1992; 257:1220–1224.
14. Long JM, Kalehua AN, Muth NJ, Hengemihle JM. Stereological analysis of astrocyte and microglia in aging mouse hippocampus. Neurobiol Aging 1998; 19: 497–.
15. West MJ, Coleman PD, Flood D, Troncoso JC. Differences in the pattern of hippocampal neuron loss in normal aging and Alzheimer's disease. Lancet 1994; 344:769–.
16. de la Torre JC, Cada C, Nelson N, Gonzalez-Lima F. Reduced cytochrome oxidase and memory dysfunction after chronic brain ischemia in aged rats. Neurosci Lett 1997; 223:165–.
17. Finch CA Neuron atrophy during aging: programmed or sporadic? Trends Neurosci 1993; 16:104–.
18. Simic G, Kostovic I, Winblad B, Bogdanovic N. Volume and number of neurons of the human hippocampal formation in normal aging and Alzheimer's disease. J Comp Neurol 1997; 379:482–.
19. Cruz-Sanchez FF, Moral A, Tolosa E, de Belleroche J, Rossi ML. Evaluation of neuronal loss, astrocytosis and abnormalities of cytoskeletal components of large motor neurons in the human anterior horn in aging. J Neural Transm 1998; 105:689–.
20. Jane JA, Francel PC. Age and outcome of head injury. In: Narayan RK, Willberger J, Povlishock JT, eds. Neurotrauma. New York: McGraw-Hill, 1996:793–804.
21. Klein M, Houx PJ, Jolles J. Long-term persisting cognitive sequelae of traumatic brain injury and the effects of age. J Nerv Ment Dis 1996; 184:459–.
22. Sulkava R, Erkinjuntti T, Palo J. Head injuries in Alzheimer's disease and vascular dementia. Neurology 1984; 35:1804–.
23. Katzman R, Aronson M, Fuld P, Kawas C. Development of dementing illness in an 80-year old cohort. Ann. Neurol 1989; 25:317–.
24. Kelly DF, Martin NA, Kordestani R. Cerebral blood flow as a predictor of outcome following traumatic brain injury. J Neurosurg 1997; 86:633–.
25. Biagas KV, Grundl PD, Kochanek PM, Schiding JK. Posttraumatic hyperemia in immature, mature, and aged rats: autoradiographic determination of cerebral blood flow. J Neurotrauma 1996; 13:189–.
26. Smith, DH, Cecil KM, Meaney DF, Chen X, McIntosh T, Gennarelli TA. Magnetic resonance spectroscopy of diffuse brain trauma in the pig. J Neurotrauma 1998; 15:665–.
27. Kotwica Z, Jakubowski JK. Acute head injuries in the elderly: an analysis of 136 consecutive patients. Acta Neurochir 1992; 118:98–.
28. Olney JW. Excitotoxin-mediated neuron death in youth and old age. Prog Brain Res 1990; 86:37–.
29. Narotam PK, Rodell TC, Nadvi SS. Traumatic brain contusions: a clinical role for the kinin antagonist CP-0127. Acta Neurochir 1998; 140:793–.
30. Roberts J, Turner N. Age-related changes in autonomic function of catecholamines. In: Rothstein M, ed. Review of Biological Research in Aging, Vol. 3. New York: Alan R, Liss 1987: 257–298.
31. Tanaka H, Dinenno FA, Hunt BE, et al. Hemodynamic sequelae of age-related increases in arterial stiffness in healthy women. Am J Cardiol 1998; 82: 1152–.
32. Van Bortel LM, Spek JJ. Influence of aging on arterial compliance. J Hum Hypertens 1998; 12:583–.
33. Martin NA, Patwardhan RV, Alexander MJ, Africk C, Lee JH, Shalmon E. Characterization of cerebral hemodynamic phases following severe head trauma: hypoperfusion, hyperemia, and vasospasm. J Neurosurg 1997; 87:9–.
34. Bonica JJ. The Management of Pain, 2nd. ed. Philadelphia: Lea & Febiger, 1989.
35. Buhler FR, Burkart F, Lutold BE, Kung M, Marbet G, Pfisterer M. Antihypertensive beta-blocking action as related to renin and age: a pharmacologic tool to identify pathogenetic mechanisms in essential hypertension. Am J Cardiol 1975; 36:653–669.
36. Bush TL, Miller SR, Criqui MH, Barrett-Connor E. Risk factors for morbidity and mortality in older population: an epidemiological approach. In: Hazzard

WR, Andres R, Bierman EL, Blass JP, eds. Principles of Geriatric Medicine and Gerontology, 2nd ed. New York: McGraw-Hill, 1990:125–137.
37. Cain WS, Stevens JC. Uniformity of olfactory loss in aging. Ann NY Acad Sci 1989; 561:29–38.
38. Carlin RK, Siekevitz P. Plasticity in the central nervous system: do synapses divide? Proc Natl Acad Sci USA 1983; 80:3517–3521.
39. Bertoni-Freddari C, Fattoretti P, Paoloni R, Caselli U, Galeazzi L, Meier-Ruge W. Synaptic Structural Dynamics and aging. In: Meier-Ruge W, ed. Gerontology. New York: Karger Publishers, 1996:170–180.
40. Coleman PD. Neuron numbers and dendritic extent in normal aging and Alzheimer's disease. Neurobiol Aging 1987; 8:521–.
41. Conroy C, Kraus JF. Survival after brain injury: cause of death, length of survival, and prognostic variables in a cohort of brain-injured people. Neuroepidemiology 1988; 7:13–.
42. Terayama Y, Meyer JS, Kawamura J. Cognitive recovery correlates with long-term increases of cerebral perfusion after head injury. Surg Neurol 1991; 36:335–.
43. Baron JC, Marchal G. Vieillessement cérébral et cardiovasculaire et metabolisme énergétique, cérébral. Presse Med 1992; 21:1231–1237.
44. Baron JC, Rougemont D, Soussaline F. Local interrelationships of cerebral oxygen consumption and glucose utilization in normal subjects and in ischemic stroke patients: a positron tomography study. J Cereb Blood Flow Metab 1984; 4:140–149.
45. Grady C. Quantitative comparison of measurements of cerebral glucose rate made with two positron cameras. J Cereb Blood Flow Metab 11:A57–A63.
46. Leenders KL, Perani D, Lammertsma AA. Cerebral blood flow, blood volume and oxygen utilization; normal values and effect of age. Brain 1990; 113:27–47.
47. Lenzi GL, Frackowiak RSJ, Jones T. CMRO2 and CBF by oxygen-15 inhalation technique. Eur Neurol 1981; 20:285–290.
48. Marchal G, Rioux P, Petit-Taboue MC. The effects of optimally healthy aging on cerebral oxygen metabolism, blood flow and blood volume in humans: a PET study. J Cereb Blood Flow Metab 1991; 11 (Suppl. 2): S785.
49. Pantano P, Baron JC, Lebrum-Grandie P, Duguesnoy N, Boussen M, Comar G. Regional cerebral blood flow and oxygen consumption in human aging. Stroke 1984; 15:635–641.
50. Yamaguchi T, Kanno I, Uemura K. Reduction in regional cerebral metabolic rate of oxygen during human aging. Stroke 1986; 17:1220–1228.
51. Itoh M, Hatazawa J, Miyazawa H. Stability of cerebral blood flow and oxygen metabolism during normal aging. Gerontology 1990; 36:43–48.
52. Frackowiak RSJ, Lenzi GL, Jones T, Heather JD. Quantitative measurement of regional cerebral blood flow and oxygen metabolism in man using 15O and positron emission tomography: theory, procedure, and normal values. J Computer Assist Tomogr 1980; 4: 727–736.
53. Frackowiak RSJ, Pozzilli C, Legg NJ. Regional cerebral oxygen supply and utilization in dementia: a clinical and physiological study with oxygen-15 and positron tomography. Brain 1981; 104:753–778.
54. Shirakura T, Kubota K, Tamura K. Blood viscosity and cerebral blood flow in the aged. Jpn J Geriatr 1993; 30:174–181.
55. Pawlik G, Heiss WD, Beil C, Wienhard K, Herholtz K, Wagner K. PET demonstrates differential age dependence, asymmetry and response to various stimuli of regional brain glucose metabolism in healthy volunteers. J Cerebr Blood Flow Metab 1987; 7 (Suppl. 1):S376.
56. de Leon M, George AE, Tomanelli J. Positron emission tomography studies of normal aging: a replication of PET III and 18F FDG using PET VI and 11-CDG. Neurobiol Aging 1987; 8:319–323.
57. Duara R, Grady C, Haxby J. Human brain glucose utilization and cognitive function in relation to age. Ann Neurol 1984; 16:702–713.
58. Junck L, Moen JG, Bluemlein I. Cerebral glucose metabolism in normal aging studied with PET. J Cerebr Blood Metab 1989; 9 (Suppl. 1):S524.
59. Kalaria RN, Harik SI. Reduced glucose transporter at the blood–brain barrier and cerebral cortex in Alzheimer's disease. J Neurochem 1989; 53:1083–1088.
60. Stewart RR, Morrazzi CA. Oxygen transport in the human brain: analytical solutions. Adv Exp Med Biol 1973; 37:843–.
61. Alavi A. Regional cerebral glucose metabolism. In: Hoyer S, ed. Aging and Senile Dementias as Determined by 18-F-deoxyglucose and Positron Emission Tomography. Berlin: Springer-Verlag, Exp Brain Res 1982; (Suppl. 5):187–195.
62. Dastur DK. Cerebral blood flow and metabolism in normal human aging, pathological aging, and senile dementia. J Cereb Blood Flow Metab 1985; 5:1–9.
63. Kuhl DE. Effects of human aging on patterns of local cerebral glucose utilization determined by the 18F fluorodeoxyglucose method. J Cerebr Blood Flow Metabol 1982; 2:163.
64. Vinters HV. Vascular diseases. In: Duckett S, ed. Pathology of the Aging Human Nervous System, 1st ed. Philadelphia: Lea & Febiger, 1991:20–76.
65. de la Torre JC. Cerebrovascular changes in the aging brain. Adv Cell Aging Gerontol 1997; 2:77–107.
66. Ajmani RS, Rifkind JM. Hemorheological changes during human aging. Gerontology 1998; 44:111–.
67. Yamaguchi T, Kanno I, Uemura K. Reduction in regional cerebral metabolic rate of oxygen during human aging. Stroke 1986; 17:1220–.
68. Teasdale G, Jennett B. Assessment of coma and impaired consciousness: a practical scale. Lancet 1974; 2:81–.
69. Gennarelli TA, Thiebault L, Adams J.H. Diffuse axonal injury and traumatic coma in the primate. Ann Neurol 1982; 12:564–.
70. Parizel PM, Ozsarlak J, Van Goethem JW, van den Hauwe L. Imaging findings in diffuse axonal injury after closed head trauma. Eur Radiol 1998; 8:960.
71. Abou-Hamden A, Blumbergs P, Scott G, Manavis J, Wainwright H, Jones N. Axonal injury in falls. J Neurotrauma 1997; 14:699–.
72. Gennarelli TA, Thiebault LE. Biomechanics of acute subdural hematoma. J Trauma 1982; 22:680–.
73. Mc Anderson R, Opeskin K. Timing of early changes in brain trauma. Am J Forensic Med Pathol 1998; 19: 1–.
74. Adams, JH, Doyle D, Ford I. Diffuse axonal injury in head injury: definition, diagnosis and grading. Histopathology 1989;15:49–.

75. Gultekin SH, Smith TW. Diffuse axonal injury in craniocerebral trauma. A comparative histologic and immunohistochemical study. Arch Pathol Lab Med 1994; 118:168–.
76. Adams JH, Doyle D, Ford I, Brain damage in fatal non-missile head injury in relation to age and type of injury. Scott Med J 1989; 34:399–.
77. Sherriff FE, Bridges LR, Sivaloganathan S. Early detection of axonal injury after human head trauma using immunocytochemistry for beta-amyloid precursor protein. Acta Neuropathol 1994; 87:55–.
78. Koszyca B, Blumbergs PC, Manavis J, Wainwright H, James R. Widespread axonal injury in gunshot wounds to the head using amyloid precursor protein as a marker. J Neurotrauma 1998; 15:675–.
79. Geddes JF, Vowles GH, Beer TW, Ellison DW. The diagnosis of diffuse axonal injury: implication for forensic practice. Neuropathol Appl Neurobiol 1997; 23:339–.
80. Bodjarian N, Jamali S, Boisset N, Tadie M. Strong expression of GFAP mRNA in rat hippocampus after a closed-head injury. Neuroreport 1997; 8:3951–.
81. Shigemori M, Kikuchi N, Tokutomi T, Ochiai S, Kuramoto S. Coexisting diffuse axonal injury (DAI) and outcome of severe head injury. Acta Neurochir Suppl 1992; 55:37–.
82. Graham DI, Adams JH, Doyle D, Teasdale GM, Lawrence AE. Ischemic brain damage is still common in fatal non-missile head injuries. J Neurol Neurosurg Psychiatry 1989; 52:346–.
83. Lee TT, Galarza M, Villanueva PA. Diffuse axonal injury (DAI) is not associated with elevated intracranial pressure (ICP). Acta Neurochir 1998; 140: 41–.
84. Ross BD, Ernst T, Kreis R. 1H MRS in acute traumatic brain injury. J Magn Reson Imaging 1998; 8: 829–.
85. Cecil KM, Hills EC, Sandel ME, Smith DH, McIntosh TK, Mannon LJ. Proton magnetic resonance spectroscopy for detection of axonal injury in the splenium of the corpus callosum of brain-injured patients. J Neurosurg 1998; 88:795–.
86. Shimokawa H. Endothelial dysfunction in hypertension. J Atheroscler Thromb 1998; 4:118–.
87. Abrahamson OR. Recent studies in the structure and pathology of basement membranes. J Pathol 1986; 149:257–.
88. de la Torre JC. Cerebrovascular changes in the aging brain. Adv Cell Aging Gerontol 1997; 2:77–.
89. de la Torre JC. Effects of aging on the human nervous system. In: Principles, Practice and Perspectives in Geriatric Surgery. New York: Springer-Verlag, (in press).
90. Hovda DA, Lee SM, Smith ML. The neurochemical and metabolic cascade following brain injury: moving from animal models to man. J Neurotrauma 1995; 12: 903–.
91. Lynch DR, Dawson TM. Secondary mechanisms in neuronal trauma. Curr Opin Neurol 1994; 7:510–.
92. Clark GD. Pharmacology of glutamate neurotoxicity in cortical cell culture: attenuation by NMDA antagonist. Clin Perinatol 1989; 16:459–.
93. Meldrum B, Garthwaite J. Excitatory amino acid neurotoxicity and neurodegenerative disease. Trends Pharmacol Sci 1990; 11:379–.
94. Orrenius S, McConkey DJ, Bellomo G, Nicotera P. Role of Ca^{2+} in toxic cell killing. Trends Pharmacol Sci 1989; 10:281–.
95. Auer RN, Siesjo BK. Biological differences between ischemia, hypoglycemia, and epilepsy. Ann Neurol 1988; 24:699–.
96. Graham DI, Ford I, Adams JH. Ischaemic brain damage associated with tissue hypermetabolism in acute subdural hematoma: reduction by a glutamate antagonist. Acta Neurochir Suppl 1990; 51:277–.
97. Graham DI. Neuropathology of head injury. In: Narayan RK, Willberger J, Povlishock JT, eds. Neurotrauma. New York: McGraw Hill, 1996:43–59.
98. Bullock R, Butcher SP, Chen MH, Kendall L. Correlation of the extracellular glutamate concentration with extent of blood flow reduction after subdural hematoma in the rat. J Neurosurg 1991; 74: 794–.
99. Zauner A, Bullock R, Kuta AJ, Woodward J, Young HF. Glutamate release and cerebral blood flow after severe human head injury. Acta Neurochir Suppl 1996; 67:40–.
100. Becker DP. Common themes in head injury. In: Becker DP, Gudeman SK, eds. Textbook of Head Injury. Philadelphia: W.B. Saunders, 1989:1–22.
101. van Dongen KJ, Braakman R, Gelpke GJ. The prognostic value of computerized tomography in comatose head-injured patients. J Neurosurg 1983; 59: 951–.
102. Gade GF, Becker DP. Surgical management of acute head injuries. In: Schmiedek HH, Sweet WH, eds. Operative Neurosurgical Techniques: Indications, Methods and Results. Philadelphia: W.B. Saunders, 1988:19–31.
103. Ribas GC, Jane JA. Traumatic contusions and intracerebral hematomas. J Neurotrauma 1992; 9 (Suppl. 1): S265–.
104. Levy ML, Masri LS, Levy KM, Johnson FL. Penetrating craniocerebral injury resulting from gunshot wounds: gang-related injury in children and adolescents. Neurosurgery 1993; 33:1018–.
105. Day JD, Levy LM, Giannotta SL. The management of penetrating vascular injuries. Neurosurg Clin. North Am 1995; 6:799–.
106. Signorini DF, Andrews PJ, Jones PA, Wardlaw J, Miller JD. Predicting survival using simple clinical variables: a case study in traumatic brain injury. J Neurol Neurosurg Psychiatry 1999; 66:20–.
107. Signorini DF, Andrews PJ, Jones PA, Wardlaw J, Miller JD. Adding insult to injury: the prognostic value of early secondary insults for survival after traumatic brain injury. J Neurol Neurosurg Psychiatry 1999; 66:26–.
108. Duthie EH, Jr. Falls. Med Clin North Am 1989; 73: 1321–.
109. Kotapka MJ, Graham DI, Adams JH, Gennarelli TA. Hippocampal pathology in fatal non-missile human head injury. Acta Neuropathol 1992; 83:530–.
110. Black DW. Subdural haematoma: a retrospective study of the 'great neurologic imitator'. Postgrad Med 1985; 78:107–.
111. Traynelis VC. Chronic subdural hematoma in the elderly. Clin Geriatr Med 1991; 7:583–.
112. O'Brien DP, Phillips JP. Chronic subdural haematomata and head injury in the elderly. Ir J Med Sci 1994; 163:162–.
113. Brooks J, Fos LA, Greve KW, Hammond JS. As-

sessment of executive function in patients with mild traumatic brain injury. J Trauma 1999; 46:158–.
114. Keefover RW. Aging and cognition. Neurol Clin 1998; 16:635–.
115. Mayeux R Ottman R, Tang M, Noboa-Bauza L, Marder K. Genetic susceptibility and head injury as risk factors for Alzheimer's disease among community-dwelling elderly persons and their first-degree relatives. Ann Neurol 1993; 33:494–.
116. Gedye A, Beattie BL, Tuokko H, Horton A. Severe head injury hastens age of onset of Alzheimer's disease. J Am Geriatr Soc 1989; 37:970–.
117. Graves AB, White E, Koepsell TD, Reifler BV. The association between head trauma and Alzheimer's disease. Am J Epidemiol 1990; 131:491–.
118. Mortimer JA, van Duijn CM, Chandra V, Fratiglioni L, Graves AB. Head trauma as a risk factor for Alzheimer's disease: a collaborative re-analysis of case-control studies. Int J Epidemiol 1991; 20(Suppl.):S28–.
119. Molgaard CA Stanford EP, Morton D. Jr, Ryden LA. Epidemiology of head trauma and neurocognitive impairment in a multi-ethnic population. Neuroepidemiology 1990; 9:233–.
120. Nemetz PN, Leibson C, Naessens JM, Beard M, Kokmen E. Traumatic brain injury and time to onset of Alzheimer's disease: a population-based study. Am J Epidemiol 1999; 149:32–.
121. Albeck MJ, Skak C, Nielsen PR, Olsen KS. Age dependency of resistance to cerebrospinal fluid outflow. J Neurosurg 1998; 89:275–.
122. Dormehl IC, Jordaan B, Oliver DW, Croft S. SPECT monitoring of improved cerebral blood flow during long-term treatment of elderly patients with nootropic drugs. Clin Nucl Med 1999; 24:29–.
123. Ng T, Graham DI, Adams JH, Ford I. Changes in the hippocampus and the cerebellum resulting from hypoxic insults: frequency and distribution. Acta Neuropathol 1989; 78:138–.
124. Pulsinelli WA. Selective neuronal vulnerability: morphological and molecular characteristics. Prog Brain Res 1985; 63:29–.
125. Gopinath SP, Robertson CS, Contant CF, Narayan RK. Early detection of delayed traumatic intracranial hematomas using near-infrared spectroscopy. J Neurosurg 1995; 83:438–.
126. Kerr ME, Marion D, Orndoff PA, Weber BB, Sereika SM. Evaluation of near infrared spectroscopy in patients with traumatic brain injury. Adv Exp Med Biol 1998; 454:131–.
127. Biestro A, Alberti R, Galli R, Cancela M, Soca A. Osmotherapy for increased intracranial pressure: comparison between mannito and glycerol. Acta Neurochir 1997; 139:725–.
128. Stuart F, Torres E, Fletcher R, Crocker D, Moore FD. Effects of single, repeated, and massive mannitol infusion in the dog: structural and functional changes in kidney and brain. Ann Surg 1970; 172:190–.
129. Wise B, Perkins R, Stevenson E. Penetratiion of 14C-labelled mannitol from serum into cerebrospinal fluid and brain. Exp Neurol 1964; 10:264–.
130. Dearden NM, Gibson JS, McDowal DG, Gibson RM. Effect of high-dose dexamethasone on outcome from severe head injury. J Neurosurg 1986; 64:81–.
131. Gudeman S, Miller J, Becker D. Failure of high-dose steroid therapy to influence intracranial pressure in patients with severe head injury. J Neurosurg 1979; 51:301–.
132. Marshall L, King J, Langfitt T. The complications of high-dose corticosteroid therapy in neurosurgical patients: a prospective study. Ann Neurol 1997; 1:201–.
133. Miller J, Leech P. Effects of mannitol and steroid therapy on intracranial volume pressure relationships in patients. J Neurosurg 1975; 42:275–.
134. Saul T, Ducker T, Salcmon M, Carro E. Steroids in severe head injury. A prospective, randomized clinical trial. J Neurosurg 1981; 54:596–.
135. Marshall LF, Maas AI, Marshall SB, Bricolo A. A multicenter trial on the efficacy of using tirilazad mesylate in cases of head injury. J Neurosurg 1998; 89:519–.
136. Young B, Runge JW, Waxman KS, Harrington T. Effects of pegorgotein on neurologic outcome of patients with severe head injury. A multicenter, randomized controlled trial. JAMA 1996; 276:538–.
137. Muizelaar JP, Marmarou A, Young HF, Choi SC, Wolf A, Kontos HA. Improving the outcome of severe head injury with oxygen radical scavenger polyethylene glycol-conjugated superoxide dismutase: a phase II trial. J Neurosurg 1993; 78:375–.
138. Shapiro HM, Galindo A, Wyte SR, Harris AB. Rapid intraoperative reduction of intracranial pressure with thiopentone. Br J Anaesth 1973; 45:1057–.
139. Clasen RA, Pandolfi S, Casey DJ. Furosemide and pentobarbital in cyrogenic cerebral injury and edema. Neurology 1974; 42:642–.
140. Ward J, Becker D, Miller J, Choi SC, Marmarov A. Failure of prophylactic barbiturate coma in the treatment of severe head injury. J Neurosurg 1985; 62:383–.
141. Schwartz M, Tator C, Rowed D, Reid SR, Meguro K. The University of Toronto Head Injury Treatment Study: a prospective, randomized comparison of pentobarbital and mannitol. Can J Neurol Sci 1984; 11:434–.
142. Eisenberg H, Frakowiak R, Contant C, Marshall L, Walker MD. Comprehensive central nervous system trauma centers: high-dose barbiturate control of elevated intracranial pressure in patients with severe head injury. J Neurosurg 1988; 69:15–.
143. Francel PC Bradykinin and neuronal injury. J Neurotrauma 1992; 9:527–.
144. Camp PE, James HE, Werner R. Acute dimethyl sulfoxide therapy in experimental brain edema: Part 1. Effects on intracranial pressure, blood pressure, central venous pressure and brain water and electrolyte content. Neurosurgery 1981; 9:28–.
145. Mullan S, Jafar J, Brown FD. Dimethyl sulfoxide in management of postoperative hemiplegia. In: Wilkins RH, ed. Cerebral Arterial Spasm. Baltimore: William & Wilkins, 1980:646–653.
146. Brown FD, Johns L, Mullan S. Dimethyl sulfoxide in experimental brain injury, with comparison to mannitol. J Neurosurg 1980; 53:58–.
147. Del Bigio M, James HE, Camp PE, Paxton HD. Acute dimethyl sulfoxide therapy in brain edema. Part 3. Effect of a 3 hour infusion. Neurosurgery 1982; 10:86–.
148. Waller FT, Tanabe CT, Treatment of elevated intracranial pressure with dimethyl sulfoxide. Ann NY Acad Sci 1983; 411:286–292.

149. Kulah A, Akar M, Baykut L. Dimethyl sulfoxide in the management of patients with brain swelling and increased intracranial pressure after severe closed head injury. Neurochirurgia 1990; 33:177–.
150. Karaca M, Bilgin U, Akar M, de la Torre JC. Dimethyl sulfoxide lowers ICP after closed head trauma. Eur J Clin Pharmacol 1991; 40:113–
151. Graham DL, McIntosh TK, Maxwell WL, Nicoll JA. Recent advances in neurotrauma. J Neuropathol Exp Neurol 2000; 59:641–651.

19. Infectious Diseases

LEILA CHIMELLI

The elderly and the very young are more susceptible to infections than individuals 10 to 60 years old. The heightened susceptibility of the elderly to infection is most likely a reflection of the age-associated decline in the competence of the immune system, particularly cell-mediated immunity and antibody response to an immunogen.[1,2] The major systemic defect accompanying the aging process that promotes infections is a loss in integrity of delayed-type hypersensitivity mechanisms that are modulated by the lymphocyte–macrophage system. This is expressed as an age-related reduction in reactivity to delayed-type intradermal antigens, such as tuberculin, streptokinase-streptodornase, and candida. A defect in polymorphonuclear leukocyte functions also occurs with aging, characterized by a reduction in percentage of polymorphonuclears performing phagocytosis when exposed to microorganisms. The population of T cells is altered with advanced age and the efficiency of the monocyte/macrophage cells to destroy microbial invaders declines.

However, other components of cell-mediated immunity may be intact and at least 25% of old individuals have immune responses as vigorous as those of young adults.[2] According to Beeson,[3] apparently no clear evidence exists to support the concepts that host defense mechanisms are less effective in the elderly, or that immune surveillance becomes defective with aging. An increased incidence of morbidity and mortality resulting from infection in the elderly does exist, however, and this stems from many of the functional and anatomical deficits that accompany the aging process and predispose the elderly to infection. Among the structural changes, prostatic hypertrophy results in urinary stasis and proclivity to infection, as may uterine prolapse. Other examples of these degenerative problems are pulmonary hypoventilation, bronchopulmonary aspiration, and decreased mucociliary clearance among older persons. In addition to respiratory and urinary tract problems, immobility, thinning of skin and mucosal surfaces, malnutrition, neoplastic diseases, digestive disorders (intestinal diverticula, gall stones), diabetes mellitus, peripheral vascular disease, and environmental exposure (from spending a greater portion of their lives in hospitals and nursing homes where they are subject to nosocomial infections) all predispose the elderly to infection by common extracellular microorganisms that are the normal flora of the mucosal and skin surfaces of the body. Older persons have a greater carriage rate of gram-negative bacteria in the oropharynx, which presumably plays a significant role in their apparent increased susceptibility to gram-negative pneumonia. Therefore, the occurrence of nidus for focal infections with subsequent spread to other organs is much more frequent in the older than in the younger population.

Poor nutrition also contributes to the vulnerability of elderly patients to infection. According to Chandra,[2] protein energy malnutrition and deficiencies of various nutrients impair several immune responses, especially cell-mediated immunity, and nutritional disorders are common in old age. Supplementation with a modest physiological amount of micronutrients improves immunity and decreases the risk of infection in old age. Such an intervention has led to a striking reduction in illness, a finding that is of considerable clinical and public health importance.

Among the infections with increased incidence in older patients, by far the most important are tuberculosis and pneumococcal pneumonia—both can complicate with meningitis. Other infections with increased incidence in the elderly that can affect the nervous system are cryptococcosis, histoplasmosis, and varicella-zoster infection. Patients who have been treated with chemotherapy and/or steroids for neoplastic disease, transplants, or other chronic diseases or who are deficient in complement or properdin also have an increased likelihood of developing central nervous system (CNS) infections.

In a series of autopsied patients in a University Hospital in Brazil over a 6-year period, 57 non-AIDS patients aged 60 years or more had infections in the CNS. Of these, 23 (40%) had bacterial acute meningitis; 20 (35%) had neurocysticercosis; 4 had micro abscesses due to infectious endocarditis, renal transplant, or septicemia; 3 had cryptococcal meningitis; 2 had cerebral abscesses due to bacterial endocarditis; 2 had neurotoxoplasmosis; 1 had lymphocytic meningitis; 1 had viral encephalitis; and 1 had neurosyphilis (L. Chimelli, unpublished observation).

BACTERIAL INFECTIONS

Meningitis

Bacterial meningitis remains one of the most feared infectious diseases because of its subtle onset and high mortality rate (38%–80% in older adults). More than 50% of all deaths from meningitis occur in persons age 60 and older. In the United States these older patients account for approximately 1000 to 3000 cases each year.[5] Although the incidence of meningitis is highest among infants during the first month of life, several large studies have documented a later peak of incidence among persons age 60 and older.

The most common bacterial pathogens responsible for the etiology of meningitis in older patients are *Streptococcus pneumoniae*, *Neisseria meningitidis*, *Listeria monocytogenes*, *Haemophilus influenza*, other gram-negative agents, *Staphylococcus aureus*, and other gram-positive agent.[5,6] Their poor prognosis is mainly due to the severity of the associated encephalitis responsible for the neurological sequelae and for mortality ranging from 20% to 30% in pneumococcal and Listeria meningitis.[6]

To assess the implications of meningitis in a more mature population, Gorse et al.[7] reviewed the records of patients with meningitis. In 71 patients aged 50 years and older, 54 (76%) had bacterial meningitis, 9 (13%) had granulomatous meningitis (7 cases were caused by *Mycobacterium tuberculosis*, 2 by fungi, *Cryptococcus neoformans* and *Coccidioides immitis*), and 8 (11%) had aseptic meningitis. Among the cases of bacterial meningitis in the older age-group, *Streptococcus pneumoniae* accounted for 24% (13/54) and enteric bacilli accounted for 17% (9/54). Serious complications occurred in 38 elderly patients (70%) with bacterial meningitis, and mortality occurred in 24 (44%).

Although meningitis typically presents with the abrupt onset of fever, headache, and meningismus, its presentation may be atypical in some older patients. When every minute counts, a delay in diagnosis has devastating consequences. Estimates of the incidence of meningitis in persons age 60 and older range from 2 to 9 per 100,000 per year.

Bacterial meningitis may result from the hematogenous spread of organisms to the CNS or from local extension to the subarachnoid space from regional colonization or local spread. It is one of the complications in the elderly with neurosurgical procedures. Once the organism reaches the cerebrospinal fluid (CSF), it encounters limited host defenses and bacteria can then proliferate markedly.

Gorse et al.[7] reviewed the underlying diseases and associated infections in 54 patients with bacterial meningitis. Neurological procedures occurred in 15 (28%), alcohol abuse in 12 (22%), sinusitis in 9 (17%), neoplastic disease and/or corticosteroid administration occurred in 9 (17%), and diabetes mellitus in 7 (13%) patients. Head trauma, cirrhosis and/or splenectomy, and a CSF leak were each identified in three patients (6%). Most of the postsurgical cases had gram-negative bacillary meningitis and two (one due to *Streptococcus agalactiae* and the other due to *Serratia marcencens*) had autopsy-proved endocarditis.

The resulting effects on the meninges and

brain lead to increased intracranial pressure and altered intracerebral vascular autoregulation. Complications may include cerebral ischemia or infarction, hydrocephalus, subdural effusion or empyema, and sagittal sinus or cortical vein thrombosis. Clinically, these intracerebral catastrophes can present as seizures, stroke syndromes, cranial nerve deficits, or persistent alteration in mental status. Among the 27 patients with bacterial meningitis who were 65 years of age or older, 12 (44%) died during the course of treatment. All 12 of these patients had one or more complication prior to death, and 11 (73%) of the 15 survivors also had complications during treatment. Thus, the complication rate in the subgroup aged 65 years or older was 85% (23/27). Complications included pneumonia, neurologic deficit, motor seizures, hydrocephalus, and urinary tract infection.[7] Therefore, prognosis is generally worse in the elderly than in the younger population. Enteric gram-negative bacillary meningitis was associated with a high mortality in the older patients. The incidence of acute and chronic morbidity is higher, partially because of the increased number of severe complications and underlying diseases.

Definitive diagnosis of meningitis relies on the interpretation of CSF studies—It is important to note the overlap in CSF findings of these meningeal syndromes. For example, early viral meningitis has findings that might be confused with early bacterial meningitis. Additionally, a lymphocytic CSF pleocytosis with an elevated protein and lowered glucose is compatible with tuberculous, fungal, or Listeria meningitis. These similarities in glucose, protein, and cell counts emphasize the need to define the causative organism by culture or serology. The CNS findings in meningitis due to various agents can be seen in Table 19–1.[5]

Macroscopically, the brain is swollen and congested. In hyperacute disease, when death occurs within 24 hrs, the exudate is very scanty. In patients who survive 2 days or longer, pus is first visible alongside meningeal veins (Fig. 19–1), and then a purulent, creamy exudate is seen over the cerebral hemispheres or the base of the brain or both.[8] The exudate associated with pneumococcal infections is particularly prominent over the cerebral convexities. The ventricles appear compressed by the swollen cerebral hemispheres or distended if the aqueduct has been obstructed by purulent material. Hemorrhagic infarcts are common and may be extensive.[9]

Histologically, the meningeal exudate contains large numbers of neutrophils, scattered macrophages, fibrin, and necrotic cellular debris. It extends along the perivascular spaces into the brain parenchyma, where bacteria are usually demonstrable (Fig. 19–2). Venous thrombosis and infarcts are often evident. Purulent material is usually seen in the choroid plexus and may also adhere to ventricular walls.[8,9]

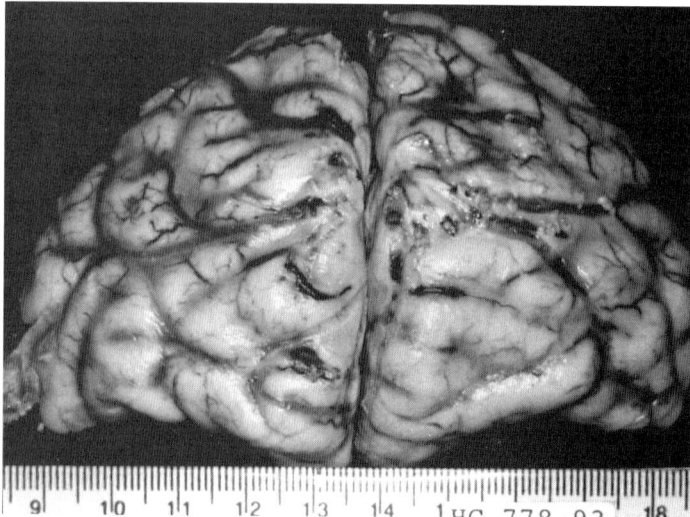

Figure 19–1. Bacterial meningitis. A purulent exudate is present alongside meningeal veins, which are severely congested.

Table 19–1. Cerebrospinal Fluid Findings in Meningitis of Various Causes, Compared with Normal Findings

Finding	Normal CSF	Acute Bacterial Meningitis	Viral Meningitis	Tuberculous Meningitis	Cryptococcal Meningitis
Opening pressure	6–20 cm H$_2$O	Usually elevated	Moderately elevated or normal	Usually elevated	Usually elevated
WBCs (per ml)	0–5 (about 85% lymphocytes)	Usually several hundred to >60,000; PMNs predominate	5 to a few hundred, only occasionally >1000; lymphocytes predominate, but may be > 80% PMNs in early stages	Usually 25–100, rarely >500; lymphocytes predominate, except in first few days, when PMNs may account for 60% of cells	Usually 0–800 (but very low or zero in patients with AIDS); usually lymphocytes predominate
Protein (mg/dl)	18–45	Usually 100–500, occasionally >1000	Normal or slightly elevated <100; may be higher in severe cases	Nearly always elevated; usually 100–200 but may be much higher in dynamic block	Usually 20–500 (average about 100)
Glucose (mg/dl)	45–80, or 0.6 times serum glucose	Usually 5–40, or <0.3 times serum glucose	Usually normal	Usually reduced; <45 in three-fourths of cases	Reduced in most cases; <30, or <0.3 times serum glucose
Other	For traumatic taps, add 1 WBC/ml and 1 mg/dl protein for each 1000 RBCs	Gram's stain positive in about 60–80% of cases	Usually not necessary to find specific causal virus	AFB-positive in <25%; culture positive in up to two-thirds of cases (but this takes 4 to 8 weeks)	CSF– or serum cryptococcal antigen–positive in about 95% of cases; India Ink–positive in 50% to 75%

AFB, acid-fast bacilli; CSF, cerebrospinal fluid; PMNs: polymorphonuclear neutrophils; WBCs: white blood cells.
Source: Adapted from Miller and Choi, 1997.[5]

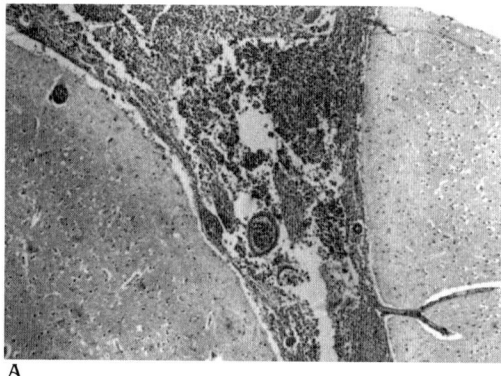

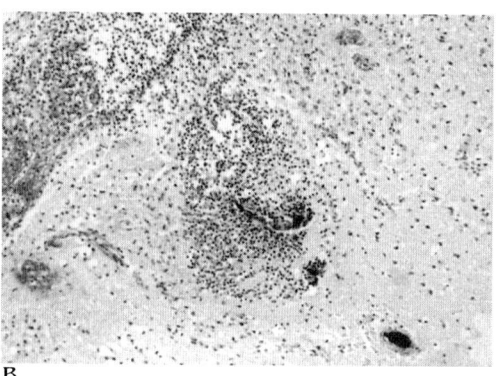

Figure 19–2. Meningeal neutrophilic exudate in a sulcus (A) and into the superficial cortex (B), where masses of bacteria can be seen. H&E.

Tuberculous Meningitis

Unquestionably, there has been a recent rise in the age at which active tuberculosis (TB) occurs. This relates in part to a greater prevalence of TB several decades ago, when today's old people were young; to some extent it reflects the higher proportion of people now living to old age. There is also a high rate of nosocomial infection with TB in elderly people residing in nursing home.[3] In fact, Stead et al.[10] reported that new infection with TB is an important risk factor for nursing home patients and that greater care should be taken to detect and treat new infections before the disease develops and the infection spreads. In developed countries where the disease is well controlled, TB is more common in adults than in children; the incidence of TB is high among ethnic groups (Asian, African, Caribbean, Latin American, American Indians), individuals who have spent time in chronic care facilities (refugee camps, prisons, nursing homes), the elderly, alcoholics, intravenous drug users, and patients whose immunity is impaired by long steroid or immunosuppressive treatment. Therefore, adults aged 65 and older of all socioeconomic backgrounds are among those most likely to develop active TB, and they may have atypical symptoms. In 1987, the TB case rate for the general U.S. population was 9.3 per 100,000, but among persons aged 65 and older it was more than twice that number—20.6 per 100,000.[11]

Potential predisposing factors for TB reactivation in the elderly are alcohol abuse, insulin-dependent diabetes mellitus, end-stage renal disease, hematological and reticuloendothelial malignant tumors, immunosuppressive therapy, prolonged corticosteroid therapy, radiation therapy to the thorax, rapid weight loss or malnutrition, sclerosis or coal worker's pneumoconiosis, and smoking. Investigations have also pinpointed the role of the human immunodeficiency virus (HIV) epidemic in the resurgence of TB. Extrapulmonary tuberculosis, including CNS disease, is considerably more frequent in the setting of HIV than it is otherwise, occurring in more than 70% of persons with TB and preexisting AIDS. No longer closer associated with primary childhood infection, most reported cases now occur in adults rather than children, with approximately equal case rates from age 20 to over age 65.[12]

Although tuberculous meningitis is not a common disease, its devastating nature and the difficulty in making a rapid diagnosis make it an important diagnosis to consider.[5] It is typically characterized by an insidious course and often a lack of frank meningeal signs. Cranial nerve deficits such as ophthalmoplegia or a facial droop may result; the clinical presentation also includes focal neurological signs, seizures, and altered mental status. Many patients have concomitant pulmonary TB. However, the clinical or radiographic presentation of TB in the older patient may be atypical or nonspecific, contributing to a delay in diagnosis and greater morbidity and mortality.

Skin testing is neither sensitive nor specific and is generally not helpful in the meningitis diagnosis. The CSF stains for acid-fast bacilli also have a low sensitivity (<25%). Multiple specimens of approximately 5 ml of CSF are recommended to increase the diagnosis yield.

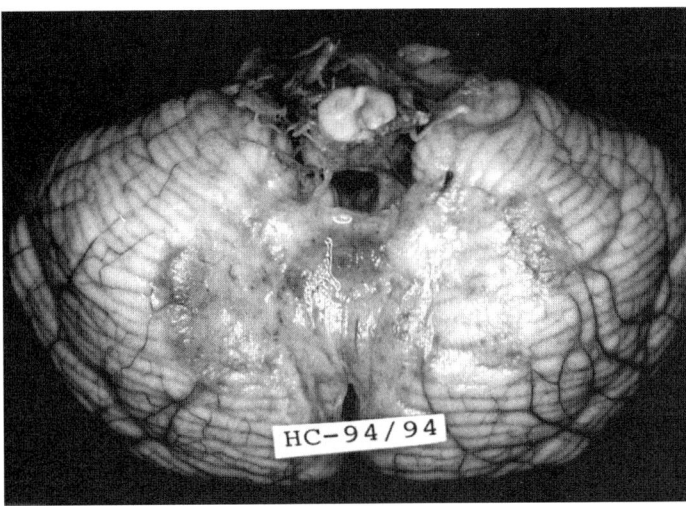

Figure 19–3. Tuberculous meningitis with thick subarachnoid exudate over the base of the cerebellum.

Cultures for the *Mycobacterium tuberculosis* usually take a minimum of 4 weeks to return, although newer diagnostic procedures, such as automated bacteriology in broth cultures, DNA probe identification, and polymerase chain reaction (PCR), may significantly decrease this interval. Mortality in most series is relatively high, reflecting both a lack of consideration of this diagnosis and a confusing early clinical course that may mimic viral, fungal, and other inflammatory disease of the CNS. Suspected cases should be treated with empiric antituberculous drugs that achieve therapeutic CSF concentrations until cultures results return.

Macroscopically, tuberculous meningitis is characterized by a gelatinous subarachnoid exudate. This may appear slightly nodular and is thickest in the Sylvian fissures, over the base of the brain (Fig. 19–3), and around the spinal cord. On sections there is similar exudate within the choroid plexus and lining the ventricles. Tubercles may be visible in the meninges, adjacent to sulcal veins and in the ventricular lining.

Microscopically, the meningeal and ventricular exudate contains lymphocytes, macrophages, and sparse plasma cells, admixed with necrotic material and fibrin. There may be accumulations of epithelioid cells and fibroblasts, multinucleated giant cells, and well-defined tuberculous granulomas with central caseous necrosis. Mycobacteria may be readily demonstrable or very sparse and may be absent in cases in which treatment has been initiated. In immunosuppressed patients the mycobacteria are usually numerous and the inflammation less granulomatous and without multinucleated giant cells. Meningeal vessels are involved by the inflammatory reaction resulting in vasculitis. The cells tend to infiltrate through the adventitia, into the media, and even the intima of the blood vessels, and granulomas can be seen in the vessel wall, which becomes thickened and even occluded by fibroblastic reaction (Fig. 19–4). Infarcts are therefore common, particularly in the superficial cortex.[8,9]

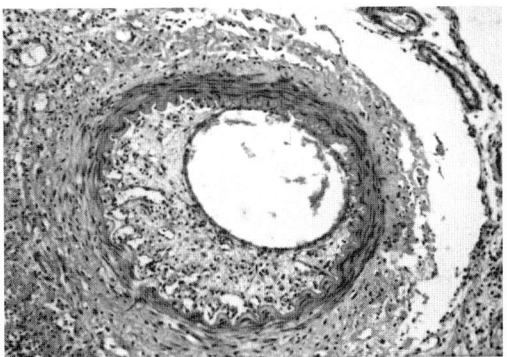

Figure 19–4. Tuberculous meningitis with mononuclear inflammatory infiltrate and fibroblastic reaction in a meningeal vessel wall. H&E.

Neurosyphilis

Although the late manifestations (gumma, aortic disease, CNS disease) usually develop in the age period between 30 and 50 years, routine serologic screening for syphilis in hospitalized patients shows a high prevalence of unsuspected infection in the elderly,[13] making unsuspected latent syphilis a common disorder in the elderly population. In addition, there is some evidence that syphilitic involvement of the CNS is more common in patients with concomitant HIV infection.

The different types of CNS involvement in syphilis are classified as follows.[8,9]

Syphilitic meningitis occurs 1–2 weeks after initial infection.

Meningovascular syphilis is due to a combination of chronic meningitis and multifocal arteritis. There is thickening and fibrosis of the leptomeninges, which rarely contain miliary gummas, and the brain may reveal infarcts. Histologically, the meninges contain scattered lymphocytes and plasma cells. The gummas, if present, resemble tubercles, and the arteritis is characterized by lymphocytic and plasma cell infiltration of the adventitia and media (Fig. 19–5) and concentric collagenous thickening of the intima, which eventually occludes the lumen.

General paresis is due to chronic meningoencephalitis. Macroscopically, the meninges are thickened and fibrotic and the underlying brain is firm and atrophic. Histologic analysis shows scanty meningeal and perivascular parenchymal aggregates of lymphocytes and plasma cells, moderate loss of cortical neurons, reactive gliosis, and striking proliferation of rod-shaped microglia. In a minority of cases, spirochetes are demonstrable in the cortex through silver impregnation.

Tabes dorsalis is due to chronic inflammatory disease of the dorsal roots and ganglia with associated degeneration of the posterior columns of the spinal cord. The peak incidence is 15 to 20 years after the initial infection. Morphologically, there is mild chronic inflammation in the fibrotic leptomeninges and dorsal root ganglia, a moderate loss of neurons from the dorsal root ganglia with an associated proliferation of satellite cells, and posterior column degeneration (Fig. 19–6). The changes are more marked in the lumbar region of the cord.

Gummatous neurosyphilis is a late manifestation of tertiary syphilis and only involves the CNS as solitary space-occupying lesions, which resemble tuberculomas. The central necrosis differs histologically because the reticulin is usually preserved.

Lyme Disease

This disease is caused by the spirochete *Borrelia burgdorferi*, which is transmitted by ticks. It is more common in northern temperate areas but has been reported in most parts of the world. Lyme disease is a multisystem disorder involving the skin, cardiovascular system, joints, and peripheral and central nervous systems. The lesions are largely caused by the inflammatory response to the spirochetes rather than the spirochetes themselves. Lymphoplasmacytic infiltrates and microglial nodules have been described in the brain. Because Lyme disease is usually not fatal, data from necropsy studies are very limited.[9]

Cerebral Complications of Infective Endocarditis in the Elderly

Subacute infectious endocarditis due to Streptococcus viridans has an early mortality rate of only 5%–10%, whereas acute prothectic valve endocarditis in an elderly patient with congestive heart failure can be fatal in up to 70% of cases. In elderly patients, neurologic manifestations tend to be more common as a

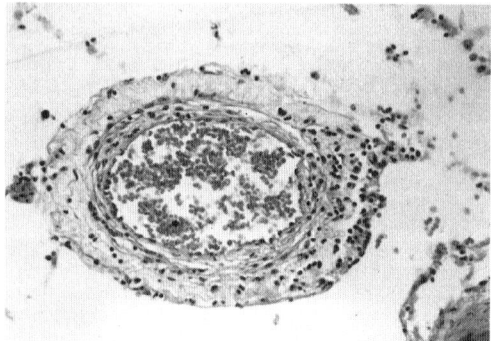

Figure 19–5. Meningovascular syphilis with lymphocytic and plasma cell infiltration of the adventitia and collagenous thickening of the meningeal vessel. H&E.

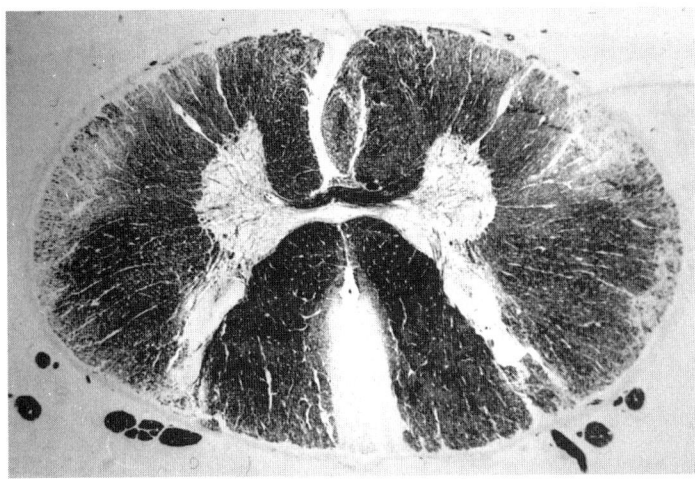

Figure 19-6. Posterior column degeneration in a case of tabes dorsalis [Courtesy of Prof. F. Scaravilli, London]

presenting clinical sign of infectious endocarditis. Purulent meningitis, parenchymal microabscesses (Fig. 19-7), and large, well-formed abscesses, usually containing clusters of bacteria, are the most frequent morphological findings.[14]

Cerebral Abscesses

These abscesses, caused by hematogenous spread in adults, are usually due to septic emboli, often from bronchiectasis, a lung abscess, or subacute endocarditis. Those caused by direct spread may be due to septic focus in the paranasal sinus, middle ear, or dental root. Other antecedents of brain abscesses include cranial trauma, neurosurgery, and immunodeficiency. Brain abscesses may present with headache, fever, epilepsy, nausea, and vomiting, altered sensorium, nuchal rigidity, or localized neurologic signs. Poor prognostic factors include extremes of age (the very young or very old), an altered sensorium at presentation, or concomitant systemic infections. The mortality rate is approximately 20%.

Abscesses caused by hematogenous spread of infection tend to occur at junctions between gray and white matter (Fig. 19-8) and are often multiple. Although any cerebral lobe can be involved, the perfusion territory of the middle cerebral arteries is usually involved. These abscesses consist of a purulent center surrounded by a capsule, which gradually thickens. Histologically, early lesions show focal suppurative encephalitis. Small foci of necrosis develop rapidly, which soon enlarge and become confluent. Early encapsulation is seen by days 5-7, characterized by early granulation tissue around the margins of the necrotic tissue, which is followed by proliferation of fibroblasts and progressive collagen deposition over subsequent weeks, thickening the capsule. The surrounding brain tissue is edematous and contains swollen astrocytes.[9]

PROTOZOAL INFECTIONS

Amebic Infections

In humans, cerebral lesions are produced by *Entamoeba histolytica* and free-living amebas.

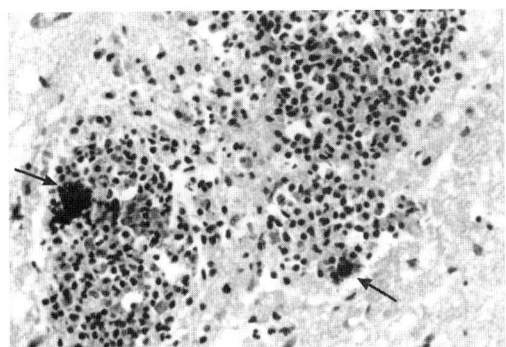

Figure 19-7. Microabscess containing masses of bacteria (arrows) in the white matter of a patient with infectious endocarditis. H&E.

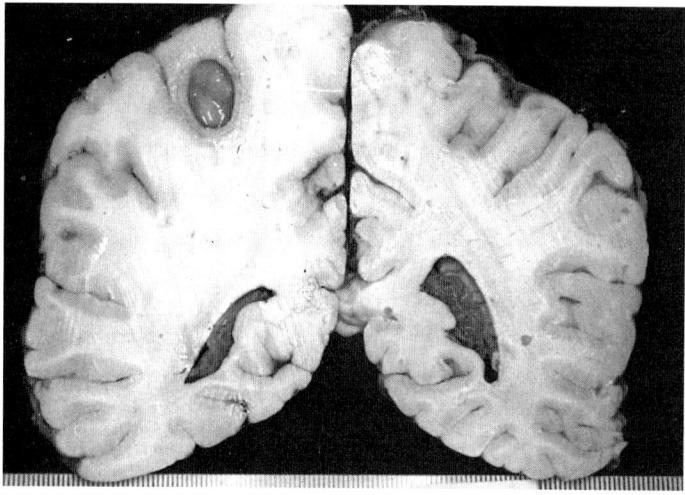

Figure 19–8. Cerebral abscess at the junction between gray and white matter in the region of the left middle cerebral artery.

After the first report by Fowler and Carter,[15] it became apparent that free-living amebas, in particular *Naegleria fowleri* and *Acanthamoeba sp*, were capable of invading the CNS in humans, producing primary amebic meningoenchephalitis and granulomatous amebic encephalitis, respectively.[16]

Primary amebic meningoencephalitis, caused by *Naegleria fowleri*, is a rare cause of severe, acute, fulminant, rapidly fatal hemorrhagic meningoencephalitis that usually affects previously healthy children and young adults with a history of swimming, diving, or water skiing in fresh water.

Granulomatous amebic encephalitis affects individuals ranging in age from 5 to 60 years. It is caused by various species of *Acanthamoeba*, which have worldwide distribution and can be found in water, soil, dust, heating ventilation and air conditioning units, and dental units. This infection is encountered predominantly in chronically ill and debilitated or immunosupressed individuals. Most of the patients have preexisting illness, including liver disease, diabetes mellitus, Hodgkin's disease, or alcoholism, or are receiving treatment, such as antibiotics, radiotherapy, or steroids.[16] It is therefore not expected that this infection occurs in elderly patients. It has also been reported in patients with AIDS.[17]

Macroscopically, there is diffuse exudate in the subarachnoid space. The cerebral hemispheres are slightly swollen and there are multiple areas of softening, hemorrhage, and necrosis, particularly in the distribution of anterior and middle cerebral arteries. Lesions are particularly severe in the cerebellum, brain stem, and thalamus, and in the anterior part of the cerebral hemispheres. Occasionally they simulate a tumor with discrete, mass-like appearance.

Histologically, there is a subacute or chronic meningitis and, within the brain substance, vasculitis involving both arteries and veins, with perivascular cuffing of lymphocytes, macrophages, and plasma cells. It is associated with a granulomatous reaction and giant cells may be present even in the walls of thrombosed vessels. Trophozoites are found in blood vessels walls and in areas free of any inflammatory reaction.

A newly recognized form of ameba that causes granulomatous encephalitis is the leptomyxid amoeba, later classified as *Balamuthia mandrillaris*.[16] It has been reported in several countries including Peru, Australia, Argentina, Brazil, Canada, Mexico, and Venezuela,[18–20] and has also been reported in patient with AIDS.[21] The lesions are morphologically indistinguishable from those described for the *Acanthamoeba* (Fig. 19–9) and it is necessary to perform immunohistochemical analysis to identify the organisms.

Cerebral amebic abscess is a rare and late complication of intestinal, pulmonary, or hepatic amebiasis due to *Entamoeba histolytica*. The abscesses present as space-occupying lesions and the symptoms vary according to their location. Meningoencephalitis can occasionally be present.

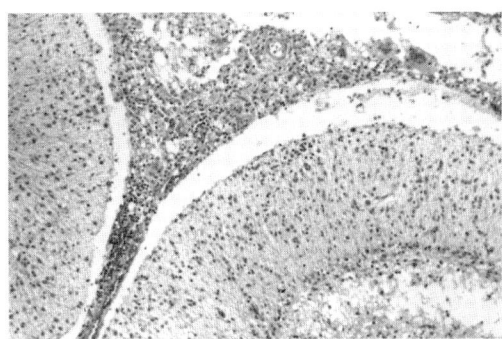

Figure 19–9. Amebic meningoencephalitis due to *Balamuthia mandrilaris* with lymphohistiocytic inflammatory infiltrate involving the leptomeninges and superficial cerebellar cortex. H&E.

In the brain, the lesion is usually single and is located predominantly in the richly vascularized cortical gray matter or basal ganglia or at the junction between cortex and white matter. Occasionally, they can be multiple and appear in the early stages as small foci of hemorrhagic necrotic neural parenchyma. Necrosis gradually becomes evident, and cavitation appears later. The contents of the cavity are yellow-green, its walls are irregular, and there is no evidence of encapsulation.

Histologically, these abscesses are composed of inflamed, necrotic tissue in which the amebas may be difficult to distinguish from macrophages. The abscess wall has an inner zone of necrotic tissue and a broad outer zone of congestion and vascular proliferation. In the surrounding brain there is gliosis and lymphoplasmacytic and histioytic inflammatory infiltrate including some polymorphs. Trophozoites (Fig.19–10) can be identified in the necrotic wall of the abscess. The overlying meninges is secondarily involved with the inflammation.[9]

Cerebral Malaria

Malaria remains a major cause of morbidity and mortality in many parts of the world. Primary cases of malaria are found in tropical and subtropical regions, but because of extensive international travel, they may be found anywhere in the world. Most of the cases occur in countries of tropical Africa. In other continents the disease is more prevalent in India, Brazil, Thailand, Sri Lanka Afghanistan, Vietnam, and China. In the Americas more than half of the cases come from Brazil, most of them from the Amazonian region.[9,22,23]

Malaria in humans is caused by four species of *Plasmodium*: *P. falciparum*, *P. vivax*, *P. malariae* and *P. ovale*. The first two are responsible for 95% of the cases. The disease is acquired by the bite of an infected *Anopheles* mosquito, which inoculates the sporozoite into humans, where the parasites penetrate hepatocytes and develop into merozoites that rupture the liver cells and enter the bloodstream, where they invade erythrocytes.

Cerebral malaria is an acute encephalopathy that occurs predominantly if not exclusively in patients infected with *P. falciparum*. The incubation period ranges from 1 to 3 weeks. It occurs most often in individuals not immune to this parasite. Cerebral involvement, which occurs in 1% to 10% of cases, accounts for the majority of fatalities from malaria.

Macroscopically, the brain is swollen, with opacity of the leptomeninges, dusky discoloration of the gray matter, and congestion. The cortex has an abnormal pink color from congestion of the leptomeninges and intracortical vessels, or a slate-gray color from the presence of abundant malarial pigment. The white matter often contains petechial hemorrhages. Histologically, small vessels are congested and contain pigment-laden and parasitized erythrocytes. The erythrocytes often appear to adhere to endothelial cells. The vessels may be surrounded by petechial ring hemorrhages (Fig. 19–11) present throughout the brain but more abundant in the white matter and may surround necrotic arterioles and veins. Patients

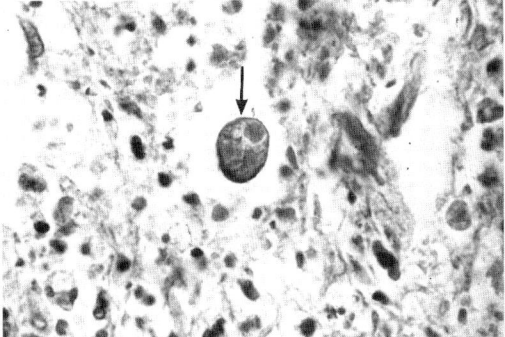

Figure 19–10. *Entamoeba histolytica* in a cerebral abscess (arrow). H&E.

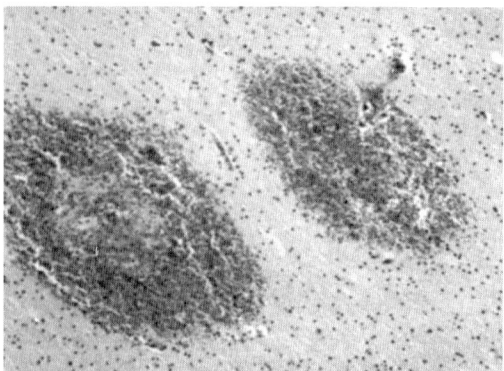

Figure 19–11. Cerebral malaria with small hemorrhages in the white matter, one of them surrounding a necrotic vessel. H&E.

with longer survival may harbor small demyelinated foci. Collections of microglial cells and astrocytes, the so-called Dürck granulomas, may be related to the ring hemorrhages and contain neutral lipids and iron pigment. Blockage of cerebral capillaries by erythrocytes, granules of dark malarial pigment (related to hematin), can be found in the lumina of capillaries. Hypoxic–ischemic changes and an inflammatory infiltrate consisting of lymphocytes and mononuclear cells with extension to the leptomeninges are also observed.[9,22,23]

Toxoplasmosis

Toxoplasmosis is caused by the coccidian *Toxoplasma gondii*. The definitive hosts for this parasite are domestic cats and other feline species. The development of toxoplasmosis in humans depends very much on the host's susceptibility and immunological status. The encysted organism can remain dormant for many years and can become reactivated and cause significant neurologic disease in immunocompromised patients, especially those with AIDS. The lesions usually appear on a computed tomography (CT) scan as multiple bilateral ring-enhancing lesions. Magnetic resonance imaging (MRI) appears to be more sensitive in detecting the multiple necrotic lesions and enables a more accurate differential diagnosis from other focal lesions that are common in the same group of patients, in particular, lymphomas.

Macroscopically, the characteristic lesions in immunosupressed patients are focal or multifocal necrotizing encephalomyelitis with minimal leptomeningeal changes. They are of variable, often large size with a necrotic center. Any region of the brain can be affected, but the basal ganglia are the most frequently involved area (Fig. 19–12a). They may be distributed in the anterior and middle cerebral arterial zones, suggesting metastatic tumors. Chronic lesions consist of small and well-demarcated cystic spaces. Brain involvement may occasionally take the form of an encephalitic process in which macroscopic lesions are unremarkable.

Histologically, necrotizing abscesses or coagulative necrosis is variously associated with infiltration by polymorphs, mononuclear cells, newly formed capillaries, astrocytes, and microglial cells. Blood vessels may sometimes undergo fibrinoid necrosis, occasionally with perivascular infiltration. They show variable amounts of hemorrhage, intimal proliferation, and thrombosis. The *Toxoplasma* organisms may be abundant and can appear as cysts (Fig. 19–12b) within or at the periphery of the necrotic areas. The free organisms are seen reasonably well when stained with hematoxylin and eosin (H&E), but their identity can be confirmed by immunoperoxidase staining techniques.[23]

American Trypanosomiasis (Chagas' Disease)

This disease is found predominantly in South America (especially Brazil) and Central America. It is caused by *Trypanosoma cruzi* and transmitted by reduviid bugs. The protozoan has a particular tropism for muscle tissue, and according to its environment, it can take a *Leishmania*-like form (amastigotes). Transmission can also occur through blood transfusion or breast-feeding, transplacentally, accidentally in laboratories, and through organ transplants.[24]

The disease is usually acquired during childhood, and may be acute or chronic. Encephalitis is more common in acute than in chronic cases, therefore it is more frequent in children than in adults.[25] Clinical manifestations of the CNS in the chronic phase are controversial. Although Chagas admitted the existence of a

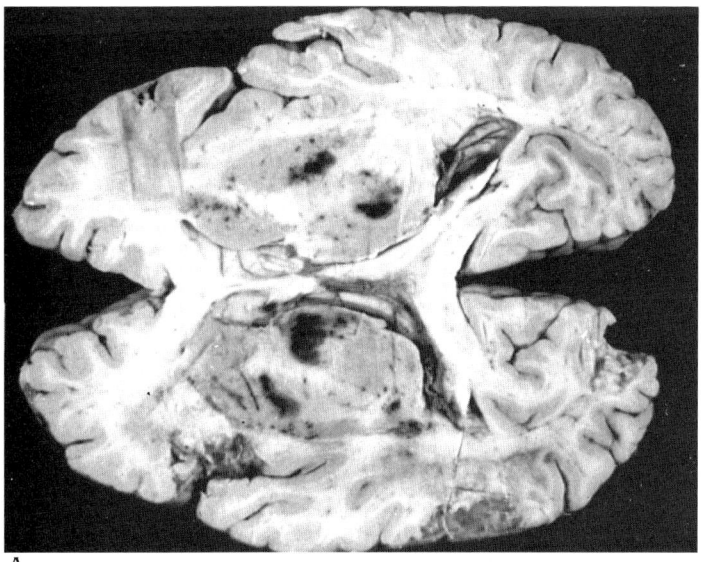
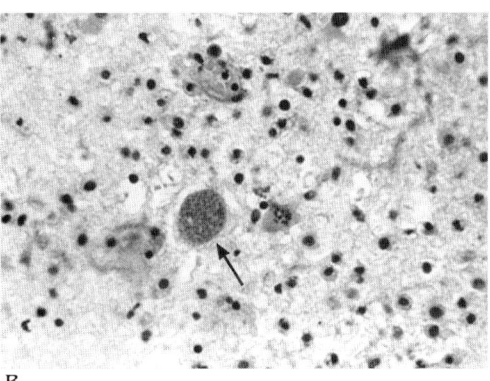

Figure 19–12. Cerebral toxoplasmosis with multiple necrohemorrhagic lesions involving the basal ganglia, cortex, and white matter (A) and a cyst filled with parasites (arrow) and surrounded by inflammatory cells (B). H&E.

chronic form affecting the CNS, this has not been well documented for a long time. Pittella[25] reported a few glial nodules and aggregates of lymphoid cells in the white matter of occasional cases, but no parasites could be identified. However, there is recent evidence of meningoencephalitis and space-occupying lesions, and multifocal necrotizing encephalitis where parasites are abundant (Fig. 19–13), in immunocompromised patients, indicating a reactivation of the disease, with severe neurological involvement.[26] In endemic areas where AIDS is prevalent, reactivation of Chagas' disease should be included in the differential diagnosis of space-occupying le-

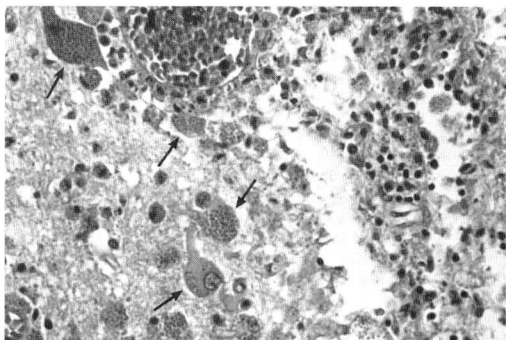

Figure 19–13. Multiple parasitized cells (arrows) in a case of reactivated *Trypanosoma cruzi* meningoencephalitis associated with immunosuppression. H&E.

sions, particularly in the elderly, who might have been infected by the *T. cruzi* during childhood.

HELMINTHIC INFECTIONS

Although any parasitic infection, such as trichinosis, schistosomosis, hidatidoses, may affect the elderly, cysticerosis deserves some comment because it is now considered the most common parasitic disease of the nervous system worldwide.

Neurocysticercosis

Although cysticercosis is relatively uncommon in the United States, it is an important infection in California and states bordering Mexico, as well as in other parts of the world, such as South America, India, and certain European countries including Portugal, Spain, and Eastern European countries, particularly Poland and Romania. Cysticercosis is caused by the *Cysticercus cellulosae*, which is the larval form of the pork tapeworm *Taenia solium*, and it develops when a human serves as its intermediate host.[27]

Macroscopically, one to several hundred cysts may be found in the neural parenchyma (especially gray matter), meninges, or ventricular system (Fig. 19–14). Intraspinal cases have been described.[28] In the meninges they appear as small, colorless structures, adherent to the pia or floating freely in the subarachnoid space, particularly in the Sylvian fissure. The basal meninges become thickened and the cysts within them tend to shrink. The viable intraparenchymal *Cysticerci cellulosae* are usually 1 to 2 cm in diameter and contain a single invaginated scolex. After degeneration they become fibrotic and represented by a firm white nodule that eventually calcifies. *Cysticerci racemosus* are large, multiloculated cysts that lack an invaginated scolex. They are usually found in the basilar cisterns and within the ventricular system, especially the fourth ventricle. Arachnoiditis and vasculitis commonly result from degeneration and death of *Cysticerci racemosus* in the subarachnoid space. Histologically, each scolex has a rostellum (Fig. 19–15A) with four suckers and a double row of hooklets. The cyst wall is sparsely cellular and consists of three distinct layers (Fig. 19–15B). While the encysted larvae are viable, the surrounded neural parenchyma shows minimal reaction. When the cisticerci degenerate and die, they elicit an intense inflammatory reaction and development of granulation tissue and foreign body giant cells in the surrounding neural parenchyma. Old nodules may be entirely fibrotic and ventricular cysticerci produce a granular ependymitis.[27]

FUNGAL INFECTIONS

Aspergillosis

This infection is caused by an organism that is usually saprophytic, growing in a debilitated host. Predisposing factors include corticosteroid and immunosuppressive therapy, prolonged antibiotic use, HIV infection, neoplasms (especially lymphomas and leukemia), collagen disorders, diabetes mellitus, chronic pulmonary disease, organ transplantation, neutropenia, hepatic failure, chronic lung disease, cavitary tuberculosis, cardiovascular surgery, alcoholism, intravenous drug abuse, marijuana use, general malnutrition, and age[29] Several species can cause CNS infection, but most cases are due to *Aspergillus fumigatus* or *Aspergillus flavus*, which are found in soil, plants, and decaying matter.[30] The fungus has a marked tendency to invade arteries and veins, producing a necrotizing angiitis, thus setting the stage for its hematogenous spread. The organs most frequently involved by metastatic propagation are the heart, brain, kidneys, gastrointestinal tract, liver, thyroid, and spleen. Direct examination and cultures are the techniques most frequently used in the diagnosis of the disease. Spinal fluid pleocytosis of under 600 cells/mm^3 is also found. The protein level is only moderarely elevated, and the sugar content is normal. Organisms are usually not found in CSF and the diagnosis of CNS involvement is infrequently established during life.

The morphological changes vary according to whether the infection is the result of hematogenous dissemination or of local spread. In the first instance, the process generally leads to multiple lesions that involve areas of the anterior and middle cerebral arterial dis-

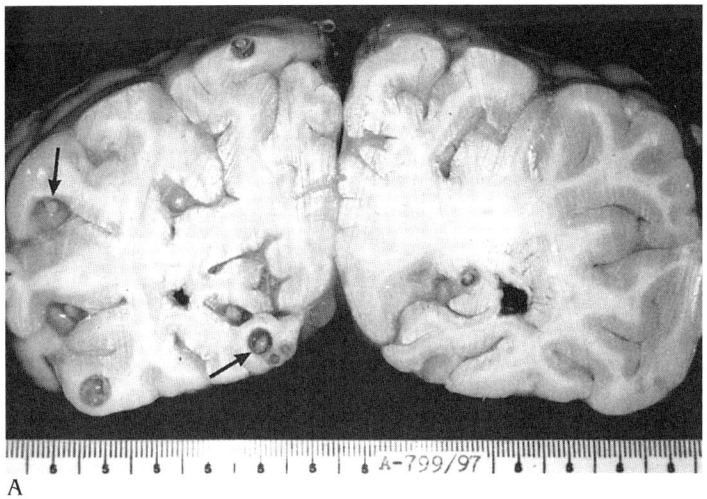

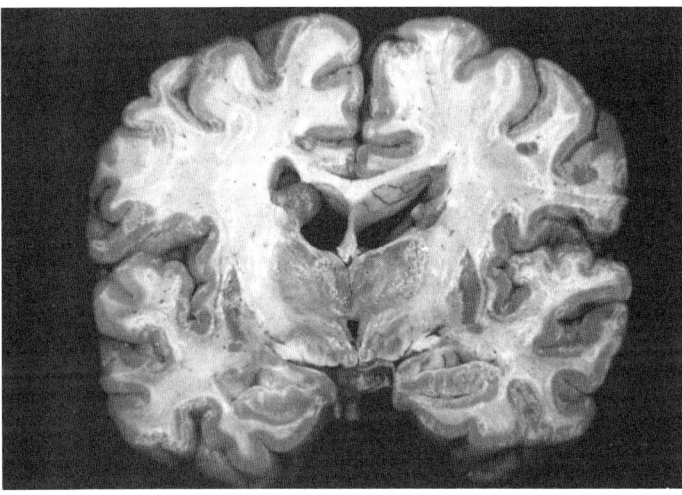

Figure 19-14. Neurocysticerosis with multiple intraparenchymal (A) and intraventricular (B) cysts some of which contain the scolex (arrows).

tributions and that tend to be acute and necrotizing or purulent. In the latter, usually the result of sino-orbital infection, they may be chronic and have a tendency toward fibrosis and granuloma formation. They involve the cerebral cortex, white matter, basal ganglia, and cerebellar hemispheres. Because the fungus is highly angioinvasive, the lesions are often foci of hemorrhagic cerebritis that resemble hemorrhagic infarcts.

Histologically, the most striking feature is the intensity of vascular invasion with thrombosis. The amount of inflammation varies according to the stage of the disease and from patient to patient; neutrophils predominate in the early phases while treated cases show no inflammatory cells. In abscesses, frank pus is seen in the center of the lesion and abundant neutrophilic infiltration at the edges, sometimes accompanied by giant and epithelioid cell granulomas. The meninges overlying both abscesses and granulomas are involved by a variable amount of exudate. Lesions of necrotizing nonsuppurative type consist of an area of coagulative necrosis with variable amounts of neutrophilic reaction and hemorrhage. In tissue, the organisms form dichotomously branching septate hyphae that are faintly visible with H&E staining and often weakly stained with periodic acid-Schiff (PAS). They are most readily demonstrated with methenamine silver stains.[29]

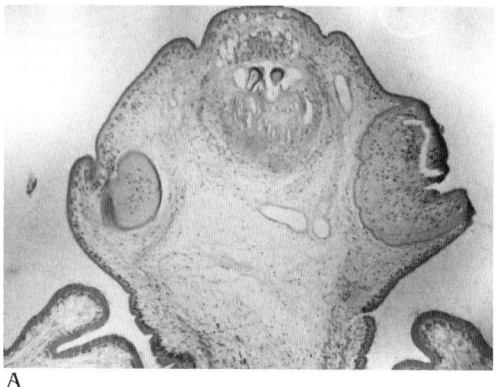

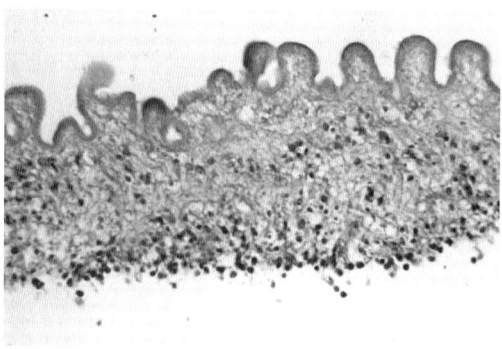

Figure 19–15. Cysticercus cellulosae: the rostellum (A) and the cyst wall (B). H&E.

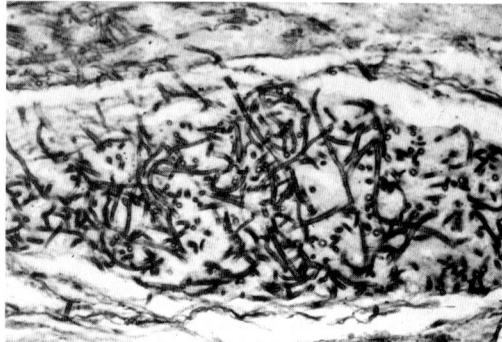

Figure 19–16. Broad hyphae in the meninges of a patient with mucormycosis. Methenamine silver.

Mucormycosis

Mucormycosis is caused by several genera that belong to the family Mucoraceae, such as *Rhizopus, Mucor,* and *Absidia* (95% of cases). The organisms are ubiquitous, are found in the soil, manure, and decaying vegetation material, and are frequently airborne. Several patterns of the disease with somewhat different predisposing conditions have been delineated. It occurs most often in diabetic patients who are ketoacidotic and patients with leukemia who are neutropenic.[30] Unlike most other mycoses, in which cerebral involvement is secondary to a primary focus in the lung, it develops most frequently from an infection of the skin of the face or in the mucosa of the nose and nasopharynx, and spreads to surround regions and to the arteries of the orbit and the internal carotid arteries, with eventual thrombosis. The illness often runs an acute, often fulminating course, with death within a few days. Even though the prognosis in this infection is usually poor, improvement can occur after treatment of the diabetic ketoacidosis. The diagnosis can be made by the appropriate clinical syndrome and examining the biopsied nasal material. The characteristic hyphae are diagnostic. The CSF is under normal pressure but may be stained with blood. Usually a minimal pleocytosis occurs, although as many as 40,000 leukocytes mm^3 have been reported. The CSF protein and sugar values are elevated. Diagnosis is usually made on the finding of the fungus in the tissue.

Macroscopically, necrotic hemorrhages occur at various sites in the brain, but mainly in the base of the frontal lobes. When the CNS involvement results from hematogenous dissemination, the lesions often produce hemorrhagic necrosis in deep gray nuclei. Thrombosis of the cavernous sinus and carotid artery commonly occurs.

The fungi are very angioinvasive and appear as broad nonseptate hyphae around and within the blood vessel walls in the meninges (Fig. 19–16) and brain. They are obstructive, causing thrombosis and associated extensive hemorrhagic infarction of the neural parenchyma, and they extend into adjacent damaged tissue. The organisms are relatively well shown with H&E staining but can be better demonstrated with PAS and methenamine silver stains.[29]

Histoplasmosis

This disorder is caused by *Histoplasma capsulatum*, which is present throughout the world. It is estimated that 25% of the population in the United States has contracted histoplasmosis; it is the most frequently observed pulmonary mycotic infection in the east central United States (Ohio, Mississippi, and St. Lawrence River valleys). All ages and races and both sexes can be affected, but there are two peaks of incidence: one in infancy and childhood, during which the disease involves the lymphoreticular system; and the other in the fifth and sixth decades, in which males are affected predominantly, probably through reinfection. Involvement of the CNS is rare, occurring in <1% of patients with active histoplasmosis.[29]

Histoplasma capsulatum is a biphasic fungus that grows as a mycelial saprophyte in the soil but converts to a yeast-like organism in infected tissue. Organisms are inhaled in infected dust contaminated by chicken, bird, or bat excreta. The portal of entry is the lung, where a primary focus is formed and commonly becomes calcified; however, primary lesions may occur in the mouth, the gastrointestinal tract, or the skin. Dissemination, especially to the CNS, is uncommon in immunocompetent individuals. The presence of CNS disease implies compromise by burns, antibiotics, steroids, HIV, or some other factor. Many of the patients with CNS involvement have AIDS, although the incidence of histoplasmosis remains low in AIDS patients.

Macroscopically, there is diffuse or basilar leptomeningitis, but discrete intraparenchymal granulomas may occur. Thickening of the leptomeninges occurs especially around the base of the brain (Fig. 19–17A) When the meningeal reaction is severe, it often consists of a thick yellow exudate with small, scattered white nodules (miliary granulomas) along the blood vessels, and focal destructive lesions. In

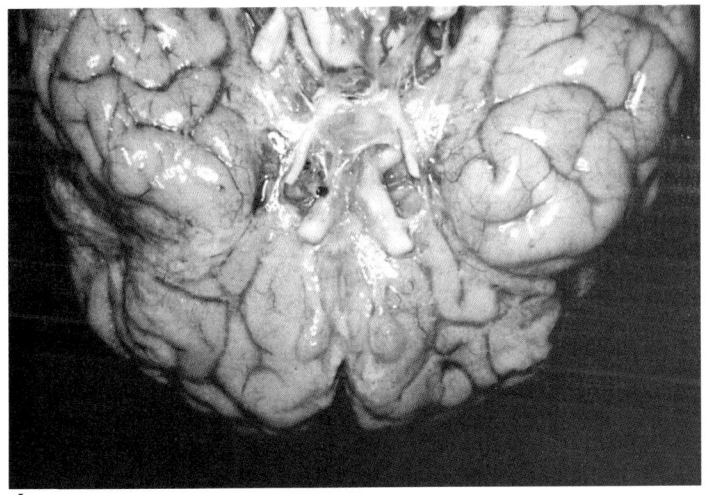

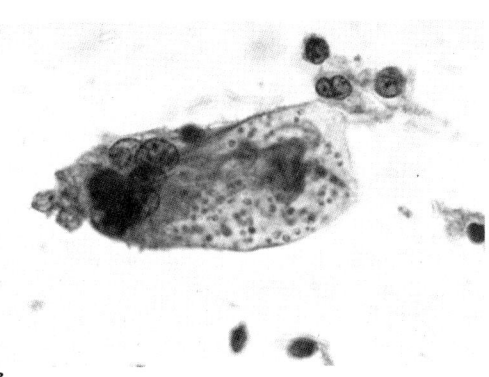

Figure 19–17. Histoplasmosis with meningeal thickening over the base of the brain of the frontal lobe and the tip of the left temporal lobe (A) and meningeal macrophage filled with *Histoplasma capsulatum* (B). Methenamine silver.

chronic cases there is meningeal fibrosis. A solitary intraparenchymal granuloma (histoplasmoma) may occur.

Histologically, a spectrum of lesions can be observed, from nodular histiocytic formations with few organisms to epithelioid cells ("tubercles") with Langhans' giant cells, the latter being indistinguishable from TB. Plasma cells and lymphocytes are found in the meninges, and granulomatous arteritis, similar to the well-known lesions in tuberculous meningitis, occurs either focally or in diffuse form. Mass lesions in the brain consist of central caseous areas surrounded by macrophages, lymphocytes, plasma cells, and giant cells. The organisms can be found within the cytoplasm of macrophages. Methenamine silver is especially useful for demonstrating the large numbers of organisms packed within macrophages (Fig. 19–17B).

Cryptococcosis

Cryptococcosis is caused by *Cryptococcus neoformans*, which is found commonly in the environment and infects humans when inhaled into the lungs. The pulmonary infection may be silent and symptoms occur only after the organism has spread to the CNS, the main target organ for infection. The disease is more frequent in the fourth to sixth decade of life and it has a propensity to occur in patients with HIV infections.[30] Classically, the CSF findings in patients with cryptococcal meningitis are lymphocytic pleocytosis, elevated protein, and decreased glucose. India ink examination of CSF may show encapsulated budding yeast, but this is not a very sensitive test. The cryptococcal antigen latex agglutination assay is more sensitive and is also very specific for the diagnosis of cryptococcal meningitis. The definite diagnosis is made by growing the organism from the CSF.

Grossly, CNS lesions may be minimal and can be overlooked. However, in most cases the leptomeninges are thickened and lose their transparency (Fig. 19–18A). The meningitic exudate may occur at any site, but is most often found over the base of the brain and cerebellum. Some cases contain myriad organisms, which give the surface of the specimen a slippery, slimy, soft consistency. On occasion, there are tubercles of 2–3 mm in diameter adjacent to the blood vessels; their similarities to tuberculous lesions have been stressed. About 50% of cases of CNS crytococcosis show meningeal involvement exclusively. Less commonly, cryptococcosis produces multiple intraparenchymal cysts related to exuberant capsular material produced by the proliferating cryptococci, especially in the basal ganglia. In rare cases, masses of fungi aggregate in an inflammatory lesion and produce large or small granulomas (cryptococcomas) in the meninges, parenchyma, ependymal surfaces, or choroid plexuses.

Histologically, the tissue reaction is pleomorphic. The cerebral lesions are of three types: a granulomatous meningitis, small granulomas or cysts within the cerebral cortex, and deeply placed solid or cystic nodules found chiefly in the gray matter of the basal nuclei. In most cases, the meningitis particularly in patients with AIDS, has minimal inflammatory reaction. However, when present, it consists of collections of lymphocytes, plasma cells, eosinophils, fibroblasts, and multinucleated giant cells, with cryptococci seen frequently within them. In the gelatinous lesions, the solid tissue is replaced by numerous organisms forming a colony, usually around a vessel. The gelatinous aspect is due to the mucinous capsular material of the numerous organisms found invading the tissue. Granulomata are rarer late reactions that can mimic tubercles. The solid granulomatous nodules are composed of fibroblasts, giant cells, and huge aggregates of organisms and areas of necrosis. The organisms are faintly stained with H&E. The cell walls are strongly stained with the PAS (Fig. 19–18B), mucicarmine, Alcian blue, and methenamine silver stains.[29]

Coccidioidomycosis

Coccidioidomycosis is a geographically restricted mycosis that occurs in regions of semiarid climate. It is endemic in the southwestern United States (especially in the San Joaquin Valley and Arizona), Mexico, and South America (particularly Argentina and Paraguay). The causative organism, *Coccidioides immitis*, is a nonbudding spherical structure with a double refractile capsule. Mature forms are filled with

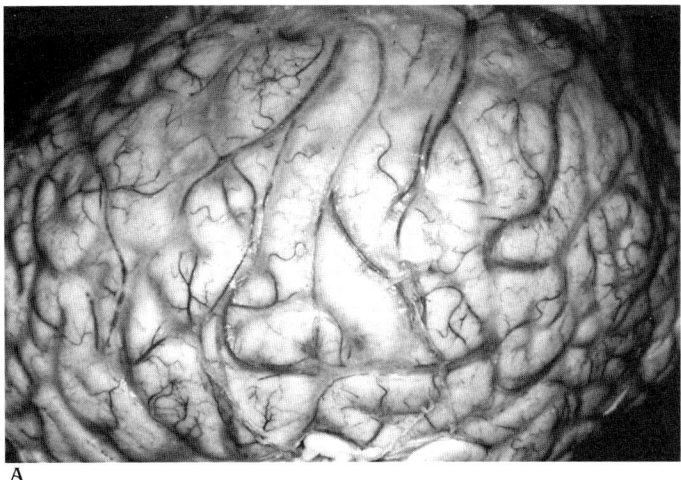

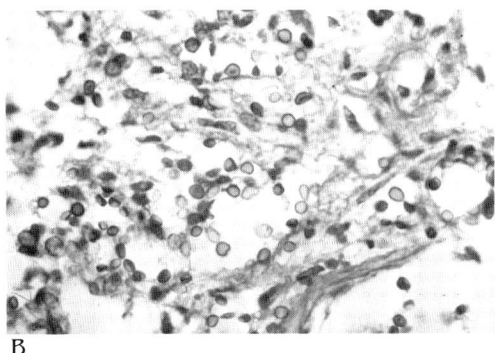

Figure 19–18. Cryptococcal meningitis with thickened opaque leptomeninges (A) containing numerous cryptococci (B). PAS.

numerous small endospores and are easily recognized on routine H&E stains. The endospores are released into the tissue after the spherules rupture.

The organism can be recognized in wet preparations of the CSF, which undergo changes similar to those occurring in tuberculous meningitis. Usually the fluid is under increased pressure and appears clear, turbid, or xanthochromic. The cell count averages several hundred per cubic millimeter, but it may be as high as 3000/mm.³ Lymphocytes predominate. Complement fixation tests on serum are helpful in recognizing this mycosis.

The pathologic findings vary with the duration of meningeal involvement. An exudate accumulates in the subarachnoid space. A thickened, cloudy leptomeninges with small nodules (caseous granulomata) is most pronounced at the base of the brain but can also occur in the cervical cord region. It may become organized and lead to fibrosis and subsequent obstructive hydrocephalus. Coccidioidal meningitis tends to concentrate in sulci rather than on a convex surface and is commonly unimpressive to naked eye examination. The disease can also produce cerebritis. Less commonly, there are larger granulomatous lesions within the brain and occasionally in the spinal cord. Histologically, the meningeal reaction resembles that of a tuberculous infection and is characterized by organisms surrounded by epithelioid cells, giant cells, lymphocytes, and plasma cells, or small abscesses with caseous necrosis. Vascular involvement may be striking. In tissue the fungi form distinctive, large sporangia (spherules). As long as the sporangia are intact, the tissue reaction is predominantly granulomatous. When the enlarging sporangia rupture, the released endospores elicit an acute inflammatory reaction. The organisms are generally basophilic when stained with H&E but are much better demonstrated with methenamine silver stain.[23,29]

Candidiasis

Candidiasis is a common mycotic infection of the CNS caused by *Candida albicans*. For these normally commensal yeast to become pathogenic, interruption of the normal defenses is necessary. Older adults are more likely to be exposed to situations that predispose them to invasive candidiasis, including treatment with broad-spectrum antibiotics, increased use of invasive monitoring devices in the intensive care unit, and aggressive chemotherapy for malignant, dermatological, and rheumatologic conditions.[31]

Gross lesions may not be apparent. Involvement of the nervous system is usually in the form of multiple microabscesses that may be accompanied by microgranulomas without central foci of necrosis. They can involve any part of the CNS, particularly in the distribution of the anterior and middle cerebral arteries. In the early stages they resemble hemorrhagic infarcts. In addition, infarcts may occur as a result of thrombosis of small blood vessels caused by filaments and budding organisms.

Histologically, the meninges contain a slight lymphocytic infiltration. Both the gray and white matter may contain acute abscesses, a granulomatous lesion (Fig. 19–19A), or merely perivascular cuffs of lymphocytes. Both yeast forms and pseudohyphae of *Candida* are encountered in the lesions. They are faintly basophilic when stained with H&E but are intensely stained by PAS and methenamine silver (Fig. 19–19B). The cellular reaction around the fungus is variable. When present, it consists of lymphocytes, plasma cells, a few polymorphs, and occasional giant cells.[29]

VIRAL INFECTIONS

Viral Meningitis

This disorder, usually caused by enterovirus, is uncommon in older adults. The diagnosis of viral meningitis can be suspected when the clinical scenario and CSF values are consistent with this infection (Table 19–1).[5] The prognosis is usually favorable without specific therapy. The meninges may be slightly opaque and inflammatory infiltrate is composed almost exclusively of lymphocytes.

Arbovirus Infections

Arboviruses are small, enveloped RNA viruses transmitted predominantly by arthropod vectors (i.e., arthropod-borne viruses). Most arbovirus infections are asymptomatic or produce only mild febrile illness and are rarely encountered in a neuropathology practice. The geographic distribution of different arboviruses reflects that of the natural hosts and insect vectors. There is marked variation in the incidence of most arbovirus infections, which are most numerous during the summer and early fall months. Some types of infection occur more frequently in children and the elderly, such as St Louis encephalitis and Eastern equine encephalitis. Japanese encephalitis

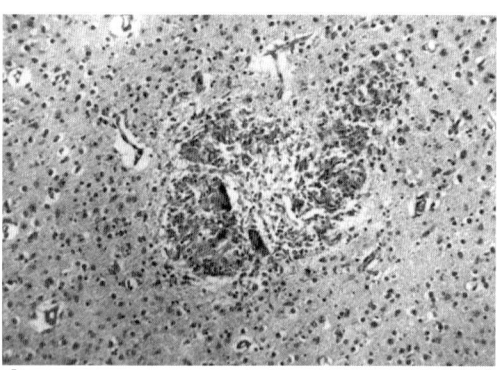
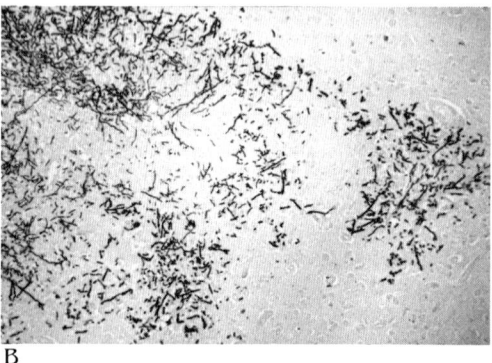

Figure 19–19. Candidiasis with granulomatous lesions containing giant cells (*A*) and numerous hyphae of *Candida albicans* (*B*). a, H&E; b, methenamine silver.

occurs in children under 10 and adults over 65 years of age, and more severe disease is evidenced by both mortality and morbidity. The seroprevalence for the Californian serogroup of viruses (especially La Crosse virus) increases with advanced age, to approximately 20% by the age of 60. The precise viral etiology is usually determined by serologic tests or by isolation of virus or specific viral RNA from the CSF. The mortality and morbidity rates vary considerably, the most serious being for Eastern equine encephalitis and Japanese encephalitis, with a mortality rate above 50% and persistent neurologic disability in a high proportion of survivors.[32]

In arboviruses the brain tends to be moderately congested and swollen. There may be petechial hemorrhages. The most severely affected areas are the basal ganglia, thalamus, and brain stem in Western or Eastern equine encephalitis, and the midbrain and thalamus in St. Louis encephalitis. In Japanese encephalitis the lesions may be widely distributed throughout the brain and spinal cord. Microscopically, there is leptomeningeal, perivascular, and parechymal infiltration, predominantly by lymphocytes and microglia or macrophages. Affected gray matter regions contain perivascular cuffs of mononuclear inflammatory cells, especially lymphocytes, perivascular hemorrhages, and microglial nodules, often surrounding degenerating neuronal cell bodies (neuronophagia). The perivascular inflammation in the white matter is associated with focal necrosis of myelinated fibers. Other features include thrombosed small blood vessels and, rarely, large regions of necrosis.[9]

Herpes Simplex Encephalitis

Classical herpes simplex encephalitis (HSV), caused by herpes simplex virus type 1 (HSV-1), is one of the most common forms of acute necrotizing encephalitis. It occurs in patients of all ages, with approximately one-third of cases being in patients younger than age 20 but over 6 months of age and approximately one-half being in patients older than 50. In older age-groups, HSV seems to be the most prevalent cause of encephalitis.[33]

Patients present with a combination of nonspecific features of encephalitis (e.g., headache, pyrexia, neck stiffness, drowsiness, coma) and focal neurological signs (e.g., dysphagia, hemiparesis, focal seizures). Without treatment, the disease progresses rapidly over the course of a few days and is usually fatal. Since the introduction of vidarabine and later acyclovir, the mortality and morbidity rates have fallen substantially, although 25%–50% of patients still die despite treatment, the risk being greater in the elderly and in those whose level of consciousness is severely depressed when treatment is started.[9]

Macroscopically, in the acute phase, most cases show obvious congestion and hemorrhagic necrosis involving the temporal lobes and, to a lesser extent, the insulae, cingulate gyri, and posterior orbital frontal cortex. The lesions are often asymmetric. The brain is usually swollen, particularly the hemorrhagic regions, but in patients dying some weeks after the onset of disease the liquefative necrosis in these regions will have progressed to cavitation and atrophy. In long-term survivors of untreated or unsuccessfully treated herpes encephalitis, the affected parts of the brain are shrunken and cavitated and show yellow-brown discoloration.

Microscopically, the earliest lesions contain relatively scanty parenchymal inflammation, although there are moderate numbers of lymphocytes and macrophages in the overlying leptomeninges. The lesions extend from the pial surface through the cerebral cortex into the white matter. The affected neurons, glia, and endothelial cells tend to have slightly hypereosinophilic cytoplasm. Many of the nuclei are pyknotic or disintegrating; others contain homogeneous eosinophilic inclusions (Fig. 19–20), which may also be visible in clumps in the

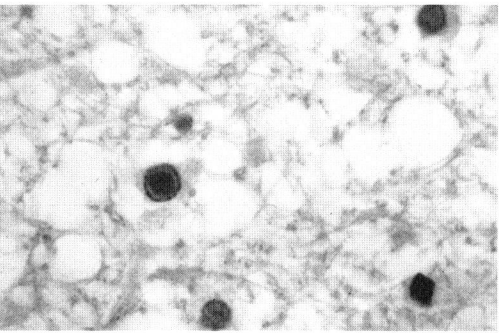

Figure 19–20. Herpes simplex intranuclear inclusion in a glial cell. H&E.

cytoplasm. In more advanced stages there are sheets of necrotic cells, foci of hemorrhage, and an intense perivascular and interstitial infiltrate of lymphocytes and macrophages. Herpesvirus nucleocapsid particles may be seen through electron microscopy. Viral antigen is readily demonstrable on immunohistochemical analysis for up to approximately 3 weeks after the onset of encephalitis, and viral DNA can be detected in frozen or paraffin sections by in situ hybridization or PCR amplification. In the chronic phase, the normal gray and white matter are replaced by cavitated glial scar tissue. Occasional clusters of lymphocytes are still seen in the meninges and brain parenchyma. At this stage, PCR is the only method that can be used to detect viral DNA.

Occasionally, herpesvirus encephalitis involves predominantly the brain stem, and both HSV-1 and HSV-2 can cause a necrotizing myelopathy, with extensive necrosis and inflammation involving the spinal gray and white matter.[9]

Herpes Zoster Virus Infection

Zoster encephalitis and myeloradiculitis usually occur in patients who are immunosuppressed, many of them with AIDS. A zosteriform skin rash usually occurs 1–2 weeks before the development of encephalitis or myeloradiculitis. Encephalitis presents nonspecifically with altered mentation, seizures, and variable neurologic deficits. Depending on the pattern of infection, visual or bulbar symptoms may predominate. In myeloradiculitis, the presenting neurologic symptoms are usually ipsilateral to the rash. Paralysis is more prominent than sensory loss.

Morphologically, several patterns have been described: multifocal lesions predominantly involving the cerebral white matter, ventriculitis, encephalitis involving the visual system, brain stem encephalitis, and myeloradiculitis. The first two patterns of infection are probably caused respectively by hematogenous and ventricular spread of virus, the third by spread of conjunctival and corneal lesions of ophthalmic zoster, and the last two by direct spread from trigeminal or dorsal root ganglia. In all cases the infection is typically necrotizing and associated with perivascular and interstitial infiltration by lymphocytes and macrophages. Intranuclear viral inclusions may be seen and viral antigen and DNA are usually demonstrable. Neuronophagia and microglial nodules tend to be prominent features of brain stem zoster encephalitis. Parenchymal infection may be associated with a necrotizing or granulomatous vasculitis involving small or large intracranial blood vessels and causing infarcts or hemorrhages, particularly in patients with AIDS.[9]

Progressive Multifocal Leukoencephalopathy

Progressive multifocal leukoencephalopathy (PML) is the result of an opportunistic infection in the brain of an immunocompromised host by the JC virus, a polyomavirus that normally infects, without obvious illness, much of the human population.

Macroscopically, the cut surface of the brain presents small foci of gray discoloration mixed with larger confluent areas of abnormal parenchyma, which may be centrally necrotic. The lesions tend to be more numerous in the cerebral white matter, but they can also involve the cerebral cortex and deep gray matter. The cerebellum, brain stem, and, much less commonly, the spinal cord may also be involved.

Microscopically, there are multiple foci of demyelination—some are small and rounded, others are confluent and irregular and occasionally centrally necrotic. These lesions contain moderate numbers of foamy macrophages (Fig. 19–21A), but only scanty perivascular lymphocytes. The presence of very large astrocytes with bizarre, pleomorphic, hyperchromatic nuclei is also common, particularly in older lesions. (Fig. 19–21B). Viral inclusions are seen toward the periphery of the foci of demyelination in the enlarged nuclei of oligodendrocytes (Fig. 19–21C). The homogeneous amphophilic inclusions largely fill the nuclei and consist of closely packed viral particles that are readily identifiable on electron microscopy.

Human T Cell Leukemia/ Lymphotropic Virus-1– Associated Myelopathy

This disorder, also known as tropical spastic paraparesis, is caused by the human T cell leu-

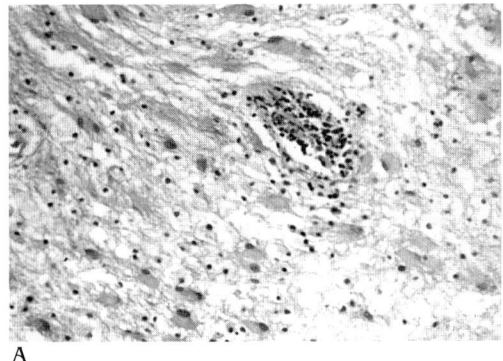

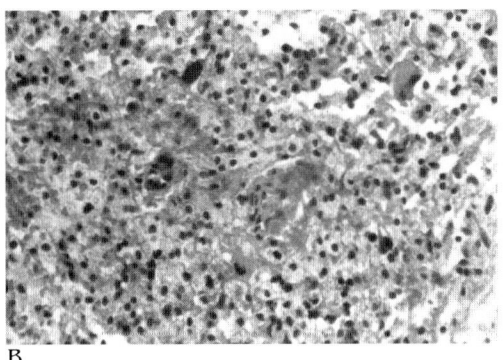

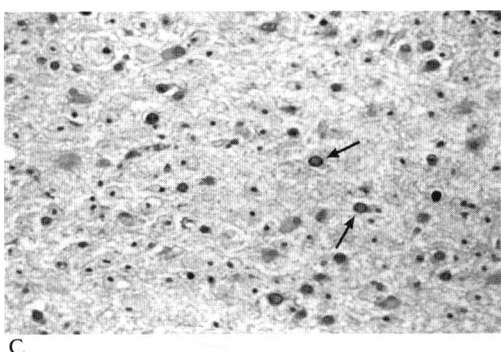

Figure 19–21. Progressive multifocal leukoencephalopathy showing areas of demyelination, gliosis, and scanty lymphocytes (*A*), collections of macrophages and bizarre astrocytes (*B*), and intranuclear inclusions (arrows) in enlarged oilgodendrocytes (*C*). H&E.

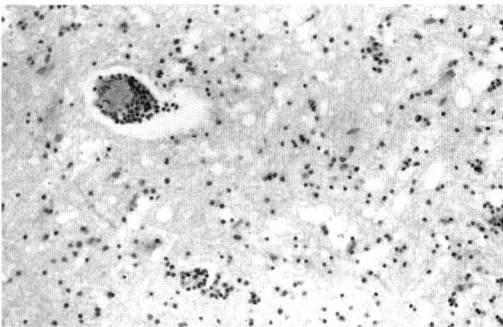

Figure 19–22. HTLV-I–associated myelopathy (HAM) with scattered and perivascular lymphocytes in the edematous spinal cord. H&E.

kemia/lymphotropic virus-1 (HTLV-1) and is endemic in the Caribbean, South America, parts of Africa, southern Japan, the Seychelles, and probably parts of India. It is transmitted through sexual contact, breast-feeding, or blood transfusion. The incubation period varies from 1 to 25 years and the age of onset is from 25 to 60 years. Symptoms of HTLV-1–associated myelopathy (HAM) include progressive spastic paraparesis and sphincter disturbance, and most patients are chair-bound within 10 years.

Macroscopically, in long-standing cases there may be meningeal thickening and atrophy of the spinal cord, particularly in the lower thoracic region. Microscopically, lymphocytes and macrophages infiltrate the leptomeninges and parenchyma of the spinal cord (Fig. 19–22), predominantly in the lower thoracic region. Hyaline thickening of the blood vessels is a prominent feature, and symmetric degeneration and gliosis of the long tracts of the spinal cord occur, particularly in the lateral columns.

Human Immunodeficiency Virus Infection and the Acquired Immunodeficiency Syndrome

In 1981 the first cases of AIDS were reported, and in 1984 the HIV, a retrovirus of the Lentivirus subfamily, was identified as the etiologic agent. HIV infection is pandemic, although the prevalence varies worldwide, the most prevalent areas being Africa, the United States, Latin America, and Southeast Asia. Transmission of infection occurs by vaginal or anal intercourse in 70% to 80% of cases intravenous drug injection in 5%–10% of cases, infection from mother to child in 5% to 10% of cases, blood transfusion in 3%–5% of cases, and health care or occupational exposure in 0.01% of cases.

Viral entry into T lymphocytes or macrophages is mediated by binding of the Env envelope glycoprotein to CD4 receptors on the cell surface. DNA provirus is synthesized from the RNA genome by the viral enzyme reverse transcryptase, which is packaged within the core particle of the virus and released on its entry into the cell. The provirus enters the nucleus and integrates at random sites in the cellular genome.

According to the Centers for Disease Control (CDC), Atlanta, in 1993, the number of CD4-positive T lymphocytes in a person with AIDS totals <200/μl, accounting for <14% of all T lymphocytes.

The number of AIDS patients over age 60 has risen steadily in the past decade.[34] Most HIV-infected patients age 60 years or older acquired their infection through sexual intercourse or blood transfusion. Intravenous drug injection and no identified risk factors comprise the remainder.[35] Disease progression appears to be more rapid in the elderly, although the observed shorter survival time may result from a delay in diagnosis. The diagnosis of HIV infection in the elderly is usually not considered by clinicians until late in the course of infection. Excess serum samples from hospitalized patients age 60 years or older without a history of HIV infection showed that 5% of the serum samples were HIV antibody positive.[36] Of these, eight had no documented identifiable risks for HIV infection. Therefore, HIV infection among elderly hospitalized patients from certain high HIV–seroprevalence communities may be a significant problem and may often remain undiagnosed during life, because this age-group has been excluded from targeted HIV testing programs.

Symptoms of HIV infection such as fatigue, anorexia, weight loss, and decreased physical and cognitive function, are often nonspecific. The diagnosis may be overlooked because older patients have a high prevalence of chronic illnesses that can cause the same symptoms. Neurological symptoms have been identified in 40% to 60% in most series whereas morphological involvement of the CNS has been found to be as high as 90% in autopsy studies.[37] These symptoms may result from direct HIV infection of the CNS or immunosupression caused by HIV infection, leading to opportunistic infections (especially cryptococcal meningitis and toxoplasmosis); neoplasm (primary brain lymphoma); and systemic factors and miscellaneous conditions related to an illness that causes cachexia, metabolic derangement, hypoxia, and other diverse abnormalities.

A syndrome of viral meningitis correlates with seroconversion or the development of symptomatic HIV-related disease. Patients will sometimes present with cranial nerve dysfunction or pyramidal signs. A dementing illness with memory and personality changes caused by the HIV may be a presenting feature of AIDS.

Neurologic dysfunction accompanied by progressive dementia should be included in the differential diagnosis of older patients with diffuse cognitive dysfunction such as Alzheimer's disease. In AIDS subcortical dementia is characterized by a decrease in attention and concentration, apathy, social withdrawal (which may be mistaken for depression), and psychomotor retardation. This dementia progresses more rapidly (over months) than that of Alzheimer's disease and is more often associated with peripheral neuropathies, myelopathies, ataxia, leg tremors, abnormal reflex, and general physical complaints (mild headache, weight loss, fatigue). The condition may progress to frank muscle weakness, paresthesia, and bladder and bowel incontinence. Unlike in Alzheimer's disease, examination of the CSF often reveals mildly elevated protein levels (mean 0.63 g/liter), and approximately 25% of patients have a mononuclear pleocytosis. HIV-associated cognitive abnormalities may improve with antiretroviral therepy.[38]

In the CNS, HIV infects mainly microglial cells or macrophages. This results in the secretion of cytokines such as tumor necrosis factor (TNF) and interleukins (e.g., IL-1, IL-6) and other potentially damaging chemicals such as nitric oxide, superoxide anion, hydroxl radical, and peroxides. The pathologic substrate of the resulting encephalopathy is the leukoencephalopathy and neocortical abnormalities such as neuron, synapse, and dendrite loss.[9]

Macroscopically, HIV encephalitis may be characterized by normal brain or diffuse atrophy with ventriculomegaly and ill-defined gray discoloration of the centrum semi-ovale. Histologically, widespread low-grade inflammation with microglial nodules and perivascular lymphocyte cuffing is apparent as well as leukoencephalopathy with patchy demyelina-

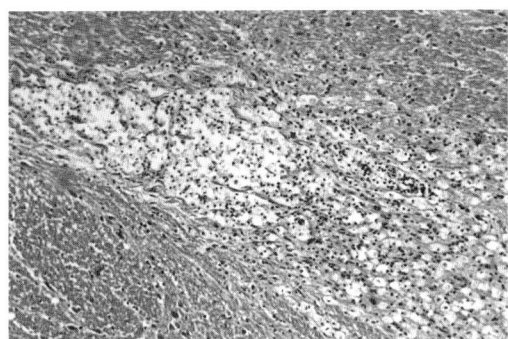

Figure 19–23. HIV pontine leukoencephalopathy showing patchy demyelination and macrophages. H&E.

tion (Fig. 19–23) and white matter gliosis and multinucleated giant cells, usually pericapillary, with scanty or abundant cytoplasm (Fig. 19–24); HIV antigen can be demonstrated in the latter with antibody to gp41 or p24. Other presentations include a necrotizing leucoencephalopathy and a vacuolar myelopathy that resembles subacute combined degeneration of the spinal cord, in addition to other less common presentations. The usual opportunistic fungal, parasitic, or bacterial infections also occur, most of which have already been described, as well as neoplastic disorders, particularly lymphoma.

REFERENCES

1. Smith PW, Roccaforte JS, Daly PB. Infection and immune response in the elderly. Ann Epidemiol 1992; 2:813–822
2. Chandra RK. Effect of vitamin and trace-element supplementation on immune responses and infection in elderly subjects. Lancet 1992; 340:1124–1127.
3. Beeson PB. Alleged susceptiblity of the elderly to infection. Yale J Biol Med 1985; 58:71–77.
4. Taylor ME, Oppenheim BA. Hospital-acquired infection in elderly patients. J Hosp Infect 1998; 38:245–260.
5. Miller LG, Choi C. Meningitis in older patients: how to diagnose and treat a deadly infection. Geriatrics 1997; 52:43–55.
6. Le Tulzo Y, Bouget J, Thomas R. Méningites bactériennes communautaires de l'adulte et du vieillard. Rev Prat 1994; 44:2165–2167.
7. Gorse GJ, Thrupp LD, Nudleman KL, Wyle FA, Hawkins B, Cesario TC. Bacterial meningitis in the elderly. Arch Intern Med 1984; 144:1603–1604.
8. Gray F. Bacterial infections. Brain Pathol 1997; 7: 629–647.
9. Ellison D, Love S. Neuropathology. A Reference Text of CNS Pathology. London: Mosby, 1998.
10. Stead WW, Lofgren JP, Warren E, Thomas C. Tuberculosis as an endemic and nosocomial infection among the elderly in nursing homes. N Engl J Med 1985; 312:1483–1487.
11. Hocking TL, Choi C. Tuberculosis: a strategy to detect and treat new and reactivated infections. Geriatrics 1997; 52:52–64.
12. Zuger A, Lowy FD. Tuberculosis. In: Scheld WM, Whitley RJ, Durak DT, eds. Infections of the Central Nervous System. Philadelphia: Lippincott-Raven, 1997; 417–443.
13. Burton AA, Flynn JA, Neumann TM, Wilson C, Quinn TC, Hook EW. Routine serologic screening for syphilis in hospitalized patients: high prevalence of unsuspected infection in the elderly. Sex Transm Dis 1994; 21:133–136.
14. Francioli PB. Complications of infective endocarditis. In: Scheld WM, Whitley RJ, Durack DT, eds. Infections of the Central Nervous System. Philadelphia: Lippincott-Raven, 1997;523–553.
15. Fowler M, Carter RF. Acute pyogenic meningitis probably due to *Acanthamoeba sp*: a preliminary report. BMJ 1965; 2:740–743.
16. Martinez AJ, Visvesvara GS. Free-living, amphizoic and opportunistic amebas. Brain Pathol 1997; 7:583–598.
17. Wiley CA, Safrin RE, Davis CE, Lampert PW, Braude AI, Martinez AJ, Visvesvara GS. Acanthamoeba meningoencephalitis in a patient with AIDS. J Infect Dis 1987; 155:130–133.

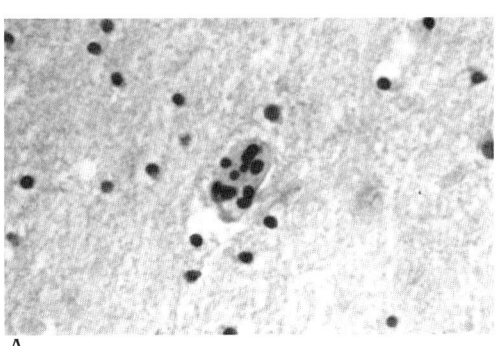

A

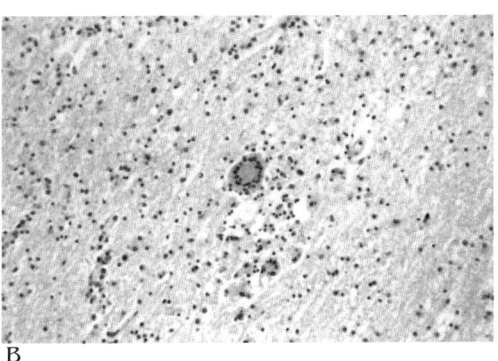

B

Figure 19–24. HIV encephalitis showing multinucleated giant cells with scanty (*A*) and abundant (*B*) cytoplasm and microglial hyperplasia (*B*). H&E.

18. Visvesvara GS, Martinez AJ, Schuster FL, Leitch G, Wallace SV, Sawyer TK, Anderson M. Leptomyxid ameba, new agent of amebic encephalitis in human and animals. J Clin Microbiol 1990; 28:2750–2756.
19. Taratuto AL, Monges J Acefe JC, Meli F, Paredes A, Martinez AJ. Leptomyxid ameba encephalitis: report of the first case in Argentina. Trans R Soc Trop Med Hyg 1991; 85:77.
20. Chimelli L, Hahn MD, Scaravilli F, Visvesvara GS. Granulomatous amebic encephalitis due to leptomyxid ameba. Report of the first Brazilian case. Trans R Soc Trop Med Hyg 1992; 86:635.
21. Anzil AP, Rao C, Wrzolek MA, Visvesvara GS, Sher JH, Koslowski PB. Amebic meningoencephalitis in a patient with AIDS caused by a newly recognized opportunistic pathogen. Leptomyxid ameba. Arch Pathol Lab Med 1991; 115:21–25.
22. Turner G. Cerebral malaria. Brain Pathol 1997; 7:569–582.
23. Scaravilli F, Cook GC. Parasitic and fungal infections. In: Graham DI, Lantos PL, eds. Greenfield's Neuropathology, Vol. 2. London: Arnold, 1997:65–152.
24. Chimelli L, Scaravilli F. Trypanosomiasis. Brain Pathol 1997; 7:599–611.
25. Pittella JEH. Brain involvement in the chronic cardiac form of Chagas's disease. J Trop Med Hyg 1985; 88:313–317.
26. Rocha A, Meneses ACO, Silva AM, Ferreira MS, Nishioka SA, Burgarelli MKN, Almeida E, Turcato Jr G, Metze K, Lopes ER. Pathology of patients with Chagas' disease and acquired immunodeficiency syndrome. Am J Trop Med Hyg 1994; 50:261–268.
27. Pittella JEH. Neurocysticercosis. Brain Pathol 1997; 7:681–693.
28. Colli BO, Assirati JA Jr, Machado HR, Santos F, Takayanagui OM. Cysticercosis of the nervous system. II. Spinal cysticercosis. Arq Neuropsiquiatr (Sao Paulo) 1994; 52:187–199.
29. Chimelli L, Malher-Araújo MB. Fungal infections. Brain Pathol, 1997; 7:613–627.
30. Kauffman CA, Hedderwick S. Opportunistic fungal infections: filamentous fungi and cryptococcosis. Geriatrics 1997; 52:40–49.
31. Hedderwick S, Kauffman CA. Opportunistic and fungal infections: superficial and systemic candidiasis. Geriatrics 1997; 52:50–59.
32. Whitley RJ. Arthropod-Borne encephalitis. In: Scheld WM, Whitley RJ, Durack DT, eds. Infections of the Central Nervous System. Philadelphia: Lippincott-Raven, 1997:147–168.
33. Koskiniemi M, Piiparinen H, Mannonen L, Rantalaiho T, Vaheri A. Herpes encephalitis is a disease of middle aged and elderly people: polymerase chain reaction for detection of herpes simplex virus in the CSF of 516 patients with encephalitis. J Neurol Neurosurg Psychiatry 1996; 60:174–178.
34. Chimelli L, Rosemberg S, Hahn MD, Lopes MBS, Barretto Netto M. Pathology of the central nervous system in patients infected with the human immunodeficiency virus. A report of 252 autopsy cases from Brazil. Neuropathol Appl Neurobiol 1992; 18:478–488.
35. Wallace JI, Paauw DS, Spach DH. HIV infection in older patients: when to suspect the unexpected. Geriatrics 1993; 48:61–70.
36. Gordon SM, Thompson S. The changing epidemiology of human immunodeficiency virus infection in older persons. J Am Geriatr Soc 1995; 43:7–9.
37. El Sadr W, Gettler J. Unrecognized human immunodeficiency virus infection in the elderly. Arch Intern Med 1995; 155:184–186.
38. Woolery WA. Occult HIV infection: diagnosis and treatment of older patients. Geriatrics 1997; 52:51–61.

20. Peripheral Neuropathies

ANNE VITAL AND CLAUDE VITAL

Individuals 55 to 75 years old constitute the largest group of any age afflicted with a peripheral neuropathy (PN) according to recorded clinical information and documented nerve biopsies in Australia, the United States, and Europe.[1-4] In a series of 519 patients with PN and nerve biopsies investigated by Mc Leod et al.,[1] 67 patients (13%) remained undiagnosed. The age of onset of symptoms in these 67 patients was 12 to 73 years (mean 50.6 years). Notermans et al.[3] investigated 75 patients with chronic polyneuropathy presenting in middle or old age (mean age 56.5 at the onset of symptoms) in whom a diagnosis could not be made even after extensive evaluation and a follow-up of 6 months. A peripheral nerve biopsy performed in 31 of these patients showed axonal degeneration.[3] Aging in itself appears to be responsible, however, for a progressive loss of and damage to nerve fibers, with great variations occurring from patient to patient, as evidenced in a personal study.[5]

The examination of the human peripheral nerve obtained at biopsy is suitably done using light and electron microscopy, immunopathology, and quantitative techniques. These methods show the nature and extent of damage to axons or myelin and surrounding tissues. In a few cases, a specific cause of the nerve damage can be seen on paraffin-embedded nerve fragments—for example, when there are amyloid deposits, necrotizing vasculitis, or certain cellular infiltrates. In certain cases of PN, anti-IgM serum binds to the myelin sheaths as demonstrated by immunopathologic study, and such cases usually display a specific myelinic alteration on ultrastructural examination. Specific Schwann cell inclusions may be disclosed in cases of PN due to certain drugs. However, most peripheral nerve biopsies do not display any specific lesion and the diagnosis is made by correlation with clinical investigations or with biologic, neurophysiologic, and molecular biology studies.

MATERIALS AND METHODS OF PERIPHERAL NEUROPATHIC STUDY

The sural nerve or the superficial peroneal nerve is usually biopsied for study. When the latter is chosen, portions of muscle tissue may be removed through the same incision for diagnostic purposes, particularly in vascular diseases that are common in elderly people. Nerve fragments taken at autopsy are of limited use because of autolytic modifications. Such specimens can be examined through light microscopy[6] or even electron microscopy, since myelin disruption begins 2 or 3 hr after death.[7] The length of nerve removed should ideally be 2 cm and divided into three fragments. The first fragment is embedded in paraffin for standard histologic techniques. The second is frozen and sections are processed for direct immunofluorescence with anti-IgA, IgG, IgM, λ and κ light-chain sera. The third fragment is immediately fixed in 2.5% glutaraldehyde and post-fixed in 1% osmium tetroxide. Plastic-embedded semi-thin and ultrathin sections are respectively prepared for light and electron microscopic examinations. In certain cases, another portion of this postfixed third fragment is prepared for examination of isolated nerve fibers by teasing.[8]

Quantitative study of myelinated fibers is usually performed by a semi-automatic method on transverse semithin sections stained with toluidine blue or paraphenylenediamine. Normally, in patients over 55 years of age, the average number of myelinated fibers is 7000 to 10000/mm^2 Their distribution according to diameter size is bimodal, with a first peak corresponding to small fibers and a second peak corresponding to large ones. In such a bimodal type histogram, at least 25% of myelinated fibers have a diameter >7 μm. Three other types of histogram may be observed according to the distribution of small and large myelinated fibers. In the unimodal type no myelinated fiber has a diameter over 7 μm. In the imbalanced-distribution type, fewer than 25% myelinated fibers have a diameter over 7 μm. In the dramatic-loss type, the number of myelinated fibers is fewer than 3000/mm^2 and there is a decrease in both small and large myelinated fibers.

ELEMENTARY LESIONS

Two main pathologic processes affect the peripheral nerve: axonal degeneration and primary demyelinating disorders.[9–14] A mixture involving both axonal degeneration and demyelination is usually found for most chronic neuropathies. Indeed, demyelination follows as a Schwann cell response to primary axonal degeneration, and in severe or sustained primary demyelination, nerve fiber loss often occurs.

Axonal Degeneration

Axonal degeneration has been thoroughly studied experimentally and reviewed in light of clinical applications.[15] Morphologic variations are well known, as is the ensuing demyelination.[16] Several types of axonal degeneration are now known.

Wallerian degeneration is the result of acute axonal damage and is typically induced by transection of a peripheral nerve. More details on this process have been obtained from ultrastructural studies.[9,10,14] Twelve hours after a crush lesion, the distal axons begin to show signs of degeneration with a paranodal accumulation of mitochondria. After 24 hr, the axoplasmic density is increased. The myelin splits at the interperiod line and lamellae peel off at the nodes. After 3 days there is extensive breakdown of myelin in the Schwann cell cytoplasm. Large ovoids consisting of myelin debris and disrupted axons are then observed. Some macrophagic histiocytes containing lipid debris are seen in the vicinity of the severely damaged fibers, which are sometimes invaded by macrophagic histiocytes. During Wallerian degeneration the basement membrane surrounding the Schwann cells remains in place and forms tubes within which the Schwann cells proliferate to form columns referred to as "bands of Büngner." On cross section, Schwann cell processes can be seen to contain various aspects of degenerated myelin, homogeneous lipid droplets, vacuoles, smooth and granular endoplasmic reticulum, Golgi complexes, microtubules, filaments, and glycogen. Regenerating axonal sprouts appear at about the fifth day and grow within the tubes derived from the Schwann cell basement membrane. The axons separate from each other to form the classic clusters that contain several rounded axons. The growing axons stay close together, although a few intervening collagen fibers can be observed. Some of these axons remyelinate and are surrounded by a myelin sheath that is too thin in relation to the axonal diameter (Fig. 20–1 and Fig. 20–2).

The technique of permanent axotomy enabled Dyck et al.[17] to study another type of axonal degeneration, the *retrograde effects* of the axonal section, which include axonal atrophy, myelin remodeling, and regeneration.

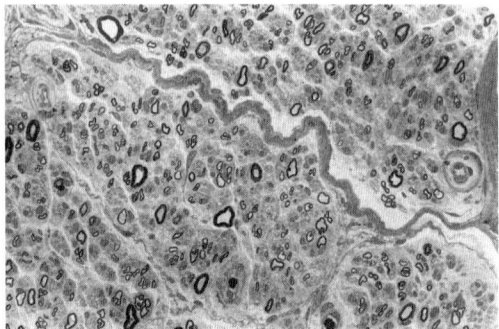

Figure 20–1. Long-standing peripheral neuropathy in a 77-year-old woman. There are numerous clusters of regenerating myelinated fibers. Semi-thin section, toluidine blue, ×430.

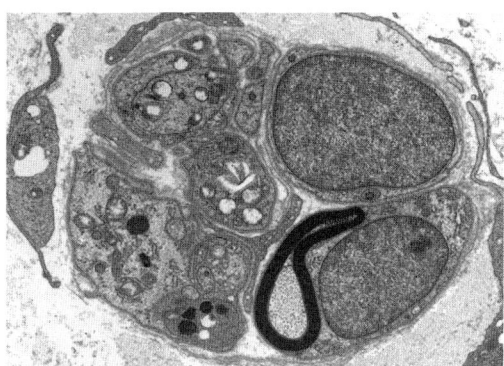

Figure 20–2. Axonal form of Guillain-Barré syndrome in a 65-year-old man. In this cluster of regenerating fibers, there is only one remyelinating axon. ×12,500.

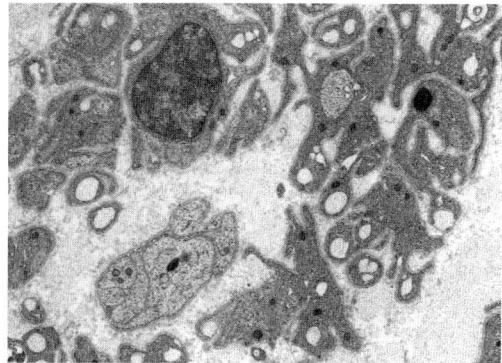

Figure 20–4. Peripheral neuropathy and IgG κ multiple myeloma in an 82-year-old woman. Several examples of collagen pockets are present and most axons are flattened. ×14,000.

Distal axonopathy corresponds to distal axonal degeneration that spreads in a progressive manner towards the cell body as the disease evolves. This "dying-back" process was studied in detail in hexacarbon-induced neuropathy.[18] This gives rise to multifocal preterminal axonal swellings with neurofilamentous accumulations. These swellings are situated on the proximal sides of several consecutive or nonconsecutive nodes of Ranvier, and the process then spreads sequentially to more and more proximal nodes. Other axoplasmic organelles may be aggregated. Axonal swelling is associated with thinner myelin sheaths and the myelin may disappear, leaving a large, naked axon (Fig. 20–3).

Peripheral nerve ischemia is a good example of *axonal dystrophy*,[19,20] which can lead to axonal swelling with aggregates of organelles.

In the early stages of *acute neuropathy*, unmyelinated axons appear enlarged and have a watery appearance due to dissolution of axoplasmic organelles. The enlarged axons then collapse, leaving flattened Schwann cell columns. In *chronic neuropathies*, some unmyelinated axons are moderately enlarged and filled with mitochondria and vesicular structures. Other axons become flattened but most axons disappear, leaving empty bands of Schwann cells. Some fibers show flattened axons and collagen pockets (Fig. 20–4). Regeneration takes place in the form of miniature axonal sprouts with Schwann cell cytoplasm rich in organelles.[21,22]

Segmental Demyelination

Segmental demyelination has been studied by electron microscopy in experimental diphteritic neuropathy.[23,24] The initial changes are widening at the node of Ranvier by retraction of the myelin paranodal loop, followed by myelin breakdown and accumulation of myelin debris in the paranodal Schwann cell cytoplasm. In some internodes this process results in complete removal of the myelin sheath. Segmental demyelination stimulates Schwann cell division, resulting in multiple Schwann cells arranged along the demyelinated internodes. Some of these daughter Schwann cells remyelinate (Fig. 20–5). On transverse semi-

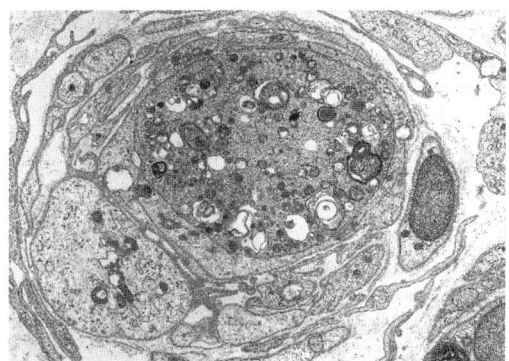

Figure 20–3. Peripheral neuropathy in a 74-year-old man with IgM monoclonal gammopathy of undetermined significance. This axon is swollen and packed with abnormal mitochondria and vesicular structures. ×18,000.

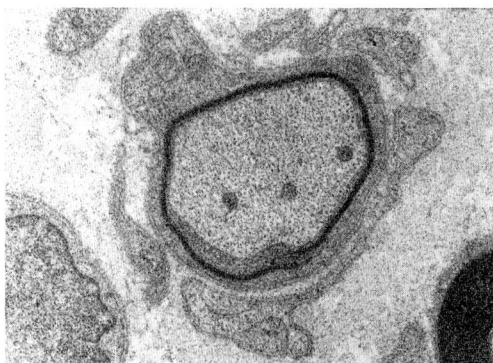

Figure 20–5. Peripheral neuropathy and IgM monoclonal gammopthy of undetermined significance in a 72-year-old man. An isolated nerve fiber is remyelinating and there are only a few myelin lamellae encircling the axon. ×33,700.

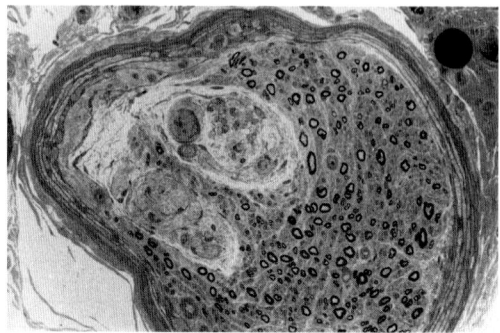

Figure 20–6. Mononeuritis multiplex in a 62-year-old man. Characteristic Renaut bodies are present in the endoneurium. Semi-thin section, toluidine blue, ×400.

thin sections, the new remyelinated fibers have a myelin sheath too thin for the axonal diameter. Macrophage-associated demyelination is described in Chronic Inflammatory Polyneuropathies, below. Atypical periodicity in myelin is dealt with in Immunoglobulin M Monoclonal Gammopathy, below. Onion-bulb formations, which are formed by concentric flattened Schwann cell processes, are believed to be secondary to successive episodes of de- and remyelination.

Interstitial Lesions

The pathology of endoneurial and perineurial capillaries, venules, and arterioles is discussed below in light of the disease concerned.

Cellular infiltrates may be inflammatory or tumoral. Various immunoperoxidase methods allow the identification of lymphomatous infiltrates, which display a monotypic lymphocytic population.

Endoneurial amorphous deposits of amyloid may indicate familial amyloidosis or be secondary to plasma cell dyscrasia. These deposits must not be confused with Renaut bodies (Fig. 20–6), which are normal structures of the endoneurium[9] but which are more frequent in people over age 80.[9,25–27]

The perineurium may appear thickened in various PN. On ultrastructural examination, hyperplastic perineurial lamellae can be seen to encase collagen fibers and a few unmyelinated fibers.[10]

ACQUIRED PERIPHERAL NEUROPATHIES IN ELDERLY PEOPLE

Acquired PN represent an important factor of disability in elderly people.[28]

Neuropathies Due to Vascular Diseases

Ischemia of the peripheral nerve may be due to microvasculitis, necrotizing vasculitis, or large artery damage. In a large series of 100 patients over 65 years of age suffering from a PN severe enough to justify performance of a peripheral nerve biopsy, Chia et al.[28] found that 35% had one form or another of vasculitic neuropathy.

MICROVASCULITIS

Microvasculitis affects vessels < 50 μm in diameter that are sometimes present in the endoneurium but mainly seen in the epineurium. Various amounts of mononuclear cells, mainly lymphocytes, are arranged in a perivascular cuff but no vessel wall necrosis is seen. Such cellular reactions can occur in a paraneoplastic process,[29–31] systemic lupus erythematosus,[9,32] essential mixed cryoglobulinemia,[9,33,34] or occasionally in multifocal and proximal diabetic neuropathy.[35] Sobue et al.[36] reported a case of chronic progressive sensory ataxic PN in a 63-year-old woman who had polyclonal gammopathy without any cryoglobulinemia. Small perivascular infiltrates were seen in peripheral nerves taken at autopsy. In a few biopsies, microvasculitis is present in peripheral nerves but without any precise cause.

NECROTIZING VASCULITIS

In this disorder segmental necrosis of the wall of epineurial arterioles and transmural inflammatory cell infiltration are combined (Fig. 20–7). The inflammatory cells are mainly T lymphocytes and macrophages,[37] mixed with a few plasma cells and polymorphonuclear leucocytes (Fig. 20–7). Iron deposits are also frequently present in the endoneurium.[38] Elderly people are particularly sensitive to necrotizing vasculitis.[28,39] Apart from cases of rheumatoid arthritis,[40] mixed cryoglobulinemia,[33] Churg and Strauss syndrome, or other connective tissue disorders[41] such as Sjögren syndrome and systemic lupus erythematosus, most cases of necrotizing vasculitis correspond to classic polyarteritis nodosa. Certain cases seem to be restricted to the peripheral nervous system and were reported as nonsystemic vasculitic neuropathy by Dyck et al.,[42] but such vascular lesions are also present in muscle specimens taken at the same time.[41]

TEMPORAL ARTERITIS

Peripheral neuropathy may occasionally be associated with temporal arteritis,[43] which typically affects people over 50; however, to our knowledge, the characteristic features of giant cell arteritis have not been reported on peripheral nerve biopsy. In a case report of a 78-year-old man with temporal arteritis, only moderate axonal degeneration and partial demyelination were observed on a sural nerve biopsy.[44]

ARTERIOSCLEROSIS

Large artery diseases correspond mainly to arteriosclerosis. We have observed cholesterol embolisms surrounded by inflammatory cellular infiltrates with macrophagic histiocytes in muscle biopsies, but we have not found these features in biopsied nerve fragments, as did Dyck.[45] Intravascular deposition of cholesterol may lead to necrotizing vasculitis.[46] Two series of patients suffering from arteriosclerosis severe enough to require amputation of the leg were studied. The first series concerned 25 arteriosclerotic diabetic patients who were all more than 60 years old,[47] and the second concerned 12 arteriosclerotic non diabetic patients, of whom 9 were more than 60 years old.[48] The nerve fiber lesions were generally more severe in the diabetic patients, highlighting the role of diabetic microangiopathy, as will be seen in the following section.

Experimental[19] and human[25,39] studies have demonstrated the relative resistance of peripheral nerve to ischemia owing to a profuse collateral circulation, and have shown that the center of a nerve fascicle seems to be more sensitive to ischemia than the periphery. However, after microsphere embolization of nerve capillaries in the rat, Nukada and Dyck[20] demonstrated that the "ischemic core" may also assume a wedge shape. The severe modification in one fascicle and the sparing of adjacent fascicles suggest an ischemic mechanism.[9] Harati and Niakan[49] found selective nerve fascicular degeneration in sural nerve biopsies of 8 patients aged 45 to 73 years (mean 58 years) out of 250 consecutive biopsies; in 6 cases this degeneration was associated with angiopathic changes. The selective sensitivity to ischemia of myelinated fibers according to their size is still debated. From our own experience in humans,[34,39] it appears that myelinated fibers of all sizes are equally affected by ischemia. Wallerian-like degenerative changes are prevalent in neuropathies due to vascular disease, especially in acute ischemic processes such as polyarteritis nodosa. Swollen axons with accumulation of various organelles have been

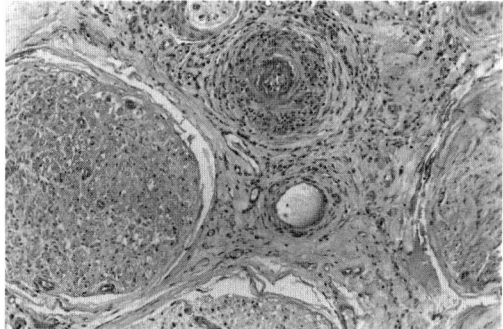

Figure 20–7. Peripheral neuropathy in a 78-year-old woman. The media of an epineurial arteriole is necrotized and invaded by inflammatory cells. Paraffin-embedded fragments, stained with hematoxylin-eosin, ×230.

observed in experimental ischemic neuropathy[19,20] as well as in humans.[39,47]

Neuropathies Due to Systemic Metabolic Disorders

DIABETES MELLITUS

Diabetes mellitus (DM) commonly causes PN, especially in the elderly. There are several syndromes associated with this disorder.

In the elderly, distal symmetric, predominantly sensory PN is most common in non insulin-dependent diabetes mellitus. In a recent study, 21 cases with a mean age 60.1 years (range 42–75) were compared with 21 younger cases with insulin-dependant diabetes.[50] In both groups, there were mainly axonal lesions on nerve biopsies with a wide range of myelinated fiber density. The relative number of regenerating fibers was significantly less in patients with non–insulin-dependent diabetes mellitus. Most clusters were surrounded by the persisting basal lamina of the original nerve fiber; this particular abnormality was described by King et al.[51] Isolated myelinated fibers possibly correspond to remyelinating ones.[52,53] Sima et al.[54,55] reported the occurrence of restricted paranodal demyelination, which was not confirmed by Thomas et al.[56]

The second major finding in diabetic patients is the presence of microangiopathy in the endoneurial capillaries, and its high frequency has been established in several series.[57,58] The main lesion of diabetic microangiopathy is the thickening of basal lamina corresponding to several concentric lamellae. In certain capillaries there are also swollen endothelial cells that sometimes almost occlude the lumen.[10,59] However, the relationship between endoneurial microangiopathy and nerve fiber lesions is not yet fully understood. Younger et al.[60] performed quantitative immunohistochemical studies of nerve biopsy specimens from 20 diabetic patients with a mean age 62 years (range 45–85). Twelve nerves had mild T-cell infiltrates in the endoneurium, mainly composed of CD8$^+$ T cells. Some had perivascular infiltrates in the epineurium. A few CD68-immunoreactive macrophages were also present in the endoneurium.

In some patients with multifocal and proximal diabetic neuropathy, Said et al.[35] observed vasculitis of epineurial blood vessels on biopsies of the intermediate cutaneous nerve of the thigh and the superficial peroneal nerve.

Acute painful neuropathy was described in nine diabetic patients by Archer et al.[61] This form is associated with severe weight loss and mainly concerns middle-aged people; two of their patients were over 55 years. In the nerve biopsies from three other patients, there was evidence of active degeneration of myelinated fibers and also degeneration of unmyelinated axons.

Subacute and chronic inflammatory demyelinating polyradiculoneuropathies are probably more frequent in diabetic patients and do not display specific myelinic lesions.[62,63]

HYPOTHYROIDISM

This disorder is sometimes associated with a distal symmetric sensorimotor PN, which recovers with the treatment of the hypothyroidism. A few cases have occurred in elderly people.[64–66] The nerve biopsy from a 61-year-old woman[65] displayed features mainly consisting of segmental demyelination and onion-bulb formations. The density of myelinated nerve fibers was slightly low (6.133/mm^2). Electron microscopic study revealed the presence of glycogen accumulations in the axons and in the Schwann cell cytoplasm. Two of the four cases reported by Meier and Bischoff[66] were over 60 years old and their nerve biopsies showed features of axonal degeneration.

NUTRITIONAL DEFICIENCIES

Polyneuropathies due to nutritional deficiencies can develop in elderly people in various conditions such as under socioeconomic difficulties or during mental impairment. Peripheral neuropathy due to vitamin B-1 deficiency (beriberi) occurs mainly in young people. In a study of nine cases of beriberi PN with sural nerve biopsy performed, one patient was 60 years old and the other eight were under 45.[67] This PN is characterized by axonal degeneration with mild, likely secondary demyelination.[67,68] Vitamin B-1 deficiency may be difficult to differentiate from alcoholic PN in some patients. Moreover, both conditions give rise to axonal modifications without characteristic lesions.[14] A few cases of PN due to vitamin B-12 deficiency presented features of axonal degeneration and no evidence of demyelination.[69] Vitamin E deficiency can cause spinocerebellar syndrome developing in the sixth and seventh decade without fat malabsorption.[70] The sural nerve biopsy of a 62-year-old patient showed a moderate loss of large myelinated fibers and dense deposits in Schwann cells and between myofibrils of quadriceps fragments.[70]

CRITICAL ILLNESS

Severe motor and sensory PN were described in critically ill patients.[71] Five cases were reported, one 66 years old. All patients had prolonged intensive care and nutritional factors may have played a role, especially since the patients improved with total parenteral nutrition. Hypoxia may also have played a role, especially at the peak of their critical illness. All nerve biopsies showed severe and acute axonal damage.

PARAPROTEINEMIC NEUROPATHIES

These conditions are encountered with significant frequency in the elderly. Most concern benign or malignant IgM monoclonal gammopathies (MG), but neuropathies associated with other forms of dysglobulinemia also occur.

IMMUNOGLOBULIN M MONOCLONAL GAMMOPATHY

Polyneuropathies associated with IgM MG have been extensively studied.[10–12,72–75] Although Waldenström's macroglobulinemia and IgM MG of undetermined significance (MGUS) are two conditions of different prognosis, peripheral nerves exhibit similar lesions.[10] In most cases, the neuropathy is demyelinating in type, with a widening of some myelin lamellae on ultrastructural examination (Fig. 20–8 to 20–10). Immunopathologic study shows IgM binding to peripheral nerve myelin and immunoblot analysis of the serum shows antibody binding to myelin-associated glycoprotein (MAG). In a study of 31 patients suffering from PN associated with IgM MG,[75] 25 were > 60 years old. Four patients had Waldenström's macroglobulinemia and 21

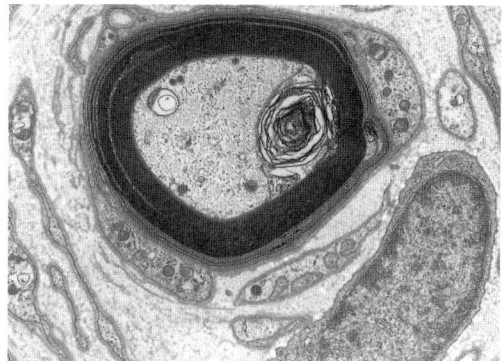

Figure 20–8. Peripheral neuropathy with IgM monoclonal gammopthy of undetermined significance in a 74-year-old man. Outer lamellae of the myelin sheath exhibit a typical widening. ×14,200.

had MGUS. In this series, features of widened myelin lamellae were observed in 20 cases: 2 Waldenström's macroglobulinemia and 18 MGUS. This characteristic and almost specific feature has been reported in cases of Waldenström's macroglobulinemia,[76,77] and in cases of MGUS.[78–81] There is usually a good correlation between the widening of myelin lamellae, the IgM binding to myelin sheaths at direct immunopathologic examination, and the presence of seric anti-MAG activity.[75] The precise localization of monoclonal IgM antibodies in widened myelin lamellae was demonstrated by immunoelectron microscopy.[82] The widening of myelin lamellae was extensively studied by King and Thomas,[83] and was present in a nerve biopsy from a patient with polyradiculoneuritis who developed an IgM MG a few months later. Onion-bulb forma-

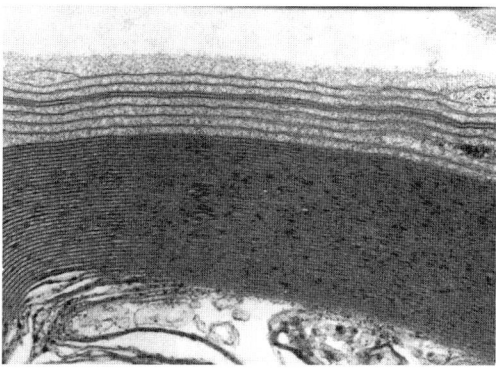

Figure 20–9. Other characteristic features of widened lamellae in the case presented in Figure 20–8. ×90,000.

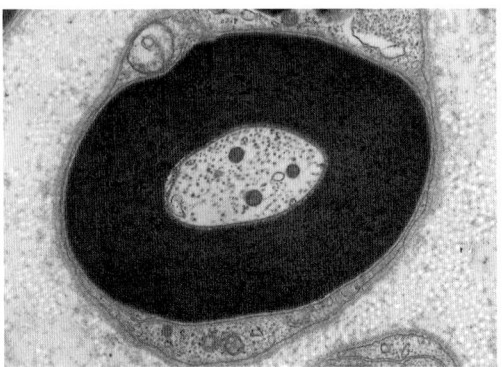

Figure 20–10. Same case presented in Figure 20–8. Only the outermost lamella is widened. ×21,000.

tions are sometimes associated with features of widened myelin lamellae. In this type of demyelinating neuropathy, lesions are mainly due to factors directed against myelin components, principally MAG. Gabriel et al. found a steady correlation between the selective loss of MAG from myelin and anti-MAG antibody titer.[84]

Other nonspecific but significant pathologic aspects include focal hypermyelination and axonal damage.[75] Some cases of PN associated with IgM MG present with a severe loss of myelinated fibers (fewer than 3000 per mm^2).[75] Endoneurial microangiopathy with thickening by reduplication of the vascular basement membrane was reported in some cases of PN with IgM MG.[85] In a few cases, plasma cells are dispersed in the endoneurium. Julien et al. reported a case with a few atypical lymphocytes in the endoneurium, but this case was unusual in that the IgM serum peak could be detected only 4 years after the widened myelin lamellae were observed on peripheral nerve biopsy when the patient was 67 years old.[86] Valldeoriola et al. reported another case with anti-MAG activity.[87] Julien et al. reported a case of PN with biclonal gammopathy in a 60-year-old man. The nerve biopsy exhibited both amyloid deposits related to an IgG-λ light-chain MG and the characteristic widened myelin lamellae related to an IgM-κ light-chain MG.[88] In some patients with a clinical presentation of chronic inflammatory demyelinating PN, an IgM MGUS is discovered. Most of these cases have seric anti-MAG activity, and on ultrastructural examination, macrophage-associated demyelination may be observed associated with the usual features of widened myelin lamellae.[89] T cells were present in 7 nerve biopsies from 19 patients with an IgM MG.[90] Busis et al. reported PN with high-serum IgM in a mother and her son.[91] The PN began when the mother was 66 years old and her son 53 years old. The son's nerve biopsy exhibited characteristic widened myelin lamellae. The authors suggested a familial disorder of immune regulation with antibody-mediated PN or a familial PN with a secondary immune response.

Some cases of PN associated with Waldenström's macroglobulinemia[10,92,93] should be considered separately because the lesions are different from those usually observed. These cases are characterized by the presence of IgM deposits in the endoneurium at by immunopathologic study. The deposits appear granular or sometimes microfibrillar on ultrastructural examination. They compress the nerve fibers, often erasing their basement membrane, and thicken the walls of the endoneurial capillaries.

IMMUNOGLOBULIN A OR G MONOCLONAL GAMMOPATHY OF UNDETERMINED SIGNIFICANCE

Some PN are associated with IgA or IgG MGUS. In the series reported by Yeung et al. there were 5 cases of IgA MGUS and 11 cases of IgG MGUS, without any specific lesion on nerve biopsies.[94] Deposition of IgG on myelin sheaths or Schwann cells has been reported in only two cases.[95] In a series of 14 cases of IgG MGUS, 5 cases presented as chronic demyelinating PN, and demyelinating lesions were observed on their peripheral nerve biopsies, with features of macrophage-associated demyelination in one case. The nine other cases presented as slowly progressive sensory or sensorimotor axonal PN and did not exhibit any specific lesion.[96] Endoneurial deposits were present in a patient investigated by Moorhouse et al.[97]

MULTIPLE MYELOMA

Peripheral neuropathy are classic in the setting of multiple myeloma and biopsies display features of chronic axonal degeneration without characteristic features.[76,98] In a few cases there are endoneurial amyloid deposits (see below).

POEMS SYNDROME

POEMS syndrome corresponds to the association of *P*olyneuropathy, *O*rganomegaly, *E*ndocrinopathy, *M*-components, and *S*kin abnormalities. Frequent in Japan, it is sometimes called "Crow-Fukase syndrome" and is frequently associated with an osteosclerotic myeloma. The monoclonal component is present in about 80% of reported cases and is IgA or IgG with a λ light chain in almost all cases. Direct immunofluorescence is usually normal and endoneurial deposits of immunoglobulins were present only in four cases reported by Adams and Said.[99] Wallerian degeneration was reported by Romas et al.,[100] but the most interesting modification is the feature of uncompacted myelin lamellae initially described by Ohnishi et al. in three cases of dysglobulinemic PN.[101] This particular feature was reported in POEMS syndrome by Bergouignan et al.,[102] Gherardi et al.,[103] and Vital et al.[104] (Fig. 20–11). It was also present in a 67-year-old Japanese case of POEMS syndrome autopsied 3 hr after death.[105] We have found it again in five other cases investigated since 1994. Uncompacted myelin lamellae can be observed in rare cases of Guillain-Barré syndrome[106] and in certain cases of Charcot-Marie-Tooth Type 1B,[107] but they are better known in POEMS syndrome. Narrowed or closed lumina of endoneurial blood vessels were present in two series from Japan[108,109] and overproduction of vascular endothelial growth factor was incriminated.[109] Gherardi et al.[110] evidenced overproduction of proinflammatory cytokines (tumor necrosis factor α, interleukin 1b and 6).

CRYOGLOBULINEMIA

Cryoglobulinemia type I features an isolated IgG or IgM MG and is rarely associated with PN.[111,112] In such cases, tubular structures identical to the cryoprecipitate extracted from the serum are observed in the endoneurium. In mixed cryoglobulinemia, type II may be identified as mixed cryoglobulins with a monoclonal component or type III as mixed polyclonal cryoglobulins.[113] These two types of cryoglobulin can cause hypersensitivity vasculitis, the patients presenting with multifocal or symmetrical PN. Most of these patients have episodes of vascular purpura of both legs. Cases with multifocal neuropathy usually show features of acute myelinoaxonal degeneration (Fig. 20–12) with numerous ovoids seen on semithin sections. Cases with symmetrical PN frequently display a dramatic loss of myelinated fibers on semithin sections. In certain cases, numerous endoneurial capillaries display swollen endothelial cells, and red blood cells and hemosiderin deposits can be seen within endoneurial macrophages. This endoneurial purpura may be considered the equivalent of the vascular purpura present in the dermis of such patients.[34] One patient had vasculitic PN, cryoglobulinemia, and anti-MAG IgM MG.[114] Cases of essential mixed cryoglob-

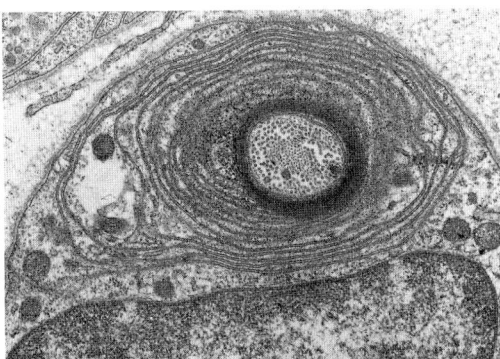

Figure 20–11. Peripheral neuropathy and POEMS syndrome in a 69-year-old woman. There is a characteristic feature of uncompacted myelin lamellae: the outer lamellae are not joined together. The diagnosis of POEMS syndrome was made 10 years after the first examination. ×21,000.

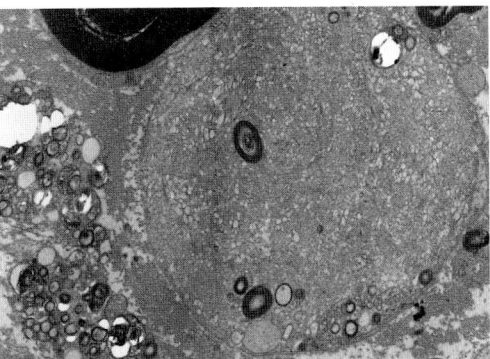

Figure 20–12. Mononeuritis multiplex with essential mixed cryoglobulinemia in a 70-year-old woman. The axon is totally destroyed and there is a vesicular disruption of the myelin sheath. ×11,000.

ulinemia associated with hepatitis C virus infection have more recently been reported, and a few presented necrotizing vasculitis on their nerve biopsy.[115,116]

Amyloid Peripheral Neuropathies

Amyloid PN may be of hereditary origin (familial amyloid polyneuropathy) or secondary to a plasma cell dyscrasia. Both conditions can be observed in elderly patients. Certain familial forms may have a late onset in countries such as the United States,[117] Portugal,[118] Spain,[119] Japan,[120,121] Ireland,[122] France and England.[123,124] In the Finnish type of familial amyloid PN, the signs and symptoms appear gradually after the age of 40 to 60 years, apart from lattice corneal dystrophy, which can be recognized after the age of 20 years.[125] Late onset of clinical symptoms was also reported in a Japanese family with the same variant.[126] Elderly people, however, are prone to present MG and amyloid PN can develop in the setting of a multiple myeloma[127,128] or in the course of Waldenström macroglobulinemia.[129] Occasionally, primary systemic amyloidosis may progress to multiple myeloma.[130] Amyloid PN developing in the course of a MGUS is rare and was related to an IgG MG in the case reported by Julien et al.[88] The amyloid origin of a PN can be strongly suspected when amyloid deposits are evidenced in another site of the body, usually in a rectal biopsy, but sometimes the nerve damage is secondary to extraneural deposition with nerve compression. This is classically observed in some cases of carpal tunnel syndrome.[9] Thus amyloid PN can truly be assessed when typical amyloid deposits are seen within endoneurial areas. Figure 20–13 shows amorphous acidophilic deposits in the endoneurium, and some endoneurial capillary walls are thickened by the same deposits. Such amyloid deposits are not to be confused with Renaut bodies. Amyloid deposits stain orange with Congo red and display typical dichroic birefringence with polarized light. On ultrastructural examination, there is a more or less severe nerve fiber loss with features of Wallerian-like degeneration. Some cases present more severe lesions of unmyelinated and small myelinated fibers.[131] Segmental demyelination is absent or

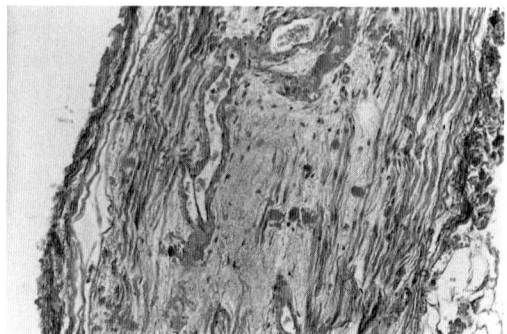

Figure 20–13. Peripheral neuropathy and IgG λ light-chain multiple myeloma in a 60-year-old woman. Round amyloid deposits are seen in the endoneurium and the capillary walls are thickened by amyloidosis. Paraffin-embedded fragments, stained with hematoxylin-eosin. ×230.

rare. The amyloid deposits are fibrillar structures (Fig. 20–14) entangled at random or more rarely bundled in parallel.[128] The basal membrane of Schwann cells is often erased by amyloid deposits. Occasionally, the diagnosis of amyloid PN can be made only on ultrastructural examination, which discloses a few small deposits located in the vicinity of endoneurial capillaries (Fig. 20–15). These minute deposits are not visible on the corresponding semithin sections.

Immunopathologic examination makes it possible to differentiate the origin of amyloid deposits.[132] In most familial cases, anti-transthyretin fixes on the deposits. However, anti-transthyretin can fix on amyloid deposits

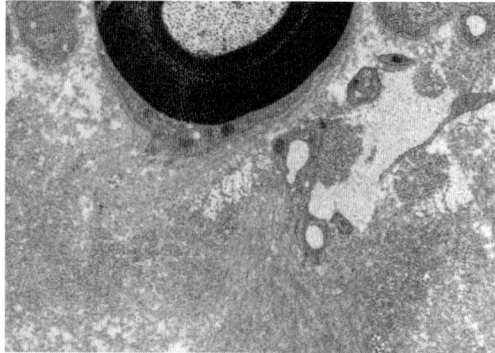

Figure 20–14. Peripheral neuropathy and IgG κ light-chain multiple myeloma in an 82-year-old woman. Fibrillar deposits, characteristic of amyloidosis, are seen close to the nerve fibers. ×16,500.

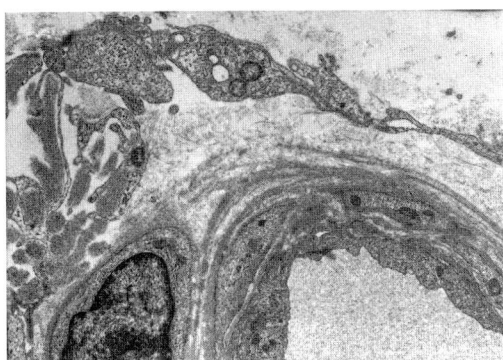

Figure 20–15. Peripheral neuropathy in a 60-year-old man. A few small bundles of amyloid fibrils are present in a perivascular location. ×18,000.

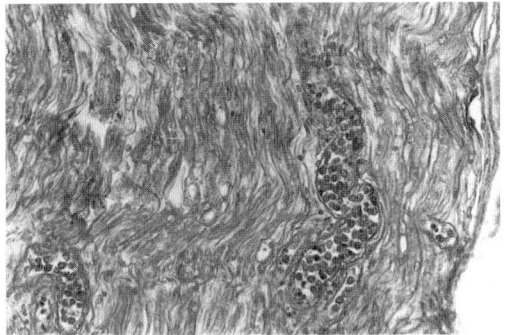

Figure 20–16. Intravascular lymphomatosis in a 62-year-old woman. Round tumoral cells are plugging the lumen of endoneurial capillaries. Paraffin-embedded fragments, are stained with hematoxylin-eosin, ×370.

from another origin.[133] To date, more than 40 mutations in the transthyretin gene have been described.[118,123] In the Finnish variant of familial amyloidosis, the deposits react with anti-gelsolin serum.[125] In cases of plasma cell dyscrasia, specific anti light-chain serum marks the deposits. Immunolabeling of amyloid fibrils can also be performed at the ultrastructural level.[134]

Lymphomatous Infiltration of Peripheral Nerve

Malignant lymphomas may invade peripheral nerves in a few cases.[135,136] Some are B-cell lymphomas, but T-cell lymphomas are also prone to invade the peripheral nervous system.[135,137] A 67-year-old woman investigated for a T-cell lymphoma had lymphomatous infiltrates in nerve and peroneus brevis muscle fragments.[135] A further study disclosed particles resembling human T-cell leukemia virus type 1 (HTLV-1) on ultrastructural examination of lymphomatous cells. In addition, polymerase chain reaction (PCR) experiments performed on deparaffinized sections demonstrated the presence of a tax sequence characteristic of HTLV-1.[138] Certain cases of malignant lymphoma invade the peripheral nervous system in unusual ways, as in the following cases. In a case of inflammatory demyelinating polyneuropathy, a 75-year-old patient with chronic lymphoid leukemia had large lymphocytic infiltrates in the epineurium. Tumoral lymphocytic cells with unusual pseudopodia and intracytoplasmic filaments had invaded the myelinated fibers and destroyed the myelin sheath.[10,135] In two cases of primary meningeal B lymphoma presenting as subacute ascending polyradiculoneuritis, lymphomatous cells were identified at cerebrospinal fluid (CSF) examination. At autopsy, lymphomatous cells were found to infiltrate several spinal roots.[139]

Intravascular malignant lymphomatosis often involves the central and rarely the peripheral nervous system.[140–142] We had the opportunity to study the superficial peroneal nerve biopsy from a 62-year-old woman who had an acute mononeuropathy of the leg. Fragments of muscle and nerve biopsies showed tumoral cells in the lumen of most blood vessels (Fig. 20–16) and tumoral markers showed a lymphomatous origin of the B type.[140] A quite similar observation concerned a 77-year-old man.[142]

Paraneoplastic Neuropathies

These are classic PN of sensory and sensorimotor type. Peripheral nerve biopsy studies have been reported, including one in elderly patients.[143] The primary pathology is axonal with secondary demyelination. Certain patients with carcinoma of the lung display features of vasculitis in the peripheral nerve.[29–31] In a 65-year-old patient with the anti-Hu syndrome, the paraneoplastic sensory neuropathy was demyelinating with evidence of microvasculitis on the sural nerve biopsy.[144] Paraneoplastic neuropathies have recently been revisited.[145]

Inflammatory Polyneuropathies

GUILLAIN-BARRÉ SYNDROME

This syndrome is the acute form of inflammatory demyelinating polyneuropathies.[146] These disorders are generally thought to have an autoimmune mechanism that damages the peripheral nervous system in various ways.[146–149]

The classic Guillain-Barré syndrome is the most frequent form in a global population. Paraffin-embedded fragments of peripheral nerve biopsies taken from cases of Guillain-Barré syndrome display only occasional and minimal endoneurial infiltrates of mononuclear cells. In our series of biopsies we have never seen the impressive features of inflammatory cells infiltrating the peripheral nervous system as reported by Asbury and Johnson[9] on fragments from spinal roots and sciatic nerves taken at autopsy. Endoneurial infiltration by macrophages has been evidenced by immunopathological study.[150,151] Ultrastructural examination is an excellent means to obtain the characteristic feature of inflammatory demyelinating polyneuropathies, i.e., macrophage-associated demyelination.[6,9–12,14,106,152,153] In the endoneurium a few histiocytes may be clustered around a myelinated fiber, even invading the Schwann cell cytoplasm (Fig. 20–17). Moreover, flattened and elongated processes from the invading histiocytes peel away certain myelin lamellae, whereas the axon remains normal or almost normal. This feature of macrophage-associated demyelination is specific in human pathology for inflammatory demyelinating polyneuropathy and has never been reported in any other condition apart from one exceptional finding in a thorough ultrastructural study of nerve biopsies from 17 patients with peroneal muscular atrophy.[154] In this case, an additional inflammatory process may have developed.

Fulminant cases of Guillain-Barré syndrome present with inexcitability of motor nerves and are not to be confused with primary acute axonal forms.[7,155–158] Most myelin

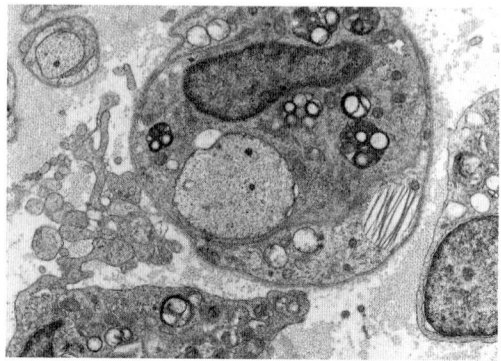

Figure 20–17. Guillain-Barré syndrome in a 66-year-old man. A histiocyte is visible inside the Schwann cell cytoplasm and the axon is totally naked. Another macrophagic histiocyte is present in the endoneurium. ×6,600.

sheaths are severely destroyed and typically present features of vesicular disruption on ultrastructural examination. Almost half of the reported cases concern the elderly: ages of these patients were 72 years,[155] 63 years,[156] 67 years,[157] and 67 years.[7] In such a severe case, demyelination and macrophage infiltration were demonstrated on the biopsy of the motor terminal branch of a musculocutaneous nerve.[159]

The acute axonal form of Guillain-Barré syndrome was described at length by Feasby et al.[160] in five patients who had electrically inexcitable motor nerves. Their first case, a 64-year-old woman, died and an autopsy study evidenced severe axonal degeneration in the nerve roots and distal nerves without inflammation or demyelination. Three other cases, aged 68, 57, and 63 years, were reported by Feasby et al.[157] and nerve biopsies showed severe axonal degeneration. The concept of acute axonal Guillain-Barré syndrome has often been challenged but is now widely recognized.[161] Griffin et al. reported three demonstrative cases aged 55, 41, and 60 years who had intra-axonal macrophages in the spinal roots studied at autopsy.[162] This macrophage-mediated attack on the axons is the most characteristic ultrastructural feature of these axonal forms and has already been described by Brechenmacher et al. in five peripheral nerve biopsies.[163] However, in most cases this axonal macrophagic invasion is not identified.[164]

Acute sensory neuropathy is rare. In a 67-year-old man who died suddenly 5 weeks after onset of symptoms, a sural nerve biopsy showed acute axonal degeneration without inflammation. At autopsy, sensory and autonomic ganglia were infiltrated by numerous CD8$_+$ T lymphocytes.[165]

CHRONIC INFLAMMATORY POLYNEUROPATHIES

Chronic inflammatory demyelinating polyneuropathies (CIDP) have a chronic progressive or relapsing course.[152,166] Endoneurial infiltration by macrophages can be evidenced by immunopathological study.[150,151,167] Periperal nerve lesions usually consist of demyelination-remyelination-ie., segmental demyelination (Figs. 20–18 and 20–19) and onion-bulb formations. The higher probability of observing macrophage-associated demyelination in Guillain-Barré syndrome[106] than in CIDP is well known.[168,169] Coexisting axonal degeneration involving both myelinated and unmyelinated fibers is usually observed, although there is some controversy about unmyelinated fiber lesions.[169–171] Focal involvement on certain nerve biopsies has been reported in a few cases of upper limb demyelinating neuropathy.[172] The possible occurrence of CIDP in association with an identified dysglobulinemic status is now recognized[89,95,96,173,174] and a causal relationship between the two has been suggested. From the previously reported data,

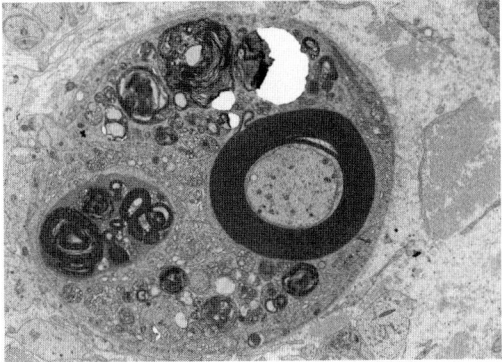

Figure 20–18. Chronic inflammatory demyelinating polyneuropathy in a 66-year-old woman. A histiocyte has invaded the Schwann cell cytoplasm and destroyed the external part of the myelin sheath. ×10,000.

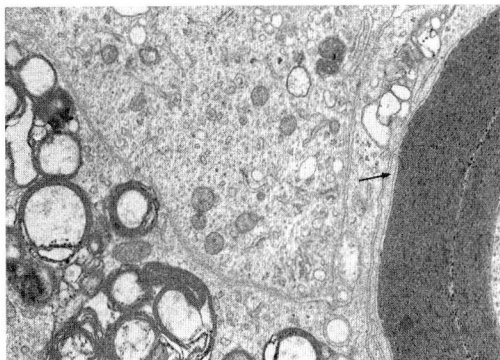

Figure 20–19. Same case as in Figure 20–18. The external part of the myelin sheath is dissociated by an elongated histiocytic process (arrow). ×45,000.

it seems that the most common association is with IgG MG and IgM MG. We had the opportunity to study 21 patients presenting with CIDP and dysglobulinemia and to have a peripheral nerve biopsy available for all of them. Seventeen were over 60 years of age. An IgG MG was identified in 8 cases, an IgM MG in 12, and an IgG-IgM biclonal gammopathy in one case. As previously reported,[95,96] the cases of CIDP with IgG MG did not differ from those without. On the contrary, all our cases with an IgM MG and the one with an IgG-IgM biclonal gammopathy had seric anti-MAG activity, and they presented widened myelin lamellae on their peripheral nerve biopsy. Additionally, macrophage-associated demyelination was also observed in six cases. This demonstrates that there is no definite gap between CIDP and polyneuropathies associated with IgM MG having anti-MAG activity.

Chronic inflammatory axonal polyneuropathies are now recognized as the corresponding forms of axonal Guillain-Barré syndrome and most cases are steroid responsive. Relapsing forms were first described,[175,176] and progressive cases have since been reported.[177] Peripheral nerve biopsies disclose primary axonal lesions and macrophages scattered in the endoneurium.

We recently reported two cases of chronic inflammatory axonal polyneuropathy presenting plasmacytoid histiocytes in the endoneurium, and a few of these were present inside the basal lamina of a myelinated fiber.[178] Such a particular cellular reaction is mainly observed in Lyme's disease[179] and in certain cases of AIDS.[180]

Multifocal motor neuropathy (MMN) with conduction block was described by Lewis et al. in 1982.[181] Certain cases present clinically as asymmetric chronic inflammatory demyelinating polyneuropathy[182–186] and the diagnosis may be difficult.[187] The nerve biopsy lesions are not characteristic and demyelinating features are few.[183,184] However, large onion-bulb formations can be seen, as well as "burnt-out" formations in other fascicles.[12] Recently, Van den Berg-Vos et al. suggested a distinct clinical entity, "multifocal inflammatory demyelinating neuropathy,"[188] which is different from both CIDP and MMN. Inflammation was present in a biopsy sample taken from the brachial plexus.[188] Ischemia has been incriminated in certain cases of PN with conduction blocks because the severity of lesions may vary among fascicles[189] and vasculitis lesions have been reported in a few cases.[190]

TICK-BITE MENINGORADICULONEURITIS (LYME DISEASE)

This disorder is suspected in patients with painful radiculoneuropathy, chronic lymphocytic meningitis, and erythema chronica migrans spreading from the bitten area.[179,191] In the series of Vallat et al.,[179] the 10 patients ranged in age from 48 to 80 years, and nerve biopsies showed infiltrates of lymphocytes and plasma cell–like histiocytes around perineurial vessels without necrosis of the vessel walls. There was a significant loss of myelinated fibers and features of axonal degeneration. A 92-year-old woman with several cranial nerve defects has been studied at length.[192]

SJÖGREN'S SYNDROME

This syndrome, characterized by dryness of eyes, mouth, and other mucous membranes, may be associated with disease of the peripheral nervous system.[193–195] As Sjögren's syndrome may be primary or secondary, it is possible that some features observed on the peripheral nerve biopsy are caused by the accompanying disease rather than by Sjögren's syndrome; this is the case for the reported necrotizing vasculitis.[193] Clinical and electrophysiological signs of PN were found in 10 of 46 patients with primary Sjögren's syndrome, and 7 of these cases were over 55 years old.[194] A peripheral nerve biopsy was performed in seven patients (five with symmetric polyneuropathy and two with sensory neuronopathy) and showed moderate remyelination and regeneration in four patients and fiber loss that was mainly extensive in three. Necrotizing vasculitis was not seen, but alterations of the endoneurial microvessels were prominent. These latter features consisted of thickening and reduplication of the basal lamina in all patients. The authors suggested that aging seems to be a critical factor for PN in Sjögren's syndrome, possibly favoring microangiopathic changes in the endoneurial vessels.[194]

OTHER DISORDERS OF INFLAMMATORY NEUROPATHY

Rheumatoid arthritis is sometimes associated with PN. Features of necrotizing vasculitis may be present in the epineurial vessels.[40]

PN may occur in the course of hypereosinophilic syndrome, which is characterized by a long-lasting increase in circulating eosinophils and manifestations of multisystem involvement. Unlike other conditions associated with hypereosinophilia (Churg-Strauss or connective tissue diseases), axonal lesions observed on the peripheral nerve biopsies in hypereosinophilic syndrome are not associated with vasculitis.[196,197] A study with well-documented ultrastructural examination in two cases pointed to an alteration of the blood nerve barrier, producing in turn an increase in the endoneurial fluid pressure.[197] Sarcoid lesions may occasionally be found in a nerve biopsy.[198] A few cases of Creutzfeldt-Jakob disease have been reported with PN. One concerned a man carrying a mutation at codon 200 of the prion protein gene.[199]

Toxic Neuropathies

Iatrogenic PN are relatively frequent in elderly people. The toxic effects of vincristine are well known. The first ultrastructural examinations of nerve biopsies disclosed axonal degeneration.[200] We studied the nerve biopsies of three cases: one case had numerous axonal modifications, a second case showed a few unmyelinated axonal modifications, and the third case showed numerous glycogen accumulations in the axons, Schwann cell cytoplasm, and even endothelial cells in the endoneurial capillaries.[10]

The effects of cisplatin on peripheral nerves were described by Thompson et al. concerning 11 patients ranging in age from 47 to 71 years.[201] Most of these patients had been treated for ovarian adenocarcinoma and all developed distal sensory PN. Morphologic studies performed on sural nerve biopsies exhibited axonal degeneration and secondary myelin breakdown.

Amiodarone is widely used in the treatment of cardiac arrythmias and angina pectoris. There may be a loss of myelinated fibers of all sizes and unmyelinated fibers show frequent features of regeneration[202,203] but segmental demyelination predominates in certain cases. Unusual inclusions are present in Schwann cells, fibroblasts, vessel walls, and perineurial cells. On ultrastructural examination, most of these inclusions are round and contain concentric membranous lamellae.

Chloroquine may cause a PN in patients treated for malaria prophylaxis, but in our experience such PN are mainly observed in patients treated for rheumatoid arthritis. The inclusions (Fig. 20–20) are almost similar to those observed in amiodarone therapy.[204] Three out of the four reported patients had features of segmental demyelination and remyelination.

Isoniazid in patients treated for tuberculosis can induce a motor and sensory PN. After interruption of isoniazid therapy, patients recover progressively. An electron microscopy study was done by Ochoa on nine patients, six of whom were over 60. Wallerian degeneration was the main pathologic process.[205]

Peripheral neuropathy secondary to disulfiram treatment is well known. In a 67-year-old man who insidiously developed a PN and encephalopathy after 30 years of disulfiram ingestion, a sural nerve biopsy showed axonal degeneration with a few swollen axons containing membranolamellar bodies, mitochondria, and bundles of neurofilaments.[206]

The neurotoxic effect of arsenic on peripheral nerve is axonal degeneration and loss of myelinated fibers.[207]

Hereditary Neuropathies

CHARCOT-MARIE-TOOTH (CMT) DISEASE

This disorder may occur in the elderly. It is now classified according to recent results of molecular genetic studies.[208–210]

Most cases of type 1A CMT disease carry a chromosome 17p11.2 duplication,[211] and three patients investigated in the Sander et al. study were over 56 years.[212] In both series there were more or less severe nerve fiber loss, hypomyelination, and numerous onion-bulb formations. Thomas et al.[213] found hypomyelination and regression of the onion bulbs in older patients. In a family presenting CMT 1 and diabetes mellitus, most onion-bulb formations consisted of very thin cytoplasmic processes.[214] Molecular genetic studies have widened the field of phenotypes associated with 17p11.2 duplication. Several cases with calf hypertrophy[211,215] have been reported as well as cases with prominent distal sensory loss resulting in acrodystrophic changes.[211] An Austrian family with Roussy-Levy syndrome is associated with a duplication on chromosome 17p11.2,[216] but the original French family carries a missense mutation on the PO gene.[217] The coexistence of proven CMT 1A and IgM MG has also been reported.[218] Peripheral myelin protein 22

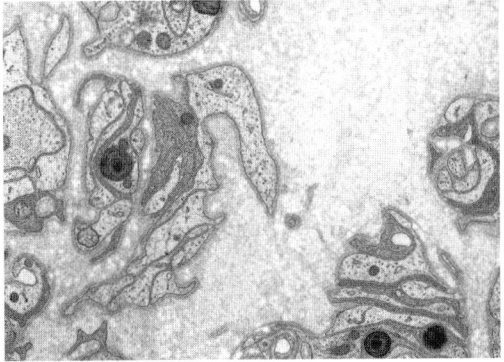

Figure 20–20. Chloroquine peripheral neuropathy in 72-year-old man. Typical multilamellar inclusions are seen in the cytoplasm of unmyelinated fibers. ×22,000.

(PMP 22) is overexpressed in myelinated Schwann cells[219,220] and is also present in the onion-bulb formations.[221]

Cases of type 1B CMT disease are not so frequent, have earlier onset, and are due to mutations on the PO gene. According to the type of mutation, features of uncompacted lamellae, or tomaculae are observed on peripheral nerve biopsy.[107,222–227] The Thr124 Met mutation is sometimes associated with a clinically distinct phenotype with late onset and marked sensory abnormalities.[228] Other atypical phenotypes can be observed, such as the original Roussy-Levy syndrome[217] and an axonal phenotype.[229]

Cases of type 1X CMT disease are relatively frequent and have been thoroughly studied.[212,230–233] An association of a normal or moderately decreased myelinated fiber density with a unimodal distribution, numerous clusters of regeneration often surrounded by flattened Schwann cell processes, and no prominent demyelinating process but discrete hypomyelination is strongly suggestive of CMT-X.[212] There is only one report showing morphological evidence of prominent demyelination in a 71-year-old CMT-X female carrier with late onset disease.[234]

Cases of type 2 CMT disease have a well-preserved motor nerve conduction velocity and a delayed onset.[208] Nerve biopsies show a marked myelinated fiber loss and a few clusters of regenerating fibers.[235] Moreover, neurofilament accumulation has been observed in certain families.[236,237]

Hereditary motor and sensory neuropathy with focally folded myelin sheaths (CMT 4B) shows genetic heterogeneity. Though first reported in a young girl,[238] this rare entity can be observed in adults.[239,240]

HEREDITARY NEUROPATHY WITH LIABILITY TO PRESSURE PALSIES

This disorder is an autosomal dominant disease and there is a PMP 22 gene deletion in most families.[241,242] This condition is characterized by focal, sausage-shaped thickening of the myelin sheaths. It was described by Behse et al.[243] and the myelin thickening was called "tomaculae" by Madrid and Bradley.[244] Though the age of onset is generally under 50, there are some patients over 60. Focal myelin thickening is seen on teased fibers, and on ultrastructural examination hypermyelination exhibits various patterns, including regular coiling of lamellae, and internal or external redundant loops. These modifications were studied in detail by Madrid and Bradley.[244] Other internodes can show demyelination or the onset of remyelination. The density of myelinated and unmyelinated fibers is normal but there is a loss of large myelinated fibers thought to be secondary to myelinic modifications. In nine cases with the characteristic chromosome 17p11.2–12 deletion, tomaculae were found at nerve biopsy.[241] Using PCR on paraffin-embedded nerve specimens, Thiex and Schröder identified the PMP 22 deletion in most cases.[245]

MACHADO-JOSEPH DISEASE

This disorder is characterized by a systemic cerebellar atrophy and a PN is sometimes present. Chronic axonal degeneration was observed in several nerve trunks taken at autopsy from three brothers aged 58, 57, and 56.[246] In a large series from Germany, electrophysiologic study demonstrated that axonal damage is mainly age related and is not determined by CAG repeat length.[247]

OTHER DISORDERS OF HEREDITARY NEUROPATHY

Neuroacanthocytosis, also called "chorea-acanthocytosis," is a rather rare entity, but a PN is sometimes observed. There were 5 cases over age 55 in a large series of 19 cases and 1 had a sural nerve biopsy.[248] Two brothers aged 69 and 62 years had a sural nerve biopsy.[249] In each case, chronic axonal degeneration was noticed.

Mc Leod syndrome can be associated with X-linked chorea-acanthocytosis. A nerve biopsy from a 55-year-old man showed a moderate loss of large fibers and a few onion-bulb formations.[250]

Diagnosis of CADASIL (cerebral *a*utosomal *d*ominant *a*rteriopathy with *s*ubcortical *i*nfarcts and *l*eukoencephalopathy) can be proved by the presence of the characteristic granular deposits in epineurial vessels.[251]

Involvement of the Peripheral Nerve in Storage Diseases

Certain storage disorders produce PN, but this occurs mainly in pediatric pathology and occasionally in young adults. We have found a few examples in patients over 55 years of age.

Tangier disease is characterized by high-density lipoprotein deficiency. Pollock et al. reported the case of a 61-year-old man[252] and Marbini et al. reported a man aged 64 years with Tangier disease.[253] Gibbels et al.[254] classified the PN of Tangier disease into three types: (1) transient or relapsing, often asymmetrical syndrome; (2) slowly progressing symmetrical PN, most marked in the lower extremities; and (3) slowly progressing symmetrical PN with a syringomyelia-like syndrome. On semi-thin sections, clear vacuoles are seen in the Schwann cell cytoplasm and are especially numerous in certain longitudinally cut fibers. On electron microscopy, there are clear, round vacuoles sometimes devoid of a limiting structure. The formation of these vacuoles is still under discussion.[254]

Metachromatic leukodystrophy may have a late onset. A 63-year-old man with this disorder was reported by Bosch and Hart.[255]

Polyglucosan body disease was described by Robitaille et al. in four patients whose age ranged from 59 to 67 years.[256] There was massive involvement of central neuronal processes. Polyglucosan bodies may also be present in the peripheral nerve.[256,257] Adult polyglucosan body disease likely has more than one biochemical basis. Glycogen branching enzyme dysfunction was evidenced in two unrelated Ashkenazi-Jewish patients having numerous intraaxonal polyglucosan bodies at sural nerve biopsy.[258] Another study on two Ashkenazi-Jewish patients, one African-American, and three Caucasian patients suffering from adult polyglucosan body disease showed that the glycogen branching enzyme activity was markedly decreased not only in the leukocytes from the two Jewish patients but also in peripheral nerve specimens, whereas it was normal in nerve tissue and leukocytes from all non-Jewish patients.[259] Moreover, this activity was normal in the muscle specimens from both Jewish and non-Jewish patients, showing that the defect is tissue specific. Vos et al. reported the case of two women who had numerous polyglucosan bodies in myelinated axons and a few in unmyelinated fibers.[260] Polyglucosan bodies can be observed occasionally in nerve biopsies from elderly patients without any specific correlation.[9,10] They are probably more frequent in intramuscular nerve twigs.[9]

Involvement of the Peripheral Nerve in Mitochondrial Encephalomyopathies

Mitochondrial disorders have recently been thoroughly revisited.[261,262] A few cases of clinically patent PN have been reported in various phenotypes of mitochondrial encephalomyopathies, and molecular analysis of mitochondrial (mtDNA) modifications is necessary to better diagnose and classify these rare cases. Interestingly, certain cases have a delayed onset and can be observed in the elderly. There were two cases of mitochondrial myopathy, encephalopathy, and stroke-like episodes (MELAS) with the characteristic 3243 mtDNA point mutation and three cases of myoclonic epilepsy and ragged-red fibers (MERFF) with the characteristic 8344 mtDNA point mutation in a recent study from Chu et al.[263] Their case 4 was a 65-year-old woman with MERFF, and the nerve biopsy showed mainly features of axonal degeneration. There were features of atypical CMT disease in a family with the 8344 MERFF mutation and a woman who was 73 years old when she was investigated.[264] This mitochondrial mutation was also evidenced in a 64-year-old man presenting with PN and multiple symmetric lipomatosis.[265] Sixteen sporadic cases of multiple symmetric lipomatosis had no mtDNA mutation.[266] The presence of PN has been reported in a few families with MERRF. We have only taken into account cases with a characteristic mtDNA: 8344 mutation[263,265–272] or the less frequent 8363 mutation.[273] In a few cases, a severe sensory PN was the prominent neurological disturbance,[264,265,271] and a case from a Cherokee Indian family was first diagnosed as an atypical CMT case.[264] A thorough morphologic study has been performed in only one case[265] and there were mainly features of axonal degeneration, but there were also conspicuous onion-bulb formations, and electrophysiologic study disclosed a chronic axonal degeneration.[265] In the nerve biopsy, a few fibers presented features of primary myelin damage probably related to mitochondrial abnormalities in the Schwann cell cytoplasm. The association of multiple symmetric lipomatosis and PN was present in several families,[264,265,267–270,272] but no lipomas were noticed in other cases.[263,271,273]

Mitochondrial encephalopathy with mtDNA deletions can present as an autosomal dominant mode of inheritance, and a PN was present in a 74-year-old man and his 73-year-old brother.[274] In a 64-year-old man reported by Sommer and Schröder, a nuclear gene mutation was probably present but the mtDNA defect was not established.[275] In a series of 20 cases with mitochondrial myopathy or with progressive external ophthalmoplegia, 3 cases were over 59 years of age and presented a PN, and one had a 8.4 kb deletion on mtDNA analysis.[276] Nerve biopsies rarely show characteristic mitochondrial modifications on ultrastructural examination of myelinated Schwann cell cytoplasm.[275] Abnormal mitochondria with paracrystalline inclusions in the cytoplasm of a few unmyelinated fibers were reported by Yiannikas et al.[277] and Schröder,[278] but their mitochondrial origin is not well established. Certain cases present accumulation of non modified mitochondria in endothelial cells of endoneurial capillaries and epineurial arterioles.[276] Intra-axonal accumulation of swollen mitochondria should not be taken into account, given that they are frequently observed in certain cases of ischemic neuropathy and especially in diabetes mellitus with severe atherosclerosis of the lower limbs.[47]

Acquired mtDNA deletions related to aging were reported by Wallace et al.[279] Toscano et al. reported three sporadic cases with ragged red fibers on muscle biopsy and loss of myelinated fibers on nerve biopsy, but without any mtDNA modifications.[280] Fadic et al.[281] reported four unrelated sporadic patients with sensory ataxic PN, dysarthria and ophthalmoparesis with multiple mtDNA deletions in muscle and peripheral nerve. Numerous ragged red fibers were present in two of them and there was a severe loss of nerve fibers on two sural nerve biopsies.[281] Molecular genetic screening of the mtDNA is justified when evaluating patients with an unusual PN.[281]

PERIPHERAL NERVE AND AGING

Clinical signs of peripheral nervous system dysfunction in the elderly are deterioration of most sensory modalities in the distal extremities, muscle wasting, decline in strength, and absence or decrease of tendon reflexes. Lascelles and Thomas[282] and Jacobs and Love[283] noticed that in humans over the age of 60, irregularities of internodal length were common on isolated fibers from the sural nerve. The authors considered these modifications to be the result of segmental demyelination and remyelination, and of regeneration after complete degeneration of nerve fibers. In a study of the normal sural nerve in humans, Ochoa and Mair have described the increase with age of myelinated fiber degeneration; however, these authors also pointed out aspects of myelinated fiber regeneration, and insisted that unmyelinated fibers are affected more markedly than myelinated ones.[21] We studied the superficial peroneal nerve biopsies of 46 patients aged 70 to 95 years.[5] Like most elderly people, these patients displayed evidence of peripheral nervous system dysfunction, but they were not suffering from any affliction known to alter the peripheral nerve. This study confirmed the possibility that myelinated fibers regenerate in elderly patients and also emphasized the large extent of unmyelinated fiber damage. Moreover, segmental demyelination was relatively rare, as were Wallerian-like degeneration and axonal organelle accumulation. Tohgi et al. studied quantitative changes with age in normal human sural nerves and noticed that myelinated fibers decreased with advancing age and that the ratio of small-to-large myelinated fibers increased with age.[284] We also found in our cases that myelinated fiber loss predominated in the large diameter group, but several patients presented a high number of small myelinated fibers, a finding that corresponds to clusters of regenerating fibers. The cause of the degeneration and decrease in peripheral nerve fibers with age is uncertain, although chronic mechanical trauma or vascular changes with age have been suggested. As reported by Jacobs and Love,[283] reduplication of the vascular basement membrane was noticed in the nerves from our cases,[5] but thickening was moderate. In fact, thickening of endoneurial capillary walls seen on semi-thin sections frequently corresponds to accumulation of collagen fibers encased by a thin fibroblastic process. Tohgi et al. reported that after 60 years there was a greater reduction in large myelinated fibers, at a time when stenosis of the vasa nervorum is more pronounced.[284] Thus, apart from neuropathies of known etiologies, the human peripheral nerve presents morphologic lesions due to aging. These consist mostly of chronic axonal lesions concerning both myelinated and unmyelinated fibers, and coexist with regeneration.

This work was supported by grants from l'Association Française contre les Myopathies (AFM, Paris), l'Institut Fédératif de Recherche en Neurosciences Cliniques et Expérimentales, and l'EA 2966: Neurobiologie des Affections de la Myéline (Bordeaux). The authors are very grateful to Marie-Hélène Canron for technical assistance, and Josiane Neveu for secretarial assistance.

REFERENCES

1. McLeod JG, Tuck RR, Pollard JD, Cameron J, Walsh JC. Chronic polyneuropathy of undetermined cause. J Neurol Neurosurg Psychiatry 1984; 47:530–535.
2. George J, Twomey JA. Causes of polyneuropathy in the elderly. Age and Ageing 1986; 15:247–249.
3. Notermans NC, Wokke JHJ, Franssen H, van der Graaf Y, Vermeulen M, van den Berg LH, Bär PR, Jennekens FGI. Chronic idiopathic polyneuropathy presenting in middle or old age: a clinical and electrophysiological study of 75 patients. J Neurol Neurosurg Psychiatry 1993; 56:1066–1071.
4. McLeod JG. Investigation of peripheral neuropathy. J Neurol Neurosurg Psychiatry 1995; 58:274–283.
5. Vital A, Vital C, Rigal B, Decamps A, Emeriau JP, Galley P. Morphological study of the aging human peripheral nerve. Clin Neuropathol 1990; 9:10–15.
6. Prineas JW. Pathology of the Guillain-Barré syndrome. Ann Neurol 1981; 9 (suppl):6–19.
7. Berciano J, Figols J, Garcia A, Calle E, Illa I, Lafarga M, Berciano MT. Fulminant Guillain-Barré syndrome with universal inexcitability of peripheral nerves: a clinicopathological study. Muscle Nerve 1997; 20: 846–857.
8. Dyck PJ, Giannini C, Lais A. Pathologic alterations of nerves. In: Dyck PJ, Thomas PK, Griffin JW, Low PA, Poduslo JF, Éds. Peripheral Neuropathy, Vol. 1. Philadelphia: Saunders, 1993:514–595.
9. Asbury AK, Johnson PC. Pathology of Peripheral Nerve. Philadelphia: W.B. Saunders, 1978.
10. Vital, C, Vallat, JM. Ultrastructural Study of the Human Diseased Peripheral Nerve, 2nd ed., New York, Elsevier, 1987.
11. Richardson EP, De Girolami U. Pathology of the Peripheral Nerve. Philadephia: W.B. Saunders, 1995.
12. Midroni G, Bilbao JM. Biopsy Diagnosis of Peripheral Neuropathy. Boston; Butterworth Heineman, 1995.
13. Thomas PK, Landon DN, King RHM. Diseases of the peripheral nerves. In: Graham D.I., Lantos PL, eds. Greenfield's Neuropathology, Vol. 2. London: Arnold, 1997, 367–487.
14. King RHM: Atlas of Peripheral Nerve Pathology. London Arnold, 1999.
15. Griffin JW, Watson DF. Axonal transport in neurological diseases. Ann Neurol 1988; 23:3–13.
16. Dyck PJ, Johnson WJ, Lambert EH, O'Brien PC. Segmental demyelination secondary to axonal degeneration in uremic neuropathy. Mayo Clin Proc 1971; 46: 400–431.
17. Dyck PJ, Lais AC., Karnes J.L, Sparks M, Hunder H, Low PA, Windebank AJ. Permanent axotomy, a model of axonal atrophy and secondary segmental demyelination and remyelination. Ann Neurol 1981; 9: 575–583.
18. Spencer PS, Schamburg HH. Ultrastructural studies of the dying-back process: III. The evolution of experimental peripheral giant axonal degeneration. J Neuropathol Exp Neurol. 1977; 35:276–299.
19. Korthals JK, Korthals MA, Wisniewski HM. Peripheral nerve ischemia. Part 2. Accumulation of organelles. Ann Neurol 1978; 4:487–498.
20. Nukada H, Dyck PJ. Microsphere embolization of nerve capillaries and fiber degeneration. Am J. Pathol 1984; 115:275–287.
21. Ochoa J, Mair WGP. The normal sural nerve in man. II. Changes in the axons and Schwann cells due to aging. Acta Neuropathol 1969; 13:217–239.
22. Behse F, Buchthal F, Carlsen F, Knappeis GC. Unmyelinated fibers and Schwann cells of sural nerve in neuropathy. Brain 1975; 98:493–510.
23. Webster de H, Spiro FD, Waksmann BH, Adams RD. Phase and electron microscopic studies of experimental demyelination. II. Schwann cell changes in guinea pig sciatic nerves during experimental diphteritic neuritis. J Neuropathol Exp Neurol 1961; 20: 5–34.
24. Weller RO. Diphteric neuropathy in the chicken: an electron microscope study. J Pathol Bacteriol 1965; 89:591–598.
25. Dyck PJ, Conn DL, Okazaki H. Necrotizing angiopathic neuropathy. Three-dimensional morphology of fiber degeneration related to sites of occluded vessels. Mayo Clin Proc 1972; 47:461–475.
26. Asbury AK. Renaut bodies: a forgotten endoneurial structure. J Neuropathol Exp Neurol. 1973; 32:334–343.
27. Bergouignan FX, Vital C. Occurrence of Renaut's bodies in a peripheral nerve. Arch. Pathol. Lab. Med. 1984; 108:330–333.
28. Chia L, Fernandez A, Lacroix C, Adams D, Planté V, Said G. Contribution of nerve biopsy findings to the diagnosis of disabling neuropathy in the elderly. A retrospective review of 100 consecutive patients. Brain 1996; 119:1091–1098.

29. Johnson PC, Rolak LA, Hamilton RH, Laguna JF. Paraneoplastic vasculitis of nerve: a remote effect of cancer. Ann Neurol 1979; 5:437–444.
30. Vallat JM, Leboutet MJ, Hugon J, Loubet A, Lubeau M, Fressinaud C. Acute pure sensory paraneoplastic neuropathy with perivascular endoneurial inflammation: ultrastructural study of capillary walls. Neurology 1986; 36:1395–1399.
31. Vincent D, Dubas F, Hauw JJ, Godeau P, Lhermitte F, Buge A, Castaigne P. Nerve and muscle microvasculitis in peripheral neuropathy: a remote effect of cancer? J. Neurol. Neurosurg. Psychiatry 1986; 49:1007–1010.
32. McCombe PA, McLeod JG, Pollard JD, Guo YP, Ingall TJ. Peripheral sensorimotor and autonomic neuropathy associated with systemic lupus erythematous. Clinical, pathological and immunological features. Brain 1987; 110:533–549.
33. Chad D, Pariser K, Bradley WG, Adelman LS, Pinn VW. The pathogenesis of cryoglobulinemic neuropathy. Neurology 1982; 32:725–729.
34. Vital C, Deminière C, Lagueny A, Bergouignan FX, Pellegrin JL, Doutre MS, Clement A, Beylot J. Peripheral neuropathy with essential mixed cryoglobulinemia: biopsies from 5 cases. Acta Neuropathol 1988; 75:605–610.
35. Said G, Goulon-Goeau C, Lacroix C, Moulonguet A. Nerve biopsy findings in different patterns of proximal diabetic neuropathy. Ann Neurol 1994; 35:559–569.
36. Sobue G, Yanagi T, Hashizume Y. Chronic progressive sensory ataxic neuropathy with polyclonal gammopathy and disseminated focal perivascular cellular infiltrations. Neurology 1988; 38:463–467.
37. Cid MC, Grau JM, Casademont J, Campo E, Coll-Vinent B, Lopez-Soto A, Ingelmo M, Urbano-Marquez A. Immunohistochemical characterization of inflammatory cells and immunologic activation markers in muscle and nerve biopsy specimens from patients with systemic polyarteritis nodosa. Arth. Rheum 1994; 37:1055–1061.
38. Adams CMW, Buk SJA, Hughes RAC, Leibowitz S, Sinclair E. Perl's ferrocyanide test for iron in the diagnosis of vasculitic neuropathy. Neuropathol Appl Neurobiol 1989; 15:433–439.
39. Vital A, Vital C. Polyarteritis nodosa and peripheral neuropathy: ultrastructural study of 13 cases. Acta Neuropathol 1985; 67:136–141.
40. Puéchal X, Said G, Hilliquin P, Coste J, Job-Deslandre C, Lacroix C, Menkès CJ. Peripheral neuropathy with necrotizing vasculitis in rheumatoid arthritis. A clinicopathologic and prognostic study of thirty-two patients. Arthritis Rheum. 1995; 38:1618–1629.
41. Said, G. Vasculitic neuropathy. Baillière's Clin. Neurol 1995; 4:489–503.
42. Dyck PJ, Benstead TJ, Conn DL, Stevens JC, Windebank AJ, Low PA. Nonsystemic vasculitic neuropathy. Brain 1987; 110:843–854.
43. Caselli RJ, Daube JR, Hunder GG, Whisnant JP. Peripheral neuropathic syndromes in giant cell (temporal) arteritis. Neurology 1988; 38:685–689.
44. Fishel B, Zhukovsky G, Alon M., Talesnic M, Joussiphov J, Fintsi Y, Yaron M. Peripheral neuropathy associated with temporal arteritis. Clin Rheumatol. 1998; 17:163–165.
45. Dyck PJ. Pathology. In: Dyck PJ, ed. Diabetic Neuropathy. Philadelphia: W.B. Saunders, 1987:223–236.
46. Bendixen BH, Younger DS, Hair LS, Gutierrez C, Meyers ML, Homma S, Jaffe IA. Cholesterol emboli neuropathy. Neurology 1992; 42:428–430.
47. Vital C, Brechenmacher C, Serise JM, Bellance R, Vital A, Dartigues JF, Boissieras P. Ultrastructural study of peripheral nerve in arteritic diabetic patients. Acta Neuropathol 1983; 61:225–231.
48. Vital A, Vital C, Brechenmacher C, Serise JM, Callen S, Nicolau H, Videau J. Quantitative, histological and ultrastructural studies of peripheral nerve in arteriosclerotic non-diabetic patients. Clin. Neuropathol 1986; 5:224–229.
49. Harati Y, Niakan E. Clinical significance of selective nerve fascicular degeneration on sural nerve biopsy specimen. Arch Pathol Lab Med 1986; 110:195–197.
50. Bradley JL, Thomas PK, King RHM, Muddle JR, Ward JD, Tesfaye S, Boulton AJM, Tsigos C, Young RJ. Myelinated nerve fibre regeneration in diabetic sensory polyneuropathy: correlation with type of diabetes. Acta Neuropathol 1995; 90:403–410.
51. King RHM, Llewelyn JG, Thomas PK, Gilbey SG, Watkins PJ. Diabetic neuropathy: abnormalities of Schwann cell and perineurial basal laminae. Implications for diabetic vasculopathy. Neuropathol Appl Neurobiol 1989; 15:339–355.
52. Ballin RHM, Thomas PK. Hypertrophic changes in diabetic neuropathy. Acta Neuropathol. 1968; 11:93–102.
53. Behse F, Buchthal F, Carlsen F. Nerve biopsy and conduction studies in diabetic neuropathy. J Neurol Neurosurg Psychiatry 1977; 40:1072–1082.
54. Sima AAF, Nathaniel V, Bril V, McEwen TAJ, Greene DA. Histopathological heterogeneity of neuropathy in insulin-dependent and non-insulin-dependent diabetes, and demonstration of axo-glial dysjunction in human diabetic neuropathy. J Clin Invest 1988; 81:349–364.
55. Sima AAF, Greene DA. Diabetic neuropathy in the elderly. Drugs Aging 1995; 6:125–135.
56. Thomas PK, Beamish NG, Small JR, King RHM, Tesfaye S, Ward JD, Tsigos C, Young RJ, Boulton AJM. Paranodal structure in diabetic sensory polyneuropathy. Acta Neuropathol 1996; 92:614–620.
57. Powell HC, Rosoff J, Myers RR. Microangiopathy in human diabetic neuropathy. Acta Neuropathol 1985; 68:295–305.
58. Giannini C, Dyck PJ. Ultrastructural morphometric abnormalities of sural nerve endoneurial microvessels in diabetes mellitus. Ann Neurol 1994; 36:408–415.
59. Johnson PC, Doll SC, Cromey DW. Pathogenesis of diabetic neuropathy. Ann Neurol 1986; 19:450–457.
60. Younger DS, Rosoklija G, Hays AP, Trojaborg W, Latov N. Diabetic peripheral neuropathy: a clinicopathologic and immunohistochemical analysis of sural nerve biopsies. Muscle Nerve 1996; 19:722–727.
61. Archer AG, Watkins PJ, Thomas PK, Sharma AK, Payan J. The natural history of acute painful neuropathy in diabetes mellitus. J Neurol Neurosurg Psychiatry 1983; 46:491–499.
62. Said G. Diabetic neuropathy: an update. J Neurol 1996; 243:431–440.
63. Stewart JD, McKelvey R, Durcan L, Carpenter S, Karpati G. Chronic inflammatory demyelinating po-

lyneuropathy (CIDP) in diabetics. J Neurol Sci 1996; 142:59–64.
64. Dyck PJ, Lambert EH. Polyneuropathy associated with hypothyroidism. J Neuropathol Exp Neurol 1970; 29:631–658.
65. Shirabe R, Tawara S, Terao A, Araki S. Myxoedematous polyneuropathy: a light and electron microscopic study of the peripheral nerve and muscle. J Neurol Neurosurg Psychiatry 1975; 38:241–247.
66. Meier C, Bischoff A. Polyneuropathy in hypothyroidism. Clinical and nerve biopsy study of four cases. J Neurol 1977; 215:103–114.
67. Takahashi K, Nakamura H. Axonal degeneration in beriberi neuropathy. Arch Neurol 1976; 33:836–841.
68. Ohnishi A, Tsuji S, Igisu H, Murai Y, Goto I, Kuroiwa Y, Tsujihata M, Takamori M. Beriberi neuropathy: morphometric study of sural nerve. J Neurol Sci 1980; 45:177–190.
69. McCombe PA, McLeod JG. The peripheral neuropathy of vitamin B12 deficiency. J Neurol Sci 1984; 66:117–126.
70. Yokota T, Wada, Y, Furukawa T, Tsukagoshi H, Uchihara T, Watabiki S. Adult-onset spinocerebellar syndrome with idiopathic vitamin E deficiency. Ann Neurol 1987; 22:84–87.
71. Bolton CF, Gilbert JJ., Hahn AF, Sibbald WJ. Polyneuropathy in critically ill patients. J Neurol Neurosurg Psychiatry 1984; 47:1223–1231.
72. Latov N, Sherman WH, Nemni R, Galassi G, Shyong JS, Penn AS, Chess L, Olarte MR, Rowland LP, Osserman EF. Plasma-cell dyscrasia and peripheral neuropathy with a monoclonal antibody to peripheral-nerve myelin. N Engl J Med 1980; 303:618–621.
73. Smith IS, Kahn SN, Lacey BW, King RHM, Eames RA, Whybrew DJ, Thomas PK. Chronic demyelinating neuropathy associated with benign IgM paraproteinaemia. Brain 1983; 106:169–195.
74. Mendell JR, Sahenk Z, Whitaker JN, Trapp BD, Yates AJ, Griggs RC, Quarles RH. Polyneuropathy and IgM monoclonal gammopathy: studies on the pathogenetic role of anti-myelin-associated glycoprotein antibody. Ann Neurol 1985; 17:243–254.
75. Vital A, Vital C, Julien J, Baquey A, Steck AJ. Polyneuropathy associated with IgM monoclonal gammopathy: immunological and pathological study in 31 patients. Acta Neuropathol 1989; 79:160–167.
76. Vital C, Vallat JM, Deminière C, Loubet A, Leboutet MJ. Peripheral nerve damage during multiple myeloma and Waldenström's macroglobulinemia:an ultrastructural and immunopathologic study. Cancer 1982; 50:1491–1497.
77. Vital C, Vital A, Deminière C, Julien J, Lagueny A, Steck AJ. Myelin modifications in 8 cases of peripheral neuropathy with Waldenström's macroglobulinemia and anti-MAG activity. Ultrastruct Pathol 1997; 21:509–516.
78. Steck AJ, Murray N, Meier C, Page N, Perruisseau G. Demyelinating neuropathy and monoclonal IgM antibody to myelin associated glycoprotein. Neurology 1983; 33:19–23.
79. Meier C, Vandevelde M, Steck A, Zurbriggen A. Demyelinating polyneuropathy associated with monoclonal IgM-paraproteinaemia. Histological, ultrastructural and immunocytochemical studies. J Neurol Sci 1983; 63:353–367.
80. Vallat JM, Jauberteau MO, Bordessoule D, Yardin C, Preux PM, Couratier P. Link between peripheral neuropathy and monoclonal dysglobulinemia: a study of 66 cases. J Neurol Sci 1996; 137:124–130.
81. Pollard JD, Young GAR. Neurology and the bone marrow. J Neurol Neurosurg Psychiatry 1997; 63:706–718.
82. Lach B, Rippstein P, Atack D, Afar DEH, Gregor A. Immunoelectron microscopic localization of monoclonal IgM antibodies in gammopathy associated with peripheral demyelinative neuropathy. Acta Neuropathol 1993; 85:298–307.
83. King RHM, Thomas PK. The occurrence and significance of myelin with unusually large periodicity. Acta Neuropathol 1984; 63:319–329.
84. Gabriel JM, Erne B, Miescher GC, Miller SL, Vital A, Vital C, Steck AJ. Selective loss of myelin-associated glycoprotein from myelin correlates with anti-MAG antibody titre in demyelinating paraproteinaemic polyneuropathy. Brain 1996; 119:775–787.
85. Powell HC, Rodriguez MM, Hughes RAC. Microangiopathy of vasa nervorum in dysglobulinemic neuropathy. Ann Neurol 1984; 15:386–394.
86. Julien J, Vital C, Vallat JM, Lagueny A, Ferrer X, Leboutet MJ. Chronic demyelinating neuropathy with IgM-producing lymphocytes in peripheral nerve and delayed appearance of «benign» monoclonal gammopathy. Neurology 1984; 34:1387–1389.
87. Valldeoriola F, Graus F, Steck AJ, Munoz E, de la Fuente M, Gallart T, Ribalta T, Bombi JA, Tolosa E. Delayed appearance of anti-myelin-associated glycoprotein antibodies in a patient with chronic demyelinating polyneuropathy. Ann Neurol 1993; 34:394–396.
88. Julien J, Vital C, Vallat JM, Lagueny A, Ferrer X, Deminière C, Leboutet MJ, Effroy C. IgM demyelinative neuropathy with amyloidosis and biclonal gammopathy. Ann Neurol 1984; 15:395–399.
89. Vital A, Lagueny A, Julien J, Ferrer X, Barat M, Hermosilla E, Rouanet-Larrivière M, Henry P, Bredin A, Louiset P, Herbelleau T, Boisseau C, Guiraud-Chaumeil B, Steck A, Vital C. Chronic inflammatory demyelinating polyneuropathy associated with dysglobulinemia: a peripheral nerve biopsy study in 18 cases. Acta Neuropathol 2000; 100:63–68.
90. Solders G, Nennesmo I, Ernerudh J, Cruz M, Vrethem M. Lymphocytes in sural nerve biopsies from patients with plasma cell dyscrasia and polyneuropathy. J Periph Nerv Syst 1999; 4:91–98.
91. Busis NA, Halperin JJ, Stefansson K, Kwiatkowski DJ, Sagar SM, Schiff SR, Logigian EL. Peripheral neuropathy, high serum IgM, and paraproteinemia in mother and son. Neurology 1985; 35:679–683.
92. Lamarca J, Casquero P, Pou A. Mononeuritis multiplex in Waldenström's macroglobulinemia. Ann. Neurol 1987; 22:268–272.
93. Vital A, Vital C. Immunoelectron identification of endoneurial IgM deposits in four patients with Waldenström's macroglobulinemia: a specific ultrastructural pattern related to the presence of cryoglobulin in one case. Clin Neuropathol. 1993; 12:49–52.
94. Yeung KB, Thomas PK, King RHM, Waddy H, Will RG, Hughes RAC, Gregson NA, Leibowitz S. The clinical spectrum of peripheral neuropathies associated with benign monoclonal IgM, IgG and IgA paraproteinaemia: comparative clinical, immunological

95. Bleasel AF, Hawke SHB, Pollard JD, McLeod JG. IgG monoclonal paraproteinaemia and peripheral neuropathy. J Neurol Neurosurg Psychiatry 1993; 56:52–57.
96. Hermosilla E, Lagueny A, Vital C, Vital A, Ferrer X, Steck A, Julien J. Peripheral neuropathy associated with monoclonal IgG of undetermined significance. Clinical, electrophysiologic, pathologic and therapeutic study of 14 cases. J Periph Nerv Syst 1996; 1:139–148.
97. Moorhouse DF, Fox RI, Powell HC. Immunotactoid-like endoneurial deposits in a patient with monoclonal gammopathy of undetermined significance and neuropathy. Acta Neuropathol 1992; 84:484–494.
98. Ohi T, Kyle RA, Dyck PJ. Axonal attenuation and secondary segmental demyelination in myeloma neuropathies. Ann Neurol 1985; 17:255–261.
99. Adams D, Said G. Ultrastructural characterisation of the M protein in nerve biopsy of patients with POEMS syndrome. J Neurol Neurosurg Psychiatry 1998; 64:809–812.
100. Romas E, Storey E, Ayers M., Byrne E. Polyneuropathy, organomegaly, endocrinopathy, M-protein and skin change (POEMS) syndrome with IgG κ paraproteinemia. Pathology 1992; 24:217–220.
101. Ohnishi A, Hirano A. Uncompacted myelin lamellae in dysglobulinemic neuropathy. J Neurol Sci 1981; 51:131–140.
102. Bergouignan FX, Massonnat R, Vital C, Barat M, Henry P, Leng B, Effroy C. Uncompacted lamellae in three patients with POEMS syndrome. Eur Neurol 1987; 27:173–181.
103. Gherardi R, Baudrimont M, Kujas M, Malapert D, Lange F, Gray F, Poirier J. Pathological findings in three non-japanese patients with the POEMS syndrome. Virchows Archiv A Pathol Anat 1988; 413: 357–365.
104. Vital C, Gherardi R, Vital A, Kopp N, Pellissier JF, Soubrier M, Clavelou P, Bellance R, Delisle MB, Ruchoux MM, Hauw JJ. Uncompacted myelin lamellae in polyneuropathy, organomegaly, endocrinopathy, M-protein and skin changes syndrome: ultrastructural study of peripheral nerve biopsy from 22 patients. Acta Neuropathol 1994; 87:302–307.
105. Sobue G, Doyu M, Watanabe M, Hayashi F, Mitsuma T. Extensive demyelinating changes in the peripheral nerves of Crow-Fukase syndrome: a pathological study of one autopsied case. Acta Neuropathol 1992; 84:171–177.
106. Brechenmacher C, Vital C, Deminière C, Laurentjoye L, Castaing Y, Gbikpi-Benissan G, Cardinaud JP, Favarel-Garrigues JP. Guillain-Barré syndrome: an ultrastructural study of peripheral nerve in 65 patients. Clin Neuropathol 1987; 6:19–24.
107. Gabreëls-Festen AAWM, Hoogendijk JE, Meijerink PHS, Gabreëls FJM, Bolhuis PA, van Beersum S, Kulkens T, Nelis E, Jennekens FGI, de Visser M, van Engelen BGM, Van Broeckhoven C, Mariman ECM. Two divergent types of nerve pathology in patients with different Po mutations in Charcot-Marie-Tooth disease. Neurology 1996; 47:761–765.
108. Saida K, Kawakami H, Ohta M, Iwamura K. Coagulation and vascular abnormalities in Crow-Fukase syndrome. Muscle Nerve 1997; 20:486–492.
109. Watanabe O, Maruyama I, Arimura K, Kitajima I, Arimura H, Hanatani M, Matsuo K, Arisato T, Osame M. Overproduction of vascular endothelial growth factor/vascular permeability factor is causative in Crow-Fukase (POEMS) syndrome. Muscle Nerve 1998; 21:1390–1397.
110. Gherardi RK., Bélec L., Soubrier M, Malapert D, Zuber M, Viard JP, Intrator L, Degos JD, Authier FJ. Overproduction of proinflammatory cytokines imbalanced by their antagonists in POEMS syndrome. Blood 1996; 87:1458–1465.
111. Vallat JM, Desproges-Gotteron R, Leboutet MJ, Loubet A, Gualde N, Treves R. Cryoglobulinemic neuropathy: a pathological study. Ann Neurol 1980; 8:179–185.
112. Vital A, Vital C, Ragnaud JM, Baquey A, Aubertin J. IgM cryoglobulin deposits in the peripheral nerve. Virchows Archiv A Pathol Anat 1991; 418:83–85.
113. Brouet J-C, Clauvel J-P. Danon F, Klein M, Seligman M. Biologic and clinical significance of cryoglobulins. A report of 86 cases. Am J Med 1974; 57:775–788.
114. Thomas FP, Lovelace RE, Ding XS, Sadiq SA, Petty GW, Sherman WH, Latov N, Hays AP. Vasculitic neuropathy in a patient with cryoglobulinemia and anti-MAG IgM monoclonal gammopathy. Muscle Nerve 1992; 15:891–898.
115. Khella SL, Frost S, Hermann GA, Leventhal L, Whyatt S, Sajid MA, Scherer SS. Hepatitis C infection, cryoglobulinemia, and vasculitic neuropathy. Treatment with interferon alfa: case report and literature review. Neurology 1995; 45:407–411.
116. Apartis E, Léger JM, Musset L, Gugenheim M, Cacoub P, Lyon-Caen O, Pierrot-Deseilligny C, Hauw JJ, Bouche P. Peripheral neuropathy associated with essential mixed cryoglobulinaemia: a role for hepatitis C virus infection? J Neurol Neurosurg Psychiatry 1996; 60:661–666.
117. Koeppen AF, Mitzen EJ, Hans MB, Peng SK, Bailey RO. Familial amyloid polyneuropathy. Muscle Nerve 1985; 8:733–749.
118. Saraiva MJM. Molecular genetics of familial amyloidotic polyneuropathy. J Periph Nerv Syst 1996; 1: 179–188.
119. Blanco-Jerez CR, Jiménez-Escrig A, Gobernado JM, Lopez-Calvo S, de Blas G, Redondo C, Garcia Villanueva M, Orensanz L. Transthyretin Tyr77 familial amyloid polyneuropathy: a clinicopathological study of a large kindred. Muscle Nerve 1998; 21:1478–1485.
120. Ikeda SI, Hanyu N, Hongo M, Yoshioka J, Oguchi H, Yanagisawa N, Kobayashi T, Tsukagoshi H, Ito N, Yokota T. Hereditary generalized amyloidosis with polyneuropathy: clinicopathological study of 65 Japanese patients. Brain 1987; 110:315–337.
121. Date Y, Nakazato M, Kangawa K, Shirieda K, Fujimoto T, Matsukura S. Detection of three transthyretin gene mutations in familial amyloidotic polyneuropathy by analysis of DNA extracted from formalin-fixed and paraffin-embedded tissues. J Neurol Sci 1997; 150:143–148.
122. Staunton H, Dervan P, Kale R, Linke RP, Kelly P. Hereditary amyloid polyneuropathy in North West Ireland. Brain 1987; 110:1231–1245.

123. Reilly MM, Staunton H. Peripheral nerve amyloidosis. Brain Pathol 1996; 6:163–177.
124. Planté-Bordeneuve V, Lalu T, Misrahi M, Reilly MM, Adams D, Lacroix C, Said G. Genotypic-phenotypic variations in a series of 65 patients with familial amyloid polyneuropathy. Neurology 1998; 51:708–714.
125. Haltia M, Ghiso J, Prelli F, Gallo G, Kiuru S, Somer H, Palo J, Frangione B. Amyloid in familial amyloidosis, Finnish type, is antigenically and structurally related to gelsolin. Am J Pathol 1990; 136:1223–1228.
126. Sunada Y, Shimizu T, Nakase H, Ohta S, Asaoka T, Amano S, Sawa M, Kagawa Y, Kanazawa I, Mannen T. Inherited amyloid polyneuropathy type IV (gelsolin variant) in a Japanese family. Ann Neurol 1993; 33:57–62.
127. Verghese JP, Bradley WG, Nemni R, McAdam PWJ. Amyloid neuropathy in multiple myeloma and other plasma cell dyscrasias. J Neurol Sci 1983; 59:237–246.
128. Vital A, Vital C. Amyloid neuropathy: relationship between amyloid fibrils and macrophages. Ultrastruct Pathol 1984; 7:21–24.
129. Bajada S, Mastaglia FL, Fisher A. Amyloid neuropathy and tremor in Waldenström's macroglobulinemia. Arch Neurol 1980; 37:240–242.
130. Rajkumar SV, Gertz MA, Kyle RA. Primary systemic amyloidosis with delayed progression to multiple myeloma. Cancer 1998; 82:1501–1505.
131. Thomas PK, King RHM. Peripheral nerve changes in amyloid neuropathy. Brain 1974; 97:395–406.
132. Li K, Kyle RA, Dyck PJ. Immunohistochemical characterization of amyloid proteins in sural nerve and clinical associations in amyloid neuropathy. Am J Pathol 1992; 141:217–226.
133. De Sousa MM, Vital C, Ostler D, Fernandes R, Pouget-Abadie J, Carles D, Saraiva MJ. Apolipoprotein AI and transthyretin as components of amyloid fibrils in a kindred with apoAI Leu178His. Am J Pathol 2000; 156:1911–1917.
134. Adams D, Said G. Ultrastructural immunolabelling of amyloid fibrils in acquired and hereditary amyloid neuropathies. J Neurol 1996; 243:63–67.
135. Vital C, Vital A, Julien J, Rivel J, de Mascarel A, Vergier B, Henry P, Barat M, Reiffers J, Broustet A. Peripheral neuropathies and lymphoma without monoclonal gammopathy: a new classification. J Neurol 1990; 237:177–185.
136. Vallat JM, De Mascarel HA, Bordessoule D Jauberteau MO, Tabaraud F, Gelot A, Vallat AV. Non-Hodgkin malignant lymphomas and peripheral neuropathies: 13 cases. Brain 1995; 118:1233–1245.
137. Gherardi R, Gaulard P, Prost C, Rocha D, Imbert M, André C, Rochant H, Farcet JP. T-cell lymphoma revealed by a peripheral neuropathy. A report of two cases with an immunohistologic study on lymph node and nerve biopsies. Cancer 1986; 58:2710–2716.
138. Vital C, Vital A, Moynet D, Broustet A, de Mascarel A, Bloch B, Guillemain B. The presence of particles resembling human T-cell leukemia virus type I at ultrastructural examination of lymphomatous cells in a case of T-cell leukemia/lymphoma. Cancer 1993; 71:2227–2232.
139. Julien J, Vital C, Rivel J, de Mascarel A, Lagueny A, Ferrer X, Vergier B. Primary meningeal B lymphoma presenting as a subacute ascending polyradiculoneuropathy. J Neurol Neurosurg Psychiatry 1991; 54:610–613.
140. Vital C, Heraud A, Vital A, Coquet M, Julien J, Maupetit J. Acute mononeuropathy with angiotropic lymphoma. Acta Neuropathol 1989; 78:105–107.
141. Glass J, Hochberg FH, Miller DC. Intravascular lymphomatosis: a systemic disease with neurologic manifestations. Cancer 1993; 71:3156–3165.
142. Roux S, Grossin M, De Bandt M, Palazzo E, Vachon F, Kahn MF. Angiotropic large cell lymphoma with mononeuritis multiplex mimicking systemic vasculitis. J Neurol Neurosurg Psychiatry 1995; 58:363–366.
143. Lamarche J Vital C. Carcinomatous neuropathy: an ultrastructural study of ten cases. Ann. Pathol 1987; 7:98–105.
144. Eggers C, Hagel C, Pfeiffer G. Anti-Hu-associated paraneoplastic sensory neuropathy with peripheral nerve demyelination and microvasculitis. J Neurol Sci 1998; 155:178–181.
145. Grisold W, Drlicek M. Paraneoplastic neuropathy. Curr Opin Neurol 1999; 12:617–625.
146. Arnason, BGW, Soliven B. Acute inflammatory demyelinating polyradiculoneuropathy. In: Dyck, PJ, Thomas PK, Griffin JW, Low PA, Poduslo JF, eds., Peripheral Neuropathy, vol 2, 3rd ed. Philadelphia: W.B. Saunders, 1993:1437–1497.
147. Hartung HP, Pollard JD, Harvey GK, Toyka KV. Immunopathogenesis and treatment of the Guillain-Barré syndrome. Muscle Nerve 1995; 18:137–164.
148. Hartung HP, van der Meché FGA, Pollard JD. Guillain-Barré syndrome, CIDP and other chronic immune-mediated neuropathies. Curr Opin Neurol 1998; 11:497–513.
149. Yuki N. Anti-ganglioside antibody and neuropathy: review of our research. J Periph Nerv Syst 1998; 3:3–18.
150. Schmidt B, Toyka KV, Kiefer R, Full J, Hartung HP, Pollard J. Inflammatory infiltrates in sural nerve biopsies in Guillain-Barré syndrome and chronic inflammatory demyelinating neuropathy. Muscle Nerve 1996; 19:474–487.
151. Kiefer R, Kieseier BC, Brück W, Hartung HP, Toyka KV. Macrophage differentiation antigens in acute and chronic autoimmune polyneuropathies. Brain 1998; 121:469–479.
152. Hughes RAC. Guillain-Barré Syndrome. London: Springer-Verlag, 1990.
153. Hughes RAC, Atkinson P, Coates P, Hall S, Leibowitz S. Sural nerve biopsies in Guillain-Barré syndrome: axonal degeneration and macrophage-associated demyelination and absence of cytomegalovirus genome. Muscle Nerve 1992; 15:568–575.
154. Madrid R, Bradley CG, Davis DJF. The peroneal muscular atrophy syndrome: clinical, genetic, electrophysiological and nerve biopsy studies: Part 2. Observations and pathological changes in sural nerve biopsies. J Neurol Sci 1977; 32:91–122.
155. Vital C, Brechenmacher C, Cardinaud JP, Manier G, Vital A, Mora B. Acute inflammatory demyelinating polyneuropathy in a diabetic patient: predominance of vesicular disruption in myelin sheaths. Acta Neuropathol 1985; 67:337–340.
156. Fuller GN, Jacobs JM, Lewis PD, Lane RJM. Pseu-

156. doaxonal Guillain-Barré syndrome: severe demyelination mimicking axonopathy. A case with pupillary involvement. J Neurol Neurosurg Psychiatry 1992; 55:1079–1083.
157. Feasby TE, Hahn AF, Brown WF, Bolton CF, Gilbert JJ, Koopman WJ. Severe axonal degeneration in acute Guillain-Barré syndrome: evidence of two different mechanisms? J Neurol Sci 1993; 116:185–192.
158. Vital C, Vital A, Arne P, Hilbert G, Gruson D, Gbikpi-Benissan G, Cardinaud JP, Petry K. Inexcitability of nerves in a fulminant case of Guillain-Barré syndrome. J Periph Nerv Syst 5: 2000; 5:111–115.
159. Hall SM, Hughes RAC, Atkinson PF, McColl I, Gale A. Motor nerve biopsy in severe Guillain-Barré syndrome. Ann Neurol 1992; 31:441–444.
160. Feasby TE., Gilbert JJ., Brown WF., Bolton CF, Hahn AF, Koopman WF, Zochodne DW. An acute axonal form of Guillain-Barré polyneuropathy. Brain 1986; 109:1115–1126.
161. Powell HC, Myers RR. The axon in Guillain-Barré syndrome: immune target or innocent bystander? Ann Neurol 1996; 39:4–5.
162. Griffin JW, Li CY, Ho TW, Tian M, Gao CY, Xue P, Mishu B, Cornblath DR, Macko C, McKhann GM, Asburry AK. Pathology of the motor-sensory axonal Guillain-Barré syndrome. Ann Neurol 1996; 39:17–28.
163. Brechenmacher C, Vital C, Laurentjoye L, Castaing Y. Ultrastructural study of peripheral nerve in Guillain-Barré syndrome: presence of mononuclear cells in axons. Acta Neuropathol 1981; (suppl.) VII: 249–251.
164. Sobue G, Li M, Terao S, Aoki S, Ichimura M, Ieda T, Doyu M, Yasuda T, Hashizume Y, Mitsuma T. Axonal pathology in Japanese Guillain-Barré syndrome: a study of 15 autopsied cases. Neurology 1997; 48:1694–1700.
165. Hainfellner JA. Kristofiritsch W, Lassmann H., Bernheimer H, Neisser A, Drlicek M, Beer F, Budka H. T cell-mediated ganglionitis associated with acute sensory neuronopathy. Ann Neurol 1996; 39:543–547.
166. Dyck PJ, Prineas J, Pollard J. Chronic inflammatory demyelinating polyradiculo-neuropathy. In: Dyck PJ, Thomas PK Griffin JW, Low PA, Poduslo JF, eds. Peripheral Neuropathy, Vol 2, 3rd ed. Philadelphia: W.B. Saunders, 1993:1498–1517.
167. Matsumuro K, Izumo S, Umehara F, Osame M. Chronic inflammatory demyelinating polyneuropathy: histological and immunopathological studies on biopsied sural nerves. J Neurol Sci 1994; 127:170–178.
168. Prineas JW, McLeod JG. Chronic relapsing polyneuritis. J Neurol Sci 1976 27:427–458.
169. Pollard JD, McLeod JG, Gatenby P, Kronenberg H. Prediction of response to plasma exchange in chronic relapsing polyneuropathy. J Neurol Sci 1983; 58:269–287.
170. Gibbels E, Kentenich M. Unmyelinated fibers in sural nerve biopsies of chronic inflammatory demyelinating polyneuropathy. Acta Neuropathol 1990; 80: 439–447.
171. Ingall TJ, McLeod JG, Tamura N. Autonomic function and unmyelinated fibers in chronic inflammatory demyelinating polyradiculoneuropathy. Muscle Nerve 1990 13:70–76.
172. Thomas PK, Claus D, Jaspert A, Workman JM, King RHM, Larner AJ, Anderson M, Emerson JA, Ferguson IT. Focal upper limb demyelinating neuropathy. Brain 1996; 119:765–774.
173. Simmons Z, Albers JW, Bromberg MB. Feldman EL. Presentation and initial clinical course in patients with chronic inflammatory demyelinating polyradiculoneuropathy: comparison of patient's without and with monoclonal gammopathy. Neurology 1993; 43:2202–2009.
174. Gorson KC, Allam G, Ropper AH. Chronic inflammatory demyelinating polyneuropathy: clinical features and response to treatment in 67 consecutive patients with and without a monoclonal gammopathy. Neurology 1997; 48:321–328.
175. Julien J, Vital C, Lagueny A, Ferrer X, Brechenmacher C. Chronic relapsing idiopathic polyneuropathy with primary axonal lesions. J Neurol Neurosurg Psychiatry 1989; 52:871–875.
176. Chroni E, Hall SM, Hughes RAC. Chronic relapsing axonal neuropathy: a first case report. Ann Neurol 1995; NN:112–115.
177. Uncini A, Sabatelli M, Mignogna T, Lugaresi A, Liguori R, Montagna P, Chronic progressive steroid responsive axonal polyneuropathy: a CIDP variant or a primary axonal disorder? Muscle Nerve 1996; 19: 365–371.
178. Vital C, Vital A, Lagueny A, Larribau E, Saintarailles J, Julien J. Subacute inflammatory polyneuropathy: two cases with plasmacytoid histiocytes in the endoneurium. Ultrastruct Pathol 1998; 22:377–383.
179. Vallat JM, Hugon J, Lubeau M, Leboutet MJ, Dumas M, Desproges-Gotteron R. Tickbite meningoradiculoneuritis: clinical, electrophysiologic, and histologic findings in 10 cases. Neurology 1987; 37:749–753.
180. Vital A, Beylot M, Vital C, Delors B, Bloch B, Julien J. Morphological findings on peripheral nerve biopsies in 15 patients with human immunodeficiency virus infection. Acta Neuropathol 1992; 83:618–623.
181. Lewis RA, Summer AJ, Brown MJ, Asbury AK. Multifocal demyelinating neuropathy with persistent conduction block. Neurology 1982; 32:958–964.
182. Oh SJ, Claussen GC, Kim DS. Motor and sensory demyelinating mononeuropathy multiplex (multifocal motor and sensory demyelinating neuropathy); a separate entity or a variant of chronic inflammatory demyelinating polyneuropathy? J Periph Nerv Syst 1997; 2:362–369.
183. Bouche P, Moulonguet A, Ben Younes-Chennoufi A, Adams D, Baumann N, Meininger V, Léger JM, Said G. Multifocal motor neuropathy with conduction block: a study of 24 patients. J Neurol Neurosurg Psychiatry 1995; 59:38–44.
184. Corse AM, Chaudhry V, Crawford TO, Cornblath DR, Kuncl RW, Griffin JW. Sensory nerve pathology in multifocal motor neuropathy. Ann Neurol 1996; 39:319–325.
185. Saperstein DS, Amato AA, Wolfe GI, Katz JS, Nations SP, Jackson CE, Bryan WW, Burns DK, Barohn RJ. Multifocal acquired demyelinating sensory and motor neuropathy: the Lewis-Sumner syndrome. Muscle Nerve 1999; 22:560–566.
186. Gorson KC, Ropper AH, Weinberg DH, Upper limb predominant, multifocal chronic inflammatory de-

187. Parry GJ. Are multifocal motor neuropathy and Lewis-Sumner syndrome distinct nosologic entities? Muscle Nerve 1999; 22:557–559.
188. Van den Berg-Vos RM, Van den Berg LH, Franssen H, Vermeulen M, Witkamp TD, Jansen GH, van Es HW, Kerkhoff H, Wokke JHJ. Multifocal inflammatory demyelinating neuropathy. A distinct clinical entity? Neurology 2000; 54:26–32.
189. Nukada H, Pollock M, Haas LF. Is ischemia implicated in chronic multifocal demyelinating neuropathy? Neurology 1989; 39:106–110.
190. Mohamed A, Davies L, Pollard JD. Conduction block in vasculitic neuropathy. Muscle Nerve 1998; 21:1084–1088.
191. Meier C, Grahmann F, Engelhardt A, Dumas M. Peripheral nerve disorders in Lyme-Borreliosis. Nerve biopsy studies from eight cases. Acta Neuropathol 1989; 79:271–278.
192. Walshe TM, Szyfelbein W. Case Records of the Massachusetts General Hospital. A 92-year-old woman with several cranial-nerve defects and weakness of the left leg. N Engl J Med 1998; 319:1654–1662.
193. Mellgren SI. Conn DL, Stevens JC, Dyck PJ. Peripheral neuropathy in primary Sjögren's syndrome. Neurology 1989; 39:390–394.
194. Gemignani F, Marbini A, Pavesi G, Di Vittorio S, Manganelli P, Cenacchi G, Mancia D. Peripheral neuropathy associated with primary Sjögren's syndrome. J Neurol Neurosurg Psychiatry 1994; 57: 983–986.
195. Grant IA., Hunder GG., Homburger HA, Dyck PJ. Peripheral neuropathy associated with sicca complex. Neurology 1997; 48:855–862.
196. Dorfman LJ. Ransom BR, Forno LS, Kelts A. Neuropathy in the hypereosinophilic syndrome. Muscle Nerve 1983; 6:291–298.
197. Monaco S, Lucci B, Laperchia N, Tezzon F, Curro-Dossi B, Nardelli E, Giannini C, Rizzuto N. Polyneuropathy in hypereosinophilic syndrome. Neurology 1988; 38:494–496.
198. Oh, SJ. Sarcoid polyneuropathy: a histologically proved case. Ann Neurol 1980; 7:178–181.
199. Antoine JC, Laplanche JL, Mosnier JF, Beaudry P, Chatelain J, Michel D. Demyelinating peripheral neuropathy with Creutzfeldt-Jakob disease and mutation at codon 200 of the prion protein gene. Neurology 1996; 46:1123–1127.
200. Bradley WG, Lassman LP, Pearce GW, Walton JN. The neuromyopathy of vincristine in man. J Neurol Sci 1970; 10:107–131.
201. Thompson SW, Davis LE, Kornfeld M, Hilgers RD, Standefer JC. Cisplatin neuropathy. Clinical, electrophysiologic, morphologic, and toxicologic studies. Cancer 1984; 54:1269–1275.
202. Pellissier JF, Pouget J, Cros D, De Victor B, Serratrice G, Toga M. Peripheral neuropathy induced by amiodarone chlorhydrate. J Neurol Sci 1984; 63: 251–266.
203. Jacobs JM, Costa-Jussa FR. The pathology of amiodarone neurotoxicity. Peripheral neuropathy in man. Brain 1985; 108:753–770.
204. Tegnér R, Tomé FMS, Godeau P, Lhermitte F, Fardeau M. Morphological study of peripheral nerve changes induced by chloroquine treatment. Acta Neuropathol 1988; 75:253–260.
205. Ochoa J. Isoniazid neuropathy in man: quantitative electron microscope study. Brain 1970; 93:831–850.
206. Borrett D, Ashby P, Bilbao J, Carlen P. Reversible, late-onset disulfiram-induced neuropathy and encephalopathy. Ann Neurol 1985; 17:396–399.
207. Goebel HH, Schmidt PF, Bohl J, Tettenborn B, Krämer G, Gutmann L. Polyneuropathy due to acute arsenic intoxication: biopsy studies. J Neuropathol Exp Neurol 1990; 49:137–149.
208. Dyck PJ, Chance P, Lebo R, Carney JA. Hereditary motor and sensory neuropathies. In: Dyck PJ, Thomas PK, Griffin JW, Low PA, Poduslo JF, eds. Peripheral Neuropathy, Vol 2, 3rd ed. Philadelphia: W.B. Saunders, 1993; 1094–1136.
209. De Jonghe P, Timmerman V, Nelis E, Martin JJ, Van Broeckhoven C. Charcot-Marie-Tooth disease and related peripheral neuropathies. J Periph Nerv Syst 1997; 2:370–387.
210. Pareyson D. Charcot-Marie-Tooth disease and related neuropathies: molecular basis for distinction and diagnosis. Muscle Nerve 1999; 22:1498–1509.
211. Thomas PK, Marques W, Davis MB, Sweeney MG, King RHM, Bradley JL, Muddle JR, Tyson J, Malcolm S, Harding AE. The phenotypic manifestations of chromosome 17p11.2 duplication. Brain 1997; 120:465–478.
212. Sander S, Nicholson GA, Ouvrier RA, McLeod JG, Pollard JD. Charcot-Marie-Tooth disease: histopathological features of the peripheral myelin protein (PMP22) duplication (CMT1A) and connexin32 mutations (CMTX1). Muscle Nerve 1998; 21:217–225.
213. Thomas PK, King RHM, Small JR, Robertson AM. The pathology of Charcot-Marie-Tooth disease and related disorders. Neuropathol Appl Neurobiol 1996; 22:269–284.
214. Thomas PK, King RHM, Bradley JL. Hypertrophic neuropathy: atypical appearances resulting from the combinaison of type I hereditary motor and sensory neuropathy and diabetes mellitus. Neuropathol Appl Neurobiol 1997; 23:348–351.
215. Uncini A., Di Muzio A., Chiavaroli F., Gambi D, Sabatelli M, Archidiacono N, Antonacci R, Marzella R, Rocchi M. Hereditary motor and sensory neuropathy with calf hypertrophy is associated with 17p11.2 duplication. Ann Neurol 1994 35:552–558.
216. Auer-Grumbach M, Strasser-Fuchs S, Wagner K, Körner E, Fazekas F. Roussy-Lévy syndrome is a phenotypic variant of Charcot-Marie-Tooth syndrome IA associated with a duplication on chromosome 17p11.2. J Neurol Sci 1998; 154:72–75.
217. Planté-Bordeneuve V, Guiochon-Mantel A, Lacroix C, Lapresle J, Said G. The Roussy-Lévy family: from the original description to the gene. Ann Neurol 1999; 46:770–773.
218. Gregory R., Thomas PK, King RHM, Hallam PLJ, Malcolm S, Hughes RAC, Harding AE. Coexistence of hereditary motor and sensory neuropathy type Ia and IgM paraproteinemic neuropathy. Ann Neurol 1993; 33:649–652.
219. Haney C, Snipes GJ, Shooter EM, Suter U, Garcia C, Griffin JW, Trapp BD. Ultrastructural distribution of PMP22 in Charcot-Marie-Tooth disease type 1A. J Neuropathol Exp Neurol 1996; 55:290–299.
220. Vallat JM, Sindou P, Preux PM, Tabaraud F, Milor

AM, Couratier P, LeGuern E, Brice A. Ultrastructural PMP22 expression in inherited demyelinating neuropathies. Ann Neurol 1996; 39:813–817.
221. Nishimura T, Yoshikawa H, Fujimura H, Sakoda S, Yanagihara T. Accumulation of peripheral myelin protein 22 in onion bulbs and Schwann cells of biopsied nerves from patients with Charcot-Marie-Tooth disease type 1A. Acta Neuropathol 1996; 92:454–460.
222. Bird TD, Kraft GH, Lipe HP, Kenney KL, Sumi SM. Clinical and pathological phenotype of the original family with Charcot-Marie-Tooth type 1B: a 20-year study. Ann. Neurol 1997; 41:463–469.
223. Komiyama A, Ohnishi A, Izawa K, Yamamori S, Ohashi H, Hasegawa O. De novo mutation ($Arg^{98}{\rightarrow}Cys$) of the myelin Po gene and uncompaction of the major dense line of the myelin sheath in a severe variant of Charcot-Marie-Tooth disease type 1B. J Neurol Sci 1997; 49:103–109.
224. Thomas FP, Lebo RV, Rosoklija G, Ding XS, Lovelace RE, Latov N, Hays AP. Tomaculous neuropathy in chromosome 1 Charcot-Marie-Tooth syndrome. Acta Neuropathol 1994; 87:91–97.
225. Tachi N, Kozuka N, Ohya K, Chiba S, Sasaki K. Tomacolous neuropathy in Charcot-Marie-Tooth disease with myelin protein zero gene mutation. J Neurol Sci 1997; 153:106–109.
226. Lagueny A, Latour P, Vital A, Rajabally Y, Le Masson G, Ferrer X, Bernard I, Julien J, Vital C, Vandenberghe A. Peripheral myelin modification in CMT1B correlates with MPZ gene mutations. Neuromusc Disord 1999; 9:316–367.
227. Ohnishi A, Yamamoto T, Yamamori S, Sudo K, Fukushima Y, Ikeda M. Myelinated fibers in Charcot-Marie-Tooth disease type 1B with Arg98His mutation of Po protein. J Neurol Sci 1999; 171:97–109.
228. De Jonghe P, Timmerman V, Ceuterick C, Nelis E, De Vriendt E, Löfgren A, Vercruyssen A, Verellen C, Van Maldergem L, Martin JJ, Van Broeckhoven C. The Thr124Met mutation in the peripheral myelin protein zero (MPZ) gene is associated with a clinically distinct Charcot-Marie-Tooth phenotype. Brain 1999; 122:281–290.
229. Chapon F, Latour P, Diraison P, Schaeffer S, Vandenberghe A. Axonal phenotype of Charcot-Marie-Tooth disease associated with a mutation in the myelin protein zero gene. J Neurol Neurosurg Psychiatry 1999; 66:779–782.
230. Hahn, AF. Hereditary motor and sensory neuropathy: HMSN type II (neuronal type) and X-linked HMSN. Brain Pathol 1993; 3:147–155.
231. Birouk N, LeGuern E, Maisonobe T, Rouger H, Gouider R, Tardieu S, Gugenheim M, Routon MC, Léger JM, Agid Y, Brice A, Bouche P. X-linked Charcot-Marie-Tooth disease with connexin 32 mutations. Clinical and electrophysiologic study. Neurology 1998; 50:1074–1082.
232. Hahn AF, Bolton CF, White CM, Brown WF, Tuuha SE, Tan CC, Ainsworth PJ. Genotype/phenotype correlations in X-linked dominant Charcot-Marie-Tooth disease. Ann NY Acad Sci 1999; 883:366–382.
233. Senderek J, Hermanns B, Bergmann C, Boroojerdi B, Bajbouj M, Hungs M, Ramaekers VT, Quasthoff S, Karch D, Schröder JM. X-linked dominant Charcot-Marie-Tooth neuropathy: clinical, electrophysiological, and morphological phenotype in four families with different connexin32 mutations. J Neurol Sci 1999; 167:90–101.
234. Tabaraud F, Lagrange E, Sindou P, Vandenberghe A, Levy N, Vallat JM: Demyelinating X-linked Charcot-Marie-Tooth disease: unusual electrophysiological findings. Muscle Nerve 1999; 22:1442–1447.
235. Berciano J, Combarros O, Figols J, Calleja J, Cabello A, Silos I, Coria F. Hereditary motor and sensory neuropathy type II. Clinicopathological study of a family. Brain 1986; 109:897–914.
236. Vogel P, Gabriel M, Goebel HH, Dyck PJ. Hereditary motor and sensory neuropathy type II with neurofilament accumulation: new finding or new disorder? Ann Neurol 1985; 17:455–461.
237. Julien J, Vital C, Lagueny A, Ferrer X. Hereditary motor and motor and sensory neuropathy type II with axonal lesions. J Neurol 1988; 235:254–255.
238. Vital A, Vital C, Riverière JP, Brechenmacher C, Marot J. Variability of morphological features in early infantile polyneuropathy with defective myelination. Acta Neuropathol 1987; 73:295–300.
239. Umehara F, Takenaga S, Nakagawa M, Takahashi K, Izumo S, Matsumuro K, Sakota S, Nishimura T, Yoshikawa H, Osame M. Dominantly inherited motor and sensory neuropathy with excessive myelin folding complex. Acta Neuropathol 1993; 86:602–608.
240. Gambardella A, Bolino A, Muglia M, Valentino P, Bono F, Oliveri RL, Sabatelli M, Brancolini V, Van Broeckhoven C, Romeo G, Devoto M, Quattrone A. Genetic heterogeneity in autosomal recessive hereditary motor and sensory neuropathy with focally folded myelin sheaths (CMT4B). Neurology 1998; 50:799–801.
241. Pareyson D, Scaioli V, Taroni F, Botti S, Lorenzetti D, Solari A, Ciano C, Sghirlanzoni A. Phenotypic heterogeneity in-hereditary neuropathy with liability to pressure palsies associated with chromosome 17p11.2–12 deletion. Neurology 1996; 46:1133–1137.
242. Dubourg O, Mouton P, Brice A, LeGuern E, Bouche P. Guidelines for diagnosis of hereditary neuropathy with liability to pressure palsies. Neuromuscular Disord 2000; 10:206–208.
243. Behse F, Buchthal F, Carlsen F, Knappeis GG. Hereditary neuropathy with liability to pressure palsies: electrophysiological and histological aspects. Brain 1972; 95:777–794.
244. Madrid R, Bradley WG. The pathology of neuropathies with focal thickening of the myelin sheath (tomaculous neuropathy): studies on the formation of the abnormal myelin sheath. J Neurol Sci 1975; 25:415–488.
245. Thiex R, Schröder JM. PMP-22 gene duplications and deletions identified in archival, paraffin-embedded sural nerve biopsy specimens: correlation to structural changes. Acta Neuropathol 1998; 96:13–21.
246. Kinoshita A, Hayashi M, Oda M, Tanabe H. Clinicopathological study of the peripheral nervous system in Machado-Joseph disease. J Neurol Sci 1995; 130:48–58.
247. Klockgether T, Schöls L, Abele M, Bürk K, Topka H, Andres F, Amoiridis G, Lüdtke R, Riess O, Lac-

cone F, Dichgans J. Age related axonal neuropathy in spinocerebellar ataxia type 3/Machado-Joseph disease (SCA3/MJD). J Neurol Neurosurg Psychiatry 1999; 66:222–224.
248. Hardie RJ, Pullon HWH, Harding AE, Owen JS, Pires M, Daniels GL, Imai Y, Misra VP, King RHM, Jacobs JM, Tippett P, Duchen LW, Thomas PK, Marsden CD. Neuroacanthocytosis: a clinical, haematological and pathological study of 19 cases. Brain 1991; 114:13–49.
249. Lantos PL, Aminoff MJ. Fine structural changes in the sural nerve of patients with acanthocytosis. Acta Neuropathol 1972; 22:257–263.
250. Malandrini A, Fabrizi GM, Truschi F, Di Pietro G, Moschini F, Bartalucci P, Berti G, Salvadori C, Bucalossi A, Guazzi G. Atypical McLeod syndrome manifested as X-linked chorea-acanthocytosis, neuromyopathy and dilated cardiomyopathy: report of a family. J Neurol Sci 1994; 124:89–94.
251. Schröder JM, Sellhaus B, Jörg J. Identification of the characteristic vascular changes in a sural nerve biopsy of a case with cerebral autosomal dominant arteriopathy with subcortical infarcts and leukoencephalopathy (CADASIL). Acta Neuropathol 1995; 89:116–112.
252. Pollock M, Nukada H, Frith RW, Simcock JP, Allpress S. Peripheral neuropathy in Tangier disease. Brain 1983; 106:911–929.
253. Marbini A., Gemignani F., Ferrarini G, Maccari S, Lucci B, Bragaglia MM, Plancher C, Vergani C. Tangier disease. A case with sensorimotor distal polyneuropathy and lipid accumulation in striated muscle and vasa nervorum. Acta Neuropathol 1985; 67:121–127.
254. Gibbels E, Schaefer HE, Runne U, Schröder JM, Haupt WF, Assmann G. Severe polyneuropathy in Tangier disease mimicking synringomyelia or leprosy. Clinical, biochemical, electrophysiological, and morphological evaluation, including electron microscopy of nerve, muscle, and skin biopsies. J Neurol 1985; 232:283–294.
255. Bosch EP, Hart MN. Late adult-onset metachromatic leukodystrophy: dementia and polyneuropathy in a 63-year-old man. Arch Neurol 1978; 35:475–477.
256. Robitaille Y, Carpenter S, Karpati G, Di Mauro S. A distinct form of adult polyglucosan body disease with massive involvement of central and peripheral neuronal processes and astrocytes. Brain 1980; 103:315–336.
257. Boulan-Predseil P, Vital A, Brochet B, Darriet D, Henry P, Vital C. Dementia of frontal lobe type due to adult polyglucosan body disease. J Neurol 1995; 242:512–516.
258. Lossos A, Barash V, Soffer D, Argov Z, Gomori M, Ben-Nariah Z, Abramsky O, Steiner I. Hereditary branching enzyme dysfunction in adult polyglucosan body disease: a possible metabolic cause in two patients. Ann. Neurol 1991; 30:655–662.
259. Bruno C, Servidei S, Shanske S, Karpati G, Carpenter S, McKee D, Barohn RJ, Hirano M, Rifai Z, DiMauro S. Glycogen branching enzyme deficiency in adult polyglucosan body disease. Ann Neurol 1993; 33:88–93.
260. Vos AJM, Joosten EMG, Gabreels-Festen AAW. Adult polyglucosan body disease: clinical and nerve biopsy findings in two cases. Ann. Neurol 1983; 13:440–444.
261. Zeviani M, Tiranti V, Plantadosi C. Mitochondrial disorders. Medicine 1998; 77:59–72.
262. Lestienne P, Bouzidi MF, Desguerre I, Ponsot G. Molecular basis of mitochondrial DNA diseases. In Lestienne P, ed. Mitochondrial Diseases. Berlin: Springer-Verlag, 1999:33–58.
263. Chu CC, Huang CC, Fang W, Chu NS, Pang CY, Wei YH. Peripheral neuropathy in mitochondrial encephalomyopathies. Eur Neurol 1997; 37:110–115.
264. Howell N, Kubacka I, Smith R, Frerman F, Parks JK, Parker WD. Association of the mitochondrial 8344 MERRF mutation with maternally inherited spinocerebellar degeneration and Leigh disease. Neurology 1996; 46:219–222.
265. Naumann M, Kiefer R, Toyka KV, Sommer C, Seibel P, Reichmann H. Mitochondrial dysfunction with myoclonus epilepsy and ragged-red fibers point mutation in nerve, muscle, and adipose tissue of a patient with multiple symmetric lipomatosis. Muscle Nerve 1997; 20:833–839.
266. Klopstock T, Naumann M, Seibel P, Shalke B, Reiners K, Reichmann H. Mitochondrial DNA mutations in multiple symmetric lipomatosis. Mol Cell Biochem 1997; 174:271–275.
267. Berkovic SF, Shoubridge EA, Andermann F, Andermann E, Carpenter S, Karpati G. Clinical spectrum of mitochondrial DNA mutation at base pair 8344. Lancet 1991; 338:457.
268. Calabresi PA, Silvestri G, DiMauro S, Griggs R. Ekbom's syndrome: lipomas, ataxia, and neuropathy with MERRF. Muscle Nerve 1994; 17:943–945.
269. Träff J, Holme E, Ekbom K, Nilsson BY. Ekbom's syndrome of photomyoclonus, cerebellar ataxia and cervical lipoma is associated with the tRNA^{Lys} A8344G mutation in mitochondrial DNA. Acta Neurol Scand 1995; 92:394–397.
270. Austin SA, Vriesendrop FJ, Thandroyen FT, Hecht JT, Jones OT, Johns DR. Expanding the phenotype of the 8344 transfer RNA^{Lysine} mitochondrial DNA mutation. Neurology 1998; 51:1447–1450.
271. Santorelli FM, Tanji K, Shanske S, Krishna S, Schmidt RE, Greenwood RS, DiMauro S, De Vivo DC. The mitochondrial DNA A8344G mutation in Leigh syndrome revealed by analysis in paraffin-embedded sections: revisiting the past. Ann Neurol 1998; 44:962–964.
272. Gamez J, Playan A, Andreu AL, Bruno C, Navarro C, Cervera C, Arbos MA, Schwartz S, Enriquez JA, Montoya J. Familial multiple symmetric lipomatosis associated with the A8344G mutation of mitochondrial DNA. Neurology 1998; 51:258–260.
273. Arenas J, Campos Y, Bornstein B, Ribacoba R, Martin MA, Rubio JC, Santorelli FM, Zeviani M, DiMauro S, Garesse R. A double mutation (A8296G and G8363A) in the mitochondrial DNA tRNA^{Lys} gene associated with myoclonus epilepsy with ragged-red fibers. Neurology 1999; 52:377–382.
274. Chalmers RM, Brockington M, Howard RS, Lecky BRF, Morgan-Hughes JA, Harding AE. Mitochondrial encephalopathy with multiple mitochondrial DNA deletions: a report of two families and two sporadic cases with unusual clinical and neuropathological features. J Neurol Sci 1996; 143:41–45.
275. Sommer C, Schröder JM. Hereditary motor and sen-

sory neuropathy with optic atrophy. Arch Neurol 1989; 46:973–977.
276. Molnar M, Neudecker S, Schröder JM. Increase of mitochondria in vasa nervorum of cases with mitochondrial myopathy, Kearns-Sayre syndrome, progressive external ophthalmoplegia and MELAS. Neuropathol Appl Neurobiol 1995; 21:432–439.
277. Yiannikas C, McLeod JG, Pollard JD, Baverstock J. Peripheral neuropathy associated with mitochondrial myopathy. Ann Neurol 1986; 20:249–257.
278. Schröder JM. Neuropathy associated with mitochondrial disorders. Brain Pathol 1993; 3:177–190.
279. Wallace DC, Shoffner JM, Trounce I, Brown MD, Ballinger SW, Corral-Debrinski M, Horton T, Jun AS, Lott MT. Mitochondrial DNA mutations in human degenerative diseases and aging. Biochim Biophys Acta 1995; 1271:141–151.
280. Toscano A, Santoro M, Vita G, Girlanda P, Sinicropi S, Fazio MC, Mazzeo A, Rodolico C, Aguennouz M, Bartolone S, Bet L, Comi GP, Messina C. Late-onset mitochondrial neuromyopathy: an age-related phenomenon? Arch Gerontol Geriatr 1996; suppl. 5: 577–583.
281. Fadic R, Russell JA, Vendanarayanan VV, Lehar M, Kuncl RW, Johns DR. Sensory ataxic neuropathy as the presenting feature of a novel mitochondrial disease. Neurology 1997; 49:239–245.
282. Lascelles RG, Thomas PK. Changes due to age in internodal length in the sural nerve in man. J Neurol. Neurosurg Psychiatry 1966; 29:40–44.
283. Jacobs JM, Love S. Qualitative and quantitative morphology of human sural nerve at different ages. Brain 1985; 108:897–924.
284. Tohgi H, Tsukagoshi H, Toyokura Y. Quantitative changes with age in normal sural nerves. Acta Neuropathol 1977; 38:213–220.

21. The Aging Autonomic Nervous System

ROBERT E. SCHMIDT

The increasing mean age of the population has widespread ramifications on disease and health care, issuing a challenge to researchers to better understand the biology of the aging nervous system and thus potentially alter it. The autonomic nervous system is charged with the maintenance and integration of visceral functions and is the substrate upon which all complex human behavior is based. Autonomic dysfunction is an increasingly recognized problem in human aging that may produce clinical symptoms directly or result in subclinical disease, decreasing the safety margin of autonomic function. Superimposition of additional metabolic (e.g., diabetes), environmental, or iatrogenic (e.g., sympatholytic antihypertensive drugs, intensive insulin therapy in diabetics) insults on an aging autonomic nervous system may produce symptomatic disease. The number of individuals with symptomatic autonomic neuropathy represents a small fraction of the number of patients with autonomic nervous system pathology, although determination of precise numbers of affected individuals depends on the sensitivity of techniques used in investigation and diagnostic criteria selected. This review concentrates on pathologic changes in the autonomic nervous system that result directly from aging and attempts to separate these changes from those that develop secondarily in response to a host of peripheral or central nervous system age-related diseases, a distinction that may be difficult to establish unequivocally in older patients.

Previously, largely anecdotal information, often contradictory and without corroboration, supported the existence of age-related autonomic dysfunction and even less was known of its neuropathologic substrate. Over the last few years, a number of investigators have contributed substantially to the understanding of clinical age-related autonomic dysfunction, and studies of aged animals have begun to address pathogenetic mechanisms and strategies for intervention.

CLINICAL STUDIES OF THE AGING HUMAN AUTONOMIC NERVOUS SYSTEM

Clinical studies (see reviews[1-4]) support a role for age-related autonomic dysfunction in a number of processes. Defective temperature regulation and abnormal sudomotor responses[5] may lead to life-threatening hypo- or hyperthermia. Abnormal bowel motility, presenting as "major gastrointestinal dysfunction" in 27% of one series of hospitalized elderly,[6] is a frequent patient complaint;[7] however, objective measures of intestinal dysmotility as a function of age alone are less compelling.[8] Although baseline gastrointestinal autonomic function may be normal in healthy elderly subjects, the motility response of the small intestine to the superimposed evocative challenge of a meal may be deficient or disorganized.[7,9] Age-related defects in the maintenance of blood pressure, resulting in orthostatic hypotension in as many as 25% of otherwise normal elderly,[10] and loss of cardiovascular reflexes[4,11] are routinely described. These apparent defects in the integrity of the aged cardiovascular sympathetic and parasympathetic nervous systems may be mimicked or exacerbated by a variety of insults including postsynaptic loss of end-organ responsiveness, reflecting alteration in the distribution, sensitivity, or number of cardiac β-receptors,[12–14] or pre- and postsynaptic α2- and possibly α1-adrenergic receptors,[15] or dysfunctional post-receptor G-protein coupled signaling.[14,16] Additionally, baroreflex impairment,[17] change in body muscle mass, altered plasma norepinephrine clearance,[18,19] or alterations in the structure of the vasculature itself (reviewed by Low[4]) may contribute to perceived age-related cardiovascular autonomic nervous system dysfunction. In a basal resting state, otherwise healthy elderly subjects may show increased muscle sympathetic nerve activity as determined by microneurography,[20] which may differ between men and women[21] and vary between end-organs, or increased plasma norepinephrine.[11,22] In addition, a variety of controlled experimental stresses to the aged sympathetic nervous system may produce an abnormally exaggerated[23,24] ("hyperadrenergic") response or result in diminished[20] or unchanged[25] responses, variations that confound a simple explanation. Power spectral analysis, a noninvasive analytic process that can be used to determine the contribution of sympathetic and parasympathetic nervous systems to heart rate control, has shown an age-related decline in both sympathetic[26] and parasympathetic[27] cardiac activity. Although cardiac vagal parasympathetic dysfunction has been well established with aging,[28] parasympathetic dysfunction may vary significantly among functional modalities. Age-related alterations in pupillary size and kinetics have been interpreted as evidence of a parasympathetic[11] and/or sympathetic deficit.[29]

Simple loss of sympathetic or parasympathetic ganglionic neurons may not underlie such complex age-related phenomena; rather, the problem may involve interference with the complex integration of autonomic functions within autonomic reflex pathways, a process known to involve prevertebral sympathetic ganglia,[30] and discrete subpopulations of neurons and neurotransmitters at various levels in the autonomic nervous system.

NEUROPATHOLOGY OF THE AGED HUMAN AUTONOMIC NERVOUS SYSTEM

Central Autonomic Pathways in Aged Human Subjects

The 5%–8% loss per decade of intermediolateral (IML) column neurons[31] and their preganglionic sympathetic axons is reported to result in symptomatic disease following the cumulative loss of 50% of IML neurons. Presumably, the segmental demyelination and Wallerian degeneration of myelinated axons in aging human paravertebral ganglia represent the involvement of preganglionic sympathetic axons.[32] The cortical and subcortical input to the control of autonomic function is widespread and systematic investigation of these sites in pure forms of aging autonomic dysfunction has not been accomplished. Damage to selected cortical regions in disease states (e.g., ventromedial frontal lobe in patients with Alzheimer's disease having autonomic dysfunction) suggests at least the possibility that similar central mechanisms could contribute to the dysfunction seen in aging.

Aged Human Sympathetic Ganglia

The identification of pathologic changes in sympathetic ganglia is complicated by the need to use autopsy- or surgically derived material, which requires that assumptions be made concerning the normal state of these ganglia. The neuronal populations of the paravertebral superior cervical ganglion (SCG) and the prevertebral celiac ganglion (CG) or superior mesenteric ganglion (SMG) are generally thought to be well preserved in aged human subjects,[33–38] although some studies[39,40] have reported age-related neuronal atrophy or degeneration. Because of the size and plexiform nature of some ganglia, neuronal density measurements (expressed as neurons/mm^2) typically have been used to approximate neuron number; however, studies in animals[41,42] using nonbiased stereological techniques suggest such density measurements may be unreliable.

In the largest series of autopsied human sympathetic ganglia,[38] actively degenerating or chromatolytic neurons or increased numbers of nodular satellite cell clusters (i.e., nodules of Nageotte, an indicator of remote neuronal loss) were not identified as a function of age. Perivascular and parenchymal lymphocytic infiltrates were frequent and nonspecific findings in this series, suggesting a cautious interpretation of the "autoimmune" infiltrates described in autopsied sympathetic ganglia in various disease states. Neurofibrillary tangles have been described in some studies of aged sympathetic ganglia[43] but not in others.[38] Decreased sympathetic perikaryal catecholamines have been reported in aged human sympathetic ganglia through the use of fluorescent histochemical techniques.[44–47] Aging sympathetic neurons show a progressive increase in neuromelanin, a by-product of catecholamine synthesis, and in lipofuscin,[47] findings of uncertain, if any, pathological significance.

Although compelling evidence for loss of sympathetic neurons with age has not been found, structural alterations in dendrites, axons, and synapses have been routinely identified in aging human sympathetic ganglia.[36–38,40,48–51] The hallmark pathologic alteration in aging prevertebral sympathetic CG and SMG and, to a much lesser degree, in the paravertebral SCG is the accumulation of markedly enlarged (5–30 μm) dystrophic axons adjacent to and compressing the perikarya of principal sympathetic neurons or their primary dendrites.[36] On modified Bielschowsky silver histochemical stains the prominent argyrophilia of most dystrophic axons and their origin from delicate preterminal axons (Fig. 21–1, arrows) appeared as a distal axonopathy or synaptic dysplasia. Ultrastructural studies[52] have identified two forms of neuroaxonal dystrophy in aged human SMG ganglia: most swollen axons contain neurofilamentous (NF) aggregates (Figs. 21–2 and 21–3); and less frequently, swollen axons contain aggregated subcellular organelles and poorly characterized vacuoles. Immunohistochemical studies have shown that NF in dystrophic axons consist chiefly of the highly phosphorylated 200 kDa NF-H isoform.[53] Immunolocalization of the nonphosphorylated epitopes of 200 kDa NF-H as well as of medium- and low-molecular-weight forms and the microtubule-associated protein

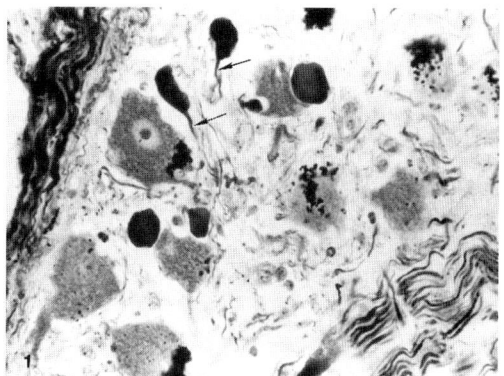

Figure 21–1. Light-microscopic appearance of neuroaxonal dystrophy in aged human superior mesenteric ganglion. Multiple large dystrophic axons arise from axons of normal dimensions (arrows) and many are located immediately adjacent to principal sympathetic neurons. Bielschowsky silver stain, ×800.

(MAP) MAP-2 labeled the perikarya and principal dendrites of sympathetic neurons but did not label dystrophic axons. Quantitative studies demonstrated a progressive increase in the frequency of dystrophic axons (expressed as lesions/principal sympathetic neuron) as a function of age (increasing particularly after the age of 60) and, surprisingly, gender (males > females). Diabetic patients developed immunohistochemically and ultrastructurally identical lesions earlier and in greater numbers than age-matched control subjects,[37] suggesting the potential for shared mechanisms.

Axons and nerve terminals in the prevertebral ganglia contain more than a dozen classical neurotransmitters and neuropeptides that reflect the contribution of neurons originating in the spinal cord, dorsal root ganglia, parasympathetic nervous system, and other sympathetic ganglia, and from retrogradely projecting alimentary tract myenteric neurons. The recognized ability of the aged autonomic nervous system to maintain normal baseline autonomic function and yet fail to respond appropriately to a variety of superimposed stresses suggests a possible abnormality of integration of visceral sympathetic reflexes, perhaps at the prevertebral ganglionic level. Dystrophic axons in aged human SMG contained dopamine-β-hydroxylase, tyrosine hydroxylase and neuropeptide Y (NPY; Fig. 21–4) as well as trk A and p75 (high- and low-affinity nerve

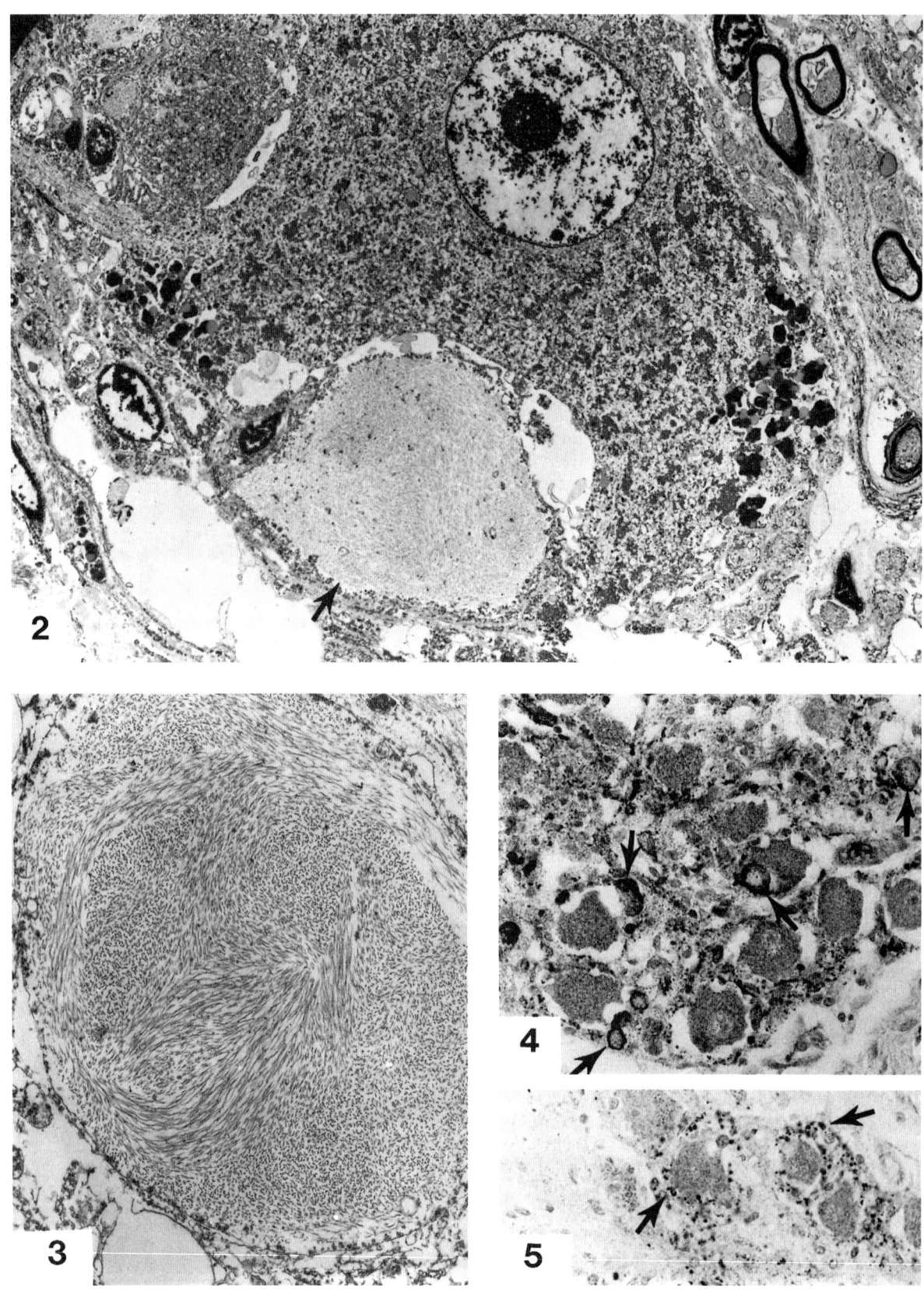

growth factor [NGF] receptors, respectively), but not substance P (Fig. 21–5), gastrin-releasing peptide (GRP)/bombesin, calcitonin gene related peptide (CGRP), or enkephalins.[36,37,54] This immunohistochemical signature is most compatible with the origin of dystrophic axons from sympathetic neurons, either located in other pre- and paravertebral ganglia or, potentially, arising within the SMG itself. The total number of NPY-containing delicate nondystrophic axons and nerve terminals actually increased in the aged SMG, a result that may reflect collateral axonal sprouting, axonal regeneration, or injury-induced altered neuropeptide synthesis. Simultaneous immunolocalization of NPY and substance P demonstrated that dystrophic NPY-containing nerve terminals targeted adjacent but often separate subpopulations of sympathetic neurons than those neurons targeted by nondystrophic substance P–containing terminals.[54] A selective age-related decrease in enkephalin containing terminals surrounding sympathetic neurons has also been described.[34]

In summary, it is generally thought that age-related sympathetic dysfunction is not the result of progressive loss of neurons in sympathetic ganglia; rather, alterations in the number and structure of presynaptic elements seem poised to interfere with sympathetic function. Apparent selective targeting of subpopulations of nerve terminals in the aging sympathetic ganglia may represent the pathoanatomic substrate of failed integration of visceral reflexes.

Aged Human Parasympathetic Ganglia

Although clinical autonomic studies suggest substantial abnormality in parasympathetic nervous system function with aging,[4] particularly altered control of heart rate, systematic studies of the vagus nerve and most cranial parasympathetic nuclei have not been accomplished in elderly human subjects. Neuron loss, however, has been reported in the aged human ciliary ganglia,[55] which may contribute to pupillomotor dysfunction.

FUNCTIONAL AND BIOCHEMICAL CHANGES IN THE AGED AUTONOMIC NERVOUS SYSTEM OF EXPERIMENTAL ANIMALS

The characterization of the pathogenetic mechanisms underlying autonomic nervous system dysfunction in aged human subjects has necessitated the development and validation of animal model systems.

Sympathetic Nervous System

A number of sympathetic functions (e.g., heart rate, arterial blood pressure) are reportedly abnormal in aged rats.[56] Sympathetic innervation of various end-organs in aged rats has been monitored by measurement of norepinephrine turnover or tyramine-induced norepinephrine release. The authors of some of these studies reported that functional changes were accompanied by structural age-related degeneration of cardiac noradrenergic innervation[57] while others showed varying tissue-specific attenuation or accentuation of norepinephrine turnover.[58–60] Cardiac synaptosomes prepared from aged rats showed decreased K^+-induced norepinephrine release, a result thought to reflect decreased numbers of functional nerve terminal Ca^{2+} channels.[61] Decreased numbers of β-adrenergic receptors

---

Figure 21–2, 21–3. Ultrastructural appearance of neuroaxonal dystrophy in aging human superior mesenteric ganglion. A dystrophic axon immediately adjacent to and distorting the perikaryon (arrow, Fig. 21–2) contains large numbers of neurofilaments, seen better at higher magnification (Fig. 21–3). Electron micrographs; Fig. 21–2, ×2920; Fig. 21–3; ×9220.

Figures 21–4, 21–5. Immunohistochemical appearance of neuroaxonal dystrophy in aging human superior mesenteric ganglion. Dystrophic axons are prominently labeled by antisera to neuropeptide Y (arrows, Fig. 21–4), but only normal, delicate substance P-containing axons (arrows, Fig. 21–5) are found in the same sections. Immunolocalization; ×350. [Figures 21–2 to 21–5 reproduced with permission from Schmidt RE, Neuropathology of human sympathetic autonomic ganglia. Microsc Res Tech 35:107–121, copyright 1996, John Wiley and Sons, Inc.]

have been reported in the aged rat pineal but not in aged myocardium, lung, and lymphocytes.[62,63] The role of the sympathetic nervous system in thermoregulation in the aged rat is similarly complex, with increased sympathetic nerve traffic to brown fat being offset by defective post-receptor signal transduction.[64] Also altered in aging rats are gastrointestinal functions, including increased colonic transit time, which, although it has been attributed to altered cholinergic function,[65] may also reflect local reflexes involving sympathetic prevertebral ganglia. In summary, no single uniform theme characterizes the distribution of changes in norepinephrine content, turnover, or receptor metabolism from end-organ to end-organ in aging rats.

In many cases baseline sympathetic functions are well maintained in aged animals; however, as in aged human subjects, superimposition of additional stresses may result in autonomic nervous system dysfunction. Immersion or immobilization stress of aged rats induced an abnormal sympathoadrenal response, which developed more slowly but continued for a longer interval than in younger adults[66] or failed to appropriately increase heart rate and blood pressure.[67] Reserpine-induced depletion of catecholamines was followed by sluggish re-synthesis and a blunted increase in β-adrenergic receptors in aged animals.[45,62,68] Finally, fasting resulted in decreased norepinephrine turnover in selected end-organs of young rats but not in aged animals, suggesting abnormal integration of sympathoadrenal function.[69]

Various biochemical measurements have also been used as monitors of ganglionic health of aged sympathetic ganglia. A variety of neurotransmitters, neurotransmitter synthesizing enzymes, or neuromodulatory substances are reportedly abnormal in sympathetic ganglia and end-organs of aging rodents, although results from different laboratories often lack consistency. Norepinephrine content has been reported to be decreased in aged rat CG, SMG, and hypogastric ganglia.[45,46,70] However, the activities of tyrosine hydroxylase (TOH) and dopamine-β-hydroxylase, two synthetic enzymes critical for norepinephrine biosynthesis, are not decreased in aged sympathetic ganglia,[68,71] and TOH mRNA is actually increased in the aged rat SCG,[72,73] although subpopulations of sympathetic neurons may be differentially affected. Choline acetyl transferase, an enzyme marker for presynaptic cholinergic elements in pre- and paravertebral sympathetic ganglia, is variously reported as unchanged or increased in aged rat SCG.[68,71] Conversely, the content of met-enkephalin, a presynaptic inhibitory neurotransmitter in sympathetic ganglia, has been reported to decrease 60% in the CG and SCG of aged rats.[74]

The monitoring of sympathetic neuron number or density of end-organ noradrenergic innervation through measurement of norepinephrine, neuropeptides, or ganglionic TOH activity may not represent an accurate measure in all settings since various pathologic processes (e.g., decentralization or axotomy induced up- or down-regulation of neurotransmitters, and especially neuropeptides) may result in decreased enzyme activity or altered neurotransmitter content without loss of sympathetic neurons or end-organ innervation. In addition, prevertebral and paravertebral ganglia differ substantially in their response to a variety of pathologic insults, thus, results with one group of ganglia may not accurately reflect changes in others.[75]

The few published metabolic studies concerning aged rat SCG and CG/SMG[76] have reported decreased metabolic activity reflected by decreased activity of succinate dehydrogenase, an important enzyme involved in oxidative phosphorylation. A 30%–40% increase in glucose utilization identified in aged rat sympathetic ganglia[56] may reflect glycolytic metabolic compensation for decreased oxidative metabolism. Recent studies[77] of aged sympathetic and parasympathetic postganglionic neurons serving the urinary bladder, however, reported no change in baseline cytochrome oxidase and succinic dehydrogenase histochemistry, a result interpreted as evidence of metabolic stability of these neurons.

Parasympathetic Function

In aged rats, mediation of reflex tachycardia becomes exclusively β-adrenergic due to decreased parasympathetic function.[78] Aging in rats is also associated with cardiac-vagal hyper- and hyporesponsiveness to chemoreflex and baroreflex, respectively.[79]

NEUROPATHOLOGY OF THE AGING AUTONOMIC NERVOUS SYSTEM OF EXPERIMENTAL ANIMALS

Central Autonomic Pathways in Aged Rat Autonomic Nervous System

Although alterations in the neuronal population of various hypothalamic nuclei have been reported as a function of age in rats,[80] findings in different laboratories have been inconsistent. The pathologic alterations of aged rat neurons of the sympathetic intermediolateral column prominently involved their dendritic structure,[81] however, their preganglionic projections to the SCG comprising the cervical preganglionic sympathetic trunk failed to show quantitative changes with age.[82]

Sympathetic Nervous System

The sympathetic autonomic ganglia of aging rodents have been typically reported to show a well-preserved complement of neurons.[41,47,83,84] Although neuronal loss was initially reported in aged rat CG/SMG, SCG,[85] and hypogastric ganglion, a mixed sympathetic and parasympathetic ganglion, recent studies using unbiased dissector methods for neuronal counting suggest that the complement of neurons in hypogastric ganglia and SCG are actually maintained with age.[41,42] A variety of ultrastructural perikaryal alterations in aged rat sympathetic ganglia including distension of perikaryal mitochondria, disarrangement of rough endoplasmic reticulum, and the Golgi apparatus have been reported;[40,70] however, their significance is unknown. The microvasculature of both SCG and CG/SMG showed decreased density of vascular profiles/area in aged animals and nearly twofold thickening of the basal lamina.[86]

Neuropathologic studies of the aging sympathetic autonomic nervous system in rats,[70,87] Chinese hamsters,[88] and, most recently, mice[89,90] have demonstrated a consistent theme of neuritic and synaptic injury. Distinctive, reproducible, markedly enlarged terminal axons and synapses with the histopathologic characteristics of neuroaxonal dystrophy (Fig.

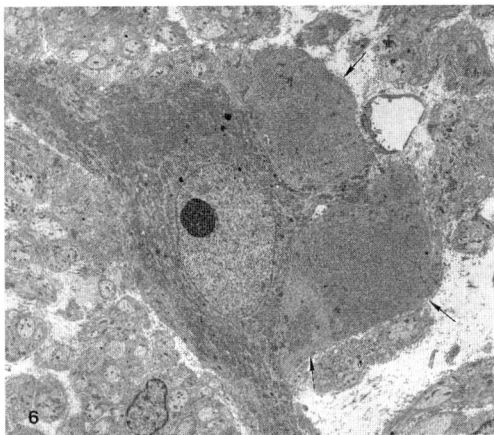

Figure 21–6. Aged rat superior mesenteric ganglion (SMG). The perikaryon and proximal dendrites of a rat SMG principal sympathetic neuron are distorted and compressed by at least three separate dystrophic axons (arrows), each containing large numbers of delicate tubulovesicular elements. Electron micrograph: ×3800 [Reproduced with permission from the Journal of Neuropathology and Experimental Neurology.]

21–6, arrows) accumulate with age and represent a pathologic hallmark of aging in the rodent sympathetic nervous system. Neuroaxonal dystrophy was infrequent within the first year of life in the rat, but increased rapidly thereafter. Sympathetic ganglia of aged rodents as well as human subjects (1) developed neuroaxonal dystrophy involving preterminal axons and synapses in sympathetic ganglia in the apparent absence of significant neuronal loss; (2) developed neuropathologic changes ultrastructurally, immunohistochemically, and anatomically identical to those in diabetics; (3) demonstrated a predilection of neuroaxonal dystrophy for prevertebral SMG and CG relative to paravertebral SCG (mouse SCG is an exception) and stellate ganglia; and, (4) demonstrated selectivity for some subpopulations of nerve terminals while completely sparing others. Although neuroaxonal dystrophy is pathologically striking, studies suggest that there also may be concomitant alterations in the numbers of normal terminals.[91] Studies of the aged rat hypogastric ganglion, which is composed of an admixture of sympathetic and parasympathetic neuronal cell bodies, showed decreased numbers of synapsin-immunoreactive nerve terminals in relation to individual sympathetic neurons but normal numbers of nerve endings on parasympathetic neurons;[91] however, in this study, paravertebral SCG, stellate and T13 sympathetic chain ganglia, as well as prevertebral CG/SMG showed no change overall in the numbers of terminals.

Enlarged dystrophic presynaptic terminal axons and synapses in the aged mouse CG/SMG were accompanied by a novel marked dilatation of neurites (mostly axons, but including dendrites as well) by numerous vacuoles ("vacuolar neuritic dystrophy," Fig. 21–7) that appeared to be confined to the aged mouse SCG.[89,90] Ultrastructural studies[90] of the cervical sympathetic trunk of aged mice (i.e., the preganglionic axons serving the SCG) failed to show dystrophic axons, as expected in distal axonopathy. Recent studies have demonstrated that there are marked differences between the frequency of vacuolar neuritic dystrophy in various mouse strains.[90] The dendritic arborization of intracellularly labeled CG/SMG neurons of young adult mice was significantly more complex and extensive than that of the SCG, and aged animals showed a relatively well-preserved CG/SMG dendritic apparatus.[89] Aged SCG neurons, however, appeared significantly smaller with regard to total dendritic length and branching than those of young animals, and exhibited short, stunted dendritic processes with large, focal, often multiple swellings along their extent.[89]

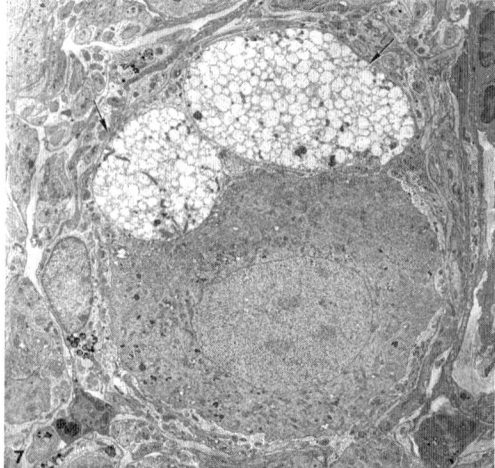

Figure 21–7. Aged mouse superior cervical ganglion (SCG). Vacuolar neuritic dystrophy consists of swollen vacuolated processes (arrows) located within the satellite cell sheath that distort the contours of individual sympathetic perikarya. ×4150.

In addition to alterations in the proximal ganglionic portions of sympathetic neurons, investigators have also reported an apparent decrease in the noradrenergic nerve terminals in a variety of target tissues including the rat heart,[57] ileum,[92] kidney,[93] bladder,[94] pineal,[95] spleen,[96] and mystacial pad,[97] and the cholinergic sympathetic innervation of sweat glands[98] but not iris and submandibular gland.[41] The reported decrease in norepinephrine in some vascular beds has been countered by no change, or even an increase, in others.[99,100] Norepinephrine turnover in various end-organs of aged rats is reportedly unchanged.[101] Interestingly, the loss of norepinephrine and serotonin innervation of aged guinea pig vasculature is accompanied by an increase in the vasodilatory neurotransmitters vasoactive intestinal peptide (VIP) and CGRP.[102] There is, therefore, no compelling evidence that aging in rats results in a generalized loss of peripheral sympathetic end-organ innervation and no single pathogenetic theme has emerged.

Three-dimensional intraneuronal injection studies of dendritic structure of aged mouse SCG neurons demonstrated focal dystrophic swellings,[89] which are poised to interfere with neuronal function since the vast majority of synapses in sympathetic ganglia terminate on dendrites. Other studies of aged rats showed dendritic atrophy of the SCG neurons innervating the middle cerebral artery (which was reversed by local application of NGF[103]), but not of those neurons innervating the iris.[103] A similar pattern of decreased neurofilament gene expression has been demonstrated for SCG neurons projecting to the middle cerebral artery but not those distributed to the iris.[104] Preganglionic neurons projecting to sympathetic neurons in aged rat hypogastric ganglia reportedly show perikaryal enlargement, proximal dendritic swelling, loss of dendritic branch points, and decreased total dendritic length,[81] similar to the appearance of sympathetic preganglionic neurons innervating the rat paracervical ganglia.[105]

Parasympathetic Nervous System

Aged parasympathetic ganglia are substantially less studied than those of the sympathetic nervous system. Relative preservation of neurons, synapses, and electrophysiologic parameters[106] in aged rat ciliary ganglion contrasts with structural changes described in neuronal perikarya and intraganglionic nerve fibers.[40] The structure of the rat cervical vagus nerve, particularly its unmyelinated axon population, showed little structural change with age,[107] however, neuron number was reportedly decreased in the aged dorsal motor nucleus of the vagus.[108] Parasympathetic neurons were relatively spared in aged rat hypogastric ganglia.[109] In contrast to preganglionic intermediolateral column neurons projecting to sympathetic neurons, neurons comprising the preganglionic parasympathetic projections to both hypogastric and paracervical ganglia showed little dendritic alteration[81,105] with aging.

Enteric Nervous System

The reported extensive loss of myenteric neurons in the rat small intestine[110] has been recently re-addressed[111] and, although select subpopulations of myenteric neurons may be decreased, the decrease in sympathetic postganglionic noradrenergic projections do not reflect simple loss of their myenteric targets. Despite the reported loss of substance P–, somatostatin- and VIP-containing intestinal nerves in aged rat small intestine,[112] functional studies are inconsistent, reporting either slowed[113] or unchanged[114] small intestinal transit. Cholinergic responses are reportedly maintained with aging in the rat small bowel, contrasting with the age-related decrease in the nitrergic contribution to nonadrenergic noncholinergic (NANC) relaxation.[115]

POSTULATED MECHANISMS OF AUTONOMIC NERVOUS SYSTEM DAMAGE WITH AGE

Although reported pathologic findings vary widely among studies, several broad themes have emerged. Most investigators agree that there is little evidence for the loss of significant numbers of neurons in aged autonomic ganglia and that significant ganglionic pathology involves dendritic alterations, changes in synapse number or structure, and neuroaxonal dystrophy that may vary significantly among different subpopulations of autonomic neurons. In the periphery, loss of axons and nerve terminals is thought to constitute the basic pathologic substrate, although site-to-site variation is prominent and some functional changes may have few structural correlates. Quantitative analysis of autonomic axons innervating target organs is difficult and catecholamine-fluorescence or neurotransmitter immunolocalization studies may confuse decreased neurotransmitter content for axon loss. The mechanisms underlying age-related damage to the peripheral nervous system remain largely unknown; however, several hypotheses have been advanced.

The Regenerative Theme

Neuroaxonal dystrophy is a structural hallmark of aging in sympathetic autonomic ganglia but it is neither confined to the sympathetic nervous system nor restricted to aging.[116–118] Although the pathogenesis of neuroaxonal dystrophy is not yet established, the ultrastructural resemblance of some dystrophic axons to growth cones,[116] the terminal motile tips of developing and regenerating axons, the frequent association of neuroaxonal dystrophy with regenerative sprouts, and its induction by frustration of peripheral axonal regeneration[88,117,119,120] suggest that the association of neuroaxonal dystrophy with axonal regeneration/collateral sprouting is more than coincidence.

The continual turnover of nerve terminals, consisting of cycles of presynaptic axonal degeneration and regeneration/collateral sprouting, has been described in normal young sympathetic ganglia in experimental animals and in various, perhaps all, end-organs as the structural equivalent of synaptic remodeling, or "plasticity."[121] It has also been identified in living autonomic ganglia and selected endorgans in situ using vital dyes.[122] Synaptic turnover may employ mechanisms shared with collateral sprouting (i.e., growth of intact uninjured axons into denervated targets) and axonal regeneration, which represent related processes with different neurotrophin dependence.[123] Axonal regeneration and, particularly, collateral sprouting of intact sympathetic axons into denervated targets have been consistently reported to be deficient in aged animals and affect the pineal,[124] hippocampus,[125] cerebral arterial vessels,[95] sweat glands,[126] the septum,[127] and hair follicles.[128] Synaptic turnover in autonomic ganglia may be further complicated in pathologic states by postganglionic axotomy, which results in the detachment, swelling, and retraction of presynaptic elements in sympathetic ganglia, a process that may represent an exaggerated form of normal synaptic turnover. The loss of SMG-derived noradrenergic terminals in the aged rat ileum[92] may involve terminal axonopathy, perhaps resulting in intraganglionic synaptic detachment and dendritic changes as described following postganglionic axotomy and, ultimately, culminating in neuroaxonal dystrophy in the SMG. Synaptic plasticity may more closely resemble collateral sprouting than axonal regeneration, particularly if turnover involves replacement of degenerated terminals with nearby uninjured axonal sprouts. The superimposition of age-related loss of synaptic plasticity on synaptic turnover or the exaggerated ganglionic response to peripheral axonal injury may eventually result in the distinctive morphologic alterations of neuroaxonal dystrophy in sympathetic autonomic ganglia. Age-related changes in cholinergic, synaptic, long-term potentiation in rat SCG,[129] in the ability to regulate expression of some synaptic vesicle proteins,[130] and in the ability to up-regulate substance P in response to decentralization in vivo and in vitro[131] have been described as indicators of loss of plasticity in aged sympathetic neurons.

Recent studies of synaptic elimination at the neuromuscular junction have provided insight into the complex mechanisms regulating synaptic plasticity.[132] Local changes in the postsynaptic muscle cell result in the loss of acetylcholine receptors beneath the synapse to be eliminated, causing the disassembly of the postsynaptic apparatus and interruption of an adhesive bond between pre- and postsynaptic elements. Ultimately, this process culminates in the loss of the overlying presynaptic axonal terminal.[133,134] The effect of the postsynaptic element on synaptic strength has been proposed to result from the elaboration of proteases or protease inhibitors with subsequent alteration of synaptic input.[135]

Although considerable attention is given to the regenerative phase of axonal growth, effective regeneration requires the process to eventually be inhibited and the synapse reconstructed and stabilized. Such a "stop" program is reported to be dependent on the proteolytic breakdown of neurofilaments as they enter the axon ending as well as on the operation of turnaround transport, which is also dependent on protease function.[136] The failure to activate a stop program appropriately by local inhibition of proteolysis[136] may result in the delivery of an excessive supply of membranes or other axonal constituents to the synapse with their accumulation as tubulovesicular elements in swollen terminals, a process that may culminate in neuroaxonal dystrophy.

Alterations in Dendritic Structure

The tertiary structure of dendrites is critical to the reception and integration of afferent signals and is markedly abnormal in aged mouse and rat SCG[89,103,137] a result that may have as much functional significance as dystrophic changes in presynaptic elements. The three-dimensional structure of dendrites[138] is dynamic and essential for the summation and integration of incoming synaptic impulses. Dendritic structure influences the extent and distribution of presynaptic axon terminals[139] and represents another potential target in aging animals. Postganglionic sympathetic axotomy results in dendritic atrophy[140] and loss of postsynaptic membrane specializations of the dendrites and cell bodies of principal sympathetic neurons, processes that may interfere with the re-formation of presynaptic axonal terminals from retracted terminal axonal swellings within sympathetic ganglia.[141] A role of neurotrophic substances in this process is proposed since atrophic dendrites of aged rats treated with NGF do increase in length but do not develop new branch points.[142] The dynamic loss of dendritic targets as part of normal turnover or regulation by the peripheral target[139] may also interfere with, and ultimately frustrate, regeneration of presynaptic axonal termini previously occupying such dendritic sites.

Neurotrophic Substances and Aging in the Peripheral Nervous System

It has been proposed that the trophic support of end-organs on their innervating neurons may decline in old age because of decreased availability of target-derived neurotrophic substances,[143,144] that have been implicated in a wide variety of developmental and pathogenetic processes in the nervous system. The response of subpopulations of aged sympathetic neurons to the neurotrophic milieu, possibly through the up-regulation or down-regulation of individual classes of receptors or the interference with neurotrophin synthesis, secretion, and uptake, may be critical to the pathogenesis and/or therapy of experimental age-related autonomic neuropathy. A deficiency of neurotrophic substances or, alternatively, excessive local production of neurotrophic substances with disorganization of axonal sprouts are theoretical possibilities.

A number of investigators have reported defects in the quantity of or neuronal responsiveness to neurotrophic substances in the aging sympathetic nervous system.[145–147] Successful transplantation of aged or young vascular muscle targets into the anterior eye chamber of young rats suggests that the age of the target tissue imposed a young or old pattern of reinnervation on collateral sprouting of host noradrenergic nerves. These results, consistent with a possible defect in age-related target-derived neurotrophic substances,[143,148] were reversed with NGF treatment,[149] and are also supported by studies reporting deficient sympathetic sprouting into the aged hippocampus.[125] Transplanted sweat glands from aged rats received a reduced density of noradrenergic innervation compared with young glands; however, there was no difference between the innervation of old and young sweat glands in their ability to induce a switch to a cholinergic phenotype, a finding that suggests that plasticity may be specific for selected functions.[148] Conversely, examination of the sprouting response of iridial nerves of aged rats in response to in oculo grafts of young and old targets showed that both ages of targets were innervated with an "old pattern" of reinnervation consistent with a neuronal defect in aging.[150] Exogenous treatment with NGF increased the innervation density on both young and old targets, although not to the same degree.[150,151] A population of SCG neurons supplying the noradrenergic innervation of the middle cerebral artery, which loses nearly half of its total innervation with age, is reported to show dendritic atrophy with age and to respond to local application of NGF with recovery of its normal structure.[142] Although NGF levels in aged SCG are reported to decrease,[152] NGF content of blood vessels, submandibular glands, and iris is generally not reduced in aged animals, nor is there a direct correlation between age-related changes in end-organ nerve density and levels of endogenous NGF.[147,148,152] Reinnervation of transplanted blood vessels by aged neurons is increased by exogenously administered NGF, but to a lesser extent than with young host neurons,[150] which may reflect decreased neuronal plasticity. Similarly, intraventricular administration of NGF to aged animals results in a prominent sprouting reaction of the axons innervating the internal carotid artery.[153] Cultured neurons from aged SCG are also reportedly less responsive to NGF in culture and develop shorter, less branched neurites than those from young SCG explants.[154] Transplanted young and old sympathetic ganglia are capable of neurite outgrowth independent of the age of the neurons.[155] The aged sympathetic nervous system may show an impaired response to NGF, but it is apparent only with reduced doses of NGF.[147] Exposure of mature and aged sympathetic neurons to anti-NGF is reported to produce atrophy of aged but not mature neurons.[156] Aged sympathetic ganglia are also reported to show decreased levels of p75 (i.e., the low-affinity neurotrophin receptor)[145] as well as mRNA for p75 and trkA, the high-affinity receptor responding primarily to NGF (and NT-3).[157]

Some of the apparent discrepancies between experiments identifying a target- or end-organ-derived defect in aged animals may reflect the differences between impaired collateral reinnervation in old animals,[150] a process that is neurotrophin sensitive, and the retained capacity for axonal regeneration in aged rats,[155] a neurotrophin-insensitive process.[123,144] In addition, increased neuronal p75 and trkA mRNA accompany collateral reinnervation but not axonal regeneration.[123] Recent studies of pilomotor innervation by noradrenergic axons have provided additional support for the neurotrophin sensitivity of collateral reinnervation, in which no direct axonal injury occurs to the neuron undergoing collateral sprouting, and the relative neurotrophin insensitivity of axonal regeneration after axotomy.[128] After experimental lesions in the septum of aged rats, collateral sprouting of sympathetic axons into the hippocampus was also diminished[158] in the presence of diminished hippocampal NGF upregulation.[146] Following extirpation of one SCG, a physiologic defect in sprouting of uninjured noradrenergic fibers within the pineal has been reported in aged but not in young rats.[124] Cycles of synaptic degeneration and regeneration may have more in common with collateral sprouting than long-distance regeneration in terms of neurotrophin sensitivity, particularly if turnover involves replacement of degenerated terminals with adjacent axonal sprouts. Synaptic maintenance, plasticity, turnover, and collateral sprouting of axons may represent multiple facets of a similar process that are differentially sensitive to neurotrophic substances.

Insulin and the insulin-like growth factors have also been shown to support the development and growth of sympathetic neurons in culture.[159] A role for insulin-like growth factor I (IGF-I) in synaptic development and axonal sprouting and regeneration has also been proposed.[160–162] Exogenously administered IGF-I enhanced the number of regenerating axons and functional recovery from sciatic nerve crush injury.[163] The increase in IGF-I in the distal stump of axotomized sciatic nerve is reportedly blunted in aging.[164] A role for IGF-I in routine synaptic turnover and its deficiency in aging and diabetes could, therefore, contribute to abnormal synaptic turnover and the development of neuroaxonal dystrophy in both conditions.

Proposed pathogenetic mechanisms may overlap. For example, axotomy-induced synaptic detachment in the young guinea pig SCG resulted in the accumulation of small numbers of organelles in detached presynaptic axon terminals but not the development of frank neuroaxonal dystrophy. These structural changes and their electrophysiologic consequences were prevented by the local application of NGF[165] or induced in normal uninjured ganglia by administration of antiserum against NGF. Nerve growth factor also controls tertiary dendritic structure, even in aged animals,[166] and may, therefore, secondarily influence presynaptic axonal structure as a response to alterations in postsynaptic dendritic targets.

Age-Dependent Alteration in Axonal Transport

Studies in somatic nerves of aging animals have consistently identified an abnormality in the rate of slow axonal transport[167] and, in particular, neurofilament transport,[168] although the rate of transport of the bulk of rapidly transported materials was reportedly unaffected by age. Turnaround transport, i.e., protease-dependent reversal of transport polarity at the nerve ending, is a specialized process that may be selectively inhibited, resulting in the accumulation of tubulovesicular elements, which are prominent constituents of dystrophic axons and may be targeted independent of either orthograde or retrograde transport. Neuroaxonal dystrophy may be initiated or exacerbated by the inhibition of the turnaround axonal transport process itself, resulting in the accumulation of large numbers of membranous organelles at axonal termini.

Synaptic Degradation of Organelles

Some materials undergo orthograde transport to the nerve terminal but are not returned and instead undergo degradation within the terminal axon. Disassembly of slowly transported neurofilaments is thought to occur in the preterminal axon in response to the activity of calcium-activated neutral proteases (calpains). Predictably, local administration of protease inhibitors resulted in the accumulation of neurofilaments in terminal axons.[169] Postsynthetic modification of neurofilaments by glycosylation and the formation of advanced glycosylation end products,[170,171] (processes that are thought to operate in both aging and diabetes) or phosphorylation may change the sensitivity of neurofilaments to calpains and could result in their excessive accumulation in axonal terminals.

Extracellular Matrix

Research into the function of the extracellular matrix has advanced rapidly over the last few years[172] and detailed studies of the normal process of removal of supernumerary neuromuscular junctions suggest a seminal role for alterations in the matrix and postsynaptic elements in the loss of presynaptic nerve terminals. Neural cell adhesion molecules (NCAM) may promote or inhibit synaptic plasticity or stability, potentially by alternative splicing or post-translational processing or by changing the level of polysialic acid.[173] Cultured aged SCG neurons exhibit reduced responsiveness to laminin in the presence of NGF,[154,174] and reduced laminin immunoreactivity is reported to correlate with reduced innervation (possibly due to reduced collateral sprouting) of middle cerebral artery walls of aging rats in vivo.[175,176] High levels of laminin may rescue NGF responsiveness of aged neurons in culture.[174] One synaptic substance, s-laminin, has been shown to affect synaptic function and structure in vitro by serving as a stop signal,[177] and s-laminin gene knockout mice develop abnormal synapses that (1) lack presynaptic specializations; (2) have dispersed synaptic vesicles; (3) have interposed Schwann cell processes; (4) have decreased levels of NCAM and synapsin; and, (5) demonstrate a decreased frequency of miniature end-plate potentials.[178,179] Laminin expression is increased in aged autonomic ganglia.[42] Age-related alterations in the extracellular matrix are thus also poised to affect nerve terminal structure, function, and plasticity.

Oxidative Injury

The relative increase in oxidative stress and alteration in free radical production or impaired free-radical scavenging has been proposed in the pathogenesis of neurologic and non-neurologic complications of aging. Lipid peroxidation of rat brain synaptosomes resulted in alterations in membrane fluidity, lipid composition, and Na^+-K^+ATPase activity, similar to changes produced by aging itself, which resulted in greater susceptibility of aged synaptic membranes to additional in vitro lipid peroxidation.[180] Chronic vitamin E deficiency resulted in the premature and exaggerated development of neuroaxonal dystrophy in aged human and rat primary sensory axon medullary terminals but, surprisingly, not in aged rat SMG.[181]

Abnormal Calcium Dynamics

In aged animals an increase in stimulation-evoked norepinephrine release and abnormal calcium handling by aged SCG neurons in culture and the noradrenergic innervation of the rat tail vasculature are thought to reflect an age-related decline in Ca^{2+} uptake by smooth endoplasmic reticulum and increased reliance on mitochondrial calcium buffering.[182] Aged rat SCG neurons in culture show a decline in Ca^{2+}ATPase in the smooth endoplasmic reticulum, which may contribute to increased stimulation-evoked release of norepinephrine in older adrenergic nerves.[183] The precise control of intracellular Ca^{2+} concentration is important for a variety of critical cellular processes, including degradative calpain-mediated cytoskeletal alterations.

CONCLUSION

Systematic studies of the autonomic nervous system of human subjects and development of well-defined animal models have begun to substantially improve our understanding of the pathogenesis of autonomic dysfunction in aging and may eventually provide strategies for intervention. A synapse-directed pathologic process represents an attack on the most significant area for neuron-to-neuron transmission of the nerve impulse. Pathologic processes that selectively target nerve terminals may have significant, protean functional consequences, particularly for integrated nervous function in which different synaptic subpopulations may subserve discrete functions. Plasticity-related synaptic remodeling could represent a preferential, highly susceptible target of the aging process. Understanding synaptic turnover and its frustration, therefore, may have far-ranging significance for understanding some of the most complex and critical processes in the peripheral and central nervous systems.

REFERENCES

1. Schmidt RE. Pathology of the sympathetic nervous system. In: Duckett S, ed. Pathology of the Aging Human Nervous System, 1st ed. Philadelphia: Lea and Febiger, 1991:431–442.
2. Amenta F. Aging of the Autonomic Nervous System. Boca Raton, FL: CRC Press, 1993.
3. Lipsitz LA. Aging and the autonomic nervous system. In: Robertson D, Low PA, Polinsky RJ, eds. Primer on the Autonomic Nervous System. San Diego: Academic Press, 1996:79–83.
4. Low PA. The effect of aging on the autonomic nervous system. In: Low PA, ed. Clinical Autonomic Disorders. Evaluation and Management. Philadelphia: Lippincott-Raven, 1997:161–175.
5. Collins KF, Dore C, Exton-Smith AN, Fox RH, MacDonald IC, Woodward PM. Accidental hypothermia and impaired temperature homeostasis in the elderly. BMJ 1977; 1:353–356.
6. Geboes K, Bossaert H. Gastrointestinal disorders in old age. Age Aging 1977; 6:197–200.
7. Anuras S, Leoning-Baucke V. Gastrointestinal motility in the elderly. J Am Geriatr Soc 1984; 32:386–398.
8. Clarkston WK, Pantano MM, Morley JE, Horowitz M, Littlefield JM, Burton FR. Evidence for the anorexia of aging: gastrointestinal transit and hunger in healthy elderly vs. young adults. Am J Physiol 1997; 272:R243–R248.
9. Anuras S, Sutherland J. Small intestinal manometry in healthy elderly subjects. J Am Geriatr Soc 1984; 32: 581–583.
10. Caird FI, Andrews GR, Kennedy RD. Effect of posture on blood pressure in the elderly. Br Heart J 1973; 35:527–530.
11. Pfeifer MA, Weinberg CR, Cook D, Best JD, Reenan A, Halter JB. Differential changes of autonomic nervous system function with age in man. Am J Med 1983; 75:249–258.
12. Dillon N, Chung S, Kelly J, O'Malley K. Age and beta adrenoceptor-mediated function. Clin Pharmacol Ther 1980; 27:769–772.
13. Lakatta EG. Cardiovascular regulation in aging. Physiol Rev 1993; 73:413–467.
14. White M, Roden R, Minobe W, Khan MF, Larrabee P, Wollmering M, Port JD, Anderson F, Campbell D, Feldman AM, Bristow MR. Age-related changes in β-adrenergic neuroeffector systems in the human heart. Circulation 1994; 90:1225–1238.
15. Docherty JR. Cardiovascular responses in aging. Pharmacol Rev 1990; 42:103–.
16. Roth GS, Joseph JA, Mason RP. Membrane alterations as causes of impaired signal transduction in Alzheimer's disease and aging. Trends Neurosci 1995; 18:203–206.
17. Laitinen T, Hartikainen J, Vanninen E, Niskanen L, Geelen G, Länsimies E. Age and gender dependency of baroreflex sensitivity in healthy subjects. J Appl Physiol 1998; 84:576–583.
18. Rubin PC, Scott PJW, McLean K, Reid JL. Noradrenaline release and clearance in relation to age and blood pressure in man. Eur J Clin Invest 1982; 12: 121–125.
19. Esler MD, Turner AG, Kaye DM, Thompson JM, Kingwell BA, Morris M, Lambert GW, Jennings GL, Cox H, Seals DR. Aging effects on human sympathetic neuronal function. Am J Physiol 1995; 268: R278–R285.
20. Iwase S, Mano T, Watanabe T, Saito M, Kobayashi F. Age-related changes of sympathetic outflow to muscles in humans. J Gerontol 1991; 46:M1–M5.
21. Ng AV, Callister R, Johnson DG, Seals DR. Age and gender influence muscle sympathetic nerve activity at rest in healthy humans. Hypertension 1993; 21:498–503.
22. Ziegler MG, Lake CR, Kopin IJ. Plasma noradrenaline increases with age. Nature 1976; 261:333–335.
23. Palmer GJ, Ziegler MG, Lake CR. Response of norepinephrine and blood pressure to stress increases with age. J Gerontol 1978; 33:482–487.
24. Rowe JW, Troen BR. Sympathetic nervous system and aging in man. Endocr Rev 1980; 1:167–179.
25. Ng AV, Callister R, Johnson DG, Seals DR. Sympathetic neural reactivity to stress does not increase with age in healthy humans. Am J Physiol 1994; 267:H344–H353.
26. Piccirillo G, Bucca C, Bauco C, Cinti AM, Michelle D, Fimognari FL, Cacciafixta M, Marigliano V. Power spectral analysis of heart rate in subjects over a hundred years old. Int J Cardiol 1998; 63:53–61.
27. Ziegler D, Laux G, Dannehl K, Spuler M, Muhlen H, Mayer P, Gries FA. Assessment of cardiovascular autonomic function: age-related normal ranges and reproducibility of spectral analysis, vector analysis, and standard tests of heart rate variation and blood pressure responses. Diabetic Med 1992; 9:166–175.
28. Low PA, Opfer-Gehrking TL, Proper CJ, Zimmerman I. The effect of ageing on cardiac autonomic and postganglionic sudomotor function. Muscle Nerve 1990; 13:152–157.
29. Bitsios P, Prettyman R, Szabadi E. Changes in autonomic function with age: a study of pupillary kinetics in healthy young and old people. Age Aging 1996; 25: 432–438.
30. Kreulen DL. Integration in autonomic ganglia. Physiologist 1984; 27:49–55.
31. Low PA, Okazaki H, Dyck PJ. Splanchnic preganglionic neurons in man. I. Morphometry of preganglionic cytons. Acta Neuropathol 1977; 40:55–61.
32. Brocklehurst JC. Ageing in the autonomic nervous system. Age Aging 1974; 4 (Suppl.): 7–17.
33. Dyck PJ, Jedrzejowska H, Karnes J, Kawamura Y, Low PA, O'Brien PC, Offord K, Ohnishi A, Ohta M, Pollock M, Stevens JC. Reconstruction of motor, sensory and autonomic neurons based on morphometric study of sampled levels. Muscle Nerve 1979; 2:399–405.
34. Jarvi R, Helen P, Pelto-Huikko M, Rapoport SI, Hervonen A. Age-related changes on enkephalinergic innervation of human sympathetic neurons. Mech Ageing Dev 1988; 44:143–151.
35. Scaravilli F. Changes in neuronal structure and cell populations with ageing. In: Thomas PK, ed. Periph-

35. eral Nerve Changes in the Elderly. New Issues in Neurosciences, Vol. 1. New York: John Wiley and Sons, 1988:95–107.
36. Schmidt RE, Chae HY, Parvin CA, Roth KA. Neuroaxonal dystrophy in aging human sympathetic ganglia. Am J Pathol 1990; 136:327–338.
37. Schmidt RE, Plurad SB, Parvin CA, Roth KA. Effect of diabetes and aging on human sympathetic autonomic ganglia. Am J Pathol 1993; 143:143–153.
38. Schmidt RE. Neuropathology of human sympathetic autonomic ganglia. Microsc Res Tech 1996; 35:107–121.
39. Botar J. Qualitative und quantitative Untersuchung der Nervenzellen des Ganglion Coeliacum im Alter. Alterserscheinungen der sympathischen Nervenzellen. Acta Anat (Basel) 1956; 28:157–206.
40. Vega JA, Calzada B, Del Valle ME. Age-induced changes in the mammalian autonomic and sensory ganglia. In: Amenta F, ed. Aging of the Autonomic Nervous System. Boca Raton, FL: CRC Press, 1993: 37–67.
41. Santer RM. Sympathetic neuron numbers in ganglia of young and aged rats. J Auton Nerv Syst 1991; 33: 221–222.
42. Warburton AL, Santer RM. The hypogastric and thirteenth thoracic ganglia of the rat: effects of age on the neurons and their extracellular environment. J Anat 1997; 190:115–124.
43. Kawasaki H, Murayama S, Tomonaga M, Izumyama N, Shimada H. Neurofibrillary-tangles in human upper cervical ganglia. Morphological study with immunohistochemistry and electron microscopy. Acta Neuropathol 1987; 75:156–159.
44. Hervonen A, Valasti A, Partanen M, Kanerva L, Hervonen H. Effects of aging on the histochemically demonstrable catecholamines and acetylcholinesterase of human sympathetic ganglia. J Neurocytol 1978; 7: 11–23.
45. Santer RM, Fluorescence histochemical evidence for decreased noradrenaline synthesis in sympathetic neurons of aged rats. Neurosci Lett 1979; 15:177–180.
46. Partanen M, Santer RM, Hervonen, A. The effect of aging on the histochemically demonstrable catecholamines in the hypogastric (major pelvic) ganglion of the rat. Histochem J 1980; 12:527–535.
47. Hervonen A, Partanen M, Helen P, Koistinaho J, Alho H, Baker DM, Johnson JE, Santer RM. The sympathetic neuron, a model of neuronal aging. In: Panulea P, Paivarinta H, Soinila S, eds. Neurohistochemistry: Modern Methods and Applications. New York: Alan R. Liss, 1986:569–586.
48. Kuntz A. Histological variation in autonomic ganglia and ganglion cells associated with age and disease. Am J Pathol 1938; 14:783–795.
49. Helen P, Zeitlin R, Hervonen A. Mitochondrial accumulations in nerve fibers of human sympathetic ganglia. Cell Tissue Res 1980; 207:491–496.
50. Helen P. Fine-structural and degenerative features in adult and aged human sympathetic ganglionic cells. Mech Aging Dev 1983; 23:161–175.
51. Hervonen A, Age related neuropathologic changes in human sympathetic ganglia. Soc Neurosci Abst 1984; 10:451.
52. Schroer JA, Plurad SB, Schmidt RE. Fine structure of presynaptic axonal terminals in sympathetic autonomic ganglia of aging and diabetic human subjects. Synapse 1992; 12:1–13.
53. Schmidt RE, Beaudet LN, Plurad SB, Dorsey DA. Axonal cytoskeletal pathology in aged and diabetic human sympathetic autonomic ganglia. Brain Res 1997; 769:375–383.
54. Schmidt RE, Dorsey DA, Roth KA. Immunohistochemical characterization of NPY and substance P containing nerve terminals in aged and diabetic human sympathetic ganglia. Brain Res 1992; 583:320–326.
55. Bigl V, Arendt T, Fischer S, Fisher M, Werner M, Arendt A. The cholinergic system in aging. Gerontolgy 1986; 33:172–180.
56. Partanen M, London ED, Rapoport SI. Glucose utilization in sympathetic ganglia of male Fischer-344 rats at different ages. J Auton Nerv Syst 1982; 5:391–398.
57. Goldberg PB, Kreider MS, McLean MR, Roberts J. Effects of aging at the adrenergic cardiac neuroeffector junction. Fed Proc 1986; 45:45–47.
58. Kregel KC. Influence of aging on tissue-specific noradrenergic activity at rest and during nonexertional heating in rats. J Appl Physiol 1994; 76:1226–1231.
59. Kregel KC. Alterations in autonomic adjustments to acute hypoxia in conscious rats with aging. J Appl Physiol 1996; 80:540–546.
60. Mazzeo RS, Grantham PA. Sympathetic response to exercise in various tissues with advancing age. J Appl Physiol 1989; 66:1506–1508.
61. Snyder DL, Johnson MD, Aloyo VJ, Eskin B, Roberts J Age-related changes in cardiac norepinephrine release: role of calcium movement. J Gerontol 1995; 50: B358–B367.
62. Weiss B, Greenberg L, Cantor E. Age-related alterations in the development of adrenergic denervation supersensitivity. Fed Proc 1979; 38:1915–1921.
63. Scarpace PJ, Decreased beta-adrenergic responsiveness during senescence. Fed Proc 1986; 45:51–54.
64. Florez-Duquet M, McDonald RB. Cold-induced thermoregulation and biological aging. Physiol Rev 1998; 78:339–358.
65. McDougal JN, Miller MS, Burks TF. Age-related changes in colonic function in rats. Am J Physiol 1984; 247:G542–546.
66. McCarty R. Sympathetic-adrenal medullary and cardiovascular responses to acute cold stress in adult and aged rats. J Auton Nerv Syst 1985; 12:15–22.
67. Chiueh CC, Nespor SM, Rapoport SI. Cardiovascular, sympathetic and adrenal cortical responsiveness of aged Fischer-344 rats to stress. Neurobiol Aging 1980; 1:157–163.
68. Partanen M, Waller SB, London ED, Hervonen A. Indices of neurotransmitter synthesis and release in aging sympathetic nervous system. Neurobiol Aging 1985; 6:227–232.
69. Rapoport EB, Young JB, Landsberg L. Impact of age on basal and diet induced changes in sympathetic nervous system activity of Fischer rats. J Gerontol 1981; 36:152–157.
70. Santer RM, Partanen M, Hervonen A. Glycoxylic acid fluorescence and ultrastructural studies of neurones in the coeliac-superior mesenteric ganglia of the aged rat. Cell Tissue Res 1980; 211:475–485.
71. Reis DJ, Ross RA, Joh TH. Changes in the activity and amounts of enzymes synthesizing catecholamines

and acetylcholine in brain, adrenal medulla, and sympathetic ganglia of aged rat and mouse. Brain Res 1977; 136:465–474.
72. Kedziedrski W, Porter JC. Quantitative study of tyrosine hydroxylase mRNA in catecholamine neurons and adrenals during development and aging. Mol Brain Res 1990; 7:45–51.
73. Kuchel GA, Richard C. Contrasting changes in neurotrophin receptor and tyrosine hydroxylase gene expression in the aged sympathetic nervous system. Soc Neurosci Abst 1995; 21:1550.
74. Govoni S, Missale C, Castelletti L, Spano PF, Trabucchi M. Decreased content of met-enkephalin like peptides in superior cervical and coeliac ganglia of aged rats. Neurobiol Aging 1983; 4:147–150.
75. Schmidt RE, McAtee SJ, Plurad DA, Parvin CA, Cogswell BE, Roth KA. Differential susceptibility of prevertebral and paravertebral sympathetic ganglia to experimental injury. Brain Res 1998; 460:214–226.
76. Baker DM, Santer RM. Development of a quantitative histochemical method for determination of succinate dehydrogenase activity in autonomic neurons and its application to the study of aging in the autonomic nervous system. J Histochem Cytochem 1990; 38:525–531.
77. Warburton AL, Santer RM. Stability of enzymatic indicators of metabolic and neuronal activity in postganglionic neurons supplying the urinary tract of aged rats. Histochem J 1998; 30:317–324.
78. Bunag RD, Krizsan D, Eriksson L. Mediation of reflex tachycardia becomes exclusively beta-adrenergic in old Fischer 344 rats. Mech Ageing Dev 1990; 52:179–194.
79. Franchini KG, Moreira ED, Ida F, Krieger EM. Alterations in the cardiovascular control by the chemoreflex and baroreflex in old rats. Am J Physiol 1996; 270:R310–R313.
80. Sartin JL, Lamperti AA. Neuronal numbers in hypothalamic nuclei of young, middle-aged and aged male rats. Experientia 1985; 41:109–111.
81. Dering MA, Santer RM, Watson AHD. Age-related changes in the morphology of preganglionic neurons projecting to rat hypogastric ganglion. J Neurocytol 1996; 25:555–563.
82. Santer RM. Quantitative analysis of the cervical sympathetic trunk in young adult and aged rats. Mech Ageing Dev 1993; 67:289–298.
83. Santer RM. Morphological evidence for the maintenance of the cervical sympathetic system in aged rats. Neurosci Lett 1991; 130:248–250.
84. Cowen T. Ageing in the autonomic nervous system: a result of nerve target interactions. A review. Mech Ageing Dev 1993; 68:163–173.
85. Baker DM, and Santer RM. Morphometric studies on pre-and paravertebral sympathetic neurons in the rat: Changes with age. Mech Ageing Dev 1988; 42:139–145.
86. Baker DM, Santer RM, Blaggan AS. Morphometric studies on the microvasculature of pre- and paravertebral sympathetic ganglia in the adult and aged rat by light and electron microscopy. J Neurocytol 1989; 18:647–660.
87. Schmidt RE, Plurad SB, Modert CW. Neuroaxonal dystrophy in the autonomic ganglia of aged rats. J Neuropathol Exp Neurol 1983; 42:376–390.
88. Schmidt RE, Plurad DA, Plurad SB, Cogswell BE, Diani AR, Roth KA. Ultrastructural and immunohistochemical characterization of autonomic neuropathy in genetically diabetic Chinese hamsters. Lab Invest 1989; 61:77–92.
89. Schmidt RE, Beaudet LN, Plurad SB, Snider WD, Ruit KG. Pathologic alterations in pre-and postsynaptic elements in aged mouse sympathetic ganglia. J Neurocytol 1995; 24:189–206.
90. Schmidt RE, Dorsey DA, Beaudet LN, Plurad SB, Parvin CA, Bruch LA. Vacuolar neuritic dystrophy in aged mouse superior cervical sympathetic ganglia is strain-specific. Brain Res 1998; 806:141–151.
91. Warburton AL, Santer RM. Decrease in synapsin I staining in the hypogastric ganglion of aged rats. Neurosci Lett 1995; 194:157–160.
92. Baker DM, Santer RM. A quantitative study of the effects of age on the noradrenergic innervation of Auerbach's plexus in the rat. Mech Ageing Dev 1988; 42:147–158.
93. Vega JA, Ricci A, Amenta F. Age-dependent changes of the sympathetic innervation of the rat kidney. Mech Ageing Dev 1990; 54:185–196.
94. Warburton AL, Santer RM. Sympathetic and sensory innervation of the urinary tract in young adult and aged rats: A semi-quantitative histochemical and immunolocalization study. Histochem J 1994; 26:127–133.
95. Kuchel GA. Alterations in target innervation and collateral sprouting in the aging sympathetic nervous system. Exp Neurol 1993; 124:381–386.
96. ThyagaRajan S, Felten SY, Felten DL. Deprenyl partially restores the age-related loss of sympathetic noradrenergic innervation in the spleens of F344 rats. Soc Neurosci Abst 1996; 22:1793.
97. Fundin BT, Bergman E, Ulfhake B. Alterations in mystacial pad innervation in the aged rat. Exp Brain Res 1997; 117:324–340.
98. Abdel-Rahan TA, Cowen, T. Neurodegeneration in sweat glands and skin of aged rats. J Auton Nerv Syst 1993; 46:55–63.
99. Santer RM. Fluorescence histochemical observations on the adrenergic innervation of the cardiovascular system in the aged rat. Brain Res Bull 1982; 9:667–672.
100. Dhall V, Cowen T, Haven AJ, Burnstock G. Perivascular noradrenergic and peptide containing nerves show different patterns of changes during development and aging in the guinea-pig. J Auton Nerv Syst 1986; 16:109–126.
101. Avakian EV, Horvath SM. Influence of aging and tyrosine hydroxylase inhibition on tissue levels during stress. J Gerontol 1982; 37:257–261.
102. Mione MC, Dhital KK, Amenta F, Burnstock G. An increase in the expression of neuropeptidergic vasodilator, but not vasoconstrictor, cerebrovascular nerves in aging rats. Brain Res 1988; 460:103–113.
103. Andrews TJ, Thrasivoulou C, Nesbit W, Cowen T. Target-specific differences in the dendritic morphology and neuropeptide content of neurons in the rat SCG during development and age. J Comp Neurol 1996; 368:33–44.
104. Kuchel GA, Poon T, Irshad K, Richard C, Julien JP, Cowen T. Decreased neurofilament gene expression is an index of selective axonal hypotrophy in ageing. NeuroReport 1996; 7:1353–1359.
105. Dering MA, Santer RM, Watson AHD. Age-related

changes in the morphology of preganglionic neurons projecting to the paracervical ganglion of nulliparous and multiparous rats. Brain Res 1998; 780:245–252.
106. Wigston DJ. Maintenance of cholinergic neurones and synapses in the ciliary ganglion of aged rats. J Physiol 1983; 344:223–231.
107. Soltanpour N, Santer RM. Preservation of the cervical vagus nerve in aged rats: morphometric and enzyme histochemical evidence. J Auton Nerv Syst 1996; 60:93–101.
108. Sturrock RR. A comparison of age-related changes in neuron number in the dorsal motor nucleus of the vagus and nucleus ambiguus of the mouse. J Anat 1990; 173:169–176.
109. Warburton AL, Santer RM. Localisation of NADPH-diaphorase and acetylcholinesterase activities and of tyrosine hydroxylase and neuropeptide Y immunoreactivity in neurons of the hypogastric ganglion of young adult and aged rats. J Auton Nerv Syst 1993; 45:155–163.
110. Santer RM, Baker DM. Enteric neuron numbers and sizes in Auerbach's plexus in the small intestine of aged rats. J Auton Nerv Syst 1988; 25:59–67.
111. Johnson RJR, Schemann M, Santer RM, Cowen T. The effects of age on the overall population and on subpopulations of myenteric neurons in the rat small intestine. J Anat 1998; 192:479–488.
112. Feher E, Penzes L. Density of substance P, vasoactive intestinal polypeptide and somatostatin-containing nerve fibers in the ageing small intestine of rats. Gerontol 1987; 33:341–348.
113. Varga F. Transit time changes with age in the gastrointestinal tract of the rat. Digestion 1976; 14:319–324.
114. Smits GJM, Lefebvre RA. Influence of aging on gastric emptying of liquids, small intestine transit and faecal output in rats. Exp. Gerontol 1996; 31:589–596.
115. Smits GJM, Lefebvre RA. Influence of age on cholinergic and inhibitory nonadrenergic noncholinergic responses in the rat ileum. Eur J Pharmacol 1996; 303:79–86.
116. Jellinger K. Neuroaxonal dystrophy: its natural history and related disorders. Prog Neuropathol 1973; 2:129–180.
117. Schmidt RE. Neuroaxonal dystrophy in aging rodent and human sympathetic autonomic ganglia: synaptic pathology as a common theme in neuropathology. Adv Pathol Lab Med 1993; 6:505–522.
118. Schmidt RE. Synaptic dysplasia in sympathetic autonomic ganglia. J Neurocytol 1996; 25:777–791.
119. Schmidt RE, Scharp DW. Axonal dystrophy in experimental diabetic autonomic neuropathy. Diabetes 1982; 31:761–770.
120. Ohara S, Beaudet LN, Schmidt RE. Transganglionic response of GAP-43 in the gracile nucleus to sciatic nerve injury in young and aged rats. Brain Res 1995; 705:325–331.
121. Cotman CW, Nieto-Sampedro M, and Harris EW, Synapse replacement in the nervous system of adult vertebrates. Physiol Rev 1981; 61:684–784.
122. Purves D, Voyvodic JT, Magrassi L, Yawo H. Nerve terminal remodeling visualized in living mice by repeated examination of the same neurons. Science 1987; 238:1122–1126.
123. Mearow KM, Kril Y, Gloster A, Diamond J. Expression of NGF receptor and gap-43 mRNA in DRG neurons during collateral sprouting and regeneration of dorsal cutaneous nerves. J Neurobiol 1994; 25:127–142.
124. Kuchel GA, Zigmond RE. Functional recovery and collateral neuronal sprouting examined in young and aged rats following a partial neural lesion. Brain Res 1991; 540:195–203.
125. Crutcher KA. Age-related decrease in sympathetic sprouting is primarily due to decreased target receptivity: implications for understanding brain aging. Neurobiol Aging 1990; 11:175–183.
126. Navarro X, Kennedy WR. Effect of age on collateral reinnervation of sweat glands in the mouse. Brain Res 1988; 463:174–181.
127. Scheff SW, Bernardo LS, Cotman DW. Decrease in adrenergic axon sprouting in the senescent rat. Science 1978; 202:775–778.
128. Gloster A, Diamond J. Sympathetic nerves in adult rats regenerate normally and restore pilomotor function during an anti-NGF treatment that prevents their collateral sprouting. J Comp Neurol 1992; 326:363–374.
129. Wu R, McKenna DG, McAffe DA. Age-related changes in the sympathetic plasticity of rat superior cervical ganglia. Brain Res 1991; 542:324–329.
130. Greif KF, Flaherty KN. Changes in expression of a synaptic vesicle antigen in aging sympathetic neurons. Neurobiol Aging 1989; 10:51–54.
131. Adler JE, Black IB. Plasticity of substance P in mature and aged sympathetic neurons in culture. Science 1984; 225:1499–1500.
132. Grinnell AD. Dynamics of nerve-muscle interaction in developing and mature neuromuscular junctions. Physiol Rev 1995; 75:789–834.
133. Balice-Gordon RJ, Lichtman JW. In vivo observations of pre-and postsynaptic changes during the transition from multiple to single innervation at developing neuromuscular junctions. J Neurosci 1993; 13:834–855.
134. Colman H, Lichtman JW. Interactions between nerve and muscle: synapse elimination at the developing neuromuscular junction. Dev Biol 1993; 156:1–10.
135. Liu Y, Fields RD, Fitzgerald S, Festoff BW, Nelson PG. Proteolytic activity, synapse elimination, and the Hebb synapse. J Neurobiol 1994; 25:325–335.
136. Liuzzi FJ. Proteolysis is a critical step in the physiological stop pathway: mechanisms involved in the blockade of axonal regeneration by mammalian astrocytes. Brain Res 1990; 512:277–283.
137. Andrews TJ. Autonomic nervous system as a model of neuronal aging: The role of target tissues and neurotrophic factors. Microsc Res Tech 1996; 35:2–19.
138. Purves D, Hadley HD, Voyvodic J. Dynamic changes in the dendritic geometry of individual neurons visualized over periods of up to three months in the superior cervical ganglion of living mice. J Neurosci 1986; 6:1051–1060.
139. Voyvodic JT. Peripheral target regulation of dendritic geometry in the rat superior cervical ganglion. J Neurosci 1989; 9:1997–2010.
140. Yawo H. Changes in the dendritic geometry of mouse superior cervical ganglion cells following postganglionic axotomy. J Neurosci 1987; 7:3703–3711.

141. Matthews RR, Nelson VH. Detachment of structurally intact nerve endings from chromatolytic neurons of rat superior cervical ganglia during the depression of synaptic transmission induced by postganglionic axotomy. J Physiol 1975; 245:91–135.
142. Andrews TJ, Cowen T. Nerve growth factor enhances the dendritic arborization of sympathetic ganglion cells undergoing atrophy in aged rats. J Neurocytol 1994; 23:234–241.
143. Gavazzi I, Andrews TJ, Thrasivoulou C, Cowen T. Influence of target tissues on their innervation in old age: a transplantation study. NeuroReport 1992; 3:717–720.
144. Gavazzi I, Cowen T. Can the neurotrophic hypothesis explain degeneration and loss of plasticity in mature and ageing autonomic nerves. J Auton Nerv Syst 1996; 58:1–10.
145. Uchida Y, Tomonaga M. Loss of nerve growth factor receptors in sympathetic ganglia from aged mice. Biochem Biophys Res Commun 1987; 146:797–801.
146. Scott SA, Liang S, Weingartner JA, Crutcher KA. Increased NGF-like activity in young but not aged rat hippocampus after septal lesions. Neurobiol. Aging 1994; 15:337–346.
147. Cowen T, Gavazzi I. Plasticity in adult and ageing sympathetic neurons. Prog Neurobiol 1998 54:249–288.
148. Cowen T, Thrasivoulou C, Shaw SA, Abdel-Rahman TA. Transplanted sweat glands from mature and aged donors determine cholinergic phenotype an altered density of host sympathetic nerves. J Auton Nerv Syst 1996; 58:153–162.
149. Thrasivoulou C, Cowen T. Regulation of rat sympathetic nerve density by target tissues and NGF in maturity and old age. Eur J Neurosci 1995; 7:381–387.
150. Gavazzi I. Collateral sprouting and responsiveness to nerve growth factor of ageing neurons. Neurosci Lett 1995; 189:47–50.
151. Gavazzi I, Cowen T. NGF can induce a 'young' pattern of innervation in transplanted old cerebral blood vessels. J Comp Neurol 1993; 334:489–496.
152. Gavazzi I, Cowen T, Crutcher KA. Lack of correlation between NGF levels and altered nerve fibre density in peripheral tissues of aging rats. Soc Neurosci Abst 1994; 20:1710.
153. Isaacson LG, Crutcher KA. Uninjured aged sympathetic neurons sprout in response to exogenous NGF in vivo Neurobiol Aging 1998; 19:333–339.
154. Jenner CS, Gavazzi I, Song GX, Cowen T. Loss of responsiveness of ageing sympathetic neurons in vitro to laminin and NGF. Eur J Neurosci (Suppl.) 1994; 7:185.
155. Gavazzi I, Cowen T. Axonal regeneration from transplanted sympathetic ganglia is not impaired by age. Exp Neurol 1993; 122:57–64.
156. Gavazzi I, Canavan REM, Cowen T. Influence of age and anti-NGF treatment on the sympathetic and sensory innervation of the rat iris. Neuroscience 1996; 73:1069–1079.
157. Kuchel GA, Rowe W, Meaney MJ, Richard C. Neurotrophin receptor and tyrosine hydroxylase gene expression in aged sympathetic neurons. Neurobiol Aging 1997; 18:67–79.
158. Milner TA, Loy R. Interaction of age and sex in sympathetic axon ingrowth into the hippocampus following septal afferent damage. Anat Embryol 1980; 161:159–168.
159. Recio-Pinto E, Rechler MM, Ishii DN. Effects of insulin, insulin-like growth factor-II, and nerve growth factor in neurite formation and survival in cultured sympathetic and sensory neurons. J Neurosci 1986; 6:1211–1219.
160. Ishii DN, Glazner GW, Whalen LR. Regulation of peripheral nerve regeneration by insulin-like growth factors. Ann N Y Acad Sci 1993; 692:172–182.
161. Ishii DN, Glazner GW, Pu SF. Role of insulin-like growth factors in peripheral nerve regeneration. Pharmacol Ther 1994; 62:125–144.
162. Cheng H-L, Randolph A, Yee D, Delafontaine P, Tennekoon G, Feldman EL. Characterization of insulin-like growth factor-I and its receptor and binding proteins in transected nerves and cultured Schwann cells. J Neurochem 1996; 66:525–536.
163. Hansson H-A. Insulin-like growth factors and nerve regeneration. Ann N Y Acad Sci 1993; 692:161–171.
164. D'Costa AP, Lenham JE, Ingram RL, Sonntag WE. Comparison of protein synthesis in brain and peripheral tissue during aging. Relationship to insulin-like growth factor-1 and type 1 IGF receptors. Ann N Y Acad Sci 1993; 692:253–255.
165. Nja A, Purves D. The effects of nerve growth factor and its antiserum on synapses in the superior cervical ganglion of the guinea-pig. J Physiol 1978; 227:53–75.
166. Ruit KG, Osborne PA, Schmidt RE, Johnson EM, Snider WD. Nerve growth factor regulates sympathetic ganglion cell morphology and survival in the adult mouse. J Neurosci 1990; 10:2412–2419.
167. Komiya Y. Slowing with age of the rate of slow axonal flow in bifurcating axons of rat dorsal root ganglion cells. Brain Res 1980; 183:477–480.
168. McQuarrie IG, Brady ST, Lasek RJ. Retardation in the slow axonal transport of cytoskeletal elements during maturation and aging. Neurobiol Aging 1989; 10:359–365.
169. Roots BI. Neurofilament accumulation induced in synapses by leupeptin. Science 1983; 221:971–972.
170. Vlassara H, Bucala R, Striker L. Pathogenic effects of advanced glycosylation: biochemical, biologic, and clinical implications for diabetes and aging. Lab Invest 1994; 70:138–151.
171. Yagihashi S, Kamijo M, Taniguchi N, Satoh K. Increased glycation of axonal cytoskeleton and preventive effect of aminoguanidine on development of experimental diabetic neuropathy. Diabetes 1991; 40 (Suppl. 1):302A.
172. Carbonetto S, Lindenbaum M. The basement membrane at the neuromuscular junction: a synaptic mediatrix. Curr Opin Neurobiol 1995; 5:596–605.
173. Doherty P, Fazeli MS, Walsh FS. The neural cell adhesion molecule and synaptic plasticity. J Neurobiol 1995; 26:437–446.
174. Cowen T, Jenner C, Xiao Song G, Santoso AW, Gavazzi I. Responses of mature and aged sympathetic neurons to laminin and NGF: an in vitro study. Neurochem Res 1997; 22:1003–1011.
175. Gavazzi I, Boyle KS, Edgar D, Cowen T. Reduced laminin immunoreactivity in the blood vessel wall of ageing rats correlates with reduced innervation in vivo and following transplantation. Cell Tissue Res 1995; 281:23–32.

176. Gavazzi I, Boyle KS, Cowen T. Extracellular matrix molecules influence innervation density in rat cerebral blood vessels. Brain Res 1996; 734:167–174.
177. Lieth E, Cardass CA, Fallon JR. Muscle-derived agrin in cultured myotubes: expression in the basal lamina and at induced acetylcholine receptor clusters. Develop Biol 1992; 149:41–54.
178. Noakes PG, Cautam M, Mudd J, Sanes JR, Merlie JP. Aberrant differentiation of neuromuscular junctions in mice lacking S-laminin/laminin beta 2. Nature 1995; 374:258–262.
179. Porter BE, Weis J, Sanes JR. A motoneuron-selective stop signal on the synaptic protein S-laminin. Neuron 1995; 14:549–559.
180. Viani P, Cervato G, Fiorilli A, Cestaro B. Age-related differences in synaptosomal peroxidative damage and membrane properties. J Neurochem 1991; 56:253–258.
181. Schmidt RE, Coleman BD, Nelson JS. Differential effect of chronic vitamin E deficiency on the development of neuroaxonal dystrophy in rat gracile/cuneate nuclei and prevertebral sympathetic ganglia. Neurosci Lett 1991; 123:102–106.
182. Tsai H, Pottorf WJ, Buchholz JN, Duckles SP. Adrenergic nerve smooth endoplasmic reticulum calcium buffering declines with age. Neurobiol Aging 1998; 19:89–96.
183. Pottorf WJ, Tsai H, Duckles SP, Buchholz J. Impact of age on smooth endoplasmic reticulum calcium buffering mechanisms in rat adrenergic nerves. Soc Neurosci Abst 1997; 23:1161.

22. Pathology of Skeletal Muscle in Aging

CYNTHIA HAWKINS AND PATRICK SHANNON

The skeletal musculature forms a very large, distributed, metabolically and structurally dynamic organ system. As such it is prone to diseases specific to the musculature, the effects of systemic illness, the demands of the nervous system, and the inherent instability of biological tissues with age. This anatomical, structural, and functional complexity endows skeletal muscle with some unique susceptibilities in the aging individual.

In clinical muscle pathology, most biopsies are performed because of clinically suspected muscle disease. Hence, the age-related changes of atrophy, degeneration, and loss of functional cellular components are rarely seen in isolation. The rigorous assessment of age-related changes is further hampered by technical considerations: the ultrastructure of skeletal muscle rapidly degenerates postmortem, so prospective collection of tissue for assessment of histochemical and ultrastructural features is difficult. Also, either myopathic or systemic disorders can lead to inactivity, so separation of the primary effects of aging from the results of disuse can be challenging to discern. The changes in muscle histopathology may therefore be best categorized into those apparently a result of aging, those related to primarily myopathic processes whose prevalence increases with age, and those secondary to age-related systemic or neurologic disease.

NORMAL HISTOLOGY

The following brief introduction is meant for those who are more familiar with the central nervous system. Skeletal muscle is composed of roughly cylindrical myocytes (or myofibers) bound together in polygonal fascicles by fine interstitial connective tissue. The fascicles are surrounded in turn by the denser perifascicular connective tissues in which travel the peripheral nerves and large vessels. The capillary bed ramifies so that in any given cross section, each myocyte is adjacent to 1–3 capillaries.

Each muscle fiber (myocyte) is surrounded by a basal lamina, underneath which lies the cell membrane (the sarcolemma) as well as the skeletal muscle regenerative cells (the myoblasts). The myocytes are syncytia; in normal muscle, over 90% of their nuclei are located at the periphery of the myofiber, while the contractile apparatus and much of the metabolic machinery fill the cylindrical sarcoplasm. The contractile apparatus is composed of sarcomeres, which display an orderly arrangement of Z-discs and associated thick and thin filaments (Fig. 22–1). The sacomeres are arranged in parallel to the long axis of the fiber, and between them are glycogen particles, mitochondria, and lipid droplets. Concentrations of these latter components, as well as of synthetic apparatus and lysosomes, are usually found in the perinuclear areas. Concentrations of mitochondria are also present in the subsarcolemmal region adjacent to capillaries and motor end plates.

Following discharge of synaptic vesicles at the motor end-plate, the postsynaptic potential travels down a system of fine tubules that originate at the cell membrane and branch around each sarcomere (the T-tubules). This postsynaptic potential triggers the release

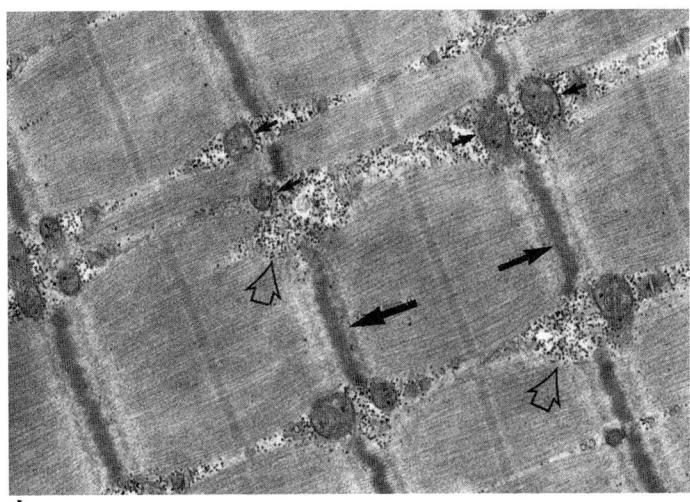
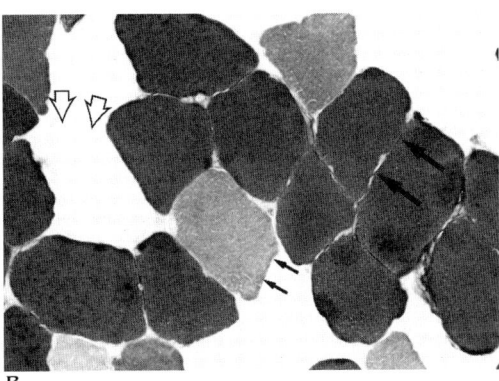

Figure 22–1. *A.* Ultrastructural view of representative human skeletal muscle sarcomeres arranged in parallel with overlapping thick and thin filaments at right angles to the electron-dense Z-bands (large arrows). Normal amounts of glycogen (open arrows) and mitochondria (small arrows) are arranged between the sarcomeres (osmium tetroxide and lead citrate). *B.* Myosin ATPase-stained section of skeletal muscle at pH 4.6, showing type I fibers (dark fibers), Type IIA fibers as unstained (open arrow) and type IIB fibers with intermediate reactivity (small arrows).

of calcium from intracellular stores within the sarcoplasmic reticulum, a system of membrane-bound cisternae and interconnecting tubules, which are arranged in pairs and course in parallel with the T-tubules (see below). Calcium release triggers the ATP-dependant conformational and structural changes in the contractile filaments to achieve contraction.

In the adult human, myofibers can be divided on the basis of their structural and functional attributes into three fiber types. The "slow twitch," or type I fibers have a myosin-associated ATPase active at low pH, are poor in glycogen, contain abundant lipid and mitochondria, and seem specialized for relatively sustained activity. By contrast, the type II fibers have a myosin-dependant ATPase that is active at high pH, are rich in glycogen and poor in mitochondria, and seem more appropriate for less sustained activity. Type II muscle fibers are further subdivided into type IIA and type IIB. Each myofiber is innervated by a single motor neuron, which determines its fiber type. Type I, IIA, and IIB fibers are distributed apparently at random with respect to each other within each fascicle. In cryostat sections of fresh–frozen biopsy tissue, the proportion and distribution of the muscle fiber types and of their mitochondrial and other metabolic enzymes can be determined using histochemical techniques.

PHYSIOLOGICAL CHANGES WITH AGING

With aging, in both humans and animals there is a decline in muscle function, including a decrease in both strength[1-6] and speed of muscle movement.[3,7–9] This loss of muscle function combined with a decline in muscle mass has been labeled "sarcopenia." It is generally agreed that there is a decline in muscle function with age, however, there is some argument as to the time course. Some studies show the decline to commence around age 30[1,2] while others demonstrate the decline beginning in the sixth decade.[3–5]

A major contributor to the loss of muscle strength with age is a decrease in muscle mass (see below). However, this decrease in mass should not affect the speed of muscle movement. In addition, some studies in both animals[10,11] and humans[12–14] have shown an age-related reduction in specific force (force/unit cross-sectional area [CSA]). This suggests that a number of other factors could also play a role, including a decrease in the number of motor neurons/motor units, resulting in denervation atrophy, excitation/contraction uncoupling, or a loss of sarcoplasmic reticulum proteins. The latter factors would more readily explain the decrease in speed of muscle movement. This section will review evidence for the various possible contributors to a decline in muscle function.

There is a general consensus that a decrease in muscle mass parallels the decline in strength, but there is some debate as to when this decline begins and the rate at which it occurs (see Table 22–1). This loss of mass may be accompanied by a decrease in both the number and size of muscle fibers. Human data indicate a loss of muscle fibers.[15,16] Lexell et al.[17] showed a loss of muscle fibers beginning at age 25 and reaching a 39% loss by age 80. Similarly, Sato et al.[18] showed a decrease beginning at age 60 and reaching a 25% reduction by age 70. Conversely, some rodent data suggest there is no loss of muscle fibers.[19–21] The reason for this discrepancy is unclear, but it may have to do with the type of muscle examined. Human studies used complex pennate muscles whereas the rodent studies used simple fusiform hind limb muscles. The decrease in human myofiber mass may be accompanied by an increase in muscle collagen.[22]

The different muscle fiber types may have different susceptabilities to attrition with aging. Several studies have shown that type II fibers are lost more readily than type I fibers.[23–28] This may be caused by denervation followed by limited reinnervation.[27] However, others have shown no change in type I–to–type II ratio with age.[29,30] With the alterations in fiber type proportion there is a corresponding shift in myosin heavy-chain expression. In very old individuals, roughly 20% of fibers expressed type I myosin heavy chain, 27% type IIa, and 29% aberrantly coexpressed types I and IIa and over 50% of all fibers expressed two or more of types I, IIa, or IIx.[31] This finding implies that the classification of fiber type may not be straightforward in aged individuals, which may explain some of the discrepancies between studies.

In contrast to the seeming controversy about changes in muscle fiber number, virtually all studies agree that there is a reduction in muscle fiber CSA with age. Most show that type II fibers bear the brunt of the age-related reduction in CSA,[17,25,26,32–34] with little change in type I fibers.[17,26,32,35] The reported reductions in type II fibers range from 13% to 30%. This reduction is seen pedominantly in type IIB fibers. A possible explanation for the predominant loss of type II fibers is the order of recruitment of motor units.[36] Type I fibers are recruited first, meaning they are in relatively regular use even in old age, whereas type II fibers, particularly type IIB, are rarely recruited and therefore subject to disuse atrophy. Consistent with this theory is a loss of motor neurons with age, particularly after age 60,[7,37–40] with preferential loss of large motor neurons.[37,40] In general, the larg-

Table 22–1. Decline in Muscle Mass with Age

Study	Start of Decline (Years)	Rate of Decline/decade (%)
Lexell et al., 1986[30]	24–50	10
	50–80	30
Danneskiold-Samsoe et al., 1984[158]	50–70	15
	70–80	30
Grimby and Saltin, 1983[159]	4th decade	8
Nair, 1995[160]	30–60	3–5
	>70	30

est motor neurons innervate type II fibers, particularly type IIB. Denervation removes the trophic influence on the fibers and leads to atrophy. In addition, in young animals and humans, when motor neurons are lost, the remaining motor neurons will sprout and reinnervate the denervated fibers. In aged animals this ability is limited.[41,42] Loss of the largest motor neurons, combined with a decreased ability to reinnervate, may help explain the preferential decrease in type II fiber size and number.

A loss of motor neurons is a likely cause of loss of fiber size and number, but for a decrease in CSA to occur there should be a decrease in contractile proteins. There is evidence to show inefficient protein synthesis with age. Elderly people have decreased synthesis rates of both the myofibrillar protein fraction,[43] myosin heavy-chain,[44] and total muscle proteins.[45]

Other muscle proteins are necessary to generate contractile force. For the muscle cell to contract, there must be an increase in the cytoplasmic concentration of calcium ions, which must then be decreased again in order for the muscle cell to relax. The major intracellular participant in this calcium flux is a closed membrane system called the "sarcoplasmic reticulum," which stores calcium, releasing it into the cytoplasm to allow muscle contraction via calcium channels (ryanodine receptors) and collecting it again to allow relaxation via energy-requiring calcium pumps. The signal to initiate this process begins when a motor neuron depolarizes, resulting in the propogation of an action potential down its axon to the neuromuscular junction. Here, acetylcholine, which is stored in vesicles at the axon terminus, is released in response to an influx of calcium through axonal membrane calcium channels that open in response to the arriving action potential. Acetylcholine then traverses the neuromuscular junction, interacting with receptors on the muscle side and opening a set of cation channels. This results in depolarization of the sarcolemmal membrane enclosing the muscle cell. Excitation of this surface membrane reaches the depths of the cell through the transverse tubule system, finally triggering calcium release from the sarcoplasmic reticulum (SR). For the muscle to relax, calcium must be removed, and the primary responsibility for removal lies with the SR Ca^{2+} pump. Problems at any of these steps can affect the function of the muscle.

If synaptic transmission at the neuromuscular junction is affected, it will affect the extent to which individual muscle fibers are recruited for normal function. Animal studies show fragmentation in the distribution of acetylcholine receptors,[46] while human studies show a decrease in acetylcholinesterase staining.[47] In rat, there is a progressive loss of synaptic contact[48] and in mice there is a 45% reduction in neuromuscular junctions that could be considered normal.[49] These results suggest a deterioration in the neuromuscular junction with age.

Coupling of sarcolemmal membrane exitation to muscle contraction involves an interaction between the sarcolemmal Ca^{2+} channel and the sarcoplasmic reticulum Ca^{2+} channel (ryanodine receptor). The dihydropyridine receptor is decreased in number in aged human muscle fibers with concomitant uncoupling of sarcolemmal excitation from SR Ca^{2+} release.[50] In addition, the caffeine threshold for calcium release from ryanodine receptors is decreased in aged rat extensor digitorum longus.[51] Studies on sarcoplasmic reticulum itself in aged animals have shown no decrease in SR protein synthesis with age.[44,52] However, calcium pump function shows a 50% decline with aging in type I fibers,[52] although some of the decline in Ca^{2+} transport is reversible with exercise.[53] Thus, in addition to a decrease in contractile protein, the ability of the muscle to both initiate and conclude a contraction is impaired with age.

Another component of muscle function, endurance, declines with age. Maximal oxygen consumption decreases by about 10% per decade.[54,55] Enzymes such as myosin ATPase, myokinase, phosphofructokinase, hexokinase, and phosphorylase, as well as resting high-energy phosphate concentration, all markers of anaerobic energy production, show little change with aging.[32,34,35,56,57] However, markers of aerobic energy production are about 25% lower in aged humans[33,37] and there is a decline in mitochondrial enzymes in human muscle with age.[58-61] This reduction in aerobic pathways decreases the production of ATP and thus the ability to resist fatigue.

There is an increase in interstitial fibrous

connective tissue with age in animals.[62–64] There are also age-related changes in muscle vasculature including reduced blood supply,[65] decreased capillary density,[33] and changes in vascular pathology.[66] The decrease in vascularity may be a factor in the decreased ability of muscle in the aged to regenerate.

Thus, muscle function is disrupted at many levels with aging. The neuromuscular junction, excitation–contraction coupling, contractile proteins, sarcoplasmic reticulum, mitochondria, and the muscular vascular supply are all affected. At the histologic level these changes lead to a number of abnormal findings in aged muscle. A major component is neurogenic atrophy, which correlates with the decrease in motor units and degeneration of neuromuscular junctions discussed above. This is manifested by type II atrophy, groups of angular atrophic fibers, target or targetoid fibers, and fiber type grouping (Fig. 22–2).[26,67–69] A wide variety of secondary changes can accompany neurogenic atrophy, especially in the indolent and chronic neuropathies that commonly accompany aging (e.g., diabetic neuropathy). These include target fibers, ring fibers, cytochrome C oxidase (Cox)–negative ragged red fibers, and rare necrotic fibers (Fig. 21–2). Target fibers are perhaps the most diagnostically important; their presence is usually thought to indicate a lesion in the peripheral nerve. Peripheral neuropathy is common in the aged, and neurogenic change can coexist with primary myopathic processes, making for both diagnostic confusion and difficulties in studying primary age-related phenomena. Other cytoarchitectural changes that tend to occur with increased frequency after the age of 70 in the absece of definable disease include cytoplasmic bodies, ring fibers, rare necrotic fibers, and increased central nuclei (Fig. 22–3A).[67,70]

The mitochondria of skeletal muscle appear uniquely susceptible to alterations with aging[71] and both ragged red and Cox-negative fibers accumulate in apparently normal aging[42,72–74] (Fig. 21–3B–E). Both the ragged red and COX-negative fibers correlate with increased mitochondrial DNA deletions with age.[75,76] In fact, individual COX-negative fibers from aged individuals have been shown to have very high levels of mutant mitochondrial DNA.[77] This is also consistent with the decline in aerobic respiration described above. The alterations in the mitochodrial genome comprise a variety of genomic deletions and point mutations, and accumulate in frequency with age, but without obvious specific mutations.[78,79] Interestingly, respiratory chain activity is not decreased in elderly athletes, suggesting that exercise has some protective effect.[80,81]

The underlying pathogenesis of most of the lesions described above is not well understood, but has often been hypothesized to be due to oxidative stress.[82] Thus lipid peroxidation, protein carbonylation, and purine hy-

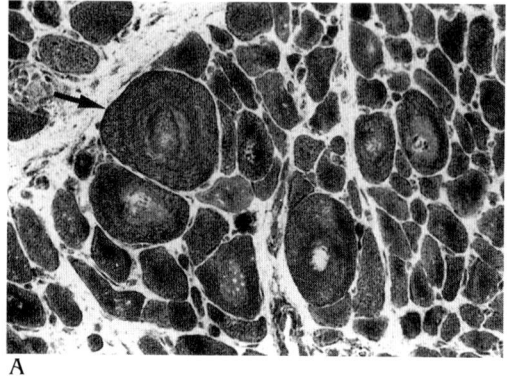

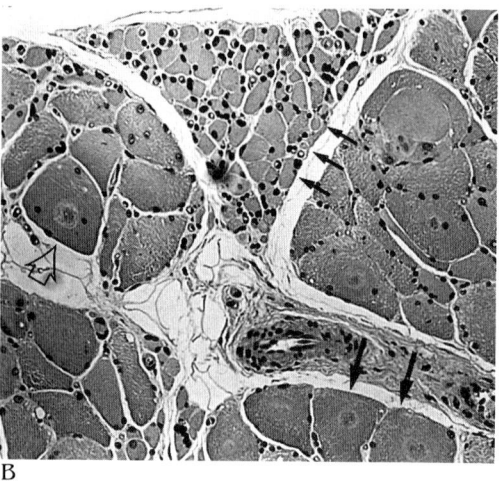

Figure 22–2. Chronic neurogenic change. *A.* Peripheral neuropathy (?CIDP) in an 81-year-old woman. Large arrow indicates one of numerous target fibers (Cryostat section, NADH-TR). *B.* Chronic neurogenic change and peripheral neuropathy, with groups of atrophic fibers (small arrows) and hypertrophic fibers (large arrows), many of which contain target figures (open arrows). Hematoxylin and eosin.

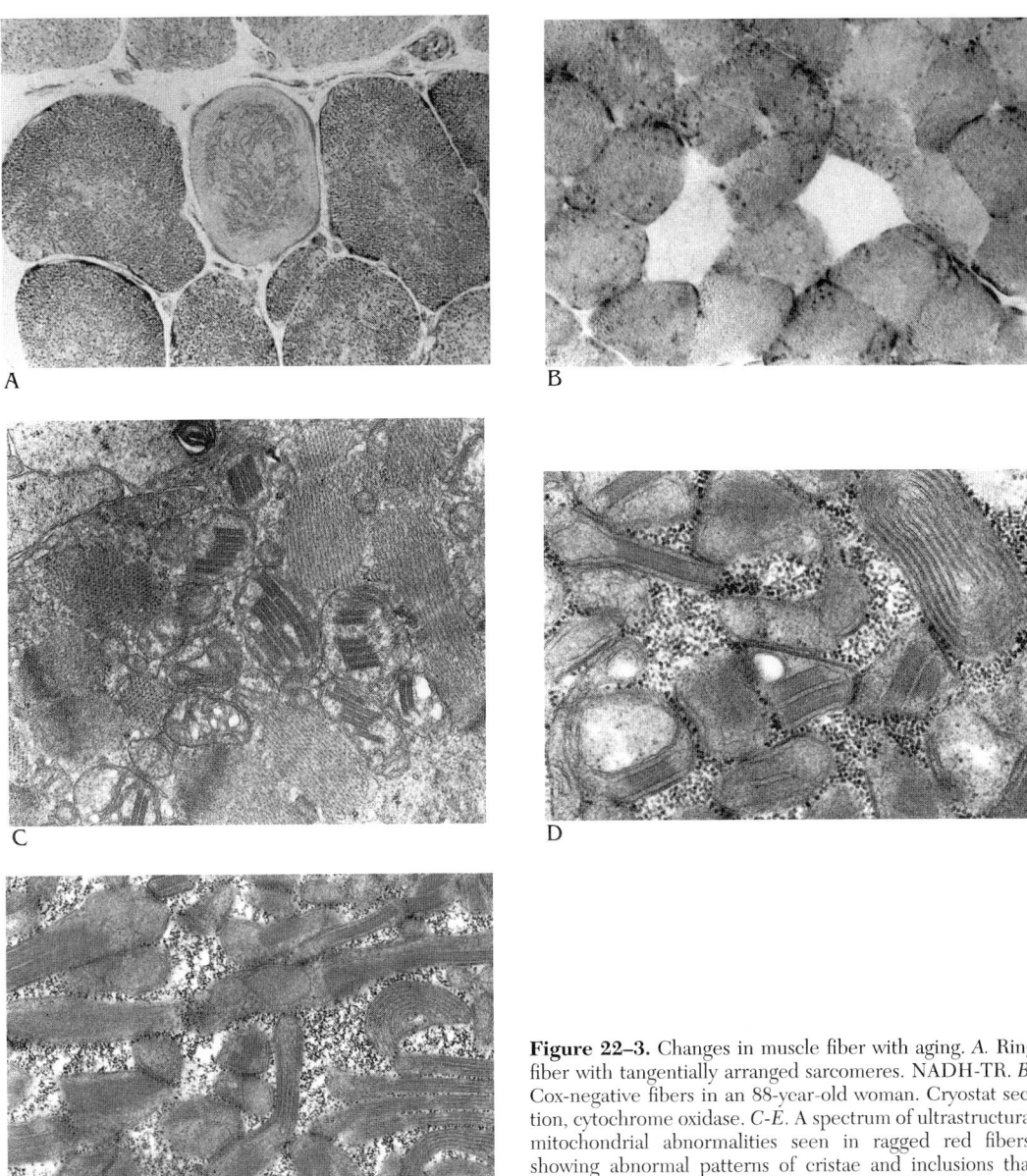

Figure 22–3. Changes in muscle fiber with aging. *A.* Ring fiber with tangentially arranged sarcomeres. NADH-TR. *B.* Cox-negative fibers in an 88-year-old woman. Cryostat section, cytochrome oxidase. *C-E.* A spectrum of ultrastructural mitochondrial abnormalities seen in ragged red fibers, showing abnormal patterns of cristae and inclusions that have been called "paracrystalline arrays" and likened to box cars, tram tracks, and parking lots. Lead citrate and osmium tetroxide.

droxylation increase with age.[83] Telomere shortening, a feature of aging in many tissues, is apparently minimal in the human muscle satellite cells from which skeletal muscle regenerates.[84] As repeatedly noted above, disuse seems to contribute to many of the age-related changes.

INFLAMMATORY MYOPATHIES

Of the primary inflammatory myopathies, dermatomyositis, polymyositis, and inclusion body myositis (IBM) are most common in aged individuals. The clinical and pathological features have been well reviewed.[85] Dermatomyositis, which may manifest as a proximal myopathy, with or without the classic skin rash, is manifest histologically by a predominantly preimysial and endomysial inflammatory infiltrate in which B cells are prominent, although in some cases, cellular inflammation is almost absent. Although myonecrosis may be common, the striking histological feature is the pattern of perifascicular atrophy accompanied by an early loss of endomysial capillaries (Fig. 22–4). Both immunoglobulin and complement can be detected on capillary endothelium. Ultrastructurally, endothelial tubuloreticular inclusions are characteristically present, although they are not pathognomonic.[86,87] Dermatomyositis is associated in some cases with the presence of anti-Mi-2 antibodies.[88] This disease has been interpreted as a primary humoral attack on the endothelium.

Polymyositis is not accompanied by an exanthem, and in contrast to dermatomyositis shows a predominantly endomysial inflammatory infiltrate in which the lymphocytes are almost wholly T cells, and cytotoxic $CD8^+$ cells predominate.[89,90] One of the histologic hallmarks is the presence of T lymphocytes invading non-necrotic myofibers (Fig. 22–5) and the widespread myocyte expression of MHC class II antigens. Ragged red fibers may be numerous. Tubuloreticular inclusions are not a feature of this myopathy, and loss of capillary density is only commensurate with loss of myofibers. A variety of auto-antibodies can be detected, but probably the most specific is the presence of anti-Jo-1 antibody.[91]

While both of these myopathies are common in younger individuals, onset of dermatomyositis in an individual over the age of 60 years warrants an investigation for systemic malignancy.[92,93] By contrast, paraneoplastic dermatomyositis is rare in childhood. The association between polymyositis and malignancy is still controversial.[94–96] A variety of other inflammatory myopathies also occur in the aged, including those associated with mixed connective tissue disease, rheumatoid arthritis, and Sjogren's syndrome; these usually resemble dermatomyositis.[97]

Inclusion body myositis is probably the most common primary myopathy among the aged. The clinical and histopathological features have been authoritatively reviewed in recent years.[98–100] It presents usually in late mid-

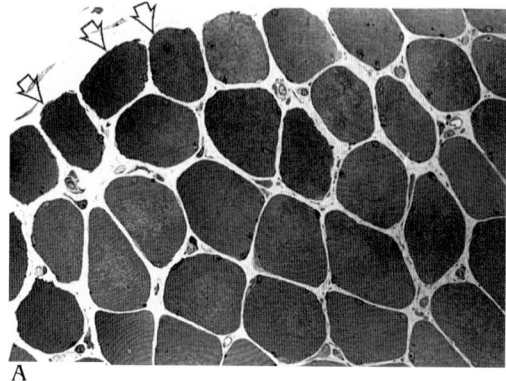
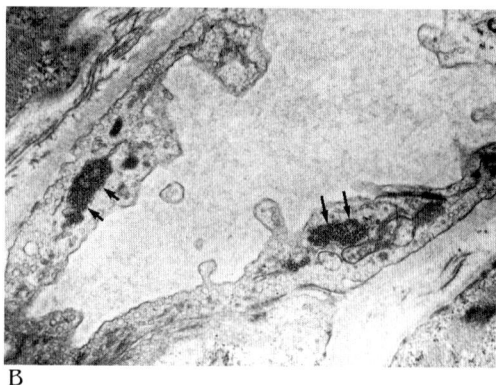

Figure 22–4. Section of muscle from 60-year-old woman with florid skin changes of dermatomyositis, including nail bed telangiectasias, Grotton's papules, and fleeting heliotrope rash. A. Inflammation is difficult to find, but the fibers near the edge of the fascicle (open arrows) are smaller than those in the center and show a paucity of surrounding capillaries. Toluidine blue on plastic embedded section. B. Endothelial tubuloreticular inclusions were numerous (arrows). Lead citrate and osmium tetroxide.

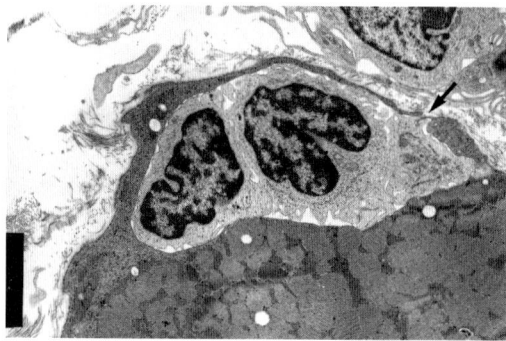

Figure 22–5. Invasion of a non-necrotic fiber by lymphocytes that have penetrated the basal lamina (arrow).

dle age or later as a steroid resistant myopathy, characteristically involving both proximal and distal muscles with particular involvement of the forearm extensors and of the quadriceps. Histologically, it shows some overlap with polymyositis, in that there is a primarily endomysial mononuclear infiltrate that contains predominantly T cells and in which B cells are usually absent. CD8+ T cells are often seen invading non-necrotic fibers. Linkage to HLA DR3 has been noted[101] (Fig. 22–6).

Histological features of chronicity are the rule, with small group atrophy and hypertrophy. As with polymyositis, ragged red fibers are not uncommon and display a wide variety of alterations in mitochondrial DNA, that are similar to those in normal aging.[102] A peripheral neuropathy may accompany IBM in the presence of the ragged red fibers.[103]

The characteristic features of IBM are the rimmed vacuoles and the intranuclear or intracytoplasmic inclusion bodies (Fig. 22–6). The rimmed vacuoles are typically located within angulated atrophic fibers and often contain amyloid, as manifest by fine congophilia under crossed polarizing filters or under flouresence microscopy. On ultrastructural examination, they correspond to membrane-bound oragnelles that are filled with myelinoid debris and are probably lysosomal. These vacuoles are often found in the same fibers as the inclusion bodies.

The inclusion bodies of IBM comprise two types. The coarse filamentous aggregates within the myonucleii are composed of tubulofilaments (Fig. 22–7). Similar aggregates of tubulofilaments are often found in the cytoplasm, are not bound by membranes, and are often surrounded by lysosomal structures. Following snap freezing, prolonged thaw, and subsequent fixation in glutaraldehyde, these filaments have a striking ultrastructural simi-

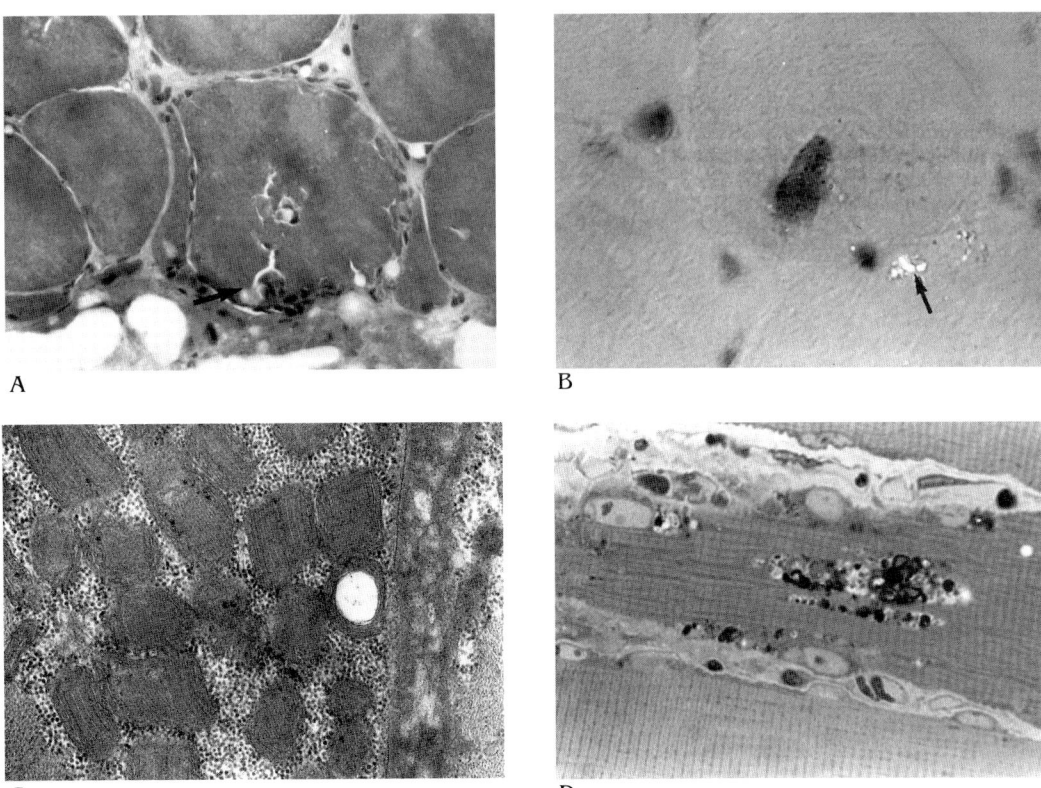

Figure 22–6. A. Inclusion body myositis. *A.* Invasion of myofiber by T lymphocytes. Modified Gomori trichrome. *B.* Birefringent amyloid inclusions (arrow). Congo red with crossed polarizing filters. *C.* Mitochondrial inclusions from a ragged red fiber. Lead citrate and osmium tetroxide. *D.* Accumulation of lysosomal debris and myelinoid figures in a rimmed vacuole. Toluidine blue on plastic embedded tissue.

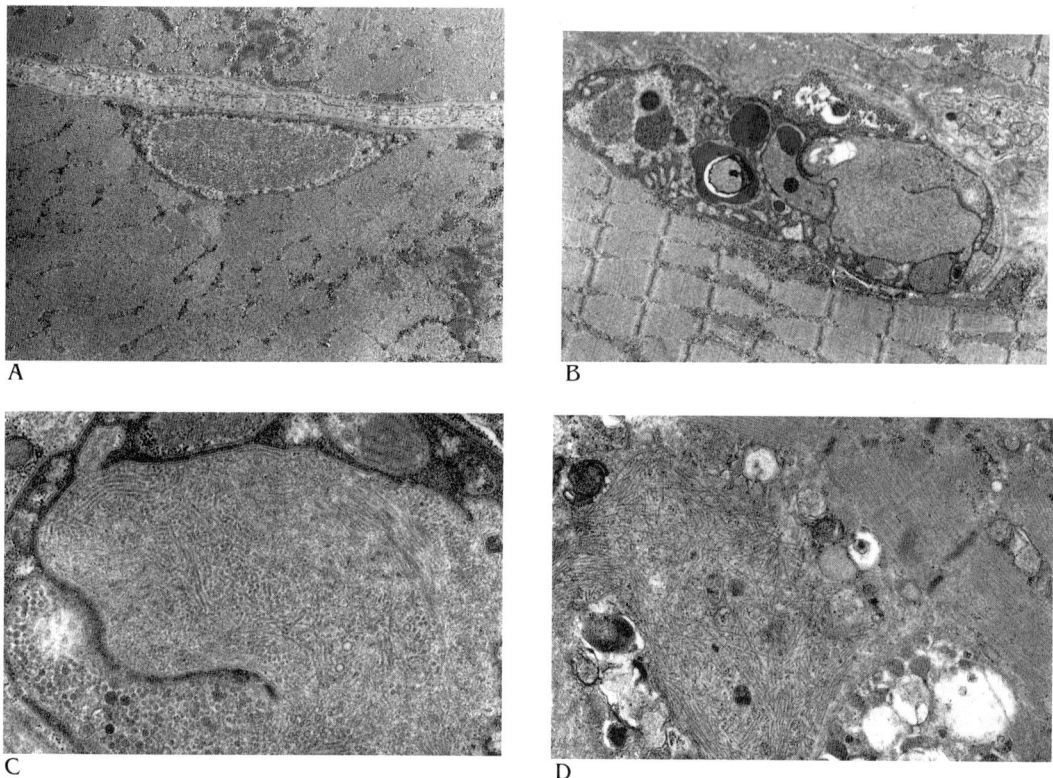

Figure 22–7. A. Nuclear accumulations of coarse filaments in inclusion body myositis (IBM). Some nuclei in IBM display aberrant morphology. (B) and prominent accumulation of hollow filaments (C) D. Cytoplasmic accumulation of coarse tubulofilaments (B–D are from the same case). Osmium tetroxide and lead citrate.

larity to the paired helical filaments (PHFs) of Alzheimer's disease (AD).[104] The second type of inclusion is a non–membrane-bound aggregate of randomly arranged fine filaments 6–10 nm in diameter. Askansas and co-workers have described immunoreactivity for tau, presenilins 1 and 2 (PS-1 PS-2), apolipoprotein E, (apo E) prion protein, and ubiquitin to the coarse tubulofilaments using a variety of techniques. α-Antichymotrypsin and prion protein have been localized to the rimmed vacuoles. The rimmed vacuoles and congophilic inclusions have also been found to show reactivity for β-amyloid.[104]

The origin of the rimmed vacuoles and tubulofilaments is not yet firmly established. Some authors, noting the perinuclear location of many of the vacuoles as well as the intranuclear location of the inclusions, have speculated that they arise from a peculiar pattern of myonuclear degeneration.[100] Ubiquitination of myonucleii is common in IBM and a protein binding single-stranded DNA has been isolated from muscle with IBM. The myonuclei can assume unusual configurations, but in our experience, actual apoptotic bodies are rare. The presence of intense reactivity for superoxide dismutase in the rimmed vacuoles has suggested that the disease may arise as a result of prolonged oxidative stress[104] perhaps as a result of chronic inflammation.

The morphology of the coarse filaments and their immunophenotype, with reactivity for tau, PS-1 and PS-2, and other epitopes have led to the suggestion that the myodegenerative process in IBM tightly parallels the neurodegenerative process in AD. In support of this theory is the finding that overexpression of β-amyloid precursor protein (β-APP) by myoblasts in culture produces a vacuolar myopathy with cytoplasmic aggregates of β-amyloid, and curiously also provokes mitochondrial paracrystalline inclusions and tubulofilament production.[104] Chronic denervation can also lead to a histological picture mimicking IBM but lacking inflammation.[105] This finding, as well as the observation that prion protein, ubiquitin, and APP normally are functional near the neuromuscular junction, points to a suggestion that the vacuolated fibers are inappropriately "junctionalized" possibly as a result of oxidative stress.[104] Interestingly, homozygosity of the prion protein for methionine at codon 129 may predispose to the development of IBM.[106]

The parallels with AD are not at all points precise. The over-representation of the apo E-4 allele in AD is not clearly present in IBM. While the tubulofilaments of IBM may resemble the PHFs of AD, their fine structure is often considerably more pleomorphic. There may be more than one type of coarse filament in IBM.[100] Further work on their protein chemistry and fine structure is needed to determine the precise degree of similarity. Along these lines, the relationship between the tubulofilaments of IBM and the tau-reactive curly fibers recently identified in muscle tissue from Alzheimer's patients has yet to be defined.[107] No increase in muscle β-APP mRNA has been detected in healthy aged subjects.[108] Finally, the prevalence of IBM in Down syndrome and familial AD needs to be determined before the proteins localized to the lesions can be accepted as fundamentally pathogenic.

The presence of apparently cytotoxic T cells actively destroying myocytes, the limited repertoire of T-cells receptor rearrangements found in the inflamed muscle, and the linkage of sporadic IBM to specific HLA haplotypes suggest that inflammation is fundamental to the disease. In one recent study, a familial variety showed a strong association with the HLA DR3 allele.[109] In this light, it should be noted that there are earlier-onset familial myopathies that mimic IBM in most ways but lack inflammation.[110] The molecular pathogenesis of these conditions is as yet obscure despite recent genetic advances. A subset of patients with a pathological diagnosis of polymyositis is refractory to steroid therapy and proves, on repeat biopsy, to have inclusion body myositis. This clinical scenario is likely a result of spatial and temporal heterogeneity and would seem to argue against the suggestion that the abnormal antigen accumulation is somehow prompting an immune response. The genesis of the structural abnormalities is likely multifactorial, with genetic, immune, and myodegenerative processes all taking part.

SYSTEMIC DISEASE AND ITS EFFECTS ON MUSCLE

The systemic diseases that affect the body with aging also affect muscle. Some of this effect is indirect and results from general debilitation and inactivity, as in congestive heart failure (CHF). In CHF the fiber cross-sectional area decreases, which is corrected by training.[111] There is also a decrease in muscle exercise capacity.[112] Similar findings apply to patients with symptomatic coronary artery atherosclerosis.[113] In addition to these findings, in CHF there is also a decrease in endomysial capillary density which is accompanied by a shift in the myosin heavy chain (MHC) composition, with an occasionally dramatic decrease in MHC I[114,115] and decreased oxidative enzyme activity.[116] Some authors have implicated a myodegenerative process in CHF with evidence of myocyte nuclear DNA injury and decreased myocyte bcl-2 expression.[117] Whether these latter changes are a response of the muscle to CHF per se or whether they partially reflect inactivity or other systemic diseases in the same population is not clear. Similarly, in chronic obstructive pulmonary disease (COPD), there is a shift in MHC composition, with a relative decrease in MHC I independent of exercise capacity,[118] although the decrease in muscle endurance in COPD seems to be largely a function of inactivity.[119]

Type II (non–insulin-dependant) diabetes is common in the elderly, and the prevalence rises with age. The changes in skeletal muscle physiology in diabetes are the subject of extensive study and review. We will concentrate on definable structural alterations in human tissue. Muscle weakness in diabetic patients is common and may be associated with mononeuropathy, polyneuropathy, amyotrophy, or involvement of the central nervous system. At the light microscopic level, histologic changes in poorly controlled diabetes mellitus are nonspecific.[120] Findings include edema, atrophy, hypernucleosis, cellular infiltration, and a decrease in periodic acid-Schiff (PAS) positivity.[121] Untrastructurally, separation of myofibrils, irregularity of Z-lines, swelling of mitochondria, dilation of sarcoplasmic reticulum, and lysosome formation can be seen.[120] Glycogen stores may or may not be depleted.[120,121] Interstitial capillaries show marked thickening of the basement membrane[120,121] and an increase in capillary density that precedes overt diabetes,[122] suggesting that muscle changes in diabetes may be secondary to capillary damage. These changes in capillary basement membrane thickness may be largely reversible with exercise training.[123] Diabetics are also predisposed to acquiring mutations of the mitochondrial genome.[124] In our experience, neurogenic change is the rule with elderly, type II diabetics.

The incidence of cancer also increases with age and with it, paraneoplastic syndromes. Paraneoplastic syndromes involving the neuromuscular junction, namely Lambert-Eaton myasthenic syndrome (LEMS) and myasthenia gravis, have been well characterized. They are thought to arise when antibodies raised against the tumor cross-react with portions of the nervous system (reviewed in Posner[125]). In the case of LEMS, the antibody is directed against a voltage-gated calcium channel found in both small cell lung cancer and at the presynaptic cholinergic synapse.[126] The antibodies bind and disrupt the normal structure of the calcium channel, resulting in the dysfunction at the neuromuscular junction observed in LEMS. In myasthenia gravis the target is the acetylcholine receptor and the associated tumor, thymoma.[125] Other paraneoplastic syndromes affecting muscle include dermatomyositis, acute necrotizing myopathy, and myotonia.[125] The inflammatory myopathies have been discussed above and do not differ from the sporadic variety. The features of paraneoplastic necrotizing myopathies have been described in a number of case reports.[127–142] The muscle weakness tends to be symmetric, with predominant involvement of the proximal muscles.[143] The CK values are routinely abnormal. The necrotic muscle fibers are usually in small or large groups, and most of these fibers do not stain for myosin ATPase, NADH-TR, or other oxidative enzymes. In addition, many regenerating fibers are seen. In contrast to the inflammatory myopathies, lymphocytic infiltrates are infrequent or absent, and necrotic fibers are more frequent.[143] Paraneoplastic necrotizing myopathy with the Jo-1 antibody has been associated with large foci of necrotic muscle fibers and prominent perimysial connective tissue inflammation.[143] In addition, serum antibody binding to a muscle protein in a patient with paraneoplastic myositis and colon cancer has been reported.[144]

Amyloidosis, leading to deposition of amyloid in muscle, also occurs more frequently with aging. It is usually clinically inapparent or presents with weakness, fatigue or autonomic symptoms; a minority of patients have a plasma cell tumor.[145,146] At the light microscopic level, amyloid deposits in muscle appear as eosinophilic amorphous material within blood vessel walls (Fig. 22–8) or, less frequently, in the endomysium. The amyloid deposits can be highlighted using the Congo red stain; they appear red under normal light and manifest an apple-green birefringence under polarized light. The peri- and endomysial collections of amyloid, while they may compress and distort muscle fibers, do not penetrate the sarcolemma.[145,147] The composition of the amyloid deposit, like those elsewhere in the body, varies with the underlying disease. The muscle fiber changes themselves, are nonspecific, and are often secondary to an accompanying peripheral neuropathy that also frequently occurs with amyloidosis.

Muscle also suffers under several other scourges of aging, namely, malnutrition and increased use of prescription drugs, with their associated side effects. Studies of protein-calorie malnutrition have been conducted on adults with chronic dietary deprivation and frequent alcoholism,[148] as well as in a group of patients with anorexia nervosa.[149,150] In both groups the predominant change was myofiber

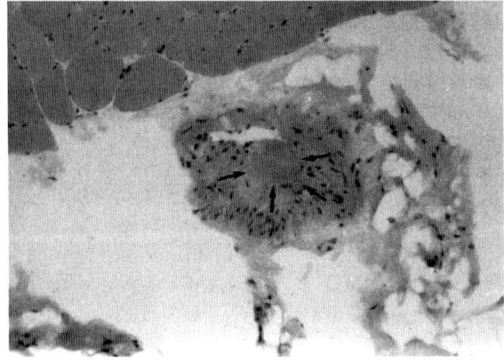

Figure 22–8. Deposit of amorphous amyloid (arrows) within a perimysial vein in a patient with rheumatoid arthritis. Hematoxylin and eosin.

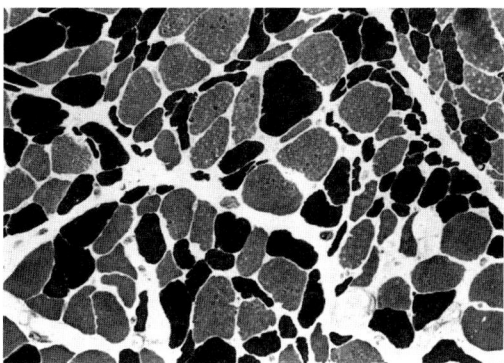

Figure 22–9. Quadriceps muscle from a house-bound 87-year-old woman with severe bilateral hip osteoarthritis who had never seen a physician. Her diet consisted largely of potatoes. Muscle wasting and bilateral, predomintly proximal upper and lower extremity weakness were noted. The clinical and electromyographic impression was that of polymyositis. The biopsy shows atrophy of type II fibers (dark fibers, myosin ATPase, pH 9.4) and is interpreted as showing the combined effects of disuse and malnutrition. The patient improved with nutrition and physiotherapy.

atrophy, which in anorexics mostly affected type II fibers (Fig. 22–9). Specific vitamin deficiencies can also affect muscle. For example, a myopathy apparently related to deficiencies in vitamin is reported in patients with chronic cholestasis and low-serum vitamin E levels, in whom large amounts of apparently lysosomal structures accumulate in the myocytes.[151,152] Weakness and wasting of the proximal limb muscles with varying degrees of pain and tenderness may also accompany vitamin D deficiency.[153] Histologically, mild, nonspecific atrophy of muscle fibers is seen. A variety of degenerative changes in the myofibrils and mitochondria, with accumulation of lipofuscin in muscle fibers, vascular endothelium, and satellite cells can also be present, depending on the clinical context of the vitamin D deficiency.

A number of drugs frequently used in the aging population are associated with muscle pathology. This topic has been extensively reviewed[154] elsewhere and the following is only intended to briefly illustrate the scope of the problem. The HMG-CoA reductase inhibitors, used in the treatment of hypercholesterolemia, are associated with necrotizing myopathy. Histologically, there is fiber necrosis, mononuclear cell infiltration with myophagocytosis, and[155,156] Hypokalemic myopathies can be caused by diuretics and laxatives, both of which are commonly used by the aging population. Three different syndromes of hypokalemic myopathy are recognized.[154] The first is a flaccid, transient, or persistent muscle weakness affecting mainly the proximal muscles, with preservation of reflexes and sensation and marked increase in serum CK levels. Histologic findings are nonspecific and consist of swelling and vacuolation, originating from T tubules, of scattered muscle fibers. In more severe cases, evidence of fiber necrosis, phagocytosis, regeneration, and type II fiber atrophy may also be present.[157] A second syndrome resembles familial periodic paralysis with areflexia. A third, rare syndrome is characterized by severe muscle necrosis and myoglobinuria. The exact mechanism by which hypokalemia causes muscle damage is not clear, but three potential culprits have been suggested: abnormally low muscle blood flow with exercise, suppression of glycogen synthesis and storage, and deranged ion transport.[154]

CONCLUSIONS

The preceding discussion can only give an incomplete picture of the spectrum of insults that skeletal muscles faces with increasing age. Skeletal muscle is structurally highly dynamic and responsive to stresses to an extent that far outstrips the remainder of the nervous system. The degree to which apparently primary muscle changes in aging can be reversed by exercise is an important question and needs further investigation. Understanding of the basic pathophysiology of aging in human muscle will require rigorous assessment of the simultaneous insults and neglect unique to each individual.

REFERENCES

1. Burke WE, Tuttle WW, Thompson CW, et al. The relationship of grip strength and grip-strength endurance to age. J Appl Physiol 1953; 5:628.
2. Kamon E, Goldfuss AJ. In-plant evaluation of muscle strength of workers. Indust Hygiene Assoc J 1978:801.
3. Larsson L, Grimby G, Karlsson J. Muscle strength and speed of movement in relation to age and muscle morphology. J. Appl Physiol 1979; 46:451.
4. Petrofsky JS, Lind AR. Aging, isometric strength and

endurance, and cardiovascular responses to static effort. J. Appl Physiol 1975; 38:91.
5. Rogers MA, Evans WJ. Changes in skeletal muscle with aging: effects of exercise and training. Exercise Sports Sci Rev 1993; 21:65.
6. Larsson L. Physical training effects on muscle morphology in sedentary males at different ages. Med Sci Sports Exercise 1982; 14:203.
7. Campbell MJ, McComas AJ, Petito F. Physiological changes in ageing muscles. J Neurol Neurosurg Psychiatry 1973; 36:174.
8. Florini JR, Ewton DZ. Skeletal muscle fiber types and myosin ATPase activity do not change with age or growth hormone administration. J Gerontol 1989; 44:B110.
9. Vandervoort AA, Hayes KC, Belanger AY. Strength and endurance of skeletal muscle in the elderly. Physiother Can 1986; 38:167.
10. Brooks SV, Faulkner JA. Contractile properties of skeletal muscle from young, adult and aged mice. J Physiol 1988; 404:71.
11. Philips SK, Wiseman RW, Woledge RC, Kushmerick MJ. Neither changes in phosphorous metabolite levels nor myosin isoforms can explain the weakness in aged mouse muscle. J Physiol 1993; 463:157.
12. Young A, Strokes M, Crowe M. The size and strength of the quadriceps muscle of young and old men. Clin Physiol 1985; 5:145.
13. Bruce SA, Newton D, Woledge RC. Effect of age on voluntary force and cross-sectional area of human adductor pollicis muscle. QJ Exp Physiol 1989; 74:359.
14. Philips SK, Rook KM, Siddle NC, Woledge RC. Muscle weakness in women occurs at an earlier age than in men, but strength is preserved by hormone replacement therapy. Clin Sci 1992; 84:95.
15. Gutmann E, Hanzlikova V. Motor units in old age. Nature 1966; 209:921.
16. Rowe RWD. The effect of senility on skeletal muscles in the mouse. Exp Gerontol 1969; 4:119.
17. Lexell J, Taylor CC, Sjostrom M. What is the cause of ageing atrophy? Total number, size and proportion of different fiber types studied in the whole vastus lateralis muscle from 15-to 83-year-old men. J Neurol Sci 1988; 84:275.
18. Sato T, Akatsuka H, Kito K, et al. Age changes in size and number of muscle fibers in human minor pectoral muscle. Mech Ageing Dev 1984; 28:99.
19. Brown M. Change in fiber size and number in aging skeletal muscle. Age Aging 1987; 16:244.
20. Eddinger TJ, Moss RL, Cassens RG. Fiber number and type composition in extensor digitorum longus, soleus, and diaphragm muscle with aging in Fisher 344 rats. J Histochem Cytochem 1985; 33:1033.
21. Alnaqeeb MA, Golspink G. Changes in fiber type, number and diameter in developing and ageing skeletal muscle. J Anat 1986; 153:31.
22. Rubinstein LJ. Aging changes in muscle. In: Bourne GH, ed. Structure and Function of Muscle, Vol. 2. New York: Academic Press, 1960:209.
23. Gollnick PD, Armstrong RB, Saubert CW, et al. Enzyme activity and fiber composition in skeletal muscle of trained and untrained men. J Appl Physiol 1972; 33:312.
24. Larsson L, Karlsson J. Isometric and dynamic endurance as a function of age and skeletal muscle characteristics. Acta Physiol Scand 1978; 104:129.
25. Gutmann E, Hanzlikova V. Basic mechanisms of aging in the neuromuscular system. Mech. Ageing Dev 1972; 1:327.
26. Larsson L, Sjodin B, Karlsson J. Histochemical and biochemical changes in skeletal muscle with age in sedentary males, age 22–65 years. Acta Physiol Scand 1978; 102:31.
27. Larsson L. Motor units: remodeling in aged animals. J Gerontol 1995; 50A:91.
28. Jakobsson F, Borg K, Edstrom L. Fiber type, composition, structure and cytoskeletal protein location of fibers in anterior tibialis muscle: comparison between young adults and physically active aged humans. Acta Neuropathol 1990; 80:459.
29. Lexell J, Henriksson-Larsen K, Winbald B, et al. Distribution of different fiber types in human skeletal muscles: effects of aging studied in whole muscle cross sections. Muscle Nerve 1983; 6:588.
30. Lexell J. Downham D, Sjostrom M. Distribution of different fiber types in human skeletal muscle: fiber type arrangement in m. vastus lateralis from three groups of healthy men between 15 and 83 years. J Neurol Sci 1986; 72:211.
31. Andersen JL, Terzis G, Kryger A. Increase in the degree of coexpression of myosin heavy chain isoforms in skeletal muscle fibers of the very old. Muscle Nerve 1999; 22:449.
32. Grimby G, Danneskold-Samsoe B, Hvid K, Saltin B. Morphology and enzymatic capacity in arm and keg muscles in 78 to 81-year-old men and women. Acta Physiol Scand 1982; 115:125.
33. Coggan AR, Spina RJ, King DS, et al. Histochemical and enzymatic comparison of the gastrocnemius muscle of young and elderly men and women. J Gerontol Sci 1992; 46:B71.
34. Coggan AR, Spina RJ, Rogers MA, et al. Histochemical and enzymatic characteristics of skeletal muscle in master athletes. J Appl Physiol 1990; 68:1896.
35. Aniansson A, Grimby G, Hedberg M, et al. Muscle morphology, enzyme activity and muscle strength in elderly men and women. Clin Physiol 1981; 1:73.
36. Henneman E, Mendell LM. Functional organization of motorneuron pool and its inputs. In: Handbook of Physiology. The Nervous System. Motor Control. Section 1, Vol. 11. Bethesda, MD: American Physiology Society, 1981: 423–507.
37. Hashimuze K, Kanda K, Burke RE. Medial gastrocnemius motor nucleus in the rat: age-related changes in the numbers and size of motorneurons. J Comp Neurol 1988; 269: 425.
38. Ishihara A, Araki H. Effects of age on the number and histochemical properties of muscle fibers and motoneurons in rat extensor digitorum longus muscle. Mech Ageing Dev 1988; 45:213.
39. Tomlinson BE, Irving D. The numbers of limb motor neurons in the human lumbosacral cord throughout life. J Neurol Sci 1977; 34:213.
40. Ansved T, Larsson L. Quantitative and qualitative morphological properties of the soleus motor nerve and the L5-ventral root in young and old rats. J Neurol Sci 1990; 96:269.
41. Rosenheimer JL. Ultraterminal sprouting in innervated and partially denervated adult and aged rat muscle. Neuroscience 1990; 38:763.

42. Pestronk A, Drachman DB, Griffin JW. Effects of aging on nerve sprouting and regeneration. Exp Neurol 1980; 70:65.
43. Welle S, Thornton C, Jozefowicz R, et al. Myofibrillar protein synthesis in young and old men. Am J Physiol 1993; 264:E693.
44. Balagopal P, Rooyackers OE, Adey DB, et al. Effects of aging on in vivo synthesis of skeletal muscle myosin heavy-chain and sarcoplasmic protein in humans. Am J Physiol 1997; 273:E790.
45. Yarasheki KE, Zachwieja JJ, Bier DM. Acute effects of resistance exercise on muscle protein synthesis rate in young and elderly men and women. Am J Physiol 1993; 265:E210.
46. Gutmann. E, Hanzlikova V. Age changes of motor endplates in muscle fibers of the rat. Gerontologia 1965; 11:12.
47. Oda K. Age changes in motor innervation and acetyl choline receptor distribution on human skeletal muscle fibers. J Neurol Sci 1989; 66:327.
48. Cordosis CA, Lafontaine DM. Aging rat neuromuscular functions: a morphometric study of cholinesterase-stained whole mounts and utrastructure. Muscle Nerve 1987; 10:100.
49. Ludatscher RM, Silberman M, Gershon D, Reznick AZ. Evidence of Schwann cell degeneration in the aging mouse motor end-plate region. Exp Gerontol 1985; 20:80.
50. Delbono O, Renganathan M, Messi ML. Excitation-Ca^{2+} release-contraction coupling in single aged human skeletal muscle fiber. Muscle Nerve 1997; 5:S88.
51. Danieli-Betto D, Betto R, Megighian A, et al. Effects of age on sarcoplasmic reticulum properties and histochemical composition of fast-and slow-twitch rat muscles. Acta Physiol Scand 1995; 154:59.
52. Narayanan N, Jones DL, Xu A, Yu JC. Effects of aging on sarcoplasmic reticulum function and contraction duration in skeletal muscles of the rat. Am J Physiol 1996; 271: C1032.
53. Hunter SK, Thompson MW, Ruell PA, et al. Human skeletal muscle sarcoplasmic reticulum Ca^{2+} uptake and muscle function with aging and strength training. J Appl Physiol 1999; 86:1858.
54. Heath GW, Hagberg JM, Ehsani AA, et al. A physiological comparison of young and older endurance athletes. J Appl Physiol 1981; 51:634.
55. Rogers MA, Hagberg JM, Martin WH, et al. Decline in $VO2_{max}$ with aging in masters athletes and sedentary men. J Appl Physiol 1990; 68:2195.
56. Moller P, Bergstrom J, Furst, et al. Effect of aging on energy-rich phosphagens in human skeletal muscles. Clin Sci 1980; 58:553.
57. Essen-Gustavsson B, Borges O. Histochemical and metabolic characteristics of human skeletal muscle in relation to age. Acta Physiol Scand 1986; 126:107.
58. Cooper JM, Mann VM, Schapira AH. Analyses of mitochondrial respiratory chain function and mitochondrial DNA deletion in human skeletal muscle: effect of ageing. J Neurol Sci 1992; 113:91.
59. Trounce I, Byrne E, Marzuki S. Decline in skeletal muscle mitochondrila respiratory chain function: possible factor in ageing. Lancet 1989; 1: 637.
60. Cardellach F, Galofre J, Cusso R, et al. Decline in skeletal muscle respiratory chain function with ageing. Lancet 1989; 2:44.
61. Boffoli D, Scacco SC, Vergari R, et al. Decline with age of the respiratory chain activity in human skeletal muscle. Biochim Biophys Acta 1994; 1226:73.
62. Marshall PA, Golspink WPE, Golspink G. Accumulation of collagen and altered fiber-type ratios as indicators of abnormal muscle gene expression in the mdx dystrophic mouse. Muscle Nerve 1989; 12:528.
63. Carlson BM, Faulkner JA. Muscle transplantation between young and old rats: age of host determines recovery. Am J Physiol 1989; 256:1262.
64. Ullman M, Ullman A, Sommerland H, Skottner A, Oldfors A. Effects of growth hormones on muscle regeneration and IGF-1 concentration in old rats. Acta Physiol Scand 1990; 140:521.
65. McCully KK, Posner JE. The application of blood flow measurements to the study of aging muscle. J Gerontol 1995; 50A:130.
66. Cooper LT, Cooke JP, Dzau VJ. The vascular pathology of aging. J Gerontol Biol Sci 1995;49:B191.
67. Jennekens FGI, Tomlinson BE, Walton JN. Histochemical aspects of five limb muscles in old age. J Neurol Sci 1971; 14:259.
68. Moore MJ, Rebeiz JJ, Holden M, et al. Biometric analysis of normal skeletal muscle. Acta Neuropath (Berl) 1971; 19:51.
69. Tomlinson BE, Walton JN, Rebeiz JJ. The effects of ageing and of cachexia upon skeletal muscle. J. Neurol Sci 1969; 9:321.
70. Jennekens FGI. Disuse, cachexia, and ageing. In: Mastaglia FL, Walton J, eds. Skeletal Muscle Pathology. Edinburgh: Churchill Livingstone, 1982: 605.
71. Liu VW, Zhang C, Nagley P. Mutations in mitochondrial DNA accumulate differentially in three different human tissues during aging nucleic acids research. 1998; 26: 1268.
72. Rifai Z, Welle S, Kamp C, et al. Ragged red fibers in normal aging and inflammatory myopathy. Ann Neurol 1995; 37:24.
73. Brierley EJ, Johnson MA, James OFW, et al. Effects of physical activity and age on mitochondrial function. Q J Med 1996; 89:251.
74. Muller-Hocker J. Cytochrom c oxidase deficient fibers in the limb muscle and diaphragm of man without muscular disease: an age-related alteration. J Neurol Sci 1990; 100:14.
75. Baumer A, Zhang C, Linnane AW, et al. Age-related human mtDNA deletions: a heterogeneous set of deletions arising at a single pair of directly repeated sequences. Am J Hum Genet 1994; 54:618.
76. Cortopassi GA, Arnheim N. Detection of a specific mitochondrial DNA deletion in tissues of older humans. Nucl Acids Res 1990; 18:6927.
77. Brierley EJ, Johnson MA, Lightowlers RN, et al. Role of mitochondrial DNA mutations in human aging: implications for the central nervous system and muscle. Ann Neurol 1998; 43:217.
78. Zhang C, Liu VW, Addessi CL, et al. Differential occurrence of mutations in mitochondrial DNA of human skeletal muscle during aging. Hum Mutat 1998; 11:360.
79. Kovaleko SA, Kopsidas G, Kelso JM, Linnane AW. Deltoid human muscle mtDNA is extensively rearranged in old age subjects. Biochem Biophys Res Commun 1997; 232:147.
80. Brierly EJ, Johnson MA, Bowman A, et al. Mito-

chondrial function in muscle from elderly athletes. Ann Neurol 1997; 41:114.
81. Barrientos A, Casademont J, Rotig A, et al. Absence of a relationship between the level of electron transport chain activities and aging in human skeletal muscle. Biochem Biophys Res Commun 1996; 229: 536.
82. Fielding RA, Meydani M. Exercise, free radical generation, and aging. Aging (Milano) 1997; 9 (1–2):12.
83. Mecocci P, Fano G, Fulle S, et al. Age-dependant increase in oxidative injury to DNA, lipids and proteins in skeletal muscle. Free Radic Biol Med 1999; 26:303.
84. Decary S, Mouly V, Hamida CB, et al. Replicative potential and telomere length in human skeletal muscle: implications for satellite cell mediated gene therapy. Hum Gene Ther 1997; 8:1429.
85. Engel AG, Hohlfield R, Banker BQ. The polymyositis and dermatomyositis syndromes. In: Engel AG, Franzini-Armstrong C, eds. Myology, Vol. 2. New York: McGraw-Hill, 1994:1333–1389.
86. Banker BQ. Dermatomyositis of childhood. Ultrastructural alterations of muscle and intramuscular blood vessels. J Neuropathol Exp Neurol 1975; 34: 46.
87. Carpenter S, Karpati G, Rothman S, Waters G. The childhood type of dermatomyositis. Neurology 1976; 26:952.
88. Duncan AG, Richardson JB, Klein JB, et al. Clinical, serologic and immunogenetic studies in patients with dermatoyositis. Acta Dermatovenerol 1991; 71: 312.
89. Arhata K, Engel AG, Arahata K. Monoclonal antibody analysis of inflammatory cells I. Quantitation of subsets according to diagnosis and sites of accumulation and demonstration and counts of muscle fibers invaded by T cells. Ann Neurol 1984; 16:193.
90. Engel AG, Arahata K. Monoclonal antibody analysis of inflammatory cells II. Phenotypes of autoinvasive cells in polymyositis and inclusion body myositis. 1984; 16:209.
91. Ehrenstein MR, Snaith ML, Isenberg DA. Idiopathic myositis: a rheumatological view. Ann Rheum Dis 1992; 51:41.
92. Marie I, Hatron PY, Levesque H, et al. Influence of age on characteristics of polymyositis and dermatomyositis in adults. Medicine 1999; 78:139.
93. Cherin P, Piette JC, Herson S, et al. Dermatomyositis and ovarian cancer: a report of 7 cases and literature review. J Rheumatol 1993; 20:1897.
94. Maoz CR, Langevitz P, Livneh A, et al. High incidence of malignancies in patients with dermatomyositis and polymyositis: an 11-year analysis. Semin Arthritis Rheum 1998; 27:319.
95. Callen JP. Myositis and malignancy. Curr Opin Rheumatol 1994; 6:590.
96. Zantos D, Zhang Y, Felson D. The overall and temporal association of cancer with polymyositis and dermatomyositis. J Rheumatol 1994; 21:1855.
97. Denko CW, Old JW. Myopathy in the Siccas syndrome (Sjogren's syndrome). Am J Clin Pathol 1969; 51:631.
98. Serratrice G. Evolving concepts of inclusion-body myositis. In: Askansas V, Serratrice G, King Engel W, eds. Inclusion Body Myositis and Myopathies. Cambridge: Cambridge University Press, 1998: 81–103.
99. Mendell JR. Sporadic inclusion body myositis: clinical and laboratory features and diagnostic criteria. In: Askansas V, Serratice G, King Engel W, eds. Inclusion Body Myositis and Myopathies. Cambridge: Cambridge University Press, 1998: 107–155.
100. Carpenter S. Inclusion body myositis: a review. J. Neuropathol Exp Neurol 1996; 55:1105.
101. Ko CC, Croager EJ, Witt CS, et al. Mapping of a candidate region for susceptibility to inclusion body myositis in the human major histocompatibility complex. Immunogenetics 1999; 49:508.
102. Horvath R, Fu K, Johns T, et al. Characterization of the mitochondrial DNA abnormalities in the skeletal muscle of patients with inclusion body myositis. J Neuropathol Exp Neurol 1998; 57:396.
103. Schroder JM, Molnar M. Mitochondrial abnormalities and peripheral neuropathy in inflammatory myopathy, especially inclusion body myositis. Mol Cell Biochem 1997; 174:277.
104. Askansas V, King Engel W. Newest approaches to diagnosis and pathogenesis of sporadic inclusion body myositis and hereditary inclusion body myopathies, including molecular-pathologic similarities to Alzheimer disease. In: Askansas V, Serratrice G, King Engel W, eds. Inclusion Body Myositis and Myopathies. Cambridge: Cambridge University Press, 1998:3–78.
105. Semino-Mora C, Dalakas MC. Rimmed vacuoles with beta-amyloid and ubiquitinated filamentous deposits in the muscles of patients with long-standing denervation (postpoliomyelitis muscular atrophy): similarities with inclusion body myositis. Hum Pathol 1998; 29:1128.
106. Lampe J, Kitzler H, Walter MC, et al. Methionine homozygosity at prion gene codon 129 may predispose to sporadic inclusion-body myositis. Lancet 1999; 353:465.
107. Miklossy J, Taddaei K, Martins R, et al. Alzheimer disease: curly fibers and tangles in organs other than brain. J Neuropathol Exp Neurol 1999; 58:803.
108. Niederwolfsgruber E, Schmitt TL, Blasko I, et al. The production of the Alzheimer amyloid precursor protein in extraneuronal tissue does not increase in old age. J Gerontol (Ser A Biol Sci Med Sci) 1998; 53:B186.
109. Sivakumar K, Semino-Mora C, Dalakas MC. An inflammatory, familial inclusion body myositis with autoimmune features and a phenotype identical to sporadic inclusion body myositis. Studies in three families. Brain 1997; 120:653.
110. Argov Z, Eisenberg I, Mitrani-Rosenbaum S. Genetics of inclusion body myopathies. Curr Opin Rheumato 1998; 10:543.
111. Tyni-Lenne R, Jansson E, Sylven C. Female related skeletal muscle phenotype in patients with moderate chronic heart failure before and after dynamic exercise training. Cardiovasc Res 1999; 42:99.
112. Okita K, Yonezawa K, Nishijima H, et al. Skeletal muscle metabolism limits exercise capacity in patients with chronic heart failure. Circulation 1998; 98:1886.
113. Ades PA, Waldmann ML, Meyer WL, et al. Skeletal muscle and cardiovascular adaptations to exercise

113. conditioning in older coronary patients. Circulation 1996; 94:323.
114. Duscha BD, Kraus WE, Keteyian SJ, et al. Capillary density of skeletal muscle: a contributing mechanism for exercise intolerance in class II–III chronic heart failure independent of other peripheral alterations. J Am Coll Cardiol 1999; 33:1956.
115. Sullivan MJ, Duscha BD, Klitgaard H, et al. Altered expression of myosin heavy chain in human skeletal muscle in chronic heart failure. Med Sci Sports Exercise 1997; 29:860.
116. Massie BM, Simonini A, Saghal P, et al. Relationship of systemic and local muscle exercise capacity to skeletal muscle characteristics in men with congestive heart failure. J Am Coll Cardiol 1996; 27:140.
117. Adams V, Jiang H, Yu J, et al. Apoptosis in skeletal myocytes of patients with chronic heart failure is associated with exercise intolerance. J Am Coll Cardiol 1999; 33:959.
118. Maltais F, Sullivan MJ, Leblanc P, et al. Altered expression of myosin heavy chain in the vastus lateralis muscle in patients with COPD. Eur Respir J 1999; 13:850.
119. Serres I, Gautier V, Varray A, Prefaut C. Impaired muscle endurance related to physical inactivity and altered lung function in COPD patients. Chest 1998; 113:900.
120. Awad EA, Kottke FJ. Changes in muscle ultrastructure in diabetes mellitus. Arch Phys Med Rehab 1970; 51:683.
121. Naccarato R, Maschio G, Sirigu F, et al. The muscle in diabetes mellitus: a histologic (light and electron microscope) and biochemical study by means of needle biopsy. Virchows Arch B Zellpathol 1970; 4:283.
122. Eriksson KF, Saltin B, Lindgarde F. Increased skeletal muscle capillary density precedes diabetes development in men with impaired glucose tolerance. A 15-year follow-up. Diabetes 1994; 43:805.
123. Williamson JR, Hoffman PL, Kohrt WM, et al. Endurance exercise training decreases capillary basement membrane width in older non-diabetic and diabetic adults. J Appl Physiol 1996; 80:747.
124. Liang P, Hughes V, Fukagawa NK. Increased prevalence of mitochondrial DNA deletions in skeletal muscle of older individuals with impaired glucose tolerance: possible marker for glycemic stress. Diabetes 1997; 46:1532.
125. Posner JB. Paraneoplastic syndromes: a brief review. Ann N Y Acad Sci 1997; 835:83.
126. Motomura M, Lang B, Johnston I, et al. Incidence of serum anti-P/Q-type and anti-N-type calcium channel autoantibodies in the Lambert-Eaton myasthenic syndrome. J Neurol Sci 1997; 147:35–42.
127. Kankelheit. Uber primare nichteitrige Polymyositis. Dtsch Arch Klin Med 1916; 120:335.
128. Bezecny R. Dermatomyositis. Arch Dermatol Syph 1935; 171:242.
129. Sheldon JH, Young F, Dyke SC. Acute dermatomyositis associated with reticulo-endotheliosis. Lancet 1939; 1:82.
130. McCombs RP, MacMahon HE. Dermatomyositis associated with metastasizing bronchogenic carcinoma: a clinicopathological conference. Med Clin North Am 1947; 31:1148.
131. Cottel CE. Dermatomyositis and malignant neoplasm. Am J Med Sci 1952; 224:160.
132. Walton JN, Adams RD. Polymyositis. Edinburgh: Livingstone, 1958:236–244.
133. Smith B. Skeletal muscle necrosis associated with carcinoma. J Pathol 1969; 97:207.
134. Holt LPJ, Azzopardi JG. A case of gastric ulcer and dermatomyositis demonstrated at the Royal Postgraduate Medical School. BMJ 1969; 4:221.
135. Urich H, Wilkinson M. Necrosis of muscle with carcinoma: myositis or myopathy? J Neurol Neurosurg Psychiatry 1970; 33:398.
136. Heffner RR. Myopathy of embolic origin in patients with carcinoma. Neurology 1971; 21:840.
137. Swash M. Acute fatal carcinomatous neuromyopathy. Arch Neurol 1974; 30:324.
138. Brownell R, Hughes JT. Degeneration of muscle in association with carcinoma of the bronchus. J Neurol Neurosurg Psychiatry 1975; 38:363.
139. Scelsi R, Pinelli P. Subclinical myopathic findings in patients affected by malignant tumours: an autopsy study. Acta Neuropathol (Berl) 1977; 30:103.
140. Yutani C, Matsuda Y, Murao S, et al. Necrotizing myopathy as a remote effect of gastric cancer accompanied with Hashimoto's thyroiditis. Acta Pathol Jpn 1978; 28:165.
141. Vosskamper M, Korf B, Frank F, et al. Paraneoplastic necrotizing myopathy: a rare disorder to be differentiated from polymyositis. 1989; 236:489.
142. Pillay PK, Estes ML. Acute necrotizing myopathy in association with carcinoma of the tongue. Ann Acad Med Singapore 1993; 22:516.
143. Levin MI, Mozaffar T, Al-Lozi MT, Pestronk A. Paraneoplastic necrotizing myopathy: clinical and pathological features. Neurology 1998; 50:764.
144. Ueyama H, Kumamoto T, Araki S. Circulating autoantibody to muscle protein in a patient with paraneoplastic myositis and colon cancer. Eur Neurol 1992; 32:281.
145. Whitaker JN, Hashimoto K, Quinones M. Skeletal muscle pseudohypertrophy in primary amyloidosis. Neurology 1977; 27:47.
146. Prayson RA. Amyloid myopathy: clinicopathologic study of 16 cases. Hum Pathol 1998; 26:463.
147. Lange RK. Primary amyloidosis of muscle. South Med J 1970; 63:321.
148. Dastur DK, Daver SM, Manghani DK. Changes in muscle in human malnutrition; with emphasis on fine structure in protein-calorie malnutrition. In: Zimmerman HM, ed. Progress in Neuropathology, Vol. 4. New York: Raven Press, 1979:299.
149. Slettebo M, Lindboe CF, Askevold F. The neuromuscular system in patients with anorexia nervosa: electrophysiological and histologic studies. Clin Neuropathol 1984; 3:217.
150. McLoughlan DM, Spargo E, Wassif WS, et al. Structural and functional changes in skeletal muscle in anorexia nervosa. Acta Neuropathol 1998; 95:632.
151. Neville HE, Ringel SP, Guggenheim MA, et al. Ultrastructural and histochemical abnormalities of skeletal muscle in patients with chronic vitamin E deficiency. Neurology 1983; 33:483.
152. Werlin SL, Harb JM, Swick H, Blank E. Neuro-

muscular dysfunction and ultrastructural pathology in children with chronic cholestasis and vitamin E deficiency. Ann Neurol 1983; 13:291.
153. Dastur DK, Gragat BM, Wadia NH, et al. Nature of muscular change in osteomalacia: light and electron microscope observations. J Pathol 1975; 117:211.
154. Victor M, Sieb JP. Myopathies due to drugs, toxins, and nutritional deficiency. In: Engel AG, Franzini-Armstrong C, eds. Myology, Vol. 2. New York: McGraw-Hill, 1994:1703.
155. Pierce LR, Wysowski DK, Gross TP. Myopathy and rhabdomyolysis associated with lovastatin-gemfibrozil combination therapy. JAMA 1990; 264:71.
156. Waclawik AJ, Lindal S, Engel AG. Experimental lovastatin myopathy. J Neuropathol Exp Neurol 1993; 52:542.
157. Comi G, Testa D, Cornelio F, et al. Potassium depletion myopathy: a clinical and morphological study of six cases. Muscle Nerve 1985; 8:17.
158. Danneskiold-Samsoe B, Kofod V, Munter J et al. Muscle strength and functional capacity in 78–81-year-old men and women European J Appl Physiol Occu Physiol 1984; 52(3):310.
159. Grimby G, Saltin B. The ageing muscle. Clin Physiol 1983; 3(3):209.
160. Nair KS. Muscle protein turnover: methodological issues and the effect of aging. J Gerontol A Biol Sci Med Sci 1995; 50:107.

23. Drug Toxicity and the Aging Brain

TERUMI A. IZUKAWA AND MICHAEL GORDON

There has been a marked shift in the demographic makeup of the populations in most western countries including the United States and Canada: a substantial increase is taking place in the percentage of elderly individuals. In Canada, currently approximately 12% of the population is, over 65 years of age, and this number is expected to increase to 17% by the year 2011 and to 21% by 2030.[1] Associated with these population shifts has been an increase in the need for treatment of the elderly for the many medical conditions that are associated with the aging process. Since many of the serious medical conditions in the elderly have an impact on the neurological system, either directly or indirectly, it is important to understand the interactions between drugs and the aging brain.

With increasing human age there is an increase in diversity of experience, physiology, and disease. Because of this, the use of medication for the prevention and management of illness becomes an increasingly complex process, and the likelihood of iatrogenic illness rises, in particular, untoward effects on neurological function. Trends in the United States suggest that those over 65 years of age account for one-third of total health care expenditures.[2] This 12% of the American population who are elderly use approximately 30% of all prescription medications.[3] Also, up to 70% of elderly individuals consume over-the-counter, nonprescription medications, the most common of which are analgesics, antacids, and anticholinergic medications such as antihistamines.[4] Approximately 15% of the elderly suffer from complex chronic medical conditions and to this can be added the effects of any intercurrent acute illness. This situation often leads to the use of polypharmacy and with it medication interactions and adverse drug reactions in this age-group.

Because of age-related changes in the anatomy and physiology of the brain as well as changes in the handling and distribution of medications as we age, the potential for drug interactions is markedly increased. Of particular concern are the cumulative effects these interactions may have on the nervous system.[5] For example, some psychotropic medications are known for their narrow therapeutic window in the elderly. While their desired effect is the improvement of function both cognitively and physically, with time they may accumulate in the system and their function may actually decrease because of side effects. In multiple studies, adverse drug reactions have been shown to be responsible for between 10% and 31% of hospital admissions of the elderly.[6-10] This does not take in to account some of the poorly studied, insidious, long-term effects of medications on the elderly.

In this chapter we review the general principles of drug prescribing in the aging individual and use several examples to illustrate some neuropathological toxic effects of medications that have been studied in the elderly. We will focus on important and clinically relevant features of geriatric prescribing and the basis for a comprehensive age-sensitive approach. We will then examine some specific examples of common geriatric neurological conditions and the interaction they have with commonly used medications.

NORMAL AGING OF THE BRAIN

It is important to emphasize that reported changes in the anatomy and physiology of the aging brain do not always have clinical implications. In particular, before the age of 75, there is usually no change in ordinary activities of daily living or occupational functioning unless there is associated pathology, despite the fact that there is an estimated 20% reduction in brain weight between the ages of 20 and 80.[11] However, these subclinical changes may have a profound effect on the brain's response to medications.

As described in more detail in Chapter 2, when we age, neurons are not replaced, but glial cells retain their ability to undergo cell division. It has been postulated that the observed dendrite proliferation seen with normal aging may be an adaptive response that allows selected neurons to maintain contact with their target cells despite neuronal loss.[12] It is fairly widely accepted that the normal aging brain undergoes atrophy in selected areas, along with a reduction in cerebral blood flow.[13] This may decrease the older brain's ability to respond in times of stress—for example, in the presence of an acute or chronic illness, predisposing to the condition we know as acute confusional state or delirium.[14]

In particular, the mild but definite decrease in cholinergic neurotransmission may make the elderly more sensitive to anti-cholinergic agents and more likely to experience adverse effects.[14] Decreases in dopaminergic neurons and dopamine D2 receptors occur with aging.[15] Also, γ-aminobutyric acid (GABA)-A receptors as well as N-methyl-D-aspartate (NMDA) receptors may be altered with age. Age-related changes in GABA-A–benzodiazepine complex numbers and subunit composition and in the processes that regulate their sensitivity have also been well described.[16,17] All of these changes can lead to altered responses to medications in the elderly, independent of disease and comorbidity, making the prescription of many medications, from anti-convulsants to benzodiazepines, a greater challenge.

CHANGES IN DRUG MANAGEMENT WITH AGING

The pharmacokinetic changes that occur as we age are well documented. The aging process, including a change in gastric pH, theoretically affects absorption, but practically speaking the main influence is that of medications that alter the rate of gastric emptying. These medications, such as anticholinergic agents, can delay the delivery of the medication to the small intestine, which is mainly where absorption occurs.[18] Concomitant ingestion of binding substances (such as calcium with bisphosphonates) may also have an effect. However, these are minor in comparison to the changes in drug distribution, metabolism, and excretion, which can be dramatically altered even in a healthy aged individual compared to in a young adult.

Aging usually alters drug distribution. With reduced albumin levels, drug binding is decreased, resulting in higher serum levels and enhanced effect, both beneficial and adverse.[19] As we age, our fat-to-water ratio increases, leading to an enhanced volume of distribution of fat-soluble drugs and lower distribution of water-soluble molecules. Drug elimination is also affected. Although there is individual variation, hepatic metabolism can be reduced by as much as one-half that of a young adult, but only becomes relevant in geriatric drug prescription for medications that are predominately handled by the liver. It is well known that renal function decreases with age, and adjustments in renally excreted medications should always be made for the elderly.[20] Toxic drug levels found, for example, in digoxin therapy for the elderly can have profound neurological effects in addition to those upon the heart.[21]

Some of the best-studied pharmacodynamic effects related to aging are those of the benzodiazepines on the aging brain, which appears to be more sensitive for a given serum level of the drug.[22,23] Warfarin is also more effective in the elderly at a given plasma level, so lower doses are required as an individual ages.[24] While taking these changes into consid-

Table 23–1. Factors Affecting Access to Drug Therapy

Type of Factor	Examples
Physical factors	Vision
	Hearing
	Motor Control
	Swallowing
Psychological	Education
	Autoageism[26]
	Cognition
	Depression, mania, or psychosis
Physician-related	Ageism
	Lack of evidence in literature
	Physician characteristics (age, gender, medical school, etc.)
Patient and caregiver relationship	Caregiver expectation
	Access to health care
Societal	Health insurance
	Socioeconomic status
	Pharmacoeconomics

Table 23–2. Principles of Drug Therapy in the Elderly

Principle of Drug Therapy	Explanation
Diagnose from symptoms.	Do not treat symptoms without first discovering their cause.
Know the drugs being used.	Know the pharmacological action of the drug, particularly the metabolism and excretion.
Start low and go slow.	Use the lowest possible dosage, monitor for adverse effects, and increase slowly to achieve desired therapeutic effect.
Avoid polypharmacy.	Minimize medications and simplify dosage regimens to improve adherence.
Do no harm	Do not prescribe if the side effects are worse than the original symptoms.
Review and rationalize regularly	Do not continue medications once they are no longer needed.

eration, the physician must also review the factors known to affect drug compliance in the elderly, including the complexity of the drug regimen, poor drug knowledge, physical limitations, poor communication with health care providers, and certain psychosocial characteristics, such as social isolation.[25] Finally, physicians must review those factors influencing access to drug therapy in the first place, so that barriers to obtaining treatment are minimized. (Table 23–1).[26]

PRINCIPLES OF PRESCRIBING FOR THE ELDERLY

By following the general principles outlined in Table 23–2, physicians can greatly decrease the chances of adverse effects of medications in the elderly. Because the elderly have atypical disease presentations, symptoms alone should not be treated, rather, first a diagnosis is needed. Clinicians should know the potential side effects and interactions of the medications they are prescribing and be alert to changes in drug excretion with aging. The lowest possible dosage should be used and patients should be closely monitored for adverse effects. Patients' medication regimen should also be frequently reviewed so as to avoid polypharmacy.

Although all medications must be prescribed very carefully in the elderly, those that are specifically targeted to the neurological system must be used with particular caution. There is often a very fine line between achieving the desired therapeutic effect and adversely affecting an aging and susceptible brain.

NEUROLEPTIC MEDICATIONS AND THE ELDERLY

Neuroleptic medications are often used in the care of the elderly, particularly in the management of schizophrenia continuing into late life, acute delirium, psychosis, and behavioral challenges in dementia. However, the benefits can be overwhelmed by the serious side effects of these agents, which range from classic anticholinergic effects (the development of drug-induced parkinsonism, tardive dyskinesia, and akathesia) to the rare neuroleptic malignant syndrome. Of these, the elderly are disproportionately prone to drug-induced parkinsonism compared to younger individuals.[27]

CASE REPORT

D.F., a 79-year-old woman living in her own home, was admitted to a general hospital with septicemia secondary to a urinary tract infection. She became delirious and agitated and was treated with antibiotics as well as haloperidol at 3 mg daily. She was unable to return home because of a decline in her mental function and was discharged to a nursing home after several weeks.

One year later she was assessed by the behavioral neurology unit at Baycrest Hospital because of continuing decline in general and mental functioning. She had lost 40 pounds, was not eating well, and was poorly motivated. Examination revealed a thin woman with parkinsonism, tardive dyskinesia, akathesia, and mild cognitive impairment.

Haloperidol was discontinued, and over the ensuing weeks of the hospitalization, she made a slow but steady recovery, with improved gait and mental performance and weight gain. She did not tolerate treatment of parkinsonism with levodopa because of an acute confusional state. At follow-up 6 months later, the patient was receiving no medications while maintaining her cognitive function with minimal gait disturbance.

This case illustrates some of the slowly developing yet lasting untoward effects of neuroleptics on the elderly. Neuroleptic medications induce parkinsonism by interfering with dopamine function in the basal ganglia. This accounts for up to 4% of all patients with parkinsonism seen in general neurology clinics.[28] In psychiatric clinics, this figure ranges from 5% to 60%.[29] The incidence increases with age, presumably because of preexisting age-related loss of dopaminergic neurons in the substantia nigra of older individuals.

Another interesting finding, that may eventually help in the understanding of the development of dementing disorders is that of increased numbers of neurofibrillary tangles in the brains of elderly schizophrenic patients treated with neuroleptics, compared to those who were not on neuroleptics. Wisniewski et. al.[30] reviewed the clinical histories and brains of 102 schizophrenic patients. Forty-one died between 1932 and 1952, and had never been treated with neuroleptics. The others died between 1954 and 1990, and had received neuroleptic medications. The authors found that the incidence of neurofibrillary tangles in these patients was twice as high and that the presence of end-stage tangles was significantly higher in the group that had received neuroleptics. They concluded that the development of neurofibrillary tangles started earlier in the treated group, and theorized that the reported increased neuronal loss seen in the brains of schizophrenics was due to treatment, not to the disease itself. The main drawback of this study was its retrospective nature, which led to some uncertainty as to the validity of the clinical diagnosis of schizophrenia. However, the authors had a unique opportunity in the examination of an unusually large number of pathological samples from the preneuroleptic era.

In a subsequent meta-analysis of eight other studies with comparison data of senile plaques and neurofibrillary tangles in the brains of schizophrenics, Baldessarini et al.[31] concluded that there was not enough data to support the contention that schizophrenics are more likely to have neuropathological changes consistent with Alzheimer's disease (AD).

Another prospective study of 71 patients with dementia (primarily AD and vascular dementia) who were treated with neuroleptics showed that the mean cognitive decline in the 16 patients who took neuroleptics was twice that of the patients who did not use them. The start of neuroleptic therapy coincided with more rapid cognitive decline. Autopsy was performed on 42 of the patients, but scant data were reported. The finding of Lewy bodies was not found to be correlated with rapid cognitive decline. Although this was a prospective, longitudinal study, it was not randomized or blinded and the numbers were small. The authors concluded that their study supports the association of cognitive decline with neuroleptic therapy in demented patients, but did not prove it.[32]

There is no doubt that there is a place for neuroleptic therapy in the care of the elderly. However, these studies reinforce the finding that careful thought must be given to the potential, insidious and long-lasting side effects of these powerful medications, and that the indications for their prolonged use in the elderly should be very clear and compelling.

LEVODOPA AND PARKINSON'S DISEASE IN THE ELDERLY

Since the 1960s, levodopa, alone or in combination with a dopa decarboxylase inhibitor, has been the mainstay of treatment for Parkinson's disease. This drug treatment revolutionized the care of patients suffering from Parkinson's disease and has provided new hope to them. However, despite the great beneficial impact of levodopa-containing medications, drug-induced complications can affect up to 50% of patients with Parkinson's disease within the first 5 years of treatment.[33] This is sometimes seen as a barrier to effective therapy. Because of the reported incidence of dyskinesias and motor fluctuations in patients treated with levodopa, there has been some controversy over whether levodopa is itself toxic to substantia nigra neurons. Not all patients develop these side effects, but they do appear to be related to the dosage of levodopa and the length of time of treatment. Of interest is the fact that individuals who were inadvertently treated with levodopa but did not have Parkinson's disease did not develop these extra movement phenomena.[34]

In tissue culture, it has been demonstrated that levodopa and dopamine undergo auto-oxidation, resulting in the production of quinones, semiquinones, hydrogen peroxide, and other oxygen radicals. According to the oxidative stress hypothesis, these by-products cause cellular damage.[35–37] Although there are endogenous antioxidants, tissues with high metabolic activity are felt to be at particularly high risk for cellular damage. The substantia nigra neurons are vulnerable because of the presence of monoamine oxidase activity and the accumulation of iron.[38] The hydrogen peroxide formed during the oxidative deamination of dopamine by monoamine oxidase in substantia nigra neurons reacts with ferrous iron and produces excess hydroxyl radicals. These hydroxyl radicals are theoretically the most reactive and cytotoxic oxidative by-products produced.[39]

Other proposed mechanisms of predisposition to cellular damage by levodopa include a demonstrated decrease in mitochondrial respiratory chain complex I activity in substantia nigra cells in Parkinson's patients.[40] This could lead to selective use of mitochondrial respiratory chain complex II, which results in release of free radicals. Also, it has recently been shown in vitro that levodopa and dopamine can induce cellular apoptosis, an abnormality that has been documented in postmortem studies of Parkinson's disease brains.

Endogenous antioxidants include retinol, ascorbic acid, and the enzymes superoxide dismutase and glutathione peroxidase. The latter catalyses the oxidation of glutathione. The reduced form of glutathione is a potent antioxidant, while the oxidated form is believed to be cytotoxic. Levels of the reduced form of glutathione have been shown to be lower in the substantia nigra neurons of patients with Parkinson's disease.[34] The oxygen radical hypothesis provides the theoretical background for the use of antioxidants such as vitamin E and monoamine oxidase inhibitors such as selegiline in the management of Parkinson's disease. It may also explain why these medications tend to be more effective in the earlier stages of the disease, perhaps before cellular damage from auto-oxidation becomes widespread.[41]

In normal animal studies, exposure to high concentrations of levodopa has not caused any toxic effect on the cells of the substantia nigra. Research in animal models of Parkinson's disease that suggested a neurotoxic effect has not been reproduced.[42] Human studies likewise do not support the contention that levodopa contributes to cellular damage.[43] Autopsy comparisons of Parkinson's disease patients treated with levodopa and those receiving no levodopa do not show any difference in the degree of damage to the substantia nigra neurons.[44]

These studies indicate that the treatment of Parkinson's disease should be carefully considered. The clinician and the patient must be convinced that the benefits outweigh the potential risks in terms of long-term, insidious damage. Special consideration should be given to low initial dosage and slow increments in treatment of the elderly in whom the risks of untoward toxic effects appear to be higher.

ALUMINUM, DIALYSIS ENCEPHALOPATHY, AND ALZHEIMER'S DISEASE

Although the neuropathology of AD is described in detail in Chapters 6 and 8, we must mention it here in the context of the aluminum etiology controversy and aluminum-containing medications such as antacids and sucralfate. The evidence leading to the assumption that aluminum is implicated in causing AD is largely epidemiological. In these studies there is an increased incidence of AD in areas with high levels of aluminum in the drinking water.[45–47] The initial association was partly based on observations of dementia developing in patients who had undergone long-term hemodialysis with chronic exposure to high levels of aluminum. However, this so-called dialysis encephalopathy is clinically and neuropathologically very unlike AD. Clinically, the patient has dysarthria, myoclonus, and seizures. Although serum levels of aluminum are elevated and there are also higher levels found in the brain, the areas in which the aluminum is deposited does not correlate with the pathological findings. The pathology lacks the classic senile plaques and tau-reactive neurofibrillary tangles of the patient with AD. Electron microscopy studies show that the neurofibrillary tangles have a straight rather than the helical structure seen in AD brains.[48]

Despite the observations related to aluminum and dialysis patients, there is currently no conclusive evidence that environmental aluminum causes AD. Perhaps more relevant to the discussion of drug toxicity is the fact that multiple longitudinal cohort studies have shown a total lack of correlation between ingestion of aluminum-containing medications and the development of Alzheimer-type dementia.[49–53]

OTHER DRUGS

The effects of ethanol on the neurological system are discussed elsewhere in this text. Many other medications are known to have neurological side effects, but the underlying neuropathology is less well documented in the elderly. Chemotherapeutic agents such as cisplatin have been associated with white matter loss.[54] Magnetic resonance imaging (MRI) studies reveal similar changes with the use of many different anti-hypertensive agents,[55] but it is difficult to separate the effects of the therapy from the effects of the disease. There are also medications that have been shown to have positive effects on the brain, such as the decrease of activated microglial cells seen in nondemented arthritic patients treated with non-steroidal anti-inflammatory drugs. It is postulated that this may be the basis for any clinical effect that non-steroidal anti-inflammatory drugs have on the development and progression of AD.[56]

There is surprisingly little literature on the neuropathological effects of other known psychotropic medications such as antidepressants. There is also very little documenting the effects of gender on the neuropathology of drug toxicity in the elderly. Clearly, as our population ages, this is an area for future research.

OTHER ILLNESSES

There are specific considerations when prescribing for the elderly who have suffered brain trauma, be it from disease such as stroke or hypertension or from acquired brain injury. In principle, monitoring for delirium, maintaining nutrition and hydration, and avoiding the development of complications such as pneumonia, pressure ulcers, and depression should be routine. Early ambulation is key to recovery, as the effects of even short-term (2 weeks) bed rest can be profound in the elderly and may significantly slow or even prevent full recovery. Early and aggressive discharge planning are important. Geriatric reactivation and rehabilitation programs may be appropriate if the goal is to return to independent living. The use of support systems, both formal and informal, are key to preventing readmission or re-injury. This includes the support of appropriate medication use.

The same general principles of prescribing for the elderly apply in all these conditions. Even so-called benign medications, such as H2 blockers, can have profound effects in the elderly who have suffered brain damage. Rational prescribing will go far in preventing complications such as delirium, falls, and further cognitive and functional decline.

PRESCRIBING FOR THE ELDERLY IN NURSING HOMES

The elderly who are admitted to a long-term care institution are at particular risk for adverse drug reactions. The use of psychotropic medications is disproportionately high, often with poorly documented reasons for the prescription and no defined end points for treatment.[57–59] These individuals are usually the frailest seniors, with few external supports and a relatively high prevalence of cognitive impairment.

Newly admitted patients should be observed for signs of withdrawal from benzodiazepines, alcohol, narcotics, and other medications that may have been used to excess because of medication errors prior to admission to a supervised setting. Conversely, they are also at risk of overdosing, as medications are suddenly being taken reliably, and compliance is no longer an issue. Admission is a good time to review every prescription medication with an eye to rationalizing prescribing, minimizing polypharmacy, and thus decreasing potential drug–drug and drug–disease interactions.

Regular medication reviews should be undertaken, and in many jurisdictions, are mandated. Dosages should be adjusted over time for changes in physical size, creatinine clearance, liver function, and cognition. It is particularly important to have identified goals of treatment so that medications are not continued beyond their usefulness, simply out of habit. For example, anti-depressants should be re-evaluated once an individual reaches end-stage dementia, when insight and higher cognitive function are lost. At that point, the benefit may no longer outweigh the risk of side effects, and a gradual attempt at withdrawal can be undertaken.

It is also important that cognitive changes, especially delirium, are not immediately attributed to medications. Other factors, such as acute or chronic illness (e.g., infection or silent myocardial ischemia), environmental changes (e.g., loss of environmental cues or personnel changes), and metabolic imbalances such as dehydration should be ruled out as well. Often the patient can give minimal history and the importance of obtaining information from other sources such as family and other staff cannot be overemphasized. Prescribing for the elderly in institutions can be very challenging and remains an example of when the art of medicine meets the science, one hopes for the overall betterment of the patients.

CONCLUSION

It is beyond the scope of this chapter to provide a comprehensive inventory of all the drugs that are known to have a real or potential negative impact on the aging neurological system. In practical terms, the most important message to medical and other practitioners is that drug therapy in the elderly is a complex and challenging undertaking. If the principles outlined above are used in the decision-making process for drug prescribing, this will minimize adverse outcomes. There must be further and more comprehensive, targeted studies that will enable us to better understand the effects of these medications at a cellular level. We can then use this knowledge clinically and ultimately improve the quality of life for those older persons for whom we provide care.

Contemporary pharmacotherapy is one of the great achievements of the modern era. With proper use, drugs can provide great relief from suffering and help older individuals to lead fuller and more productive lives. The risks to the aging body in general and to the neurological system in particular must always be high on our agenda when decisions are made to prescribe drugs for our elderly patients.

REFERENCES

1. Goel V, Iron K, Willimas JI. Indicators of health determinants and health status. In: Goel V, Willimas JI, Anderson GM, et al., eds. Patterns of Health Care in Ontario. The ICES Practice Atlas, 2nd ed. Ottawa: Canadian Medical Association, 1996:27–42.
2. Kane RL, Ouslander JG, Abrass IB. Essentials of Clinical Geriatrics, 3rd ed. New York: McGraw-Hill, 1994.
3. Lamy PP. Pharmacotherapeutics in the elderly. Md Med J 1989; 38:144–148.

4. Lowenthal DT, Nadeau SE. Drug induced dementia. South Med J 1991; 84(IS):24–31.
5. Atkin PA, Veitch PC, Veitch EM, Ogle SJ. The epidemiology of serious adverse drug reactions among the elderly. Drugs Aging 1999; 14(2):141–152.
6. Seidl LG, Thornton GF, Smith JW, Cluff, LE. Studies on the epidemiology of adverse drug reactions. III. Reactions in patients on a general medical service. Bull Johns Hopkins Hosp 1966; 119:299–315.
7. Hurwitz N. Predisposing factors in adverse reactions to drugs. 1969; BMJ 1:536–539.
8. Learoyd BM. Psychotropic drugs and the elderly patient. Med J Austr 1972; 1:1131–1133.
9. Williamson J, Chopin JM. Adverse reactions to prescribed drugs in the elderly: a multicentre investigation. Age Ageing 1980; 9:73–80.
10. Grymonpre RE, Mitenko PA, Sitar DS, Aoki FY, Montgomery PR. Drug-associated hospital admissions in older medical patients. J Am Geriatr Soc 1988; 36:1092–1098.
11. Turnheim K. Drug treatment in the elderly. Pharmacokinetic and pharmacodynamic considerations. In: Mallarkey G, ed. Drug Treatment Considerations in the Elderly. Hong Kong: Adis International, 1999:35–59.
12. Coleman PD, Flood DG. Neuron numbers and dentritic extent in normal aging and Alzheimer's disease. Neurobiol Aging 1987; 8:521–545.
13. Dekaban AS, Sadowsky BS. Changes in brain weight during the life span of human life: relation of brain weight to body heights and body weight. Ann Neurol 1978; 4:345–356.
14. Moore AR, O'Keeffe ST. Drug-induced cognitive impairment in the elderly. Drugs Aging 1999; 15(1):15–28.
15. Wong DF, Young D, Wilson PD, Meltzer CC, Gjedde A. Quantification of neuroreceptors in the living human brain. D2-like dopamine receptors: theory, validation and changes during normal aging. J Cereb Blood Flow Metab 1997; 17:316–330.
16. Lanius RA, Pasqualotto BA, Shaw CA. Age-dependent expression, phosphorylation and function of neurotransmitter receptors: pharmacological implications. Trends Pharmacol Sci 1993; 14:403–408.
17. Gutierrez A, Khan ZU, Miralles CP, et al. $GABA_A$ receptor subunit expression changes in the rat cerebellum and cerebral cortex during aging. Mol Brain Res 1997; 45(1):59–70.
18. Bender AD. Effect of age on intestinal absorption: Implications for drug absorption in the elderly. J Am Geriatr Soc 1968; 16:1331–1339.
19. Montamat SC, Cusack BJ, Vestal RE. Management of drug therapy in the elderly. N Engl J Med 1989; 321(5):303–309.
20. Greenblatt DJ, Sellers EM, Shader RI. Drug Disposition in old age. N Engl J Med 1982; 306:1081–1088.
21. Roberts J, Tumer M. Pharmacodynamic basis for altered drug action in the elderly. Clin Gerlatr Med 1988; 4(1):127–149.
22. Castleden CM, George CF, Mercer D, Hallet C. Increased sensitivity to nitrazepam in old age. BMJ 1977; 1:10–12.
23. Greenblatt DJ, Divoll M, Harmatz JS, MacLaughlin DS, Shader RI. Kinetics and Clinical effects of flurazepam in young and elderly noninsomniacs. Clin Pharmacol Ther 1981; 30:475–486.
24. Shepherd AM, Hewick DS, Moreland TA, Stevenson IH. Age as a determinant of sensitivity to warfarin. Br J Clin Pharmacol 1977; 4:315–320.
25. Ascione F. Medication compliance in the elderly. Generations 1994; 28–33.
26. Dombrower H, Izukawa TA, Veinish SL. Factors affecting access to drug therapy in the elderly. Drugs Aging 1998; 13(4):303–309.
27. Burns RJ, Schultz DW. Drug-induced neurological disorders. Med J Austr 1993; 159:624–626.
28. Stacy M, Jankovic J. Differential diagnosis of Parkinson's disease and the parkinsonism plus syndromes. Neurol Clin 1992; 10:341–345.
29. Gershanik OS. Drug-induced parkinsonism in the aged. Drugs Aging 1994; 5(2):127–132.
30. Wisniewski HM, Constantinidis J, Wegiel J, Bobinski M, Tarnawski M. Neurofibrillary pathology in brains of elderly schizophrenics treated with neuroleptics. Alzheimer Dis Assoc Disord 1994; 8(4):211–227.
31. Baldessarini RJ, Hegarty JD, Bird ED, Benes FM. Meta-analysis of postmortem studies of Alzheimer's disease-like neuropathology in schizophrenia. Am J Psychiatry 1997; 154(6):861–863.
32. McShane R, Keene J, Gedling K, Fairburn C, Jacoby R, Hope T. Do neuroleptic drugs hasten cognitive decline in dementia? Prospective study with necropsy follow-up. BMJ 1997; 314:266–270.
33. Fahn S. Adverse effects of levodopa. In: Olanow CW, Lieberman AN, eds. The Scientific Basis for the Treatment of Parkinson's Disease. Carnforth: Parthenon, 1992:89–122.
34. Simuni T, Stern MB. Does levodopa accelerate Parkinson's disease? Drugs Aging 1999; 14(6):399–408.
35. Carlsson A, Fornstedt B. Possible mechanisms underlying the special vulnerability of dopaminergic neurons. Acta Neurol Scand 1991; 84(S136):16–18.
36. Pardo B, Mena MA, Casarejos MJ, Paino CL, De Yebenes JG: Toxic effects of L-DOPA on mesencephalic cell cultures: protection with antioxidants. Brain Res. 1995; 682:133–143.
37. Mytinineou C, Han S, Cohen G. Toxic and protective effects of L-DOPA on mesencephalic cell cultures. J Neurochem. 1993; 61(4):1470–1478.
38. Fahn S, Cohen G. The oxidant stress hypothesis in Parkinson's disease: evidence supporting it. Ann Neurol 1992; 32:804–812.
39. Hirsh EC, Francheux BA. Iron metabolism and Parkinson's disease. Mov Disord 1998; 13(Suppl 1):39–45.
40. Przedborski S, Jackson-Lewis V, Fahn S. Antiparkinsonian therapies and brain mitochondrial complex I activity. Mov Disord 1995; 10(3):312–317.
41. Mena MA, Pardo B, Casarejos MJ, Fahn S, De Yebenes JG. Neurotoxicity of levodopa on catecholamine-rich neurons. Mov Disord 1992; 7(1):23–31.
42. Melemed E, Rosenthal J. Can chronic levodopa therapy accelerate degeneration of dopaminergic neurons and progression of Parkinson's disease? In: Nagatsu T, Fisher A, Yoshida M, eds. Basic, Clinical and Therapeutic Aspects of Alzheimer's and Parkinson's Diseases. New York: Plenum Press, 1990:253–256.
43. Rajput AH, Fenton ME, Dhand A. Is levodopa toxic to non-degenerating substantia nigra cells? Clinical evidence [abstract]. Neurology 1996; 46 Suppl:A371.
44. Rajput AH, Fenton ME, Birdi S, et al. Is levodopa

45. McLachlan DRC, Bergeron C, Smith JE, Boomer D, Rifat SL. Risk for neuropathologically confirmed Alzheimer's disease and residual aluminum in municipal drinking water, employing weighted residential histories. Neurology 1996; 46:401–405.
46. Neri LC, Hewitt D. Aluminum, Alzheimer's disease and drinking water. Lancet 1991; 338:390.
47. Forbes WF, Lessard S, Gentleman JF. Geochemical risk factors for mental functioning, based on the Ontario Longitudinal Study of Aging (LSA), V: comparison of the results, relevant to aluminum water concentrations, obtained from the LSA and from death certificates mentioning dementia. Can J Aging 1955; 14:642–656.
48. Munoz-Garcia D, Pendlebury WW, Kessler JB, Perl DP. An immunocytochemical comparison of cytoskeletal proteins in aluminum-induced and Alzheimer-type neurofibrillary tangles. Acta Neuropathol (Berl) 1986; 70:243–248.
49. Forster DP, Newens M, Kay DW, Edwardson JA. Risk factors in clinically diagnosed presenile dementia of the Alzheimer type: a case–control study in northern England. J Epidemiol Commun Health 1995; 49:253–258.
50. The Canadian Study of Health and Aging: risk factors for Alzheimer's disease in Canada. Neurology 1994; 44:2073–2080.
51. Graves AB, White E, Koepsell TD, Reifler BV, van Belle G, Larson EB. The association between aluminum-containing products and Alzheimer's disease. J Clin Epidemiol 1990; 43:35–44.
52. Flaten TP, Glattre E, Viste A, Sooreide O. Mortality from dementia among gastroduodenal ulcer patients. J Epidemiol Commun Health 1991; 45:203–206.
53. Colin-Jones D, Langman MJ, Lawson DH, Vesley MP. Alzheimer's disease in antacid users. Lancet 1989; 1:1453.
54. Brown MS, Stemmer SM, Simon JH, Stears JC, Jones RB, Cagnoni PJ, Sheeder JL. White matter disease induced by high-dose chemotherapy: longitudinal study with MR imaging and proton spectroscopy. Am J Neuroradiol 1998; 19(2):395–396.
55. Heckbert SR, Longstreth WT, Psaty BM, Murros KE, Smith NL, Newman AB, Williamson JD, Bernick C, Furberg CD. The association of antihypertensive agents with MRI white matter findings and with modified mini-mental state examination in older adults. JAGS 1997; 45:1423–1433.
56. Mackenzie IRA, Munoz DG. Nonsteroidal anti-inflammatory drug use and Alzheimer-type pathology in aging. Neurology 1998; 50:986–990.
57. Ray WA, Federspiel CF, Schaffer W. A study of antipsychotic drug use in nursing homes: epidemiologic evidence suggesting misuse. Am J Public Health 1980; 70:485–491.
58. Avorn J, Dreyer P, Connelly K, Soumerai SB. Use of psychoactive medication and the quality of care in rest homes: findings and policy implications for a statewide study. N Engl J Med 1989; 320:227–232.
59. Beers MH, Ouslander JG, Fingold SF, Morgenstern H, Reuben DB, Rogers W, Zeffren MJ, Beck JC. Inappropriate medication prescribing in skilled-nursing facilities. Ann Intern Med 1992; 117:684–689.

24. Forensic Neuropathology

JAN E. LEESTMA

Medical–legal issues associated with aging that have been recognized and addressed to some degree are end-of-life disease management and the hospice movement; assisted suicide and euthanasia issues; the problem of the elderly demented individual and competence to manage affairs; elder abuse and neglect; motor vehicle operation and licensure; right of access and special needs and vulnerabilities of the aged individual; and medical malpractice arising out of failure to diagnose and appropriately treat a patient, delays in diagnosis, misdiagnosis and mistreatment, and neglect and negligence. In recent years, issues of forensic importance have arisen in connection with virtually all of these categories, often involving pathologists and neuropathologists.

PHYSICAL INJURY AND THE AGING BRAIN

While the bulk of cranial trauma occurs in the young from vehicular and pedestrian accidents or violence, most cranial trauma incidents in the elderly are accidental and occur at the rate of about 200 cases per 100,000 population, or about one-third the prevalence rate for individuals between 10 and 30 years of age.[1] Accepted as a part of aging are diminished physical strength and endurance, lessened coordination and balance, tremor and/or rigidity, circulatory and cardiovascular deficits; sensory deficits (vision, hearing, attention, position sense), and cognitive impairments that alone or in combination can predispose that individual to increased likelihood of physical injury by accidental means. Commonly elderly individuals are subjected to polypharmacy, and reactions to medications can contribute to the spectrum of medical problems they already face. Drug reactions due to an underdose or overdose or during interactions may also contribute to or cause neurological symptoms and pathology.

The most common form of accidental injury to affect the elderly person is a fall,[2] which most likely occurrs at home and then most commonly on a stairway or in the bathroom. Sometimes even minor falls or bumps have major consequences for the individual, perhaps setting into motion a subdural hematoma that may or may not be discovered and appropriately treated. More severe impacts may cause brain contusions and diffuse traumatic lesions that may have profound clinical and functional consequences. The legacy of old brain injury in the elderly is significant—those who have suffered serious head injury when younger have a shortened life span and seem to suffer from more cerebrovascular disease and its complications than those who have no history of head trauma in the past.[3] Frequently, falls mark the beginning of the end for the afflicted elderly individual because of medical complications and the underlying fragile state of health. There are ample opportunities for medical–legal interplay in relation to the cause, detection, treatment, and consequences of head trauma in the elderly and the effects of prior head injury on longevity and quality of life.

Scalp and Skin Injuries

The skin as well as the scalp in the aged individual is often thinner and more delicate than in younger individuals, thus it is more likely to bruise and show injury. Since the scalp is a major protective barrier for the underlying skull and brain, absorbing up to 90% of kinetic energy from blow-type impacts, atrophy of this structure deprives the aged individual of a significant element of protection from brain injury.[4] Furthermore, from a forensic point of view, interpretations of scalp and facial skin injuries in the elderly require more discrimination than such interpretations in younger individuals, because of to the fragility of the elderly skin and its propensity to make superficial injuries look worse than they are, implying that their cause had to have been due to more physical force than was actually involved. It is vital to interpret superficial physical injuries to the skin in light of the individual's medication history (specifically anticoagulants), medical treatment, circumstances, and behavior and in terms of the chronology of events. All of these secondary issues can cause or modify the appearances of skin lesions and may cause erroneous interpretations that may have important forensic or legal consequences.

As in other contexts, caution should be exercised in attempting to precisely age and date skin bruises on the basis of their color;[5,6] contrary to one's intuition, this is not a simple matter. By the same token, microscopic examination of skin bruises is also anything but an exact science. The presence or absence of a so-called vital reaction may be difficult to ascertain, and there is a tendency to think that skin bruises are more superficial in the integument than they actually are. Furthermore, there appear to be significant variances among individuals with respect to the rapidity and degree of leukocyte responses to physical injury in the skin. At autopsy, proper documentation by photography makes later interpretation possible and provides the opportunity for demonstrative evidence in court. When specific pattern injuries are found, it may be quite useful to examine scene photographs and/or the actual scene environment in an effort to match up objects that could have produced the pattern injuries. Such correlations may provide valuable information to investigating officials in the case of criminal investigations.

Epidural Hematoma

Epidural hematomas in adults are usually the result of head trauma, most often with an associated skull fracture (85% of cases).[7] Conversely, about 25% of skull fractures and about 10% of major cases of closed head trauma are attended by an epidural hematoma. The branches of the middle meningeal arteries are easily sheared or avulsed when there has been significant in-bending of the skull with or without skull fracture. Bleeding from an injured meningeal artery may be brisk and lead to rapid accumulation of a hematoma that may compress the brain faster than cerebrospinal fluid (CSF) can be absorbed. This may lead to rapid development of unconsciousness and brain stem herniation, Duret hemorrhages, coma, and death.[8] When bleeding is episodic or partially tamponaded, the evolution of the epidural hematoma may progress more leisurely, permitting gradual accommodation and an increased likelihood for clinical detection and intervention.[9] Delayed or "latent" epidural hematomas may present significant forensic issues.[10–13] These arise out of superficial or hurried, apparently normal examinations of elderly head injury victims in emergency rooms, followed by no period of observation or inadequate instructions to caregivers or the patient regarding important symptoms that may signal the need for immediate medical consultation. When epidural hematomas resolve, they are converted into dense connective tissue that may become mineralized or contain bone.

Subdural Hematoma

In the young individual, the greatest percentage of subdural hematomas is associated with an obvious traumatic physical event (e.g., motor vehicle accident, violence); in the elderly, this association is much less certain (possibly <50%).[14] Often in retrospect, a history of minimal trauma is obtained and can consist of a minor fall in the home or out of doors; a minor traffic accident; a minor scuffle or altercation; a history of severe coughing, perhaps associated with a cold or asthma attack; or a history of constipation and straining at stool. Because of the prevalence of cerebral atrophy in the elderly patient, subdural hematomas in this group tend to be five times larger at discovery than in younger persons.[2] Thus an important issue for elderly individuals who are taking anticoagulant medication is the risk of subdural hemorrhage, where even minor trauma may lead to a fatal hemorrhage. There appears to be a predilection in such cases for midline/falcian subdural hemorrhage.[15] Immediate symptoms of a subdural hematoma may be entirely absent and may be misinterpreted or missed clinically and not interpreted by the affected individual as a serious problem, to their peril.

ACUTE SUBDURAL HEMATOMA

Individuals who suffer subdural hemorrhage, regardless of age, experience one of the following clinical scenarios: (1) unconscious throughout (17%); (2) unconscious to lucid (12%); (3) unconscious to lucid to unconscious (13%) (4) conscious throughout (29%); (5) lucid to unconscious (17%).[16] It is likely that the fourth scenario will assume greater importance in an elderly population than in a younger one. It has been estimated that as many as 20% of victims of subdural hematomas die undiagnosed.[11] A leading confusional factor is the role of drugs and alcohol that may give the false impression that the victim is intoxicated.

From a forensic point of view, when subdural hematomas are evacuated, it is very useful that the material removed be sent for pathological and histological examination and that the intraoperative appearance of the clot be described in the operative note for later reference, should questions arise about aging and dating of the lesion. If the hematoma is discovered at autopsy, it should be standard practice, that photographs be taken and that the entire cranial dura be stripped and fixed before sectioning, and that topography of the hematoma be documented by diagrams or drawings.

SUBACUTE SUBDURAL HEMATOMA

A unique phenomenon of blood clots that form in the subdural compartment is that they have a time course of reaction and resolution that occurs nowhere else in the body. This process was recognized and and described in detail by Munro and Merritt in the 1930s.[17,18] This seminal work, a histological study of 105 cases of subdural hemorrhages in adults, the ages of which were documented, has formed the basis for histological aging and dating of subdural hematomas ever since. Comparatively little of consequence has been added to these data over the past 60 years. The scheme described by Munro and Merritt is illustrated in chart form[14] in Table 24-1.

Because there are fibrinolytic and thrombolytic factors as well as inflammatory mediators in the clot, the tiny organizing capillaries bleed spontaneously, adding a new, acute component to the clot to in effect start the process all over again, repeatedly.[19,20] This process causes expansion of the original clot and increases its mass effect, sometimes rapidly, with clinical consequences. At one time it was thought that subdural hematomas expanded because of osmotic pressures within the clot compartment, but studies have shown that hematoma fluid is isosmolar and that the capillary re-bleed phenomenon is most likely the generative force behind expansion.[19]

It bears repeating that along with all phases of hematoma healing and red cell lysis that fresh, intact red cells may be admixed with any or all components of the hematoma. This fact is often misunderstood or is confusing to lay people such as jurors or attorneys and even to some pathologists who may not have fully conceptualized the dynamic character of the hematoma.

CHRONIC SUBDURAL HEMATOMA

As discussed above, by common clinical and pathological usage, a chronic subdural hematoma is one that has been in existence 2 to 3 weeks and thus is completely enclosed by neomembranes. These are hematomas that have passed through the acute and the subacute phases, often without detection, only to declare themselves at some temporal distance from the event that caused them, which may have been trivial or unappreciated. While there are cases that have gone on for many months or even years, chronic subdural hematomas are usually detected before 3 months have elapsed from inception. From a symptomatic point of view, the elderly, patient with

Table 24–1. Aging and Dating of Subdural Hematomas

Interval	Clot	Dural Side	Arachnoid Side
24 hr	Intact RBCs	Thin-layer fibrin	Thin layer fibrin
36 hr	Intact RBCs	Early fibroblastic activity	Thin layer fibrin
4 days	Loss of RBC sharp contour and variability of staining	2–4 layers of fibroblasts	Thin layer fibrin
5 days	Loss of RBC sharp contour and variability of staining	3–5 layers of fibroblasts; first siderophages appear at edges of the clot	Thin layer fibrin
7–8 days	Laked RBCs, clot liquefies, fibroblasts enter clot	12–14 layers of fibroblasts; neomembrane visible grossly when clot scraped away	Thin layer fibrin
11 days	Broken up into islands by capillaries and fibroblasts and thick strands of fibrin	Fibroblasts migrate around the edges of the clot	Siderophages are visible on arachnoid side
15–17 days	Most original RBCs lysed; capillary formation obvious	Membrane ½ to ⅓ dural thickness	Variably thin, earliest complete neomembrane; clot may be completely enveloped
18–26 days	Clot completely liquefied, larger vessels permeate clot	Membrane same thickness as dura; siderophages in membranes	Membrane up to ½ dural thickness; siderophages in membranes
27–36 days	Large capillaries	Well-formed membrane	Well-formed membrane
1–3 months	Giant capillaries, secondary bleeding and fresh RBCs	Hyalinization of membranes, less cellular, more collagen	Hyalinization of membranes, less cellular, more collagen; nearly thickness of dura
3–6 months	No original RBCs and only focal re-bleeding	Hyalinized neomembrane	Hyalinized neomembrane
>1 year	No RBCs	Resembles dura	Resembles dura

Source: RBC, red blood cell. Compiled from data collected and compiled by Munro and Merritt[17,18] and previously published.[14] Used with permission.

chronic subdural hematoma may show few if any symptoms that suggest the lesion. Symptoms are often subtle and slowly evolving and are often mistaken for something else. Imaging studies are often dramatic. The medical–legal issue here is that often no imaging or follow-up studies have been performed for various reasons, leading to a missed therapeutic opportunity. Often, when a subdural hematoma is eventually discovered and treated, there are sequelae that can compromise the individual and render him or her incapable of resuming whatever life standard had been enjoyed previously. The medical–legal issues arising out of these circumstances often lead to litigation and large financial settlements or judgments.

Subarachnoid Hemorrhage

Subarachnoid hemorrhage is a relatively common finding in autopsies performed at a medical examiner's or coroner's facility. It is important to divide such cases into those in which trauma is suspected and those in which bleeding appears to have been spontaneous (or without known cause).

SPONTANEOUS SUBARACHNOID HEMORRHAGE

According to a large study on subarachnoid hemorrhage, Locksley[21] reported that 22% of subarachnoid hemorrhage cases occurred in individuals over the age of 60 years. With respect to etiology, 27% of subarachnoid hemorrhages in the over 60 age-group were due to bleeding from aneurysms, 7% were due to bleeding vascular anomalies (usually arteriovenous malformations), and 38% were due to other lesions, chiefly hypertensive hemorrhages but including a very long list of other etiologies. These can include hemorrhage from neoplasms, vasculitis, amyloid vascular disease, bleeding disorders, drug reactions, or infections. In spontaneous, nonfatal subarachnoid hemorrhage cases, with all ages combined, no obvious source for the hemorrhage could be found in up to 25% of cases. This troublesome group of cases is also encountered among the elderly.

A common forensic issue, relative to ruptured cerebral aneurysms, is the possible or probable linkage to some external circumstance or event. Typical situations include being the victim of an assault or vehicular, workplace, or other trauma; suffering a stressful situation without physical injury such as a robbery or mugging; and undergoing medical or surgical treatment or anticoagulant medication and then suffering a rupture of a cerebral aneurysm. Correlation of aneurysm rupture with such events to a reasonable degree of medical certainty, the standard that must be applied in a forensic situation for a medical expert, is always difficult and may be impossible. Historical information may be helpful regarding previous symptoms, and pathological study of the aneurysm may provide information about possible recent or past pathological reactions in the aneurysm or the tissue around it that could have been exacerbated by some recent event.

Analysis of the circumstances of rupture in a series of more than 2000 aneurysm cases has shown that 36% of aneurysm ruptures occurred during sleep; 12% occurred during bending, lifting, or stooping; 4.4% occurred during emotional stress or strain; 8.4% occurred during presumed Valsalva maneuver (straining at stool, coughing, urinating); 3.8% occurred during coitus; 2.8% were associated with an episode of physical trauma; fewer than 1% occurred during childbirth; and 32% of cases had no known special circumstance associated with rupture.[21] These data are helpful but hardly definitive in the forensic arena. Other circumstances of life style modes that may be related to higher-than-expected incidences of aneurysm rupture include heavy alcohol use; those who abuse alcohol may experience twice the rate of aneurysm rupture as a nondrinking population.[22] Cigarette smoking in both males and females raises the risk for aneurysm rupture by a factor of nearly 4 over the nonsmoking control population.[23] Cocaine use has also been known to be associated with fatal aneurysm rupture.[24,25]

Central Nervous System Hemorrhage

All forms of hemorrhages into the substance of brain, brain stem, cerebellum, and spinal cord occur in the elderly. In many cases, there are no special characteristics or issues regarding these hemorrhages that are particularly relevant or restricted to the elderly. The situations discussed below are those that do or may have relevance to the elderly, especially in a forensic sense.

"HYPERTENSIVE" INTRACEREBRAL HEMORRHAGE

Intracerebral hemorrhage (hemorrhage into the brain itself) occurs in about 10% of all strokes, with most of the victims being older than 50 years of age.[26] Furthermore, the incidence of intracerebral hemorrhage rises dramatically with advancing age, from about 17/100,000 population at age 50–59 to 350/100,000 by age 80.[27] The major causative factor is hypertension, which, by age 85, is present or was present historically in up to 89% of cases in some series, but is considerably less prevalent in other series, with as low as 26% of cases having a clinical history of hypertension.[27–29] Sometimes it is an important forensic and medical–legal issue in cases of so-called hypertensive intracerebral hemorrhage, regardless of whether the victim was actually clinically hypertensive or not, since even good clinical records may indicate no significant departure from normal blood pressure readings. It seems likely that allegedly normotensive individuals may actually have hypertension with a pattern that does not declare itself by usual measures[30] but may reflect its presence by collateral pathology at autopsy, such as increased heart weight and histological evidence of renal pathology.[31]

Not infrequently, an elderly individual may be the victim of an assault (robbery, burglary, sexual assault/rape, altercation) and later suffer a cerebral hemorrhage or other form of stroke. Naturally, the antecedent event is often implicated and may have forensic importance. Just as stress can play a role in rupture of cerebral aneurysms,[32] intracerebral hemorrhage has been linked to similar antecedent events, even in apparently normotensive individuals, but only in about 10% of cases.[30,33] The mechanism often invoked is elevated blood pressure, probably associated with catecholamine release. There are no reliable pathological means of definitively establishing a link between stress and subsequent stroke, except that underlying vascular disease pathology may represent fertile soil for complications with an external event and aggravating circumstances may represent a logical causative event. Expert opinions on such difficult matters inevitably rest upon the individual's experience, accompanying and collateral evidence, and sound judgment.

A major medication-related form of intracerebral hemorrhage, especially in the elderly, is anticoagulant-related hemorrhage. Since a larger percentage of anticoagulated individuals are elderly and attention to drug compliance and laboratory follow-up of coagulation status may be spotty, this population is inherently at risk. When these risk factors are coupled with a high incidence of falling and other forms of accident-related trauma, this problem becomes a major one. Another factor that has forensic significance is the tendency of anticoagulant-related brain hemorrhages to evolve in a subtle fashion, with waxing and waning of symptoms and signs, sometimes over many hours or even days,[30,34] before deterioration occurs. This situation provides ample opportunity for misdiagnosis, delays in treatment, and horrific clinical outcomes. It goes without saying that individuals who are anticoagulated and are the victims of assaults or accidents may suffer brain hemorrhages that they might not otherwise have suffered.

Delayed Post-traumatic Cerebral Hemorrhage

This phenomenon, first noted by Bollinger in 1891,[35] was described then and now as a sudden hemorrhage into the substance of the brain, hours, days, or even weeks or longer after a head injury, often with a fatal result in individuals who otherwise had few if any symptoms or underlying disease processes.[36] A number of case reports and series, reviewed by Cooper,[37–39] take into account the vastly improved detection of such lesions by newer imaging studies that may show small hemorrhagic lesions that would otherwise never have been detected. Fukamachi et al.[40] have developed the following classification for traumatic intracranial hemorrhages: type I, hematomas present on initial imaging studies but which decreased in size with time; type II, small or medium-sized hematomas that increased in size on later examinations; type III, hematomas that developed in previously clear areas; and type IV, hematomas that developed from or in connection with cortical contusions. These authors have coined the acronym DTICH (Delayed Traumatic Intracerebral Hematoma) to apply to the latter two types of lesions.[40,41]

The incidence of the DTICH phenomenon (a new hemorrhagic lesion) appears to be highly variable, ranging from 50% to <1% of head-injured individuals. Lipper et al.[42] estimate that about 16% of severely head-injured patients will develop DTICH. It most likely occurs in individuals who have some other form of intracerebral traumatic lesion and is rather rare in individuals having no obvious imaging study evidence of an intracerebral lesion. The degree of delay in the development of DTICH is usually <48 hr after injury, but instances of DTICH (usually prescanning period) have been alleged even months after injury.[43] The location of most DTICH lesions is subcortical and probably usually in association with a cortical contusion rather than a more deeply seated lesion. The cause of such lesions is not known but may involve subtle or field effects of nearby injury to vessels that takes many hours to develop, vascular autoregulation dysfunction, regional ischemia and vasospasm with necrosis, disorders of coagulation,[44] and other factors.[39] Mortality is variable and may reach 75%, but probably averages about 50%.[37,38]

Traumatic Intraventricular Hemorrhage

Intraventricular hemorrhage can occur in conjunction with any form of major head trauma but is uncommon in the absence of significant associated traumatic lesions in the brain. Occasionally, one can encounter cases in which there is little or no or minimal external or internal evidence of head trauma (contusions), yet the individual has a fatal intraventricular and subarachnoid hemorrhage. Such lesions are not confined to any particular age-group, but they do affect the elderly in some special circumstances.

The typical situation involves an individual who may be found in extremis beside the roadway, in a pedestrian walkway, in bed, or in a care facility (in the case of elderly victims). Histories are often vague but can include being tangentially struck by a car or truck, bicycle, or roller board, or by a skater, or being slapped or cuffed on the side of the head. The elderly may be particularly vulnerable to these incidents because of their walking on pathways favored by young cyclists, skate boarders, roller blade skaters, and runners who may be oblivious of others or act out their rage by side-swiping a vulnerable elderly pedestrian. Furthermore, slapping and cuffing of elderly and demented patients in care facilities by attendants may also give rise to such lesions.

While there may be bruising or some other sign of skin injury (especially if motor vehicles were involved), there is usually a subgaleal hemorrhage present. There may or may not be a skull fracture and there may or may not be any sign of cerebral contusion. The cerebral ventricles are usually filled with blood and there is usually an extensive subarachnoid hemorrhage. The site of origin of the hemorrhage usually appears to be at the root of the choroid plexus/tela choroidea, the septum pellucidum/fornix region. Here, avulsion of one or more of the previous structures may be seen.[14,45] The likely mechanism is that of a tangential application of force to the head that results in shearing or torsional forces in the middle of the brain that are sufficient to tear off the root of the choroid plexus or nearby structures, causing rapid and fatal bleeding.

Avulsion Injuries of Cerebral Vessels

Occasionally, one is faced with a victim who has no or minimal evidence of external or internal trauma, yet has a diffuse, subarachnoid hemorrhage with no obvious source. These cases pose a major challenge to the neuropathologist or forensic pathologist since, unless great care and expertise are exercised, the source of such bleeding can easily be missed. In rare instances a small rent or actual avulsion of one or more vessels at the base of the brain can be demonstrated. This issue has been exhaustively reported upon and reviewed by Krauland,[46] few other authors have devoted themselves to this problem. In fairness, it is extremely difficult to demonstrate conclusively a vascular avulsion in and around the circle of Willis at autopsy, as there is always the possibility that removal artifact was responsible for any loose vessel found. However, in the absence of an aneurysm or other cause for subarachnoid hemorrhage, vessel avulsion should be considered. Vessel avulsion may occur in conjunction with virtually any form of head injury but seems to occur most often in fist fights in which a forceful lateral punch results in torsion of the head or in other instances in which rotation of the head occurs. In the elderly individual, vessels may have a longer course or may be damaged or weakened by atherosclerosis compared to in younger persons, making older people more vulnerable to this form of injury, rare though it may be.

BRAIN CONTUSIONS

Coup Contusions

Coup contusions are classically thought of as those brain injuries that occur beneath or otherwise topographically proximate to the major axis of force in impacts to the cranium caused by blows. Generally for a coup contusion to occur, objects of sufficient mass and velocity to in-bend and/or fracture the skull are required.[47] The consequence of in-bending upon the brain is probably minimal; rather, it is likely the rebound out-bending of the skull that produces a momentary drastic decrease in ambient hydrostatic pressure, causing water in CSF and blood vessels to cavitate (enter gaseous phase) and damage neural parenchyma and capillaries.

Coup contusions are generally thought to occur from blows that tend not to accelerate the head to a sufficient degree so as to induce contracoup contusions. Thus, they can occur in the immobile head from in-bending of the overlying skull. Since the degree to which the skull is in-bent is a function of the force transmitted to it, overlying structures and materials that absorb or dissipate energy are added variables to be considered in any given case. Part of the forensic analysis in alleged blow cases is to determine if there are epidermal pattern injuries that might be correlated with possible objects employed in the blow.[14] While objects are routinely looked for in blow-contusion cases, extremely forceful blows with a fist may rarely produce coup-type contusions.

Contracoup Contusions

Contracoup contusions arise as a consequence of accelerative trauma to the cranium in which the major brain injury occurs 180° away from the impact site. The etiology of contracoup contusions is still subject to controversy even after more than 200 years of discussion and experiments.[14,48] The most likely scenario for this seemingly counterintuitive phenomenon is as follows: on impact, the moving head and brain come together at the impacting surface to produce a spike of positive and then damped oscillations (negative and positive) in the ambient hydrostatic pressure that may be insufficient to damage the brain in an obvious way in that location, but on the opposite side of the cranium, the impact produces an initial, pronounced, negative pressure spike, again followed by damped oscillations in pressure. The internal ambient pressure is transiently low enough that local water, deprived of forces that keep it in liquid form at body temperature, momentarily vaporizes (cavitate) distending small capillaries, momentarily swelling neural parenchyma that subsequently damages the blood–brain barrier and capillary integrity. This leads to edema, hemorrhage, and ultimately, necrosis.

The clinical effect of contracoup contusion injuries is highly variable and rests not so much on the mere presence of contracoup lesions but on associated injuries deep in the brain, often referred to as "diffuse axonal injury" or "inner cerebral trauma."[47] The clinical and, potentially, the forensic importance of these observations is that certain individuals may suffer head injuries that appear less severe than they ultimately turn out to be. An instance that occurs very frequently and often involves an elderly person is as follows: a disheveled male presents to an emergency room smelling of ethanol and reportedly having either fallen or been assaulted. The victim may have gotten to the care facility under his own power or been brought there by police. There may be signs of facial or scalp injury, and the victim is semicoherent and apparently drunk. An imaging study may or may not be performed and interpreted as normal, and the patient is released or leaves the facility on his own, perhaps against medical advice, only to return some hours later moribund. When imaging studies are again performed, extensive contracoup contusions with or without subdural hematomas are found, or these same lesions are noted at autopsy.

Always at issue is the possibility of additional trauma, which may not ever be resolved; yet the conundrum here is, how could this individual who apparently injured his brain and eventually showed evidence of contracoup contusions (usually of the frontal lobes) have been conscious and able to leave with the observed degree of brain pathology that ultimately proved fatal? This phenomenon has been described by others as the "talk-and-die syndrome" (TADS).[49–52] Such cases illustrate the dynamic and multifaceted character of traumatic brain injuries, where one or more processes evolving independently of each other ultimately produce sufficient mass effect through edema and hemorrhage as well as alterations of cerebral blood flow and other intracranial processes to cause decompensation and death. The medical–legal and forensic implications of TADS are significant: what happened, and who is or could be responsible for the outcome? There is no simple pathway toward truth in such cases; only careful analysis of what is known can shed light on the circumstances and help determine the pathology.

Fracture Contusions

When the skull is fractured, it may simply split when its elastic limit has been exceeded, or the edges of the fracture, especially in cases of complex fractures, may vibrate or see-saw onto the brain surface, directly traumatizing it. This may produce a contusion on the brain that follows the fracture lines. Fracture contusions of the upper portion of the cerebrum may certainly occur but are not commonly seen at autopsy. Basilar skull fractures, possibly because of the greater forces involved in producing them than those producing a simple linear parietal fracture, are very prone to produce obvious and sometimes extensive contusions of the brain and in cerebellum when the fracture lines pass through the posterior fossa.[14,53] The temporal evolution of fracture contusions is probably not dissimilar from that of coup or contracoup contusions.

"Gliding" Contusions

As previously defined, gliding contusions occur primarily at the base of the brain in major accelerative head trauma due usually to falls or high-velocity impacts. The mechanism of these contusions is said to arise from the brain gliding or sweeping back and forth over bony ridges during the course of the impact(s). Precisely how this occurs biomechanically is not clear. Nevertheless, such contusions may be seen separate from contracoup or other forms of contusions in severe head trauma but may also be seen blending into them.

BRAIN STEM INJURY

In the same way that a pedestrian may be side-swiped or struck under circumstances that can produce traumatic intraventricular hemorrhages, an impact may be more directly posterior such that the individual suffers a high G-force whip-lash to the head and neck. Under these circumstances, which usually involve rear impacts by motor vehicles to pedestrians but can involve the driver or passenger in a motor vehicle struck from behind, a collective of typical injuries may be seen. These include an avulsion injury of the pontomedullar junction, cervical-medullary junction, with or without associated ring fractures of the base of the skull, and fracture-subluxations of the upper cervical spine. In rare instances, while attempting to restrain struggling and disoriented patients, attendants have caused hyperextension injuries to the cervical region that have resulted in pontomedullary avulsions. Most instances of pontomedullary avulsion are immediately fatal, probably due to immediate respiratory paralysis and/or brain stem neural shock.[14,54] However, occasional victims have survived 'stretch' injuries of the pontomedullary junction for varying periods of time.[55] Pathologically these injuries appear as a complete or partial avulsion of the medulla from the pons at their junction. There is usually some degree of subarachnoid and fourth ventricular bleeding present, which differentiates such an avulsion from an accidental separation during brain removal.

SPINAL CORD HEMORRHAGE/INJURY

Spinal cord injuries can occur at any age but are most common in individuals under 40 years of age. In the elderly the causes of spinal cord injury are most often due to falls, assaults, vehicular accidents, or therapeutic misadventures, rather than to swimming or diving or motorcycle and sports-related accidents more prevalent among the young.

Traumatic spinal cord injury may or may not be associated with spinal fractures, regardless of etiology. Very commonly, especially when the patient may be or appear to be intoxicated and traumatized, spinal fracture with or without spinal cord trauma may be missed in emergency room situations, with varying consequences in up to 30% of cases.[56] Though it might seem hard to understand how a spinal cord-injury could be missed, spinal cord injured patients may appear to have had a stroke or be hemiplegic or paretic due to supposed intracranial pathology rather than intraspinal pathology,[56] such as a Brown-Sequard syndrome. At issue is often the allegation of failure to diagnose and properly treat such patients and the consequences of such alleged lapses. Individuals who are frequently targets of such professional misjudgments often include emergency medical technicians, ambulance attendants, first aid workers, and emergency room physicians and personnel. Also, even though an individual initially appears to have no neurological injury, frequently instability of the spine due to fracture and/or ligamentous injuries, may later lead to spinal cord injury—particularly in cervical injury scenarios but also in the lower spine where myelopathy may be missed, and thus a window of opportunity for therapeutic intervention may likewise have passed.

Therapeutic misadventures may also lead to or directly cause spinal cord injuries. These include vigorous or ill-considered chiropractic manipulations and related procedures,[57–60] and malpositioning of needles or catheters in the spine for the treatment of pain or for radiological imaging so that these instruments actually penetrate into the spinal cord. Injuries to the spinal cord can also occur through excessive force in intubation during anesthesia (hyperextension of the neck); malpositioning for surgery; vascular injury due to positioning or manipulation; and as a consequence of surgery in the neck, cervical, thoracic, or lumbar spine or intrathoracic or intrabdominal surgery.[61] These latter occurrences may damage the spinal cord by interfering with radicular arterial blood flow producing infarction of the cord, by obstruction and/or dissecting injuries to vertebral arteries and their end-vessel territories, may also cause myelopathy.[57]

While allegedly common during abuse in infancy, whiplash–shaking also can occur among adults[62] and the elderly, sometimes with a fatal result. Reported instances are rare but they can occur. An elderly, perhaps weakened and debilitated or demented individual may so frustrate caregivers that, in what seems to be an unthinking response, the victim may be shaken with sufficient force that either cervical spine/cord or vessel injuries may result in addition to subdural hematomas. The pathology of such shaking–whiplash trauma is not unexpected: soft tissue injury to the muscles and ligaments of the cervical region; epidural and/or subdural hematomas of the cervical region; subdural hematomas; and associated injuries (scalp hematoma and skull fracture when impacts are involved). It is not known if retinal hemorrhages are found under such circumstances, for no pathological studies speak to this point. In addition to the above injuries, there may be associated grip mark bruising and hemorrhage of upper extremities and shoulders, and/or there may be signs of gripping of the neck with underlying stigmata of strangulation (strap muscle and anterior neck soft tissue hemorrhage, and hyoid bone and/or thyroid cartilage fracture).

CASE REPORT: Case 1

An 81-year-old female with severe dementia attributed to Alzheimer's disease had been a resident of a nursing home. Her past medical history included falls with various injuries and a history of seizures attributed to a small falcian meningioma for which she was receiving phenytoin. She was diabetic and had cardiovascular disease as well. Because of her propensity to fall and her disoriented state, physician orders had been placed for side rails to be installed on her bed. This order was not carried out. The patient fell from her bed one afternoon, striking her head. She sustained bruises and a laceration to the left side of her forehead and was transported to a hospital emergency room for evaluation and treatment. Upon admission, the patient was conscious but agitated. A CT scan (Fig. 24–1) was performed that showed soft tissue injury to the left forehead but no skull fracture or other acute process. Her forehead laceration was sutured and bandaged and she was returned to the nursing home, again with instructions for side rails to be placed on her bed.

A few hours later the patient fell again from her bed, striking her head in the same location as before. She was found unconscious beside her bed by an aide. No side rails had been placed on her bed. Following her return from the hospital the first time she had been conscious and showed no change in neurological status. Upon admission to the hospital the second time, the patient was unconscious and was placed on a ventilator. Another CT scan (Fig. 24–2) was performed that showed a large intracerebral hemorrhage in the right parietal and basal temporal region as well as a thin, acute subdural hematoma on the right side and midline shift was noted. Clinical assessment by a neurosurgical consultant indicated that brain stem reflexes were absent and that her prognosis was poor; after several hours, life support was terminated.

An autopsy was performed that revealed multiple contusions (Fig. 24–3) primarily to the left side of the face and forehead. There were soft tissue injuries to the right hand as well. There were scalp

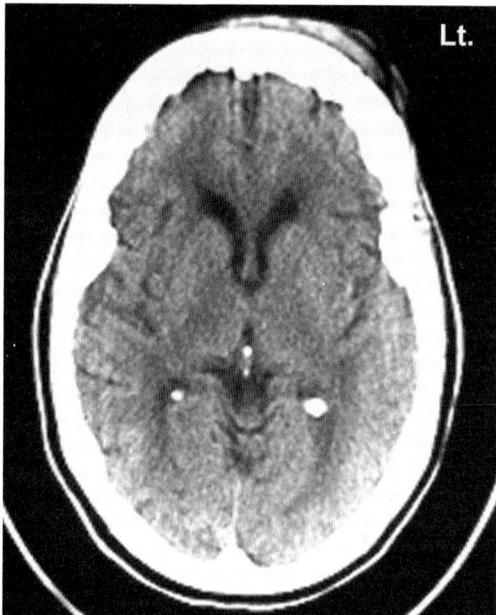

Figure 24–1. Case 1. This CT image was taken at the first hospital admission after a fall from bed by an 81-year-old woman in a nursing home. No obvious injury is noted other than a soft tissue density in the left frontal region.

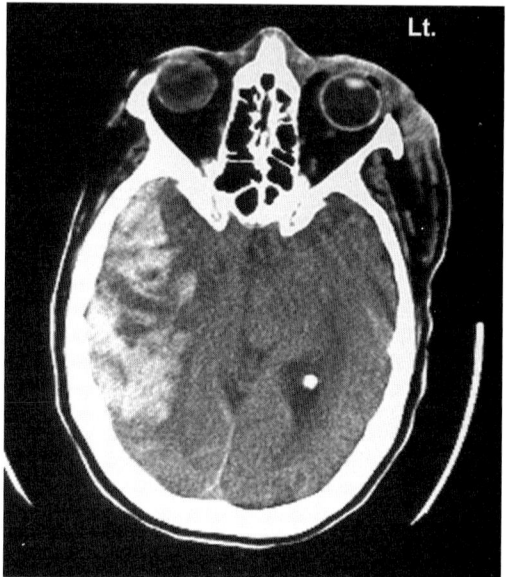

Figure 24–2. Case 1. This CT image was taken several hours after the first hospital admission following a second fall from bed resulting in unconsciousness in the same patient. Note the extensive cortical and subcortical density on the right side of the brain with midline shift and a thin density of the falx that may represent an early subdural hematoma. There is a pronounced soft tissue density in the left frontal region as well.

hemorrhages in the left frontal and anterior parietal regions. No skull fractures were noted. The brain weighed 1260 g. The brain was swollen and there was a large area of hemorrhage on the right side of the brain and right temporal region that was said to extend into the basal ganglia. Brain vessels appeared free of atheromata. There was an incidental meningioma along the falx that was 2.5 × 1.0 cm. Microscopic examination of the brain showed a moderate degree of lacunar state and numerous senile plaques throughout the cortex. Some penetrating arterioles in the cortex may have been affected with amyloid deposits (Fig. 24–4)

The issue in this case posed by the attorneys defending the nursing home was the following: was this woman's intracerebral hemorrhage due to her falling out of bed or was it a spontaneous intracerebral hemorrhage due to a stroke or amyloid vasculopathy with the facial trauma incidental?

The author's interpretation, and that sustained by the Court during litigation on the matter was that this woman had injured herself by falling out of bed while disoriented. Despite orders to place side railings on her bed, this was not done. It was determined that had these precautions been exercised, it is more likely than not that she would not have sustained these ultimately fatal injuries.

CASE REPORT: Case 2

A 79-year-old widow lived alone in her home and was assaulted by a burglar. The day following the assault, a physician was notified by friends who examined the woman. She appeared alert and oriented but refused to be extensively examined or taken to the hospital. She had numerous abrasions and bruises on her face from the assault. Six days later, the woman was examined in her home again and found to have a large fungating carcinoma in an area of previous radical mastectomy and to be deteriorating somewhat. She still refused medical treatment. Twenty-five days after the assault she was found dead in her home.

An autopsy revealed multiple metastases from her recurrent breast carcinoma, including one in the dura associated with a right-sided chronic subdural hematoma (Fig. 24–5) with underlying compression and molding of the brain (Fig. 24–6). Controversy developed over the age of the subdural hematoma and its relationship to the assault and the underlying dural metastasis. This was a major issue during the trial of the offender who had been apprehended and charged with felony murder.

FORENSIC ASPECTS OF DEMENTIA

The state of higher brain function in the elderly individual is often a forensic issue that may involve the neuropathologist. Typical circumstances involve assessment of cognition and determination of competence of an individual at a given point in time in relation to that person having executed a legal document such as a will, a deed, bill of sale, or documentation of some other financial transaction. Another instance is evaluation of the competence of an elderly individual who may be accused of a crime of or another act that has harmed another person.

The pathology of dementing illnesses are well known to neuropathologists. It may fall to the neuropathologist to examine the brain of an allegedly affected individual to determine to what degree, at a specific point in time, the individual might or could have been or was (within a reasonable degree of medical certainty) compromised in so far as the individual's capability to make judgments, remember them, and know the limits of their bounty and the significance of their acts. To be sure, this is not the usual task of the neuropathologist, and it may not be possible to comply with a request for this sort of interpretation. Nevertheless, it may be possible for the neuropathologist, given his or her knowledge of the above disease states, to determine the limits of a possible interpretation and to work with others to reconstruct or formulate a matrix of information that may be useful to answer questions of competence. One can easily confront the limits of knowledge regarding the topography of lesions and their functional significance with respect to memory acquisition, storage, and retrieval.[63,64]

Certain technologies and practices have evolved that enable the neuropathologist to delve into the difficult realm of functional–

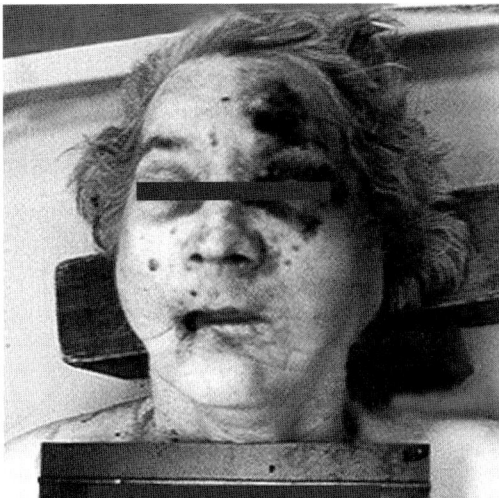

Figure 24–3. Case 1. This photograph was taken at the time of autopsy and shows multiple bruises and abrasions of the left forehead, eyebrow region, and mouth as well as bilateral black eyes that resulted from two falls from bed separated by a few hours in time, prior to final hospitalization and death.

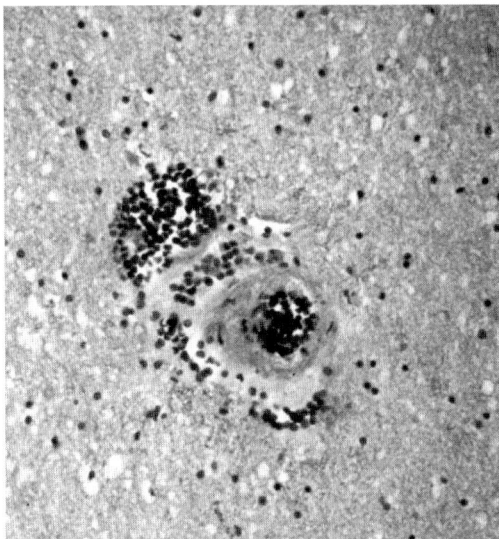

Figure 24–4. Case 1. This H&E–stained section of subcortical white matter showed a perivascular hemorrhage as well some thickened arterioles. Staining for amyloid was equivocal for this and other penetrating cortical vessels. ×160.

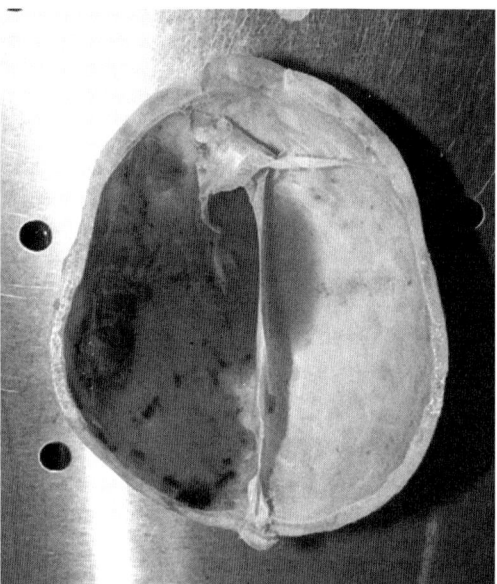

Figure 24–5. Case 2. This view of the interior of the vertex cranial vault shows the dura and falx. On the right side is a large subdural hematoma that originally had a light, chocolate-brown color with obvious membrane formation, and a lumpy more hemorrhagic density laterally that was found to represent a metastasis from a recurrent breast carcinoma.

anatomic correlations if one has the time, interest, and technical support to do so. A great deal of work has been done, chiefly on clinical–pathological correlations in Alzheimer's disease, that is valuable in a forensic sense.[65] The work embodied in the Khachaturian protocol for the neuropathological diagnosis of Alzheimer's disease is typical in this regard.[66] Other related protocols have also been described.[67] The work of Terry and others[68–71] has shown that loss of synapses, primarily between the frontal and parietal cortical regions, correlates significantly with the severity of the dementia in Alzheimer's disease. Using these methods and others that are evolving, one may be able to formulate some sort of severity index of dementia, if one has sufficient brain material to work with and the supporting technologies available. This information can be applied to clinical observations by others regarding the state of the individual at or prior to death, possibly with historical information over a significant time period prior to death, to create a curve of deterioration or functioning for a given individual. Unfortunately, the state of knowledge of the pathological–clinical progression of Alzheimer's disease is poorly understood, since relatively few cases have been studied in which at least one prior tissue sample (brain

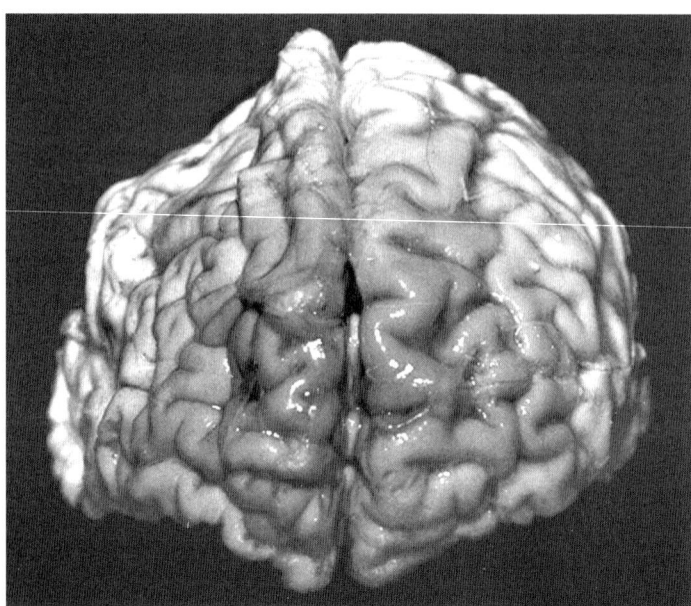

Figure 24–6. Case 2. This frontal view of the brain reveals obvious molding on the right side due to the presence of a chronic subdural hematoma and metastasis shown in Figure 24–5.

biopsy) is comparable to the postmortem specimen, thus there will be inherent limits to interpretation and analysis.

REFERENCES

1. Kraus JF. Epidemiology of head injury. In: Cooper PR, ed. Head Injury, 3rd ed. Baltimore: Williams & Wilkins, 1993:1–25.
2. Howard MA, Gross AS, Dacey RG Jr, Winn HR. Acute subdural hematomas: an age dependent clinical entity. J Neurosurg 1989; 71:858–863.
3. Weiss GH, Caveness WF, Einsiedel-Lechtape H, McNeel ML. Life expectancy and causes of death in a group of head-injured veterans of World War I. Arch Neurol 1982; 39:741–743.
4. Gurdjian ES. Impact Head Injury. Mechanistic, Clinical and Preventive Correlations. Springfield, IL: CC Thomas, 1975.
5. Langlois NEI, Gresham GA. The aging of bruises: a review and study of the colour changes with time. Forensic Sci Int 1991; 50:227–238.
6. Janssen W. Forensic Histopathology. Berlin: Springer-Verlag, 1984:81–97.
7. Kvarnes TL, Trumpy JH. Extradural hematomas: report of 132 cases. Acta Neurochir 1978; 41:223–231.
8. Cordobes F, Lobato RD, Rivas JJ, Munoz MJ, Chillon D, Portillo JM, Lamas E. Observations on 82 patients with extradural hematoma: comparison of results before and after the advent of computerized tomography. J Neurosurg 1981; 54:179–186.
9. Hirsh LF. Chronic epidural hematomas. Neurosurgery 1980; 6:508–512.
10. Borovich B, Braun J, Guilburd JN, Zaaroor M, Michich M, Levy L, Lemberger A, Grushkiewicz I, Feinsod M, Schachter I Delayed onset of traumatic extradural hematoma. J Neurosurg 1985; 63:30–34.
11. Galbraith S, Teasdale G. Misdiagnosis and delayed diagnosis in traumatic subdural hematoma. BMJ 1976; 1:1438–1439.
12. Iwakuma T, Brunngraber CV. Chronic extradural hematomas: a study of 21 cases. J Neurosurg 1973; 38:488–493.
13. Poon WS, Rehman SU, Poon CYF, Li AKC. Traumatic extradural hematoma of delayed onset is not a rarity. Neurosurgery 1992; 30:681–686.
14. Leestma JE. Impact injuries to the brain and head. In: Forensic Neuropathology. New York: Raven Press, 1988:200–222.
15. Houtteville JP, Toumi K, Theron K, Theron J, Derlon JM, Benazza A, Hubert P Interhemispheric subdural haematomas: seven cases and review of the literature. Br J Neurosurg 1988; 2:357–368.
16. Jamieson KG, Yelland JDN. Surgically treated traumatic subdural hematomas. J Neurosurg 1972; 37:137–149.
17. Munro D, the diagnosis and treatment of subdural hematomata. N Engl J Med 1934; 210:1145–1160.
18. Munro D, Merritt HH. Surgical pathology of subdural hematoma. Based on a study of one hundred and five cases. Arch Neurol Psychiatry 1936; 35:64–78.
19. Weir B. The osmolality of subdural hematoma fluid. J Neurosurg 1971; 34:528–533.
20. Weir B, Gordon P. Factors affecting coagulation: fibrinolysis in chronic subdural fluid collections. J Neurosurg 1983; 58:242–245.
21. Locksley HB. Natural history of subarachnoid hemorrhage: intracranial aneurysms and arteriovenous malformations. Based on 6368 cases in the cooperative study. In: Sahs AL, Perret GE, Locksley HB, Nishioka H, eds. Intracranial Aneurysms and Subarachnoid Hemorrhage. A Cooperative Study. Philadelphia: Lippincott, 1969:35–108.
22. Hillbom M, Kaste M. Does alcohol intoxication precipitate aneurysmal subarachnoid haemorrhage? J Neurol Neurosurg Psychiatry 1981; 44:523–526.
23. Bell BA, Symon L. Smoking and subarachnoid haemorrhage. BMJ 1979; 1:577–578.
24. Lundberg GD, Garriott JC, Reynolds PC, Cravey RH, Shaw RF. Cocaine-related death. J Forensic Sci 1977; 22:402–408.
25. Kaufman MJ, Levin J, Ross MH, et al. Cocaine-induced cerebral vasoconstriction detected in humans with magnetic resonance angiography. JAMA 1998; 279:376–380.
26. Kunitz SC, Gross CR, Heyman A, Kase CS, Mohr JP, Price TR, Wolf PA. The pilot study stroke data bank: definition, design and data. Stroke 1984; 15:740–746.
27. Brott T, Thalinger K, Hertzberg V. Hypertension as a risk factor for spontaneous intracerebral hemorrhage. Stroke 1986; 17:1078–1083.
28. Calandre L, Arnal C, Ortega JF, Bermejo. F, Felgeroso B, del Ser T, Vallejo A. Risk factors for spontaneous cerebral hematomas. Case control study. Stroke 1986; 17:1126–1128.
29. Stemmermann GN, Hayashi T, Resch JA, Chung CS, Reed DM, Rhoads GG. Risk factors related to ischemic and hemorrhagic cerebrovascular disease at autopsy. The Honolulu Heart Study. Stroke 1984; 15:23–28.
30. Wityk RJ, Caplan LR. Hypertensive intracerebral hemorrhage. Epidemiology and clinical pathology. In: Spontaneous Intracerebral Hemorrhage. Batjer HH, ed. Neurosurg Clini North Am, Philadelphia: W.B Saunders, 1992; 3:521–532.
31. Bahemuka M. Primary intracerebral hemorrhage and heart weight: a clinicopathologic case–control review of 218 patients. Stroke 1987; 18:531–536.
32. Caplan LR, Mohr JP: Intracerebral hemorrhage: an update. Geriatrics 1978; 33:42–45, 48–52.
33. Garcia JH, Mena H. Vascular diseases. In: Garcia JH, Budka H, McKeever PE, Sarnat HB, Sima AAF, eds. Neuropathology. The Diagnostic Approach. St. Louis: Mosby, 1997:263–320.
34. Kase CS, Robinson RK, Stein RW, DeWitt LD, Hier DB, Harp DL, Williams JP, Caplan LR, Mohr JP. Anticoagulant-related intracerebral hemorrhage. Neurology 1985; 35:943–948.
35. Bollinger O. Über traumatische Spät-Apoplexie, ein Beitrag zur Lehre von der Hirnerschütterung. Festschrift Rudolf Virchow, 70 Lebensjahr. Int Beitr Wiss Med 1891; 2:457–470.
36. Baratham G. Dennyson WG. Delayed traumatic intracerebral hemorrhage. J Neurol Neurosurg Psychiatry 1972; 35:698–706.
37. Cooper PR. Delayed brain injury: secondary insults. In: Povlishock JT, Becker DP, eds. Bethesda, MD: Central Nervous System Trauma Status Report—

1985, Vol. 31. National Institutes of Neurological Communicative Diseases and Stroke, 1987:217–228.
38. Cooper PR. Delayed traumatic intracerebral hemorrhage. In: Cooper PR, ed. Head Injury, 3rd Baltimore: Williams & Wilkins, 1993:659–665.
39. Cooper PR. Post-traumatic intracranial mass lesions. In: Cooper PR, ed. Head Injury, 3rd Baltimore: Williams & Wilkins, 1993:275–329.
40. Fukamachi A, Nagaseki Y, Kohno K, Wakao T. The incidence and developmental process of delayed traumatic intracerebral haematomas. Acta Neurochir 1985; 74:53–39.
41. Diaz FG, Yock DH Jr, Larson D, Rockswold GL. Early diagnosis of delayed posttraumatic intracerebral hematomas. J Neurosurg 1979; 50:217–223.
42. Lipper MH, Kishore PRS, Girevendulis AK, Miller JD, Becker DP. Delayed intracranial hematoma in patients with severe head injury. Radiology 1979; 133:645–649.
43. Young HA, Gleave JRW, Schmidek H, Gregory S. Delayed traumatic intracerebral hematoma: report of 5 cases operatively treated. Neurosurgery 1984; 14:22–25.
44. Kaufman HH, Moake JL, Olson JD, Miner ME, du Cret RP, Pruessner JL, Gildenberg PL. Delayed and recurrent intracranial hematomas related to disseminated intravascular clotting and fibrinolysis in head injury. Neurosurgery 1980; 7:445–449.
45. Grcevic N. Traumatic tears of the tela choroidea: a hitherto unrecognized cause of post-traumatic hydrocephalus. Acta Neurochir (Suppl.) 1983; 32:79–85.
46. Krauland W. Verletzungen der intrakranieallen Schlagadern. Berlin: Springer-Verlag, 1982.
47. Gennarelli TA, Thibault LE. Biological models of head injury. In: Central Nervous System Trauma Status Report–1985. Bethesda MD: National Institute of Neurological and Communicative Disorders and Stroke, National Institutes of Health, 1985:391–404.
48. Dawson SL, Hirsch CS, Lucas FV, Sebek BA. The contrecoup phenomenon. Reappraisal of a classic problem. Hum Pathol 1980; 11:155–166.
49. Lobato RD, Rivas JJ, Gomez PA, Castaneda M, Canizal JM, Sarabia R, Cabera A, Munoz MJ. Head-injured patients who talk and deteriorate into coma: analysis of 211 cases studied with computerized tomography. J Neurosurg 1991; 75:256–261.
50. Marshall LF, Toole BM, Bowers SA. The National Traumatic Coma Data Bank: II. Patients who talk and deteriorate: implications for treatment. J Neurosurg 1983; 59:285–288.
51. Reilly PL, Graham DI, Adams JH, Jennett B. Patients with head injury who talk and die. Lancet 1975; 2:375–377.
52. Rockswold GL, Leonard PR, Nagib MG. Analysis of management in the thirty-three closed head injury patients who 'talked and deteriorated'. Neurosurgery 1987; 21:51–55.
53. Lindenberg R. Mechanical injuries of brain and meninges. In:Spitz WU, Fisher RS, eds. Medicolegal Investigation of Death. Guidelines for the Application of Pathology to Crime Investigation. Springfield IL: Charles C. Thomas, 1973:420–469.
54. Leestma JE, Kallelkar MF, Teas SS. Ponto-medullary avulsion associated with cervical hyperextension. Acta Neurochir 1983; 32 (Suppl):69–73.
55. Pilz P, Strohecker J, Grohouschek M. Survival after traumatic ponto-medullary tear. J Neurol Neurosurg Psychiatry 1982; 45:422–427.
56. Bohlman HH. Acute fractures and dislocations of the cervical spine: an analysis of 300 hospitalized patients and a review of the literature. J Bone Joint Surg 1979; 61:1119–1142.
57. Davidson KD, Weiford ED, Dixon GD. Traumatic vertebral artery pseudoaneurysm following chiropractic manipulation. Radiology 1975; 115:651–652.
58. Pratt-Thomas HR, Berger KE. Cerebellar and spinal injuries after chiropractic manipulation. JAMA 1947; 133:600–603.
59. Easton JD, Sherman DG. Cervical manipulation and stroke. Stroke 1977; 8:594–597.
60. Heros RC. Cerebellar infarction resulting from traumatic occlusion of a vertebral artery: case report. J Neurosurg 1979; 51:111–113.
61. Ebel W, Hegewald G, Heese R. The Zieve syndrome. Z Gesammte Intern. Med 1972; 27:805–808.
62. Pounder J. Shaken adult syndrome. Am J Forensic Med Pathol 1997; 18:321–324.
63. Baddeley A. Working memory. In: Gazzaniga MS, ed. The Cognitive Neurosciences. Cambridge, MA: MIT Press, 1995:755–764.
64. Markowitsch HJ. Intellectual Functions and the Brain. Toronto: Hogrefe and Huber, 1992.
65. Crystal H, Dickson D, Fuld P, Masur D, Scott R, Mehler M, Masdeu J, Kawas C, Aronson M, Wolfson L. Clinico-pathologic studies in dementia: nondemented subjects with pathologically confirmed Alzheimer's disease. Neurology 1988; 38:1682–1687.
66. Khachaturian ZS. Diagnosis of Alzheimer's disease. Arch Neurol 1985; 42:1097.
67. Ball MJ, Griffin-Brooks S, MacGregor JA, Nagy B, Ojalvo-Rose E, Fewster PH. Neuropathological definition of Alzheimer disease: multivariate analyses in the morphometric distinction between Alzheimer dementia and normal aging. Alzheimer Dis Assoc Disord 1988; 2:29–37.
68. Hof PR, Morrison JH. The cellular basis of cortical disconnection in Alzheimer disease and related dementing conditions. In: Terry RD, Katzman R, Bick KL, eds. Alzheimer Disease. New York: Raven Press, 1994:197–229.
69. Terry RD. The pathogenesis of Alzheimer disease: an alternative to the amyloid hypothesis. J Neuropath Exp Neurol 1996; 55:1023–1025.
70. Masliah E, Terry RD, Mallory M, Alford M, Hansen LA. Diffuse plaques do not accentuate synapse loss in Alzheimer disease. Am J Pathol 1990; 137:1293–1297.
71. Masliah E, Terry RD, DeTeresa RM, Hansen LA. Immunohistochemical quantification of the synapse-related protein synaptophysin in Alzheimer disease. Neurosci Lett 1989; 103:234–239.

Appendix 1
Support Groups for the Neurologically Impaired Patients and Their Caretakers

UNITED STATES
American Association of Retired Persons (AARP)
601 E Street, NW
Washington, DC 20049
Tel: 800-424-3410
Internet: www.aarp.org

ALS Association
National Office
27001 Agoura Road, Suite 150
Calabasas Hills, CA 91301-5104
Tel: 800-782-4747
Internet: www.alsa.org

Alzheimer's Association
919 North Michigan Avenue
Suite 1100
Chicago, IL 60611-1676
Tel: 800-272-3900 or 312-335-8700
Internet: www.alz.org

American Brain Tumor Association
2720 River Road, Suite 146
Des Plaines, IL 60018
Tel: 800-886-2282
Internet: www.abta.org

American Chronic Pain Association
PO Box 850
Rocklin, CA 95677
Tel: 916-632-0922
Internet: www.theacpa.org

American Diabetes Association National Service Center
1701 North Beauregard Street
Alexandria, VA 22311
Tel: 800-342-2383
Internet: www.diabetes.org

American Heart Association
7272 Greenville Avenue
Dallas, TX 75231
Tel: 800-242-8721 or 214-373-6300
Internet: www.americanheart.org

American Pain Society
4700 West Lake Avenue
Glenview, IL 60025
Tel: 847-375-4715
Fax: 847-375-6315
Internet: www.ampainsoc.org

American Parkinson Disease Association (APDA)
1250 Hylan Blvd., Suite 4B
Staten Island, NY 10305-1946
Tel: 800-223-2732 or 718-981-8001
Internet: www.apdaparkinson.com

CDC National Prevention Information Network
PO Box 6003
Rockville, MD 20849-6003
Tel: 800-458-5231
Internet: www.cdcnpin.org

Charcot-Marie-Tooth Association
2700 Chestnut Street
Chester, PA 19013-4867
Tel: 800-606-CMTA
Internet: www.charcot-marie-tooth.org

Christopher Reeve Paralysis Association
500 Morris Avenue
Springfield, NJ 07081
Tel: 800-223-0292 or 201-379-2690
Internet: www.apacure.com

Clearinghouse on Disability Information
Office of Special Education and Rehabilitation Services

US Department of Education
Switzer Building, 330 C Street, SW, Rm. 3132
Washington, DC 20202-2524
Tel: 202-732-1723 or 202-732-1241

Congress of Organizations of the Physically
Handicapped
16630 Beverly Avenue
Tinley Park, IL 60477-1904
Tel: 708-532-3566

Daniel Heumann Fund for Spinal Cord Research
6878 Fleetwood Road, Suite D
McLean, VA 22101
Tel: 703-442-8797
Internet: www.heumannfund.org

Department of Health and Human Services
Administration on Developmental Disabilities
200 Independence Avenue, SW
HHH Building, Room 325D
Washington, DC 20201
Tel: 202-245-2890

Epilepsy Foundation
4351 Garden City Drive
Landover, MD 20785
Tel: 800-EFA-1000 or 301-459-3700
Internet: www.efa.org

Family Survival Project for Brain Damaged Adults
425 Bush Street, Suite 500
San Francisco, CA 94108
Tel: 800-445-8106 or 415-434-3388

Fibromyalgia Network
PO Box 31750
Tucson, AZ 85751
Tel: 800-853-2929
Internet: www.fmnetnews.com

Foundation Fighting Blindness
National Retinitis Pigmentosa Foundation, Inc.
Executive Plaza I, Suite 800
Hunt Valley, MD 21031-1014
Tel: 800-683-5555 or 410-785-1414
Internet: www.libertyresources.org/ffb.html

Guillain-Barre Syndrome Foundations
International
PO Box 262
Wynnewood, PA 19096
Tel: 610-667-0131
Internet: www.webmast.com/gbs

Helen Keller International World Headquarters
90 West Street, 2nd Floor
New York, NY 10006
Tel: 212-766-5266
Internet: www.hki.org

Hereditary Disease Foundation
11400 West Olympic Blvd., Suite 855
Los Angeles, CA 90064-1560
Tel: 310-575-9656
Internet: www.hdfoundation.org

Huntington's Disease Society of America (HDSA)
158 West 29th Street, 7th Floor
New York, NY 10001-5300
Tel: 800-345-HDSA or 212-239-3430
Internet: www.hdsa.org

Hydrocephalus Association
870 Market Street, Suite 705
San Francisco, CA 94102
Tel: 415-732-7040
Internet: hydroassoc.org

Hydrocephalus: News and Notes
1670 Green Oak Circle
Lawrenceville, GA 30243
1670 Green Oak Circle
Lawrenceville, GA 30243
Tel: 404-995-95870

Inclusion Body Myositis Association, Inc.
1420 Huron Court
Harrisonburg, VA 22801
Tel: 703-433-7935

International Tremor Foundation (ITF)
7046 West 105th Street
Overland Park, KS 66212-1803
Internet: www.essentialtremor.org

Learning Disabilities Association of America
4156 Library Road
Pittsburgh, PA 15234-1349
Tel: 412-341-1515
Internet: www.Idnatl.org

Lighthouse, International
111 East 59th Street
New York, NY 10022-1202
Tel: 800-829-0500 or 212-821-9200

Les Turner ALS Foundation
8142 North Lawndale Avenue
Skokie, IL 60076-3322
Tel: 888-ALS-1107 or 847-679-3311
Internet: lesturnerals.org

Multiple Sclerosis Association of America
National Headquarters
706 Haddonfield Road
Cherry Hill, NJ 08002
Tel: 800-LEARN MS
Internet: www.msaa.org

Multiple Sclerosis Foundation, Inc.
6350 North Andrews Avenue
Fort Lauderdale, FL 33309-2130
Tel: 800-441-7055 or 305-776-6805
Internet: www.msfacts.org

Muscular Dystrophy Association
810 Seventh Avenue

New York, NY 10019
Tel: 212-586-0808

Muscular Dystrophy Association-USA
3300 East Sunrise Drive
Tucson, AZ 85718
Tel: 800-572-1717
Internet: mdausa.org

Myasthenia Gravis Foundation of America
National Office
123 West Madison Street, Suite 800
Chicago, IL 60602
Tel: 800-541-5454 or 312-853-0522
Internet: www.myasthenia.org

Myoclonus Families United
1564 East 34th Street
Brooklyn, NY 11234
Tel: 718-252-2133

Myoclonus Research Foundation
200 Old Palisade Road, Suite 17D
Fort Lee, NJ 07024
Tel: 201-585-0770
Internet: www.myoclonus.com

Myositis Association of America (MAA)
755 Cantrell Avenue, Suite C
Harrisonburg, VA 22801
Tel: 540-433-7686
Fax: 540-432-0206
Internet: www.myositis.org

Narcolepsy and Cataplexy Foundation of America
445 East 68th Street, Suite 121
New York, NY 10021
Tel: 212-628-6315

Narcolepsy Network
10921 Reed Hartman Highway
Cincinnati, OH 45242
Tel: 513-891-3522
Internet: www.narcolepsynetwork.org

National Association for Visually Handicapped
22 West 21st Street, 6th Floor
New York, NY 10010
Tel: 212-889-3141
Internet: www.navh.org

National Ataxia Foundation
2600 Fernbrook Lane
Suite 119
Minneapolis, MN 55447
Tel: 763-553-0020
Fax: 763-553-0167
Internet: www.ataxia.org

National Brain Research Association
110 Irving Street, NW, Room 256
George Hyman Research Building
Washington, DC 20010

National Brain Injury Research Group, Inc.
1730 M Street, NW
Washington, DC 2003
Tel: 800-447-8445 or 202-331-8445

National Center for Learning Disabilities
381 Park Avenue South, Suite 1401
New York, NY 10016
Tel: 888-575-7373 or 212-545-7510
Internet: www.ncld.org

National Center for Stuttering
200 East 33rd Street
New York, NY 10016
Tel: 800-221-2483 or 212-532-1460
Internet: www.stuttering.com

National Chronic Pain Outreach Association
7979 Old Georgetown Road, Suite 100
Bethesda, MD 20814-2429
Tel: 301-652-4948
Internet: neurosurgery.mgh.harvard.edu/ncpainoa.htm

National Head Injury Foundation
Houston, TX
Tel: 888-222-5287 or 713-774-6110
Internet: www.nhif.org

National Head Injury Foundation
1776 Massachusetts Ave, NW, Suite 100
Washington, DC 20036
Tel: 800-444-6443 or 202-296-6443

National Headache Foundation
428 W. St. James Place, 2nd Floor
Chicago, IL 60614-2750
Tel: 888-NHF-5552
Internet: www.headaches.org

National Health Council
1730 M Street, NW, Suite 500
Washington, DC 20036
Tel: 202-785-3910
Internet: www.nhcouncil.org

National Health Education Committee, Inc.
865 United Nations Plaza
New York, NY 10017
Tel: 212-421-9010

National Hydrocephalus Foundation
1670 Green Oak Circle
Lawrenceville, GA 30243
Tel: 404-995-95870

National Institute on Deafness and Other Communication Disorders (NICDC)
31 Center Drive, MSC, 2320
Bethesda, MD 20892-2320
Tel: 800-241-1044 (Voice)
800-241-1055 (TDD/TTY)
Internet: www.nih.gov/nicdcd

National Institute on Disability and Rehabilitation Research (NIDRR)
400 Maryland Avenue, SW
Washington, DC 20201-2572
Tel: 202-205-8134 (Voice)
202-205-9433 (TTY)
Internet: www.ed.gov/offices/OSERS/NIDRR

National Institute of Neurological Disorders and Stroke
31 Center Drive MSC 2540
Building 31, Room 8A16
Bethesda, MD 20892
Tel: 800-352-9424
Internet: www.ninds.nih.gov

National Institutes of Health
9000 Rockville Pike
Building 31, Room 2B10
Bethesda, MD 20892
Tel: 301-496-1766
Internet: www.nih.gov

National Mental Health Association
1021 Prince Street
Alexandria, VA 22314
Tel: 800-969-NMHA or 703-684-7722
Internet: www.nmha.org

National Multiple Sclerosis Society
733 Third Avenue
New York, NY 10017
Tel: 800-344-4867 or 212-986-3240
Internet: www.nmss.org

National Neurofibromatosis Foundation
95 Pine Street, 16th Floor
New York, NY 10005
Tel: 800-323-7938 or 212-344-6633
Internet: www.nf.org

National Organization for Rare Disorders, Inc.
PO Box 8923
New Fairfield, CT 06812-8923
Tel: 800-999-6673 or 203-746-6518
Internet: www.rarediseases.org

National Parkinson Foundation, Inc.
1501 NW 9th Avenue (Bob Hope Road)
Miami, FL 33136-1494
Tel: 800-327-4545 or 305-547-6666
Internet: www.parkinson.org

National Rehabilitation Information Center
1010 Wayne Avenue, Suite 800
Silver Spring, MD 20910
Tel: 800-346-2742 or 301-562-2400
Internet: www.naric.com

National Scoliosis Foundation
5 Cabot Place
Stoughton, MA 02072
Tel: 800-673-6922 or 781-341-6333
Internet: www.scoliosis.org

National Sleep Foundation
1522 K Street, NW, Suite 500
Washington, DC 20005
Internet: www.sleepfoundation.org

National Spasmodic Torticollis Association Inc.
9920 Talbert Avenue, #233
Fountain Valley, CA 92708
Tel: 800-487-8385
Internet: www.torticollis.org

National Spinal Cord Injury Association
8701 Georgia Avenue, Suite 500
Silver Spring, MD 20851
Tel: 800-962-9629 or 301-588-6959
Internet: www.spinalcord.org

National Spinal Cord Injury Hotline
Montibello Rehabilitation Center
2201 Argonne Drive
Baltimore, MD 21218
Tel: 800-526-3456

National Stroke Association
9707 E. Easter Lane
Englewood, CO 80112-3747
Tel: 800-787-6537 or 303-649-9299
Internet: www.stroke.org

National Stuttering Association
5100 East La Palma, Suite 208
Anaheim Hills, CA 92807
Tel: 800-364-1677
Internet: www.nsastutter.org

Neurofibromatosis, Inc.
8855 Annapolis Road, Suite 110
Lanham, MD 20706-2824
Tel: 800-942-6825 or 301-577-8984
Internet: www.nfinc.org

Paralyzed Veterans of America
National Office
801 18th Street, NW
Washington, DC 20006
Tel:800-424-8200 or 202-872-1300
Internet: www.pva.org

Parkinson's Disease Foundation
Columbia-Presbyterian Medical Center
710 West 168th Street
New York, NY 10032-9982
Tel: 800-457-6676 or 212-923-4700
Fax: 212-934-4778
Internet: www.pdf.org

Parkinson's Education Programs, USA
3900 Birch Street, Suite 105
Newport Beach, CA 92660
Tel: 800-344-7872 or 714-250-2975

Parkinson's Support Groups of America
11376 Cherry Hill Road
Beltsville, MD 20705
Tel: 301-957-1545

Prevent Blindness America
500 East Remington Road
Schaumburg, IL 60173-4557
Tel: 800-331-2020 or 708-843-2020
Internet: www.prevent-blindness.org

Research to Prevent Blindness, Inc.
645 Madison Avenue, 21st Floor
New York, NY 10022
Tel: 800-621-0026 or 212-752-4333

Restless Legs Syndrome Foundation, Inc.
819 Second Street SW
Rochester, MN 55902-2985
Tel: 507-287-6465
Internet: www.rls.org

Speech Foundation of America
PO Box 11749
Memphis, TN 3811

Trigeminal Neuralgia Association
PO Box 340
Barnegat Light, NJ 08006
Tel: 609-361-6250
Internet: www.tna-support.org

United Parkinson Foundation
833 W. Washington Boulevard, Suite 401
Chicago, IL 60617

Vestibular Disorders Association
PO Box 4467
Portland, OR 97208-4467
Tel: 503-229-7705
Internet: www.vestibular.org

Von Hippel–Lindau Foundation
PO Box 733
Toms River, NJ 08754
Tel: 908-244-7635

Wilson's Disease Association
4 Navaho Drive
Brookfield, CT 06810
Tel: 800-399-0266 or 203-775-9666

BELGIUM
European Charcot-Marie-Tooth Consortium
Laboratory of Neurogenetics
University of Antwerp
B-2610 Antwerp, Belgium
Fax: 32-3-820-2541
E-mail: gisele@uai.ua.ac.be

BRAZIL
Parkinson Association of Brazil
Av. Bosque da Saúde, 1155

São Paulo-SP, Brazil
Tel: 11-55-578-8177
Internet: www.parkinson.org.br

FRANCE
Association Francaise de Recherche Genetique
Alain Bouvet
5, rue Casimir Delavigne
75006 Paris, France
Tel: 01 43 25 0 00
Fax: 01 42 54 32 56

Association France-Parkinson
37, bis rue La Fontaine
75016 Paris, France
Tel:01 45 20 22 20
Fax: 01 40 50 16 44

Association Huntington France
42, rue du Château des Rentiers
75013 Paris, France
Tel: 01 53 60 08 79
Fax: 01 53 60 08 99

Association pour la Recherche sur la Sclérose La
téral Amyotrophique
245, rue Lacharrière
75011 Paris, France
Tel: 01 43 38 99 89
Fax: 01 43 38 31 59

France Alzheimer
21, bld Montmartre
75002 Paris, Paris
Tel: 01 42 97 52 41
Internet: orphanet.infobiogen.fr/associations/FA

Ligue Francaise contre la Sclerose en Plaque
40, rue Duranton
75015 Paris, France
Tel: 01 53 98 98 80
Fax: 01 53 98 98 88
Internet: www.handinews.com/lfsep

GERMANY
Deutsche Alzheimer Gesellschaft e.V.
Kantstrasse 152
D-10623 Berlin, Germany
Tel: 030 31 50 57 33
Email: deutsche, alzheimer.ger@t-online.de
Internet: www.deutsche-alzherimer.de

Deutsche Parkinson-Vereinigung-Bundesverband,
e.V.
Moselstrasse 31
41464 Neuss 1
Tel: 021 31 41 01 6/7
Internet: uni-ulm.de/klinik/expneuro/dpv

ITALY
World Parkinson Disease Association
via Zuretti, 35

20125 Milano, Italy
Tel: 39-02-66713111
Internet: www.wpda.org

JAPAN
The Japan Stroke Association
E-mail: jsasq@mbox2.inet-osaka.or.jp

UNITED KINGDOM
Alzheimer's Society
Gordon House
10 Greencoat Place
London SW1P 1PH, UK
0207 306 0606
Internet: www.alzheimers.org.uk

The Muscular Dystrophy Campaign
Nattrass House
7–11 Prescott Place
London SW4 6BS, UK
Tel: +44 (0) 20 7720 8055
Fax: +44 (0) 20 17498 0670
Internet: www.muscular-dystrophy.org.uk

Parkinson Disease Society
215 Vauxhall Bridge Road
London SW1V 1EJ, UK
Tel: +44 (0) 207 932 1304
Fax: +44 (0) 207 233 9226

The Stroke Association
Stroke House
123 Whitecross Street
London EC1Y 8JJ, UK
0207566 0300
Internet: www.stroke.org.uk

Appendix 2
The Diagnosis of the Creutzfeldt-Jakob Concept

SERGE DUCKETT, EDITOR

Names based on unproven speculations about causation should be avoided, since evidence for any of these is at least inadequate.

—J. G. Scadding[1]

In August 2000, there appeared a report[2a] that forecast that between 63 and 135,000 United Kingdom (UK) residents would be afflicted with the "new variant" of Creutzfeldt-Jakob disease (vCJD) in the next decades; these numbers are less than the previous projected figures of up to 500,000 and possibly millions, published in December 1999.[2b] Only 84 cases have been reported so far—at this writing—all occurring in the UK plus two possible cases in France—and nowhere else in the world. If these predictions materialize, then vCJD would become the most frequent fatal dementing illness, affecting all age groups, in the UK. This predilection for vCJD in the UK is explained by the proposition that the abnormal prion which causes bovine spongiotic encephalopathy (BSE) was transmitted to humans by the 750,000 prion infected or presumed infected cattle slaughtered in the UK between 1980 and 1996.[2a,2b]

Such an epidemic of vCJD has been predicted since at least 1996. Again, in 1999 *The Lancet*[3] and *British Medical Journal*[4], reported a "statistically significant" increase in the number of cases of vCJD—that is, nine cases reported in a 3-month period from November 1998 to March 1999 by the National CJD Surveillance Unit in Edinburgh.[5] *The Lancet* described this increase as a "disquieting change in notification rate" in an editorial entitled "Tragedy of Variant Creutzfeldt-Jakob Disease," which begins as follows:

The unfinished tragedy of variant Creutzfeldt-Jakob disease (CJD) in the UK begins with a distasteful practice; progresses through protracted scientific investigation, hampered by political farce; and culminates in continued uncertainty—is there to be a massive epidemic of variant CJD that was predicted in 1996, or is the scare a product of an imaginative diagnostic definition and doom-mongering statistical prognostication.[5]

More recently it was noted in *The Lancet* that "[t]he realization of an epidemic of vCJD would be a nightmare-scenario for UK healthcare planners,"[6] as well as for others, one might add.

The qualified neuropathologist, after consultation with other specialists, and in the light of her/his professional judgment, is the only physician who can sign the pathology report that professionally informs the patient and his entourage via the attending physician, that he or she is afflicted with a fatal mental and neurological disease; an important moral responsibility for which the neuropathologist is legally accountable. Today, that diagnosis is confirmed by the demonstration of the presence of an abnormal prion in cerebral tissues.[7,8] The treating physician or the neurologist depend wholly on that report to confirm the diagnosis of vCJD or any other prion disease.

However, some neuropathologists feel uneasy, some even refuse to make that diagnosis because there is no proof—at this time—that any prion causes vCJD or any other disease; other reasons are that the incubation periods of any prion disease are unknown, that there is no evidence of the presence of any type of inflammatory reaction, a response of any prion in any type of prion so-called "infection," and no therapy. This follows nearly four decades of a well-funded though unsuccessful search for the proven cause of the "slow-viral cum prion" diseases. However, this search has led to the discovery of the normal and so-called abnormal prions and thus raised the possibility of new frontiers in human neural biology, which hopefully will lead to the effective treatment of human and animals diseases.

There are also materialistic down to earth realities about making potentially doubtful diagnoses, which concern money and a job. Many neuropathologists have been sued and or dismissed for signing an incorrect pathology report, sometimes based upon misleading scientific or clinical information, thus the need to be heavily insured at great expense to them or their employer, to practice their profession. This incidentally, may be an added reason for the marked decrease in recent years in the number of trained full-time neuropathologists and trainees.

In response to these reports of a potential major epidemic of vCJD, the difficulty in assigning a correct diagnosis to CJD and other "prion diseases" to everyone's satisfaction, the confusion concerning the identity of the CJ concept (i.e., disease [CJD] or syndrome [CJS]?), this review has been added to inform interested readers of the origins of CJ concept and of the proposed pathogenesis of Kuru in the development of the modern interpretation of that concept, namely CJD, and its diagnosis.

THE CREUTZFELDT-JAKOB SYNDROME[9]

In the early 1920s, Hans Creutzfeldt[10,11] and Alfons Jakob[12–15] described a neuropathological syndrome consisting of a widespread destruction of neurons throughout the central nervous system (CNS) of six patients afflicted with syphilis, malaria, alcoholism, or herpes zoster. This global polioencephalopathy or poliodystrophy involved primarily the frontal cortex and, to a varying degree, the basal ganglia, thalamus, and the cortex of other cerebral regions, the cerebellum, brain stem, and spinal cord. Cortical laminar necrosis was present in all cases. All of their patients were demented with a varied and complicated neurological presentation and died 6 to 18 months later. Both authors had originally assumed that this entity might be a new disease, but upon further study they concluded that their patients were afflicted with a neuropathological syndrome, namely a widespread destruction of neurons, which complicated various other diseases. All patients were demented and the variability of the associated clinical picture varied in accordance with the CNS region most acutely involved. Creutzfeldt thought "[i]t is best to do without a clinical label altogether as the comparative diversity of the picture makes a symptomatological name more difficult, whereas the knowledge of the characteristic histological findings guide us securely and unambiguously [to the diagnosis]."[16] They each gave this syndrome a neuropathological name, albeit cumbersome and different, "degeneratio grisei focularis et diffusa progressiva"[16] and "spastic pseudosclerosis encephalopathy with disseminated foci of degeneration."[12] Both names are replaced in this text by that of the Creutzfeldt-Jakob syndrome (CJS). The differentiation between a syndrome, which is common to several diseases, and a disease, which has a known and identified cause, is crucial in the search for a diagnosis and treatment.[1,17–19]

The first case of CJS was a 20-year-old woman named Bertha, who was admitted in June 1913 with multiple neurological signs and symptoms of dementia and herpes zoster to the neurological service of Alois Alzheimer, in the care of his assistant, Creutzfeldt. She died 2 months later; an autopsy was done, including a thorough neuropathological study. Both physicians studied this patient in great detail. With Alzheimer's approval, Creutzfeldt decided to publish the case. One year later, World War I began, and Creutzfeldt joined the navy. In 1915 Alzheimer died. After the war in 1919, Creutzfeldt worked in Walther Spielmeyer's neuropathology laboratory where, under Spielmeyer's guidance, he studied and described the clinical and pathological findings of Bertha's case. His study, approved by Spielmeyer, was first published in 1920[10] and in more detail the following year.[11] Spielmeyer was Alzheimer's chosen heir in Munich when the latter resigned to go to Breslau, and it is to Spielmeyer's credit that he insisted that that this study indicate that it originated in Alzheimer's Breslau laboratory and that Creutzfeldt be the only author. Creutzfeldt described the case, but prudently did not make any claims at this time as to whether it was a neuropathological syndrome or disease. He concluded: "I have restricted myself to a simple statement of the findings because I believe that in a single case all of the possible manifestations of the disease group to which it belongs cannot be developed, and primarily I do not want, by ill-based attempt at interpretation, to lead similar cases into all too narrow a track" (p. 25).[10]

The next year, 1921, Jakob described cases,[12] all with different diagnoses, including syphilis, malaria, and alcohol intoxication, to which he added Creutzfeldt's case, all presenting with the same neuropathological syndrome, namely a polioencephalopathy characterized by cortical laminar necrosis (CLN). Jakob, who was primarily a neuropathologist, toyed with the idea that these cases were examples of a "disease caused by another disease," and as an example he described the case of a man with syphilis and amyotrophic lateral sclerosis (pp. 202–209).[12] He proposed that "spastic pseudosclerosis" was similar to Wilson's disease. Wilson's response was direct: "[T]he syndrome has nothing whatever to do with hepatolenticular degeneration [Wilson's disease]," to which he added strong criticisms of Jakob's confused efforts to change a poorly defined syndrome into a disease.[20]

In 1922, Spielmeyer used the term "disease" in relation to the Creutzfeldt Jakob (CJ) concept.[21] The decision to do so was not scientific and has resulted in a great deal of confusion. Jakob's pupils[9] felt that it was he who had really described the CJ concept and they denigrated Creutzfeldt's contribution as incidental. Spielmeyer was disturbed by these allegations and, inspired by loyalty rather than by fact, he coined the eponym "Creutzfeldt-Jakob disease" in defense of his pupil's contribution:

The peculiar focal disorder of the cerebral cortex reported by Creutzfeldt has not remained solitary. Clinically it is above all characterized by spasms, hyperalgesias and psychiatric symptoms. In his material studied with exceptional care A. Jakob has discovered a whole series of cases of this disease. Thus we may hope that the clinical and anatomical characteristics of Creutzfeldt-Jakob disease will be well demarcated.[21]

No matter how well intentioned he was, it was not possible for Spielmeyer to justify the use of the term "disease" in this case as he did on the basis of hope. He is said to have eventually repudiated this opinion. Even Jakob never directly referred to the CJ concept as a disease, he had merely raised the possibility, which he eventually repudiated, as we shall see below. Creutzfeldt strongly objected to the use of the term "disease."[16] He agreed that the neuropathological picture of their cases was similar. Creutzfeldt's criticisms were echoed by leading English and French neurologists of the day, such as Kinnier Wilson: "The indeterminate character of this syndrome... makes nomenclature difficult" (p. 1044).[20] Jean Lhermitte and Douglas MacAlpine wrote, "it is questionable whether one can accept it as a definite clinical entity."[22] Two leading neuropathologists, William McMenemey and Alfred Meyer, a pupil of Jakob's, as well as others referred to CJD as a syndrome that represented "a convenient dumping ground for several instances of atypical senile dementia."[23,24] Jakob eventually dropped his proposal that the CJ concept was, or might be, a disease and stated during his American tour in 1924: "I agree with most authors, especially S. A. K. Wilson, that nearly all problems in connections with it[the CJ concept] are still unsolved."[25] He never again proposed that their cases or their concept represented a disease, and he now accepted the view that the CJ concept was a neuropathological syndrome (CJS), a neurological complication common to a variety of diseases.

Spielmeyer,[21] Scholz,[25a] and others proposed soon after the description of CJS that the cause of polioencephalopathy and cortical laminar necrosis was interference with the energy needs of the neurons, be it the vascular or hematological purveyance of oxygen, glucose and other energy sources to the neuron, or genetically or acquired structural neuronal anomalies that hampered the use of those nutrients, resulting in hypoxia and hypoglycemia. The neuropathological changes caused by hypoxia are similar to those described in CJS, which is the result of survival after an insult to the brain, and the varied distribution of neuronal destruction is manifested by a variety of clinical pictures identifying the region affected. Thus the patient may present with a cerebellar variant of CJS (Brownell-Oppenheimer) or an occipital variant (Heidenhain) or a thalamic variant (Stern), but all patients also present with involvement of the frontal cortex, which is invariably involved.

Experimental and Clinical Evidence of Creutzfeldt-Jakob Syndrome

In 1930, E. F. Gildea and Stanley Cobb produced CJS, polioencephalopathy, cortical laminar necrosis, and abnormal behavior in cats ("mad cats") by partial strangulation.[26] In 1934, Lhermitte and Barrelet[27] and Alajouanine et al.[28] described the complete clinicopathological details of humans presenting rather suddenly with dementia as well as a complex neurological and psychiatric picture and the classic neuropathology of CJS, polioencephalopathy, and CLN caused by air embolism, introduced intravenously, during surgery. In 1958, Courville, an experienced neuropathologist and expert on cerebral anoxia, cited 30 cases presenting with CJS and dementia caused by hypoxia, drugs, respiratory and cardiovascular problems, epilepsy, anesthetics, asthma, and other agents.[29]

CORTICAL LAMINAR NECROSIS

In 1925 Jakob wrote a study explaining the diagnostic importance of cortical laminar necrosis (CLN) in CJS.[30] This disorder can involve large areas of the cerebral cortex as in CJS, or it can be limited to one area.[31] The distribution of neuronal pathology in CJS always involves the frontal lobe of the cerebral cortex, often the temporal, and less frequently, the occipital cortex (Heidenhain variant). The most frequently involved portion of the cerebral cortex is the region of the third and adjacent laminae. The successive stages of CLN are (1) the destruction of neurons; (2) the edematous stage and appearance of phagocytes 24–48 hr later; (3) a hyperplasia of astroglial cells; (4) the appearance of spongiosis; and, finally, (5) tissue scarring and atrophy. These stages indicate approximately the age of the insult. The process of CLN, from beginning to end, takes approximately 6 to 8 weeks.[29] Thus the examiner sees the stage of development of the CLN prevalent at the time of the biopsy or demise. Jakob noted spongiosis in only one of his cases and Kirschbaum reported the presence of spongiosis in 59 of the first reported 150 cases of CJS/CJD.[32] However, spongiotic artifact is so easily produced in the brain by decomposition, late fixation, and the handling of tissues for eventual histological examination that its diagnostic value is often contested.[8,23,33] The type of spongiosis, i.e., intercellular or extracellular, the identity of the cells affected, and its site, i.e., focal or laminar, may be useful in identifying its cause and distinguishing artefact. In fact, it is not possible to prove that spongiosis exists in vivo, since all methods of tissue preparation, including paraffin or celloidin embedding, or freezing, modify the tissue—the method influences the result.

The diagnostic importance of CLN has been underlined in the last decade by radiologists who, with magnetic resonance imaging (MRI), have identified CLN, even when sometimes clinically unsuspected, in a variety of diseases afflicting all ages, such as CJD,[34,35] genetic and metabolic disorders[36–39] and hypoxia.[40] A Medline search concerning the diagnosis of CJD with MRI between January 1997 and January 2000 brought up 35 publications. Physiologists and biochemists have confirmed and developed the proposition that the CJS-type polioencephalopathy and CLN are caused by a reduction in the supply of energy of neurons through interference with the means of transport or production of nutrients, such as oxygen and glucose, and/or through morphological, physiological, or biochemical defects at the site of reception of that delivery at the blood–neuron barrier. The response and topographical distribution of the neurons to such injury vary according to the intensity or character of the interference, and the clinical manifestations indicate the region of the CNS affected, since neurons with similar physiological, morphological, and chemical characteristics tend to be grouped regionally.[8,41] Interference with the means of production or delivery of energy can take place in red blood cells (RBCs) (volume, quality, hematopoiesis, biochemical) in components of the cardiovascular system (cardiac disease, blood pressure, thrombosis, trauma, emboli), and at the blood–neuron point of contact—that is, the site of transfer of that energy (morphological, chemical).[42–44] A major point here is that Creutzfeldt and Jakob did describe a neuropathological syndrome but never described the disease that today bears their name.

CREUTZFELDT-JAKOB DISEASE[8] (SEE CHAPTER 7).

In the decades following World War II, the United Kingdom was the leading center for neuropathological studies, led by J. G. Greenfield, Alfred Meyer, Dorothy Russell, R. M. Norman, W. McMenemey, J. A. N. Corsellis, L. Rubinstein, Wendy Grant, William Mair, L. Crome, J. B. Cavanagh, J. B. Brierley, S. Stritch, C. E. Lumsden, among others. They were not particularly interested in the CJ concept, disease, or syndrome, because it was rare and ill defined until the mid-1950s when the members of the Maida Vale school of neuropathology, Sam Nevins and William McMenemey, and their colleagues began to study the CJ concept in depth. They proposed that there were different types of CJD, which they referred to as "spongiform encephalopathies" caused by vascular pathology, trauma, and uremia.[45–50] They noted the presence of the spongiform changes, which they associated with vascular pathology. Spongiosus was not a pathological feature particularly associated with the disease.

However, spongiotic encephalopathy had been of great interest before World War I (Probst, 1903; Fischer, 1911; see review[9]) but soon thereafter, neuropathologists lost interest in this disorder because of the frequently artefactual nature of spongiosus. The members of the Maida Vale school, sometimes erroneously referred to as the "Queen Square" school, and their supporters were named the "dualists" because they believed that the CJ concept represented several nosological entities.[51] In contrast to them were the "unicists," who were mostly neurologists from the European continent, thus referred to as the "Continental" school, who believed that there was but one CJD, even if its cause was unknown.

There were heated debates between the dualists and unicists, thus an international meeting was held in 1967 to clarify matters.[51] No agreement was reached at that meeting. Nevins, Barnard, and McMenemey proposed that, because of the confusion, there should be an in-depth review of the concept, beginning with the original studies of Creutzfeldt and Jakob:

When an eponym such as Jakob-Creutzfeldt is given to disease of unknown nature, it is essential that the clinical and pathological findings in cases so designed must correspond exactly with what these authors have described; to add or detract will render their definition imprecise, create confusion, hinder the spread of knowledge and delay the progress of research.[52]

In 1968, W. R. Kirschbaum, Jakob's pupil, reviewed the first 150 published cases of CJD/CJS.[32] Seventy-four of these reports were identified by title as cases of CJS or as neuropathological cases, 49 were identified by title as cases of CJD particularly; most of the latter were described after 1945. For those who believed that spongiosus was an important marker of CJD, he pointed out that there were no spongy changes in the neural tissue of 91 of these 150 cases. Kirschbaum concluded his book, in agreement with Creutzfeldt and Jakob by stating: "Multiple causative factors lead to the particular histopathological changes of the J-C type. The available neuropathological information supports the conclusion that J-C disease is not a unified disease concept."[32]

Kuru, Creutzfeldt-Jakob Disease, Transmission Studies, and the Slow Virus Theory[53]

The present interpretation of the CJ concept began in the Eastern Highlands of New Guinea. In 1954, an Australian Patrol-Officer,

J. R. MacArthur, saw and reported a case of a disease known locally as kuru, the local word for "trembling." Victor Zigas, the local Public Health officer, whose wartime German medical qualifications had not been accredited by the Australian medical authorities, diagnosed it as hysteria: "So where is the trouble," said he, after examining the patient (p. 156).[54] Later, C. J. Gajdusek, a visiting American pediatrician, joined Zigas and diagnosed Kuru as Sydenham's chorea, then "Wilson's disease–like Parkinsonism" and "paralysis agitans" (pp. 59, 70).[55] Kuru had decimated exclusively one primitive tribe, the Fore people, among the many tribes that inhabit New Guinea. According to Gadjusek and Zigas, this disease was transmitted by endocannibalism, that is, the eating of the brain of members of one's family afflicted with kuru, a view that was strongly contradicted by American anthropologists doing fieldwork in the highlands of New Guinea.[56,56a] Even the famous photograph published in the Nobel lecture,[57] the only photo documenting cannibalism in New Guinea, purporting to show a family eating the remains of a dead kuru-afflicted family member was later found to be erroneous; as Gadjusek admitted—in fact, they were eating pork.[56] Gadjusek's explanation for this error was that the real pictures were "too offensive."[56] Concerning cannibalism, his answer to the anthropologists' comments was: "The whole of Australia knows these people are cannibals. It is 100% documented."[56] As for the anthropologists who questioned the cannibalism data, they were "desk anthropologists sitting around in chairs. If they would just get off their asses and go to New Guinea, they would find hundreds of cases."[56]

Gajdusek and Zigas wrote an article that was turned down by the editors of *Science*[55] and by the *New England Journal of Medicine*, where it met "unexpected opposition to its acceptance" by its editorial board, according to the editor, J. Garland, who told his friend and Gajdusek's boss at the National Institutes of Health (NIH), J. Smadel, that "[s]ome of my associates and I are greatly impressed by Dr. Gajdusek's description of "Kuru" and the picturesque background of his studies." (p. 201).[55] Two weeks later, this same study was accepted by Garland's temporary editorial replacement, Ted Ingalls, with the addition of a very short neuropathological description by Drs. Milton Shy and Igor Klatzo of the NIH, who asked that their names not be mentioned (p. 202).[55] Basically the same article was published within a 6-month span in three medical journals—two of them 9 days apart—in the United States, Australia, and Europe,[58–60] and shortly thereafter the same article with the same title appeared in two other medical journals.[61,62] Just before these publications, *Time* magazine had written a lengthy story about Gajdusek and kuru. In short, the topic was well publicized.

The Australian authorities who governed New Guinea were concerned about the activities of Gadjusek and Zigas, and a pair of professional neurologists, Donald Simpson and Harry Lander, were sent out to New Guinea from Australia. They discarded the medical labels proposed by Gajdusek and Zigas, including that of "paralysis agitans."[59] They diagnosed kuru as a subacute cerebellar disease[63] and incidentally taught neurology and neuroanatomy to Zigas and Gajdusek, who, by their own admission, were not neurologists. In his biography, Zigas writes: "Being near amateurs in neurological pedantry, Donald (Simpson) supplied a good deal of neurological training.... When the top of the cranium had been sawn off, Donald motioned me closer. ... Now, here is the dura matter. . . . Here we have the Sylvian fissure with its two branches. ... here the fissure of Rolando." (p. 262–263)[54] Gajdusek wrote: "Simpson has given me a good deal of neurological training, corrected my numerous neurological errors, pointed out my neurological blunders and oversights, and straightened out all the neurological pedantry of the Kuru situation with me." (p. 338).[55] This letter was written December 19, 1957, 1 month after the *New England Journal of Medicine* publication. It is interesting to note that they both referred to neurologic professionalism as pedantic.

The diagnosis of subacute noninflammatory cerebellar pathology was confirmed by NIH-visiting neuropathologists J. G. Greenfield, Webb Haymaker, and E. G. Robertson (pp. 304–308),[55] who examined the brain of a case of kuru, and by a subsequent study by Fowler and Robertson, who examined five cases.[64] At this point, Smadel recruited Igor Klatzo to study the neuropathology of 12 cases of kuru. Klatzo, an eminent NIH experimental neuroscientist, not a clinical neuropathologist, was reluctant to do this work.[65] He did and his conclusion was that these cases of Kuru presented a pathological picture similar to that of "Creutzfeldt-Jacob disease" without specifying which one of the 100+ variants of CJD, and thus misspelling Jakob's name.[66] This was not a typographical error, for Klatzo uses this appellation throughout his text and he underlines this choice by citing a study of H. Jacob, concerning the hereditary form of CJD, the famous Baker family.[66a] Moreover Klatzo 'corrected' the references by replacing Jakob's name by that of Jacob. Neither the name nor the studies of Alfons Jakob, nor those of Hans Creutzfeldt the original authors are mentioned in Klatzo's study, including the references. It happens that in 1958, the year before Klatzo's publication, Jacob had described a disease "subacute presenile spongiform atrophy with terminal dyskinesia" which he differentiated from CJD.[66b] This raises the possibility that Klatzo may indeed have been referring to "Jacob's disease" not to CJD, otherwise it would appear that he confused the worksand names of Jacob and Jakob. In any event, ever since then Klatzo's study has been the biblical reference of the association of CJD and Kuru and the neuropathological basis for the assumption that both diseases are caused by an abnormal prion. Unfortunately for review purposes, the tissues and histological slides of all of Klatzo's cases have been lost.

Elizabeth Beck and Peter Daniels, professional neuropathologists and close associates of Gajdusek, examined the tissues of cases of Kuru and did not agree with Klatzo that the neuropathological picture of Kuru closely resembled that of CJD nor its cerebellar variant (Brownell-Oppenheimer).[67] The general consensus of opinion of neuropathologists and neurologists who examined the cases of Kuru, diagnosed it as primarily a subacute cerebellar degenerative process.[55] [pp. 304–308][63,64,67,68].

The New Concept of Creutzfeldt-Jakob Disease

The early 1970s marked the end of UK hegemony in human neuropathological matters and the end of the dualist view of the CJ concept; the unicists, headed by Gajdusek, now led the way. On the basis of his work with Kuru, Gajdusek, proposed that the CJ concept was a disease caused by a virus with a long incubation period—a "slow virus"—a concept previously proposed by Sigurdson et al.,[69] but a real virus, nonetheless. As discussed below, Gajdusek eventually proposed that his virus was not a typical virus. Masters and Gajdusek borrowed Jakob's original material from Hamburg University, destained and restained the histological slides, and found that Jakob had "failed" to note the presence of spongiosis in one case. They concluded that four of the six original cases of Creutzfeldt and Jakob were not cases of CJD.[70] Incidentally, all of Jakob's material received back by the Neuropathology Department at Hamburg University, thus there is no possibility for review (private communication, Pr. D. Stavrou, Director of Neuropathology, Hamburg University).

The Neuropathology of Creutzfeldt-Jakob Syndrome and Creutzfeldt-Jakob Disease

The neuropathological diagnosis of CJS as described by Creutzfeldt and Jakob was a global polioencephalopathy, a widespread neuronal destruction, a complication common to many different diseases.[10–16] The neuropathological picture of CJD as described today consists basically of neuronal loss, gliosis, and spongiosis, with emphasis on the latter, and the presence of plaques of PrPsc.[7,8] "While delicate spongiform change may be pathognomonic of CJD, the other forms of degeneration described therein are not. Nor are astrogliosis, activation of microglia, or neuronal loss of significant diagnostic value, because they occur in many other neurodegenerative disorders."[71], p. 915.[8] The pathogenesis of CJD remains to be defined. It is not clear what element of the neural tissue is primarily targeted by PrPsc, what cells are affected, what the type of spongiosis is, whether intra- or extracellular, or what the cause of the spongiosus is.

It is a classical neuropathological rule that every neuropathological anomaly, be it gliosis, demyelination, partial or widespread neuronal loss, activation of microglia etc, is crucial for a correct diagnosis, because the pathology and the many clinical manifestations of diseases of the human nervous system are expressed by a very limited number of tissue anomalies.[72,73] However a neuropathological syndrome, as described by Creutzfeldt and Jakob, can occur as a complication of numerous neurological diseases.

The Link between CJD and Kuru

The link between CJD and Kuru was based on Klatzo's observation that the neuropathological picture of the two diseases was similar.[66] As noted above, this observation was a minority view. The sequence of steps that led from the proposition of the "resemblance" of Kuru and CJD to the identification of the "cause" of CJD, as described by Gajdusek and colleagues, is as follows:

1. The neuropathological similarity between CJD and Kuru was noted.[66]
2. Cerebral tissue from a case of Kuru was injected into the brain of a chimpanzee, which was said to eventually present with the typical clinical and pathological signs of Kuru.[74]
3. Cerebral tissue from a case of CJD was injected into the brain of a chimpanzee, said to eventually present with the typical clinical and pathological signs of CJD, including the dementia.[75] Gajdusek and colleagues concluded that these experiments demonstrated the similarity between Kuru and CJD.
4. Gajdusek proposed that Kuru was caused by a slow virus.[57]
5. Consequently, concluded Gajdusek, CJD is caused by a slow virus.

All of this work was done without the demonstration of the proposed transmitting agent—a slow virus in the donor tissue or in the injected animal. Eventually, the slow virus theory was replaced by the prion theory proposed by Prusiner and Hsaio.[76] The transition from the term slow virus to that of abnormal prion has been described as follows:

This 'slow virus', however, was remarkably resistant to inactivation, appeared to possess no nucleic acid, and seemed to consist entirely of some sort of unusual protein. It was quite unlike any other virus described and many began referring to it as an "unconventional" virus or transmissible agent. The term "prion" (proteinaceous infectious particle) was coined by Prusiner in 1982 to describe this "unconventional agent."[77]

The prion theory has produced a great deal of interesting information but the role of normal or abnormal prions remains unknown. Leading prion experts now tell us:

The causative transmissible agent (the "prion") has tenaciously eluded attempts at definitive identification.... The physiological function of the normal prion has so far resisted elucidation.[78] "The causative agents of all the TSEs (transmissible spongiotic encephalopathies) remain an enigma.... Prions continue to be vaguely defined, and for the most part this term is used as an operational term for the transmissible agent, but without structural imp.[79]

CONCLUSION

The recent announcement by a group of eminent scientists of the Welcome Trust Center at Oxford University, that the toll of cases of prion diseases in the UK will explode from one elderly human in a million to up to 163,000 humans of all ages, within the next decades, has received universal attention.[2a] But as questioned by *The Lancet* concerning a previous similar threat,[3] will it materialize or is it "a product of an imaginative diagnostic definition and doom-mongering statistical prognostication." The reputation of the source warrants that these statistical projections be accepted as proposed, adequate diagnostic methods developed, and a treatment discovered. Sadly enough, it would appear that the die is cast, that these victims are already infected by prions, doomed to dementia and death, a disease untreatable at present.

At present the number of professional neuropathologists who are expert priontologists is very limited because of the extremely small number of cases—but if the proposed epidemic materializes, every neuropathologist will become an expert. However, can one make the diagnosis of a prion induced disease without any knowledge of the role of that cause, nor any proof that it is the cause? Such a diagnosis based upon the presence of a prion is so firmly established presently, that too frequently, it terminates the search for another cause.

These questions and doubts, still lingering after decades of research, demonstrate the need for a review of the whole topic beginning with a review of the circumstances of the original descriptions of the CJS and Kuru, both said to be prion induced, which shows that both ailments have been the subject of considerable corrective interpretation with time. The change in qualification of the Creutzfeldt-Jakob concept from that of a syndrome to that of a disease, has resulted in a great deal of literature and confusion but no cause, no therapy. Incidentally, it should be noted that there is no original or princeps page-and-verse description of CJD in the literature, as there is, for example, for Alzheimer's, Wilson's, Parkinson's. This review raises the possibility that Hans Creutzfeldt and Alfons Jakob were right in claiming that there is no Creutzfeldt-Jakob disease with a single cause, but that there is a Creutzfeldt-Jakob syndrome, a neurological complication that occurs in different diseases, a proposition that does not contradict the possible role of a prion and includes the possibility of successful treatment?

REFERENCES

1. Scadding JG. Essentialism and nominalism in medicine: logic of diagnosis of disease terminology. Lancet 1996; 348:594–596.
2a. Ghani AC, Ferguson NM, Donnelly CA, Anderson RM. Predicted vCJD mortality in Great Britain. Nature 2000; 406:583–584.
2b. Opinion of the Scientific Steering Committee on the Human Exposure Risk (HER) via Food with respect to BSE. Presented at European Union Scientific Steering Committee, 10 December 1999.
3. Editorial. Tragedy of variant Creutzfeldt-Jakob disease. Lancet 1999; 353:939.
4. Jones J. Deaths from nvCJD rise sharply. BMJ 1999; 318:829.
5. Wills RG, Cousens SN, Farrington CP, Smith PG, Knight RSG, Ironside JW. Death from variant nvCJD. Lancet 1999; 353:979.
6. Boon D. Future uncertainties for reliable vCJD screening test. Lancet 2000; 356:228.
7. Budka H, Agguzi A, Brown P, Brucher JM, Bugiani O, Gullota F, Haltia M, Hauw JJ, Ironside JW, Jellinger K, Kretzschrmar HA, Lantos PL, Masullo C, Schlote W, Tateishi, Weller R. Neuropathological diagnostic criteia for Creutzfeldt-Jakob disease (CJD) and other human spongiform encephalopathies (Prion Diseases). Brain Path 1995; 5:459–466.
8. Kretschmar HA, Ironside JW, DeArmond SJ, Tateichi J. Diagnostic criteria for sporadic Creutzfeldt-Jakob disease. Arch Neurol 1966; 53: 913–920.
9. Duckett S, Stern J. Concerning the original Creutzfeldt-Jakob concept. J Hist Neurosci 1999; 8: 21–34.
10. Creutzfeldt HG. Uber eine eigenartige herdformige Erkrankung des Zentralnervensystems. Z Ges Neurol Psychiatrie 1920; 57:1–18.
11. Creutzfeldt HG. Uber eine eigenartige herdformige Erkrankung des Zentralnervensystems. In: Nissl R, Alzheimer A, eds. Histologische und Histopathologische Arbeiten uber die Grosshirnrinde. Jena: Gustav Fischer, 1921: 1–48.
12. Jakob A. Uber eigenartige Erkrankungen des Zentralnervensystems mit bemerkenswerten anatomischen Befunden (spastische Pseudosklerose Encephalomyclopathie mit disseminierten Degenerationherden). Dtsch Z Nervenheilkd 1921; 70:132–146.
13. Jakob A. Uber eigenartige Erkrankungen des Zentralnervensystems mit bemerkenswerten anatomischen Befunden (spastische Pseudosklerose Encephalomyelopathie mit disseminierten Degenerationsherden. Z Ges Neurol Psychiatrie 1921b; 64: 147–228.
14. Jakob A. Über eine der multiplen Sklerose klinisch nahestehende Erkrankung des Zentralnervensystems (spastische Pseudosklerose) mit bemerkenswerten anatomischen Befunden. Med Klin 1921; 13:372–376.
15. Jakob A. Die extrapyramidalen Erkrankungen (spastische Pseudosklerose). In: Foerster O, Willmanns K, eds. Monographien aus dem Gesamtgebiete der Neurologie und Psychiatrie 37/8. Berlin: Springer-Verlag, 1923: 215–315.
16. Creutzfeldt HG. Review. Z Ges Neurol Psychiatrie 1921; 25:321–322.
17. Fagot-Largeault A. Aproche médicale de la causalité dans les systêmes complexes. Arch Intern Physiol Bioch (Liège) 1986; 94(4): C85–C94.
18. Campbell EJM, Scadding JG, Roberts RS. The concept of disease. Lancet 1979; 2:757–762.
19. Cohen MM. Syndromes, associations and sequences. In: The Child with Multiple Birth Defects, 2nd ed. New York: Oxford University Press, 1997: 3–14.
20. Wilson SAK. Syndrome of Jakob cortico striatospinal degeneration. In: Bruce AN, ed. Neurology, Vol. 2. Baltimore: Williams & Wilkins, 1955: 1044–1047.
21. Spielmeyer W. Die histopathologische Forschung in der Psychiatrie. Klin Wochenschr 1 (37) 1992; 1817–1819.
22. Lhermitte J, McAlpine D. A clinical and pathological resume of combined disease of the pyramidal extrapyramidal systems with special reference to a new syndrome. Brain 1926; 19:157–176.
23. McMenemey WH. Critical review. Dementia in middle age. J Neurol Psychiatry 1941; 4:48–70.
24. Meyer A, Leigh D, Bigg CE. A rare presenile dementia associated with cortical blindness. J Neurol Neurosurg Psychiatry 1954; 17:129–133.
25. Jakob A. The anatomy, clinical syndromes and physiology of the extrapyramidal system (lecture given at Columbia University, April 1924). Arch Neurol Psychiatry 1925; 13:596–620.
25a. Scholz H. Zur Frage der shiftformigen Veränderungen der Gehirnrinde. Zentratlblat Ges Neurol Psychiat 1926: 57; 312–360.
26. Gildea ED, Cobb S. Effect of anemia on cerebral cortex of cat. Arch Neurol Psychiatry 1930; 23:876–903.
27. Lhermitte J, Barrelet H. Embolie gazeuse cérébrale d'origine péripherique. Étude anatomique. Rev Neurol (Paris) 1934); ii. 851–857.
28. Alajouanine T, Hornet T, Thurel R. L'aspect fenêtre

de l'écorce cérébrale étude des troubles circulatoires localisés à certaines couches céllularies du cortex. Rev Neurol (Paris) 1936; 65:819–857.
29. Courville CB. Etiology and pathogenesis of laminar cortical necrosis. Arch Neurol Psychiatry 1958; 79:7–30.
30. Jakob A. Über die regionäre (areale) and Laminäre Prozessocalisation bein des Geisteskrankheiten. Allg Z Psychiatrie 1927; 102:343–349.
31. Nishimura M, Mochizuki H, Tavahi M, Tavobe H, Odo M. Thrombosis of the superior cerebral vein with hemorrhagic cerebral infarction—serial MRI and pathological study of a case. Rinho Shinkeigaku. 1990; 30:864–868.
32. Kirschbaum WR. Jakob-Creutzfeldt Disease (Spastic Pseudosclerosis. A Jakob Heidenhain Syndrome: Subacute Spongiform Encephalopathy). New York: Elsevier, 1968.
33. Lindenberg R. Tissue reaction in the gray matter of the central nervous system. In: Haymaker W, Adams R, eds. Histology and Histopathology of the Nervous System. Springfield, MA: Charles C. Thomas, 1982; 973–980.
34. Falcone S, Quencer RM, Bowen B, Bruce JH, Naidich TP. Creutzfeldt-Jakob disease: focal symmetrical cortical involvement demonstrated by MR imaging. Am J Neurol 1992; 13:403–406.
35. Iwasaki Y, Ikeda K. Tagaya N, Kinoshuta M. Magnetic resonance imaging and neuropathological findings in two patients with Creutzfeldt-Jakob disease. J Neurol Sci 1994; 126:228–231.
36. Shyu W, Lee CC, Hsu YD, Lih JC, Lee JT, Lee WH, Tsao WL. Panencephalitic Creutzfeldt-Jakob disease. Unusual presentation of magnetic resonance spectroscopy. J Neurol Sci 1996; 138:157–160.
37. van der Knapp MS, Smit LS, Lauta JJP, Lteber HN, Valk J. Cortical laminar abnormalities—occurrence and clinical significance. Neuropediatrics 1993; 24:143–148.
38. Isozumi K, Fukuushi Y, Tanaka O, Nogawa S, Ishihara T, Sakuta R.A MELAS (mitochondrial myopathy, encephalopathy, lactic acidosis and stroke-like episodes) mt DNA mutation that indices subacut dementia which mimics Creutzfeldt-Jakob disease. Int Med 1994; 33:543–546.
39. Kinoshita T, Takahashi S, Ishii K, Higano S, Matsumoto K, Haginaga K, Lunuma L. Reye's syndrome with cortical laminar necrosis: MRI. Neuroradiology 1996; 38:269–272.
40. Takahashi S, Hano S, Ishii K, Matsumoto K, Sakamoto K, lwasaki Y. Hypoxic brain damage: cortical laminar necrosis and delayed changes in white matter at sequential MR imaging. Radiology 1993; 189:449–456.
41. Vogt C, Vogt O. Erkrankungen der Grossirrinde im Lichte der Topistik, Pathoklise und Pathoarchitectonik. Jahresber Psychiatr Neurol 1922; 28:1–27.
42. Skoog I. The relationship between blood pressure and dementia: a review. Biomed Pharmacol 1997; 51:367–375.
43. Ramp FL. Intermittent oxygen deficiency as the cause of dementia. Med Hypotheses 1999; 53: 175–176.
44. Arbelarg A, Castillo M, Mukhaji SK. Diffusion—weighed MR imaging of global cerebral anoxia. Am J Neuroradiol 1999; 20:999–1007.
45. Jones D, Nevin S. Rapidly progressive cerbral degeneration subacute vascular encephalopathy with mental disorder, focal disturbances and myoclonic epilepsy. J Neurol Psychiatry 1954; 17:148–159.
46. Nevin S, McMenemey WH, Behrmann S, Jones DP. Subacute spongiform encephalopathy. A subacute form of encephalopathy attributable to vascular dysfunction (spongiform cerebral atrophy). Brain 1960; 83:519–564.
47. McMenemey WH, Pallis C. Spongiform encephalomyelopathy in a case of treated chronic uraemia. In: Livre Jubilaire en l'Honneur du Professeur L van Bagaert. Acta Med (Belg) 1962; 556–561.
48. Behrmann S, Mandybar T, McMenemey WH. Un cas de maladie de Creutzfeldt-Jakob a la suite d'un traumatism cranien. Rev Neurol (Paris) 1962; 107:453–459.
49. Crompton R. A case of subacute spongiform encephalopathy supporting a vascular pathogenesis. Acta Neuropathol (Berl) 1963; 2:291–296.
50. McMenemey WH, Grant HC, Behrmann S. Two examples of presenile dementia (Pick's disease and Stern-Garcin syndrome) with a history of trauma. Arch Psychiatr Z Ges Neurol 1965; 207:128–140.
51. van Bogaert L. Preface: Symposium on presenile spongiform encephalopathies. Venice (June 1965). Acta Neuropath (Berl) Suppl 1967; III:1–2.
52. Nevin S, Barnard RO, McMenemey WH. Different types of Creutzfeldt-Jakob disease. In: Symposium on Presenile Spongy Encephalopathies, Venice. Acta Neuropathol (Berl) Suppl 1965; III: 7–1.
53. Duckett S. L'Histoire de la Maladie du Kuru. (The History of the Disease Kuru). Thèse de Doctorat. Ecole des Hautes Études Pratiques, Sorbonne, Université de Paris (in preparation).
54. Zigas V. Laughing Death. The Untold Story of Kuru. Clifton, NJ: Humana Press, 1990.
55. Correspondence on the Discovery and Original Investigations on Kuru. Smadel-Gajdusek Correspondence. 1955–1958. US Department of Health & Welfare, NIH, 1976, 62C.
56. Kolata G. Anthropologists suggest cannibalism is a myth. Science 1985; 232:1497–1500.
56a. Steadman LB, Merbs CF. Kuru and cannibalism? Am Anthropol 1982; 84:611–617.
57. Gajdusek DC. Unconventional viruses and the origin and disappearance of kuru. Science 1966; 197(4307): 943–960.
58. Gajdusek DC, Zigas V. Degenerative disease of the central nervous system in New Guinea. The endemic occurrence of kuru in the native population. N Engl J Med 1957; 257:974–978.
59. Zigas V, Gajdusek CD. Kuru: clinical study of a new syndrome resembling paralysis agitans in natives of the Eastern Highlands of Australian New Guinea. Med J Aust 1957; 2:745–754.
60. Gajdusek CD, Zigas V. Untersuchungen über die Pathogenese von Kuru: eine klinische, pathologische und epidemiologische Untersuchung einer chronischen und unter den Eigeboronen der Eastern Highlands von New Guinea epidemischen Ausmasse erreichenden Erkrankung des Zentralnervensystems. Klin Wochnschr 1958; 36:445–459.
61. Zigas V, Gajdusek DC. Clinical, pathological and epidemiological study of a recently discovered acute progressive degenerative disease of the central ner-

vous system reaching epidemic proportions among natives of the Eastern Highlands of New Guinea. Papua New Guinea Med J 1959; 3:1–31.
62. Zigas V, Gadjusek DC. Clinical, pathological and epidemiological study of a recently discovered acute progressive degenerative disease of the central nervous system reaching epidemic proportions among natives of the Eastern Highlands of New Guinea. Am J Med 1959; 26:442–469.
63. Simpson DA, Lander H, Robson HN. Observations on kuru. II. Clinical features. Aust Ann Med 1959; 8: 8–15.
64. Fowler M. Robertson EG. Observations on kuru. III. Pathological features in five cases. Aust Ann Med 8: 16–26. 1959;
65. Goodfield J. Quest for Killers. Boston: Birkhauser, 1985: 19–20.
66. Klatzo I, Gajdusek DC, Zigas V. Pathology of Kuru. Lab Invest 1959: 8 (4): 799–847.
66a. Jacob H, Pyrkosch W, Strube H. Die erbliche Form der Creutzfelt-Jakobischen Krankheit (Familie Backer). Arch Psychiat u Nervenkr 1958; 184: 653–674.
66b. Jacob H, Eicke W, Orthner H. Zur Klinik und Neuropathologie der subakuten praesenilen, spongiosën Atrophien mit dyskinetischen Endstadium. Dtsch Z Nervenheilk 1958; 178: 330–357.
67. Beck E, Daniels PM. Neuropathological changes in Kuru compared and contrasted with tose of some other neurological disease. In: Hornabrook R. ed. Essays on Kuru. Farrington, Berks. EW Classey Ltd. 1976:117–124.
68. Hornabrook RW. Kuru—a subacute cerebellar degeneration. The natural history and clinical features. Brain 1968; 91:53–74.
69. Sigurdson B, Pallson PA, Grimson H. Visna. A demyelinating transmissible disease of sheep. J Neuropath Exp Neurol 1957; 389–403.
70. Masters CL, Gajdusek DC. The spectrum of Creutzfeldt-Jakob disease and the virus-induced spongiform encephalopathies. In: Smith WT, Cavanagh JB, eds. Recent Advances in Neuropathology, Vol. 2. Edinburgh: Churchill-Livingstone, 1982:139–163.
71. Hamilton RL, Wiley CA. Prion protein encephalopathies. In: Davis RL, Robertson DM, eds. Textbook of Neuropathology, 3rd ed. Baltimore: Williams & Wilkins, 1997:1030.
72. Crome L. Neuropathological changes in diseases caused by inborn errors of metabolism. In: Holt KS, Milner J, eds. Neurometabolic Diseases in Children. London: Livingstone, 1966: 50.
73. Grunthal E. Die Pathologische Anatomie der Senilen Demenz und der alzheimerschen Krankheit. Handbuch der Geisteskrankheiten, Pt 7. Berlin: Springer-Verlag, 1930.
74. Gajdusek DC, Gibbs CJ, Alpers MP. Experimental transmission of a Kuru-like syndrome to chimpanzees. Nature 1966; 209:794–796.
75. Gibbs CJ Jr, Gajdusek CD, Asher DM, Alpers MP, Beck E, Daniels SB, Matthews WB. Creutzfeldt-Jakob disease (spongiform encephalopathy). Transmission to a chimpanzee. Science 1968; 161:388–389.
76. Prusiner SB, Hsiao KK. Human prion diseases. Ann Neurol 1994; 135:385.
77. DeArmond SJ, Dickson DW, DeArmond B. Creutzfeldt-Jakob disease and Kuru. In: Davis RL, Robertson DM, eds. Textbook of Neuropathology, 3rd ed. Baltimore: Williams & Wikins, 1997:1112.
78. Aguzzi A, Weissmann C. Prion research: the next frontier. Nature 1997; 389:795–798.
79. Smith Chesebro B. BSE and prions: uncertainties about the agent. Science 1998; 279:42–43.

Index

Abetalipoproteinemia, 398
Acetylcholine, 549
Acquired immunodeficiency syndrome (AIDS), 495–497, 497f
Activity-dependent neurotrophic factor (ADNF), 27–28, 28f
AD. *See* Alzheimer's disease
Adams, John, 3
Adams, John Quincy, 3
ADCA. *See* Autosomal dominant cerebellar ataxia
ADLBV. *See* Alzheimer's disease Lewy body variant
ADNF (activity-dependent neurotrophic factor), 27–28, 28f
Adrenoleukodystrophy, 431–432, 432f
Adrenomyeloneuropathy, 431–432, 432f
Advanced glycation end products (AGEs), 142
Age-related diseases. *See also specific age-related diseases*
    free-radical disease and, 127
AGEs (advanced glycation end products), 142
Aging
    activity-dependent neurotrophic factor and, 27–28, 28f
    alcohol and, 400
    autonomic nervous system, clinical studies of, 527–528
    brain. *See* Brain, aging
    markers, 19
    neuronal loss during, 458–459
    parasympathetic ganglia, 531
    pathological hallmarks
        ballooned neurons or Pick cells, 164, 165f
        cerebral atrophy, 159–160
        granulovacular degeneration, 161, 162f
        Hirano bodies, 162, 162f
        Lewy bodies, 162–163, 162f, 163f
        Marinesco bodies, 163, 163f
        neuritic plaques, 160–161
        neurofibrillary changes, 161
        Pick bodies, 164, 164f
        status spongiosus *vs.* spongiform changes, 164, 165f, 166
        ventricular enlargement, 160
    peripheral nerves and, 516–517
    pharmacokinetic changes, 564–565, 565t
    skeletal muscle and, 547–551, 548t, 550f, 551f
    sympathetic ganglia, 528–529, 529f–531f, 531
    vs. Alzheimer's disease, 208

AIDS (acquired immunodeficiency syndrome), 495–497, 497f
AIE (anoxic/hypoxic-ischemic encephalopathy), 59–60, 61f
Air embolism, 72
Alcoholic myopathy, 405
Alcoholism
    brain volume and, 400–401, 401f, 402f
    premature aging from, 403–404, 404f
    white matter loss, reversibility of, 404–405
Allocortex, in dementia, 157
ALS. *See* Amyotrophic lateral sclerosis
Aluminum, Alzheimer's disease and, 242
Aluminum-containing medications, Alzheimer's disease and, 568
Alzheimer's disease (AD)
    amino acid deficits, 238–239
    amyloid-β peptide-associated alterations
        amyloid angiopathy. *See* Cerebral amyloid angiopathy
        protein aggregation, 23–24, 23t
        senile plaques. *See* Plaques, neuritic
    amyloid hypothesis, 141
    Apo E-ε4 allele and, 134
    apoptosis, 7, 213–216, 216
    brain
        aluminum accumulation, 242
        astrocytosis, 234
        capillaries, 138, 139f, 140, 140f
        Golgi apparatus fragmentation, 234
        granulovacuolar degeneration, 233, 233f
        gray matter changes, 233–234, 233f
        gross examination, 209
        Hirano bodies, 233–234
        leukoaraiosis, 235
        Lewy bodies, 234
        neuronal loss, 234–235
        nucleolus volume decrease, 234
        spongiform changes, 234
        weight/volume, 209
        white matter changes, 234–235
    calcium in, 32–33
    case report, fall-related injury, 581–582, 582f, 583f
    caspase activation, 24, 25f
    cell loss in, 127
    central nervous system atrophy in, 126
    cerebral amyloid angiopathy, 229–232, 230f

Alzheimer's disease (AD) *(continued)*
  cerebral atrophy, 160, 209–210, 210f–213f, 213
  cerebral blood vessels, molecular abnormalities in, 133–135, 135f
  cerebral perfusion, 135–138, 136t
  cognitive impairments
    cholinergic neurotransmission defects and, 237
    risk factors for, 136, 136t
  dementia, 123
  dendritic changes, 232–233
  development, traumatic brain injury and, 466–467
  diagnosis, 207–209
    criteria for, 235–236
  Down syndrome and, 240
  etiologic hypothesis, 241–243
  genetic factors, 132–133, 143–144
    Apo E genotype, 241–242
    mutations, 32–33, 32f
    susceptibility gene, 137
    symptoms, 207
    synaptic disconnection in, 130–131
    synaptic loss, 232–233
    tau-associated alterations. *See also* Neurofibrillary tangles, morphology of, 216–218, 217f, 218f
    twin studies, 242
    with vascular dementia, 239–240
    vascular dementia and, 116–117
    vascular dementia treatment and, 138
    vs. dementia with Lewy bodies, 282
    vs. normal aging, 208
  with Huntington disease, 382, 384–385, 384t
  incidence, 207, 241
  inflammation and, 226–227
  Lewy body variant, 241
  magnetic resonance imaging hypersignals, 235
  mitochondrial dysfunction, 29–30, 30f
  neuritic pathology in, 130–131
  neurochemical deficits
    cholinergic hypothesis of, 236–237
    in dopaminergic system, 238
    in noradrenergic system, 237
    in serotonergic system, 237–238
  neurodegeneration, 123
  neuronal cytoskeleton alterations, 17f, 18
  neuronal glucose depletion in, 140–141
  neuronal loss, 213–216
  neuropathology, 124
    aluminum-containing medications, 568
    dialysis encephalopathy, 568
  neuropeptide deficits, 238
  neurotransmitter signaling alterations, 25–27, 26f
  oxidative phosphorylation in, 140
  oxidative stress, 22, 23
  Par-4 expression, 20–21, 20f
  pathogenesis, 136, 137–138, 139f
  perikaryal atrophy, 213–216
  postmortem studies, apoptosis, 126
  presenilins in, 232
  prevalence, 156, 207
  protective factors, 242
  risk factors, 136t, 241–242
Alzheimer's disease Lewy body variant (ADLBV)
  brainstem in, 159, 160f
  definition, 170
  demographics, 170, 170t
  vs. dementia with Lewy bodies, 171
Alzheimer's disease/senile dementia of Alzheimer's type, 66
Alzheimer type I glia, 442, 442f
American trypanosomiasis (Chagas' disease), 484–486, 485f
Amino acids deficits, in Alzheimer's disease, 238–239
Amiodarone peripheral neuropathy, 513
Amoebic infections, 481–483, 483f
Amygdala, in dementia, 159
Amyloid argyrophilic plaques. *See* Plaques, neuritic
Amyloid-β peptide
  age-related changes, 19
  in Alzheimer's disease, 23–24, 23t
  apoptosis and, 129
  associated alterations
    amyloid angiopathy. *See* Cerebral amyloid angiopathy
    protein aggregation, 23–24, 23t
    senile plaques. *See* Plaques, neuritic
  in cerebral amyloid angiopathy, 66
  cerebral constriction and, 138
  deposits
    in cerebral amyloid angiopathy, 231–232
    in Creutzfeldt-Jakob disease, 181
  distribution, 227–228
  forms, 225–226
  functions, 24
  neuronal injury, 24
  non-Aβ component, 226
  nonamyloid deposits
    in dementia, 141–142
    diffuse, 227
    fleecy, 227
    focal or dense, 227
    granular, 227
    lake-like, 227
  in plaques, 222, 223f, 224–226
Amyloid hypothesis, of Alzheimer's disease, 141
Amyloidosis, 556, 556f
Amyloid peripheral neuropathies, 508–509, 508f, 509f
β-Amyloid precursor protein (APP)
  in age-related neurodegenerative disease, 23, 23t
  in senile plaques, 224–226
Amyloid precursor protein mutations, 32–33, 32f
Amyotrophic lateral sclerosis (ALS)
  animal models, 361
  central nervous system atrophy in, 126
  cytoskeleton alterations, 18
  diagnosis
    immunocytochemical analysis, 360
    neuropathological, 360

familial, 360–361
   pathogenesis, astrocytes in, 365
   SOD1 mutation and, 364, 365–366
gene mutations, 33
genetic factors, 365–366
historical aspects, 360
immunocytochemical analysis, 365
incidence, 365
mortality rates, 365
neuropathology, 125, 361, 361*f*, 362*f*
   Bunina bodies, 362, 362*f*
   Golgi apparatus fragmentation, 362–363, 363*f*
   intaneuronal Lewy body-like hyaline inclusions, 364, 364*f*
   neurofilaments, 361–362
   ubiquitin inclusions, 363–364, 363*f*
oxidative stress, 22–23
pathogenesis, 365–366
protein aggregates, 23*t*
sporadic, 360
Aneurysms
   berry/saccular, 81–83, 82*f*–85*f*
   Charcot-Bouchard, 78
   dissecting, 85
   fusiform, 86, 87*f*
   inflammatory, 83, 85
   mycotic, 83, 85
Angiitis. *See* Vasculitis
Angioendotheliomatosis, neoplastic, 116
Animals, experimental
   age-related changes
      in parasympathetic nervous system, 532
      in sympathetic nervous system, 531–532
   neuropathology
      central pathways, 533
      parasympathetic pathways, 534–535
      sympathetic pathways, 533–534, 533*f*, 534*f*
ANNA-1 (antineuronal nuclear antibody), 453
Anoxia-ischemia, central nervous system and, 59–60, 60*f*
Anoxic/hypoxic-ischemic encephalopathy (AIE), 59–60, 61*f*
Anthony, Susan B., 3
Anticholinergic agents, elderly and, 564
Anticipation phenomenon, 286
Antigens, 447–448
Antigen spreading, 448
Antioxidants, apoptosis prevention, 24
Anti-Ri antibodies, 454
Anti-Yo antibodies, 454
Antoni A and B type tissue, 423, 424*f*
Aphasia, subcortical, 51, 52*f*
Apolipoprotein E (ApoE)
   E-ε2 allele, 32
   E-ε4 allele, 32
      Alzheimer's disease etiology and, 241–242
      Alzheimer's disease risk and, 134
      dementia with Lewy body risk and, 241
   in plaques, 226

Apoptosis
   DNA fragmentation and, 24, 126
   free radicals and, 127
   molecular mechanisms, 128–130
      amyloid-β, 129
      heme oxygenase-1, 130
      nitric oxide synthase-3, 130
      presenilins, 129
      superoxide dismutase I, 129–130
   in neurodegenerative diseases, 123, 125–126
      age-related, 20
      Alzheimer's disease, 7, 123, 216
      Creutzfeldt-Jakob syndrome, 7
      glial cells and, 132
   oxidative stress and, 24
   prevention, 24
APP. *See* β-Amyloid precursor protein
APP gene overexpression, in Down syndrome, 125
Arbovirus infections, 492–493
Arteriopathies
   large artery, 61*t*
   small artery, 61*t*
Arteriosclerosis, 18, 503–504. *See also* Atherosclerosis
Arteriovenous malformation (AVM), intraparenchymal hemorrhage and, 92, 92*f*
Arylsulphatase A deficiency, in metachromatic leukodystrophy, 431
Aspartame, brain tumors and, 410–411
Aspergillosis, 486–487
Astrocytes
   in familial amyotrophic lateral sclerosis pathogenesis, 365
   tuft-shaped, 276, 277*f*
Astrocytoma, 417–418, 417*t*
Astrocytosis, Alzheimer's disease, 234
Asymmetrical lesions, in vascular dementia, 114–115
Ataxia-telangiectasia, genetics, 331, 332*t*
Ataxin-1, 288
Atheroembolus, 62, 65*f*
Atherosclerosis
   of carotid artery, 62, 64*f*
   of circle of Willis, 62, 63*f*
   microscopic features, 63, 65–68, 65*f*–68*f*
   neuropathology, 18
   pathogenesis, 62
   plaques. *See* Plaques
Atherosclerotic Parkinsonism, 295
ATP synthesis, reduced substrate delivery for, 136–137
Atrophy, panlaminar, 196, 196*t*
Autonomic nervous system
   age-related damage, 535, 539–540
      axonal transport and, 538
      calcium dynamics and, 539
      dendritic structural alterations and, 536
      extracellular matrix and, 539
      neurotrophic substances and, 537–538
      oxidative injury and, 539

Autonomic nervous system (*continued*)
    regeneration and, 535–536
    synaptic organelle degradation and, 538–539
  aging, clinical studies of, 527–528
  central pathways
    in aged human subjects, 528
    neuropathology in animals, 533
  dysfunction, 527
  enteric pathways, neuropathology in animals, 535
  of experimental animals, age-related changes, 531–532
  neuropathology
    in aged population, 528–529, 529f–531f, 531
    parasympathetic ganglia, 531
    sympathetic ganglia, 528–529, 529f–531f, 531
  parasympathetic pathways, neuropathology in animals, 534–535
  sympathetic pathways, neuropathology in animals, 533–534, 533f, 534f
Autoregulation, 44, 44t
Autosomal dominant cerebellar ataxia (ADCA)
  prevalence, 331
  types, 286–287
Autosomal recessive early-onset parkinsonism with diurnal fluctuation, 311
Axonal degeneration, 500–501, 500f, 501f
  retrograde effects, 500
  Wallerian, 500, 500f
Axonal dystrophy, 501
Axonal retraction balls, 462, 462f
Axonal swelling, 501, 501f
Axonal transport, age-dependent alterations, 538

BACE (β-site APP cleaving enzyme), 225
Bacterial infections
  cerebral abscesses, 481, 482f
  endocarditis, 480–481, 481f
  Lyme disease, 480
  meningitis, 475–476, 476f, 477t, 478–479, 478f, 479f
  neurosyphilis, 479–480, 480f, 481f
Balamuthia mandrillaris, 482
Ballooned neurons (Pick cells)
  histologic features, 164, 165f, 199t, 200
  historical aspects, 191–192
Bands of Büngner, 500
Barbiturate therapy, for head injury, 468
Barton, Clara, 3
Basal ganglia
  in neurodegenerative disease
    Huntington disease, 370–372
    with Parkinsonian symptoms, 271–272, 272f–275f, 274–276, 278–279
  nomenclature, 370–371
  pathways
    input compartment, 371
    output compartment, 371
  striosome-matrix compartments, 371
Basic fibroblast growth factor (bFGF), 20
  age-related changes, 27

Basket cell neurons, 326
BDNF (brain-derived neurotrophic factor), age-related changes, 20, 27–28, 28f
Bellini, Giovanni, 3
Benzodiazepines, aging brain and, 564–565
Bergmann astrocytes, 326
Beriberi, 393
Bernhardt, Sarah, 3
Berry/saccular aneurysms, 81–83, 82f–85f
Bilateral lesions, in vascular dementia, 112
Binswanger disease
  associated disorders, 107
  contributing factors, 109–110
  differential diagnosis, 110–112, 111f, 113f
    CADASIL, 110–111, 113f
    cerebral amyloid angiopathy, 110, 111f
  morphology, 106–107, 108f, 109f
  neuroimaging, 107, 109
Binswanger's subcortical leukoencephalopathy (BSLE), 77
Blood-brain barrier, 18019
Blood vessels
  cerebral, molecular abnormalities in Alzheimer's disease, 133–135, 135f
  small, abnormalities, in vascular dementia, 116, 116f
Border infarct (watershed), 76–77, 77f
Borrelia burgdorferi, 480
Bovine spongiform encephalopathy (BSE), 178
Boyd, William, 3
Braak and Braak staging, 220
Bradycor (CP-0127), for head injury, 468
Brain. *See also specific brain regions*
  aging
    histologic examination, 6
    in Huntington disease, 382–384, 383t
    morphology, 5
    neurogenesis of, 6–7
    normal, 1, 564
    physical injury and, 572–575, 575t
    radioimaging, 5–6
    "use-it-or-lose-it" hypothesis, 29, 29f
  capillary degeneration, 137
  cells
    anoxia susceptibility, 59
    histology in normal aging, 6
  hyperperfusion, 137
  infarct. *See also* Cerebral infarct
    incidence, 58
    ischemic. *See* Ischemic brain infarct
  normal, physiology/pathophysiology, 43–44
  perfusion, 18
  protein content, 19
  size, 5
  trauma. *See* Brain trauma
  volume
    age-related changes *vs.* alcoholism, 400–404, 402t, 403t, 404f

alcoholism and, 400–401, 401f, 402f
  in Alzheimer's disease, 209
  in cerebral hemispheres, alcoholism and, 401–404, 402t, 403t, 404f
 weight
  alcoholism and, 400–401, 400t, 401t
  in Alzheimer's disease, 209
  in Pick disease, 195
 white matter. *See* White matter
Brain contusions
 contracoup, 579–580
 coup, 577–578
 fracture, 580
 gliding, 580
Brain-derived neurotrophic factor (BDNF), age-related changes, 20, 27–28, 28f
Brainstem
 in dementia, 159, 160f
 injury, 580
 neuronal loss, in Alzheimer's disease, 214
Brain trauma, 458
 cerebral hemodynamics after, 460–462, 460f
 from closed head injuries, 464–465, 464f, 465f
 diffuse axonal injury, 462–463, 462f
 excitotoxicity after, 464
 intracerebral hematomas, 467–468
 neurodegeneration and, 459–460
 pathological sequelae, age and, 459
 primary impact injury, 462
 secondary injury, 462
 treatment, 468–469
Brain tumors
 age and, 408
 etiology, 409–411, 412t, 413, 413t
 extrinsic, 408
 imaging strategies, 413–415, 414f, 415f
 incidence, 408, 409, 409t
 intrinsic, 408
 management, 425
 palliative care, 425
 primary intrinsic, 416–417
  astrocytoma, 417–418
  classification of, 417
  glioblastoma multiforme, 418–421, 418f–420f
  malignant lymphoma, 423–425, 424f
  meningioma, 421–422, 421f– 423f
  schwannoma, 423, 424f
  secondary carcinoma/melanoma, 422–423
  survival rates, 417, 417t
 risk factors, 408
 secondary metastatic, 415–416, 416f
BSE (bovine spongiform encephalopathy), 178
Buffon, G.L., 3–4

CAA. *See* Cerebral amyloid angiopathy
CADASIL
 dementia, 159
 diagnosis, 514

differential diagnosis, 110–111, 113f
 genetic factors, 33–34
CAG expansion repeat disorders, 286, 332–334, 333t. *See also specific disorders*
Cajal, Santiago Ramon y, 322, 324f
Calcium
 abnormal dynamics, age-related autonomic nervous system damage and, 539
 age-related changes, 27
 in Alzheimer's disease, 32–33
 extracellular, in anoxia-ischemia, 59
 homeostasis, in dementia, 141
Calcium-ion channels, 27
Calpains, 24
Candida albicans, 492
Candidiasis, 492, 492f
Capsase activation, 126
Carbon monoxide poisoning, secondary Parkinsonian syndromes, 294
Cardiac surgery, unintentional embolization, 72–73, 73f, 74f
Carotid artery atherosclerosis, 62, 64f
Carotid endarterectomy, for stroke prophylaxis, 62, 64f, 65f
CATCH hypothesis, 136
Cavernous hemangiomas, 93, 93f, 95
Cavernous sinus thrombosis, 79
CD15 cell adhesion molecule, brain tumors and, 416
CD4$^+$ cells, 447
Cell death, programmed. *See* Apoptosis
Centenarians, 2
Central nervous system
 anoxia-ischemia and, 59–60, 60f
 atrophy, in neurodegenerative disease, 126
 hemorrhage, 576–583, 582f, 583f
 impairment, in neurodegeneration, 124–125
 involvement in neurosyphilis, 479–480
 neuroimmunologic diseases of, 455–456
Central pontine myelinolysis (CPM), 396, 396f, 441–442, 441f
Cerebellopontine acoustic neuroma, MRI scan, 415t
Cerebellum
 afferents, 323
  climbing fibers, 323
  mossy fibers, 323
 anatomy
  macroscopic, 322–323
  microscopic, 322, 325–326
 atrophy, in Huntington disease, 378–379
 chemical neuroanatomy, 328
 cortex
  circuitry, 326, 328, 328f
  degeneration, 398–399, 399f
  neurons, 326, 327f
 degeneration, 286–293, 398–399, 399f
 degenerative diseases
  classification, 330
  clinical features, 329–330, 331

Cerebellum *(continued)*
    epidemiology, 330–331
    genetics, 331–334, 332*t*, 333*f*
    neuropathology, 331–334
  functional domains, 322–323
  functional neuroanatomic connections
    afferent, 323
    efferent, 323–325
Cerebral abscesses, 481–482, 482*f*
Cerebral amyloid angiopathy (CAA)
  amyloid deposits, 231–232
  associated disorders, 65–66
    age-related disease, 230–231
    intraparenchymal hemorrhage, 90, 91*f*, 92
  blood vessel abnormalities, 134, 135*f*
  differential diagnosis, 110, 111*f*
  familial, 66–67
  histologic features, 66–68, 66*f*–68*f*, 229–230, 230*f*
  in Huntington disease, 383, 383*t*
  incidence, 231
  pathogenesis, 67–68
Cerebral atrophy, 5, 159–160
  Alzheimer's disease, 209–210, 210*f*–213*f*, 213
  granular, 102–103, 105*f*, 106*f*
  Huntington disease, neostriatal pathology and, 378
Cerebral blood flow, after brain trauma, 459
Cerebral cortex
  age-related changes, in Huntington disease, 382–384, 383*t*
  allocortex, 157
  atrophy. *See* Cerebral atrophy
  blood vessels, molecular abnormalities in Alzheimer's disease, 133–135, 135*f*
  causes of dementia
    neuroanatomical, 157, 158*f*
    neurodegenerative disease involvement, 279–280, 282–284, 285*f*, 286
  degeneration, 1, 7
  embolism. *See* Embolism, cerebral
  neocortex, 157, 158*f*
Cerebral hemisphere volume, alcoholism and, 401–404, 402*t*, 403*t*, 404*f*
Cerebral hemorrhage, delayed post-traumatic, 576–577
Cerebral infarct
  definition, 59
  hemorrhagic, 73
  lacunar, 77–78, 78*f*
  macroscopic features, 73, 75*f*
  microscopic features, 73–76
  nonhemorrhagic or bland, 73
  watershed or border, 76–77, 77*f*
Cerebral malaria, 483–484, 484*f*
Cerebral metabolic rates, after brain trauma, 461
Cerebral perfusion
  after brain trauma, 460–461
  in Alzheimer's disease, 135–138, 136*t*, 139*f*
  in vascular dementia, 135–138, 136*t*

Cerebral perfusion pressure (CPP), hemodynamic/metabolic changes, 44, 44*t*
Cerebral vascular disease. *See also* Arteriosclerosis; Atherosclerosis; Cerebral amyloid angiopathy
  classification, 61–62, 61*t*
  microangiopathy, 62–63, 63*f*, 64*f*
Cerebral vessels, avulsion injuries of, 577
Cerebrovascular disease
  classification, 58
  risk factors, 18
Cerebrovascular resistance (CVR), 460
Cerebrum, contralateral effects, in stroke, 51
Cervantes, Saavedra, Miguel De, 4
^{11}C-flumazenil, 43
  as neuronal loss marker, 53
Chagas' disease (American trypanosomiasis), 484–486, 485*f*
Charcot-Bouchard aneurysms, 78
Charcot-Marie-Tooth disease (CMT), 513–514
ChAT (choline acetyltransferase), in Alzheimer's disease, 236–237
Chemotherapeutic agents, white matter loss, 568
CHF (congestive heart failure), 555
Chloroquine peripheral neuropathy, 513, 513*f*
Choline acetyltransferase (ChAT), in Alzheimer's disease, 236–237
Cholinergic hypothesis, 236–237
Choline transport, deficits, 25
Chorea-acanthocytosis, 514
Chronic inflammatory demyelinating polyneuropathies (CIDP), 454–455, 511–512, 511*f*
Chronic obstructive pulmonary disease (COPD), 555
Churchill, Winston, 4
CIDP (chronic inflammatory demyelinating polyneuropathies), 454–455, 511–512, 511*f*
Circle of Willis
  aneurysmal dilatation, 62
  atherosclerosis, 62, 63*f*
Circulatory disturbances, in vascular dementia, 115–116
Clemenceau, Georges, 4
Cobalamine deficiency, 397–398, 398*f*
Coccidioidomycosis, 490–492, 491*f*
Cognition, estrogen and, 31
Cognitive impairment, in Alzheimer's disease, 124
Computed tomography (CT)
  aging brain, 5–6
  brain tumors, 413–414
  diffuse axonal injury, 463, 463*f*
Congestive heart failure (CHF), 555
Congophilic amyloid angiopathy. *See* Cerebral amyloid angiopathy
COPD (chronic obstructive pulmonary disease), 555
Corot, J.B., 4
Corpus striatum, 370–371
Cortical-basal ganglionic degeneration (corticobasal degeneration), 278–279, 280*f*–281*f*
Cortical hypometabolism, behavioral stroke recovery and, 53

Cortical laminar necrosis, in Creutzfeldt-Jakob disease
    diagnosis, 596–597
Cortical Lewy body disease. See Dementia with Lewy
    bodies
Cortical ribbon thickness/length, in Alzheimer's disease,
    210, 213, 213f
Corticobasal degeneration (CBD)
    differential diagnosis, 279
    macroscopic examination, 278
    microscopic examination, 278–279, 280f–281f
    symptoms, 278
    tau protein, 279
Corticodentatonigral degeneration (corticobasal
    degeneration), 278–279, 280f–281f
Coup contusions, 577–578
CP-0127 (Bradycor), for head injury, 468
^{11}C-PK 11195, 43, 54
CPM (central pontine myelinolysis), 396, 396f, 441–442,
    441f
Creutzfeldt-Jakob disease
    brainstem in, 159, 160f
    central nervous system atrophy in, 126
    clinical course, 179
    concept, new, 599
    cortical laminar necrosis and, 596–597
    diagnosis, 596–597, 600
    familial, 177, 179
    genetics, 177–179
    historical aspects, 594–596, 597
    iatrogenic form, 177
    incidence, 179
    incubation period, 178
    kuru and, 597–599, 600
    neuropathology, 179–182, 180f, 181f, 599–600
        amyloid deposits, 181–182
        fibrillary astrocytosis, 181
        spongiform changes, 177, 180–181, 180f
    Parkinsonian syndrome in, 294
    plaques, 181–182, 181f
    prevalence, 179
    prion protein and, 177–179
    slow virus theory, 598–599
    sporadic, 177, 179
    symptoms, 177, 179
    synonyms, 177
    transmission, 178, 597–599
    variants, 177, 596
        Heidenhain, 596
        new, 593–594
    vs. syndrome, 597
Creutzfeldt-Jakob syndrome
    apoptosis, 7
    experimental/clinical evidence, 596
    historical aspects, 594–596
    neuropathology, 599–600
    vs. disease, 597
Critical illness, peripheral neuropathy from, 505
Crossed cerebellar hypometabolism (diaschisis), 50–51, 51f

Crow-Fukase syndrome, 507, 507f
Cryoglobulinemia, 507–508, 507f
Cryptococcal meningitis, 477t
Cryptococcosis, 490, 491f
CT. See Computed tomography
Cysticercosis, 486, 487f, 488f
Cytochrome oxidase, in Alzheimer's disease, 140
Cytokines, inflammation and, 143

DAI (diffuse axonal injury), 462–463, 462f
DDE (dichlorodiphenyl-dichloroethylene), brain tumors
    and, 411, 412t, 413, 413t
DDT (dichlorodiphenyl-trichloroethylene), brain tumors
    and, 411, 412t, 413, 413t
Delayed traumatic intracerebral hematoma (DTICH),
    576–577
Dementia. See also specific dementing diseases
    Alzheimer's. See Alzheimer's disease
    brainstem in, 159, 160f
    causes, 156
    clinical features, 156
    diagnosis, 156
    forensic aspects, 583–584
    frontal. See Frontal lobe dementia; Frontotemporal
        dementia
    lacking distinctive histology, 189
    metabolic factors, 138, 139f, 140–141
    mixed, 239–240
    neuroanatomical basis, 157
        cerebral cortex, 157, 158f
        cerebral white matter, 157, 159
        subcortical nuclei, 159
        substrate for, 124–125
    neurodegeneration in, 123
    neuroleptics for, 566
    pathogenesis
        calcium homeostasis and, 141
        free radicals, 142
        genetic factors, 143–144
        inflammation, 142–143
        non-amyloid-β component of AD amyloid, 141–142
    pathological hallmarks
        ballooned neurons or Pick cells, 164, 165f
        cerebral atrophy, 159–160
        granulovacular degeneration, 161, 162f
        Hirano bodies, 162, 162f
        Lewy bodies, 162–163, 162f, 163f
        Marinesco bodies, 163, 163f
        neuritic plaques, 160–161, 161f
        neurofibrillary changes, 161
        Pick bodies, 164, 164f
        status spongiosus vs. spongiform changes, 164, 165f,
            166
        ventricular enlargement, 160
    thalamic, 52
    vascular. See Vascular dementia
    vs. depression, 156
Dementia pugilistica, 459

Dementia with Lewy bodies (DLB)
  brain, microscopic features, 282–283
  brainstem in, 159, 160f
  central nervous system atrophy in, 126
  cerebral atrophy, 160
  clinical presentation, 280, 282
  cortical Lewy bodies, 270
  demographics, 170, 171t
  diagnostic classification, neuropathological, 171
  differential diagnosis
    vs. Alzheimer's disease, 282
    vs. Alzheimer's disease Lewy body variant, 171
    vs. Parkinson's disease, 171
  genetics, 170–171
  historical aspects, 170, 279–280
  incidence, 170
  neuropathology, 125
    gross examination, 171, 171t, 172f
    microscopic examination, 171–173, 172f, 173f
  risk, 241
  symptoms, 170
Dendrites
  in Alzheimer's disease, 232–233
  structural alteration, 536
Dentatorubral degeneration, 355
Dentatorubral pallidoluysian atrophy
  clinical manifestations, 349
  genetic factors, 311, 332t
  molecular genetics, 349–350
  neuropathology, 349–350
Depression, vs. dementia, 156
Dermatomyositis, 449–450, 551–552, 552f
Diabetes mellitus
  non-insulin or type II, skeletal muscle and, 555–556
  peripheral neuropathy from, 504
Dialysis encephalopathy, 568
Diaschisis
  crossed cerebellar, 50–51, 51f
  definition, 50
  thalamo-cortical, 52
Dichlorodiphenyl-dichloroethylene (DDE), brain tumors and, 411, 412t, 413, 413t
Dichlorodiphenyl-trichloroethylene (DDT), brain tumors and, 411, 412t, 413, 413t
Diet restrictions, for slowing age-related nervous system changes, 34–35, 35f
Diffuse axonal injury (DAI), 462–463, 462f
Diffuse Lewy body disease. See Dementia with Lewy bodies
Dimethyl sulfoxide, for head injury, 468
Disinhibition-dementia-Parkinsonism-amyotrophy complex, 311
Disraeli, Benjamin, 4
Distal axonopathy, 501
Diuretic agents, for head injury, 468
DLB. See Dementia with Lewy bodies
DLBD. See Dementia with Lewy bodies
DNA damage, free-radical mediated, 21–22, 23
Dopamine receptors, age-related impairments, 26

Dopaminergic system
  neurochemical deficits, in Alzheimer's disease, 238
  in Parkinson's disease, 312–313
Dopa-responsive dystonia (Segawa's disease), 310–311
Down syndrome
  Alzheimer's disease and, 240
  Alzheimer-type neurodegeneration in, 124–125
  central nervous system atrophy in, 126
  neurofibrillary tangles, 221
Drug-induced Parkinsonism, 293
Drugs. See also specific drugs
  aluminum-containing, Alzheimer's disease and, 568
  neuroleptic, elderly and, 565–567
  prescribing principles for elderly, 565, 565t
  skeletal muscle and, 557
  therapeutic access, elderly and, 564–5665, 565t
DTICH (delayed traumatic intracerebral hematoma), 576–577
Dystrophic neurites, 223

EAE (experimental allergic encephalomyelitis), 455
Eastern equine encephalitis, 492–493
Edison, Thomas A., 4
Edrophonium test, 450–451
EGFR (epidermal growth factor receptor), 419
Elderly. See also Aging
  accomplishments of, 3–5
  alcohol consumption, 400
  causes of death, 7, 8t–9t
  cerebrovascular disease in. See Cerebrovascular disease
  drug usage
    neuroleptic, 565–567
    in nursing homes, 569
    prescribing principles for, 565, 565t
    prescription considerations, 568–569, 569
    trends, 563
  population demographics, 563
Ellington, Edward Kennedy (Duke), 4
Embolism, cerebral
  air, 72
  diagnosis, 70–71
  sources, 70, 70t
    infective endocarditis, 71–72
    noncardiogenic/nonatheromatous, 72–73, 73f
    unintentional after cardiac surgery, 72–73, 73f, 74f
Encephalitis, granulomatous amoebic, 482
Encephalopathy
  anoxic/hypoxic-ischemic, 59–60, 61f
  hepatic, 442, 442f
  hypoglycemic, 393
  uremic, 442, 442f
  Wernicke's, 393–396, 394f, 395f, 395t
Endocarditis, infectious, cerebral complications, 71, 480–481, 481f
Energy metabolism, mitochondrial, age-related alterations, 29–31, 30f
Entamoeba histolytica, 481–483, 483f
ENU (ethylnitrosourea), brain tumors and, 410
Epidermal growth factor receptor (EGFR), 419

Epidural hematoma, 573
Epidural hemorrhage, 79–80
Episodic ataxia type 2, 347
Estrogen
  age-related changes, 31–32, 31f
  Alzheimer's disease and, 242
État criblé, 105
Excitatory neurotransmitters, accumulation after head injury, 460
Excitotoxicity
  after brain trauma, 464
  oxidative stress and, 316
Experimental allergic encephalomyelitis (EAE), 455
Extracellular matrix, age-related autonomic nervous system damage and, 539
Extrapontine myelinolysis, 441–442

Fabry disease, 433
Fall-related injuries
  brain trauma from, 465–466
  case report, in Alzheimer's disease, 581–582, 582f, 583f
  elderly and, 572
Familial Alzheimer's disease, 143–144
Familial neuronal intranuclear hyaline inclusion disease (NIHID), 292–293, 292f
Familial progressive subcortical gliosis, 311
Fatal familial insomnia, 179
Fat emboli, 72
Fibrillary astrocytosis, in Creutzfeldt-Jakob disease, 181
Fibromuscular dysplasia, 116
Foamy macrophages, 65, 65f
Forensic neuropathy
  case reports, 581–583, 582f, 583f
  central nervous system hemorrhage, 576–583, 582f, 583f
  dementia, 583–584
  physical injury and aging brain, 572–575, 575t
Fracture contusions, 580
Franklin, Benjamin, 4
Free radicals
  damage mediated by, 21–22, 21f
  definition, 21
  definition of, 315
  in dementia, 142
Friedreich's ataxia
  atypical forms, 350
  clinical manifestations, 350
  genetics, 331–334, 332t, 333f
  molecular genetics, 350–351
  neuropathology, 350–351, 351f–354f, 354–355
  prevalence, 330–331
Frontal lobe dementia
  genetics, 184–185
  neuropathology
    categorization, 189
    gross examination, 185–186, 186f, 187f
    microscopic examination, 186–187, 188f
  vs. Pick disease, 188–189
Frontocingular lesions, in vascular dementia, 114
Frontotemporal dementia (FTD)
  with amyotrophic lateral sclerosis, 184
  clinical features, 283
  genetic factors, 184–185, 283–284
  motor neuron disease and, 284, 285f
  neuropathology
    categorization, 189
    macroscopic examination, 185–186, 186f, 187f, 283
    microscopic examination, 186–187, 188f
    neurofibrillary tangles, 221–222
  symptoms, 184
  synonyms, 283
FTD. See Frontotemporal dementia
Fungal infections
  aspergillosis, 486–487
  candidiasis, 492, 492f
  coccidioidomycosis, 490–492, 491f
  cryptococcosis, 490, 491f
  histoplasmosis, 488–490, 489f
  mucormycosis, 488, 488f

GABA. See Gamma-aminobutyric acid
β-Galactosidase deficiency, 433
Galanin deficits, in Alzheimer's disease, 238
Galilei, Galileo, 4
Gamma-aminobutyric acid (GABA)
  in Alzheimer's disease, 238–239
  in normal aging, 20, 27
GAPDH (glyceraldehyde-3-phosphate dehydrogenase), 381–382
GBM (glioblastoma multiforme), 418–421, 418f–420f
Gene expression, age-related alterations, 19–21, 20f
Gerstmann-Sträussler-Scheinker syndrome (GSSS)
  amyloid deposits, 181
  brainstem in, 159, 160f
  cerebellar ataxia, 179
  plaques, 181–182, 181f
GFAP (glial fibrillary acidic protein), 19, 417
Giant cell arteritis/angiitis, 69–70, 69f, 450
Gladstone, W.E., 4
Glasgow Coma Scale
  age and, 460, 460f
  open head injuries and, 465, 467t
Glial cells
  age-related changes, 16–17
  in neurodegenerative diseases, 132
  proliferation, marker or, 54
Glial cytoplasmic inclusions, in oligodendrocytes, 272, 274–275, 275f
Glial fibrillary acidic protein (GFAP), 19, 417
Glial fibrillary tangles, 276, 277f
Gliding contusions, 580
Glioblastoma multiforme (GBM), 418–421, 418f–420f
Globoid cell leukodystrophy, 431
Globus pallidus (paleostriatum)
  anatomy, 370–371
  atrophy, in Huntington disease, 377–378

Glucose
  cerebral metabolic rate, after brain trauma, 461
  metabolism, in dementia, 138, 139f
  neuronal depletion, in Alzheimer's disease, 140–141
  utilization, in MPTP model of Parkinson's disease, 313–314
Glucose transport proteins, age-related changes, 20, 30–31
Glutamate, excitotoxicity after brain trauma, 464
Glutamate receptors, age-related changes, 27–28
Glyceraldehyde-3-phosphate dehydrogenase (GAPDH), 381–382
Glycogenoses, 438–439, 439f, 439t
GM1 gangliosidoses, 433
Goeth, Wolfgang van, 4
Golgi apparatus fragmentation
  Alzheimer's disease, 234
  in amyotrophic lateral sclerosis, 362–363, 363f
Goodwin, J., 322, 325f
G protein-coupled receptors, in Huntington disease, 372
Granulovacuolar degeneration
  in Alzheimer's disease, 233, 233f
  in dementia, 161, 162f
Gray Panther revolution, 2–3
GSSS. See Gerstmann-Sträussler-Scheinker syndrome
GTP-binding proteins, age-related alterations, 25–26, 26f
GTP cyclohydrolase gene mutations, 311
Guerilla cells, 415–416
Guillain-Barré syndrome, 454–455, 510–511, 510f
Gummatous neurosyphilis, 480
Gyral atrophy, Alzheimer's disease, 209–210, 210f–212f

Hallervorden-Spatz disease, genetic factors, 311
Hals, Franz, 4
Hardy, Thomas, 4
H_2 blockers, 568–569
HD. See Huntington disease
Head injuries. See also Brain trauma
  aging brain and, 572–575, 575f
  Alzheimer's disease risk and, 242
  closed, 464–465, 464f, 465f
  epidural hematoma, 573
  open, 464f, 465–467
  skin/scalp, 573
  subarachnoid hemorrhage, 575–576
  subdural hematoma, 573–575, 575t
  treatment, 468–469
Health costs, for elderly, 10–11, 11t–13t, 13–14
Heat-shock protein 70 (HSP-70), 19–20
Helminthic infections, 486, 487f, 488f
Hematomas
  delayed traumatic intracerebral, 576–577
  epidural, 573
  hypertensive, 90
  intracerebral, 467–468
  subdural, 573–575, 575t
Heme oxygenase-1, apoptosis and, 130
Hemianopia, 52

Hemodynamic failure
  mapping, 44, 47
  stages, 44, 44t, 45f, 46f
Hemodynamic reserve impairment, 42, 43f
Hemorrhage
  central nervous system, 576–583, 582f, 583f
  delayed post-traumatic cerebral, 576–577
  epidural, 79–80
  hereditary cerebral with amyloidosis, 66, 230
  hypertensive intracerebral, 576–577
  intraparenchymal. See Intraparenchymal hemorrhage
  intraventricular traumatic, 577
  spinal cord, 580–581
  subarachnoid. See Subarachnoid hemorrhage
  subdural, 80–81, 80f
Hereditary ataxias. See also Spinocerebellar ataxia
  epidemiology, 330–331
  genetics, 331–334, 332t, 333f
Hereditary cerebral hemorrhage with amyloidosis
  Dutch type, 66, 230
  Icelandic type, 66
Hereditary neuropathies, 513–514
Herpes simplex infections, 493–494, 493f
Herpes zoster infection, 494
Hexosaminidase A deficiency, 433
Hexosaminidase B deficiency, 433
Hippocampus
  age-related changes, 157
  neuronal loss, after traumatic brain injury, 467
Hirano bodies
  aging and, 162, 162f
  Alzheimer's disease, 233–234
  in dementia, 162, 162f
  formation, 157
  in Huntington disease, 383, 383t
Histoplasma capsulatum, 488–489
Histoplasmosis, 488–490, 489f
HIV infection (human immunodeficiency virus), 495–497, 497f
HMG-CoA reductase inhibitors, side effects, 557
Holmes, O.W., 4
HTLV-1-associated myelopathy, 494–495, 495f
Hugo, Victor, 4
Human immunodeficiency virus infection (HIV), 495–497, 497f
Human T cell leukemia/lymphotrophic virus-1-associated myelopathy, 494–495, 495f
Huntingtin protein
  biochemical characteristics, 380
  in Huntington disease, 23t, 24
  mutant, 369, 380–381, 381f
  pathogenic mechanisms, 381–382
  wild-type, 380–381
Huntingtin protein gene, 370
Huntington disease (HD)
  age of onset, 370
  with Alzheimer's disease, 382, 384–385, 384t
  brain
    age-related changes in, 382–384, 383t

basal ganglia of, 370–372
cerebral atrophy in, 159
clinical features, 369–370
diagnosis, 369
genetic features, 33, 311, 369–370, 370t
grading system in research, 380
huntingtin protein. See Huntingtin protein
neostriatal pathology, 377
    cerebellum atrophy and, 378–379
    cerebral cortex atrophy and, 378
    globus pallidus atrophy and, 377–378
    neurons, relative vulnerability of, 379–380
    substantia nigra atrophy and, 378
    subthalamic nucleus atrophy and, 378
    thalamus atrophy and, 378
neuropathology, 125
    historical view, 372–373
    macroscopic examination, 373–374, 373f–375f
    striatal, grading of, 374–377, 375f–377f
nonagenarians with, 385–3836, 386t
nuclear inclusions, 381, 381f
oxidative stress, 22, 23
prevalence, 331, 369
protein aggregates, 23t
4-Hydroxynonenal, 22
Hypereosinophilia, 512
Hypersensitivity vasculitis, 68
Hypertension
    intracerebral hemorrhage, 576–577
    intraparenchymal hemorrhage, 87, 89f, 90
Hypoglycemic encephalopathy, 393
Hypokalemic myopathies, 557
Hypothyroidism, peripheral neuropathy from, 504
Hypotonia, 329–330
Hypoxia. See Anoxia-ischemia

IgA MGUS (immunoglobulin A monoclonal gammopathy of undetermined significance), 506, 511
IGFs. See Insulin-like growth factors
IgG MGUS (Immunoglobulin G monoclonal gammopathy of undetermined significance), 506
Ig M monoclonal gammopathy, 505–506, 505f, 506f
Imaging techniques. See specific imaging techniques
    physiologic variables, 42, 43t
    radiotracers, 43
    types of, 42–43
Immune system
    age-related changes, 31–32, 31f
    bypass mechanisms, 447, 447t
    host defenses in elderly, 474
    nervous system targets, 448–449, 448t, 449t
    organization, 446–448, 447t
    polyclonal activation, 447–448
Immunoglobulin A monoclonal gammopathy of undetermined significance (IgA MGUS), 506, 511
Immunoglobulin G monoclonal gammopathy of undetermined significance (IgG MGUS), 506

Immunoglobulin M monoclonal gammopathy, 505–506, 505f, 506f
Immunologic diseases
    differential diagnosis, 446
    of nervous system. See Neuroimmunologic diseases
Inclusion body myositis, 552–554, 553f, 554f
Infectious disease
    bacterial
        cerebral abscesses, 481, 482f
        endocarditis, 480–481, 481f
        Lyme disease, 480
        meningitis, 475–476, 476f, 477t, 478–479, 478f
        neurosyphilis, 479–480, 480f–482f
        tuberculous meningitis, 477t, 478–479, 479f
    fungal, 486–492, 488f, 489f, 491f, 492f
        aspergillosis, 486–487
        candidiasis, 492, 492f
        coccidioidomycosis, 490–492, 491f
        cryptococcosis, 490, 491f
        histoplasmosis, 488–490, 489f
        mucormycosis, 488, 488f
    helminthic, 486, 487f, 488f
    incidence, in elderly, 474–475
    protozoal, 481–486, 483f–485f
        American trypanosomiasis, 484–486, 485f
        amoebic, 481–483, 483f
        cerebral malaria, 483–484, 484f
        toxoplasmosis, 484, 485f
    susceptibility, age and, 474–475
    viral, 492–497, 493f, 495f, 497f
        AIDS, 495–497, 497f
        arbovirus, 492–493
        herpes simplex, 493–494, 493f
        herpes zoster, 494
        HIV, 495–497, 497f
        human T cell leukemia/lymphotrophic virus-1-associated myelopathy, 494–495, 495f
        progressive multifocal leukoencephalopathy, 494, 495f
Infective endocarditis, 71–72
Inflammation
    Alzheimer's disease and, 226–227
    in dementia, 142–143
Inflammatory aneurysms, 83, 85
Inflammatory myopathies, 551–555, 552f–554f
Inflammatory polyneuropathies, 510–512, 510f
Ingres, J.A.D., 4
Insulin, 538
Insulin-like growth factors (IGFs)
    age-related changes, 27
    synaptic development and, 538
Intellectual deficit, senile plaques and, 228–229
Interleukin-6, synthesis, 143
Intracerebral hematomas, 467–468
Intracerebral hemorrhage, hypertensive, 576–577
Intracranial hemorrhage
    extra-/epidural, 79–80
    subarachnoid, 81–83, 82f–85f
    subdural, 80–81, 80f

Intranuclear neuronal inclusions, 291–292, 292f
Intraparenchymal hemorrhage
  causes, 86–87
    cerebral amyloid angiopathy, 90, 91f, 92
    hypertension, 87, 89f, 90
    systemic/miscellaneous factors, 94f, 95
    vascular malformations, 92–93, 92f, 93f, 95
  histologic features, 88f
Intraventricular hemorrhage, traumatic, 577
Iron, in Parkinson's disease, 316
Ischemic brain infarct
  pathophysiology
    cerebral embolism, 70–73, 70t, 71f, 73f–76f
    vascular disease, 61–63, 63f–69f, 65–70
  patterns, 62
Ischemic necrosis, 44, 46f
Ischemic penumbra, 44, 45f, 49
Ischemic stroke
  acute stage
    clinical correlates, 45f, 46f, 48
    irreversibly damaged tissue, 46f, 47–48
    penumbral tissue, 45f, 48
    spontaneous hyperperfusion, 46f, 48
  imaging studies
    management and, 50
    positron emission tomography, 47–49
    single-photon emission computed tomography, 49–50
    xenon-computed tomography, 49–50
  recovery, alleviation of penumbra in, 49
Isocortex
  amyloid-β peptide distribution, 228
  neuronal loss, in Alzheimer's disease, 214–215
  thickness/length, in Alzheimer's disease, 210, 213, 213f

Japanese encephalitis, 492–493
Jefferson, Thomas, 4

Kearns-Sayre syndrome, 440
Ki-67 labeling index, 417
Korsakoff's psychosis, 394
Korsakoff syndrome, 113
Kufs' disease, 434
Kuhn, Maggie, 4
Kuru
  clinical course, 179
  Creutzfeldt-Jakob disease and, 597–599, 600

Lacunae, types, 103, 105–106, 107f
Lambert-Eaton myasthenic syndrome (LEMS), 451, 556
LANP (leucine-rich acidic nuclear protein), 335
Lateral ventricular volume, in Pick disease, 195
LBD. See Dementia with Lewy bodies
LDL (low-density lipoprotein), 18
Leigh syndrome, 440–441
LEMS (Lambert-Eaton myasthenic syndrome), 451, 556
Leucine-rich acidic nuclear protein (LANP), 335
Leukoaraiosis, Alzheimer's disease, 235

Leukodystrophies
  globoid cell, 431
  metabolic, 430
  metachromatic, 430–431, 430f, 515
Levodopa
  for MPTP parkinsonism, 314
  for Parkinson's disease in elderly, 567–568
Lewy bodies
  in Alzheimer's disease, 234
  brainstem or classical
    histologic features, 162f, 163, 171–172
    localization of, 266
  components, 18
  cortical
    histologic features, 163, 163f, 172–173, 172f
    in Parkinson's disease, 241
    staining, 270
  in dementia, 162–163, 162f, 163f, 241
  historical aspects, 162
  in Huntington disease, 383, 383t
  localization, 270
  molecular biology, 267–268, 269f
  in Parkinson's disease
    cortical type, 241
    historical aspects, 265–267
    idiopathic, 268, 269f, 270
Lewy body dementia. See Dementia with Lewy bodies
Lewy-related neurites, 173, 270
Lipid peroxidation
  in anoxia-ischemia, 59
  in dementia, 142
  DNA damage and, 21
  in Parkinson's disease, 316
Lipofuscin, 19
Lipohyalinosis, 65. See also Atherosclerosis
Long-term potentiation (LTP), 28–29
Low-density lipoprotein (LDL), 18
LTP (long-term potentiation), 28–29
Luxury perfusion, 44, 46f
Lyme disease, 512
Lymphoma, malignant
  peripheral neuropathies from, 509, 509f
  primary, 423–425, 424f

Machado-Joseph disease (SCA type 3)
  clinical manifestations, 289, 338, 340, 514
  genetic factors, 289–290, 311
  histologic features, 289, 289f
  molecular genetics, 340–341, 341f–342f, 343
  neuropathology, 340–341, 341f–342f, 343
  prevalence, 331
Macroangiopathy, 62–63, 63f–65f
Madison, James, 4
MAG (myelin-associated glycoprotein), 505–506
Magnetic resonance imaging (MRI)
  aging brain, 5–6
  brain tumors, 413–415, 414f, 415f
  diffuse axonal injury, 463
  hypersignals, Alzheimer's disease, 235

Malaria, cerebral, 483–484, 484f
Malnutrition
  causes, 392
  diseases associated with, 393
    central pontine myelinolysis, 396, 396f
    cerebellar cortical degeneration, 398–399, 399f
    hypoglycemic encephalopathy, 393
    Marchiafava-Bignami disease, 396–397, 397f
    peripheral neuropathies, 400
    vitamin deficiencies, 397–398, 398t
    Wernicke-Korsakoff syndrome, 393–396, 394f, 395f, 395t
  prevalence, 392
  skeletal muscle and, 556–557, 557f
Malondialdehyde, 22
Mamillary body shrinkage, in Wernicke-Korsakoff syndrome, 394, 395f
Manganese poisoning, Parkinsonian syndromes from, 294–295
Mannitol, for head injury, 468
Mantegna, Andrea, 4
MAPs (microtubule-associated proteins), 17–18, 529
Marchiafava-Bignami disease, 396–397, 397f
Marinesco bodies
  histologic features, 163, 163f
  in Huntington disease, 383, 383t
MBP (myelin basic protein), 455
McLeod syndrome, 514
Medicaid, 11, 132
Medicare, 11, 11t, 13
MELAS (mitochondrial encephalopathy with lactic acidosis and stroke-like episodes), 116, 440, 440f, 441f, 515–516
Meningioma, 421–422, 421f–423f
Meningitis
  bacterial, 475–476, 476f, 477t, 478f
    complications, 476
    diagnosis, 476, 477t
    incidence, 475
    pathogens, 475
  cryptococcal, 477t
  syphilitic, 479
  tuberculous
    diagnosis, 477t, 478–479
    epidemiology, 478
    macroscopic examination, 479, 479f
    predisposing factors, 478
  viral, 477t
Meningoencephalitis, amoebic, 482
Meningovascular syphilis, 479–480
MERRF (myoclonic epilepsy with ragged red fibers), 440, 515–516
Metabolic leukodystrophies, 430
Metachromatic leukodystrophy, 430–431, 430f, 515
Methylnitrosourea (MNU), 410
1-Methyl-4-phenyl-1,2–3,6- tetrahydro pyridine model of Parkinson's disease, 313–315
Michaelangelo, Buanarroti, 4
Microangiopathy, 63, 65–68, 65f–68f

Microglia, 31
Microglioma, 424–425
Microtubule-associated proteins (MAPs), 17–18, 529
Microvasculitis, 502–503
Miller Fisher syndrome, 454
Mitochondria
  age-related changes, 550–551, 551f
  DNA damage, 127–128, 128f
  function, age-related alterations, 29–31, 30f
  hereditary disorders, 439–441, 440t
Mitochondrial encephalomyopathies, peripheral nerve involvement, 515–516
Mitochondrial encephalopathy with lactic acidosis and stroke-like episodes (MELAS), 116, 440, 440f, 441f, 515–516
Mitochondrial neurogastrointestinal encephalomyopathy (MNGIE), 441
Mitochondrial respiratory chain, oxygen free radicals, 127
Mitral annular calcification, 72
Mitral valve prolapse (MVP), 72
MMN (multifocal motor neuropathy), 512
MNGIE (mitochondrial neurogastrointestinal encephalomyopathy), 441
MNU (methylnitrosourea), 410
Molecular mimicry, of antigens, 448
Monoclonal gammopathy of undetermined significance (MGUS), 505–506, 505f, 506f
Motor neuronopathy
  differential diagnosis, 453
  frontotemporal dementia and, 284, 285f
MPS (mucopolysaccharidoses), 436–437, 437f, 437t
MPTP model of Parkinson's disease, 313–315
MRI. *See* Magnetic resonance imaging
MSA. *See* Multisystem atrophy
Mucopolysaccharidoses (MPS), 436–437, 437f, 437t
Mucormycosis, 488, 488f
Multifocal motor neuropathy (MMN), 512
Multi-infarct dementia, 101. *See also* Vascular dementia
"Multiple-hit" hypothesis, 123
Multiple-infarct dementia, 102, 103f, 104f
Multiple myeloma, 506
Multiple sclerosis, 455–456
Multisystem atrophy (MSA)
  brain
    macroscopic examination, 271, 272f, 273f
    microscopic examination, 271–272, 274–275, 274f, 275f
  central nervous system atrophy, 126
  incidence, 271
  neuropathology, 125
  types, 271, 355
Muscle
  fibers
    age-related changes, 548–549
    types, 547, 547f
  neuroimmunologic diseases of, 449–450
Myasthenia gravis, 450–451
Mycotic aneurysms, 83, 85

Myelin-associated glycoprotein (MAG), 505–506
Myelin basic protein (MBP), 455
Myoclonic epilepsy with ragged red fibers (MERRF), 440, 515–516
Myocyte, histologic features, 546–547, 547f
Myopathy, alcoholic, 405

NBTE (nonbacterial thrombotic endocarditis), 71–72
Necrotizing vasculitis, 503, 503f
Neocortex
  in dementia, 157, 158f
  neuronal loss, in Alzheimer's disease, 214
Neostriatum
  atrophy, in Huntington disease, 374–377, 375f–377f
  in dementia, 159
  neurons
    classification of, 371–372
    dark, 376, 376f
    relative vulnerability in Huntington disease, 379–380
Nerve growth factor (NGF), age-related changes, 20, 27, 537
Nervous system
  age-related changes, 16
    hormonal, 31–32, 31f
    immunological, 31–32, 31f
    immunologic diseases and, 446–447, 447t
    parasympathetic, 531, 532
    slowing, dietary restriction for, 34–35, 35f
    structural, 16–19, 17f
    sympathetic, 528–529, 529f–531f, 531–532
  arterial diseases of, 61–62, 61f
  autonomic. See Autonomic nervous system
  central. See Central nervous system
  cerebellum cortex circuitry, 326, 328, 328f
  immune system targets, 448–449, 448t, 449t
  oxidative stress, 21–22, 22t
Neuraminic acid-related disorders, 438
Neurites, Lewy-related neurites, 173, 270
Neuroacanthocytosis, 514
Neurocysticercosis, 486, 487f, 488f
Neurodegeneration
  in Alzheimer's disease, 145
  apoptosis, molecular mechanisms of, 128–130
  brain trauma and, 459–460
  central nervous system impairment and, 124–125
  in dementia, 123
  in Down syndrome, 124–125
  mitochondrial DNA damage and, 126–128, 128f
  non-Alzheimer, 131–132, 145
Neurodegenerative diseases
  age-related changes, 34–35, 35f
  Alzheimer's disease. See Alzheimer's disease
  cell death pathways in, 125–126
  dietary restrictions for, 34–35, 35f
  gene abnormalities, 132–133
  involving cerebral cortex and causing dementia, 279–280, 282–284, 285f, 286
  non-Alzheimer. See Huntington disease; Parkinson's disease

  with Parkinsonian symptoms, involving basal ganglia, 271–272, 272f–275f, 274–276, 278–279
  protein aggregates in, 23–24, 23t
Neuroendocrine system, age-related changes, 31–32, 31f
Neurofibrillary changes, 161
Neurofibrillary lesions
  constituents, 219
  morphology, 216–218, 217f, 218f
  tau-associated. See Neurofibrillary tangles
Neurofibrillary tangles (NFTs)
  constituents, 218–219
  distribution, 219–220
  in elderly schizophrenics, 566
  histologic/morphologic features, 18, 216–218, 217f, 218f
  in non-Alzheimer diseases, 221–222
  in postencephalatic Parkinsonism, 294
  prevalence, 220–221
  in progressive supranuclear palsy, 276, 277f
  significance, 220–221
Neurogenesis, 6–7
Neurogenic atrophy, peripheral neuropathy with, 550, 550f
Neuroimmunologic diseases. See also specific neuroimmunologic diseases
  of central nervous system, 455–456
  of muscle, 449–450
  of neuromuscular junction, 450–451
  of peripheral nervous system, 451–455, 452t
  safety factor, 449
  symptoms, timing of, 449
Neuroleptic medications, elderly and, 565–567
Neurometabolic disorders
  acquired
    central pontine myelinolysis, 441–442, 441f
    extrapontine myelinolysis, 441–442
    hepatic encephalopathy, 442, 442f
    uremic encephalopathy, 442, 442f
  in adults, 429–430
  in children, 429
  classification, 429
  hereditary
    adrenoleukodystrophy, 431–432, 432f
    adrenomyeloneuropathy, 431–432, 432f
    globoid cell leukodystrophy, 431
    glycogenoses, 438–439, 439f, 439t
    metabolic leukodystrophies, 430
    metachromatic leukodystrophy, 430–431, 430f
    mitochondrial disorders, 439–441, 440t
    mucopolysaccharidoses, 436–437, 437f, 437t
    neuraminic acid-related disorders, 438
    neuronal ceroid-lipofuscinosis, 433–436, 434t, 435f, 436f
    Niemann-Pick disease, 437–438
    oligosaccharidoses, 438
    sialic acid-related disorders, 438
    spingolipidoses, 432–433, 433f
Neuromuscular junction, neuroimmunologic diseases of, 450–451

Neuronal ceroid-lipofuscinosis, 433–436, 434t, 435f, 436f
Neuronal loss
 age-related, 402, 403t
 during aging, 458–459
 in alcoholism, 402, 403t
 Alzheimer's disease, 213–216
 dopaminergic, 564
 hippocampal, after traumatic brain injury, 467
 marker for, 53–54
 motor, 548–549
 neostriatal, in Huntington disease, 374–377, 375f–377f
Neurons. See also Neuronal loss
 age-related changes, 16–18, 17f
 amyloid β peptide-induced injury, 24
 argyrophilic, 187
 in cerebral cortex, 326
 noradrenergic, 26
Neuropathy
 adrenomyeloneuropathy, 431–432, 432f
 alcohol-related, 400
 forensic. See Forensic neuropathy
 hereditary, with pressure palsies, 514
 multifocal motor, 512
 peripheral. See Peripheral neuropathies
Neuropeptide deficits, in Alzheimer's disease, 238
Neuropil threads, morphology, 218
Neurosyphilis, 479–480, 480f, 481f
Neurotransmission, striatal, in Huntington disease, 372
Neurotransmitters, in senile plaques, 224
Neurotransmitter signaling system, age-related alterations, 25–27, 26f
Neurotrophic factor signaling systems, alterations in, 27–29
Neurotrophic substances, age-related autonomic nervous system and, 537–538
Newton, Sir Isaac, 4
NF-κB, 19
NGF (nerve growth factor), age-related changes, 20, 27, 537
NG2 transmembrane chondroitin sulphate proteoglycan, in glioblastoma multiforme, 418–419
Niacin deficiency, 397
Niemann-Pick disease, 437–438
Nitric oxide (NO), 21, 21f, 59
Nitric oxide synthase (NOS)
 formation, 21, 21f
 peroxynitrite formation, 59
 type-3, apoptosis and, 130
Nitrosocompounds, brain tumors and, 410
Nonagenarians, 2
Nonamyloid amyloid-β peptide deposits, 141–142, 227
Nonbacterial thrombotic endocarditis (NBTE), 71–72
Non-Friedreich's recessive ataxias, 331
Nonsteroidal antiinflammatory agents, Alzheimer's disease development and, 143
Noradrenergic system neurochemical deficits, in Alzheimer's disease, 237
Norepinephrine receptors, 26

NOS. See Nitric oxide synthase
Nucleolus volume decrease, Alzheimer's disease, 234
Nucleus basalis of Meynert, 224
Nursing home patients, drug prescription considerations, 569
Nutritional deficiencies, peripheral neuropathy from, 504–505
Nystagmus, 329

Occipital lesions, in vascular dementia, 112–113
Old age, definition, 1
Oligemia, 44, 45f
Oligodendrocytes, glial cytoplasmic inclusions, 272, 274–275, 275f
Oligosaccharidoses, 438
Olivocerebellar fibers, 323
Olivopontocerebellar atrophy (SCA type 1)
 brain
  intranuclear inclusions, 291–292, 291f
  microscopic examination, 271–272, 273f, 287–288, 288f
 chromosome abnormality, 288
 clinical features, 287, 334–335
 differential diagnosis, 335, 336f–338f
 historical aspects, 271
 molecular genetics, 335
 neuropathology, 335, 336f–338f
 nomenclature, 286–287
Opalski cells, 442
Opsoclonus-myoclonus syndrome, 454
Osmotic diuretic agents, for head injury, 468
Oxidative injury, age-related autonomic nervous system damage and, 539
Oxidative stress
 definition of, 316
 in dementia, 142
 mechanisms, 21–22, 22t
 in neurodegenerative disorders, 22–23
 Parkinson's disease pathogenesis and, 315–317
Oxygen
 cerebral metabolic rate, after brain trauma, 461
 consumption, age-related changes, 549
Oxyradicals, 21–22, 21f

PACNS (primary angiitis of central nervous system), 68–69, 69f
Paired helical filaments (PHFs)
 morphology, 217–218
 tau proteins in, 218–219
Pale bodies, 266
Paleostriatum. See Globus pallidus
Paraneoplastic limbic encephalitis
 causes, 175
 neuropathology
  gross examination, 175–176, 175f
  microscopic examination, 176, 176f
Paraneoplastic syndromes
 neurologic, 453–454
 skeletal muscle and, 556
Paraproteinemic neuropathies, 505

Parasympathetic nervous system
  age-related changes
    in experimental animals, 532
    in humans, 531
  ganglia, age-related changes, 531
Paresis, general, 480
Par-4 expression, 20–21, 20f
Parkin gene, 268
Parkinsonian syndromes
  atherosclerotic, 295
  in Creutzfeldt-Jakob disease, 294
  drug-induced, 293
  epidemiology, 309
  genetics, 309–310
    with known genetic loci, 310–311
  from manganese poisoning, 294–295
  neuroleptic-induced, 566–567
  postencephalitic, 293–294
  post-traumatic, 295–296
  secondary to carbon monoxide poisoning, 294
  tumors and, 295
Parkinsonism-dementia complex of Guam, 284, 286
Parkinson's disease (PD)
  epidemiology, 309
  genetics, 267–268, 309–310
    autosomal dominant, 309–310
    autosomal recessive, 310
    mutations, 33
  historical aspects, 264–265, 265f–268f
  idiopathic
    neuroanatomical connections, 312
    neuropathology of, 268, 268f, 269f, 270
  incidence, 264
  levodopa for, 567–568
  Lewy bodies, 18, 265–267
    Alzheimer's disease and, 240–241
    α-synuclein and, 267–268, 269f
  mitochondrial enzyme dysfunction, 29
  neuropathology, 125
    central nervous system atrophy, 126
    neurofibrillary tangles, 221–222
    neuronal cytoskeletal alterations, 18
    neuronal loss, 270
  pathogenesis, 264
    MPTP model, 313–315
    neuroanatomical connections and, 311–313
    oxidative stress and, 22, 23, 315–317
    α-synuclein and, 23t, 24, 267–268, 269f
  prevalence, 264
  sporadic, 310
  symptoms, 315
  treatment, 270, 567–568
  vs. dementia with Lewy bodies, 171
PCBs (polychlorinated biphenyls), brain tumors and, 411, 412t, 413, 413t
PcD. See Pick disease
PD. See Parkinson's disease
PEG-SOD (polyethylene-glycol-conjugated superoxide dismutase), for head injury, 468

Pericerebal space, calculation, 400–401, 401f
Perikaryal atrophy, Alzheimer's disease, 213–216
Peripheral nervous system
  age-related changes, neurotrophic substances and, 537–538
  neuroimmunologic diseases of, 451–455, 452t
Peripheral neuropathies
  acquired
    due to systemic disorders, 504–508, 505f–507f
    due to vascular disease, 502–504, 503f
  age of onset, 499
  aging and, 516–517
  amiodarone, 513
  amyloid, 508–509, 508f, 509f
  chloroquine, 513, 513f
  chronic, 501, 501f
  from critical illness, 505
  from diabetes mellitus, 504
  diagnostic studies, 499–500
  elementary lesions, 500
    axonal degeneration, 500–501, 500f, 501f
    interstitial, 502, 502f
    segmental demyelination, 501–502, 502f
  etiology, 400
  hereditary, 513–514
  from hypothyroidism, 504
  inflammatory polyneuropathies, 510–512, 510f
  from lymphomatous infiltration, 509, 509f
  with mitochondrial encephalomyopathies, 515–516
  with neurogenic atrophy, 550, 550f
  from nutritional deficiencies, 504–505
  paraneoplastic, 509–510
  with storage diseases, 515
  toxic, 512–513, 513f
  from vitamin B-1 deficiency, 504–505
Peroxynitrite, 21, 21f, 59, 316
Pesticide residues, brain tumors and, 411, 412t, 413, 413t
PET. See Positron emission tomography
PHFs (paired helical filaments), 217–219
Picasso, Pablo, 4
Pick, Arnold, 190, 191f
Pick bodies
  argyrophilic perinuclear ring, 198–199, 198f
  histologic features, 164, 164f, 197–200, 198f
  historical aspects, 191–192
  sites of predilection, 199
Pick cells (ballooned neurons)
  histologic features, 164, 165f, 199t, 200
  historical aspects, 191–192
Pick disease (PcD)
  ballooned neurons. See Pick cells
  brainstem in, 159, 160f
  clinical features, 193–194
  diagnostic criteria, neuropathological, 200–202, 201t
  differential diagnosis
    vs. Alzheimer's disease, 193–194
    vs. frontal lobe dementia, 188–189
  genetics, 194

historical aspects, 190–193, 191f
neuropathology, 125
   brain weight, 195
   central nervous system atrophy, 126
   gross examination, 195–197, 195f, 196f, 196t, 197t
   lateral ventricular volume, 195
   microscopic examination, 197–200, 197f–199f
   neurofibrillary tangles, 221
   Pick bodies. *See* Pick bodies
   Pick cells. *See* Pick cells
   status spongiosus, 197f, 200
symptoms, 193–194
types, 200–202, 201t
without Pick bodies. *See* Frontotemporal dementia
Plaques
   astrocytic, 229
   burned out or cored, 227
   compact fibrillar form, 23
   Creutzfeldt-Jakob disease, 181–182, 181f
   development, 160
   diffuse or pre-amyloid, 23, 161, 222, 227
   formation, 62
   GSSS, 181–182, 181f
   immature, 161
   kuru, 181–182, 181f
   morphologic stages, 160–161, 161f
   neuritic, 160–161, 161f
      components, 222–226, 223f, 226
      core, 224–226
      crowns, 218, 223–224
      distribution, 227–228
      intellectual deficit and, 228–229
      morphology, 218
      processes, 223–224
      staining, 222–223, 223f, 224f
   in non-Alzheimer disease, 229
   rupture, 62
   unstable, 62
   variants, 224f, 227
Plasma cell dyscrasia, 452–453
Plasmatic viscosity, 110
POEMS syndrome, 507, 507f
Polychlorinated biphenyls (PCBs), brain tumors and, 411, 412t, 413, 413t
Polyethylene-glycol-conjugated superoxide dismutase (PEG-SOD), for head injury, 468
Polyglucosan body disease, 438, 515
Polymyalgia rheumatica, 450
Polymyositis, 450, 552, 552f
Positron emission tomography (PET)
   of hemodynamic failure, 44, 45f, 46f
   ischemic stroke, 47–49
   materials/methods, 42
Postencephalatic Parkinsonism, 293–294
Post-traumatic Parkinsonian syndromes, 295–296
Presenilin-1 gene mutations, 32–33, 32f
Presenilins
   in Alzheimer's disease, 232
   apoptosis and, 129

Pressure palsies, hereditary neuropathy with, 514
Primary angiitis of central nervous system (PACNS), 68–69, 69f
Prion diseases. *See* Creutzfeldt-Jakob disease
Programmed cell death. *See* Apoptosis
Progressive multifocal leukoencephalopathy, 494, 495f
Progressive supranuclear palsy (PSP)
   brain
      macroscopic examination, 276
      microscopic examination, 276, 277f
   central nervous system atrophy in, 126
   diagnosis, 275–276
   incidence, 275
   neuropathology, 125
   prevalence, 275
   tau protein, 279
Prosthetic heart valves, emboli from, 72
Protein. *See also specific proteins*
   aggregation, 23–24, 23t
   mitochondrial, 29–31, 30f
   oxidation, 21–22
Protein-calorie malnutrition, 392
Protein-energy malnutrition, 392
Protozoal infections
   American trypanosomiasis, 484–486, 485f
   amoebic, 481–483, 483f
   cerebral malaria, 483–484, 484f
   toxoplasmosis, 484, 485f
PSP. *See* Progressive supranuclear palsy
PTEN gene, 419, 420
Purkinje cell, histology, 326, 327f

Radiation exposure, brain tumors and, 411
Radiotracers, 43
Reactive oxygen species (ROS), 315–316
Reticulocerebellar fibers, 323
Retirement, 1–2
Rheumatic heart disease, 72
Rheumatoid arthritis, 512
ROS (reactive oxygen species), 315–316
Rossini, G.A., 4

St. Louis encephalitis, 492–493
St. Saens, C.c., 4
Salla disease, 438
Sandhoff disorder, 433
Sarcopenia, 548
Sarcoplasmic reticulum, age-related changes, 549
S-100β
   astrocyte activation in aging and, 19
   overexpression in Down syndrome, 125
SCA. *See* Spinocerebellar ataxia
Scalp injuries, aging brain and, 573
Schwannoma, 423, 424f
SDAT (senile dementia of Alzheimer type), 6, 208. *See also* Alzheimer's disease
Segawa's disease (dopa-responsive dystonia), 310–311
Senile dementia of Alzheimer type (SDAT), 6, 208. *See also* Alzheimer's disease

Senile dementia of Lewy body type. *See* Dementia with Lewy bodies
Senile plaques. *See* Plaques, neuritic
Serotonergic system neurochemical deficits, in Alzheimer's disease, 237–238
Serotonin, age-related changes, 26
Shaw, G.B., 4
Sialic acid-related disorders, 438
Single-photon emission computed tomography (SPECT)
  of brain trauma, 467
  of ischemic stroke, 49–50
  materials/methods, 42–43
Sjögren's syndrome, 512
Skeletal muscle
  age-related changes, 547–551, 548*t*, 550*f*, 551*f*
  histology, normal, 546–547, 547*f*
  inflammatory myopathies, 551–555, 552*f*–554*f*
  systemic disease and, 555–557, 556*f*, 557*f*
Skin injuries, aging brain and, 573
Skull fractures, 465
Slow virus diseases. *See* Creutzfeldt-Jakob disease
SNCA (α-synuclein gene), Parkinson's disease and, 310
SOD-1 gene overexpression, in Down syndrome, 125
Sophocles, 4
SPECT. *See* Single-photon emission computed tomography
Spinal cord hemorrhage/injury, 580–581
Spingolipidoses, 432–433, 433*f*
Spinocerebellar ataxia (SCA)
  genetics, 331–333, 332*t*, 333*f*
  type 1. *See* Olivopontocerebellar atrophy
  type 2, 288
    clinical manifestations, 335, 337
    molecular genetics, 337–338
    neuropathology, 337–338, 339*f*–340*f*
  type 3. *See* Machado-Joseph disease
  type 4
    clinical manifestations, 343
    molecular genetics, 343, 343*f*–346*f*
    neuropathology, 343, 343*f*–346*f*
  type 5
    clinical manifestations, 343
    molecular genetics, 343, 343*f*–346*f*
    neuropathology, 343, 343*f*–346*f*
  type 6, 347
  type 7, 290–291, 290*f*
    clinical manifestations, 347
    molecular genetics, 347–349
    neuropathology, 347–349, 348*f*–349*f*
Spinocerebellar degeneration
  classification, 286–287
  in spinocerebellar ataxias. *See* Spinocerebellar ataxia
  in trinucleotide repeat expansions, 286–287
Spongiform changes
  in Alzheimer's disease, 234
  in Creutzfeldt-Jakob disease, 177, 180–181, 180*f*
  in dementia with Lewy bodies, 173, 173*f*
  vs. status spongiosus changes, 164, 165*f*, 166

Spongiform encephalopathies. *See* Creutzfeldt-Jakob disease
Sporadic ataxias, 355
Status spongiosus
  Pick disease, 197*f*, 200
  vs. spongiform changes, 164, 165*f*, 166
Steele-Richardson-Olszewski syndrome. *See* Progressive supranuclear palsy
Stellate cells, 326
Storage diseases, peripheral neuropathies with, 515
Stroke
  causes, vascular disease, 61–63, 63*f*–69*f*, 65–69
  incidence, 58
  ischemic. *See* Ischemic stroke
  metabolic effects, 50–53, 51*f*
    contralateral cerebral, 51
    crossed cerebellar diaschisis, 50–53, 51*f*
    ipsilateral, 52–53
    subcortico cortical, 51–52, 52*f*
  mortality, 58
  recovery, cortical hypometabolism and, 53
  white matter, 53
Subacute sclerosing panencephalitis, neurofibrillary tangles, 222
Subarachnoid hemorrhage
  berry/saccular aneurysms, 81–83, 82*f*–85*f*
  dissecting aneurysms, 85
  fusiform aneurysms, 86, 87*f*
  inflammatory aneurysms, 83, 85
  mycotic aneurysms, 83, 85
  spontaneous, 576
  trauma and, 575–576
Subcortical aphasia, 51, 52*f*
Subcortical dementia, white matter stroke and, 53
Subcortical neglect, 52
Subcortical nuclei, 159
Subdural hematoma
  acute, 574
  aging/dating, 574, 575*t*
  case report, 583, 584*f*
  causes, 573–574
  chronic, 574–575, 575*t*
  subacute, 574, 575*t*
Subdural hemorrhage, 80–81, 80*f*
Substantia innominata, amyloid-β peptide distribution, 228
Substantia nigra
  atrophy, in Huntington disease, 378
  in Parkinson's disease, 265, 268*f*
Subthalamic nucleus
  atrophy, in Huntington disease, 378
  functional anatomy, 312
Superficial peroneal nerve biopsy, 499–500
Superoxide anion radical, 21, 21*f*
Superoxide dismutase (SOD), 21, 21*f*
Superoxide dismutase 1 gene
  apoptosis and, 129–130
  mutation, in amyotrophic lateral sclerosis, 363, 364, 365–366

Support groups, for neurologically impaired patients, 587–592
Sural nerve biopsy, 499–500
SV40, oncogenicity, 411
Sympathetic ganglia, aging, 528–529, 529f–531f, 531
Sympathetic nervous system, age-related changes
  in experimental animals, 531–532
  in humans, 528–529, 529f–531f, 531
Synapse
  age-related changes, 18
  disconnection, in Alzheimer's disease, 130–131
  loss, in Alzheimer's disease, 232–233
  plasticity, 536
  turnover, in automatic ganglia, 536
Synaptic organelle degradation, age-related autonomic nervous system damage and, 538–539
α-Synuclein
  in dementia, 141–142
  Parkinson's disease and, 267–268
α-Synuclein gene (SNCA), Parkinson's disease and, 310
Systemic disease, skeletal muscle and, 555–557, 556f, 557f

Tabes dorsalis, 480, 481f
Talk-and-die syndrome (TADS), 579–580
Tangier disease, 515
Tau gene mutations, 124
Tau protein
  age-related neurodegeneration and, 19
  in Alzheimer's disease, 218–219
  biochemical characteristics
    in corticobasal degeneration, 279
    in progressive supranuclear palsy, 279
  hyperphosphorylation, 18
Tay-Sachs disorder, 433
T cells, 447
Temporal arteritis, 450, 503
Temporal lesions, in vascular dementia, 113
Tennyson, A., 4
Thalamo-cortical diaschisis, 52
Thalamus
  atrophy, in Huntington disease, 378
  in dementia, 159
  hypometabolism, 53
  lesions, in vascular dementia, 113–114, 114f
Thiamin, for Wernicke-Korsakoff syndrome, 393–394
Tick-bite meningoradiculoneuritis, 512
Tirilazad, for head injury, 468
Titan (Tiziano, V.), 5
Transmissible spongiform encephalopathies. See Creutzfeldt-Jakob disease
Trinucleotide mutations, 332–334, 333t
Trinucleotide repeat expansions, 286
T-tubules, 546–547
Tuberculous meningitis
  diagnosis, 477t
  macroscopic examination, 479, 479f
  microscopic examination, 479, 480f

Tubman, Harriet, 5
Tumors, Parkinsonian syndromes and, 295

Ubiquitin inclusions, in amyotrophic lateral sclerosis, 363–364, 363f
Undernutrition, causes, 392
Unilateral lesions, in vascular dementia, 115
United States population
  causes of death, 7, 8t–9t
  growth, 7, 10, 10f, 10t
  over age 65, 1
  over age 90, 2
"Use-it-or-lose-it" hypothesis of brain aging, 29, 29f

Vascular dementia
  with Alzheimer's disease, 239–240
  Alzheimer's disease and, 116–117
  cerebral perfusion in, 135–138, 136t
  classification, 101–102
  definition, 101–102
  diffuse forms
    Binswanger disease, 106–107, 108f, 109–110, 109f
    cortical granular atrophy, 102–103, 105f, 106f
    lacunae, 103, 105–106, 107f
    multiple infarcts, 102, 103f, 104f
  focal forms, 112–115, 114f
  historical aspects, 101
  incidence, 102
  neuroimaging, 102
  pathogenesis, 115–116, 115f
  risk factors, causing cerebral perfusion impairment, 136t
  treatment, Alzheimer's disease and, 138
Vascular disorders. See also specific vascular disorders
  peripheral neuropathies from, 502–504, 503f
  receptor studies, 53–54
Vascular endothelial growth factor (VEGF), 418
Vasculitis, 68–70, 69f
Vasoactive intestinal polypeptide (VIP), in Alzheimer's disease, 238
VEGF (vascular endothelial growth factor), 418
Venous angiomas, 93
Venous thrombosis, 78–79
Ventricles
  dilation/enlargement
    in Alzheimer's disease, 213
    in dementias, 160
  size, age-related changes and, 5
Verdi, G., 5
VIP (vasoactive intestinal polypeptide), in Alzheimer's disease, 238
Viral infections
  AIDS, 495–497, 497f
  arbovirus, 492–493
  herpes simplex, 493–494, 493f
  herpes zoster, 494
  HIV, 495–497, 497f
  human T cell leukemia/lymphotrophic virus-1-associated myelopathy, 494–495, 495f

Viral infections *(continued)*
  meningitis, 477t
  progressive multifocal leukoencephalopathy, 494, 495f
Viruses, oncogenic, 411
Vitamin deficiencies
  B1. *See* Wernicke-Korsakoff syndrome
  B12, 397–398, 398f
  E, 398
  niacin, 397
Voltaire, J.F.A., 5

Waldenström's macroglobulinemia
  clinical features, 452–453
  widened myelin lamellae, 505–506, 505f, 506f
Wallerian degeneration, 500, 500f
Watershed infarct, 76–77, 77f
Wernicke-Korsakoff syndrome
  brain volume and, 402
  clinical features, 393–394
  distribution/severity of lesions, 395, 395t
  histologic features, 394–396, 394f, 395f
  peripheral neuropathy from, 504–505
White matter
  density, Alzheimer's disease, 235
  lesions, risk factors, 135
  loss
    chemotherapeutic agents and, 568
    reversibility with alcoholism, 404–405
  volume, Alzheimer's disease, 235
White matter stroke, subcortical dementia and, 53
Wilson's disease, genetic factors, 311

Xenon-computed tomography, 43
  ischemic stroke, 49–50
X-linked dystonia-Parkinson's disease complex, 311

Z-discs, 546, 547f